CURRENT THERAPY IN
HEMATOLOGY-ONCOLOGY

MEDICAL TITLES
IN THE CURRENT THERAPY SERIES

CURRENT THERAPY IN HEMATOLOGY-ONCOLOGY

FOURTH EDITION

MICHAEL C. BRAIN, D.M., F.R.C.P., FRCPC

Professor of Medicine
McMaster University Faculty of Medicine
Hamilton, Ontario, Canada

PAUL P. CARBONE, M.D., D.Sc. (Hon.), F.A.C.P.

Professor
Departments of Human Oncology and Medicine
University of Wisconsin Medical School
Director
University of Wisconsin Clinical Cancer Center
Madison, Wisconsin

B.C. Decker
An Imprint of Mosby–Year Book

Publisher

B.C. Decker
320 Walnut Street
Suite 400
Philadelphia, Pennsylvania 19106

Sales and Distribution

United States and Puerto Rico
Mosby–Year Book, Inc.
11830 Westline Industrial Drive
Saint Louis, Missouri 63146

Canada
Mosby–Year Book Limited
5240 Finch Avenue E., Unit 1
Scarborough, Ontario M1S 5A2

Australia
McGraw–Hill Book Company Australia Pty. Ltd.
4 Barcoo Street
Roseville East 2069
New South Wales, Australia

Brazil
Editora McGraw–Hill do Brasil, Ltda.
rua Tabapua, 1.105, Itaim–Bibi
Sao Paulo, S.P. Brasil

Colombia
Interamericana/McGraw–Hill de Colombia, S.A.
Carrera 17, No. 33–71
(Apartado Postal, A.A., 6131)
Bogota, D.E., Colombia

Europe, United Kingdom, Middle East and Africa
Wolfe Publishing Limited
Brook House
2–16 Torrington Place
London WC1E 7LT England

Hong Kong and China
McGraw–Hill Book Company
Suite 618, Ocean Centre
5 Canton Road
Tsimshatsui, Kowloon
Hong Kong

India
Tata McGraw–Hill Publishing Company, Ltd.
12/4 Asaf Ali Road, 3rd Floor
New Delhi 110002, India

Indonesia
Mr. Wong Fin Fah
P.O. Box 122/JAT
Jakarta, 1300 Indonesia

Japan
Igaku–Shoin Ltd.
Tokyo International P.O. Box 5063
1-28-36 Hongo, Bunkyo-ku,
Tokyo 113, Japan

Korea
Mr. Don-Gap Choi
C.P.O. Box 10583
Seoul, Korea

Malaysia
Mr. Lim Tao Slong
No. 8 Jalan SS 7/6B
Kelana Jaya
47301 Petaling Jaya
Selangor, Malaysia

Mexico
Interamericana/McGraw–Hill de Mexico, S.A. de C.V.
Cedro 512, Colonia Atlampa
(Apartado Postal 26370)
06450 Mexico, D.F., Mexico

New Zealand
McGraw–Hill Book Co. New Zealand Ltd.
5 Joval Place, Wiri
Manukau City, New Zealand

Portugal
Editora McGraw–Hill de Portugal, Ltda.
Rua Rosa Damasceno 11A–B
1900 Lisboa, Portugal

Singapore and Southeast Asia
McGraw–Hill Book Co.
21 Neythal Road
Jurong, Singapore 2262

South Africa
Libriger Book Distributors
Warehouse Number 8
''Die Ou Looiery''
Tannery Road
Hamilton, Bloemfontein 9300

Spain
McGraw–Hill/Interamericana de Espana, S.A.
Manuel Ferrero, 13
28020 Madrid, Spain

Taiwan
Mr. George Lim
P.O. Box 87–601
Taipei, Taiwan

Thailand
Mr. Vitit Lim
632/5 Phaholyothin Road
Sapan Kwai
Bangkok 10400
Thailand

Venezuela
Editorial Interamericana de Venezuela, C.A.
2da. calle Bello Monte
Local G–2
Caracas, Venezuela

NOTICE

The authors and publisher have made every effort to ensure that the patient care recommended herein, including choice of drugs and drug dosages, is in accord with the accepted standards and practice at the time of publication. However, since research and regulation constantly change clinical standards, the reader is urged to check the product information sheet included in the package of each drug, which includes recommended doses, warnings, and contraindications. This is particularly important with new or infrequently used drugs.

Current Therapy in Hematology-Oncology, Fourth Edition

ISBN 1–55664–263–6
ISSN 0899–6857
D–21227

92 93 94 95 96   GW/MY/MY   9 8 7 6 5 4 3 2

CONTRIBUTORS

MARK R. ALBERTINI, M.D.

Oncology Fellow, University of Wisconsin Clinical Cancer Center, Madison, Wisconsin

RICHARD H. ASTER, M.D.

Clinical Professor of Medicine and Pathology, Medical College of Wisconsin; President, Blood Center of Southeastern Wisconsin, Milwaukee, Wisconsin

LAURENCE H. BAKER, D.O.

Professor of Medicine, Wayne State University School of Medicine; Director, Division of Hematology and Oncology, Detroit Medical Center, Detroit, Michigan

CHARLES M. BALCH, M.D., F.A.C.S.

Professor and Head, Division of Surgery, and Chairman, Department of General Surgery, The University of Texas M.D. Anderson Cancer Center; Associate Chairman, Department of Surgery, The University of Texas Medical School at Houston, Houston, Texas

MICHAEL J. BARNETT, B.M.

Clinical Assistant Professor of Medicine, University of British Columbia; Member, Leukemia and Bone Marrow Transplantation Program of British Columbia, Vancouver, British Columbia, Canada

WILLIAM R. BELL, M.D., Ph.D.

Professor of Medicine and Radiology, The Johns Hopkins University School of Medicine; Director, Special Coagulation Laboratory, The Johns Hopkins University Hospital, Baltimore, Maryland

ANN M. BENGER, M.D., FRCPC

Associate Professor of Medicine, Department of Medicine, McMaster University School of Medicine; Hematologist, Hamilton Civic Hospitals, Henderson General Division, Hamilton, Ontario, Canada

AMY LOUISE BILLETT, M.D.

Instructor in Pediatrics, Harvard Medical School; Clinical Associate in Pediatrics, Dana-Farber Cancer Institute, and Assistant in Medicine (Hematology/Oncology), The Children's Hospital, Boston, Massachusetts

MORRIS A. BLAJCHMAN, M.D., FRCPC

Professor, Departments of Pathology and Medicine, McMaster University School of Medicine; Chief of Hematology Service, McMaster University Medical Center, Hamilton, Ontario, Canada

ANTHONY J. BLEYER, M.D.

Fellow, Department of Medicine, The Johns Hopkins University School of Medicine, Baltimore, Maryland

GIANNI BONADONNA, M.D.

Professor of Hematology, University of Milan School of Medicine; Chief, Division of Medical Oncology, National Tumor Institute, Milan, Italy

THEODORE A. BRAICH, M.D.

Assistant Professor, Mayo Medical School, Rochester, Minnesota; Consultant in Hematology/Oncology, Mayo Clinic Scottsdale, Scottsdale, Arizona

MICHAEL C. BRAIN, D.M., F.R.C.P., FRCPC

Professor of Medicine, McMaster University Faculty of Medicine, Hamilton, Ontario, Canada

KYRAN BULGER, M.D.

Assistant Professor of Medicine, Boston University School of Medicine; Physician, Section of Medical Oncology, Boston University Medical Center, Boston, Massachusetts

ROBERT F. BURROWS, M.D., FRCSC

Associate Professor, Obstetrics and Gynecology, McMaster University School of Medicine; Obstetrician, Chedoke-McMaster Hospitals, McMaster Division, Hamilton, Ontario, Canada

GEORGE P. CANELLOS, M.D.

William Rosenberg Professor of Medicine, Harvard Medical School; Chief, Division of Clinical Oncology, Dana-Farber Cancer Institute, and Physician, Brigham and Women's Hospital, Boston, Massachusetts

ROBERT L. CAPIZZI, M.D.

Charles L. Spurr Professor of Medicine and Chief, Section of Hematology/Oncology, Bowman Gray School of Medicine, and Director, Comprehensive Cancer Center of Wake Forest University; Attending Physician, North Carolina Baptist Hospital, Winston-Salem, North Carolina

PAUL P. CARBONE, M.D., D.Sc. (Hon.), F.A.C.P

Professor, Departments of Human Oncology and Medicine, University of Wisconsin Medical School; Director, University of Wisconsin Clinical Cancer Center, Madison, Wisconsin

PETER A. CASSILETH, M.D.

Professor of Medicine, University of Pennsylvania School of Medicine; Associate Director for Clinical Research, University of Pennsylvania Cancer Center, Philadelphia, Pennsylvania

ANN-LII CHENG, M.D.

Attending Physician, Department of Internal Medicine, National Taiwan University Hospital, Taipei, Taiwan

CHARLES S. CLEELAND, Ph.D.

Professor of Neurology, University of Wisconsin Medical School; Director, Pain Research Group, Madison, Wisconsin

BERNARD A. COOPER, M.D.

Professor, Departments of Medicine and Physiology, McGill University Faculty of Medicine; Director, Hematology/Medical Oncology, Royal Victoria Hospital, Montreal, Quebec, Canada

DONALD H. COWAN, M.D., FRCPC

Professor, Department of Medicine, and Associate Dean, University of Toronto Faculty of Medicine; Physician, Department of Medicine, Sunnybrook Health Sciences Centre, Toronto, Ontario, Canada

CHRISTINE DEMERS, M.D., FRCPC

Research Fellow, McMaster University Medical Centre, Hamilton, Ontario, Canada

RUSSELL F. DeVORE, M.D.

Assistant Professor of Medicine, Division of Medical Oncology, Vanderbilt University School of Medicine; Medical Oncologist, Vanderbilt University Medical Center, Nashville, Tennessee

RALPH R. DOBELBOWER, M.D., Ph.D., F.A.C.R.

Professor and Chairman of Radiation Therapy, and Professor of Neurological Surgery (Radiation Therapy), Medical College of Ohio, Toledo, Ohio

WILLIAM L. DONEGAN, M.D.

Professor of Surgery, Medical College of Wisconsin; Chairman of Surgery, Sinai Samaritan Medical Center, Milwaukee, Wisconsin

JOHN D. EARLE, M.D.

William H. Donner Professor of Oncology, Mayo Medical School; Consultant, Mayo Clinic, Rochester, Minnesota

ALLEN C. EAVES, M.D., Ph.D., FRCPC

Professor and Head, Division of Hematology, Department of Medicine, University of British Columbia; Director, Terry Fox Laboratory, British Columbia Cancer Agency, and Head, Division of Hematology, British Columbia Cancer Agency and Vancouver General Hospital, Vancouver, British Columbia, Canada

CONNIE J. EAVES, Ph.D.

Professor, Department of Medical Genetics, University of British Columbia; Staff Scientist, Terry Fox Laboratory, British Columbia Cancer Agency, Vancouver, British Columbia, Canada

RICHARD S. EISENSTAEDT, M.D.

Professor and Associate Chairman, Department of Medicine, Temple University School of Medicine, Philadelphia, Pennsylvania

DAVID S. ETTINGER, M.D.

Associate Professor of Oncology, The Johns Hopkins University School of Medicine; Active Staff, Medical Oncology, The Johns Hopkins Hospital, Baltimore, Maryland

LLOYD K. EVERSON, M.D.

Clinical Associate Professor of Medicine, Section of Oncology/Hematology, Department of Medicine, Indiana University School of Medicine; Director, Indiana Regional Cancer Center, Community Hospitals Indianapolis, Indianapolis, Indiana

CLARENCE L. FORTNER, M.S.

Head, Drug Management and Authorization Section, Investigational Drug Branch, Cancer Therapy Evaluation Program, Division of Cancer Treatment, National Cancer Institute, National Institutes of Health, Bethesda, Maryland

MELVIN H. FREEDMAN, M.D., FRCPC

Professor, Department of Pediatrics, University of Toronto Medical School; Head, Clinical Hematology, Hospital for Sick Children, Toronto, Ontario, Canada

MICHAEL A. FRIEDMAN, M.D.

Associate Director, Cancer Therapy Evaluation Program, Division of Cancer Treatment, National Cancer Institute, National Institutes of Health, Bethesda, Maryland

LILLIAN M. FULLER, M.D.

Professor of Radiotherapy, The University of Texas M.D. Anderson Cancer Center, Houston, Texas

PAUL S. GAYNON, M.D.

Professor of Pediatrics and Director, Clinical Pediatric Hematology/Oncology, University of Wisconsin Clinical Cancer Center, Madison, Wisconsin

JEFFREY S. GINSBERG, M.D., FRCPC

Assistant Professor of Medicine and Director, Thromboembolism Unit, McMaster University Medical Centre, Hamilton, Ontario, Canada

ROBERT L. GOODMAN, M.D.

Professor of Radiation Oncology, University of Pennsylvania School of Medicine; Chairman, Department of Radiation Oncology, Hospital of the University of Pennsylvania, Philadelphia, Pennsylvania

F. ANTHONY GRECO, M.D.

Professor of Medicine and Chief of Medical Oncology, Vanderbilt University School of Medicine, Nashville, Tennessee

PETER GREENWALD, M.D., Dr.P.H.

Director, Division of Cancer Prevention and Control, National Cancer Institute, National Institutes of Health, Bethesda, Maryland

LEONARD L. GUNDERSON, M.D., M.S.

Professor of Oncology, Mayo Medical School; Chairman of Radiation Oncology, Mayo Clinic, Rochester, Minnesota

JOHN D. HAINSWORTH, M.D.

Associate Professor of Medicine, Vanderbilt University School of Medicine; Director, Oncology Inpatient Unit, Vanderbilt University Medical Center, Nashville, Tennessee

MICHAEL J. HAWKINS, M.D.

Chief, Investigational Drug Branch, Cancer Therapy Evaluation Program, Division of Cancer Treatment, National Cancer Institute, National Institutes of Health, Bethesda, Maryland

JOHN D. HINES, M.D.

Professor of Medicine, Case Western Reserve University School of Medicine; Director, Division of Hematology/Oncology, MetroHealth Medical Center, Cleveland, Ohio

A. VICTOR HOFFBRAND, D.M., F.R.C.P., F.R.C.Path.

Professor of Haematology, Royal Free School of Medicine; Honorary Consultant Haematologist, Royal Free Hospital, London, England

HERBERT C. HOOVER, Jr., M.D.

Associate Professor of Surgery, Harvard Medical School; Chief, Surgical Oncology Research, Massachusetts General Hospital, Boston, Massachusetts

JOHN HORTON, M.B., Ch.B., F.A.C.P.

Professor of Medicine, Albany Medical College; Attending Physician, Albany Medical Center, Albany, New York

NEIL IRICK, M.D.

Clinical Assistant Professor, Indiana University School of Medicine, and Adjunct Professor of Nursing, Indiana University School of Nursing; Director, Pain Resource Center, Indianapolis, Indiana

KAREN ISEMINGER, C.R.N.P., M.S.N., O.C.N.

Manager, Patient and Family Supportive Care, Indiana Regional Cancer Center, Indianapolis, Indiana

VINAY JAIN, M.B., B.S.

Visiting Associate, Pediatric Branch, National Institutes of Health, Bethesda, Maryland

DAVID H. JOHNSON, M.D.

Associate Professor of Medicine, Division of Medical Oncology, Vanderbilt University School of Medicine; Medical Oncologist, Vanderbilt University Medical Center, Nashville, Tennessee

TIMOTHY J. KINSELLA, M.D.

Professor and Chairman, Department of Human Oncology, and Director of Radiation Oncology, University of Wisconsin Medical School, Madison, Wisconsin

PETER C. KOHLER, M.D., Ph.D.

Assistant Professor, Department of Human Oncology, University of Wisconsin Medical School; Staff Physician, Meriter Hospital, Madison, Wisconsin

GEORGE J. KONTOGHIORGHES, Ph.D.

Senior Research Fellow, Royal Free Hospital School of Medicine, University of London, London, England

RICHARD A. LARSON, M.D.

Associate Professor of Hematology/Oncology, Department of Medicine, University of Chicago Pritzker School of Medicine, Chicago, Illinois

HILLARD M. LAZARUS, M.D.

Associate Professor of Medicine, University Ireland Cancer Center, and Director, Bone Marrow Transplant Program, Case Western Reserve University, Cleveland, Ohio

GEORGE C. LEWIS, Jr., M.D.

Professor Emeritus, Obstetrics and Gynecology, Jefferson Medical College, Philadelphia, Pennsylvania

PATRICK J. LOEHRER, Sr., M.D.

Associate Professor of Medicine, Indiana University School of Medicine, Indianapolis, Indiana

CHARLES L. LOPRINZI, M.D.

Assistant Professor, Mayo Medical School; Consultant in Medical Oncology, Mayo Clinic, Rochester, Minnesota

JUDITH A. LUCE, M.D.

Assistant Clinical Professor of Medicine, University of California San Francisco School of Medicine; Director, Oncology Services, San Francisco General Hospital, San Francisco, California

JEANNE M. LUSHER, M.D.

Marion I. Barnhart Hemostasis Research Professor, Wayne State University School of Medicine; Director, Division of Hematology/Oncology, Children's Hospital of Michigan, Detroit, Michigan

IAN MAGRATH, M.B., B.S., F.R.C.P., F.R.C.Path.

Chief, Section of Lymphoma Biology, Pediatric Branch, National Institutes of Health, Bethesda, Maryland

DENNIS G. MAKI, M.D.

Ovid O. Meyer Professor of Medicine and Head, Section of Infectious Diseases, Department of Medicine, University of Wisconsin Medical School; Attending Physician, Center for Trauma and Life Support, Madison, Wisconsin

GEORGE D. MALKASIAN, Jr., M.D.

Senior Consultant and Professor, Department of Obstetrics and Gynecology, Mayo Medical School; Staff Physician, Mayo Clinic, Rochester, Minnesota

JAMES A. MARTENSON, M.D.

Assistant Professor in Oncology, Mayo Medical School; Consultant in Radiation Oncology, Mayo Clinic, Rochester, Minnesota

ROBERT J. MAYER, M.D.

Associate Professor of Medicine, Harvard Medical School; Associate Professor, Dana-Farber Cancer Institute, Boston, Massachusetts

J. A. McBRIDE, M.B., F.R.C.P. (Edin.), FRCPC, F.R.C.P.

Professor, Department of Pathology, McMaster University Faculty of Medicine; Head, Haematology Laboratory, Henderson General Hospital, Hamilton, Ontario, Canada

RONALD P. McCAFFREY, M.D.

Professor of Medicine, Boston University School of Medicine; Chief, Section of Medical Oncology, Boston University Medical Center, Boston, Massachusetts

MINESH P. MEHTA, M.D.

Assistant Professor, University of Wisconsin School of Medicine; Staff Physician, University of Wisconsin Hospital, William S. Middleton Veterans Affairs Hospital, and Beloit Memorial Hospital, Madison, Wisconsin

HOLLIS W. MERRICK III, M.D.

Professor of Surgery, Medical College of Ohio, Toledo, Ohio

EDWARD M. MESSING, M.D., F.A.C.S.

Associate Professor of Surgery and Human Oncology, Division of Urology, University of Wisconsin School of Medicine; Staff Urologist, University Hospital, Madison, Wisconsin

HANS A. MESSNER, M.D., Ph.D., FRCPC

Associate Professor, Department of Medicine, University of Toronto Faculty of Medicine; Staff Physician and Director, Bone Marrow Transplant Team, Princess Margaret Hospital, Toronto, Ontario, Canada

RALPH M. MEYER, M.D., FRCPC

Associate Professor, Department of Medicine, McMaster University School of Medicine; Hematologist, Hamilton Civic Hospitals and Hamilton Regional Cancer Centre, Hamilton, Ontario, Canada

PAUL F. MILNER, M.D., F.R.C.Path.

Professor of Pathology and Medicine, Medical College of Georgia; Physician in Charge, Adult Sickle Cell Clinic, Division of Hematology, Department of Medicine, Medical College of Georgia Hospital and Clinics, Augusta, Georgia

MARK MINDEN, M.D., Ph.D., FRCPC

Associate Professor, Department of Medicine, University of Toronto Faculty of Medicine; Staff Physician, Princess Margaret Hospital, Toronto, Ontario, Canada

JOEL L. MOAKE, M.D.

Professor of Medicine, Baylor College of Medicine, and Associate Director, Biomedical Engineering Laboratory, Rice University; Director, Medical Hematology Section, The Methodist Hospital, Houston, Texas

PETER B. NEAME, M.D., FRCPC, F.A.C.P., F.R.C.Path.

Professor of Pathology and Medicine, McMaster University School of Medicine; Head of Service, Haematology Laboratory, Hamilton Civic Hospitals, General Division, Hamilton, Ontario, Canada

G. H. NEILD, M.D., F.R.C.P.

Professor of Nephrology, Institute of Urology, University College and Middlesex School of Medicine; Consultant Physician, St. Philip's Hospital, London, England

PAUL M. NESS, M.D.

Associate Professor of Pathology and Medicine, The Johns Hopkins University School of Medicine; Director, Blood Bank, The Johns Hopkins Hospital, Baltimore, Maryland

PAMELA A. O'HOSKI, A.R.T.

Chief Technologist, Blood Bank, Henderson General Hospital, Hamilton, Ontario, Canada

STANLEY E. ORDER, M.D., Sc.D., F.A.C.R.

Williard and Lillian Hackerman Professor of Oncology and Radiological Sciences, The Johns Hopkins University School of Medicine; Director, Radiation Oncology, The Johns Hopkins Hospital, Baltimore, Maryland

ROBERT F. OZOLS, M.D., Ph.D.

Chairman, Department of Medical Oncology, Fox Chase Cancer Center, Philadelphia, Pennsylvania

THOMAS W. PATON, Pharm.D.

Associate Professor, Faculty of Pharmacy, University of Toronto Faculty of Medicine, Toronto; Director, Department of Pharmacy, Sunnybrook Health Science Centre, North York, Ontario, Canada

GORDON L. PHILLIPS, M.D.

Professor of Medicine, University of British Columbia; Director, Leukemia and Bone Marrow Transplantation Program of British Columbia, Vancouver, British Columbia, Canada

LORI J. PIERCE, M.D.

Assistant Professor, Department of Radiation Oncology, University of Pennsylvania School of Medicine; Staff, Radiation Oncology, Hospital of the University of Pennsylvania, Philadelphia, Pennsylvania

LEONIDAS C. PLATANIAS, M.D.

Fellow, Department of Medicine, Section of Hematology/Oncology, University of Chicago Pritzker School of Medicine, Chicago, Illinois

ARTHUR I. RADIN, M.D.

Attending Physician, The Johns Hopkins Oncology Center and The Johns Hopkins Hospital, Baltimore, Maryland

KANTI R. RAI, M.D., F.A.C.P.

Professor of Medicine, Albert Einstein College of Medicine; Chief, Division of Hematology/Oncology, Long Island Jewish Medical Center, New Hyde Park, New York

GUILLERMO RAMIREZ, M.D., F.A.C.P

Professor of Human Oncology, University of Wisconsin Clinical Cancer Center, Madison, Wisconsin

MARK J. RATAIN, M.D.

Assistant Professor of Medicine and Clinical Pharmacology, University of Chicago Pritzker School of Medicine, Chicago, Illinois

JAY J. REDINGTON, M.D.

Fellow, Section of Infectious Diseases, University of Wisconsin Medical School, Madison, Wisconsin

SCOT C. REMICK, M.D.

Assistant Professor of Medicine and Director of Clinical Research, AIDS Treatment Center, Division of Medical Oncology, Albany Medical College, Albany, New York

HAROLD R. ROBERTS, M.D.

Sarah Graham Kenan Professor of Medicine, The University of North Carolina School of Medicine; Attending Physician, The University of North Carolina Hospitals, Chapel Hill, North Carolina

H. IAN ROBINS, M.D., Ph.D.

Associate Professor, Departments of Human Oncology, Medicine, and Neurology, University of Wisconsin School of Medicine; Director, Medical Oncology, Department of Human Oncology, and Section Chief, Medical Oncology, Department of Medicine, University of Wisconsin Clinical Cancer Center, Madison, Wisconsin

GAIL ROCK, Ph.D., M.D.

Clinical Assistant Professor of Medicine, and Chairman, Canadian Apheresis Study Group, University of Ottawa Faculty of Medicine, Ottawa, Ontario, Canada

REY RODRIGUEZ, M.D.

Resident, Radiation Oncology, University of Wisconsin Medical School, Madison, Wisconsin

VIRGIL L. ROSE, M.D.

Hematology Fellow, The University of North Carolina School of Medicine; Attending Physician, The University of North Carolina Hospitals, Chapel Hill, North Carolina

COLEMAN ROTSTEIN, M.D., FRCPC

Associate Professor of Medicine, Division of Infectious Diseases, McMaster University Faculty of Medicine, Hamilton, Ontario, Canada

JACK M. ROZENTAL, M.D., Ph.D.

Assistant Professor, Department of Neurology, University of Wisconsin Medical School; Staff Neurologist and Head of Neurology Service, William S. Middleton Veterans Affairs Hospital, Madison, Wisconsin

ZAVERIO M. RUGGERI, M.D.

Associate Member, Scripps Clinic and Research Foundation, La Jolla, California

YOUCEF M. RUSTUM, Ph.D.

Deputy Director, Grace Cancer Drug Center, Roswell Park Memorial Institute, Buffalo, New York

STEPHEN E. SALLAN, M.D.

Professor of Pediatrics, Harvard Medical School; Clinical Director, Department of Pediatric Oncology, Dana-Farber Cancer Institute, Boston, Massachusetts

WILLIAM T. SAUSE M.D.

Clinical Professor of Radiology, University of Utah School of Medicine; Director, Radiation Therapy Center, LDS Hospital, Salt Lake City, Utah

ANDREW I. SCHAFER, M.D.

Professor and Vice-Chairman, Department of Medicine, Baylor College of Medicine; Chief, Medical Service, Houston Veterans Affairs Medical Center, Houston, Texas

JOAN H. SCHILLER, M.D.

Assistant Professor, University of Wisconsin Clinical Cancer Center, Madison, Wisconsin

DAVID A. SEARS, M.D.

Professor of Medicine, Baylor College of Medicine; Attending Physician, Harris County Hospital District, Houston, Texas

MICHAEL V. SEIDEN, M.D., Ph.D.

Clinical Fellow in Oncology, Dana-Farber Cancer Institute, Boston, Massachusetts

SANDOR S. SHAPIRO, M.D.

Director, Cardeza Foundation for Hematological Research, Jefferson Medical College, Philadelphia, Pennsylvania

DALE SHOEMAKER, Ph.D.

Chief, Regulatory Affairs Branch, Cancer Therapy Evaluation Program, Division of Cancer Treatment, National Cancer Institute, National Institutes of Health, Bethesda, Maryland

S. EVA SINGLETARY, M.D.

Assistant Professor, The University of Texas Medical School at Houston; Associate Surgeon, The University of Texas M. D. Anderson Cancer Center, Houston, Texas

BEN SISCHY, M.D., F.A.C.R., D.M.R.T. (Edin.)

Clinical Professor of Radiation Oncology, University of Rochester School of Medicine and The Daisy Marquis Jones Radiation Oncology Center at Highland Hospital; Attending Physician, Highland Hospital, Rochester, New York

PRANITI SOAMBOONSRUP, B.Sc., M.T. (A.S.C.P.), S.H.

Chief Technologist, Haematology Laboratory, Hamilton Civic Hospitals, General Division, Hamilton, Ontario, Canada

PAUL M. SONDEL, M.D., Ph.D.

Professor, Departments of Pediatrics, Human Oncology, and Genetics, University of Wisconsin Medical School, Madison, Wisconsin

MICHAEL SPIRITOS, M.D.

Adjunct Assistant Professor of Medicine, University of Pennsylvania School of Medicine, Philadelphia, Pennsylvania

GARY B. STILLWAGON, Ph.D., M.D.

Assistant Professor of Oncology and of Radiology and Radiologic Sciences, The Johns Hopkins University School of Medicine; Director, Radiation Oncology, St. Agnes Hospital, Baltimore, Maryland

WENDY STOCK, M.D.

Fellow, Section of Hematology/Oncology, Department of Medicine, University of Chicago Pritzker School of Medicine, Chicago, Illinois

RICHARD M. STONE, M.D.

Instructor in Medicine, Harvard Medical School; Staff Physician, Dana-Farber Cancer Institute, Boston, Massachusetts

F. KRISTIAN STORM, M.D., F.A.C.S

Professor of Surgery and Human Oncology, and Chairman, Division of Surgical Oncology, University of Wisconsin School of Medicine, Madison, Wisconsin

IH-JEN SU, M.D., Ph.D.

Associate Professor and Attending Physician, Department of Pathology, National Taiwan University Hospital, Taipei, Taiwan

MALCOLM S. TRIMBLE, M.D., FRCPC

Clinical Fellow in Pathology, McMaster University Faculty of Medicine, Hamilton, Ontario, Canada

WILLIAM N. VALENTINE, M.D.

Professor Emeritus, Department of Medicine, University of California Los Angeles School of Medicine, Los Angeles, California

ALONZO P. WALKER, M.D.

Assistant Professor of Surgery, Medical College of Wisconsin; Staff, Milwaukee County Medical Complex, Milwaukee, Wisconsin

PHIL WELLS, M.D., FRCPC

Chief Resident, Haematology Service, McMaster University Faculty of Medicine, Hamilton, Ontario, Canada

DOUGLAS R. WHITE, M.D.

Associate Professor of Medicine, Section of Hematology/Oncology, Bowman Gray School of Medicine and Comprehensive Cancer Center of Wake Forest University; Attending Physician, North Carolina Baptist Hospital, Winston-Salem, North Carolina

GEORGE WILDING, M.D.

Assistant Professor, Department of Human Oncology, University of Wisconsin Clincial Center Center; Chief, Oncology Section, William S. Middleton Veterans Affairs Hospital, Madison, Wisconsin

JAMES S. WILEY, M.D.

Director of Haematology, Austin Hospital, Heidelberg, Victoria, Australia

WILLIAM E. C. WILSON, M.D., C.M., FRCPC, F.A.C.P.

Clinical Professor, Department of Medicine, McMaster University Faculty of Medicine; Service of Clinical Haematology, Department of Medicine, Hamilton Civic Hospitals, Hamilton, Ontario, Canada

SHIAO Y. WOO, M.D.

Assistant Professor of Radiotherapy and of Pediatrics, The University of Texas Medical School at Houston; Radiotherapist and Pediatrician, University of Texas M. D. Anderson Cancer Center, Houston, Texas

JEROME W. YATES, M.D., M.P.H.

Professor of Medicine, State University of New York at Buffalo School of Medicine and Biomedical Sciences; Associate Director for Clinical Affairs, Roswell Park Cancer Institute, Buffalo, New York

NEAL S. YOUNG, M.D.

Chief, Cell Biology Section, Clinical Hematology Branch, National Heart, Lung, and Blood Institutes, National Institutes of Health, Bethesda, Maryland

MARK M. ZALUPSKI, M.D.

Assistant Professor of Medicine, Division of Hematology and Oncology, Wayne State University School of Medicine, Detroit, Michigan

RALPH ZALUSKY, M.D.

Professor of Medicine, Mount Sinai School of Medicine; Chief, Division of Hematology/Oncology, Beth Israel Medical Center, New York, New York

JOHN L. ZIEGLER, M.D.

Professor of Medicine, University of California San Francisco School of Medicine; Director, AIDS Clinical Research Center, and Associate Chief of Staff for Education, Veterans Affairs Medical Center, San Francisco, California

THEODORE S. ZIMMERMAN, M.D. (deceased)

Former Professor, Department of Basic Clinical Research, Director, Coagulation Laboratory, and Staff, Division of Hematology/Oncology, Scripps Clinic and Research Center, La Jolla, California

PREFACE

The fourth edition of *Current Therapy in Hematology-Oncology*, as all the prior editions, is designed to provide the primary physician, oncology fellow, and practicing oncologist with a comprehensive and concise review of management approaches to a variety of cancers. It gets at the key essentials and avoids stereotypical, stylized repetition of detail that will not be useful to the busy practitioner. The chapters are designed to find therapeutic answers to both common and rare hematologic and oncologic problems. The primary purpose of this edition is to provide the practicing physician or trainee with the experience and advice of experts working in their subspecialty fields. The authors are well recognized internationally and offer their expert opinions as to how best to manage specific problems. Their chapters focus on precise therapeutic options, detailing the benefits and risks. A brief list of readings at the end of each chapter is offered for those who need to know more.

We are grateful to our many colleagues who have taken the time to write their thoughts and approaches. We also want to thank our secretaries, Sue Parman and Audrey Moffett, for their invaluable help in sending out letters and reminders to the authors. We also want to thank the editors and staff of B.C. Decker for their excellent editing and support of our efforts.

Michael C. Brain
Paul P. Carbone

CONTENTS

ONCOLOGY

HEMATOLOGY

APLASTIC ANEMIA

NEAL S. YOUNG, M.D.

The infrequency of aplastic anemia (incidence = 2 to $6/10^6$) does not allow most hematologists to have comfortable familiarity with its treatment. Aplastic anemia is often fatal, but more than half of patients with severe bone marrow failure can be cured. All forms of definitive therapy require adequate supportive care; these are the subject of this chapter.

Before a therapeutic strategy is decided on, the diagnosis must be exactly established and an estimate made of the patient's prognosis.

Differential Diagnosis. Despite the clarity of the clinical presentation of aplastic anemia—pancytopenia with an "empty" bone marrow—many patients with low blood counts are misdiagnosed because of inadequate tissue sampling, mistaken pathologic interpretation, or ignorance of pathophysiologic mechanisms. Careful examination of the aspirate smear and judgment of cellularity from a 1-cm core biopsy are the minimal diagnostic requirements. Idiopathic aplastic anemia should be especially distinguished from (1) Fanconi's anemia or congenital aplastic anemia (by cytogenetic analysis of peripheral blood mononuclear cells cultured in the presence of mitomycin C or diepoxybutane); (2) paroxysmal nocturnal hemoglobinuria, which may develop from or into aplastic anemia (by Ham's test); (3) aleukemic acute leukemia and lymphoma restricted to the bone marrow (by attention to blast cells that can be nestled close to spicules in an otherwise hypocellular specimen); (4) myelofibrosis (by remembering that failure to aspirate marrow, or a dry tap, is unusual in aplasia); and (5) dysmyelopoietic syndromes, which may be hypocellular and associated with chromosomal abnormalities restricted to marrow cells.

Prognosis. Blood counts at presentation are the major determinants of survival, whereas age, sex, toxic exposures, and other historical features have had no important prognostic role in patient populations analyzed retrospectively. Patients with aplastic anemia are generally categorized as having severe disease if at clinical presentation they fulfill two of three blood count criteria: polymorphonuclear cell number less than 500 per cubic millimeter; platelets less than 20,000 per cubic millimeter; reticulocytes less than 1 percent (corrected) or less than 60,000 per cubic millimeter (absolute). Very low neutrophil counts have a particularly dire significance. Severity implies a poor prognosis, with mortality for disease untreated at 1 year of 80 to 90 percent; patients with moderate disease have a better outlook, although many ultimately die of the complications of pancytopenia or transfusional hemosiderosis. Unfortunately, blood count criteria are not infallible. Some patients with virtually absent granulocytes or platelets survive for years. Conversely, a patient's blood count may fall following presentation, refractoriness to platelet transfusions may permit fatal hemorrhage, or a trivial untreated infection may become established. Nevertheless, patients with severe aplastic anemia require immediate definitive therapy, usually either bone marrow transplantation or horse antithymocyte globulin therapy.

Initial Evaluation. The rapidity of the initial clinical and laboratory evaluation is intrinsic to the appropriate care of the aplastic anemia patient. Severely pancytopenic patients can deteriorate rapidly as a result of sepsis or bleeding, and the initiation of curative therapy is then postponed in order to treat cascading complications. These complications and their treatments can further diminish the probability of success of the definitive treatment. For example, avoidance of transfusions enhances the survival of the patient undergoing bone marrow transplantation. For either replacement therapy in the form of transplantation or immunologic therapy with horse antiserum to human lymphocytes, the patient in good general medical condition has the best opportunity of immediate survival and ultimate recovery. Table 1 summarizes the crucial laboratory studies that should be completed within the first several days of presentation.

BONE MARROW TRANSPLANTATION

Transplantation in the form of bone marrow infusion can restore normal blood counts and can decrease acute mortality in aplastic anemia. The procedure itself

Table 1 Initial Evaluation

Complete blood counts, with differential, reticulocytes × 2
Bone marrow aspiration and 1-cm biopsy
If < 30 years old, cytogenetics of peripheral blood leukocytes
Ham's test
Liver enzymes
HLA typing

carries a significant risk of death, acute and delayed morbidity, and expense. Patients with histocompatible family members (four identical human leukocyte antigens [HLA] plus absence of mixed lymphocyte reactivity), almost always siblings, should always be considered for bone marrow transplantation. Although occasional patients have successfully received transplants across HLA barriers from relatives or from HLA-identical unrelated donors, the overall success rate using nonidentical or unrelated donors is very low. Fewer than half of patients have identical sibling donors.

The major factors that contribute to the outcome of bone marrow transplantation in bone marrow failure are: (1) patient age, (2) transfusion history, and (3) infection at time of transplant. The incidence of graft-versus-host disease (GVHD), one of the major complications of bone marrow transplantation, increases with age and is more than 90 percent in patients over 30 years of age. Untransfused (actually meaning no transfusions within 72 hours before conditioning therapy begins) patients have a lower incidence of graft rejection because their lymphocytes have not been sensitized by prior antigen exposure.

Good candidates—young, untransfused, and uninfected—have an excellent prospect of hematopoietic recovery when undergoing transplants at experienced centers, as high as 75 percent long-term survival with hematopoietic engraftment. Statistics almost as good for transfused patients have been reported in some studies, although survival rates of 40 to 65 percent are more common. Death immediately following transplantation usually results from acute GVHD or interstitial pneumonitis. Chronic GVHD, even if not fatal, can be a serious multisystem disease and is not always responsive to immunosuppressive therapy. There is a roughly inverse relationship between graft rejection and GVHD. Success at reducing the rejection rate to about 10 percent by intensifying immunosuppression preconditioning has been accompanied by an increased incidence of GVHD, and efforts, at least to date, to reduce GVHD by in vitro T-cell depletion of donor bone marrow have resulted in higher rates of graft rejection.

Delayed complications of marrow transplantation for any indication result from the effects of irradiation and chemotherapy: diminished pulmonary function, endocrine dysfunction and infertility, cognitive disorders and leukoencephalopathy, and secondary malignancies. Patients with Fanconi's anemia have undergone successful transplants using a necessary reduced conditioning regimen; already at risk for malignancy, they have exaggerated long-term effects.

Patients with aplastic anemia may experience graft rejection because of the underlying pathophysiology of bone marrow failure. Simple infusions of marrow from syngeneic twins, without immunosuppressive therapy of the host, fail about half the time. Recurrence of aplasia in identical twins who were immunosuppressed prior to transplantation is further evidence of an inhospitable environment for stem cells in some patients with bone marrow failure.

ANTITHYMOCYTE GLOBULIN

Mathé, who first noted recovery of autologous bone marrow function in some patients in whom rejection of marrow grafts had occurred, suggested that aplastic anemia might be immunologically mediated. This clinical demonstration of functionally quiescent stem cells in aplastic patients indicated that the empty bone marrow contains cells capable of rescue with nonreplacement therapy. Laboratory experiments in general have supported the hypothesis of suppression of hematopoiesis by T cells and their soluble products, but when applied to individual patients, these tests are inadequate to predict clinical response to immunologic therapy. The decision to employ antilymphocyte sera is therefore clinical.

Two types of horse serum preparations are in wide use. Antithoracic duct lymphocyte globulin (ALG or ATDLG) is European and is manufactured by the Swiss Serum Institute or Institut Merieux of Lyons; despite extensive experience with these agents, they have not been approved for use in the United States. Antithymocyte globulin (ATG, ATGAM), manufactured by Upjohn, is commercially available. Although it is a controversial subject, there is little convincing laboratory or clinical evidence of important differences between ATG and ALG preparations or among lots. Regimens have also varied, ALG usually being administered in higher doses over shorter periods of time than ATG. Because the foreign proteins are rapidly cleared once the patient produces antihorse IgG antibodies at about 1 week, briefer treatment is probably more rational. We currently administer ATG, 40 mg per kilogram per day for 4 days.

About half of patients treated with ATG recover hematopoiesis, often not to completely normal blood counts but sufficient to be free of infection and the need for transfusion of red cells and platelets. Hematopoietic recovery rates in different studies have ranged from 25 to 85 percent; this is possibly related to differences among centers in patient selection and supportive care. Recovery rates are not apparently related to age, sex, or the etiology of bone marrow failure. Patients with very severe neutropenia (< 200 neutrophils per cubic millimeter) may not survive to benefit from ATG. Hematopoietic improvement is usually apparent within a few months of ATG therapy. Later improvement can occur, although specific therapeutic benefit due to ATG is then harder to distinguish from the effects of subsequent therapy and spontaneous late remission in well-supported aplastic anemic patients. Perhaps 10 percent of patients who have remissions with ATG subsequently relapse, and they may respond to a second course of ATG.

The complications of ATG therapy are best managed by a hematologist experienced in its use; however, patients do not require routine transfer to intensive care units for ATG therapy. Although rare, anaphylaxis due to horse protein allergy is the most serious consequence and has been fatal. Skin testing may predict susceptible patients. We currently test by epicutaneous prick testing with undiluted ATG. A wheal and flare reaction would indicate the need for desensitization before ATG administration. More common allergic symptoms are fever, chills, and urticaria with the first few infusions. Serum sickness at about day 10 of therapy is also common and manifests usually as a flu-like illness with a characteristic maculopapular eruption, fever, arthralgia and myalgia, and gastrointestinal symptoms. Serum transaminase and creatinine levels may be transiently increased, and the albumin value may be depressed. Although it is generally tolerated when corticosteroids are administered at high doses (60 to 80 mg methylprednisolone in divided daily doses), serum sickness can be temporarily incapacitating; myositis and myocarditis have been observed. Finally, as ATG binds to circulating blood elements as well as lymphocytes, lower platelet and granulocyte

counts during ATG therapy should be expected and may necessitate increased numbers of transfusions or antibiotic administration; the result on Coombs' test may become positive during ATG therapy.

CYCLOSPORINE

Cyclosporine, which interferes with T-cell function more specifically than ATG, is effective in about 40 percent of patients in whom conventional immunosuppressive therapy has failed; preliminary European data suggest that cyclosporine added to ALG may increase the initial response rate in severe disease. We administer cyclosporine at 12 mg per kilogram per day in adults and 15 mg per kilogram per day in children and adjust dosage for nephrotoxicity and blood levels (tests obtained every 2 weeks). Aplastic anemia patients receiving cyclosporine can resemble patients with acquired immunodeficiency syndrome and are susceptible to infection with unusual agents such as *Pneumocystis carinii*.

ANDROGENS

Often disparaged but often used, androgens have a mixed reputation, mainly because only trials from Europe have supported their use. Nonetheless, most hematologists have had at least one aplastic patient who has clearly responded to hormone therapy. Androgens may work best in patients with some residual hematopoiesis. Dosage is also probably important. Choice of androgen is largely individual: oxymetholone, fluoxymesterone, and nandrolone decanoate are among the more popular formulations. We employ nandrolone decanoate at 2 to 5 mg per kilogram per week, given intramuscularly (injection is well tolerated even in thrombocytopenic patients if followed by 15 minutes of pressure); parenteral androgens avoid the hepatotoxicity associated with oral preparations. With any androgen, a fair clinical trial is 3 to 6 months.

HEMATOPOIETIC GROWTH FACTORS

A few patients have been reported to respond to granulocyte macrophage colony–stimulating factor (GM-CSF) and interleukin-3 in early trials, usually with neutrophil improvement but occasionally with increased platelets and reticulocytes. In general, the best responses have been in cases with residual hematopoiesis or chronic disease; GM-CSF has not been shown to be helpful in severe neutropenia associated with serious infection. Cytokine flu and a capillary leak syndrome are the major toxicities of GM-CSF. Interleukin-3 and also GM-CSF appear to be much less toxic. Future trials will test factors that act at the primitive hematopoietic stem cell level (interleukin-1 and interleukin-3) and combinations of growth factors.

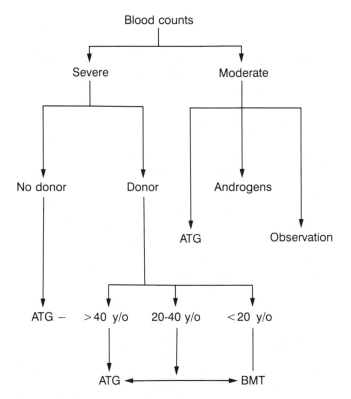

Figure 1 Treatment alternatives in aplastic anemia. BMT = bone marrow transplant.

SUPPORTIVE THERAPY

Infections

Febrile episodes and serious infections are common in severely affected patients and represent the major cause of death in aplastic anemia. Fever, local infections, and even vague symptoms such as generalized malaise suggestive of early sepsis must be regarded with extreme seriousness in the setting of neutropenia. Suspicion of sepsis should initiate administration of broad-spectrum, full-dose parenteral antibiotic therapy (ceftazidime or a combination of a cephalosporin, semisynthetic penicillin, and an aminoglycoside). Unless a nonbacterial cause of fever becomes obvious (e.g., serum sickness, viral infection), therapy should be continued for 10 to 14 days, even with negative blood culture results. More important is the prompt institution of antibiotics rather than the precise choice of agents prescribed.

With the first episodes of infection, neutropenic patients defervesce and improve symptomatically within a few days of treatment. Persistent or recurrent fever despite antibiotics occasionally responds to addition of a more specific drug that broadens bacterial coverage, such as vancomycin (for resistant *Staphylococcus*) or clindamycin (for anaerobes). More usually, persistent fever in the repeatedly treated patient signifies fungal infection and demands amphotericin B therapy; empiric antifungal therapy should be started in a patient who has fever after 7 days of antibacterial antibiotics. Infections caused by resistant organisms, rare bacterial species, and *Pneumocystis* are uncommon in aplastic anemia patients.

Delaying administration of antibiotics may lead to seeding of organisms, a virtually intractable problem in aplastic patients. Surgical approaches tend to spread infection across fascial planes, and concentrated collections of bacteria, even sensitive *Escherichia coli* and *Pseudomonas,* may not be eradicated even with prolonged antibiotic treatment. The role of granulocyte transfusions, which may be employed in the deteriorating patient with a seated infection, is uncertain.

Bleeding and Platelet Transfusions

Bleeding is common in bone marrow failure but is rarely fatal. Thrombocytopenia alone usually results in mucocutaneous hemorrhage and manifests as petechiae, ecchymoses, and gingival oozing. Spontaneous intracranial hemorrhage is the most feared complication; it is often, but not invariably, fatal. Major gastrointestinal, genitourinary, or pulmonary bleeding is not usually due to diminished platelet numbers alone but occurs in the setting of infection, stress, and corticosteroid therapy.

Serious bleeding is treated by platelet transfusions administered as often as required for clinical effect. Four units of platelets or the donation from a single cytophoresed donor may raise the platelet count above 30,000 to 40,000 and may stem hemorrhage; transfusions as often as three times daily may be required in other circumstances. Life-threatening hemorrhage is customarily treated with platelet transfusions even in the absence of satisfactory increments in peripheral blood platelet numbers in the hope of homing to bleeding sites.

Platelets administered prophylactically can prevent hemorrhage, although there are no data indicating improved survival as a result of prophylaxis as compared with platelets on demand. A convenient goal is to maintain platelet counts at over 5,000 per cubic millimeter. There is no rationale for prophylactic transfusion in patients whose disease has become refractory because of alloantibody formation. Bleeding in these patients may respond to Amicar, an oral antifibrinolytic agent. Patients should, of course, be advised not to take aspirin or aspirin-like drugs, and abnormalities of coagulation factors, induced by inanition and antibiotic therapy, must be corrected.

Erythrocytes and Hemochromatosis

Blood should be transfused regularly to permit comfortable physical activity, usually achieved with a normal cardiovascular state at a hemoglobin concentration of over 7 to 8 g per deciliter and in the presence of coronary disease at a hemoglobin concentration over 9 g per deciliter. Complete replacement of erythropoiesis in an adult requires transfusion of about 1 unit per week of packed red blood cells. Hemochromatotic damage to the heart, liver, and endocrine glands can be expected once the transfusion burden exceeds 100 U, a good point at which to start desferrioxamine chelation in patients with chronic disease.

ALTERNATE, EXPERIMENTAL, AND FUTURE THERAPIES

Immunosuppression

Very-high–dose corticosteroid therapy has had success rates comparable to those of ALG in Europe, although it probably is most effective in patients treated within a few weeks of diagnosis. Methylprednisolone therapy has aimed at infusion of 100 mg per kilogram during the first week, 50 mg per kilogram during the second week, and gradual tapering of the dose over 30 to 40 days. Toxic effects are common, including salt and water retention, hypertension, diabetes, electrolyte imbalance, occult infection, and aseptic joint necrosis. High-dose corticosteroids should be reserved for treatment of patients when or where ATG is unavailable.

Antiviral Therapy

Some cases of aplastic anemia follow infectious mononucleosis, and in other patients, Epstein-Barr virus can be found in the bone marrow despite a negative clinical history. Remissions have followed acyclovir therapy. Acyclovir is not very toxic and can be given to patients with herpesvirus associated with aplasia at 15 mg per kilogram per day in three divided, intravenous doses.

SUGGESTED READING

Hathorn JW, Pizzo PA. Infectious complications in the pediatric cancer patient. In: Pizzo PA, Poplack DG, eds. Pediatric oncology. Philadelphia: JB Lippincott, 1989.

Kurtzman G, Young N. Aplastic anemia. In: Masur H, Parrillo J, eds. The critically ill immunosuppressed patient. Rockville, MD: Aspen, 1987.

Leonard EM, Raefsky E, Griffith P, et al. Cyclosporine therapy of aplastic anaemia, congenital and acquired aplastic anemia. Br J Haematol 1989; 72:278–284.

O'Reilly RJ. Allogeneic bone marrow transplantation: Current status and future directions. Blood 1983; 62:941–964.

Young NS, Alter BA. Bone marrow failure. In: Handin RI, Lux SE, Stossel TP, eds. Blood: Principles and practice of hematology. Philadelphia: JB Lippincott, in press.

Young N, Speck B. Antithymocyte and antilymphocyte globulins: Clinical trials and mechanism of action: In: Young N, Levine A, Humphries PK, eds. Aplastic anemia: stem cell biology and advances in treatment. New York: Alan R. Liss, 1984:221.

MEGALOBLASTIC ANEMIA

BERNARD A. COOPER, M.D.

Megaloblastic anemia is characterized by megaloblastic morphology in bone marrow smears, caused by either (1) relatively specific and undefined defects in nucleotide metabolism induced by antimetabolites or deficiency of certain coenzymes, or (2) equally undefined metabolic abnormalities in erythroid precursors in some clonal hematologic diseases, such as the leukemias. Although morphologic features in peripheral blood (such as macrocytosis or multilobed neutrophils) and some biochemical abnormalities (such as elevations of levels of iron or LDH in serum, abnormal deoxyuridine suppression test in stimulated lymphocytes, methylmalonate excretion in urine, or low levels of folate or vitamin B_{12} in serum or blood) correlate with megaloblastic morphology. They do not invariably predict it.

DIAGNOSIS

The effectiveness of therapy is often determined by how effectively diagnostic procedures are selected when the patient is first seen. Initial examination should include detailed history for evidence of nutritional deficiency, intestinal disease, dysphagia, ingestion of antimetabolic drugs, alcohol, or other medications that might predispose to deficiency, and previous episodes of anemia and their response to therapy. Careful examination may reveal evidence of weight loss, hepatic cirrhosis, reflex changes, loss of vibration sense, glossitis, or petechiae and/or ecchymosis. Blood samples should be taken for determinations of levels of vitamin B_{12} and folate in serum and of erythrocyte folate. The former utilizes serum from clotted blood, and commercially available vacutainers (red top) are appropriate. The latter requires unclotted blood and should be taken into either citrate (blue top) or EDTA (purple top) vacutainers. It is recommended that 5 ml of serum be provided to the laboratory so that the remaining unclotted specimen can be sent for determination of plasma methylmalonic acid and total homocysteine if this is required. Routine hematologic studies including reticulocyte count, platelet count, and peripheral smear are required, and prothrombin time determination may aid in recognition of intestinal malabsorption.

Bone marrow aspiration should be performed before therapy is instituted. For most cases, aspiration and smear are adequate, and biopsy is not required.

GENERAL THERAPY

Anemia. If life-threatening, anemia should be treated by blood transfusion sufficient to provide adequate peripheral oxygenation and cardiac function. Patients seeking medical aid because of anemia often do so because the reflex increase of cardiac output caused by the anemia exceeds the capacity of their myocardium. In such cases, cardiac failure responds to transfusion of a single unit of packed erythrocytes, together with appropriate therapy for cardiac failure. Cardiac failure responds to diuretic therapy, and so in the uncomplicated patient, furosamide, 20 mg, should be injected as transfusion is begun or as soon as the patient is seen. Further diuretic therapy should be selected on the basis of central venous pressure observation and standard clinical criteria.

Leukopenia. Seldom is leukopenia of sufficient degree to cause susceptibility to infection.

Thrombocytopenia. Occasionally, thrombocytopenia may cause life-threatening hemorrhage: although in uncomplicated megaloblastic anemia, it usually is associated with severe anemia, thrombocytopenia may appear without anemia, and its cause may thus be obscure. Severe thrombocytopenia with evidence of petechiae and ecchymoses or bleeding should be treated with platelet transfusion.

Other Somatic Manifestations. These include

glossitis, dysphagia, anorexia, diminished levels of circulating immunoglobulins, and decreased lymphocyte reactivity; they are probably never dangerous and require no specific therapy.

Severe Psychologic Depression. This has been described in association with pernicious anemia and possibly with folate deficiency. There is evidence that the depressive features are corrected when diagnosis is made and may thus be reactive. Specific therapy is thus not required. For serious depression, sedation and antidepressive therapy are identical with those used in depressive disorders of other causes. The organic brain syndrome and loss of intellectual function associated with deficiency of vitamin B_{12} respond only to replacement therapy with vitamin B_{12}.

SPECIFIC THERAPY

Clinical Situation I

In this case, bone marrow is megaloblastic, with macrogranulocytes present, and clinical examination is consistent with nutritional megaloblastic anemia. Based on clinical information and the presence or absence of neurologic signs or symptoms, a presumptive diagnosis of deficiency of vitamin B_{12} or folate is made.

If the anemia is presumed to be the result of vitamin B_{12} deficiency, treatment consists of subcutaneous injections of vitamin B_{12} (cyanocobalamin), 5 μg per day for 2 days, followed by 100 μg per day if the patient is in the hospital, or weekly if not.

If the presumption is that the anemia is due to folate deficiency, treatment consists of oral folic acid as follows: 200 μg per day for 2 days followed by 2 mg per day for 1 week.

Monitoring Response

The classic *reticulocyte response* to therapy may be monitored, and some response will be observed, even if anemia is partially corrected by transfusion. *Neutrophil count* increases by the third or fourth day following initiation of therapy, simultaneously with the earliest increase of reticulocytes. *Serum iron,* if elevated, decreases to deficient levels within 24 hours of initiation of specific therapy, and erythropoiesis in the *bone marrow* becomes morphologically normoblastic within 48 hours of initiation of appropriate therapy (macrogranulocytosis persists for 10 to 14 days). With this recommended dosage schedule for vitamin B_{12}, serum iron may not decrease to very low levels before 72 hours after therapy. If response is not observed in the peripheral blood, demonstration of conversion to normoblastic bone marrow morphology confirms the selection of correct therapy. It is well established that infection and iron deficiency obscure response to therapy in the peripheral blood, but do not prevent conversion of bone marrow to normoblastic.

Follow-Up Therapy

One week after the first injection of 100 μg of vitamin B_{12}, vitamin B_{12} absorption should be tested by the *Schilling test* if deficiency of vitamin B_{12} has been confirmed. If deficiency of vitamin B_{12} is confirmed by serum level and malabsorption of the vitamin confirmed by the Schilling test, therapy should be continued for life with 100 μg of vitamin B_{12} monthly. If vitamin B_{12} malabsorption is shown to be caused by a lack of intrinsic factor by correction of absorption with a source of intrinsic factor, no further investigation is required. If intestinal malabsorption is suggested by the Schilling test, and the reliability of the test used is confirmed, further investigation is required, but therapy should be continued as above. If blind loop syndrome is recognized, surgical correction is required if vitamin B_{12} injections are to be discontinued. Antibiotic therapy produces only a transient improvement in malabsorption of vitamin B_{12} caused by bacterial infestation of segments of the small bowel.

Variant of Clinical Situation I

In this case, neurologic manifestations strongly suggestive of those caused by deficiency of vitamin B_{12} (subacute combined degeneration of the spinal cord, or dementia) are present without macrocytosis, anemia, or serum vitamin B_{12} level that is diagnostic of deficiency. There is now increasing awareness that such patients may comprise 30 to 40 percent of all patients with symptomatic deficiency of vitamin B_{12}, and in 5 percent serum B_{12} level may be within the normal range. In most of these, bone marrow is megaloblastic and the investigation described in Clinical Situation I will suffice. In such patients, serum should be analyzed for total homocysteine and for methylmalonic acid, which if elevated will diagnose deficiency of vitamin B_{12} and if absent will exclude it as a cause of the patient's symptoms. After treatment with vitamin B_{12}, changes should be recorded in laboratory parameters listed under Clinical Situation I, and the elevated homocysteine and methylmalonic acid levels will disappear.

Clinical Situation II

In this case bone marrow is megaloblastoid, and macrogranulocytes usually are not observed. Deficiency of vitamin B_{12} or folate is clinically improbable.

Atypical morphology in bone marrow usually is not caused by nutritional deficiency, and so specific therapy may be withheld until investigation suggests the presence of deficiency of vitamin B_{12} or folate. A few cases of sideroblastic anemia with megaloblastic changes have responded to large doses of pyridoxine (100 mg per day by mouth) or other nutrients (viz, thiamine); a few cases have been corrected by discontinuing drugs usually considered innocuous (e.g., analgesics), but most of these are caused either by antimetabolic drugs or by stem cell defects, some of which terminate as acute leukemia.

General therapy should be instituted depending on the clinical situation. Anemia and thrombocytopenia, which may threaten survival, should be treated as already described. In the absence of exposure to antimetabolites, no effective therapy is available for these conditions. Diagnosis must thus be precise, and nutritional causes must be excluded. Most observers verify that the cause is not nutritional deficiency by *therapeutic trial* of vitamin B$_{12}$ and folate over several weeks. Although it is possible that treatment with these vitamins may augment the development of early neoplastic disease, the evidence for this is weak, and thus such therapeutic trials should not be withheld. A normal *deoxyuridine suppression test* on cells obtained from a bone marrow aspirate also may be used as strong evidence against nutritional deficiency as cause of the megaloblastic morphology.

Treatment consists of the following:

1. Manage life-threatening anemia or thrombocytopenia as above.
2. Exclude nutritional deficiency by either (a) treating with vitamin B$_{12}$ and folate in the doses listed above, and verifying the persistence of megaloblastoid morphology in bone marrow after 3 days, or of failure of hematocytopenias to improve over 2 to 3 weeks, or (b) doing a deoxyuridine suppression test on cells obtained from a bone marrow aspirate and demonstrating that this is normal.
3. Exclude the taking of antimetabolic drugs, especially those with antifolate activity.

If evidence is obtained that the patient has taken a drug known to interfere with intracellular metabolism, this usually should be discontinued. Following discontinuation of some antimetabolites such as 6-mercaptopurine, megaloblastoid features may persist for several weeks with only very slow correction of hematocytopenia. There is no evidence that administration of purines, amino acids, or other nutrients accelerate the correction of these drug-related diseases except that megaloblastic features and hematocytopenia induced by folate antagonists respond to administration of folates. Included in this category are: methotrexate, trimethoprim (often administered with sulfonamide), pyrazinamide and certain other antimalarials, triampterin, and a variety of antineoplastic agents that are modifications of methotrexate.

Treatment includes discontinuation of the drug and treatment with either folic acid, 5 mg per day by mouth, or a reduced (tetrahydro-) folate (folinic acid), which may be administered orally at 3 mg per day or by injection at similar dose. It is apparent that in patients receiving large doses of antifols for treatment of neoplastic disease, the usual therapeutic considerations for these are required, including monitoring of plasma methotrexate level and therapy with folinic acid until plasma level approaches 0.1 micromolar (10^{-6} M). In situations in which antifol therapy should not be discontinued (e.g., high-dose trimethoprim-sulfonamide treatment of *Pneumocystis* infection), treatment with folic acid, 5 mg per day for 3 to 4 days, should revert the megaloblastic change without neutralizing the beneficial effects of the antimicrobial therapy because most organisms inhibited by this type of preparation do not effectively accumulate folate. However, following initial therapy of the anemia, it probably is prudent to limit daily folic acid intake to 200 to 500 μg per day—a dose that should prevent megaloblastic anemia without affecting antimicrobial activity.

Most megaloblastoid anemias without macrogranulocytes in the bone marrow and in which bone marrow morphology is not typical of megaloblastic change are due to clonal diseases of the bone marrow and may terminate as acute leukemia. Megaloblastic morphology also is observed in some congenital and acquired aplastic anemias. Macrocytosis in peripheral blood and neutropenia and thrombocytopenia often coexist. In a minority of these, bone marrow morphology is typically megaloblastic, and their differentiation from nutritional anemias is more difficult. Bone marrow biopsy in these cases often reveals hypoplasia with islands of erythroid hyperplasia in contrast to the generalized hyperplasia in classic megaloblastic anemia.

NUTRITIONAL MEGALOBLASTIC ANEMIA: ADDITIONAL OBSERVATIONS

Treatment with Large Doses of Vitamin B$_{12}$ and Folate

Patients deficient in either vitamin respond to such therapy. The availability of assays for vitamin B$_{12}$ and folate in blood make therapeutic trials rarely useful. Most patients with pure deficiency of folate do not respond to usual doses of vitamin B$_{12}$, although in some, reticulocytosis is observed. Although all patients with pure deficiency of vitamin B$_{12}$ show some hematologic response to large doses of folic acid, conversion of the bone marrow to normoblastic by folic acid alone is probably not complete. Complete conversion of bone marrow to normoblastic after therapy with one or the other vitamin thus is reasonable evidence that deficiency was caused by that vitamin. The latter is little justification for single therapy, however, since second bone marrow aspirations, although useful, are rarely performed in practice.

The major justification for treating with small doses of a single vitamin relates to possible dangers of too rapid conversion of bone marrow to normoblastic. Sudden death has occurred during therapy of pernicious anemia—especially in patients with severe anemia. Some of these deaths have been ascribed to severe hypokalemia, relatively refractory to prophylaxis with potassium supplements, and more severe in severely anemic patients with thrombocytopenia and neutropenia. Thrombotic and embolic episodes also have been reported in patients treated for megaloblastic anemia with large doses of vitamins. It is not known whether these catastrophic episodes during therapy are caused by abrupt conversion of megaloblastic to normoblastic bone marrow with arrest of potassium leak from cells, changes of lipids in the plasma, thrombocytosis, correction of platelet defects observed in megaloblastic anemia, or another cause.

It has been demonstrated that single doses of vitamin B_{12} in excess of 80 μg completely converts megaloblastic bone marrow to normoblastic with correction of the anemia, whereas single doses less than 15 μg never completely correct the abnormality.

Because of the possibility that abrupt conversion of megaloblastic to normoblastic maturation may be dangerous, and the observations that the rate of correction of anemia is not significantly decreased by treating with small doses of the deficient vitamin, it would seem prudent to initiate therapy with small doses of vitamin B_{12} or folate, which would convert megaloblastic to normoblastic maturation over 3 to 4 days. This can be accomplished with the treatment regimen recommended above, which is best applied using single nutrients for therapy. It must be emphasized, however, that the advantage of this approach has not been tested.

Vitamin B_{12} Absorption Test (Schilling Test) as Initial Therapy

Flushing radioactivity into the urine in this test requires injection of 1000 μg (1 mg) of vitamin B_{12}. As previously indicated, it is possible that this may be dangerous. Such an approach also may produce erroneous data with misdiagnosis and inappropriate duration of therapy. A proportion of patients with megaloblastic anemia due to deficiency of vitamin B_{12} or folate develop transient malabsorption of vitamin B_{12}, which is corrected after therapy. Although this correction may occasionally be delayed for several weeks, it probably is corrected in most subjects over one cycle of intestinal epithelial cells—about 3 days. A patient might thus have transient malabsorption of vitamin B_{12} secondary to folate deficiency, with malabsorption observed in the first stage of the test, and with apparent correction with intrinsic factor in a later test because of correction of the intestinal defect by therapy. In tests of vitamin B_{12} absorption using simultaneous administration of free and intrinsic factor (IF)-bound vitamin B_{12}, an intestinal malabsorption pattern is observed. Thus, it is recommended that replacement therapy should be continued for at least 3 to 4 days before absorption of vitamin B_{12} is tested.

Repletion of Stores of the Deficient Vitamin

Vitamin B_{12} stores in the liver are repleted slowly following depletion and may require many months to reach normal levels. The anemia caused by deficiency of vitamin B_{12} does not respond to therapy more quickly when large doses are administered—maximum rate of hemoglobin rise being achieved by 2 to 5 μg of vitamin B_{12} per day. Patients treated with larger doses of vitamin B_{12} (e.g., 30 to 100 μg per month by injection) require longer to relapse when therapy is discontinued than do patients treated with smaller doses (e.g., 20 μg per month). The benefit of the slower relapse is unknown.

There is no evidence that injections given more frequently produce better health, although many patients insist that they feel fatigued immediately before their next injection. There is no evidence that this represents deficiency of vitamin B_{12}, as serum levels are not depleted, and stores remain high. It is the impression of most physicians that these symptoms are psychologic.

Folate stores are small and are depleted to levels associated with megaloblastic anemia within 4 months of stopping folate intake. Thus, there is no benefit to treating with more folate than is required to correct clinical and chemical manifestations of deficiency.

Treatment of Subacute Combined Degeneration of the Spinal Cord

Neurologic lesions similar to human subacute combined degeneration of the spinal cord have been produced in monkeys and bats made deficient in vitamin B_{12} or treated with nitrous oxide. In these animals, folate supplementation appears to aggravate the lesions, and methionine supplementation appears to prevent them. Clinical studies appear to indicate that small doses of vitamin B_{12} arrest neurologic disease in pernicious anemia, and neither clinical studies nor animal experiments have demonstrated benefit with larger doses of vitamin B_{12}. Single injections of vitamin B_{12} of less than 50 to 100 μg do not increase spinal fluid cobalamin level within a few hours of injection, and this might support use of large doses of vitamin B_{12} in neurologic disease. Despite this indirect evidence, treatment with standard doses of vitamin B_{12}, as described above, should be considered adequate.

In nutritional anemia in adults, the aforementioned commercial forms of vitamin B_{12} and folate are adequate and probably represent the preferred therapy because of their stability and purity. Although the frequency of injections of vitamin B_{12} required to maintain normal levels of serum vitamin B_{12} is less when hydroxocobalamin is used, the trivial clinical advantage is probably offset by the periodic development of antibodies against hydroxocobalamin during such therapy. Because reduced folates are transported 100 times better into most mammalian cells than is folic acid, reduced folate is preferable to folic acid when counteracting antifols, and so folinic acid is used routinely.

In infants and children with inherited intracellular defects of folate or cobalamin metabolism, the inherited defect may prevent optimal utilization of these forms of the vitamins. In children with intracellular defects of cobalamin metabolism, treatment with hydroxocobalamin is more effective than that with cyanocobalamin, and treatment usually requires large doses (500 to 1,000 μg per day) of this material. In children with deficiency of transcobalamin 2, either cobalamin may be used, but because cyanocobalamin is more effectively absorbed when fed, these children usually are maintained on oral cyanocobalamin (500 μg, 2 to 7 times per week). In children with defective intracellular folate enzymes (e.g., 5 to 10 methylene tetrahydrofolate reductase), folinic acid probably represents better therapy than does folic acid, but optimal therapy would be provided by injections of 5-methyl tetrahydrofolate, if available. Such children also should receive methionine supplements. Note that such children usually do not have megaloblastic anemia.

In inherited metabolic defects, efficacy of therapy should be monitored by disappearance of homocystinuria or methyl malonic aciduria, and by restoration of normal levels of plasma methionine.

SUGGESTED READING

Cooper BA, Rosenblatt DS. Inherited defects of vitamin B_{12} metabolism. Ann Rev Nutr 1987; 7:291–320.

Hall CA. Pernicious anemia: diagnosis and treatment. Geriatrics 1967; 22:109–118.

Reizenstein P, Ljunggren G, Drougge E. Quality of diagnosis and managing anemia in four countries. Biomed Pharmacother 1984; 38:194–198.

IRON-DEFICIENCY ANEMIA

THOMAS W. PATON, PHARM.D.
DONALD H. COWAN, M.D., FRCPC

Iron deficiency is a manifestation of an imbalance between intake and absorption of iron, and a loss or increase of utilization. A normal adult man loses about 1 mg per day of iron, mostly in the stool. To achieve balance, the same amount must be absorbed from dietary sources. An average North American diet contains 10 to 20 mg of iron, and approximately 10 percent of this is absorbed. It is obvious that the probability of negative iron balance is high with menstruation or chronic blood loss from any site; in infancy, with a milk diet low in iron; or during periods of increased utilization, such as pregnancy. In these conditions, a normal diet may not contain sufficient dietary iron to achieve balance, and iron depletion, with or without anemia, commonly occurs. Further, when iron-deficiency anemia is treated, it is necessary to prescribe elemental iron because, at best, 3 to 5 mg of iron per day can be absorbed from dietary sources.

The diagnostic approach to a patient with suspected iron deficiency involves two distinct steps. First, one must establish that lack of iron is the cause of the anemia. The clinical situation and a few simple tests often make the diagnosis obvious; however, not infrequently one must consider a broader range of possibilities and more testing is required. One should remember that a variety of inflammatory or malignant disorders can decrease the serum iron, decrease the total iron-binding capacity, increase the serum ferritin, and consequently may confuse the interpretation of these test results. Further, the ingestion of an iron-containing preparation before blood is drawn for a serum iron test may increase the result to normal levels; thus, no oral iron should be taken for at least 24 hours before the test. Treatment with oral iron for a period of 2 to 3 weeks may also increase ferritin levels to the point that the test is not useful in the diagnosis of iron deficiency. In any of these situations, a low serum ferritin level is diagnostic of iron deficiency. Occasionally, a bone marrow specimen, stained for iron, is necessary to establish the diagnosis. Second, one must determine the cause of the iron lack. These two steps should be carried out in sequence in order to guard against unnecessary investigation in a patient who has an anemia that is not due to iron deficiency.

The objective of therapy is not only to return the hemoglobin to normal levels but also to replenish the body's iron stores. At the same time, measures must be taken to correct the cause of the iron deficiency. Therapy is almost always administered in the oral form; in rare instances, parenteral therapy may be necessary, and occasionally transfusion of red cells may be required as an adjunct to treatment with iron.

ORAL IRON THERAPY

The treatment of patients with iron deficiency with oral elemental iron is specific, economical, effective in almost all instances, and acceptable to patients. A large number of oral iron preparations is available on the market. In Canada, there are more than 30 products. A number of these consist of combinations of drugs, including potential enhancers of absorption (vitamin C), other hematinics (folic acid, vitamin B_{12}, and liver extract), and other vitamins. The dose of elemental iron varies between preparations; in addition, some products are in a slow-release form, whereas others are enteric-coated. The extensive variety of preparations has led to confusion in the selection of the most appropriate product.

One should keep several points in mind when considering which preparation is appropriate for replacement of iron: (1) Because iron is absorbed in the ferrous form, successful therapy depends on the administration of a preparation that contains a ferrous salt. (2) The medication must be in solution, or dissolved in the stomach or upper gastrointestinal tract, in order to be available for absorption in the duodenum and upper jejunum, which are the sites of optimal iron absorption. (3) The preparation must contain sufficient elemental iron. A total dose of 150 to 200 mg of elemental iron each day is recommended for adults. (4) Finally, in selecting a preparation, one should focus on single-ingredient products that contain only an iron salt. Unfortunately, pharmaceutical companies have provided a large number of preparations that contain multiple hematinics and vitamins along with the iron. These are expensive, unnecessary, and can be dangerous. Folic acid, particularly, may mask coincidental pernicious anemia and allow the development of neurologic abnormalities. Dosage forms that contain ascorbic acid are purported to increase the absorption of iron, but the same result can be achieved by increasing the dose of iron; the combination only adds to the cost of treatment. Iron deficiency should be treated specifically, with iron alone. There is no indication for combination products, and they should be avoided.

The dosage forms of oral iron consist of solutions, conventional film-coated tablets, enteric-coated tablets, and slow-release products. Optimal absorption is provided by the solution and the film-coated tablets. Although the solution provides a reliable form of iron and is useful in the rare individual who cannot swallow tablets, the potential for staining the teeth makes it undesirable for routine use. Absorption of the slow-release products is unpredictable and unreliable; they may bypass the site of absorption in the duodenum and jejunum before dissolving and releasing the iron. Recent work suggests that iron from enteric-coated tablets results in incomplete and unpredictable absorption in the majority of users. This is best illustrated by Figure 1, which demonstrates conclusively that the solution and film-coated tablets of ferrous sulfate are well absorbed and to the same extent. The enteric-coated products are virtually nonabsorbable (Fig. 1). There are well-documented cases of poor or no response to both slow-release and enteric-coated products followed by prompt response to liquid iron or film-coated tablets. Although some patients exhibit a rise in hemoglobin on taking these products, there is no indication for their use.

Ferrous sulfate is the most widely prescribed form of oral iron. This is due in part to the drug's excellent solubility and the fact that it is the least expensive iron preparation. The ferrous gluconate, fumarate, and succinate salts are also acceptable forms of treatment, although one should appreciate that the amount of elemental iron provided by each of these tablets differs. The ferrous sulfate and fumarate tablets generally contain 60 mg of elemental iron, whereas the ferrous gluconate and succinate tablets contain 35 mg (Table 1).

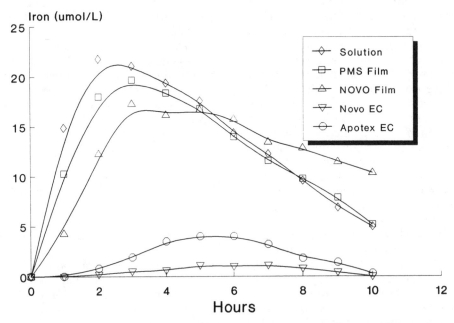

Figure 1 Mean serum iron concentration–time profile for five ferrous sulfate preparations given to healthy normal volunteers. Diamonds = oral solution, squares = Pharmascience film-coated tablet, triangles = Novopharm film-coated tablet, inverted triangles = Novopharm enteric-coated tablet, circles = Apotex enteric-coated product. (Adapted from Walker SE, Paton TW, Cowan DH, et al. Bioavailability of iron in oral ferrous sulfate preparations in healthy volunteers. Can Med Assoc J 1989; 141:543; with permission.

Table 1 Amount of Elemental Iron in the Ferrous Salts

Salt	Dose of Salt (mg)	Dose of Elemental Fe^{++} (mg)
Sulfate	300	60
Gluconate	300	35
Fumarate	200	60
Succinate	100	35

The cost also differs and can vary from as little as 2 dollars per month to as high as 30 dollars per month, depending on the preparation and whether or not there is a generic form of the iron salt (Table 2). The cost of the combination products is considerably higher.

It has long been recognized that optimal therapy consists of 150 to 250 mg of elemental iron daily. This is equivalent to 300 mg of ferrous sulfate (60 mg of elemental iron), 3 to 4 times a day, or 600 mg of ferrous gluconate (70 mg of elemental iron), 3 to 4 times daily. Patients will respond to smaller doses, but because the rate of response is dose-dependent, the rise in hemoglobin will be slower. Because certain foods interfere with iron absorption, maximal absorption occurs when the iron tablet is taken on an empty stomach; therefore, it is recommended that the medication be taken 1 to 2 hours before meals and at bedtime. At this dosage level, one would anticipate a rise in the hemoglobin level of approximately 1 to 2 g per liter per day. Compared to the brisk reticulocyte response seen after vitamin B$_{12}$ therapy for pernicious anemia, the reticulocytosis after iron therapy is lower in magnitude, occurs later, and is more drawn out. Most clinicians do not follow the reticulocyte count but rather utilize the rising hemoglobin level as a measure of response to iron therapy. The hemoglobin level usually takes 6 to 10 weeks to return to normal. It is then necessary to continue treatment for a further 4 to 6 months in order to replenish the iron stores.

Gastrointestinal symptoms, including nausea, epigastric discomfort and pain, diarrhea, and constipation, have all been attributed to oral iron therapy. Many conclude that a large portion of these symptoms is of a psychological nature, or at least not specific to the iron content of the medication. It may be that the widespread expectation that oral iron will cause gastrointestinal side effects contributes to the problem. Nevertheless, it is clear that a proportion of patients do have symptoms attributable to iron. The lower gastrointestinal complaints are not dose-related and can be managed with symptomatic treatment. The upper gastrointestinal symptoms, however, appear to become more severe with increasing doses of elemental iron. With appropriate manipulation of dose and timing of medication, it would be unusual that these side effects prevent the adequate therapy of iron deficiency with oral medication. When prescribing iron, it is wise to avoid suggesting the occurrence of side effects. If upper gastrointestinal symptoms do occur, one can advise that the medication be taken after meals. This often resolves the problem.

Table 2 Comparative Monthly Costs of Oral Iron Products*

Product	Range ($)
Tablets	
Ferrous sulfate	1.97–2.11 (generic)
	23.00–30.00 (brand)
Ferrous gluconate	3.80–7.30 (generic)
	7.65 (brand)
Ferrous fumarate	2.46–3.33 (generic)
	23.00 (brand)
Ferrous succinate	27.37 (brand)
Solution	
Ferrous sulfate	6.75 (syrup)

*Equivalent to ferrous sulfate—three tablets per day

Another approach is to reduce the dose by changing from a medication such as ferrous sulfate, which contains 60 mg of elemental iron, to one such as ferrous gluconate, which contains 35 mg. This has the added advantage of changing to a medication with a different external appearance. The number of tablets given each day can also be reduced. Frequently, when symptoms abate, the dose can be increased gradually. Both of these strategies decrease the amount of iron that is absorbed and delay the rate of response. It is preferable, however, to accept this slower response rate than to stop therapy. At the same time, note that slow-release and enteric-coated preparations to reduce gastrointestinal symptoms do so by reducing the amount of iron available for absorption in the gut and therefore add nothing to the simple strategy of dose reduction.

If patients fail to respond after appropriate oral iron therapy, then the following questions should be raised:

1. Is the diagnosis of iron-deficiency anemia correct? Thalassemia syndromes and a variety of chronic inflammatory and malignant disorders may result in a blood picture that can be confused with iron deficiency.
2. Are there other factors, including chronic diseases or concomitant deficiencies of either vitamin B$_{12}$ or folic acid, that might retard the response to therapy?
3. Has the patient been compliant? Lack of compliance is a very common cause of poor response. Tablet counts, the use of a personal diary, or merely asking the patient to tick a calendar when each tablet is taken may help resolve the problem.
4. Is the patient taking a satisfactory dose of iron in an appropriate form? It is important under these circumstances for the physician to have the patient bring the medication for identification. Unfortunately, most physicians and pharmacists are not aware of which preparations are enteric-coated, and even if a prescription specifies "non–enteric-coated," there is a risk that patients

will in fact receive an enteric-coated product. In some regions, the commonly available generic preparation of ferrous sulfate is enteric-coated. Pharmacists should become aware of which products are enteric-coated, and physicians should choose and prescribe a product that is not enteric-coated. At the same time, pharmaceutical companies should be encouraged to abandon the enteric-coated products and, in particular, not to coat the generic form of ferrous sulfate. An additional factor for consideration is the fact that many forms of iron are available as over-the-counter products. Not infrequently, patients, for a variety of reasons, purchase one of these products or take "iron tablets" that have been used by other family members. These may contain inadequate amounts of elemental iron or be a form that does not favor optimal absorption.

5. Is there evidence of continued bleeding? Aside from the usual methods of detecting blood loss, the presence of a persistent reticulocytosis without a concomitant rise in hemoglobin along with a blood film showing a mixed picture of normochromic, normocytic cells and a residual population of hypochromic, microcytic cells suggests that iron is being absorbed and utilized for red cell production, while significant blood loss continues.

6. Malabsorption of elemental iron is a rare cause of poor response. Patients with a partial gastrectomy usually absorb medicinal iron, although those with a complete gastrectomy may have significant impairment of absorption. Abnormalities of the upper intestine such as extensive resection, chronic inflammatory bowel disease, or gluten enteropathy may cause malabsorption of iron; these conditions are usually obvious. Gluten enteropathy may be more occult, but once a diagnosis is established, a gluten-free diet will restore the ability to absorb medicinal iron.

PARENTERAL IRON THERAPY

The necessity for the use of parenteral iron is unusual, and its routine use is not justified. Owing to the potential toxicity of iron given by the parenteral route, one must be certain about the failure of oral iron therapy. If, after what appears to be an appropriate therapeutic trial, there has not been an adequate response and the clinician is satisfied that the aforementioned reasons for failure of therapy have been identified and eliminated as far as possible, then consideration of parenteral iron therapy is appropriate. Therefore, in the presence of malabsorption, intractable gastrointestinal intolerance to oral therapy, continued uncontrolled blood loss that cannot be compensated for by oral iron, and for the unusual patient who is uncooperative, one is justified in using parenteral iron.

At present in Canada and the United States, iron dextran is the only commercially available product for parenteral use. Each milliliter of the solution contains 50 mg of elemental iron. Iron dextran can be administered by either the intramuscular or intravenous route. In either circumstance, it is important to note that the correction of the iron deficiency with parenteral iron is no more rapid than with an optimal regimen of oral iron. Anaphylactic reactions have been reported both with the intravenous route of administration and more rarely with intramuscular injection. The manufacturer recommends a test dose at the beginning of a course of therapy. It follows that medication and equipment for the management of anaphylaxis should be readily available.

When the intramuscular route is chosen, the drug is given by deep intramuscular injection in the upper quadrant of the buttock in doses of 50 to 250 mg per injection site at a frequency ranging from daily to weekly until the required amount of iron has been administered. It has been suggested that one should start with a small dose of 0.5 ml (25 mg of iron) and gradually increase with subsequent injections to the maximum dose of 5 ml (250 mg of iron). This mode of administration is often associated with staining of the skin and a moderate degree of pain at the injection site. Rarely, muscle necrosis has been reported. In addition to the occasional rare severe allergic reactions, systemic symptoms consisting of fever, flushing, nausea, vomiting, and arthralgias may occur.

Whereas iron dextran can be given as an undiluted solution in a series of repeated intravenous injections, a preferred method is the single total-dose intravenous infusion technique, in which the total iron requirement is calculated and diluted in 250 to 1,000 ml of normal saline immediately prior to starting the infusion. The initial rate of infusion should not exceed 5 drops per minute for 10 minutes, and the patient must be observed closely for anaphylaxis. If this test dose is well tolerated, the rate may be progressively increased to 45 to 60 drops per minute and continued at this rate until the infusion is completed. Following the administration, the patient should remain in bed for at least 30 minutes to prevent orthostatic hypotension. Local phlebitis of the infused vein is usually transient and responds to analgesic and anti-inflammatory measures. Systemic reactions, including arthralgia, muscle pain, and fever, may occur but usually subside spontaneously in several days. Iron dextran should not be used in patients with rheumatoid arthritis because it is known to cause a flare up of synovitis.

A simple method for determining the total dose of parenteral iron is as follows. Because total blood volume is approximately 65 ml per kilogram and the iron content of hemoglobin is 0.34 percent by weight, the total dose of iron for correction of anemia can be derived as follows:

$$D_{Fe} \text{ (g)} = (D_h \div 1000) \times W_{kg} \times 65 \times 0.0034$$
$$D_{Fe} \text{ (mg)} = D_h \times W_{kg} \; x \; .22,$$

where D_{Fe} = total hemoglobin iron deficit, D_h = whole blood hemoglobin deficit (grams per liter), and W_{kg} = body weight in kilograms. For example, if one assumes a normal hemoglobin concentration of 150 g per liter, an individual weighing 70 kg with a hemoglobin concentration of 70 g per liter would require $(150 - 70) \times 70 \times 0.22 = 1,230$ mg of iron to correct the anemia. In addition, an arbitrary amount of 600 mg for a woman and 1,000 mg for a man is added in order to replace the iron stores.

BLOOD TRANSFUSION

Transfusion of blood should not be considered a primary form of therapy for iron deficiency. In the majority of cases, there has been a slow onset of anemia, patients have adapted physiologically, and it is preferable to treat with iron and wait for a normal response to the medication. There are, however, situations in which transfusion is necessary to maintain adequate circulating blood volume and oxygen-carrying capacity. Transfusion is indicated when there is actual or threatened acute blood loss, superimposed on chronic iron-deficiency anemia, that might lead to an acute and dangerous decrease in circulating blood volume with consequent threat to organ function or life. On rare occasions, in the face of very severe anemia without continued significant blood loss, careful transfusion with packed red blood cells may be indicated if organ function is at risk. In this situation, one must keep in mind the dangers of circulatory overload associated with transfusion, particularly in individuals with compromised cardiac function. Finally, if an immediate surgical procedure is necessary, transfusion may be required to correct a low hemoglobin concentration.

SUGGESTED READING

Boggs DR. Fate of a ferrous sulfate prescription. Am J Med 1987; 82:124–128.

Callender ST. Treatment of iron deficiency. Clin Hematol 1982; 11:327–338.

Harju E. Clinical pharmacokinetics of iron preparations. Clin Pharmacokinet 1989; 17(2):69–89.

Walker SE, Paton TW, Cowan DH, et al. Bioavailability of iron in oral ferrous sulfate preparations in healthy volunteers. Can Med Assoc J 1989; 141:543–547.

SECONDARY ANEMIA: THE ANEMIA OF CHRONIC DISEASE

DAVID A. SEARS, M.D.

The etiology, mechanisms, and pathogenesis of the anemia of chronic disease (ACD) are still ill-defined. Thus, ACD is a syndrome that is defined by its major clinical and laboratory features. Traditionally, these features have included (1) the exclusion of other possible etiologies, like renal or endrocrinologic disease; (2) the presence of certain characteristic features of iron distribution and metabolism; and (3) the existence of an underlying infectious, inflammatory, or neoplastic disease. The characteristic pattern of iron distribution in ACD includes a low value for the serum iron and normal or increased amounts of storage iron, as measured by stainable iron in bone marrow samples or by serum ferritin levels. Recently, it has been observed that there are many patients who have the abnormalities of iron distribution characteristic of ACD but lack an apparent infectious, inflammatory, or neoplastic disease. Some patients with renal or endocrinologic diseases may also have the abnormalities of iron distribution typical of ACD and may thus have both disorders. Furthermore, iron deficiency may coexist with ACD and alter some of the characteristic iron measurements. Until etiologies and mechanisms of ACD are better defined, an inclusive view of the disorder seems appropriate.

CHARACTERISTICS

The clinical characteristics of ACD are not specific and depend more on the patient's other disease(s) than on the anemia. The major laboratory features of ACD are listed in Table 1. The features that define ACD are a subnormal level of serum iron and a normal or elevated level of serum ferritin. The latter criterion could be substituted for by the finding of stainable iron stores in the bone marrow. The level of serum ferritin one chooses to define ACD depends on how stringently one wishes to exclude patients with coexisting iron deficiency. Setting the "diagnostic" serum ferritin level at greater than 50 ng per milliliter excludes almost all patients with iron deficiency.

The level of anemia in ACD is usually moderate, but as many as one-fifth of patients have hematocrits below 25 percent. Most patients have normocytic red cells, but red cells are microcytic in 20 percent to 25 percent of patients. When the reticulocyte count is converted to a red cell production index by appropriate corrections, red cell production is not significantly above basal levels. Serum total iron-binding capacity (TIBC) is usually in the low normal to normal range. Coupled with the low serum iron level, this results in a low percent saturation

Table 1 Laboratory Characteristics of ACD

Characteristics defining ACD:
  Serum iron <60 μg/dl
  Serum ferritin >50 ng/ml

Other characteristics:
  Anemia usually moderate (hematocrit >25% in 4/5 of patients)
  Red cells normocytic to microcytic
  Reticulocyte count normal to slightly elevated
  Serum total iron-binding capacity normal
  Percent saturation of serum iron-binding capacity low
  Stainable storage iron present in bone marrow
  Sideroblasts absent from the bone marrow

Table 2 Possible Mechanisms in ACD

Impaired reutilization of hemoglobin iron
Decreased red cell lifespan
Ineffective erythropoiesis
Relative erythropoietin deficiency
Impaired responsiveness of erythroid marrow to erythropoietin

of serum iron-binding capacity. Bone marrow iron stains show ample storage iron but no stainable iron in developing erythroid cells, i.e., no sideroblasts.

DIAGNOSIS

The diagnosis of ACD is made according to the definition of the disorder as described previously. Because iron-deficiency anemia and ACD are the only diseases in which the serum iron value is low, the problem in diagnosis is usually differentiating these two disorders or identifying their coexistence. The level of the serum TIBC is, on the average, higher in iron-deficiency anemia than in ACD, and the percent saturation is lower, but these distinctions are not helpful in an individual case because of the marked overlap of these values in the two conditions. The serum ferritin level may be helpful in defining the situation in the hypoferremic patient. Patients with a subnormal ferritin level (e.g., <20 ng per milliliter) most likely have iron deficiency alone. When the serum ferritin level is in the range of 20 to 50 ng per milliliter, coexistent iron deficiency and ACD should be suspected. A serum ferritin level above 50 ng per milliliter suggests ACD alone. There is, however, overlap in each of these ranges, and they are given as guidelines, not rules. When coexistent iron deficiency and ACD are suspected, a therapeutic trial with oral iron is appropriate. Obviously, a source of blood loss causing the iron deficiency must also be sought.

When a patient with renal insufficiency has serum iron and ferritin values that meet the criteria for ACD, it is likely that the anemia of renal failure and ACD are both present because the patient with pure anemia of renal failure should have a high, rather than a low, serum iron level. In this setting, the presence of iron deficiency may be difficult to diagnose without direct examination of iron stores in the bone marrow or a therapeutic trial of iron.

MECHANISMS AND PATHOGENESIS

A number of mechanisms for ACD have been proposed based on studies of various groups of patients

(Table 2 and Figure 1). Experiments in human subjects using two isotopes of iron have demonstrated that reutilization of red cell (hemoglobin) iron for new hemoglobin synthesis is impaired in comparison to the utilization of transferrin-bound iron. Because 95 percent of the iron used in the production of new red cells comes from the hemoglobin of destroyed senescent red cells, even a small "block" in the mobilization of this iron from reticuloendothelial cells could have important consequences. This mechanism could explain the common clinical findings in ACD of low serum iron, increased bone marrow storage iron, increased serum ferritin, and reduced bone marrow sideroblasts (red cell precursors containing stainable iron). It could account for some of the similarities of ACD to iron-deficiency anemia because it would predict iron-deficient erythropoiesis. A second proposed mechanism is reinduced red cell survival. When red cell lifespan has been studied in ACD, it has commonly been found to be mildly reduced owing to extracorpuscular factors. It has been suggested that stimulated macrophages are overactive in the destruction of red cells. This slightly accelerated removal of red cells would not be sufficient to produce anemia unless the ability of the bone marrow to increase its red cell production was also impaired. A third mechanism, ineffective erythropoiesis, has been stated to occur in ACD but is not described as a mechanism in most reports. Finally, in many patients studied, there has been a failure of adequate bone marrow erythropoietic response to the anemia in ACD. This has been attributed in some cases to a relative deficiency of erythropoietin; i.e., the increase in erythropoietin is not as great as one would expect for the degree of anemia. In other cases, the erythropoietin level has been found to be increased appropriately, but the bone marrow erythropoietic response is less than anticipated for the level of erythropoietin. Mechanisms involving erythropoietin are of particular interest in view of recent evidence that exogenously administered erythropoietin can correct the anemia of ACD (see the section on treatment).

Further speculations about the pathogenesis of ACD have been developed as the role of the cytokine, interleukin-1 (IL-1), in mediating the acute-phase response has been elucidated. One such hypothesis is presented in Figure 1. It suggests that a stimulus, such as inflammation, causes macrophages to secrete IL-1. Interleukin-1 stimulates neutrophils to release lactoferrin. Lactoferrin, which has greater avidity for iron than transferrin, particularly in an acid milieu, as might exist in a locus of inflammation, "captures" iron from transferrin and transfers it directly to macrophages. Iron thus bypasses the bone marrow, and the abnormalities of

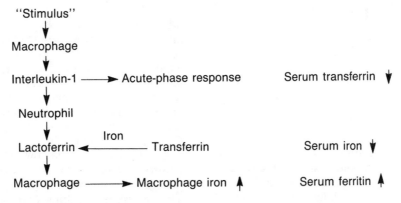

Figure 1 Proposed mechanisms for the abnormalities of iron distribution in anemia of chronic disease (ACD).

iron distribution characteristic of the ACD ensue. In addition, IL-1 has been shown to inhibit the action of erythropoietin on erythroid precursor cells; thus, this hypothesis could explain some of the observations related to erythropoietin that were discussed previously. However, other data do not support the hypothesis. For example, low serum iron levels are observed when neutropenic patients develop infection or inflammation despite low plasma lactoferrin levels. This is the case, for example, in the leukemia patient with bacterial sepsis. Thus, the lowering of the serum iron in ACD does not require normal numbers of circulating neutrophils or normal plasma levels of lactoferrin. Furthermore, animal studies have shown that administration of IL-1 produces hypoferremia even in the presence of neutropenia. Thus, the importance of IL-1 in mediating ACD remains incompletely defined.

TREATMENT

There is no proven effective specific therapy for ACD. It is clear, however, that if the underlying disease can be treated successfully, the anemia will resolve. Although decreased availability of iron for new hemoglobin synthesis may be a pathogenetic mechanism in ACD, it has not been convincingly demonstrated that iron therapy can ameliorate the anemia. Theoretically, if one were able to administer iron in a manner that would bypass the reticuloendothelial system or overwhelm the

apparent block in mobilization of iron from that source, the anemia might be improved. It has been claimed that a single large dose of intravenous iron can alleviate the anemia in ACD, but these studies require confirmation.

The anemia in the patient with ACD is usually not so severe as to require transfusion, but occasionally, in severely affected patients with other serious diseases, transfusions may be required as a temporary expedient. Recently, recombinant human erythropoietin has been administered to a few patients with ACD in doses similar to those used for the treatment of the anemia of renal failure, and the hematocrits of the ACD patients have improved. It seems unlikely that this form of therapy will be utilized widely because of the mild degree of the anemia in ACD and because of the expense, but this form of therapy deserves further evaluation and may help us better understand the mechanisms of ACD.

SUGGESTED READING

Birgens HS, Kristensen LØ, Borregaard N, et al. Lactoferrin-mediated transfer of iron to intracellular ferritin in human monocytes. Eur J Haematol 1988; 41:52–57.

Cash JM, Sears DA. The anemia of chronic disease: Spectrum of associated diseases in a series of unselected hospitalized patients. Am J Med 1989; 87:638–644.

Lee GR. The anemia of chronic disease. Semin Hematol 1983; 20:61–80.

Means RT, Olsen NJ, Krantz SB, et al. Treatment of the anemia of rheumatoid arthritis with recombinant human erythropoietin: Clinical and in vitro studies. Arthritis Rheum 1989; 32:638–642.

MYELODYSPLASTIC SYNDROMES

WENDY STOCK, M.D.
RICHARD A. LARSON, M.D.

The myelodysplastic syndromes (MDS) are a heterogeneous group of hematopoietic stem cell disorders that are characterized by cytologic dysplasia in the bone marrow and blood and by various combinations of anemia, neutropenia, and thrombocytopenia. The natural history of these syndromes varies widely, ranging from chronic anemias with a low propensity for leukemic conversion to syndromes with severe hematologic disturbances and a high risk of progression to acute myeloid leukemia (AML). The management of this generally elderly group of patients has primarily consisted of supportive care, although more specific therapeutic intervention can be considered in certain subsets of patients.

DEFINITIONS AND CLINICAL FEATURES

A variety of terms, including preleukemia, smoldering or subacute leukemia, dysmyelopoietic syndrome, and myelodysplasia, have all been used to describe this group of patients. In 1982, the French-American-British (FAB) cooperative group attempted to standardize the classification of these patients using criteria based on cytology and the number of blast cells in the marrow and peripheral blood. The FAB subsets of MDS include refractory anemia (RA), refractory anemia with ring sideroblasts (RARS), refractory anemia with excess blasts (RAEB), refractory anemia with excess blasts in transformation (RAEB-T), and chronic myelomonocytic leukemia (CMML) (Table 1). There is a natural progression of disease between categories as cellular maturation becomes more arrested and blast cells accumulate.

Ineffective hematopoiesis with multilineage dysplasia dominates the bone marrow picture in patients with MDS. The marrow is usually hypercellular or normocellular but rarely can be hypocellular. These latter cases must be distinguished from aplastic anemia. The anemia is usually macrocytic. The most prominent red cell abnormalities are erythroid hyperplasia with megaloblastoid features. Platelets are usually decreased in number and may be poorly granulated. Megakaryocytes are often normal or increased in number and have dysplastic features with small size and a low ploidy. Granulocytic abnormalities include an increase in early myeloid cells in the marrow, whereas peripheral blood neutrophils exhibit the Pelger-Huet anomaly, with hyposegmented nuclei and poorly condensed chromatin. The neutrophilic granules are often decreased in number. Functional abnormalities are present in addition to the morphologic abnormalities; these include decreased neutrophil chemotaxis and phagocytosis, an increased red cell membrane sensitivity to complement lysis, and impaired platelet adherence.

Myelodysplastic syndromes occur in the late middle-aged to elderly population; the median age is 65 years or older. Myelodysplastic syndrome is rarely seen in patients younger than 50 years old. The disorder is more common in men. Initial symptoms are weakness, easy bruisability, and infection, which reflect the peripheral pancytopenia. Ninety percent of patients are anemic at diagnosis, and approximately 50 percent are pancytopenic. Splenomegaly or hepatomegaly is uncommon.

A secondary form of myelodysplasia occurs in an often younger group of patients who have been previously treated with cytotoxic chemotherapy, usually containing alkylating agents, or with radiotherapy for either a malignant tumor or a nonneoplastic disease. Marrow hypocellularity and fibrosis are more commonly seen in therapy-related MDS (t-MDS) than in the primary (de novo) form of the disease. In those patients who survive the preleukemic period, t-AML usually occurs 7 to 12 months after recognition of the secondary MDS.

PROGNOSTIC FACTORS

Unfortunately, survival is short for the majority of patients with MDS (Table 2). Myelodysplastic syndrome is a life-threatening disorder owing to persistent and

Table 1 FAB Classification of Myelodysplastic Syndromes

	Peripheral Blood	Bone Marrow
RA	<1% Blasts	<5% Blasts
RARS	<1% Blasts	<5% Blasts with ≥15% ring sideroblasts
CMML	<5% Blasts with ≥1,000 monocytes/μl	1%–20% Blasts
RAEB	<5% Blasts	5%–20% Blasts
RAEB–T	>5% Blasts	20%–30% Blasts or presence of Auer rods

Table 2 Prognosis in Myelodysplastic Syndromes and Probability of Transformation to Acute Leukemia

	Frequency (%)	Survival Median (Mo)	Range	Transformed to AML (%)
RA	28	50	18–64	12
RARS	24	51	14–76+	8
CMML	16	11	9–60+	14
RAEB	23	11	7–16	44
RAEB–T	9	5	2–11	60

profound cytopenias regardless of whether transformation to leukemia occurs. Morphologic classification has been limited in its ability to predict the natural history of the disease. Several scoring systems, including the Bournemouth score and the FAB classification, are based on the severity of cytopenia in conjunction with the bone marrow blast count and the degree of granulocytic and megakaryocytic dysplasia. Multilineage dysplasia and a higher blast cell count are associated with the more rapid development of acute leukemia and thus decreased survival, but most patients die from infection or bleeding or a transfusion-related complication prior to developing AML.

Cytogenetic abnormalities may also be an important prognostic factor in MDS. Certainly, the detection of an abnormal karyotype in a patient's bone marrow cells clearly establishes a neoplastic diagnosis and removes any doubt about a possible nutritional deficiency or drug toxicity as a cause for cytopenia. Half of patients with MDS have detectable karyotypic abnormalities, most commonly deletion (del) of the long arm of chromosome 5 [del(5q)], monosomy 7 or del (7q), trisomy 8, and del (20q). These chromosomal abnormalities are also common in AML. Complex cytogenetic abnormalities correlate with short survival. Abnormalities of chromosomes 5 and/or 7 are common in t-MDS and denote a poor prognosis. Importantly, however, a subset of primary MDS patients with an isolated del(5q) abnormality, characterized by refractory anemia with small hypolobulated megakaryocytes, has a relatively good prognosis with a low propensity for evolution to AML. The use of one or more of these prognostic factors may be useful to the clinician in establishing the appropriate treatment approach to this heterogeneous group of diseases.

SUPPORTIVE CARE

No specific, generally effective therapy currently exists for MDS. Clinical prognostic factors, including bone marrow morphology and cytogenetics, should be evaluated at diagnosis. A period of observation with close follow-up of serial peripheral blood counts is recommended for initial management, and a second bone marrow examination after several months is useful to assess the rapidity of disease progression.

Patients with RA or RARS often have a clinically indolent course and may need no treatment for variable lengths of time. However, patients who are severely anemic (hemoglobin < 7 to 8 g per deciliter), should receive red blood cell transfusions to maintain the hemoglobin concentration at 9 to 10 g per deciliter or greater. Washed red blood cell units are rarely necessary. Patients with peripheral vascular or coronary artery disease who are symptomatic should also receive red cell transfusions to ameliorate their symptoms. Commonly, the recurrence of fatigue or angina is a more useful indicator of the need for the next red blood cell transfusion than any particular hemoglobin level. Transfusion require-

ments increase as MDS progresses, and iron overload and hemochromatosis may occur when the transfusion burden exceeds 80 to 100 units of red blood cells. This is not a common problem because most patients with MDS are elderly and die first of intercurrent illnesses or from other complications of MDS, including infection, hemorrhage, or acute leukemia. In younger patients, however, iron overload can lead to cardiac, hepatic, or endocrine disease. In these patients, iron stores can be estimated by measurement of serum iron concentration, transferrin saturation, and serum ferritin. Chronic chelation therapy with subcutaneously administered desferroxamine can delay the development of hemochromatosis.

Prophylactic platelet transfusions should not routinely be administered to thrombocytopenic patients with MDS because of the expense, inconvenience, and risk of alloimmunization. This risk increases with the frequency of platelet transfusion and may limit future treatment options. Platelet support should be reserved for treatment of acute hemorrhage or for prophylaxis prior to surgery. In patients who become refractory to platelet transfusions with random donor units, single donor apheresis units or cross-matched or HLA-matched platelets may be effective. Patients with MDS who have thrombocytopenia should be carefully instructed to avoid aspirin, aspirin-containing products, and other nonsteroidal anti-inflammatory agents that can interfere with platelet function.

Infections are a common problem in patients with MDS and can be life-threatening. Fever, localized infections, or even general malaise should be seriously evaluated in these patients who have quantitative as well as functional neutropenia. Prompt institution of broad-spectrum antibiotic coverage while trying to locate the source of infection is critical, and therapy should continue for 10 to 14 days even without an obvious source or positive blood cultures. Chronic outpatient antibacterial suppression with a quinolone derivative or another broad-spectrum oral antibiotic can be considered for those patients who have required frequent hospitalization for fevers presumed to be due to bacterial infections. If a neutropenic patient fails to respond to antibacterial agents or has repeated episodes of fever without an obvious source, a fungal infection should be suspected, and treatment with amphotericin B or fluconazole should be initiated. Atypical mycobacteria, *Pneumocystis carinii*, and other opportunistic infections are not commonly found in patients with MDS.

HEMATINICS, ANDROGENS, AND CORTICOSTEROIDS

Despite the megaloblastoid appearance of the bone marrow, there is no evidence that vitamin supplementation with folic acid or cyanocobalamin (vitamin B_{12}) is beneficial in MDS unless a measurable deficiency exists. The anemia of MDS is characteristically refractory to iron supplements. A small subset of patients with sideroblastic anemias will respond to pyridoxine (50 mg per day), but the response rarely lasts for more than a few months. Most patients with MDS do not respond to pyridoxine.

Although androgens may stimulate erythropoiesis in patients with aplastic anemia or myelofibrosis, the evidence that androgens are beneficial in the treatment of MDS is largely anecdotal. Clinical trials including all FAB subtypes have clearly demonstrated their lack of efficacy. A possible exception to these failures is the synthetic attenuated androgen, danazol, which may prove useful in some thrombocytopenic patients with platelet-associated immunoglobulin. Improvement in platelet and reticulocyte counts has been reported in some patients with MDS who were treated with danazol at 600 to 800 mg orally on a daily basis for periods of 8 to 12 weeks. The drug is usually well tolerated except for rashes. The mechanism of action is not completely understood but may involve inhibiting the binding of antibody-coated platelets to the Fc receptors on macrophages. Glucocorticosteroids at varying dosages have not been helpful in most patients with MDS, and may lead to further immunosuppression. A small number of patients who may benefit can be identified by marrow cell cultures that show a hematopoietic response to corticosteroids in vitro.

CYTOTOXIC CHEMOTHERAPY

The role of cytotoxic drugs in the treatment of MDS is uncertain for the majority of patients and should only be considered for the younger and healthier patients with more aggressive forms of disease, such as those with RAEB, RAEB-T, and the secondary MDS. In general, cytotoxic therapy with standard regimens used in the treatment of AML (containing daunorubicin and standard or high doses of cytarabine, e.g.) have had limited success in extending the survival for the majority of patients with MDS. This is not surprising for a number of reasons: (1) most MDS patients are elderly and poorly able to tolerate aggressive treatment; (2) the number of normal hematopoietic stem cells available to regenerate the marrow following therapy-induced hypoplasia is probably reduced; and (3) because the majority of effective antileukemia drugs act primarily during cell division, they may be relatively ineffective in the low proliferative states seen in MDS. For these reasons, intensive chemotherapy has been associated with complete response rates in the 10- to 30-percent range, with durations of remissions generally lasting less than 1 year. In older patients, the toxicity of the therapy and the prolonged hypoplasia and cytopenia that it produces may actually shorten their lives. It is, therefore, important to direct this treatment option primarily to the younger group of patients with MDS, who are better able to tolerate it.

More recently, allogeneic bone marrow transplantation has been tested as curative therapy in the very small group of patients with MDS who are younger than 50 years of age (approximately 10 percent of all patients with MDS) and who have a histocompatible donor.

Several clinical trials have been published that describe a variety of preparative regimens using combinations of cyclophosphamide and busulfan, or etoposide and cytarabine, or total body irradiation. Results show disease-free survivals ranging from 1 to 7 years in approximately 40 percent of patients transplanted. These data suggest that appropriately chosen patients can respond to bone marrow transplantation with prolonged remissions and can probably be cured.

DIFFERENTIATING AGENTS

Because the majority of patients with MDS are not candidates for bone marrow transplantation, and the outcome with conventional cytotoxic therapy has generally been poor, attention has been focused on agents that can induce differentiation of acute leukemia cell lines in vitro, slowing proliferation and restoring apparently normal maturation and function. Many such "differentiating agents" have been tested in clinical trials of MDS.

Low doses of cytarabine can induce differentiation in leukemia cell lines in vitro together with inhibition of proliferation. There are reports of small groups of patients who were treated with an average cytarabine dose of 20 mg per square meter per day, given subcutaneously in single or divided daily doses or by continuous intravenous infusion over 14 to 21 days. Individual patients have had considerable improvement in peripheral blood counts, with reductions in red blood cell and platelet transfusion requirements. A review of 170 patients with MDS treated with low-dose cytarabine in a large number of small trials revealed that the overall response rate was 37 percent and the median duration of response was 10.5 months. Responses are rarely complete remissions, but significant improvement in blood counts can occur. Patients who respond to an initial cycle can be retreated with a second or third cycle of cytarabine; in some cases, similar good responses lasting a few months can be achieved with each cycle. A recently reported randomized prospective trial compared low-dose cytarabine at 10 mg per square meter administered subcutaneously every 12 hours over a 21-day cycle to supportive care alone. Results indicated that low-dose cytarabine delayed progression of MDS to acute leukemia and was most effective for patients with RAEB-T. The overall survival, however, was not significantly improved in the treated group of patients.

Low-dose cytarabine treatment does have toxicity, particularly in elderly patients; it uniformly causes an initial decline in platelets that then recover after several weeks. Treatment-related deaths have been reported in about 15 percent of patients. Two lines of evidence suggest that low-dose cytarabine may act via a cytotoxic mechanism rather than as an inducer of differentiation: first, bone marrow hypoplasia frequently occurs, and second, cytogenetically abnormal metaphase cells have been detected after therapy despite concurrent improvement in peripheral blood counts. In either case, low doses of cytarabine do not appear to improve survival in the majority of patients with MDS and thus cannot be broadly recommended for general use.

13-*Cis*-retinoic acid and other retinoids can inhibit tumor cell growth in vitro and induce differentiation in a variety of tumor cell lines, including human leukemia. Oral *cis*-retinoic acid has been used in several MDS trials testing various doses, and some improvement in hematopoiesis has been reported in up to 30 percent of patients. Toxicities include dry skin, cheilitis, stomatitis, lethargy, arthralgias, headache, thrombocytopenia, and hepatotoxicity, and these are common when higher doses of the drug (> 100 mg per square meter per day) are used.

In a randomized trial restricted to patients with RA or RARS, treatment with a daily dose of 20 mg *cis*-retinoic acid was well tolerated. Treated patients had a marked improvement in survival at 1 year compared to control patients, but no accompanying increases in peripheral blood counts were noted. Unfortunately, the survival for the untreated control group of patients was unusually poor in this trial. Another trial randomized 68 patients with various MDS subtypes to either 13-*cis*-retinoic acid at 100 mg per square meter daily or to oral placebo. Treatment continued for up to 6 months, with almost all patients receiving therapy for at least 8 weeks. No significant differences in hematologic responses or progression-free survival were noted, but a possible benefit to those with early stage disease could not be excluded because fewer than 15 percent of patients had RA or RARS. Case reports of individual patients receiving retinoids have described clinical and cytogenetic responses occurring slowly after several months of treatment. Despite this, the literature suggests that the majority of patients with MDS do not benefit from *cis*-retinoic acid.

Another agent that can induce myeloid differentiation in vitro is 1,25-dihydroxy vitamin D_3, the active metabolite of vitamin D. In trials evaluating daily oral doses between 2 μg and 4 μg, significant improvements in hematopoietic parameters have not been noted, although occasional patients have been reported to have transient improvements in peripheral blood counts. The potential benefit to be gained by escalating the dose of vitamin D_3 further is limited by hypercalcemia, which occurs in the majority of patients receiving greater than 4 μg per day.

Other potential differentiating agents that have been reported to improve hematopoiesis in small numbers of patients with MDS include alpha or gamma interferons and haem-arginate, an enhancer of erythroid precursor activity. 5-Azacytidine has proved useful when given by continuous intravenous infusion, and studies examining the efficacy of subcutaneously administered 5-azacytidine are currently in progress. Limited data are available on the usefulness of sodium butyrate, all-*trans*-retinoic acid, homoharringtonine, or hexamethyl-bis-acetamide (HMBA). At this time, none of these differentiating agents can be recommended for MDS patients except within the setting of a clinical trial.

HEMATOPOIETIC GROWTH FACTORS

Recombinant human hematopoietic growth factors have recently become available for use in clinical trials in patients with various states of bone marrow failure, including those with MDS. Both recombinant human granulocyte-macrophage colony-stimulating factor (GM-CSF) and granulocyte colony-stimulating factor (G-CSF) have demonstrated potent stimulation of hematopoiesis in patients with MDS in phase I and phase II trials. Prolonged intravenous infusions or daily subcutaneous injections of GM-CSF elicit dose-related increases in peripheral neutrophils, eosinophils, and monocytes in almost all patients. A GM-CSF dose of 3 μg per kilogram per day is sufficient to produce a granulocyte count of 5,000 to 10,000 per microliter in most patients with RA and RAEB. The useful dose range of G-CSF is also about 1 to 3 μg per kilogram per day. The drugs have been generally well tolerated even in elderly patients, and tachyphylaxis or neutralizing antibodies have not yet been observed with repeated administration. Unfortunately, despite the multilineage potency of GM-CSF in vitro, improvements in anemia or thrombocytopenia have only occasionally been observed in treated patients. An additional concern regarding the clinical use of GM-CSF or any other myeloid growth factor is the possibility that treatment may actually accelerate the rate of progression to acute leukemia, particularly in those MDS patients with high initial blast percentages. Nevertheless, GM-CSF and G-CSF have important therapeutic potential, and their impact on the natural history of MDS and its associated morbidity needs further evaluation in the large randomized phase III trials that are currently underway. Other recombinant growth factors with potential for multilineage stimulation are IL-3 (interleukin-3 or multi-CSF) and IL-1, and these have recently entered clinical trials.

Anemic patients with MDS who have normal renal function usually have very high physiologic levels of endogenous erythropoietin. As yet, there are no data indicating that additional erythropoietin in pharmacologic doses will provide any clinical benefit for these patients.

SUGGESTED READING

Appelbaum FR, Bariall J, Storb R, et al. Bone marrow transplantation for patients with myelodysplasia. Ann Intern Med 1990; 112: 590–597.

Cheson BD, Jasperse DM, Simon R, et al. A critical appraisal of low-dose cytosine arabinoside in patients with acute non-lymphocytic leukemia and myelodysplastic syndromes. J Clin Oncol 1986; 4:1857–1864.

Koeffler HP, Heitjan D, Mertelsmann R, et al. Randomized study of 13-*cis*-retinoic acid versus placebo in the myelodysplastic disorders. Blood 1988; 71:703–708.

Koeffler HP. Myelodysplastic syndromes (preleukemia). Semin Hematol 1986; 23:284–299.

Vadhan-Raj S, Keating M, Le Maistre A, et al. Effects of recombinant human granulocyte-macrophage colony-stimulating factor in patients with myelodysplastic syndromes. N Engl J Med 1987; 317:1545–1552.

HEREDITARY SPHEROCYTOSIS, ELLIPTOCYTOSIS, AND RELATED DISORDERS

JAMES S. WILEY, M.D., F.R.A.C.P., F.R.C.P.A.

The hereditary hemolytic anemias considered here all result from a defect in the erythrocyte membrane, which gives rise to a characteristic red cell morphology on blood smear. In the five hemolytic anemias listed, the spleen is the major site of red cell destruction, and splenic enlargement is invariable when the hemolysis is clinically significant. Anemia and signs of hemolysis as well as gallstones may be present, and all these features can be found in asymptomatic relatives of affected family members. In hereditary spherocytosis there is an absolute deficiency in erythrocyte spectrin, an elongated fibrous protein that is the major component of the cytoskeleton. A defect in spectrin dimer–tetramer self-association in some patients with hereditary elliptocytosis as well as hereditary pyropoikilocytosis weakens the cytoskeleton and leads to red-cell fragmentation. In contrast, hereditary xerocytosis or stomatocytosis are disorders of red cell hydration in which excessive dehydration or overhydration, respectively, lead to erythrocyte destruction, primarily in the spleen.

HEREDITARY SPHEROCYTOSIS

Splenectomy was performed in occasional cases of splenic anemia by Spencer Wells in the 1880s, but the operation did not gain wide acceptance until the turn of the century, when osmotic fragility testing made diagnosis more certain and numerous case reports documented cure of anemia by removal of the spleen.

Splenectomy is indicated in all patients with hereditary spherocytosis except at the extremes of age or if associated medical conditions contraindicate surgery. In general, splenectomy should be deferred in young children with hereditary spherocytosis until after the age of 2 because of the increased risk of fulminant bacterial septicemia in young asplenic children. The spleen has a central role in host defenses against blood-borne microorganisms, both by sequestration and phagocytosis of bacteria and by rapid synthesis of specific antibody after exposure to intravenous antigen. *Pneumococcus (Diplococcus pneumoniae)* is most often associated with fatal septicemia after splenectomy in children, but the incidence of other septicemias from *Meningococcus (Neisseria meningitidis)* and *Haemophilus influenzae* is also increased. For these reasons, the best time for elective splenectomy in children is around the age of 6 to 7, when administration of anesthesia is facilitated by the growth in airway size and the immune system has fully matured. Despite these considerations children of any age who present with erythroid aplasia secondary to parvovirus infection should have transfusion support and be considered for earlier splenectomy. At the other extreme of age, splenectomy is not generally indicated in those over 60 because of the increased operative and anesthetic risks.

A definite contraindication to splenectomy is an immunodeficiency state such as hypogammaglobulinemia or lymphopenia (either congenital or acquired). The spleen is an important site of antibody production in the primary immune response, and this organ should be preserved when other components of the immune system are defective. Splenectomy should not generally be performed in patients with hereditary spherocytosis and coexisting polycythemia vera or essential thrombocythemia. In these diseases the enlarged spleen contains a substantial platelet pool, and splenectomy may produce sustained and hazardous rises in the platelet count. In contrast, splenectomy may be beneficial in hereditary spherocytosis with congestive heart failure or ischemic heart disease provided anesthesia can be given safely. Splenomegaly causes plasma volume expansion as a result of arteriovenous shunting of blood, and the fall in blood volume associated with splenectomy may alleviate cardiac symptoms.

There is controversy over whether splenectomy is indicated in patients with mild hereditary spherocytosis, i.e., those with low-normal hemoglobin, reticulocytosis less than 2 percent, and median erythrocyte osmotic fragility barely above the normal range. Such patients often have an impalpable spleen and may show significant signs of hemolysis only in association with bacterial or viral infections (which increases the phagocytic activity of splenic macrophages). In this group of patients splenectomy should be recommended only when definite splenomegaly is detected by clinical examination or by radionuclide liver–spleen scan.

Finally all patients with significant hemolysis should receive folic acid supplements, a point of particular importance with coexistent pregnancy which further increases folate requirements.

PREOPERATIVE AND OPERATIVE CONSIDERATIONS

All patients recommended for splenectomy should receive polyvalent pneumococcal vaccine approximately 1 month before operation. Vaccination against the 14 most virulent serotypes of pneumococcus confers substantial (about 75 percent), but not complete, protection against subsequent pneumococcal infections. For vaccination to be optimally effective it should be given at least 1 week before operation because splenectomy attenuates the primary immune response. Unfortunately, pneumococcal vaccine produces a suboptimal immune response in children, particularly those younger than 2 years of age. If splenectomy is necessary before school age, oral penicillin should be given as prophylaxis against infection. Adults recommended for splenectomy should have abdominal ultrasound or radiographic examination to establish if gallstones are present.

Simple splenectomy is usually performed through a left upper quadrant abdominal incision, whereas combined splenectomy and cholecystectomy is performed through a midline abdominal approach. At operation the surgeon should check for the presence of splenunculi, which occur in 10 percent of patients and should be removed along with the spleen. Manual palpation of the gallbladder should be performed to check the ultrasonic findings. Cholecystectomy is indicated if stones are proven, and this procedure is usually performed at the same time as splenectomy. It may be safer, however, to defer cholecystectomy if the patient has any risk factors, such as emphysema, which predispose to postoperative pneumonia.

Splenectomy is nearly always followed by a sustained thrombocytosis, and low-dose heparin (5,000 U, every 12 hours subcutaneously) should be given in the perioperative and postoperative period as prophylaxis against deep venous thrombosis and pulmonary embolism. This low-dose heparin should be continued until the patient is fully ambulant. Surgery is accompanied by an abrupt fall in the reticulocyte count and serum iron, and it may take weeks to several months for the hemoglobin to attain normal values. The success of splenectomy should be judged after 3 to 6 months, and most patients experience an increased feeling of well-being as well as rise in hemoglobin and normalization of reticulocytes. After splenectomy some patients with extremely high erythrocyte osmotic fragility do not normalize their laboratory parameters of hemolysis. Careful measurement of erythrocyte survival in such patients confirms mild persistent hemolysis. In this subgroup, however, splenectomy is still beneficial because of the marked amelioration in hemolytic rate.

The factors that should be considered for and against the use of splenectomy are outlined in Table 1. Surgical intervention avoids a number of potential complications that may be lethal, e.g., aplastic crisis, traumatic rupture of an enlarged spleen, cholecystitis, and pancreatitis (resulting from gallstones). Because patients have had lifelong hemolysis, they are often unable to anticipate the better health that will result from a splenectomy, a procedure that not only increases hemoglobin values but also removes a major arteriovenous shunt from the circulation and improves exercise tolerance. Erythrocyte 2,3-diphosphoglycerate increases slightly after splenectomy, and this factor also may improve exercise tolerance. Hemosiderosis is now recognized as a rare, but preventable, complication of many hereditary hemolytic anemias, including hereditary spherocytosis. This complication occurs in patients who are heterozygous for the gene causing hemochromatosis and leads to excessive iron absorption in patients with hemolytic anemia.

Several risks must be weighed against the clear benefits of splenectomy. With an experienced surgeon the immediate risks of splenectomy are small and can be further minimized if one surgeon performs all such operations for a hematology unit. The long-term increase in the incidence of pneumococcal septicemia in asplenic patients is well-recognized, but can be minimized by pneumococcal vaccination given before splenectomy. Long-term prophylaxis against pneumococcal infection is also provided by oral penicillin V, 250 mg daily, although this alternative is usually offered only to young children in whom successful vaccination has not been possible. In some centers both vaccination and penicillin V are given routinely post-splenectomy.

HEREDITARY ELLIPTOCYTOSIS

Several forms of hereditary elliptocytosis have been recognized—a common type, a spherocytic variety, and Melanesian elliptocytosis—but in all, hemolysis is mild and anemia is usually absent. A number of patients may have only intermittent hemolysis coinciding with viral or bacterial infections. In some patients with homozygous hereditary elliptocytosis there is evidence of red-cell fragmentation, and in this more severe variant moderate to severe hemolysis is present. This heterogeneity in clinical severity has a parallel at the molecular level, where several spectrin variants as well as a deficiency of other membrane proteins (band 4.1, membrane sialoglycoprotein) have all been described in elliptocytic red cells.

All patients with hereditary elliptocytosis should receive folic acid. For those with homozygous elliptocytosis and severe hemolysis, a splenectomy should be considered, because this operation mitigates or cures all signs of hemolysis. Hemolytic anemia severe enough to require transfusions is an indication for splenectomy. For the reasons outlined earlier, splenectomy should not be performed before the age of 2. An additional reason for postponing splenectomy is that some children with hereditary elliptocytosis who have severe hemolysis in the neonatal period show marked clinical improvement after the first year of life.

Table 1 Factors to Consider Concerning Splenectomy in Hereditary Spherocytosis

Benefits	Increases well-being of patient (from rise in hemoglobin, and slight increase in erythrocyte 2,3-diphosphoglycerate)
	Prevents hemolytic or aplastic crises
	Prevents cholelithiasis and its complications
	Abolishes risk of traumatic rupture of the spleen
	Removes the low incidence of hemosiderosis
Risks	Fulminant bacterial sepsis in asplenic patients (usually pneumococcal)
	Surgical risks associated with splenectomy

HEREDITARY PYROPOIKILOCYTOSIS

The rare hemolytic syndrome of hereditary pyropoikilocytosis demonstrates striking abnormalities on blood smear, which shows poikilocytes, microspherocytes, and fragmented red cells. Of particular note is the microcytosis with mean corpuscular volume (MCV) as low as 50 fl, despite increased reticulocytes. Hemolysis is often severe in this syndrome, and the severity of anemia can be correlated with one of two characteristic defects on the tryptic digest of the spectrin molecule. When hemolysis is severe, splenectomy should be performed, preferably after the child reaches the age of 2 years.

HEREDITARY XEROCYTOSIS AND STOMATOCYTOSIS

Xerocytosis describes the dehydrated target cells seen on blood smears of patients with this hemolytic syndrome, which presents with abdominal pain, splenomegaly, or cholelithiasis. A unique feature of this syndrome is that most patients show normal or near-normal hemoglobin values, despite clinical and laboratory evidence of hemolysis. Occasional patients with severe erythrocyte dehydration may be markedly anemic. Splenectomy should be performed in those with persistent anemia or abdominal pain. Splenectomy, however, may only partially correct the anemia and reduce the reticulocytosis only slightly. One possible explanation is that dehydrated erythrocytes can lyse intravascularly with the increased shear stresses induced by exercise, and this mechanism of hemolysis may be as important as erythrocyte destruction in the spleen. At present it is not established whether splenectomy is beneficial for patients without anemia.

The rare hemolytic syndrome of hereditary stomatocytosis often presents with severe anemia in childhood, with stomatocytes on blood film. Splenectomy confers benefit but does not completely cure the hemolytic process. Splenectomy is indicated for moderate or severe anemia requiring transfusion, but if possible operation should be delayed until the patient is over the age of 2 years.

HEMOLYTIC ANEMIA DUE TO RED CELL ENZYME DEFICIENCIES

WILLIAM N. VALENTINE, M.D.

The nonnucleated human erythrocyte is metabolically underprivileged. Beyond the reticulocyte stage of maturation, it contains no ribosomes, mitochondria, or other cellular organelles, cannot synthesize proteins or lipids or generate adenosine triphosphate (ATP) from small molecular precursors, and possesses only ineffectual vestiges of the enzymatic machinery necessary for oxidative phosphorylation. Nonetheless, it normally survives some 120 days in the circulation, transporting oxygen and carbon dioxide to and from every tissue of the body, a function that neither requires nor expends energy. Despite the fact that some 95 percent of its dry weight is hemoglobin, it must also possess the capacity to protect this crucial protein from oxidative denaturation, pump cations in and out against electrochemical gradients, preserve its shape and the deformability of its membrane, incorporate plasma adenosine into its adenine nucleotide pool, and carry out other metabolic functions essential to its integrity. The energy supporting these functions is derived solely from the conversion of glucose to lactate, a glycolytic process that normally generates a net gain in high-energy ATP. Given its metabolic limitations, it is not surprising that genetically determined deficiencies in essential enzymatic machinery, when severe, are associated with grossly shortened red cell survival and, hence, clinically significant hemolytic anemia.

Red cell enzymopathies associated with hemolytic syndromes fall into three main categories:

1. Enzymopathies of the hexosemonophosphate shunt and related glutathione metabolism. The hexosemonophosphate (HMP) shunt requires oxygen, and it is the only significant pathway in the red cell cycling NADP$\longleftrightarrow$NADPH. Six carbon glucose is converted to pentose and then into intermediates re-entering the main pathway of glycolysis. To function, this pathway requires two dehydrogenases and the enzymatic capacities to synthesize, oxidize, and reduce glutathione. Glutathione oxidation occurs in the course of the enzyme-mediated reactions converting peroxides to harmless water or alcohols. In the red cell, the HMP shunt serves to protect hemoglobin and other proteins from noxious oxidant stresses in the environment and to provide the reducing power of NADPH.

2. Enzymopathies of the anaerobic (Embden-Meyerhof) glycolytic pathway. Anaerobic glycolysis supplies the conversion of glucose to lactate and a net gain in ATP that serves to fuel the energy needs of the erythrocyte. This net gain in ATP is diminished by virtue of a portion of glucose being diverted into 2,3-diphosphoglycerate (2,3-DPG), which has regu-

latory effects on the oxidative dissociation curve of hemoglobin. The Embden-Meyerhof pathway, by virtue of the cycling of its pyridine nucleotide co-factor NAD$\longleftrightarrow$NADH, is also essential for the conversion of any unwanted methemoglobin to functional hemoglobin.

3. Enzymopathies of certain enzymes of nucleotide metabolism. Severe deficiencies (and, in one instance, a striking, genetically determined excess) of certain enzymes in this category are associated with aberrations in metabolism that are sufficiently severe to be manifested as a hemolytic anemia.

THERAPY OF ERYTHROENZYMOPATHIES OF THE HMP SHUNT

X chromosome–linked deficiency of G6PD, the first dehydrogenase of the HMP shunt, is the prototype. This erythroenzymopathy is perhaps the most common enzyme deficiency afflicting man, and the clinical manifestations as well as their underlying molecular lesions are extremely pleomorphic. More than 300 variants may affect some 400 million people worldwide. In most patients, hemolysis is episodic and induced by medications, infection, or ingestion of fava beans. In members of the black population of the United States manifesting the common A-variant, there is impunity to favism, whereas the so-called Mediterranean G6PD mutant common in Sardinia and elsewhere is associated with potentially severe and even fatal hemolysis if fava beans are ingested. In a small percentage of subjects who are severely deficient in G6PD, nonspherocytic hemolytic anemia is constantly present. Episodic hemolysis is of variable severity, associated with hemoglobinuria and hemosiderinuria, and accompanied by red cell inclusions consisting of oxidatively denatured hemoglobin derivatives known as Heinz bodies. Clinical manifestations include drug-induced hemolysis, infection-induced hemolysis, favism, neonatal jaundice, and nonspherocytic hemolytic anemia. Prevention of hemolytic episodes due to medications requires that the physician pay special attention to the interdiction of agents known to precipitate attacks and instruct the patient as to the nature of the disorder and the potential hazards of inadequately supervised treatment regimens. Table 1 lists agents that have been incriminated in the induction of hemolysis in G6PD-deficient subjects. The list is incomplete, and the medical literature contains references to many additional agents that have been postulated to induce hemolysis. The reasons for inaccurate, doubtful, or uncertain documentation are evident. Many hemolytic episodes occur in subjects taking multiple medications, lending difficulties to critical incrimination of the offender. In other instances, medications have been taken in the course of infections that themselves may be the true culprits. A further complication lies in the variable severity of deficiency states and the consequent widely varying

Table 1 Drugs and Chemicals That Should Be Avoided by Persons with G6PD Deficiency

Acetanilid	Phenylhydrazine
Doxorubicin	Primaquine
Furazolidone (Furoxone)	Sulfacetamide
Methylene blue	Sulfamethoxazole (Gantanol)
Nalidixic acid (NeGram)	Sulfanilamide
Naphthalene	Sulfapyridine
Niridazole (Ambilhar)	Thiazolesulfone
Nitrofurantoin (Furadantin)	Toluidine blue
Phenazopyridine (Pyridium)	Trinitrotoluene (TNT)

From Beutler E. Glucose-6-phosphate dehydrogenase deficiency. In: Williams WJ, Beutler E, Ersley AJ, et al, eds. Clinical hematology, 4th ed. New York: McGraw-Hill, 1990:598; with permission.

susceptibility to agents that produce hemolysis in some patients and not in others. If a hemolytic episode supervenes, *all* suspect offending medications should be withdrawn. As with any hemoglobinuric syndrome, adequate urinary output must be maintained. Transfusions are discussed subsequently, but should be used judiciously and most often are not required for self-limited hemolytic episodes. In cases in which favism is suspected or documented, it should be made clear to the patient and family that ingestion of the beans is to be completely interdicted in the future. Fava beans are a staple item of diet in certain ethnic populations and, although most dangerous to susceptible subjects when fresh, can also produce hemolysis even when dried or canned.

Infections and sometimes other stresses, including surgery and metabolic derangements such as diabetic acidosis, may also result in a hemolytic episode. Infections must be treated with appropriate agents, and hemolytic anemia should be monitored and treated with transfusion only when necessary. Viral infections, particularly hepatitis, have also been implicated as precipitating causes of hemolysis.

Neonatal jaundice requires special mention. It is not uncommon in infants with G6PD deficiency, and it constitutes a potential threat of kernicterus. Neonatal jaundice must be monitored carefully; exchange transfusions of non–G6PD-deficient blood should be utilized if necessary, and conventional treatment of threatening hyperbilirubinemia with phenobarbitol or other measures must be employed if indicated. Some physicians have advocated administration of supplementary vitamin E to the newborn because of its properties as an antioxidant, although its efficacy is not well documented.

Other documented enzymopathies involve HMP shunt enzymes responsible for glutathione synthesis as well as glutathione reductase and, possibly, glutathione peroxidase. Although rare, they may be associated with hemolysis and, in certain cases, neurologic deficits. In one syndrome involving deficient glutathione synthetase, severe metabolic acidosis and hemolytic anemia are components of multisystem disease. In these rare enzymopathies, medication interdictions pertinent to G6PD-deficient subjects are also applicable.

NONSPHEROCYTIC HEMOLYTIC ANEMIA DUE TO ERYTHROENZYMOPATHIES

Nonspherocytic hemolytic anemia characterizes severe deficiencies of many enzymes of anaerobic glycolysis and nucleotide metabolism as well as the episodic and chronic hemolytic syndromes discussed previously. These include severe deficiencies of the glycolytic enzymes hexokinase, glucosephosphate isomerase, phosphofructokinase, aldolase, triosephosphate isomerase, phosphoglycerate kinase, and pyruvate kinase. All are encoded on autosomes except for X chromosome–linked phosphoglycerate kinase. Deficiency in the latter is fully expressed in hemizygous men, whereas heterozygous women possess two red cell populations, one normal and one deficient and subject to premature destruction. In addition to hemolytic anemia, deficiency of phosphofructokinase is also characterized by myopathy. Deficiency of triosephosphate isomerase gives rise to severe multisystem disease, with devastating neurologic dysfunction and other features in addition to hemolytic anemia. Phosphoglycerate kinase deficiency in hemizygous men likewise is associated with an array of neurologic abnormalities not observed in heterozygous women. In addition, two glycolytic pathway enzymes are not associated with hemolysis when severely deficient. In one type of lactate dehydrogenase deficiency, myopathy, but not hemolysis, is present. In 2,3-diphosphoglycerate mutase deficiency, there is near-total lack of 2,3-DPG and modest, asymptomatic erythrocytosis, but hemolysis is lacking.

The most common enzyme deficiency of nucleotide metabolism associated with hemolytic anemia (and very prominent basophilic stippling on stained blood films) is that of pyrimidine nucleotidase. A second unusual enzymopathy is that of dominantly transmitted adenosine deaminase excess, in which the apparently normal enzyme is 50 to 100 times more active than normal. Rarely, hemolytic anemia may be associated with adenylate kinase deficiency.

All of the preceding enzyme deficiencies are relatively rare except for pyruvate kinase deficiency, which, next to G6PD deficiency, is the most common erythroenzymopathy associated with hemolysis. Precise diagnosis may require assistance from research laboratories working in the field. A screening test is available in many clinical laboratories for G6PD and pyruvate kinase deficiency. In the latter, false-negative results may be obtained if contaminating leukocytes are not eliminated from the blood specimen prior to running the test. The following discussion applies to the chronic nonspherocytic hemolytic anemias due to red cell enzyme deficiencies.

TRANSFUSIONS

Transfusions should be kept to the minimum compatible with maintaining a reasonable quality of life, avoiding as much as possible the attendant hazards of reactions, hepatitis, development of anitbodies that may potentially hinder future transfusion therapy, and eventual iron overload. The latter, in particular, may compromise vital functions of the pancreas, liver, and heart. Many patients do not require transfusions or, if they do, they require them only sporadically. In any event, therapy in affected subjects is directed at the patient and not the hemoglobin level. (This is particularly true of pyruvate kinase deficiency, in which the increase in 2,3-DPG that results from the enzyme defect lowers hemoglobin-oxygen affinity, thereby enhancing oxygen delivery to tissues despite the low hemoglobin level.) The objective of treatment is a stable, reasonable quality of life and not the maintenance of normal hematologic parameters. Transfusion is indicated when anemia is rapidly worsening; when anemia-induced angina, electrocardiographically documented myocardial ischemia or high-output cardiac failure is present; when obtundation or chronic debilitation is believed to be associated with anemia; and sometimes when infectious complications exist or surgery is contemplated. Exchange transfusion of the newborn is indicated when kernicterus is threatened. Note that the marrow in compensated hemolytic syndromes is producing cells at the maximal possible rate. Any complication that is even partially marrow-suppressive or may increase peripheral hemolysis (such as infection, surgery, and other clinically "stressful" circumstances) is reflected in increasing anemia and a falling hemoglobin level. As with all chronic, ongoing hemolytic anemias, so-called aregenerative crises, which are usually induced by myelosuppressive, "flulike," viral illnesses, and are often ascribed to a parvovirus, occasionally occur. These are self-limited, usually last around 7 to 12 days, and may be associated with worsening anemia, sometimes requiring transfusion, and, temporarily, with diminishing reticulocytosis and icterus.

FOLATE

Folate administration (1 to 2 mg per day) is indicated in chronic hemolytic syndromes of any severity. Folate requirements of an intensely hyperactive marrow are not well delineated. Many believe that hemoglobin levels are often slightly better maintained and the incidence of "aregenerative crises" reduced by daily folate therapy.

SPLENECTOMY

In pyruvate kinase deficiency, it is clear that splenectomy provides only modest benefit. After surgery, hemolysis continues and reticulocytosis may even increase. Nonetheless, there is slight to moderate improvement in the anemia, and this may be life-saving in the most severe syndromes; in others, it may serve to diminish or even eliminate transfusion requirements. Splenectomy should be considered only in patients with ongoing transfusion requirements and the accompanying severe clinical manifestations. Whereas data are more sketchy for hemolytic anemias due to enzymopathies other than that of pyruvate kinase, in these, too, splenectomy should be seriously considered if transfusion requirements are chronic.

IRON

Iron therapy is contraindicated unless, for some entirely unrelated reason, iron deficiency is clearly documented. In the chronic nonspherocytic hemolytic anemias, there is no renal loss of iron because hemoglobinuria and hemosiderinuria are absent.

STEROIDS

There is no evidence that steroid therapy has any place in the management of hemolytic syndromes associated with these enzymopathies.

COMPLICATIONS

With all chronic hemolytic syndromes, hyperbilirubinemia carries with it the increased risk of early onset of cholelithiasis due to pigment stones. The treatment, however, does not differ from that of cholelithiasis of other etiology. If surgery is indicated, we favor transfusion to essentially normal hemoglobin levels prior to the procedure.

Rare patients develop ulcers in the region of the ankles. This is not a common complication, but, if present, it should be managed by transfusion, bed rest and avoidance of stasis, and, rarely, skin grafting, should this prove necessary.

SUGGESTED READING

Beutler E. Hemolytic anemia in disorders of red cell metabolism. New York: Plenum, 1978.
Luzzatto L, Mehta A. Glucose-6-phosphate dehydrogenase deficiency. In: Scriver CR, Beaudet AL, Sly, WS, et al, eds. The metabolic basis of inherited disease, 6th ed. New York: McGraw-Hill, 1989: 2237–2265.
Valentine WN, Tanaka KR, Paglia DE. Pyruvate kinase and other enzyme deficiency hemolytic anemias. In: Scriver CR, Beaudet AL, Sly WS, et al, eds. The metabolic basis of inherited disease, 6th ed. New York: McGraw-Hill, 1989:2341–2365.

AUTOIMMUNE HEMOLYTIC ANEMIA

PAUL M. NESS, M.D.

The autoimmune hemolytic anemias (AIHA) are a group of disorders in which the patient produces autoantibodies directed against his or her own red cell antigens. These antibodies recognize attachment sites on the erythrocyte membrane, often activating the complement cascade, which leads to intravascular red cell destruction or extravascular red cell sequestration, with subsequent destruction in the reticuloendothelial system (bone marrow, spleen, liver, or lymph nodes). The erythrocyte life span is decreased by antibody-induced hemolysis, and the bone marrow reserve is often incapable of compensating for the increased red cell destruction, resulting in anemia.

Autoimmune hemolytic anemias can be classified as idiopathic or secondary, depending on whether a primary disorder known to be associated with AIHA is present. The most common causes of secondary AIHA are collagen vascular disorders or the many varieties of lymphoproliferative diseases. Other systems of classifying AIHA depend on the antibody class (IgG or IgM) that typically causes autoimmune hemolysis in man. Warm AIHA is typically associated with antibodies of the IgG class, which react optimally at 37°C. Cold AIHA syndromes are usually associated with IgM autoantibodies, which are optimally reactive at 4°C. Because the antibody class is predictive of the pathogenesis of the hemolytic disorder, it is important to distinguish which class of autoantibody is involved in each case; the clinical course resulting from the site and time course of red cell destruction, the response to therapy, and the overall prognosis generally can be anticipated by the distinction of warm and cold AIHA caused by IgG and IgM antibodies, respectively.

Another large category of AIHA is associated with adverse reactions to drugs. In most cases, the drug induces antibody formation and the drug-antibody immune complex attaches to the red cell, with subsequent hemolysis. In other cases, the antibody reacts with drug-coated red cells in patients on high doses of the culprit drug (e.g., penicillin). Other drugs, such as alpha-methyldopa, stimulate the production of red cell autoantibodies and are associated with an illness that is clinically and serologically undistinguishable from idiopathic warm AIHA. Because any drug can be associated with AIHA, even in the absence of previous documented cases, it is prudent practice to obtain a comprehensive drug history in all cases and stop any medication that appears to be involved in AIHA of recent onset.

GENERAL INDICATIONS FOR THERAPY

In many patients with warm or cold AIHA, no therapy is required because the hemolysis may be mild and fully compensated. If AIHA is secondary to an underlying disorder, control of the primary disease often results in resolution of the immune hemolysis. If the patient has significant anemia attributable to the hemolysis, therapeutic intervention may be necessary. The target of therapy is not the normalization of the direct antiglobulin test (DAT). Patients may have positive DAT without hemolysis and anemia, or, alternatively, patients may have symptomatic AIHA with a negative DAT. In addition, the common forms of therapy may correct the anemia without any quantifiable difference in the DAT.

THERAPY OF WARM AIHA

Corticosteroids

Corticosteroids are the therapy of first choice for patients with idiopathic or secondary forms of AIHA. The clinical response to corticosteroids is a result of three basic mechanisms. First, corticosteroids have been shown in vitro and in vivo to block IgG and complement receptors on tissue macrophages so that the clearance of IgG or C3-coated cells is much less efficient. This mechanism accounts for the earliest therapeutic effects of corticosteroids, and it is one reason why the anemia may improve with no change in DAT. Corticosteroids also decrease the production of the IgG autoantibody. This effect does not occur until several weeks of corticosteroid therapy have been administered. A third effect of corticosteroids impairs the attachment of autoantibody to red cells or hastens the elution of antibody from coated cells; whether this effect has a clinical benefit is unclear.

The initial regimen of corticosteroids of choice is 1 to 1.5 mg per kilogram per day of oral prednisone. Other equivalent corticosteroid preparations can be used but have no advantage over prednisone and may have more adverse effects. Parenteral administration can be used, but no specific advantage has been documented. The initial dose is usually maintained for 2 to 3 weeks. Most patients have a response with a stabilization of hematocrit or a loss of transfusion requirements within that time. As patients begin to respond, the DAT may become weaker and serum autoantibody may fade or disappear; despite these trends, the DAT cannot be relied upon to monitor clinical activity of the disease. Patients with no response in hematocrit or reticulocyte index after a 3-week trial are considered steroid failures.

When the steroid-responsive patient begins to stabilize, usually after 3 to 4 weeks of the initial prednisone regimen, it is prudent to begin a progressive tapering of the dose. One schedule that is useful is to reduce the dose by 10 mg per day each week until a dose of 30 mg per day is achieved and then continue to reduce the dose by decrements of 5 mg per day each week. When a dose of 15 to 20 mg of prednisone per day is achieved, several therapeutic options can be exercised. One possibility is to begin an alternate-day schedule (20 to 30 mg every other day) to minimize the adverse side effects of corticosteroids. Another option is to continue the slow tapering process by dose reductions of 2.5 mg per day with weekly steps. The overall tapering scheduling should be slow. For the occasional patient with a clinically severe relapse, one can return to the previous successful dose or re-institute the initial regimen of 1 to 1.5 mg per kilogram of prednisone.

Although 75 percent to 80 percent of patients respond to corticosteroids, the majority of patients will relapse as the dose is tapered. Many patients can be maintained on lower doses of prednisone, but daily prednisone levels of 15 to 20 mg place the patient at considerable risk of steroid side effects, including peptic ulcer disease, hypertension, myopathy, osteoporosis, and susceptibility to infection. If a dose of more than 15 mg of prednisone per day is required to maintain a stable hematocrit, other therapies should be considered. Permanent remissions in adults treated with corticosteroids that have been tapered and eventually stopped do occur, but the vast majority of patients will require reinstitution of prednisone with or without other therapies.

Splenectomy

In patients whose response to corticosteroids is incomplete, splenectomy is the next therapy to be considered. The spleen is the major site of sequestration of IgG-coated erythrocytes, in part due to its unique architecture, where red cells can be concentrated in close proximity to tissue macrophages. When radiolabeled red cells coated with autoantibody are injected, the spleen is the major site of clearance, and the liver plays a secondary role. Because the spleen has also been shown to have a role in autoantibody production, splenectomy may also be effective in AIHA by removing the autoantibody production capacity of the larger lymphoid network of splenic B lymphocytes.

Approximately 50 to 60 percent of patients will have a good therapeutic response to splenectomy, with marked improvement in hematocrit or complete hemologic remission. Late relapses do occur, however, most likely as a result of increased antibody synthesis and a shift to hepatic red cell sequestration. Many patients have a partial response to splenectomy and a stable hematocrit can subsequently be maintained with less than 15 mg per day of prednisone. For these reasons, patients who have no initial response to corticosteroids, patients who require unacceptable high doses of corticosteroids for maintenance, and patients with intolerance to the corticosteroid side effects should be offered splenectomy. Red cell survival or sequestration studies are not predictive of a clinical response to splenectomy and cannot be recommended because of their cost and time requirements.

Splenectomy is usually well tolerated, with low morbidity and mortality, because most patients with

AIHA are in reasonable health and massive splenomegaly is uncommon. There is a low risk of developing the overwhelming postsplenectomy sepsis syndrome, which is usually caused by *Streptococcus pneumoniae*; this risk can be reduced by the administration of pneumococcal vaccine to all patients undergoing splenectomy and the prompt use of antibiotics for febrile episodes in these patients.

Immunosuppressive Agents

Because transient or partial remissions are common in patients undergoing splenectomy for warm AIHA, immunosuppressive agents may be administered as a third line of therapy. The general indications for these agents include their use in patients with symptomatic anemia who have failed splenectomy or relapsed after a transient remission, patients who are not acceptable surgical candidates for splenectomy, or patients who have serious side effects from corticosteroids.

A number of agents have been used, but azathioprine and cyclophosphamide are the most common drugs of choice. The mode of action of these agents is to reduce the synthesis of the IgG autoantibody. At least 2 weeks of therapy are required for a response, and a trial of several months may be required to determine the effectiveness of a chemotherapeutic agent. A dose of oral cyclophosphamide, 50 to 100 mg per day, is usually begun with small dose increments—often several weeks of 25 mg per day each week—until a clinical benefit is noted or side effects become intolerable. Marrow suppression with leukopenia, hemorrhagic cystitis, and gastrointestinal symptoms are the major adverse effects of cyclophosphamide. Patients on cyclophosphamide should increase their fluid intake and be monitored with weekly blood counts so that dosage can be adjusted to maintain granulocyte counts higher than 1,000 per microliter and platelet counts greater than 50,000 per microliter. In patients who respond to cyclophosphamide, a successful dose level should be maintained for 6 months and then tapered over several months. Because of the long-term potential of alkylating agents to increase the risk of leukemia or other malignancies, chronic administration should be avoided.

Other Therapies

Danazol, an attenuated synthetic androgen, has been used with clinical benefit in some patients with refractory warm AIHA. Typical doses of 600 to 800 mg per day have been used, most commonly with prednisone as part of an initial therapeutic regimen or after corticosteroids when single agents have proved ineffective. Responders will often improve within 1 to 3 weeks of the onset of therapy, permitting the reduction of corticosteroids administered concomitantly. If remission becomes sustained, the danazol dose is usually reduced to 200 to 400 mg per day. Because long-term side effects are uncommon, the most serious being hepatic dysfunction, it is likely that danazol may be used more frequently in the future in an attempt to corroborate initial enthusiastic reports.

Intravenous immunoglobulin (Ig) has also been used in patients with AIHA, usually in combination with other therapies for patients who are refractory. It is typically given for 5 days at dosage levels of 400 mg per kilogram daily. Its suggested mode of action is binding to and blocking Fc receptors on macrophages to reduce the clearance of circulating red cells coated with IgG antibodies. A recent series of patients with secondary AIHA and lymphoproliferative diseases demonstrated some long-term benefit and reduction in antibody titer with a maintenance schedule of intravenous Ig. Other case reports suggest temporary benefit or no benefit from intravenous Ig regimens.

Plasma exchange has been used in AIHA patients with acute hemolytic episodes, and some stabilization may be noted. The efficacy of plasma exchange is limited in warm AIHA because the autoantibody production is not inhibited and IgG has a large extravascular volume that rapidly repletes the serum levels to preapheresis levels, unless autoantibody production is diminished by other therapies. Despite these concerns, nominal drastic responses have been noted that may provide temporary relief before corticosteroids or splenectomy becomes effective.

THERAPY OF COLD AGGLUTININ SYNDROMES

The therapeutic approach to patients with cold agglutinin disease or cold AIHA depends on the severity of this process, the serologic characteristics of the autoantibody, and whether the cold AIHA is idiopathic or secondary to an underlying lymphoproliferative disorder. Many cases present with mild to moderate anemia and require no therapy other than avoiding exposure to cold, which can precipitate hemolytic episodes. Corticosteroids are generally ineffective in most cases unless the thermal amplitude is very high; in cases in which corticosteroids are effective, the concomitant presence of an IgG antibody along with the IgM antibody diagnostic of cold AIHA should be suspected. In addition, splenectomy is usually not effective because the liver is the predominant site of red cell sequestration of complement-coated red cells.

Patients with severe anemia can be treated with oral alkylating agents. Chlorambucil is often used at a dose level of 4 mg per day, which can be increased by increments of 2 mg per day at monthly intervals until a response is noted or toxicity becomes intolerable. Blood counts should be monitored at weekly intervals. Therapy is more likely to be useful in patients with a lymphoproliferative disorder and is only occasionally successful in patients with idiopathic cold AIHA. When the presence of cold autoantibodies is a feature of a B-lymphocyte malignancy, clinical responses to therapy for the malignancy tend to correlate with improvement in hemolysis.

Plasma exchange has a more logical role in cold AIHA than in warm AIHA because IgM is predominantly intravascular. It can be an effective therapy in acute hemolytic episodes but the benefit is only transient. The use of blood warmer is advisable to avoid hemolysis in the extracorporeal circuit. Some patients may require elevating the ambient temperature of their environment to avoid hemolytic exacerbation. A recent report of the use of a temperature-regulated space suit obtained from the National Aeronautics and Space Administration to reduce hemolysis in cold AIHA indicates that this therapy is worthy of further trials.

TRANSFUSION THERAPY

Blood transfusion may be required for patients with AIHA who present with fulminant hemolysis or patients with chronic hemolysis who become symptomatic while awaiting response to primary modes of therapy. The presence of red cell autoantibody coating the patient's red cells or appearing as a panagglutinin in the serum adds additional risks of blood transfusion to the general risks of infectious disease transmission or transfusion reaction from alloantibodies to red cells, white cells, platelets, or serum proteins. The autoantibody can make it difficult to detect coexisting red cell alloantibodies, which can cause severe hemolytic transfusion reactions; in addition, the red cell autoantibody will cause increased destruction of the donor red cells. Despite these concerns, transfusion may be required in AIHA and may be life-saving. A recent report documented a series of patients with AIHA and reticulocytopenia despite intense erythroid hyperplasia in the bone marrow. In all five cases, transfusions were required as a life-sustaining measure for profound anemia in patients transferred from other hospitals where transfusions had been withheld because of serologic incompatibilities. Reticulocytopenia persisted from 4 to 160 days before the onset of adequate erythropoiesis or control of the hemolytic process with corticosteroids or splenectomy. These cases emphasize that transfusion should not be avoided in AIHA, despite old dogma to the contrary.

The transfusion management of patients with AIHA requires careful communication between the clinician and the transfusion service. It is important to know the capabilities of the transfusion service for performing specialized immunohematologic procedures as well as where these procedures may be available on a referral basis. It is also critical for the clinician to assess the patient's history of pregnancies and previous transfusions with great care; it is unlikely that a previously untransfused man will have alloantibodies in his serum.

When the decision has been reached to begin transfusions, several additional steps can enhance patient safety. In some cases, transfusions of small aliquots of blood may be sufficient to provide relief of symptoms while avoiding the complications of fluid overload. The use of leukocyte-poor red blood cells is useful to avoid febrile, nonhemolytic transfusion reactions whose initial presentation can suggest a hemolytic reaction with more severe consequences. In cases of transfusion for patients with cold agglutinin disease, blood warmers are often suggested, but there are limited data to support or refute this recommendation.

In view of the complications that can arise in patients with AIHA who may require transfusion, measures can be taken during remissions to enhance patient safety. One reasonable approach involves the use of predeposit autologous transfusions with frozen storage for patients who are likely to relapse in the future or who may require transfusions in the event that a splenectomy is required. Another measure to be considered is extended red cell phenotype analysis while the patient remains in remission.

SUGGESTED READING

Conley CL, Lippman SM, Ness PM, et al. Autoimmune hemolytic anemia with reticulocytopenia and erythroid marrow. N Engl J Med 1982; 301:281–286.
Frank MM, Schreiber AD, Atkinson JP, et al. Pathophysiology of immune hemolytic anemia. Ann Intern Med 1987; 87:210–220.
Petz LD, Garratty G. Acquired immune hemolytic anemias. New York: Churchill Livingstone, 1980.

HEMOLYTIC UREMIC SYNDROME

G.H. NEILD, M.D., F.R.C.P.

The hemolytic uremic syndrome (HUS) is a clinicopathologic syndrome in which thrombocytopenia and a microangiopathic hemolytic anemia occur together with acute renal failure and a characteristic renal vascular pathology. It most commonly affects children under 5 years of age. In children, the renal failure usually recovers. In adults, HUS is a very rare condition and is commonly associated with irreversible renal failure. Hemolytic uremic syndrome is not a single disease. The etiology varies, and until recently the cause was usually unknown. A diarrheal infection due to a verocytotoxin producing *Escherichia coli* is now known to be the usual cause of HUS. Whatever the cause, the end result is extensive endothelial injury of the renal microvasculature.

In the closely related syndrome of thrombotic thrombocytopenic purpura (TTP), a similar vascular injury occurs simultaneously in many organs, and the associated hematologic findings are correspondingly more severe. Is there any point in distinguishing between HUS and TTP? By and large, nephrologists call the syndrome HUS and hematologists call it TTP, and partly for this reason renal failure is found to be milder in TTP. There is, however, a homogeneous subset of TTP in which a recurring illness characteristically affects adult women, and renal failure is rarely a major problem. In other respects, HUS and TTP are on a continuum, with TTP representing a more systemic disease.

Hemolytic uremic syndrome can be divided into the following three clinical groups:

1. There is an epidemic or diarrhea-associated form, which typically has an acute presentation with bloody diarrhea. Although dialysis may be required, there is usually a complete recovery.
2. There is an endemic or sporadic form, which has a less acute onset. Severe hypertension is common, and the kidneys may be irreversibly damaged. This is the form usually seen in adults, and it may occur postpartum.
3. In some sporadic cases, there is a family history of HUS.

A number of conditions may either lead to or can be associated with HUS (Table 1). It is intriguing to speculate what the common factors may be.

The etiologic causes can be broadly divided into diarrhea-associated and noninfectious causes. Other causes of HUS are generally unknown, but various conditions predispose to HUS. In adults, it may be seen either postpartum, in women taking the contraceptive pill, or in those who are already hypertensive. Increasingly, an association with immunosuppressive drugs has been described. These drugs include cyclosporin and several cytotoxic drugs, including mitomycin-C and 5-fluorouracil. In some cases, there is a family history, often with the syndrome occurring postpartum.

PATHOGENESIS

The initial injury is so severe that injury to the endothelium is conspicuous, and platelet involvement is not just morphologically visible but can be measured in the circulation. Thrombocytopenia is believed to be due to both platelet activation and consumption at sites of endothelial injury. In some cases, the endothelial "injury" might be no more than loss of the normal negative charge on the endothelial cell surface due to the action of bacterial or viral neuraminidase.

Failure of vascular prostacyclin synthesis may also be involved. In 1978, Remuzzi and his colleagues showed that vascular tissue taken from patients with HUS and TTP generated abnormally low levels of prostacyclin. Furthermore, when plasma from these patients was incubated with either normal endothelial cells in culture or washed rings of aortic tissue (which no longer

Table 1 Etiology and Predisposing Factors

Infections
  Diarrhea-associated (*Escherichia coli* verotoxin)
  Shigella-associated
  Neuraminidase-associated
  Others (campylobacter, viruses)

Sporadic, nondiarrheal causes
  Idiopathic
  Familial
  Drugs (e.g., cyclosporin, mitomycin)
  Tumors
  Pregnancy
  Systemic lupus erythematosus
  Transplantation
  Scleroderma
  Malignant/accelerated hypertension
  Superimposed on glomerulonephritis

produced prostacyclin), it was unable to stimulate the normal prostacyclin synthesis by these tissues. The factor in plasma that "stimulated" prostacyclin synthesis was called prostacyclin-stimulating factor (PSF).

The origin of PSF remains unknown. It has been characterized as a very polar compound with a molecular weight of 300 to 400 that appears to act by prolonging or protecting the action of cyclo-oxygenase, probably by acting as a reducing co-factor for cyclo-oxygenase peroxidase. Lack of PSF activity represents either a relative deficiency of this substance or antagonism of its action by an inhibitor. During oxidant injury, peroxides and free radicals are produced that can inhibit or inactivate cyclo-oxygenase. Thus, this factor appears to act as an antioxidant. Other defects of normal prostacyclin biology have also been described in HUS.

DIFFERENTIAL DIAGNOSIS

Both HUS and TTP are characterized by localized microvascular thrombosis, or "localized intravascular coagulation," and it is unusual for coagulation factors to be consumed sufficiently for clotting times to be prolonged. In contrast, a generalized or disseminated intravascular coagulation (DIC), which may cause a very similar hematologic and clinical state, is associated with consumption of clotting factors and prolongation of clotting times. Disseminated intravascular coagulation in this context is usually caused by infection, but it can occur with certain neoplasms.

It is therefore imperative that one question the patient closely about travel, environment, and occupation and seek a cause or predisposing factor for HUS. If the clotting is abnormal, one must search carefully for infection (usually septicemia) and sometimes neoplasia.

PATHOLOGY

Blood vessels have a limited number of ways in which they may respond to injury. Hemolytic uremic syndrome and TTP are part of a group of conditions in which thrombosis and necrosis of intrarenal vessels occur in the absence of cellular inflammation. Synonyms for this histopathologic constellation include malignant nephrosclerosis, thrombotic microangiopathy, and proliferative arteriopathy. In HUS, two different histopathologic patterns are seen, although they may overlap. In the diarrhea-associated variety of HUS, there is predominantly glomerular capillary thrombosis with some arteriolar necrosis. With other forms of HUS, particularly in adults, arterioles and small arteries commonly show intimal proliferation with luminal stenosis, i.e., a preglomerular pathology. With the former pattern, recovery is to be expected, but not with the latter.

OUTCOME

The natural history of HUS, when preceded by a diarrheal illness and associated with glomerular thrombi, is one of spontaneous recovery, although there may be some residual injury. In idiopathic cases, particularly in adults, there is often major preglomerular vascular pathology and irreversible renal failure.

A study from the Hospital for Sick Children in London reported on prognostic features in 72 children admitted between 1969 and 1980. Seventy-eight percent required dialysis, and of these, 37 (66 percent) recovered within 2 weeks. Seventy percent of the children made a complete recovery. Three (4 percent) died during the acute phase, 16 percent remained dependent on dialysis, and 11 percent had residual injury in the form of hypertension or renal insufficiency. Recovery was associated with a younger age and presentation in the summer with a diarrheal illness — features now known to be associated with verotoxin from *E. coli*. In a Belgian study, 46 children who developed HUS between 1970 and 1976 were followed up 10 years later. Seventy percent had no sign of renal disease, but 14 patients had at least one stigmata, usually inability to concentrate fully. Three had both hypertension and proteinuria. However, a more aggressive disease was reported in 1986 from an outbreak in the West Midlands of Britain involving 35 children. Twenty three children (66 percent) required dialysis; 3 patients died, and 6 (17 percent) developed chronic renal failure. Twelve children had seizures (associated with a plasma sodium level < 126 mmol per liter), and 4 had long-term neurologic sequelae.

Hemolytic uremic syndrome occurring postpartum was initially described as "idiopathic postpartum renal failure." It occurs between 1 day and several weeks after what is often an entirely uneventful pregnancy. Very rarely, there is a family history of HUS. The management is entirely similar to HUS. Unfortunately, often due to late presentation of patients who have already gone home, there may be severe preglomerular vascular injury, irreversible renal failure, and the development of severe hypertension.

In summary, a worse prognosis may be anticipated when there is either no diarrheal prodrome, family history, severe central nervous system involvement, or severe hypertension at presentation, or no recovery of renal function after 7 days.

GENERAL MANAGEMENT APPROACH

Because of the differing modes of presentation and the understandable delays in referral to renal centers, patients will often be seen well after the onset of the illness. This is important to appreciate when trying to evaluate hematologic changes and response to therapy. For example, adults presenting late with severe hypertension may already have irreversible renal damage that could not be expected to respond to any treatment.

Standard Supportive Therapy

As with any case of acute renal failure, blood volume should be assessed and hypovolemia corrected as quickly as possible. Volume depletion may be a consequence of diarrhea and vomiting. In very severe cases, the endothelial injury may lead to increased capillary permeability, and both crystalloid and colloid are lost from the circulation. In such cases, there will be a rapid fall in plasma albumin, and initially the hematocrit may even be increased.

The plasma sodium level is frequently reduced, and hyponatremia may be a factor in any central nervous system disturbance. The plasma sodium level should be normalized, and this will occur with dialysis.

If the patient is seen early and is still passing urine, he or she should be managed in a conventional way. After correction of the circulating volume with crystalloid, bolus doses of furosemide or an infusion of low-dose dopamine (2.5 to 5.0 µg per kilogram per minute) may be started to try to initiate, or maintain, the diuresis.

It is reasonable to hope that a prostacyclin infusion might help. A dose of 2.5 ng per kilogram per minute can be started and gradually increased to 5 ng per kilogram, or higher, if the drug is well tolerated. There is no evidence, however, that prostacyclin affects the outcome, and reports claim only limited success. However, failures may represent late cases in which vascular injury was too advanced to expect recovery.

It has also been suggested that the striking hyperuricemia that may occur can lead to a urate nephropathy, and that vigorous therapy with crystalloids and high-dose intravenous furosemide may convert such patients to a polyuric phase and avoid the need for dialysis. In support of this is the observation that patients on dialysis may have several days of complete anuria and then have a rather sudden return of function.

Acute Tubular Necrosis. When the patient is first seen, acute tubular necrosis may not be established. Apart from hypovolemia, there may be a nephrotoxic insult from hemoglobinemia or hyperbilirubinemia.

A vigorous attempt should be made to establish a diuresis.

Hypertension. This may be a problem, but it can usually be controlled in conventional ways. It may be due in part to salt and water retention, and this should be dealt with promptly by either diuretics or dialysis. The blood pressure sometimes falls following plasma infusions.

Anemia. A microangiopathic hemolytic anemia occurs. Red cell morphology shows fragmented and deformed cells (schistocytes, spherocytes). Depending on the degree of hemolysis, there will be an increase in reticulocytes, and increase in unconjugated bilirubin and plasma lactic dehydrogenase (LDH) and its heat-stable isoenzyme hydroxybutyrate dehydrogenase (HBD) (from red cells), and a decrease in haptoglobin levels. Hemolysis may occur from 1 to 3 weeks, with the cells being removed by the spleen. If the patient is admitted early in the clinical course of the disease, the hematocrit may be increased owing to hypovolemic hemoconcentration.

The hemoglobin level may fall rapidly to as low as 3 g per deciliter, but the median values are 7 to 9 g per deciliter. The degree of anemia is not related to acute renal failure and vice versa. Blood transfusions should be given as clinically indicated. We prefer to keep the hemoglobin around 10 g per deciliter in patients who are being dialyzed. Continuing disease activity can be monitored by examining red cell morphology of peripheral blood and the plasma LDH or HBD concentration.

Thrombocytopenia. Thrombocytopenia with less than 100×10^9 platelets per liter occurs at some point in the illness, although at presentation 50 percent of patients will have levels above 100×10^9 per liter. Counts may fall to 5 to 20×10^9 per liter, but more usually to around 50×10^9 per liter.

Red cell fragments may falsely raise "automated" platelet counts. Thrombocytopenia lasts from 7 to 20 days, but the severity and duration do not correlate with the severity of the illness. Platelet transfusions are not required and should not be given.

Dialysis. Both peritoneal and hemodialysis are equally effective. In renal units, peritoneal dialysis is now infrequently used for acute renal failure. There is a risk of bleeding if the platelet count is very low, which would deter one from peritoneal dialysis; for this reason, vascular access should be obtained via internal jugular or femoral veins.

Specific Strategies

Besides the standard management of severe anemia and renal failure, several specific strategies may be tried to inhibit the vascular injury.

Plasma Infusions. Fresh frozen plasma has been tried with considerable success. This might be expected to help for several reasons: (1) replacement of prostacyclin-stimulating factor (PSF) activity and von Willebrand factor (vWF) multimer degrading factor, (2) inhibition of platelet aggregating factors, (3) replacement of fibronectin, which has been consumed in the removal of products of thrombosis, and (4) neutralization of any factors that may be toxic to endothelium.

The required dose has not been established. Remuzzi's group used a loading dose of 30 to 40 ml per kilogram and then a daily dose of 15 to 20 ml per kilogram. In the absence of any definitive information, I usually recommend around 1 L per day of fresh frozen plasma until the platelet count has returned to normal values and red cell hemolysis has ceased. In our experience, we usually see a response (i.e., rise in platelet count and decreases in hemolysis), after 3 to 4 days.

Plasmapheresis. Plasma exchange may not have any special advantages, except that in cases with oliguria, it may be the only way of infusing sufficient fresh frozen plasma. It is often advocated, however, and there are cases in which it has been successful after all other remedies have failed.

Antioxidants. Because vitamin E levels are low in HUS and lipid peroxidation contributes to the pathology, therapy with vitamin E has been proposed. In an uncontrolled trial of HUS in children, vitamin E appeared to improve the prognosis, but a larger study showed no benefit.

Antiplatelet Therapy. Antiplatelet drugs have not been shown to be of benefit, but this may also reflect the timing of the treatment. Drugs such as dipyridamole may potentiate the action of prostacyclin and might be used in combination with prostacyclin infusions.

Anticoagulants. Similarly, anticoagulants have not been shown to be of benefit. Heparin does not improve the outcome and is not recommended on theoretical grounds because (1) there is usually little or no evidence of classical pathway coagulation, (2) it antagonizes prostacyclin synthesis, and (3) it neutralizes the inhibiting effect of prostacyclin on platelet aggregation and makes platelets hyperaggregable.

SUGGESTED READING

Karmali MA, Petric M, Lim C, et al. The association between idiopathic haemolytic uraemic syndrome and infection by verotoxin-producing E. coli. J Infect Dis 1985; 151:775–782.

Neild GH. Haemolytic uraemic syndrome. Q J Med 1987; 63:367–376.

Remuzzi G. HUS and TTP: Variable expression of a single entity. Kidney Int 1987; 32:292–308.

SICKLE CELL DISEASE

PAUL F. MILNER, M.D., FRC, PATH

The sickle cell diseases are inherited anemias in which hemoglobin S (Hb S) replaces all, or most, of the normal hemoglobin A (Hb A). In North America, the Hb S mutation is present in about 1 in 12 people of African descent. Such subjects are said to have sickle cell trait (A/S), and under normal conditions, this does not cause anemia or symptoms. Symptoms may occur, however, at altitudes above 8,000 feet (2,500 meters). About 3 percent of patients with sickle cell traits may experience one or more episodes of painless hematuria during their normal life span.

Sickle cell anemia (S/S) can occur in the offspring of parents who are both A/S; the chance is one in four. Similarly, if one parent is A/S and the other has a trait for Hb C (A/C), or a β-thalassemic gene (A/β⁰thal or A/β⁺thal), there is a one in four chance of their having an offspring with S/C, S/β⁰thal, or S/β⁺thal. All these conditions can cause various degrees of symptoms and anemia (Table 1). The concomitant inheritance of an α-thalassemic gene (α-thal), which is present in about 30 percent of patients in the black population, can modify the clinical expression of sickle cell disease, particularly of the S/S genotype. These patients are less anemic and often have a better physique, but they may get more frequent acute pain crises and bone infarcts. Finally, persistance of fetal hemoglobin (Hb F) in a high proportion of the red cells, which occurs in some patients, can also modify the clinical expression. The combination of both α-thalassemia and a high level of Hb F in an S/S patient is particularly beneficial.

Because of the broad spectrum of clinical expression of these inherited defects, some patients will need a lot of care, whereas others need only to be seen for routine "keep well" check-ups. As the disease tends to have different symptoms and complications in childhood than in adult life, it is useful to discuss their management under separate headings.

THE PEDIATRIC PATIENT

Ideally, the diagnosis should be made at birth by hemoglobin electrophoresis of cord blood, but many patients will not present to a physician until they are several years old. Because of the high mortality from pneumococcal sepsis secondary to hyposplenism, infants should be placed on prophylactic penicillin

Table 1 Some Clinical Effects and Laboratory Results in Sickle Disease

Genotype	Major Clinical Effects	Average Hematologic Profile	Hemoglobin Electrophoresis Results %
S/S	Severe hemolytic anemia Stroke in childhood Splenic sequestration crises Aplastic crises Vaso-occlusive crises Avascular necrosis of the femoral and humeral heads Gallstones Ankle ulcers	Hb 6–9 g/dl* PCV 18–30 g/dl* MCV 90–120 fl*	A 0 S 80–95 A$_2$ 2–3.5* F 2–20
S/β⁰thal	Moderate to severe anemia Vaso-occlusive crises Highest incidence of femoral head necrosis	Hb 7–10 g/dl PCV 20%–35% MCV 65–80 fl	A 0 S 80–95 A$_2$ 3–6 F 1–1
S/C	Proliferative retinopathy Occasional vaso-occlusive crises Aseptic necrosis of femoral head in about 5% of cases Mild splenomegaly	Hb 10–14 g/dl PCV 30%–35% MCV 75–95 fl	A 0 S 50 C 50
S/β⁺thal	Mild anemia Rare vaso-occlusive crises Avascular necrosis in about 5% of cases Risk of proliferative retinopathy	Hb 10–14 g/dl PCV 35%–45% MCV 65–80 fl	A 10–30 S 55–75 A$_2$ 3.5–6 F 1–15
S/δβ⁻thal	Mild anemia Rare vaso-occlusive crises Rare complications	Hb 10–12 g/dl PCV 36%–40% MCV 75–85 fl	A 0 S 70–80 A$_2$ 1–3 F 15–30

*S/S patients with concomitant α-thal have Hb A$_2$ levels of 4–5 percent, to a decreased mean corpuscular volume (MCV) of 75 to 85 fl, and a slightly higher hemoglobin (Hb) and packed cell volume (PCV).

(amoxicillin 125 mg, chewable tablets are most practical) until they are at least 3 years old. Standard immunization schedules should be followed, and polyvalent pneumococcal vaccine should be added at age 2 to 3 years. Some pediatricians would advise continuing penicillin at 250 mg (Penicillin V tablets) twice a day until age 5 years.

Counseling Parents: Prenatal Diagnoses

Parents of infants and small children need counseling regarding the genetic origin of their child's sickness. They might want to discuss the chances of having another affected child. This is probably the best opportunity the physician will have to discuss prenatal diagnosis.

The genotype of a fetus can now be established as early as 8 weeks' gestation by examining DNA obtained by aspiration of trophoblast from chorionic villi. Trophoblast biopsy may be safely performed on outpatients without anesthesia. The risk to the fetus is said to be less than 3 percent. In counseling the parents, it should always be made clear that not all S/S children are severely ill and that there is no way of predicting the clinical course at the present time.

Routine Care

Children should have a physical examination every 2 to 3 months until about age 5 years, and then three to four times a year depending on severity. A hematologic profile, including a reticulocyte count, should be obtained at each visit. It is important to educate the parents about the possible complications (see Table 1) and how to look for them. They should be encouraged to take the child's temperature, feel for its spleen, and watch for lassitude, dizziness, or evidence of pain; as far as possible, however, the child should lead a normal life and have a normal nutritious diet. Folic acid, 1 mg a day, may be prescribed if there is doubt about the diet, as requirements are increased by the hemolytic anemia.

The spleen is often palpable in small children and may persist in Hb S/C and S/β-thalassemia. Gross splenomegaly is uncommon but may occur in S/β^0thal or S/S with α-thal. If hypersplenism develops, splenectomy is indicated. Some pediatricians would consider splenectomy after one or more acute splenic sequestration crises, especially if emergency medical care is not available close to the child's home. In older S/S children, the spleen becomes fibrotic and is no longer palpable, but it may appear as a faintly calcified shadow on abdominal radiograph and bone scintigraphy.

About 14 percent of S/S children younger than 10 years of age and about 30 percent of teenagers have gallstones, so it is important to remember to inquire about symptoms. Elective cholecystectomy should be considered if symptoms persist. Children improve after surgery, gain weight, and have fewer acute episodes that require attention.

Nocturnal enuresis has been shown to occur much more frequently in children with sickle cell anemia, particularly boys, than it does in normal controls of similar racial or economic background. Management is no different from that of children with Hb A.

Teachers should be aware that the child has sickle cell anemia and may need to leave the classroom frequently to urinate. Home-tutoring teachers should be arranged for children who are out of school through illness so that they do not fall behind. Summer camps for children with sickle cell anemia are an excellent way to encourage an optimistic coping attitude through association with peers with similar health problems.

Pain Control at Home

Small prescriptions for narcotic pain medication may be given for use at home under the parents' control. Usually all that is needed is aspirin or acetaminophen with 15 to 30 mg of codeine every 4 to 6 hours. In older children, however, 2.5 mg of oxycodone (Percodan-demi) may be occasionally necessary. A daily fluid intake of at least 3.5 L (6 pints) should be encouraged.

Pain and swelling of one limb or extremity may be handled on an outpatient basis with nonsteroidal analgesics such as tolmetin, 400 mg every 8 hours, or, in an older child, indomethacin, 25 mg every 8 hours. Although uncommon, the possibility of osteomyelitis, particularly that caused by *salmonellae*, should always be considered, and suitable follow-up visits should be arranged to check for persistent or increased swelling or the onset of fever.

A fever about 38.3°C (101°F), a fall in hemoglobin level or obvious mucosal pallor, acute enlargement of the spleen, abdominal pain or vomiting, or generalized severe pain in the extremities, back, or chest are all indications for immediate hospital admission.

Treatment of Acute Events

Inpatient care differs little from that for any other sick child. Fever above 39°C (102.2°F) calls for blood cultures and intravenous broad-spectrum antibiotics until results are available. Pain is best controlled by morphine sulfate given intravenously in doses of 1.0 to 0.15 mg per kilogram every 3 hours over the first 2 to 3 days. As the condition improves, the dose can be reduced, without changing the interval between doses. Intravenous fluid is essential at 1.5 to 2 times maintenance requirements, given as D5W for the first liter, then D5⅓NS. Small "butterfly" needles should be used for venous access for patients of all ages, and sites should be changed every 2 to 3 days. It is very important to preserve venous access. Potassium and magnesium supplements are given as indicated by the results of laboratory tests. Oxygen is unnecessary unless pulmonary complications give rise to decreased oxygen saturation, as documented by arterial blood gas results. Although severe acidosis should be corrected, routine use of bicarbonate or citrate solutions is contraindicated.

Blood Transfusion

Splenic sequestration is a medical emergency that requires immediate blood transfusion. In aplastic crises (reticulocytes < 1.0 percent) or hemolytic crises (hemoglobin < 5.0 g per deciliter), transfusion is indicated, with the goal of raising the hemoglobin to around 10 g per deciliter. Exchange transfusions should be reserved for patients with severe bilateral pneumonia, severe sepsis, or acute renal failure. Blood transfusions should otherwise be used sparingly and only when severe anemia is likely to lead to further complications. In a patient confined to bed, transfusion is probably unnecessary if the hemoglobin level is above 5.0 g per deciliter, especially if the reticulocyte count is above 10 percent (150,000 absolute count). There is no evidence to show that transfusion aborts or shortens an uncomplicated vaso-occlusive (VOC) crisis.

About 18 percent of frequently transfused patients will develop one or more alloantibodies to red cell antigens by the time they reach adult life unless measures are taken to prevent this. Although somewhat costly, it is important to match the patient for blood groups other than just A,B,O, and D (C,E, and Kell should always be checked) and to provide appropriately matched blood. This will greatly reduce the development of alloantibodies that can cause so much difficulty later on, as well as life-threatening delayed transfusion reactions.

Treatment of Stroke Victims

Stroke is a serious manifestation of sickle cell anemia that usually occurs in children younger than 10 years of age. The most common cause is cerebral infarction, which is due to narrowing of the lumen of the internal carotid arteries and its branches. Rapid evaluation (computed tomography [CT] without contrast may be helpful) and close monitoring of progression of symptoms are necessary. Partial exchange transfusion should be performed as soon as possible and will help prevent progression. The chance of the child having another stroke is fairly high, but stroke can be prevented by a chronic transfusion regimen to keep the level of Hb S below 30 percent. The optimal duration of transfusion therapy is not known, but the risk of recurrence is greatest in the first 3 years after the initial event, so continuation for at least 5 years is the usual practice. It is important to prevent hemosiderosis by employing an iron chelation program using desferoxamine by the subcutaneous route via syringe pump.

Prophylactic Transfusions

Occasionally, a young patient who is having repeated acute episodes requiring frequent medical attention or hospital admission will benefit from a limited chronic transfusion program. This will require two units of washed, packed red cells every 3 to 4 weeks to maintain a hemoglobin level of 9 to 11 g per deciliter and

reduce the proportion of Hb S-containing cells. An initial exchange may be necessary if the starting Hb level is above 8 g per deciliter. The program should be continued for at least 1 year.

THE TEENAGE PATIENT

The early teens are often surprisingly free of symptoms. Healthy exercise and noncompetitive sports should be encouraged as tolerated, but activities that precipitate crises, such as swimming, should be avoided. Independence should be encouraged and parental overprotection avoided. The normal growth spurt is often delayed, as is puberty, but this should not cause anxiety. Height charts may show a gradual fall away from the childhood percentile, sometimes to below the fifth, but a late growth spurt usually places the child back on the original percentile, or a slightly higher one, by age 18 to 20 years. Hormones are contraindicated unless there is another cause for the delayed growth.

Contraception and Pregnancy

This is the time to provide proper counseling for the patient with sickle cell disease regarding the clinical course of the disease. The use of oral contraceptives is not contraindicated in sickle cell disease. Low-estrogen preparations should be used and adjusted as necessary to prevent breakthrough bleeding or amenorrhea, which may occur more frequently in girls with sickle cell anemia.

Teenage pregnancy should be avoided, but maternal mortality is too low to be considered a contraindication to pregnancy and, despite anecdotal reports, most Hb S/C women have an uneventful pregnancy and delivery. Most young women will want to have one or two children and, with modern methods of fetal monitoring and careful prenatal care, they should be able to carry a fetus to maturity. Symptoms may increase during pregnancy, and care of the patient should ideally be shared by the physician and the obstetrician. Blood transfusions should be given only as clinically indicated. Early induction of labor or cesarean section will often be needed to prevent fetal distress.

Priapism

Attacks of priapism in boys and young men can be distressing but should be managed conservatively as far as possible. These attacks are usually self-limiting but may occur frequently. Attacks sometimes respond to nefedipine, 10 mg, in repeated doses. If an acute attack persists for more than 24 hours, surgical procedures should be considered. The most successful is a corpora spongiosum shunt (Winter procedure), which should be carried out by a urologist. The procedure, which can be done under local anesthesia, involves inserting a needle or fine scalpel through the glans into one of the corpora cavernosa and aspirating the viscous blood. After removing the instrument, a communication remains that permits continued drainage of cavernous blood from the penis to the systemic circulation. Subsequent erectile function should not be affected. Blood transfusion has little place in treatment, but it is often tried.

THE ADULT PATIENT

The transition from teenage dependence to adult self-reliance is difficult for the patient with sickle cell anemia, and the frequency of symptoms often increases in early adult life, especially for men. Problems with getting or holding a job, or poor attendance at college due to episodes of illness, need medical and social service support. Hospital bills become a growing anxiety as discontinuance from parents' insurance coverage or other childhood medical support occurs. Medical insurance policies at work may be inadequate. Many patients, however, can go for long periods without acute or severe exacerbation of their sickle cell disease; many patients will live a full life, some S/S patients even reach the sixth or seventh decade.

Routine Care

The frequency of doctors' visits or physical examinations depends very much on the type of sickle cell disease. Patients with Hb S/C or β^+ thal or mild sickle cell anemia may not need to be seen more than once a year. Some S/S patients, however, require pain medication fairly frequently and will need to be seen every 2 to 3 months. At routine visits, it is important to question the patient for possible symptoms that can be caused by complications such as gallstones, osteonecrosis of the hips or shoulder joints, gout, or renal disease. On each occasion, a thorough physical examination should be performed while keeping these complications in mind, and blood should be drawn for a hematologic profile, including a reticulocyte count, and chemistries for liver and kidney function. Some clinical investigations should be ordered on a routine basis (see section on complications).

Pain Control at Home

Only about 40 percent of S/S patients, and fewer S/C or S/β-thal patients, experience pain crises severe enough to require emergency room treatment or hospital admission. Episodes of moderate pain lasting several days are not, however, uncommon. These episodes may involve the joints—mainly the wrists, knees, and ankles—and are best treated with nonsteroidal analgesics. Acetaminophen with 30 to 60 mg of codeine or 7.5 mg of hydrocodone or 100 mg of propoxyphene napsylate, can all be tried. Knee effusions respond well to indomethacin, 25 mg three times daily, and should never be tapped unless a septic arthritis is strongly suspected. Bone pains may also respond to nonsteroidals but fre-

quently require a narcotic preparation such as acetaminophen or aspirin with 5 mg of oxycodone. Oral demerol and more addictive narcotics, such as diamorphine or methadone, are best avoided.

Narcotic Abuse

Prescriptions for narcotics should always be written for small amounts, 25 to 30 tablets at most. If more are required, the patient should return to be further evaluated. Although habituation to narcotics may occur in a few patients, it is wrong to consider all patients who need narcotic pain medicine as addicts. With supporting care and continuity, narcotics can be used constructively. Emotional state and chronic anxiety are also important factors. Antidepressants, such as amitriptyline or nortriptyline, 25 mg three times daily, can be useful in reducing narcotic usage. Interestingly, biofeedback-assisted relaxation methods can reduce the frequency of self-pain dosing at home while not changing the frequency of emergency room visits or hospitalizations.

The Pain Crisis

Contrary to popular belief, pain crises in adults are seldom associated with infection; even severe infections, such as pneumococcal sepsis with high fever, may not precipitate the typical symptoms of the painful crisis. Severe pain is most frequently felt in the spine, the sternum, the ribs, and the long bones of the extremities. It is usually abrupt in onset, intense, and frightening. It is unpredictable and may go away within a few hours or a few days, but frequently it persists and gets worse until it cannot be tolerated. The patient who is used to these attacks will already have taken oral narcotics before seeking medical assistance, and now requires further treatment for pain relief.

The essentials of treatment are intravenous fluid and adequate pain medication (Table 2). When managing these patients, one should allow for tolerance to narcotics, which results in a decrease in the duration of the analgesic effect. Although meperidine is the most popular narcotic, it is not the best. It tends to produce heavy sedation, but the aroused patient still complains of pain. It has a short half-life and is metabolized to an inactive but toxic product, normeperidine, which can cause dysphoria, central nervous system excitation, and seizures. Morphine is a better narcotic. More hospitals are now using patient-controlled analgesic (PCA) pumps. These are ideal for patients with sickle cell disease because their pain often comes in spasms, and with PCA they have more control over its relief. It is important, whatever schedule is used, to gain the patient's confidence and provide efficient pain relief from the outset. As the patient's condition improves, the dosage can be gradually reduced and changed to an oral preparation. In anxious patients, hydroxizine (50 mg three times daily), amitriptyline, or nortriptyline (25 mg three times daily) may be added. If there are joint effusions or swelling over bones, indomethacin (25 mg

Table 2 Treatment of the Adult Patient in
Vaso-occlusive crisis

In the Emergency Room
  Hydration: Intravenous D5W at 200–250 ml/hr for the first
    2 L, then D5¼ NS at 100–150 ml/hr. If patient's condition
    has not improved after 8–12 hr, arrange admission to the
    hospital. If discharged, give 2 days supply of oxycodone,
    5–10 mg q4h.
  Pain Medication: Bupremorphine,* 0.3 mg by slow IV push
    (over 1 min) into IV fluid line. If pain is not relieved in 30
    min, repeat 0.3 mg deep IM injection. Pain will usually be
    relieved for 4–6 hr. If necessary, repeat 0.3 mg IM after 4
    hr. Phenergan, 25 mg IM or IV, prevents nausea and
    vomiting.
  Morphine, 4 mg IM or slow IV push into fluid line. If there is
    no relief in 30 min, add 2–4 mg. Repeat the total dose after
    3 and 6 hr if necessary.
  Meperidine, 75–100 mg IM. If there is no relief in 60 min,
    repeat with 25 mg or add 100 mg to the IV bag to deliver
    over 4 hr. Maximum dose is 200 mg.
  Drugs of the nalorphine type (pentazocine, nalbuphine,
    butorphanol) are best avoided, unless the patient's previous
    drug history is well known, because they can produce
    withdrawal symptoms in patients who have been taking
    opiates chronically.

In the Hospital
  Hydration: Continue D5W, alternating with D½ NS, at 100–150
    ml/hr. Discontinue when the patient is able to drink and eat
    a normal diet.
  Pain Medication: Morphine, 0.1–0.15 mg/kg (4–10 mg) into IV
    line every 2–3 hr†. If using an IV pump set to deliver at a
    fixed rate, the drug can be added to the infusion fluid and
    the dose titrated, e.g., 2.5–5 mg/hr.
  PCA‡: A 1 mg/ml solution of morphine: continuous infusion
    of 0.5–1.5 mg/hr to which the patient can add a bolus of
    0.5–1.5 mg within a preset interval of 5–15 min. Maximum
    dose, 20–30 mg over 4 hr. Adjust the bolus dose and interval
    every 12 hr.
  Aspirin, acetaminophen (650 mg), ibuprofen (600 mg), or
    indomethacin (25 mg) PO q8h enhance analgesic effect.
  Hydroxizine, 50 mg IM or PO, is also effective with little extra
    sedation.
  Phenergan, 25 mg q8h, prevents nausea and vomiting.

---

*For patients who use narcotics regularly, bupremorphine may not be
effective.
†When using the IV route with small doses at frequent intervals, less
drug is needed and unpredictable absorption and peak levels are avoided.
‡Patient–controlled analgesia.

three times daily) is very effective. Although informative,
bone scans do not alter treatment and are usually
unnecessary.

If peripheral venous access has been compromised,
the external jugular vein is preferable to a central line,
which carries the risk of pneumothorax. Some patients
who have frequent hospitalizations and "no veins" will
benefit from insertion of a Port-A-Cath. This can be
placed in the external jugular vein under local anesthesia, and the subcutaneous access port can be placed just
below the clavicle. It will require flushing with heparin/
saline every 4 to 6 weeks.

On admission, hemoglobin and hematocrit levels
may be slightly higher than steady-state levels, only to
fall below these after a few days. When the crisis is over,
the hemoglobin level will return to the steady-state level.
Blood transfusion is rarely required. Fever is unusual in
the first 24 hours or so, but as the crisis worsens, a mild
fever frequently develops without obvious cause and is
accompanied by leukocytosis.

Acute Chest Syndrome

Normal-appearing lungs on initial chest radiograph
may subsequently show typical basal infiltrates as the
crisis worsens. Occasionally, pleurisy is a presenting
symptom, and a lung infiltrate with effusion is present
on admission. Sputum production, however, is often
minimal, and this may help distinguish the sickle cell
lung, which is due to sequestration of sickle cells or
small lung infarcts, from true bacterial or viral pneumonia. Secondary infection may occur, requiring a
broad-spectrum antibiotic. Oxygen should be administered if blood gases show deterioration in arterial Po_2
or oxygen saturation. In the rare case of a deteriorating
patient, exchange transfusion is indicated and may be
life-saving.

COMPLICATIONS

Proliferative Sickle Retinopathy

Patients with Hb S/C of S/β^+ thal or mild sickle cell
anemia are at risk for proliferative retinopathy, even in
their early twenties, and should be referred to a retinal
specialist and be followed at least every 2 years. Ablative
laser therapy or cryotherapy is indicated for grade 3
disease to prevent vitreous hemorrhage and subsequent
retinal detachment. Patients with sickle cell anemia are
at a much lower risk for serious eye complications, but
should ideally get an initial retinal examination and a
follow-up every few years, particularly if they have a
relatively high hematocrit.

Gallstones

Almost 80 percent of S/S patients and 50 percent of
S/C patients will develop gallstones. They consist of
dessicated bilirubin or calcium bilirubinate, and only
about 50 percent will be visible on a plain x-ray film. It
is, therefore, good practice to get a routine ultrasound
examination of the upper abdomen. If gallstones are
present, their significance should be discussed with the
patient.

Vague right upper quadrant pain and discomfort
after meals can be relieved by antispasmodics such as
dicyclomine, 10 mg, or hyoscyamine sulfate, 0.125 mg per
5 ml. By avoiding dietary excesses and restricting
consumption of fried and fatty food, some patients will
remain symptom-free for many years. When symptoms
recur or become chronic, elective cholecystectomy is
advisable, but surgery is not indicated in the asymptomatic patient.

Osteonecrosis of the Femoral Head

Patients should be questioned about hip pain, and the joint should be put through its full range of movement. Pain on internal rotation is an early sign that indicates the need for a radiograph. If the radiograph is reported as normal and pain persists, a bone scan or magnetic resonance imaging (MRI) examination is indicated. New orthopedic techniques are available for the treatment of osteonecrosis at an early stage, thus avoiding, or delaying for many years, the necessity for total hip arthroplasty. Many patients become less symptomatic over time and have a minimal disability despite the appearance of the femoral head on radiograph.

Osteonecrosis of the Humeral Head

As with the head of the femur, this can occur in late teens, or later, and cause persistent shoulder pain. The radiograph may show destruction of the humeral head. Most cases will settle down with nonsteroidal therapy, but, if pain is persistent and narcotics are required on a chronic basis, arthroplasty may be advised.

Leg Ulcers

These rarely occur before the late teens, but continue to occur in patients over 40 years of age and seem to be more common in the more anemic patients. They are essentially infarcts in the subcutaneous fat, with death of overlying dermis, and are most frequently seen on the lateral or medial side of the ankle. They occasionally occur higher up on the shin. The necrotic tissue becomes easily infected, and, like a bed sore, they are difficult to heal.

The first goal of treatment is to eradicate the infection. The foot or leg should be immersed for 30 minutes in a tub of warm water to each gallon of which has been added a tablespoon of salt and one or two tablespoons of hypochlorite solution (household Clorox). This should be done at least twice a day and the ulcer covered with a wad of gauze soaked in the same solution and kept in place with a bandage.

Once the ulcer is clean, healing can begin. If there is a very deep slough, a proteolytic enzyme preparation, such as Elase, may be applied every evening under the dressing. A zinc oxide–impregnated bandage (Unna's boot) should then be applied to cover the ulcer and a generous area above and below. The boot can be cut up one side and removed and replaced every week until healing has occurred. Recently, we have found the preparation Duoderm, from ConvaTec, to be very effective in speeding up healing when applied to a clean ulcer. It is left in place for several days, and a new piece is applied after bathing as described previously.

Elevation of the leg and the avoidance of prolonged standing are essential for a successful outcome. Blood transfusion is unnecessary if the preceding regimen is followed. Topical antibiotics often cause allergic dermatitis and are best avoided.

Renal Insufficiency

Most patients with sickle cell disease have a low urinary specific gravity and an inability to concentrate urine normally on fluid deprivation. The resulting polyuria and nocturia may be a precipitating cause of vaso-occlusive crises if fluid intake is restricted. Proteinuria is a common finding, and about 30 percent of S/S patients have more than a trace. Most of this is probably attributable to papillary necrosis, as it is frequently associated with microscropic hematuria. At routine visits, blood urea nitrogen (BUN) and creatinine levels are usually below the normal ranges for age. A BUN level of 15 mg per deciliter and a creatinine level of 1.5 mg per deciliter are three times the average for sickle cell anemia and may indicate an early progressive renal insufficiency. Mild hyperuricemia is not uncommon. If the level rises to over 10 mg per deciliter, it may be controlled with probenecid, 0.5 mg twice daily. A few patients require allopurinol, 100 to 300 mg per day.

Increasing renal insufficiency, ultimately leading to renal failure, is an important cause of poor health in S/S patients over 40 years, and occasionally in younger subjects. An early feature is worsening anemia with hemoglobin levels below 5.0 g per deciliter. Some patients can tolerate this for long periods of time, but others will need intermittent blood transfusion. This prolonged predialysis phase is a difficult time for these patients. The careful administration of erythropoietin may make a tremendous difference to the quality of life for these people, but there is little experience with it at this time. Vaso-occlusive crises could be precipitated by raising the hematocrit too high. This has been seen to occur in renal transplant patients, but further developments in the therapy of sickle cell disease may help to deal with this problem.

SURGERY AND ANESTHESIA

No single measure can replace good clinical judgment as to whether it is necessary to transfuse a patient prior to surgery. The risk of hypoxia during induction is the same as for a normal patient because sickling does not occur instantaneously. There is no clinical basis for the much advocated formulae that call for a certain level of hemoglobin or reduction of Hb S for safe anesthesia, but there is clear evidence that the lower the whole blood viscosity, the less likely are VOC events. Blood viscosity is largely a function of the hematocrit. Also, anesthetic gases such as halothane, forane, and ethrane have been shown to have antisickling properties, and under anesthesia the patient is getting oxygen and intravenous hydration. Clinical studies have confirmed that anesthesia does not precipitate a "crisis" if it is properly handled.

Patients are transfused preoperatively only if the hemoglobin is below 8.0 g per deciliter, giving two units of packed cells to raise the hemoglobin to about 10.0 g per deciliter. Otherwise, for most surgery, blood loss is simply replaced. Exceptions are cardiothoracic surgery or brain surgery in which hypothermia or extracorporeal procedures will be used. In these cases, exchange transfusion to remove most of the patient's red cells (about 10 percent to 15 percent Hb S in the posttransfusion sample) is advisable. This may require two exchanges with an interval of a few days in between. If possible, the procedure should be carried out using a cell-separating machine, with attention given to maintaining an adequate platelet count.

The difficult decisions involve the Hb S/C and Hb S/β^+ thal patients who have a normal or above-normal hematocrit preoperatively. The S/β^+ thal patient has 10 percent to 35 percent Hb A in every red cell and does not need an exchange transfusion. The Hb S/C patient can be phlebotomized down to a hematocrit of about 35 percent preoperatively, and blood loss simply can be replaced at surgery. This should be satisfactory for prolonged and bloody procedures such as total hip surgery.

When planning exchange transfusions requiring many units of blood, the risks of unexpected incompatibility must be considered. All major blood group antigens should be matched between the patient and the donors. A delayed transfusion reaction in an extensively exchanged patient may be fatal, and becomes a tragedy if the exchange transfusion was not really necessary.

PROGNOSIS

With good regular clinical care, the outlook for patients with sickle cell disease is better now than at any other time, but frequent prolonged VOC, severe hemo-lysis, or renal insufficiency is an indicator of a poor prognosis.

Several experimental approaches are currently being explored that may reduce hemolysis and decrease the frequency of VOC events that cause organ damage. The most promising of these is the use of hydroxyurea to increase the proportion of red cells containing fetal hemoglobin. Hb S polymers cannot form so easily in these cells, so the red cell life span is increased. Anemia is improved, and the frequency of VOC events is decreased. For the severely affected child, bone marrow transplantation from a compatible sibling may be a feasible proposition if advances in posttransplantation management can reduce the mortality. Unfortunately, most patients with sickle cell disease come from a poor socioeconomic background, and finding financial resources for adequate care is perhaps as important as new therapeutic approaches, which will almost certainly be expensive.

SUGGESTED READING

Charache S, Lubin B, Reid CD, eds. Management and therapy of sickle cell disease. US Department of Health and Human Services, NIH Publication No. 89–2117, Revised 1989.

Foley KM. The practical use of narcotic analgesics. Med Clin North Am 1982; 66:1091–1104.

Shapiro BS. The management of pain in sickle cell disease. Pediatr Clin North Am 1989; 36:1029–1045.

White PF. Use of patient-controlled analgesia for management of acute pain. JAMA 1988; 259:243–247.

PRIMARY AND SECONDARY POLYCYTHEMIA

MALCOLM S. TRIMBLE,
MICHAEL C. BRAIN

A relatively constant red cell mass is maintained by the control exercised by erythropoietin (Ep), a glycoprotein hormone produced mainly in the kidney and to a lesser extent in the liver. The production of Ep is regulated through control of Ep gene expression. Expression of the Ep gene is induced by anemia or hypoxia and results in increased Ep synthesis, which stimulates red cell production. The increase in Ep production results from the recruitment of more Ep-producing renal interstitial cells. A heme protein may be the renal oxygen sensor. Following secretion, Ep binds to receptors on the primitive erythroid cells, allowing erythroid differentiation to proceed.

Polycythemia is an excess number of red cells per unit volume of blood. *Absolute* polycythemia is the result of an increase in the red cell mass and is reflected in the elevation of hemoglobin, hematocrit, and red cell count. *Relative* polycythemia is the apparent elevation of the red cell mass by plasma volume depletion. A classification of polycythemia is presented in Table 1.

The absolute polycythemias can be classified as Ep-independent (primary polycythemia and erythemia) or Ep-dependent (secondary polycythemias). In second-

Table 1 Classification of Polycythemia

Absolute Polycythemia

Primary
    Polycythemia vera
    Primary erythrocytosis
Secondary
    Cyanotic congenital heart disease
    Hypoxic pulmonary disease
    Neonatal polycythemia
    High affinity hemoglobin
    High altitude hypoxia
    Autonomous erythropoietin production

Relative Polycythemia

Dehydration
Capillary Leak
Decreased oncotic pressure/third space
Stress
Hypertension
Hypoxia
Pheochromoctyoma

Table 2 Investigations for the Patient with Polycythemia

Test	Rationale
History and physical examination	Evidence of a specific cause
^{51}Cr RBC mass study	Confirm absolute polycythemia
^{125}I Albumin plasma volume	Confirm relative polycythemia
Complete blood count	Thrombocytosis, leukocytosis in PRV
Blood film	Basophilia, eosinophilia, in PRV
Oxygen saturation blood gases	Low in secondary causes
Bone marrow examination	Fibrosis in some PRV
Cytogenetic studies	Rarely abnormal in PRV
Abdominal radiology (CT scan, Ultrasound)	Splenomegaly in PRV Exclude secondary tumors
Carboxy-hemoglobin concentration	High in smokers
P_{50}	Low in abnormal hemoglobins
Leukocyte alkaline phosphatase	High in PRV
Serum erythropoietin concentration	If elevated, suggests secondary causes

ary polycythemias the Ep may be produced either autonomously or as an excessive response to physiologic stimulation. Determination of Ep levels by radioimmunoassay is particularly useful in distinguishing between the primary and secondary polycythemias. Functional assays for Ep can be performed by measurement of the incorporation of radiolabelled iron into the red cell precursors of polycythemic mice.

Red cell mass and plasma volume are determined with ^{51}Cr-labeled red blood cells and ^{125}I-labeled albumin. Acute states of reduced plasma volume are usually obvious, and measurement of red cell mass is not necessary. Investigations for the classification of polycythemia are listed in Table 2 along with the rationale for their use. In absolute polycythemia, the diagnosis of polycythemia rubra vera is made by excluding all secondary causes of polycythemia and documenting splenomegaly. Occasionally, a definitive diagnosis may not be possible if the polycythemia is multifactorial or if there is no secondary cause. The symptoms and adverse effects of polycythemia are caused by an increase in whole blood viscosity.

MANAGEMENT

Viscosity is the measure of resistance to the flow of fluid when it is subjected to a force. In whole blood, red cells are the major determinant of viscosity; thus, viscosity reflects the total number of red blood cells and the deformability of each cell. When the hematocrit rises above 0.50, the increase in viscosity becomes exponential. This results in reduced blood flow particularly in the microcirculation (where shear rates are low) and the appearance of clinical features of hyperviscosity

(Table 3). Many of the features are nonspecific, and although their frequency and relationship to the hematocrit are variable, in severe polycythemia (hematocrit >0.60) symptoms are usually present.

Absolute Polycythemia

Primary Polycythemia

Most primary polycythemia is caused by polycythemia rubra vera, a clonal stem cell disorder. The diagnosis and treatment of this condition is covered in the following chapter. Some patients with an increased red cell mass will not fit the diagnostic criteria of the polycythemia rubra vera study group yet a secondary cause for their erythrocytosis is not evident. The typical features of polycythemia rubra vera usually develop, but in a few patients unexplained, absolute erythrocytosis persists, a form of primary polycythemia that has been termed erythemia.

Erythemia may require treatment to return the hematocrit to normal, and phlebotomy is the treatment of choice for young or middle-aged patients. Phlebotomy avoids the potential long-term risk of leukemia that is associated with some forms of myelosuppressive therapy such as ^{32}P. These long-term risks are of less concern in older patients (> 70 years); therefore, myelosuppressive therapy can be considered. In younger patients whose disease cannot be controlled with phlebotomy alone, hydroxyurea (500 to 1500 mg per day) should be used because this agent has not yet been shown to be leukemogenic. Recombinant interferon alpha has recently demonstrated efficacy in controlling the elevated red cell mass in polycythemia rubra vera when given

Table 3 Signs and Symptoms of Hyperviscosity

Constitutional
  Weakness
  Fatigue
  Exercise intolerance
  Weight loss
Hemostasis
  Bleeding
  Bruising
  Elevated bleeding time
Neurological
  Disturbance of vision
  Papilledema
  Engorged retinal veins; hemorrhage, thrombosis
  Stroke, transient ischemic attack
  Encephalopathy, dementia
Cardiopulmonary
  Heart failure
  Angina, myocardial infarction
  Thromboembolism
  Hypertension
Peripheral vascular
  Erythromelagia
  Arterial occlusion
  Rubor

subcutaneously (3 to 5 $\times$ 10^6 U) three times a week. The presumed absence of any leukemogenic side effects may make interferon a future option for treatment of erythemia.

Secondary Polycythemia

Ectopic Erythropoietin Production

Autonomous production of Ep by a variety of benign and malignant lesions, including renal cysts, renal cell carcinoma, uterine leiomyoma, cerebellar hemangioblastoma, and hepatomas, has been described. In renal cell carcinoma, the presence of Ep mRNA has confirmed that the tumor is a site of ectopic synthesis of Ep. The polycythemia may be incidental or part of the symptom complex that brings the patient to medical attention. Removal of the tumor leads to resolution of the polycythemia. Polycythemia also may be an early indicator of tumor recurrence. Phlebotomy to return the hematocrit to normal preoperatively may reduce operative risk, and if required, the blood can be used for autologous donation. If more rapid reduction of the hematocrit is needed, the phlebotomy can be accompanied by the infusion of an equal volume of isotonic saline.

Post-Renal Transplant Erythrocytosis

Polycythemia occurs in approximately 10 percent of patients undergoing renal transplantation. It has been associated with renal transplant artery stenosis, hypertension, graft rejection, hydronephrosis, diuretic use, and erythropoietin overproduction from residual renal tissue, especially in polycystic disease. A reasonable diagnostic approach is to exclude obstruction and renal artery stenosis with an ultrasound examination and renal flow scan. Decreased plasma volume from diuretics can be managed by altering the antihypertensive therapy. Phlebotomy can be used to treat absolute polycythemia, particularly if the hematocrit is above 0.60. Theophylline was shown to be helpful in reducing the hematocrit by attenuation of Ep production.

High-Altitude Polycythemia

Acute or chronic exposure to high altitude results in a shift in the oxygen dissociation curve and increased erythropoiesis to maintain oxygen delivery. The hematocrit will rise initially as a result of intravascular fluid loss followed by expansion of the red cell mass. In some individuals, alveolar hypoventilation, particularly during sleep, will further worsen the hypoxia and lead to a marked rise in the hematocrit. Venesection is of benefit for severe polycythemia and should be accompanied by the infusion of equal volumes of isotonic saline. Return to a lower altitude is the definitive treatment.

Hypoxic Lung Disease

Chronic hypoxia can lead to progressive pulmonary hypertension as a result of hypoxic pulmonary vasoconstriction and fatal cor pulmonale. The hypoxia also stimulates Ep production, however, the benefit of an elevated hematocrit is uncertain because the improvement in oxygen delivery may be offset by a reduction in cardiac output. Chronic oxygen therapy will reduce the erythropoietic stimulation, and because thromboembolic events may be increased when the hematocrit is above 0.60, phlebotomy can normalize the hematocrit. The concurrent infusion of isotonic saline may avoid a drop in cardiac output during phlebotomy.

Cyanotic Congenital Heart Disease

In adults with cyanotic congenital heart disease, phlebotomy is best reserved for the treatment of symptomatic hyperviscosity, particularly if hematocrit levels exceed 0.65. It can occasionally be difficult to distinguish the symptoms of iron deficiency from those of polycythemia. Symptomatic iron deficiency is more likely if the hematocrit is less than 0.65. Isovolumetric phlebotomy by removal of 500 mL of blood over 45 minutes followed by replacement with isotonic saline avoids a reduction in cardiac output. If the symptoms are caused by hyperviscosity, improvement is evident in 24 hours. The relationship between the hematocrit and thromboembolic events is uncertain; therefore, the role of routine phlebotomy is not clear. Preoperatively the hematocrit should be reduced by the removal of 500 mL of blood and infusion of isotonic saline daily until the hematocrit is less than 0.65. The units can be reserved for intraoperative autologous donation. Phlebotomy may result in improved hemostasis in addition to its beneficial effects on the cardiopulmonary status.

High-Affinity Hemoglobin

Several hemoglobin variants are characterized by a very low P_{50} resulting in diminished oxygen delivery. This may result in polycythemia, although the hematocrit is not usually greater than 0.60. Phlebotomy can be performed for relief of symptoms.

Neonatal Polycythemia

The normal hematocrit at birth is 0.51 to 0.56, which reflects the much larger neonatal red blood cell. Neonatal polycythemia is seen predominantly in two clinical settings. The first is late clamping of the umbilical cord (more than 30 seconds), which can increase the hematocrit by as much as 30 percent owing to the transfusion of placental blood. This form of polycythemia can be prevented by early umbilical cord clamping. Second, conditions associated with placental dysfunction may lead to intrauterine hypoxia and increased fetal erythropoiesis. Newborns who are small for gestational age or infants of diabetic mothers are particularly at risk for polycythemia.

Symptoms of polycythemia in newborns are nonspecific and include lethargy, poor sucking, poor feeding, tachypnea, and cyanosis. These same symptoms are seen with cardiopulmonary disease. A useful diagnostic approach is to perform a heelstick hematocrit 2 to 3 hours after birth in those newborns at risk or who have symptoms that suggest polycythemia. If the heelstick hematocrit is 0.70 or more, a venous hematocrit is obtained at 4 to 6 hours of life. If the venous hematocrit is 0.65 or greater, polycythemia is present. Isovolumetric phlebotomy should be performed in symptomatic newborns using either albumin or plasma replacement. Aliquots of 5 to 10 mL of whole blood are removed via an umbilical vein catheter. The blood volume (85 mL per kg) is multiplied by the ratio of the observed hematocrit minus the desired hematocrit (usually 50%) and is then divided by the observed hematocrit. This will give the exchange volume required. If the symptoms are caused by the polycythemia, improvement should be evident within hours.

Relative Polycythemia

Dehydration

Fluid loss or inadequate intake may elevate the hematocrit. The cause of dehydration is usually evident, and the treatment is volume replacement.

Stress Polycythemia

In 1905, Gaisbock described patients with polycythemia who had features of hypertension, obesity, and psychological stress but who lacked the splenomegaly characteristic of a myeloproliferative disorder. He hypothesized that the elevated hematocrit was a result of hemoconcentration. Today we know that the features described by Gaisbock (as well as smoking, alcohol, and diabetes) can all cause a reduction in the plasma volume. The role of stress in the pathogenesis of the depletion is still uncertain. Primary vascular constriction from increased adrenergic tone can diminish venous capacitance and secondarily deplete the plasma volume. Treatment includes correction of the increased viscosity by volume repletion and possibly phlebotomy and the removal or correction of contributing factors. Hypertension is best treated with vasodilators rather than diuretics.

SUGGESTED READING

Danish EH. Neonatal polycythemia. Prog Hematol 1986; 55–98.
Da Silvia J-L, Lacombe C, Bruneval P, Casadevall N, et al. Tumor cells are the site of erythropoietin synthesis in human renal cancers associated with polycythemia. Blood 1990; 75:577–582.
Isbister JP. The contracted plasma volume syndromes (relative polycythemias) and their hemorrheological significance. Balliere's Clin Hematol 1987; 1:665–693.
Pearson TC. Rheology of the absolute polycythemias. Bailliere's clinical hematology 1987; 1:637–664.
Perloff JK, Rosove MH, Child JS, Wright GB. Adults with cyanotic congenital heart disease: hematologic management. Ann Intern Med 1988; 109:406–413.
Silver RT. A new treatment for polycythemia vera: recombinant interferon alfa. Blood 1990; 76:664–665.
Thorling EB. Paraneoplastic erythrocytosis and inappropriate erythropoietin production. Scand J Hematol 1972; Suppl 17:1–166.

POLYCYTHEMIA RUBRA VERA

ARTHUR I. RADIN, M.D.

Polycythemia rubra vera (PRV) is a low-grade malignancy of the hematopoietic stem cell. The primary manifestation of this disease is an expansion of the red cell mass. However, its identity as a stem cell disorder is expressed in the clinical manifestations and natural history of the disease.

Polycythemia rubra vera progresses through a number of well-recognized clinical phases. It most commonly presents in the proliferative stage, which is characterized by the excessive production of erythrocytes, granulocytes, and platelets. Typically, the onset is insidious, and the elevated hematocrit is discovered as an incidental finding on blood tests drawn for unrelated reasons. Patients with more advanced peripheral blood abnormalities may present with symptoms suggesting impaired circulation to the heart, central nervous system, or extremities. Approximately 30 percent of patients report a hemostatic complication at some time during their course. Pruritus, often made worse by bathing, and splenomegaly are characteristic of this disorder.

An appreciable minority of patients will enter the stable phase, during which essentially normal blood counts are maintained for months or years without specific therapy. Approximately 10 percent of patients will progress to postpolycythemic myeloid metaplasia with myelofibrosis, more commonly referred to as the "spent" phase of the disease. This stage is characterized by extensive marrow fibrosis, hepatosplenomegaly, and peripheral cytopenias, which resemble agnogenic myeloid metaplasia clinically and pathologically. Generally, the spent phase develops from 2 to 13 years after the polycythemia has been manifest; rarely, however, myelofibrosis may precede, or appear coincident with, the erythrocytosis.

DIAGNOSIS

The first obligation of the physician who has assumed responsibility for a patient with "polycythemia" is to determine its cause. Polycythemia rubra vera must be distinguished from relative (or stress) polycythemia, in which the red cell mass is in the normal or high-normal range but the plasma volume is reduced; and from secondary polycythemia, a heterogeneous group of disorders in which the red cell mass has increased in response to factors originating beyond the bone marrow. Polycythemia rubra vera can be differentiated from these other conditions, in most cases, without difficulty, using the diagnostic criteria set forth by the Polycythemia Vera Study Group (PVSG) (Table 1). These

Table 1 Diagnostic Criteria for Polycythemia Rubra Vera of the Polycythemia Vera Study Group

Category A
  A1. Increased red cell volume
       (by ^{51}Cr-labeled red cell determination)
       Men $\geq$ 36 ml/kg
       Women $\geq$ 32 ml/kg
  A2. Arterial oxygen saturation $\geq$ 92%
  A3. Splenomegaly

Category B
  B1. Thrombocytosis: platelets $\geq$ 400,000/mm^3
  B2. Leukocytosis: WBC $\geq$ 12,000/mm^3
       (in the absence of fever or infection)
  B3. Elevated leukocyte alkaline phosphatase score: > 100 (in the absence of fever or infection)
  B4. Serum B$_{12}$ > 900 pg/ml or unbound B$_{12}$-binding capacity >2200 pg/ml

Criteria for Diagnosis:
  PRV is diagnosed when
  1. All three conditions in category A are present (A1 + A2 + A3); or
  2. The combination of an elevated red cell mass and normal oxygen saturation is present, along with any two conditions in category B (A1 + A2 + any two from B).

standards are quite stringent, and may exclude patients with early disease or mild manifestations of the illness. At a minimum, however, the diagnosis of PRV requires confirmation of an elevated red cell mass and evidence of stem cell involvement.

In equivocal cases, a number of laboratory tests may help to establish the diagnosis (Table 2). Cytogenetic analysis may reveal clonal chromosomal abnormalities in approximately one-fifth of cases at presentation—most frequently, complete or partial trisomy of chromosomes 1, 8, or 9, or deletions of the long arm of chromosome 20. Serum erythropoietin levels in PRV should be normal or depressed; elevated erythropoietin levels suggest secondary erythrocytosis. In selected patients, in vitro culture of erythroid progenitors (BFU-E) may be useful. The hematopoietic stem cell in PRV is extremely sensitive to erythropoietin and will grow in culture without the addition of this growth factor, whereas normal erythroid precursors will not. In vitro bone marrow culture techniques are not ordinarily available, however, and this test is rarely necessary for diagnosis.

CONTROL OF THE RED CELL MASS

The principal symptoms of polycythemia vera, and many of its more serious complications, can be related directly to the overproduction of red blood cells. This has three major effects: the total blood volume expands; the red cell mass, and, therefore, the hematocrit, increases beyond safe limits; and the metabolic demands on the patient rise. Because whole blood viscosity increases, approximately, as the third power of the hematocrit, even a small change in the red cell mass can have a significant effect on hemodynamics. Moreover, the greater blood volume in these patients distends their veins and increases the cross-sectional area of their blood vessels. This can result in a reduction in the mean linear rate of blood flow, so that in some vessels, blood may be virtually stagnant. Together, these effects more than offset the potential benefit of the increased hemoglobin in transporting oxygen to the tissues. Circulation is impaired, and the relative oxygen transport capacity of the blood is decreased.

Table 2 Tests Recommended for the Evaluation of an Elevated Hematocrit

Complete blood count with WBC differential and quantitative platelet count
Leukocyte alkaline phosphatase
Serum B$_{12}$ and B$_{12}$ binders
Radionuclide determination of red cell mass and plasma volume
Arterial oxygen saturation (for smokers, obtain carboxyhemoglobin level)
Hemoglobin P$_{50}$ to exclude a high oxygen-affinity hemoglobinopathy
Erythropoietin assay
Imaging of the kidneys—intravenous pyelogram, CT scan, or ultrasonogram
Imaging of the liver, spleen, and brain, as clinically indicated
Bone marrow examination with cytogenetics
Bone marrow colony growth

The most direct way to reduce the red cell mass is simply to remove blood by phlebotomy. In fact, phlebotomy has proven itself to be the safest and most reliable means of treating patients with this disease. Prompt reduction of the hematocrit speedily relieves symptoms and substantially reduces the patient's risk of catastrophic complications. Depending on the urgency of treatment and the ability of the patient to tolerate rapid changes in blood volume, phlebotomies of 1 unit of blood should be performed daily, or two to three times per week, until the hematocrit is within normal range. Traditionally, it has been said that the hematocrit should be maintained below 46 percent. However, vascular complications appear to be more frequent as the hematocrit approaches this limit, and cerebral blood flow may be impaired even at this level. Therefore, it appears prudent to set the hematocrit somewhat lower, nearer to 40 percent.

Advanced age is not a contraindication to this therapy, although, in elderly patients and those with cardiovascular disease, smaller volumes of blood (e.g., 200 to 300 ml) may be removed at each treatment. Some physicians prefer to treat their more fragile patients by infusing fluids in one arm while withdrawing blood from the other, in order to avoid dehydration and rapid hemodynamic changes. In crises, such as in preparation for emergency surgery, intensive phlebotomy with plasma replacement can be life-saving.

Patients managed by phlebotomy will rapidly deplete their iron stores, and red cell production will be impaired. Because iron absorbed from dietary sources will be used almost exclusively to produce red blood cells, patients should be advised to avoid iron supplements or medicines that contain iron. The induced iron deficiency rarely causes clinical symptoms; however, severe iron deficiency can make the red blood cell more rigid and may exacerbate the thrombotic tendency in some patients. Thus, although mild iron deficiency can facilitate the management of the red cell mass and may be desirable, severe iron deficiency should be avoided. Iron supplementation at reduced doses may be considered for those patients who develop symptoms or hematologic signs of severe iron deficiency (e.g., a mean corpuscular hemoglobin less than 22 pg). Vigilant monitoring of the patient is necessary during iron treatment in order to avoid potentially dangerous elevations in the hematocrit.

MYELOSUPPRESSION

Although phlebotomy satisfactorily controls the foremost symptoms of PRV, it does not address the underlying disease process. Myelosuppressive agents, directed against the malignant clone itself, are often required in order to manage the other distressing and potentially life-threatening complications of the illness. First, these agents further suppress erythropoiesis, facilitating the management of the red cell mass. Between 50 percent and 80 percent of patients treated with myelosuppressive agents are relieved of the need for phlebotomy. In addition, myelosuppression has proven effective in checking the hypermetabolic state in most patients, controlling the leukocytosis and thrombocytosis characteristic of this stem cell disorder, shrinking the size of the spleen, and reducing the risk of thromboembolic complications. However, because of the potential risks of these drugs, most notably that of secondary malignancies, myelosuppressive therapy cannot be recommended for all patients. Therapy must be tailored to the individual, balancing the patient's risk of morbidity from the disease against the potential immediate and long-term complications of this form of treatment.

Present recommendations for use of myelosuppressive agents are based principally on the experience of the PVSG. In a landmark multi-institutional study, 431 patients meeting strict criteria for PRV were randomized to treatment by phlebotomy alone, or by phlebotomy plus myelosuppression, using either radioactive phosphorus (^{32}P) or chlorambucil. During the first 5 years of treatment, the mortality rates among the three groups were similar; however, the incidence of nonfatal thrombotic episodes was significantly higher in the group managed by phlebotomy alone. Risk factors for the occurrence of thrombosis included older age, a history of prior thrombotic events, and a greater-than-average requirement for phlebotomy. During the following 10 years, however, the mortality rate of patients treated with myelosuppressive agents exceeded that of the phlebotomy group. The increase in mortality was due primarily to an increased incidence of secondary malignancies, including acute leukemias, lymphoblastic lymphomas, and various carcinomas, particularly those of the skin and gastrointestinal tract. Acute leukemia developed earlier in patients treated with chlorambucil than in patients treated with ^{32}P: the median time to the development of leukemia in these two groups was approximately 5 years and 6 to 10 years, respectively.

Based on these observations, general recommendations for the treatment of PRV have emerged. In patients under age 50 with no history of prior thrombosis, and relatively low phlebotomy requirements, myelosuppressive therapy appears ill-advised. The risk of thromboembolic complications is low in these patients, and their overall survival may be diminished by the development of secondary malignancies. Phlebotomy alone appears to be the most appropriate management. In patients over age 70, the incidence of thrombotic events is considerably greater. Considering the advanced age of these patients and the long interval required for secondary malignancies to evolve, myelosuppression appears justified. In patients between 50 and 70 years of age, the decision to embark on myelosuppressive therapy should be based on an assessment of that individual's symptoms and risk of thrombotic complications.

Chlorambucil is no longer considered to be an appropriate myelosuppressive medicine in PRV because of its inordinate carcinogenic properties. Rather, the myelosuppressive agents most commonly employed in this illness include ^{32}P, busulfan, and hydroxyurea. Recently, hydroxyurea has emerged as the agent of choice owing to its low carcinogenic potential. However, ^{32}P or busulfan may be suitable for patients who fail to achieve adequate disease control with hydroxyurea, who experience untoward effects from this drug, or in whom compliance is doubtful.

Radioactive phosphorus is given intravenously as a bolus at 2.3 to 3.0 mCi per square meter, with no single dose to exceed 5 mCi. Occasionally, additional doses of ^{32}P may be required to achieve optimal disease control. To avoid excessive myelosuppression, these treatments should be repeated no more frequently than every 3 to 6 months. Hematologic improvement is obtained in 75 to 85 percent of cases, with maximum effects evident approximately 10 weeks after therapy. The chief advantage of ^{32}P is its long duration of action: a single treatment may control the disease for 6 to 24 months. Thus, patient compliance is not an issue. Untoward effects of ^{32}P include unpredictable degrees of myelosuppression, subtle alterations in immune function, and secondary leukemias.

Busulfan is an alkanesulfonate ester with pharmacologic properties distinct from the "classic" alkylating agents such as chlorambucil and the other nitrogen mustards. Usually, it is administered at 4 to 6 mg daily for 4 to 6 weeks, or until the platelet count is below 300,000 per cubic millimeter. Remissions may be obtained with this regimen in approximately 50 percent of cases. In a European cooperative group study comparing busulfan to ^{32}P as a supplement to phlebotomy, busulfan induced longer remissions and resulted in a longer median survival than ^{32}P. The leukemogenic potential of the two agents was similar. However, the potential for cumulative, irreversible myelosuppression, and a variety of nonhematologic toxicities, including pulmonary fibrosis, an Addisonian-like syndrome of asthenia, and cutaneous hyperpigmentation undermine the attractiveness of this agent.

Hydroxyurea is an inhibitor of ribonucleotide reductase, an enzyme required for the synthesis of deoxyribonucleotides and, ultimately, of DNA. Because it does not interact with DNA directly, its mutagenic potential is considerably less than that of the alkylating agents. At doses of 15 to 30 mg per kilogram daily, approximately 70 to 80 percent of patients will achieve long-term control of their disease. The chief shortcoming of this drug is its relatively brief duration of action, which may cause peripheral blood counts to be erratic. Also, it appears to affect the production of white blood cells to a relatively greater degree than red blood cells. Therefore, mild leukopenia may be unavoidable, and supplemental phlebotomies may be required. Other untoward effects include gastrointestinal discomfort, fevers, rash, stomatitis, hepatitis, and, possibly, renal dysfunction. Experience with this drug in PRV is relatively limited, and additional long-term studies will be necessary in order to determine its appropriate role in therapy.

HEMOSTATIC COMPLICATIONS

Hemorrhagic and thrombotic events are the leading cause of morbidity in this disease, and are reported as the cause of death in 20 percent to 40 percent of patients. The prevention of hemostatic complications is the most appropriate therapeutic strategy. Fortunately, this goal can be achieved, in most cases, with proper management. Control of the red cell mass is of primary importance, using phlebotomy or myelosuppression as suitable. In one study, the rate of thrombotic episodes was more than 10 times greater for patients with hematocrits greater than 60 percent than for patients with hematocrits maintained between 40 percent and 44 percent.

Unfortunately, the published studies were not designed to examine the contribution of thrombocytosis or platelet dysfunction to the hemostatic diathesis, and the impact of these factors on the incidence of thrombotic events remains controversial. Neither in vitro tests of platelet function nor the bleeding time has correlated with the risk of hemostatic complications, and neither has been of value in directing therapy. For these reasons, a comprehensive evaluation of the patient's platelet function cannot be recommended in asymptomatic patients; nor should modest elevations in the platelet count cause undue concern. It is reasonable, however, to consider severe thrombocytosis (greater than 1,000,000 per cubic millimeter) as another possible risk factor for thrombotic events when considering the institution of myelosuppressive therapy.

Antiplatelet therapy should not be recommended for antithrombotic prophylaxis, regardless of the patient's platelet count. In a PVSG study, aspirin at 300 mg three times daily and dipyridamole at 75 mg three times daily as a supplement to phlebotomy failed to reduce the incidence of thrombosis. However, the incidence of significant gastrointestinal hemorrhages increased significantly. Antiplatelet therapy may be appropriate as short-term treatment for patients who have suffered recent microvascular occlusive episodes. However, myelosuppressive therapy, as described previously, remains the best therapeutic option for the prevention of thrombohemorrhagic complications.

Hemostatic complications that do arise should be treated in the usual manner, with particular attention to the correction of any pre-existing coagulation disorders. Acquired abnormalities in von Willebrand factor (vWF) and deficiencies of clotting factors V and XII are common in PRV, and should be considered in the patient's evaluation. Low-grade disseminated intravascular coagulation (DIC) should also be excluded. Infusions of DDAVP or plasma fractions may be of benefit. Platelet transfusions also may be justified, even in the face of a normal or elevated platelet count, because the patient's own platelets are frequently dysfunctional. Acute thrombotic episodes can be treated with heparin, followed by warfarin anticoagulation. Patients with severe thrombocytosis may appear relatively resistant to heparin anticoagulation, however, owing to the antiheparin effect of platelets.

Recent advances in our understanding of PRV may improve our ability to prevent and manage these hemostatic complications. It has been reported that patients with the greatest reduction in platelet serotonin content exhibit the greatest prolongation in their bleeding times following a test dose of aspirin. These patients may be at the greatest risk of complications should antiplatelet therapy be initiated. Similarly, it has been reported that individuals with PRV who additionally have abnormalities of vWF, particularly deficiencies of the high molecular weight multimers, are at an increased risk of hemorrhage. In one study, fully 75 percent of patients with vWF abnormalities reported a bleeding tendency. As our ability to determine which patients are at the greatest risk of hemorrhage or thrombosis improves, therapy can be fashioned more appropriately to the individual.

PRURITUS

Pruritus is one of the more common, and troublesome, symptoms of PRV, affecting 14 percent to 52 percent of patients in different reports. Too commonly, this symptom is dismissed by the physician as unimportant, for it has little impact on the prognosis or clinical course of the disease. To the afflicted patient, however, it is one of the more distressing, and even disabling, aspects of the illness.

Pruritus in these patients appears to be multifactorial in origin, and no single therapeutic approach has proved uniformly successful. Two-thirds of patients with uncontrolled PRV have elevated plasma or urine histamine levels, suggesting an etiologic role for this factor. Serotonin and prostaglandins released by the neoplastic platelets may also mediate the itch. Customarily, the first agents employed are antihistamines, because these are relatively free of side effects. In most cases, treatment is started with an H_1 blocker, such as diphenhydramine hydrochloride or hydroxyzine. H_1 blockade alone, however, is ineffective in the majority of patients, and the addition of an H_2 blocker such as cimetidine may improve the response. Combined histamine and serotonin blockade using doxepin hydrochloride, trifluoperazine hydrochloride, and cyproheptadine also has been used with success. Aspirin, although frequently effective, cannot be recommended because of the associated risk of life-threatening hemorrhagic complications.

If these measures fail, iron supplementation may be considered. The pathogenesis of pruritus in iron deficiency is unknown, but the association is well documented, even in otherwise normal individuals with iron-deficiency anemia. Iron supplements invariably accelerate erythropoiesis, however, and the patient must be monitored closely to prevent a rapid and unacceptable rise in hematocrit. Once the pruritus is controlled, the dose of iron should be reduced as much as possible to limit erythropoiesis.

Anecdotal reports in the literature suggest that ultraviolet light, photochemotherapy using psoralens combined with ultraviolet A light (PUVA therapy), and cholestyramine may benefit some patients. These therapies have not been studied sufficiently to predict their response rates. When all else fails, myelosuppression

may be considered. However, myelosuppression is not reliably effective, and most physicians do not consider pruritus alone sufficient reason to embark on this treatment.

MANAGEMENT OF THE SPENT PHASE

Treatment during the spent phase is largely supportive. As is standard in the management of bone marrow failure of any etiology, an attempt should be made to correct any reversible causes of pancytopenia. Deficiencies of iron, folic acid, or vitamin B_{12} should be considered and corrected if present. If these measures are ineffective, it is reasonable to try to stimulate hematopoiesis with androgens. Oxymetholone, fluoxymesterone, and nandrolone decanoate are the most commonly used preparations. Overall, androgens are modestly effective in 50 percent of cases. In some patients, red cell survival may be improved and the anemia ameliorated by glucocorticoids. Unfortunately, red cell survival studies have not proved useful in predicting which patients will respond to steroids, and a therapeutic trial of prednisone may be necessary. As hematopoiesis fails, blood transfusions may be required. The median survival of patients in the spent phase is approximately 2 years, and the long-term consequences of transfusions, such as hemochromatosis, are rarely of concern.

Massive splenomegaly may cause discomfort for the patient and exacerbate the peripheral cytopenias. Moreover, massive splenomegaly has been associated with a significant increase in portal blood flow, resulting in portal hypertension and esophageal varices. During the proliferative phase of the illness, splenomegaly usually can be controlled with myelosuppressive agents. However, these medicines are relatively contraindicated during the spent phase, as hematopoiesis already is compromised and further myelosuppression may produce dangerous cytopenias. Radiotherapy will provide relief of splenic pain in the majority of patients. However, the benefits of radiation generally last for only 3 to 4 months.

Splenectomy may improve the quality of life in patients who do not respond to more conservative management. It is virtually 100 percent effective in alleviating the mechanical discomfort associated with a large abdominal mass and in relieving the pain associated with recurrent splenic infarctions. Its success in treating hypersplenism, refractory thrombocytopenia, and portal hypertension ranges from 30 percent to 80 percent in different series. Hematologic improvements following splenectomy may persist for 2 to 70 months, with a median improvement of 10 months. Although splenectomy may palliate symptoms, it is a formidable undertaking in this debilitated group of patients. In several single institution reviews published since 1977, the immediate postoperative mortality has ranged from 0 percent to 18 percent, and postoperative morbidity, primarily hemorrhage and infection, was reported in 35 percent to 75 percent of patients. Because splenectomy has not been shown to affect survival, it should be considered with extreme caution for symptomatic patients who do not respond to more conservative treatment.

Foci of extramedullary hematopoiesis may arise in organs other than the spleen. Most commonly, the liver and lymph nodes are affected, but myeloid metaplasia also may develop in the lungs, kidneys, gastrointestinal tract, peritoneum, or central nervous system. Masses of hematopoietic tissue may compromise the function of these organs, simulating abscesses, disseminated carcinoma, or thrombotic events. Extramedullary hematopoiesis within the meninges has presented as increased intracranial pressure, hemiparesis, and spinal cord compression, whereas peritoneal involvement has caused ascites. It is important to recognize the nature of these lesions because radiotherapy or surgical decompression is highly effective in alleviating symptoms.

TREATMENT OF ASSOCIATED CONDITIONS

Hypermetabolism

Hypermetabolic manifestations are common during the proliferative phase of the illness, and include fevers, heat intolerance, or hyperuricemia. Some patients may present with renal colic or hematuria caused by uric acid concretions within the urinary tract or with acute gouty arthritis. Once infection has been excluded, fevers or heat intolerance may be treated effectively with myelosuppression. Acute gouty arthritis is managed, as in primary gout, with colchicine, nonsteroidal anti-inflammatory drugs, or glucocorticoids. To prevent recurrences, the patient should be started on allopurinol. Although myelosuppression will also reduce the incidence of gout, allopurinol is safer and generally is sufficient. Because acute gout occurs in only 10 percent of patients, the use of allopurinol for asymptomatic patients with hyperuricemia is debatable.

Erythromelalgia

Erythromelalgia is a rare complication of PRV characterized by intense burning pain, erythema, and elevated skin temperature in a localized, acral distribution. These attacks may last from minutes to days, although between attacks, the extremity seems entirely normal. This syndrome appears to be caused by platelet-mediated vascular injury, but alterations in the innervation of the skin have been implicated as well. As may be expected for a disease of the vasculature, complications of erythromelalgia include osteoporosis of the affected extremity, nonhealing skin ulcers, gangrene, and multiple cerebral infarctions. Erythromelalgia is generally treated with antiplatelet agents, particularly those that inhibit cyclo-oxygenase (aspirin, indomethacin), and with cytotoxic drugs to lower the platelet count. Phlebotomy alone has been effective in some cases of erythromelalgia secondary to PRV. Other therapeutic modalities that have been used, with varying success, include vasodilators (nitroprusside, propranolol), surgical sympathectomy, and biofeedback.

Leukemic Transformation

Acute leukemia evolves in 2 percent to 15 percent of patients with PRV, generally arising 8 years or more after the onset of the primary disease. These leukemias are almost always nonlymphocytic, but occasional cases of acute lymphocytic or biphenotypic leukemia are reported. The treatments that have been tried are similar to those used in de novo cases, and generally include cytosine arabinoside, daunomycin, and a third agent, such as 6-thioguanine, etoposide, or amsacrine. Treatment usually is ineffective, however, and survival is short. In elderly patients, it may be appropriate to provide palliative and supportive care only, rather than embarking on aggressive chemotherapy. However, this decision must be made on an individual basis.

INVASIVE PROCEDURES

Invasive procedures, including surgery and angiography, are dangerous in uncontrolled polycythemia, primarily because of the greatly increased risk of hemorrhagic and thrombotic complications. In an analysis of 81 major operations in patients with PRV, the perioperative mortality was seven times higher in patients with uncontrolled polycythemia (hematocrits greater than 52 percent) than in those with controlled disease. Interestingly, the duration of disease control prior to surgery affected the incidence of both fatal and nonfatal complications. There were no deaths, and a morbidity rate of only 5 percent, in patients with a normal hemoglobin value for 4 months or longer before their operation. However, the mortality and morbidity rates were 15 percent and 42 percent, respectively, for patients whose hemoglobin was normal for less than 1 week prior to surgery. Therefore, elective procedures should be postponed until the blood count has been controlled for several months. When immediate intervention is necessary, intensive isovolemic phlebotomy prior to the procedure may reduce the risk.

FUTURE DIRECTIONS

Antiplatelet Agents

Anagrelide is a new imidazo-quinazolin compound that is under investigation as an antiplatelet agent. At low doses, the drug has been shown to produce thrombocytopenia in humans. At higher concentrations, it also demonstrates potent antiaggregating activity. Anagrelide has been tested in 20 patients with chronic myeloproliferative disorders and thrombocytosis greater than 800,000 per cubic millimeter; 18 of these 20 patients responded, with a decrease in their platelet counts to normal levels within 12 days. Side effects included nausea, headache, and mild hypotension. Importantly, anagrelide is not a general myelosuppressive agent. No significant effect was noted on the leukocyte count or hemoglobin level, nor on the in vitro growth characteristics of the neoplastic clone. The carcinogenic potential of the drug remains unknown, but it lacked mutagenicity in preclinical tests.

Ticlopidine is another antiplatelet agent presently being evaluated in clinical trials. This drug is believed to act during megakaryopoiesis to alter the platelet membrane, thereby reducing platelet reactivity. In initial studies, ticlopidine proved superior to aspirin in preventing recurrent strokes and myocardial infarctions, but its efficacy in the chronic myeloproliferative disorders is still untested. Side effects of ticlopidine include reversible neutropenia and gastrointestinal distress.

These drugs may prove to be important additions to our therapeutic armamentarium, enabling us to reduce the incidence of hemostatic complications without the leukemogenic risk associated with ionizing radiation or alkylating agents.

Biologic Response Modifiers

The most promising of the biologic response modifiers in the treatment of PRV is interferon-alpha$_2$. In a recent report, interferon-alpha$_2$ was administered subcutaneously, three times a week, to three patients with PRV in the proliferative phase of the illness. All three achieved good disease control, with reduced phlebotomy requirements and decreased spleen size. In a second study, the ability of interferon to achieve long-term control of thrombocytosis was evaluated in 31 patients with chronic myeloproliferative disorders. Complete responses, defined as a platelet count of 440,000 per cubic millimeter or less for at least 4 consecutive weeks, were achieved in 71 percent of patients, and the number of disease associated symptoms, including venous and arterial thromboses, were diminished in almost all cases. Most encouraging, these responses also included improved erythropoiesis, control of leukocytosis, and improvement in bone marrow histology. The basis for this activity is uncertain, although a general antiproliferative effect, the induction of differentiation, and potentiation of the host's immune surveillance system have been implicated. Side effects were those typical of interferon therapy, including a flulike syndrome, fevers, weight loss, myalgias, alopecia, and gastrointestinal upset. Larger, prospective studies are in progress to confirm these results and to determine the proper role of interferon-alpha$_2$ in the treatment of this disease.

SUGGESTED READING

Berk PD, Goldberg JD, Donovan PB, et al. Therapeutic recommendations in polycythemia vera based on polycythemia vera study group protocols. Semin Hematol 1986; 23:132–143.

Brenner B, Nagler A, Tatarsky I, et al. Splenectomy in agnogenic myeloid metaplasia and postpolycythemic myeloid metaplasia: A study of 34 cases. Arch Intern Med 1988; 148:2501–2505.

Gisslinger H, Ludwig H, Linkesch W, et al. Long-term interferon therapy for thrombocytosis in myeloproliferative diseases. Lancet 1989; 1(8639):634–637.

Hocking WG, Golde DW. Polycythemia: Evaluation and management. Blood Rev 1989; 3:59–65.

Lofvenberg W, Wahlin A. Management of polycythemia vera, essential thrombocythaemia and myelofibrosis with hydroxyurea. Eur J Haematol 1988; 41:375–381.

Silverstein MN, Petitt RM, Soldberg LA, et al. Anagrelide: A new drug for treating thrombocytosis. N Engl J Med 1988; 318:1292–1294.

CHRONIC MYELOGENOUS LEUKEMIA

KYRAN BULGER, M.D.,
RONALD P. MCCAFFREY, M.D.

Chronic myelogenous leukemia (CML) is characterized, in its initial presentation as stable phase disease, by a ten- to greater than a hundred-fold increase in the leukocyte mass and splenomegaly. Leukocytosis, with a spectrum of immature myeloid forms, eosinophils, and basophils, together with mild anemia and thrombocytosis are characteristic presenting findings. The differential diagnosis at this point usually poses little difficulty. In 90 to 95 percent of patients with CML, the characteristic cytogenetic marker, the Philadelphia (Ph[1]) chromosome, will be identified in hematopoietic cells, a finding that can be helpful in resolving rare diagnostically ambiguous cases. Clinical symptoms during the stable phase may be absent, or limited to nonspecific complaints of a hypermetabolic state, or to symptomatic splenomegaly. About 30 percent of patients are asymptomatic at diagnosis and are discovered to have CML during routine blood studies performed for unrelated reasons.

Over a variable period of time, the stable phase of CML evolves to an acute leukemic phase. The time to evolution of the acute leukemic phase (blast crisis) can be as short as several weeks to as long as two decades; the median time to blast crisis is 3.5 years. Blast crisis is assumed to have supervened when the blast cell percentage, in either bone marrow or peripheral blood, exceeds 25 percent. As this crisis approaches, there is progressive splenomegaly, anemia, thrombocytopenia, and general overall clinical deterioration. Signs suggestive of a transition from the stable phase to the acute leukemic phase include increasing basophilia and eosinophilia, worsening anemia, and the development of additional cytogenetic abnormalities, particularly a second Ph[1] chromosome. By multimarker analyses the blast cells, although usually myeloid, can be lymphoid (30 percent of cases) or, less frequently, erythroid, megakaryocytoid, or of mixed lineage. The factors regulating this phenotypic variation in blast crisis are presently obscure. As noted later, it may be important to select lymphoid-specific therapy for those patients whose blast phase is characterized by cells with lymphoblastic markers.

Overall, the appropriate effective management of CML in the 1990s remains problematic. Bone marrow transplantation is at present the only curative therapy, and should be considered in all patients with newly diagnosed cases of CML. However, bone marrow transplantation is a treatment option appropriate for only a minority of patients with CML. One is thus left, for the majority of patients, with treatment options that can control only disease symptoms or delay the pace of disease progression, but cannot effect a cure.

THERAPY

Stable Phase Disease

White blood cell counts in the range of 50,000 to 100,000 cells per mm^3, platelet counts above 500,000 cells per mm^3, or the development of symptoms are usually considered indications for the commencement of treatment. Initial therapy usually consists of single-agent chemotherapy, either busulfan or hydroxyurea, given orally. Although such therapy is not curative, it delays the time to disease progression and achieves good symptomatic disease control during the chronic phase. The mean survival of treated patients is currently 40 months as compared to 19 months for untreated patients. Specific directions on the use of these single agents are presented. The role for splenic irradiation, splenectomy, leukapheresis, and intensive combination chemotherapy is reviewed. Interferon therapy and bone marrow transplantation are discussed separately.

Busulfan

Busulfan (Myleran) is traditionally the therapy of first choice for chronic phase CML. It is relatively inexpensive, has a 98 percent response rate, and can produce long remissions as defined by control of leukostasis, thrombocytosis, and reduction in symptomatic complaints. The usual starting dose is 3 mg per m^2 given once daily before breakfast. Doses of more than 8 mg per day are rarely required, and the need for progressive dose incrementation implies disease progression. Blood counts are checked weekly; the dose is reduced when the white cell count begins to decline, and therapy discontinued when the count falls to 20,000 cells per mm^3. When the white cell count begins to rise again, a lower maintenance dose is employed for several additional weeks. Once the cell concentration is stabilized, therapy can often be discontinued for a variable period, usually 6 to 12 months. A decrease in the white cell count can be expected between 10 to 14 days, and the platelet response follows within 2 to 6 weeks. Resolution of organomegaly, however, takes several months.

The main toxicity of busulfan is prolonged and sometimes fatal marrow aplasia when it is given in excess. Busulfan acts at the level of the stem cell, so it has a delayed effect on the peripheral white cell count. It is therefore essential not to continue busulfan when the white cell count falls below 20,000 cells per mm^3. Rarely after busulfan-induced pancytopenia, selective erythroid hypoplasia can persist despite return of the white cell and platelet count to normal. Affected patients can benefit from androgenic steroids.

With prolonged use, busulfan can produce pulmonary fibrosis, which is clinically evident in 1 percent of patients and significantly increases the incidence of interstitial pneumonitis after bone marrow transplantation. Other side effects include skin pigmentation, hypogonadism, cataract formation, and a wasting syndrome clinically resembling Addison's disease.

Hydroxyurea

Hydroxyurea (Hydrea) is now considered the drug of first choice for stable phase CML by most practitioners. It has a rapid (less than 24 hours) effect on reducing the white cell count, and, as compared to busulfan, is relatively platelet sparing. It does not produce prolonged bone marrow suppression and even when given in excess, bone marrow recovery is rapid. It should be used in preference to busulfan in all patients for whom bone marrow transplantation is considered, because the incidence of interstitial pneumonitis is increased after bone marrow transplantation if there has been prior exposure to busulfan. Disadvantages of hydroxyurea include a relatively higher cost and the need for continuous therapy with frequent monitoring of the blood count. The initial dose is usually 1 g bid orally. The blood count is checked weekly and the dose adjusted to maintain a white cell count of 10,000 to 20,000 cells per mm^3. Once stabilized, the blood counts can be monitored monthly, and an average dose of 1 to 1.5 g per day is given continuously. Relative drug resistance can be seen during the stable chronic phase but more commonly the need for dose incrementation indicates disease progression. Side effects are uncommon and usually occur when the daily dose exceeds 2 g per day. Nausea and stomatitis, especially of the tongue, can occur. Skin rashes, hyperkeratosis, and impaired liver function are less common. Megaloblastic erythropoiesis is noted in most patients, but significant anemia is not a limiting toxic effect.

Other Single-Agent Chemotherapeutic Regimens

Melphalan, uracil mustard, mercaptopurine, thioguanine, thiotepa, chlorambucil, and cyclophosphamide are all active in chronic phase CML, but none shows a clear advantage over busulfan or hydroxyurea. Only melphalan is equal to busulfan in its ability to establish and maintain disease control, and prolonged bone marrow aplasia occurs less commonly with this drug than with busulfan. Mercaptopurine is relatively platelet sparing and is useful in conjunction with hydroxyurea in the terminal phases of the disease when busulfan therapy is associated with severe thrombocytopenia.

Splenic Irradiation

Before the advent of busulfan chemotherapy in the 1950s, splenic irradiation was the standard therapy for chronic phase CML. When given as 15 Gy over 2 to 6 weeks, it produced good disease control for several months, after which time therapy could be repeated. When compared with busulfan chemotherapy, however, treatment is considerably more inconvenient and expensive. Prolonged periods of marrow aplasia can occur after radiation. In one randomized control trial of splenic irradiation against busulfan, irradiated patients had a significantly shorter survival. Splenic irradiation is now reserved for CML therapy during pregnancy, where the deleterious effects of chemotherapy on the fetus are to be avoided, and in those patients with refractory hypersplenism in whom splenectomy is contraindicated.

Splenectomy

Despite occasional reports of blastic CML transformation arising in the spleen and conjecture on the growth promoting effects of the splenic derived factors on the malignant clone, splenectomy has not been shown to improve response to therapy or to prolong patient survival. Its use should be restricted to those cases of refractory cytopenias secondary to hypersplenism. However, in the terminal phases of CML, when massive splenomegaly and hypersplenism are most common, splenectomy is associated with inordinate morbidity and mortality rates, and splenic irradiation is usually the preferred management. However, it is well appreciated that patients who present with massive splenomegaly frequently suffer severe morbidity from splenomegaly in the terminal phase. A case may be made for elective splenectomy during the stable chronic phase in such patients.

Leukapheresis

Leukostasis is unusual in chronic phase CML because the mature myeloid cells are readily deformable and do not significantly contribute to blood viscosity. When the white cell count exceeds 300,000 cells per mm^3 or at lower counts with a high blast count, leukostasis can occur. Prompt institution of leukapheresis with concomitant chemotherapy (hydroxyurea, 1 g every 4 hours) usually results in symptom resolution. Vigorous hydration, and allopurinol, 600 to 800 mg daily are necessary to avoid the complications of a tumor lysis syndrome. Hydroxyurea chemotherapy alone also is effective, albeit

with several hours' delay, and can be used in settings where leukapheresis is not available.

Intensive Combination Chemotherapy

Several intensive chemotherapy regimens have been investigated in stable phase CML, including cytosine arabinoside and 6-thioguanine with or without daunorubucin or L-asparaginase; cytosine arabinoside, vincristine, and prednisone with or without rubidazone or cyclophosphamide; cytosine arabinoside, 6-thioguanine, vincristine, and doxorubicin. Despite achieving a small percentage of cytogenetic complete remissions, these regimens have not yet been shown to result in significantly prolonged survival. Currently they represent no advantage over single-agent chemotherapy, which can achieve similar disease control with much less morbidity. Their use, therefore, cannot be recommended outside the setting of an investigative study.

Therapy During the Accelerated and Blast Phase

Disease control becomes increasingly difficult as CML evolves into an accelerated and blast phase. If the patient is eligible for bone marrow transplantation, it should be carried out as soon as possible, although ideally this should have been performed during the chronic phase. At this late stage of disease, busulfan often cannot be given without producing unacceptable cytopenias, and hydroxyurea often with mercaptopurine or thioguanine is usually the preferred management. Supportive therapy with blood products is frequently required. Indomethacin and steroids can help alleviate the hypermetabolic symptoms of night sweats and fever.

When CML has progressed to blast crisis, phenotypic analysis of the blast cells is important to identify the 30 percent of patients with lymphoid blast crisis. Such patients have an initial response rate of 80 percent with the nontoxic regimen of vincristine and prednisone. Maintenance therapy in such responders with an anti-ALL maintenance regimen (see the chapter, *Acute Leukemia*) may achieve prolonged disease control. The prognosis for patients with nonlymphoid blast crisis is currently extremely dismal. Only 30 percent of patients show a transient response to standard aggressive ANLL induction chemotherapy, and survival, with or without therapy, is usually less than 5 months.

Therapy with Interferons

There are now several reports, encompassing several hundred patients, on the use of interferon alpha in stable phase CML. Overall, a complete hematologic response is achieved in 50 to 80 percent of patients, and 15 to 25 percent of patients become cytogenetically negative for the Ph^1 chromosome. It should be emphasized that in very late stage disease (the accelerated or preblast crisis stage) interferon alpha as a single agent has markedly diminished activity. Both interferons, but especially interferon gamma, have been shown to be effective in refractory thrombocytosis associated with chronic phase CML. Studies with the recombinant gamma interferon documented its definite but lower activity compared with alpha interferon.

The effectiveness of interferon alpha has been shown to be dose dependent, with the best response seen at 5 million units per m^2 per day given continuously either subcutaneously or intramuscularly. The dose is adjusted to maintain a white cell count of 3000 to 4000 cells per mm^3. Therapy is usually undertaken for at least 1 year. The response is delayed and return of the bone marrow to normal occurs in approximately 9 months. At these high doses of interferon the majority of patients experience an influenza-like syndrome. This can be diminished by slow dose incrementation and addition of acetaminophen. The flu-like illness usually resolves within 6 to 8 weeks. However, severe anorexia and lassitude can persist. Other side effects include impaired liver function, pancytopenia, and neurotoxicity manifested by a frontal lobe-type syndrome.

The achievement of cytogenetic remissions with interferon in CML holds the promise that this therapy will result in prolonged freedom from disease progression and improved survival. The clinical studies are not yet mature enough to allow this conclusion to be drawn. Therapy with the interferons is considerably more toxic and difficult to administer than the current standard single-agent chemotherapy; therefore, their use should be reserved for patients with refractory thrombocytosis and for participants in clinical trials until their value is fully established by these trials.

Bone Marrow Transplantation

Bone marrow transplantation using normal donor marrow is the only known curative therapy for CML. Unfortunately, bone marrow transplantation is applicable to only a minority of patients with CML. Determinants of eligibility for transplant include age and the presence of a suitably matched donor. Patients older than 45 to 50 years have an unacceptably high mortality rate from graft versus host disease (GVHD) and conditioning chemotherapy. Approximately 40 percent of otherwise eligible CML patients have a suitably matched sibling donor. It has been demonstrated recently that unrelated donor and partially matched sibling donor bone marrow transplantation can be used successfully in the treatment of CML. Optimal donor/recipient matching criteria have yet to be determined but it seems clear that more than one site of mismatch at the HLA-DR locus is associated with prohibitive GVHD and graft rejection. The procurement of suitably matched unrelated donors has been improved by the development of a national and international bone marrow donor registry.

Transplantation should be performed in the chronic phase of disease. When results of transplants performed in chronic, accelerated, and blast crisis disease phases are compared, estimates of 5-year survival are 0 to 10 percent for blast crisis, 15 to 30 percent for accelerated phase, and 55 to 65 percent for chronic phase patients. Advanced age is a recipient characteristic also associated with poor outcome; there is a significant decrease in survival for recipients older than 30 years of age. The International Bone Marrow Transplant Registry data suggest that survival is decreased for chronic phase patients over 20 years compared with younger recipients. Concerns that splenomegaly may hinder engraftment and harbor sites of advanced or refractory disease have not been justified. Although time to bone marrow engraftment is shorter in splenectomized individuals, splenectomy is not indicated in anticipation of bone marrow transplantation.

Some controversy exists over the timing of bone marrow transplant for stable phase CML. Many CML patients enjoy several years of good health and easily controlled disease, whereas transplant recipients experience a 20 to 25 percent peritransplant mortality. It is impossible to predict accurately the time of disease progression for an individual patient. It is clear that delay of transplantation beyond the chronic phase of CML has dramatic effects on the outcome. In addition, it has been recently reported that chronic phase recipients transplanted within 1 year of diagnosis have significantly better survival (> 70 percent) than recipients transplanted at a longer interval from diagnosis. It seems reasonable, therefore, to recommend early transplantation, i.e., within 1 year of diagnosis, for all eligible patients.

Autologous bone marrow transplantation using bone marrow cryopreserved during the chronic phase has, with few exceptions, been unsuccessful. For the future, innovative approaches for the use of autologous bone marrow transplantation in CML, may include the use of patient bone marrow cells harvested after conversion to a Ph^1-negative state by in vivo interferon therapy. It is also possible that bone marrow grown in long-term liquid culture or treated ex vivo with chemotherapeutic agents will be suitable as a source of autologous marrow for transplantation. Studies to address these issues are now in progress.

SUGGESTED READING

Donnall TE, Clift RA. Indications for marrow transplantation in chronic myelogenous leukemia. Blood 1989; 73:861–864.

Ozer H. Biotherapy of chronic myelogenous leukemia with interferon. Semin Oncol 1988; 15:14–20.

Talpaz M, Kurzrock R, Kantarjian HM, Gutterman JU. Recent advances in the therapy of chronic myelogenous leukemia. Important Adv Oncol 1988; 297–321.

CHRONIC LYMPHOCYTIC LEUKEMIA

KANTI R. RAI, M.D., F.A.C.P.

The most common type of leukemia found in a population aged 50 years and over is chronic lymphocytic leukemia (CLL). The classic form of CLL is the B-cell type (B-CLL); only about 5 percent of cases manifest as the T-cell type of CLL or as prolymphocytic leukemia. These latter two variants exhibit certain phenotypic and morphologic characteristics and they are generally not responsive to therapy. However, there are no therapeutic approaches for these variants that are distinct from those applied in B-CLL. This discussion focuses on management of patients with B-CLL. As is the case with many other malignancies, approach to treatment differs considerably in different centers. The treatment plan practiced in my clinic is detailed here.

OBSERVATION PHASE

It is our practice not to institute any cytotoxic therapy immediately upon making a diagnosis of CLL. A period of observation after diagnosis is advisable to determine if any treatment is indicated.

Clinical Staging of Chronic Lymphocytic Leukemia

It is first necessary to establish the clinical stage of a patient newly diagnosed as having CLL. The criteria of staging are as follows:

Stage 0. This stage manifests only with lymphocytosis in the peripheral blood and the bone marrow. Although an absolute lymphocyte count of 5,000 per cubic millimeter is an acceptable definition of lymphocytosis in peripheral blood, in most instances this count is over 15,000. Bone marrow aspirate must show 30 percent or more mature-appearing lymphocytes upon differential count of all nucleated cells, or a biopsy specimen must show lymphocytic infiltration. It should be noted that bone marrow is normocellular or hypercellular (i.e., not hypocellular) at the time of diagnosis of CLL.

Stage I. This stage exhibits lymphocytosis with evidence of enlarged lymph nodes.

Stage II. This stage exhibits lymphocytosis with evidence of enlargement of the spleen and/or the liver. Lymph nodes may or may not be enlarged.

Stage III. This stage is characterized by lymphocytosis with anemia (hemoglobin < 11 g per deciliter). The nodes, spleen, and liver may or may not be enlarged.

Stage IV. This stage exhibits lymphocytosis with thrombocytopenia (platelets < 100,000 per cubic milli-

meter). Anemia and enlargement of nodes, spleen, and liver may or may not be present.

When we examine the actuarial survival curves of patients with CLL, we recognize that there are three distinct patterns rather than five. Therefore, in accordance with the survival curves, I recently recommended that stage 0 be called low-risk group, stages I and II combined be called intermediate-risk group, and stages III and IV combined be called high-risk group. This modified Rai staging system is being used in all clinical trials in the United States.

After the clinical stage is determined, I try to find out if symptoms (e.g., weakness, weight loss, night sweats, fever, and increased susceptibility to infections) are present. In addition, blood counts are serially monitored at intervals of 2 to 4 weeks to determine the rate of increase of blood lymphocyte count, whether lymphocyte doubling time (actual or projected) is long (> 12 months) or short (≤ 12 months). The latter is associated with an aggressive clinical course in the low and intermediate risk groups.

INDICATIONS FOR THERAPEUTIC INTERVENTION

After an observation period of about 4 to 6 months, during which time the patient is seen regularly in the clinic, a decision is made whether therapeutic intervention is necessary. I use the following indications as guidelines and institute therapy if any one of these is present:

1. Progressive, disease-related symptoms.
2. Evidence of progressive marrow failure (i.e., worsening anemia, thrombocytopenia, and recurrent sepsis associated with hypogammaglobulinemia).
3. Autoimmune hemolytic anemia or immune thrombocytopenia.
4. Massive splenomegaly with or without evidence of hypersplenism.
5. "Bulky" disease, as evidenced by large lymphoid masses.
6. Progressive hyperlymphocytosis. The rate of increase of blood lymphocyte count is a more persuasive indicator than the absolute number. I generally do not withhold therapy when the count is higher than 150,000 per cubic millimeter. Leukostasis, which is associated with a high leukocyte count in other leukemias, is seldom encountered in CLL, but complications from hyperviscosity syndrome from hyperleukocytosis have been reported in CLL.

On rare occasion, however, the patient is markedly symptomatic at the time of initial diagnosis of CLL. It may not be advisable to withhold therapy under such a circumstance; I do not go through an observation period but institute therapy immediately in these patients.

THERAPEUTIC PLAN FOR SPECIFIC INDICATIONS

Progressive Disease-Related Symptoms

Usually such symptoms are controlled with chlorambucil and prednisone. I prefer to give intermittent bursts of treatment at intervals of 3 to 4 weeks rather than to treat by continuous daily regimens throughout the month. Chlorambucil is given, 0.7 mg per kg body weight by mouth in a single dose on day 1, day 28, and so forth. Prednisone is given, 0.5 mg per kg body weight by mouth, in one dose or divided in two doses daily for 7 days (days 1 through 7) in each monthly cycle. Concomitantly, allopurinol, 300 mg daily by mouth, is prescribed for 7 days of each cycle. Usually, symptoms (e.g., weakness, night sweats, fever) are controlled within 6 to 8 months after institution of therapy, at which time such therapy may be discontinued and the observation phase resumed.

Evidence of Progressive Marrow Failure

Progressive marrow failure is treated in the same manner as detailed above, by intermittent chlorambucil and prednisone.

Autoimmune Hemolytic Anemia or Immune Thrombocytopenia

Prednisone alone is given for these complications. Prednisone is started at 0.8 mg per kg body weight per day by mouth for 2 weeks, and if the anemia or the thrombocytopenia has started to improve, the prednisone dose is reduced by 50 percent at each 2-week interval for an overall continuous therapy time of 6 weeks' duration. Thereafter, prednisone may be given for 1 week every month at 0.5 mg per kg body weight per day for an additional 4- to 6-month period.

It should be emphasized that patients with CLL are generally elderly people with a somewhat high incidence of diabetes mellitus. Therefore, special attention must be given to the control of hyperglycemia, which may be exaggerated with prednisone therapy.

Massive Splenomegaly With or Without Evidence of Hypersplenism

Radiation therapy of the spleen is our first choice of treatment. Usually total doses of between 250 and 1,000 rad, delivered in 5 to 10 fractions, are adequate to reduce spleen size and control hypersplenism. However, if there is inadequate control with radiation therapy or the spleen again enlarges to significant proportions or hypersplenism remains a major problem, splenectomy is advisable. Even elderly patients (with good cardiopulmonary status) withstand this surgery without undue morbidity. However, it should be noted that if massive splenomegaly is not a solitary feature of a patient's disease (i.e., if adenopathy of a significant degree is also present), chemotherapy should be the initial therapeutic choice. If hypersplenism and splenomegaly persist after an adequate trial, splenic irradiation or splenectomy should be considered.

"Bulky" Disease of Large Lymphoid Masses

Most often chlorambucil therapy (without prednisone) at the dosage already detailed is adequate to reduce the size of large lymphoid masses. Such therapy is usually necessary for a period of 1 to 2 years on an intermittent monthly schedule. However, if the lymphoid masses are not generalized but are present at only one or two sites, or such masses are causing or likely to cause symptoms by pressing on adjacent vital organs (e.g., on a bronchus or the superior vena cava), local irradiation therapy is recommended. The total dose necessary under these circumstances ranges between 500 and 1,500 rad delivered in 5 to 15 fractions.

Progressive Hyperlymphocytosis

Usually chlorambucil at the dosage already detailed is adequate to reduce the blood lymphocyte count. If resources are available, it is recommended that leukapheresis be the first step in therapy when the starting blood count is in excess of 600,000 per cubic millimeter; chlorambucil therapy is initiated immediately after three to four treatments on a cell-separator machine. Side effects of chlorambucil are usually mild nausea and minimal suppression of bone marrow function. Allopurinol should always be added while treating hyperlymphocytosis.

THERAPEUTIC GUIDELINES BASED ON CLINICAL STAGING

Low-Risk Group (Stage 0). Patients in this stage are generally without any symptoms, and no cytotoxic agent is prescribed. However, patients should be seen in the clinic at intervals of 1 to 3 months. Median life expectancy is in excess of 12 years.

Intermediate-Risk Group (Stages I and II) A. Asymptomatic. There is no evidence that cytotoxic therapy is necessary or beneficial in these patients. I continue to observe them at monthly intervals. The median life expectancy of these patients ranges between 6 and 8 years and is probably not changed with therapy.

Intermediate-Risk Group (Stages I and II) B. Symptomatic. I recommend chlorambucil on an intermittent, monthly schedule at the dosage already detailed. The median life expectancy of these patients is about 5 years. It is not yet known whether therapy increases life expectancy.

High-Risk Group (Stages III and IV). Patients in these stages have a median life expectancy of 1.5 years. I give chlorambucil and prednisone to these patients as per the dosage already detailed. The therapeutic objective is to achieve a partial (PR) or a complete remission (CR). Usually it takes 8 to 10 months of therapy to achieve a partial remission. Patients achieving either a CR or a partial remission have prolongation of median survival time to about 5 years, whereas those patients achieving less than a partial remission have a 1.5-year median survival.

Alternative to Chlorambucil

I use cyclophosphamide in lieu of chlorambucil if the patient cannot tolerate the latter drug or is no longer showing a satisfactory response to it. Cyclophosphamide is administered by mouth or by intravenous injection. The dose of cyclophosphamide, on intermittent schedule, is 200 mg per square meter per day by mouth for 5 days in cycles that repeat at 3-week intervals or 750 mg per square meter on day 1 by intravenous injection every 3 weeks. Toxicity of this drug consists of controllable nausea and vomiting, hair loss, bone marrow suppression, and chemical cystitis.

Second-Line Therapy

When single-agent therapy (chlorambucil or cyclophosphamide) with or without prednisone fails to control CLL-related problems, I use fludarabine phosphate, a new drug recently approved by the U.S. Food and Drug Administration, for patients with CLL who have become refractory to alkylating agents. Fludarabine phosphate is administered intravenously daily, for 5 days every month, at a dosage of 25 mg per square meter per day. If a beneficial response is to result, it occurs within 6 to 8 cycles (6 to 8 months) of therapy—usual responses are PR and occasionally CR. Toxicities are dose related and generally avoidable. The second promising new drug, 2-chlorodeoxyadenosine (2cdA), is currently under experimental trials. If a physician has access to a 2cdA protocol, a patient with refractory CLL has a good likelihood of benefitting from this therapy. If none of these new drugs are available, combination chemotherapy protocols are the options to be considered. These are combinations that are usually administered in treatment of non-Hodgkin's lymphoma or multiple myeloma, e.g., cyclophosphamide, vincristine, and prednisone (COP), COP with doxorubicin (CHOP), and COP with carmustine (BCNU), and melphalan (M-2 protocol). The dosages utilized in each drug combination are decided on after considering each patient's bone marrow reserve, previous exposure to and level of tolerance of cytotoxic therapy, and the overall medical status.

Assessment of Therapeutic Response

I define a CR when there are no symptoms and no abnormal findings on physical examination, and hemogram and bone marrow study reveal normal values. If all these criteria are fulfilled but serum immunoglobulin levels are still lower than normal or there is persistence of increased B lymphocytes, I would rate such a response as a CR. Achievement of even such a CR is a rather

unusual occurrence in CLL, and it is my belief that our target must be to increase the incidence of CR according to this clinical definition before we can aim to achieve a CR that would include normalization of immune function and lymphocyte subpopulations ratios as well. A partial remission is defined as a 50 percent decrease in absolute lymphocyte count in peripheral blood, hemoglobin more than 11 g per deciliter, platelets more than 100,000 per cubic millimeter, or improvement in these values by 50 percent of their deviation from normal and decrease in palpable lymph nodes and spleen by at least 50 percent.

SUPPORTIVE THERAPY

In order to control signs and symptoms of anemia, transfusion of packed red cells is given as supportive therapy. Transfusions of platelets and granulocytes are rarely given in CLL. High-dose gamma globulin therapy by intravenous route, 400 mg per kilogram body weight every 21 days, is of benefit to those patients who have marked hypogammaglobulinemia or have recurrent bacterial infections. There are no contraindications to giving pneumococcal vaccine or flu vaccine, but the usefulness of such vaccines is in doubt in patients with CLL. Analogues of androgens have been effective on a few occasions by stimulating erythropoiesis in patients with significant anemia. However, such therapy may be associated with adverse side effects of hepatotoxicity, fluid retention, exacerbation of symptoms of prostatic hypertrophy in men, and masculinizing effects in women. I have observed beneficial responses to cyclosporine therapy in those patients with CLL whose severe anemia is found to be from pure red cell aplasia.

TERMINAL PHASE

In CLL, death occurs most often from infectious complications secondary to disease-induced or therapy-induced neutropenia and immunodeficiency. Complications are especially difficult to control in advanced stages of CLL. The next most common causes of morbidity and mortality are bleeding complications, hepatic failure, and inanition and wasting. On rare occasions, CLL is transformed into a large cell lymphoma (Richter's syndrome) or a prolymphocytoid cell leukemia. Such cases receive aggressive chemotherapy generally used in high-grade lymphoma, but there is little evidence that any regimen is effective in prolonging life. Even less frequently, CLL transforms into acute myelocytic leukemia, which is also refractory to intensive therapy that is currently used successfully in de novo acute leukemia.

Supported by grants from Aaron Diamond Foundation, Helena Rubinstein Foundation, Denis Klar Leukemia Fund, Rosenstiel Foundation, Doyle Dane Bernbach, National Leukemia Foundation, United Leukemia Fund, and Wayne Goldsmith Leukemia Fund.

Cheson BD, Bennett JM, Rai KR, et al. Guidelines for clinical protocols for chronic lymphocytic leukemia: Recommendations of National Cancer Institute-sponsored Working Group. Am J Hematol 1988; 29:152–163.

Cooperative Group for the Study of Immunoglobulin in Chronic Lymphocytic Leukemia. Intravenous immunoglobulin for the prevention of infection in chronic lymphocytic leukemia. A randomized controlled clinical trial. N Engl J Med 1988; 319:902–907.

Foon KA, Rai KR, Gale RP. Chronic lymphocytic leukemia: New insights into biology and therapy. Ann Intern Med 1990; 113: 525–539.

French Cooperative Group on Chronic Lymphocytic Leukemia. Effects of chlorambucil and therapeutic decision in initial forms of chronic lymphocytic leukemia (Stage A): Results of a randomized clinical trial on 612 patients. Blood 1990; 75:1414–1421.

International Workshop on Chronic Lymphocytic Leukemia. Chronic lymphocytic leukemia: Recommendations for diagnosis, staging, and response criteria. Ann Intern Med 1989; 110:236–238.

Keating MJ, Kantarjian H, Talpaz M, et al. Fludarabine: A new agent with major activity against chronic lymphocytic leukemia. Blood 1989; 74:19–25.

Piro LD, Carrera CJ, Beutler E, Carson DA. Chlorodeoxyadenosine: An effective new agent for the treatment of chronic lymphocytic leukemia. Blood 1988; 72:1069–1073.

Rai KR. A critical analysis of staging in chronic lymphocytic leukemia. In: Gale RP, Rai KR, eds. Chronic lymphocytic leukemia: Recent progress and future directions. New York: Alan R. Liss, 1987:253.

Shustik C, Mick R, Silver R, et al. Treatment of early chronic lymphocytic leukemia: Intermittent chlorambucil versus observation. Hematol Oncol 1988; 6:7-12.

ACUTE LYMPHOBLASTIC LEUKEMIA IN ADULTS

RALPH M. MEYER, M.D.

Acute lymphoblastic leukemia (ALL) is a disease involving the malignant proliferation of primitive lymphoid progenitor cells. The disease is usually recognized by the appearance of these cells in peripheral blood and bone marrow. Additional involvement of the central nervous system and nodal, extranodal, and thymic tissues may occur in some patients. Marked variation of incidence with age is noted; the peak occurrence of disease is in children younger than 5 years. The incidence of ALL in patients older than 15 years does not vary with age, except that a second peak is observed in the ninth decade of life. Patients with ALL account for more than 75 percent of children with leukemias, and more than 25 percent of all children with cancer. In contrast, only 20 percent of all newly diagnosed cases of adult acute leukemia are classified as ALL.

The outcome from therapy for adult patients is also much different from that observed in children. Although the proportion of patients entering remission may be comparable in some series, curative potential is now realized in as many as 75 percent or more of children, whereas only one-third of adults appear to have durable remissions. This difference appears to be due primarily to variation of disease biology rather than to treatment choice or tolerance. Children 10 years old and older are often considered as having "high-risk" ALL, implying that all adults must have high-risk disease. In fact, in adults (usually considered as age older than 15 years), age is a continuous variable that influences achievement of remission and long-term survival. This must be remembered when analyzing results of therapeutic trials in adult patients. Although the incidence of ALL does not vary significantly between the ages of 15 and 70 years,

a median age of 20 to 30 years is reported in most case series, suggesting a bias of entry of younger patients into such protocols.

It is apparent that significant improvements in the treatment of adults with ALL have occurred over the past 15 years. These advances have, in part, resulted from a better understanding of the use of chemotherapy gained in treating childhood ALL as well as from improvements in supportive care. Additional understanding of molecular biology has improved our ability to determine disease status and prognosis. These components of specific and supportive therapy, diagnostic testing, and determination of prognosis are organized in Table 1 into a format of phases of management for adults with ALL.

INITIAL EVALUATION

Prompt management of initial complications and commencement of definitive therapy are necessary to prevent further deterioration of the patient's status. At initial presentation it is necessary to complete baseline assessments to confirm the diagnosis, identify disease complications, and later allow determination of prognosis. Further requirements of the initial evaluation period include implementation of treatments to correct disease complications and to prepare the patient for chemotherapy. Entry of the patient into clinical trials of therapy should be attempted whenever possible.

Confirmation of Diagnosis

Laboratory studies for diagnosis and prognosis include a complete blood count with examination of the peripheral blood smear and bone marrow studies including morphology, cytochemistry, immunophenotyping, and cytogenetics. Investigations of research interest that may be of future importance include determination of clonal gene re-arrangement and assessment of oncogene activity.

Studies of the peripheral blood reveal a variable

Table 1 Phases of Management of ALL

Initial evaluation
  Confirmation of diagnosis
  Management of complications
  Preparation for chemotherapy
Induction therapy
  Chemotherapy
  Management of complications
Post induction therapy
  Assessment of prognosis
  Continued therapy
    Consolidation/maintenance therapy
    Central nervous system therapy
    Bone marrow transplantation
Management of long-term complications
Management of relapsed leukemia

degree of anemia, neutropenia, and thrombocytopenia. Most patients will demonstrate the presence of leukemic blast cells in the peripheral blood with counts of greater than 100×10^9 cells per L noted in 10 to 20 percent of patients. Bone marrow aspirate studies demonstrate a hypercellular marrow with a diffuse increase in blast cells. The morphology of the blast cells using Wright staining can be classified using French-American-British (FAB) nomenclature. Sixty-five percent of adults will have FAB L2 morphology with large blast cells of a heterogeneous appearance. Nuclear clefting is observed in some of these cells. The typical FAB L1 morphology of childhood ALL, with small homogeneous cells containing regularly shaped nuclei, is seen in 20 to 30 percent of adult patients. Fewer than 10 percent of patients will have FAB L3 ALL, in which cells identical to those seen in Burkitt's lymphoma are observed. Testing for the presence of the intracellular enzyme terminal deoxynucleotidyl transferase (TdT) and immunophenotyping using a panel of monoclonal antibodies will delineate lymphoblastic from myeloblastic leukemia and will determine cell lineage and maturation stage of lymphoid blast cells. Cytogenetic studies may be helpful in assessing prognosis. For example, the 15 to 25 percent of adults who have the presence of a Philadelphia chromosome (t[9;22]) have a particularly adverse prognosis. These studies, including those now considered to be of research interest, may subsequently prove useful in assessing for residual disease.

Management of Complications

Initial complications requiring attention may include anemia, infection, bleeding, and a number of potential metabolic disturbances. Initial assessment should include a thorough history and physical examination; particular attention should be paid to the state of hydration, features of infection and bleeding, and evidence of nodal and extranodal involvement, which may be referred to as leukemia–lymphoma syndrome.

Significant deficiencies of hemoglobin level and platelet count should be corrected. Transfusion support is recommended for hemoglobin values of less than 100 g per L and for platelet counts of fewer than 20×10^9 cells per L. Transfusion of single donor or HLA-matched platelets does not appear to offer any advantage over pooled platelet concentrates. Reactions to these blood products can consist of fever, chills, and rigors, and these reactions can be alleviated with acetaminophen and diphenhydramine. Meperidine can be used for more severe reactions.

Although the presenting feature of fever may be directly caused by leukemia cell proliferation, careful assessment for septic processes is necessary. In patients with neutropenia, defined as neutrophil counts of less than 1.0×10^9 cells per L, fever of 38.0° C or higher requires initiation of broad-spectrum antibiotic therapy. These should include an aminoglycoside, such as tobramycin, and a semisynthetic penicillin derivative with a spectrum of activity against *Pseudomonas* such as piperacillin. Choice of antimicrobials may vary depending on institutional infection patterns. Specific assessment for infection of the oropharynx, skin, chest, urinary tract, and perianal area should be undertaken.

Although multiple abnormalities of hemostatic mechanisms may be present at the time of diagnosis, it is uncommon for bleeding of a life-threatening nature to occur during the phase of initial evaluation. The most common manifestation of an increased bleeding tendency is the presence of cutaneous petechiae secondary to thrombocytopenia. Bleeding from the gastrointestinal or urinary tract is a less common problem and intracranial bleeding before the initiation of therapy is rare. Twenty-five percent of patients will present with platelet counts of fewer than 20×10^9 cells per L; prophylactic platelet transfusions are warranted as indicated earlier.

A second cause of bleeding, and a major risk for intracranial hemorrhage, is hyperleukocytosis. In this situation, peripheral blood blast counts of 100×10^9 cells per L or higher are seen. The marked increase in blast cell number results in stasis of cerebral blood flow and perivascular blast cell infiltration, leading to loss of integrity of vessel structure. Subsequent rupture and hemorrhage may then result. Appropriate therapy consists of establishment of an alkaline diuresis, administration of allopurinol, and commencement of chemotherapy as soon as metabolic parameters allow. Intravenous fluids consisting of two-thirds dextrose in water, one-third normal saline with the addition of 100 mL of 7.5 percent sodium bicarbonate (44.6 mEq per 50 mL ampule) per liter of intravenous fluid should be administered. This solution should be administered at a rate of 3 L per square meter of body surface area per day. Allopurinol should be prescribed as 300 mg twice daily for the first 2 days and then maintained at 300 mg per day. When diagnostic difficulties prevent the prompt initiation of definitive chemotherapy, hydroxyurea, 2 to 3 g per square meter per day can be given to assist in lowering the blast count. The use of emergency leukophoresis and cranial irradiation has been reported in case series, but consistent evidence that these modalities improve short- or long-term outcome is not available.

Disorders of the coagulation system, including disseminated intravascular coagulation (DIC), are the third cause of an increased bleeding risk. DIC of a clinically significant nature is less common in ALL than in acute nonlymphocytic leukemia. Results of coagulation tests may suggest increased thrombin activation (positive protamine sulfate and D-D dimer tests, increased fibrinopeptide A levels) but hypofibrinogenemia requiring replacement therapy is relatively uncommon. When fibrinogen values of less than 1.0 g per L are noted, prophylactic replacement with cryoprecipitate is indicated. Less severe degrees of hypofibrinogenemia should be treated only in actively bleeding patients.

Metabolic complications include alterations of fluid and electrolyte balance, hyperuricemia, abnormalities of calcium and phosphate metabolism, and renal dysfunction. Dehydration may be a presenting complication owing to poor oral intake, vomiting, and excessive losses due to renal tubular dysfunction. Sodium losses are usually proportionate to water losses, resulting in normal sodium concentrations. Hypokalemia may be observed and is of multifactorial origin, including resulting from excessive renal tubular losses. Hyperuricemia results from an increased rate of cell lysis and DNA catabolism. Similarly, increased cell lysis may lead to hyperphosphatemia, although this complication is more commonly a feature of the tumor lysis syndrome seen after the initiation of therapy. A variety of abnormalities of calcium metabolism may occur in patients with ALL. Hypercalcemia may result from leukemia cell–induced osteoclast activation. Calcium values will usually return to normal with the standard measures of rehydration and subsequent initiation of chemotherapy. Profound hypercalcemia with lytic bone disease suggests the diagnosis of HTLV-1–related T-cell leukemia–lymphoma and will require additional measures for control. When rapid tumor lysis results in hyperphosphatemia, hypocalcemia caused by precipitation of calcium with phosphorus may occur. These problems of dehydration, hyperuricemia, and abnormal calcium–phosphate metabolism may induce renal dysfunction.

The treatment of all of the above-mentioned metabolic derangements requires appropriate rehydration with minimum expectations of 100 mL per hour of urine output. Allopurinol should be given to all patients on a prophylactic basis. Potassium supplementation and the use of phosphate binders such as aluminum hydroxide will depend on the results of investigations in individual patients. Resistent or severe hypercalcemia (greater than 3.0 mmol per L) also will require specific therapeutic measures, including more aggressive fluid administration and the use of agents such as calcitonin.

Preparation for Chemotherapy

In addition to instituting measures to correct the previously discussed problems and prevent tumor lysis syndrome, interventions to deal with anticipated difficulties are required. Specific issues include prevention of infection, maintenance of venous access, and attention to psychological ramifications resulting from the diagnosis and proposed treatment.

Prevention of *Pneumocystis carinii* infection with cotrimoxazole has been shown to be possible in children with ALL and is thus recommended for adults. Prophylactic use of other antibacterial and antifungal agents remains under study but has not yet been demonstrated to be of benefit to adult ALL patients. Measures such as reverse isolation and sterilization of food are unnecessary.

The use of an indwelling venous catheter simplifies treatment and is found by most patients to be more convenient than continued use of peripheral venous access. Although septic complications related to these catheters remain a significant problem, it is likely that similar infection problems would result from use of peripheral access. Five to ten percent of patients who require long-term catheter use will develop thrombotic problems such as axillary or subclavian vein thrombosis. These diagnoses should be confirmed by venography and treated by anticoagulation if the patient is not severely thrombocytopenic. Ideally, the catheter should be removed if alternate venous access is available. There are no consistent data to indicate superiority of an external system, such as the Hickman catheter, or a closed indwelling port system; choice of catheter will depend on institutional and patient preferences.

Psychological issues related to diagnosis, therapy with associated toxicities, and prognosis are a major concern throughout the treatment course. Discussion with the patient and his or her family of the nature of the illness and treatment, including the rationale for aspects of therapy, is exceedingly important. Such discussion should take place as soon as possible after confirmation of the diagnosis. Patients may not recall much of the content of these initial conversations, but the development of a trusting relationship between the patient and members of the health care team will depend on compassionate and honest discussion early in the relationship.

INDUCTION THERAPY

Chemotherapy

Determination of optimal treatment ultimately requires the completion of randomized controlled trials. The feasibility of completing such trials in adult patients with ALL is made difficult because of the uncommon incidence of this illness. Most reports of therapy in adult ALL patients are case series; occasionally authors have compared outcomes to those of a historically treated cohort. Case series reports cannot be confidently compared because variation in factors other than treatment regimen may influence outcome. Patient factors such as age and performance status, disease factors such as blast count and immunophenotype, and trial methodologies such as single or multi-institutional design may differ between published reports. Thus, knowledge of what constitutes the optimal regimen of chemotherapy remains speculative.

Despite these reservations, improved treatment results have been observed over the past decade, and portions of therapy can be uniformly regarded as essential. Past studies of childhood ALL have established that vincristine and prednisone are crucial components of an induction regimen. These agents result in achievement of remission in 90 percent of children, but only 50 percent of adults. The addition of L-asparaginase (500 IU per kg for 10 to 14 days) to adult induction regimens has not been shown to influence this outcome. Improved remission rates in case series were reported more than a decade ago when daunorubicin was added to induction protocols. This was later confirmed in a randomized trial comparing vincristine, prednisone, and L-asparaginase with and without daunorubicin. The use of these four agents will lead to achievement of remission in 65 to 85 percent of patients.

As the specifics of various regimens are complex, the drug dose and schedule of a chosen protocol should be examined in original publications. Some recent reports are indicated in Table 2. As trial designs, including eligibility criteria differ, these reports cannot be directly compared. This fact is emphasized by the variable results observed with a given protocol administered in different settings.

Management of Complications

Problems caused by both underlying disease and complications from therapy are numerous and require daily review of all organ systems. These assessments include an appropriate history, thorough physical examination with attention to evidence of infection, and routine laboratory studies. Management of some complications has already been discussed in the section dealing with initial evaluation; blood product support should be continued on a prophylactic basis, and an adequate state of hydration should be maintained.

Additional problems accumulate during the treatment period, with complete resolution of many not occurring until remission is achieved. Sepsis continues to be the major cause of morbidity and mortality. Twenty-five to 50 percent of patients will require broad-spectrum antibiotic therapy. Deaths due to infection occur in 5 to 15 percent of patients. The risk of death from infection increases with advancing age. Initial management of the febrile, neutropenic patient has been discussed previously. With prolonged periods of neutropenia, secondary infections occur and usually require empiric antibiotic modifications. The management of persistent fever should include cultures of the blood, urine, throat, and the central venous access site. If diarrhea occurs, cultures of stool, including specimens for *Clostridium difficile,* should be obtained. A chest radiograph should be reviewed to assess for opportunistic lung infections, including interstitial pneumonia. Antimicrobial agents to consider for treatment of continued fever while neutropenia persists are vancomycin for resistant Staphylococcal infections and amphotericin B for invasive fungal infections.

Common metabolic complications can include hyperglycemia, hypokalemia, and renal dysfunction. Older patients are particularly susceptible to developing hy-

Table 2 Clinical Trials of Therapy: Induction Regimens

Author/Reference	Drug	Dose (mg/m²)	Schedule	Remission (%)
Schauer et al, J Clin Oncol, 1983	Vincristine	2.0 mg	d 1, 8, 15, 22, 29	84
	Prednisone	60 mg	d 1–35	
	Doxorubicin	20 mg	d 17–19	
		30 mg	d 36	
	Cyclophosphamide	600 mg	d 36	
Hussein et al, Blood, 1989	Vincristine	2.0 mg	d 1, 8, 15, 22, 29	68
	Prednisone	60 mg	d 1–35	
	Doxorubicin	20 mg	d 17–19	
		30 mg	d 36	
	Cyclophosphamide	600 mg	d 36	
Hoelzer et al, Blood, 1984*	Vincristine	1.5 mg	d 1, 8, 15, 22	74
	Prednisone	60 mg	d 1–28	
	Daunorubicin	25 mg	d 1, 8, 15, 22	
	L-asparaginase	5000 U	d 1–14	
Linker et al, Blood, 1987	Vincristine	1.4 mg	d 1, 8, 15, 22	94
	Prednisone	60 mg	d 1–28	
	Daunorubicin	50 mg	d 1–3, ± 15†	
	L-asparaginase	6000 U	d 17–28	
Radford et al, J Clin Oncol, 1989	Vincristine	1.4 mg	d 1, 8, 15, 22	75
	Prednisone	60 mg	d 1–7, 15–21	
	Doxorubicin	30 mg	d 1–3, ± 15–17†	
	L-asparaginase	10000 U	d 22–31	

*A second phase of induction therapy consisting of cyclophosphamide, cytarabine, methotrexate, and 6-mercaptopurine was given to all patients.

†Additional dose(s) are given depending on results of bone marrow studies during induction therapy.

perglycemia. This problem is exacerbated by the use of steroids and may necessitate administration of insulin. Hypokalemia also may result from steroid use as well as from the co-existent use of antibiotics and amphotericin B, which leads to increased renal losses of potassium. Intravenous replacement is usually required. Renal dysfunction is most commonly attributed to the use of antibiotics and amphotericin B. Maintenance of antibiotic drug levels within a therapeutic range and avoidance of dehydration aid in preserving renal function.

Gastroenterologic problems include nausea, vomiting, and anorexia. Subsequent deficiencies of protein and calorie intake, coupled with a catabolic state induced by corticosteroids and sepsis, may necessitate enteral or parenteral feeding. Caloric intake should be monitored and ongoing input from a dietician obtained. A specific intestinal complication of the chemotherapeutic agent vincristine is the development of autonomic nervous system dysfunction leading to hypomotility and constipation. High doses of vincristine, for example, 2 mg per m^2 to a maximum of 2 mg, may induce a paralytic ileus requiring nasogastric suction and subsequent attenuation of the vincristine dose. The prophylactic use of stool softeners and laxatives may assist in prevention of this syndrome.

POST-INDUCTION THERAPY

Assessment of Prognosis

The determination of prognosis may prove to be an important part of choosing therapy in adults with ALL. In general, studies of prognostic factors should include several qualities. Of greatest importance is the description of an "inception cohort" of all patients with a given disease diagnosed within a geographic area in a defined time period. If this criterion is not completely satisfied, careful assessment of referral method and patient eligibility criteria is required. Reports can then be analyzed for potential biases that influence outcome and assignment of prognostic significance. It remains necessary to have complete follow-up of all patients entered into the inception cohort with objective measures used to assess both the prognostic factor(s) and outcome. In a disease such as adult ALL in which interactions of multiple prognostic factors might exist, multivariate analyses should be performed. In addition, it should be remembered that prognostic factors may be protocol dependent: the development of a new very effective treatment may negate the influence of previously determined predictors of outcome.

Results of case series have consistently shown that success of remission induction is influenced by patient age. Multiple "cut-off" values, such as 25 to 35 years of age, have been described above which remission proportions diminish. It is likely, however, that age is a continuous variable. Older patients are both more likely to suffer fatal complications during induction therapy and to demonstrate resistant disease. Not unexpectedly, studies that exclude older patients fail to demonstrate these associations. No other factors have consistently been observed to influence attainment of remission. Patients with FAB L3 morphology (and expression of surface immunoglobulin) are described as having decreased remission proportions. This observation does not usually reach statistical significance because of the rare incidence of this ALL subtype. Alteration of induction therapy based on pretreatment prognostic assessment has not been shown to result in more efficacious therapy, although some protocols do employ augmented anthracycline administration during induction based on bone marrow findings assessing initial response to treatment.

The discussion of prognostic assessment is included in this section on post-induction therapy for three reasons. First, choice of induction therapy has not yet been shown to be dependent on pretreatment prognosis. Second, important prognostic determinants for long-term outcome may not be known before the achievement of remission. Finally, there is greater speculation that long-term outcomes may be improved by therapeutic alterations of post-induction therapy based on prognostic factors. Specifically, the potential role of bone marrow transplantation may be influenced by these factors.

Young age is described in most series as being predictive for prolonged duration of remission and overall survival. Parameters of disease biology also impact on duration of remission. Most consistently, increased pretreatment white blood cell count and prolonged time to disease response predict short remission durations. As with the effect of age, pretreatment white blood cell count appears to be a continuous variable, with cut-off values of 15 to 35 $\times$ 10^9 cells per L described. Disease response is usually described as time to complete remission; lack of remission by the 28th day of therapy is predictive of less durable remissions.

Influence on remission duration has been attributed to a number of other factors, but these observations have been inconsistent. Specifically, the role of immunophenotype remains uncertain. Most series have described prolonged remissions in patients expressing the common acute leukemia (CD 10) or T-cell antigens. Patients with null-ALL appear to have a poorer prognosis. Conflicting results, however, have been reported. The additional finding of "dual markers" with myeloid-positive disease has usually been associated with inferior outcomes. The "leukemia–lymphoma" syndrome and cytogenetic abnormalities other than the Philadelphia chromosome have a variable impact on prognosis.

In summary, increased age, increased pretreatment white blood cell count, prolonged time to achieve remission, and possibly null-ALL predict for shorter remission durations. A recent report of a multicenter German study concluded that 62 percent of patients achieving remission and possessing none of these adverse prognostic features remain in remission at 5 years after treatment. In contrast, remission durations of 5 years were seen in 33 percent of patients with one adverse factor, 22 percent of patients with two adverse factors, and 11 percent of patients with three adverse factors. These observations may allow stratification of patients into groups in which alternate forms of post-remission therapy can be given. Because age is a factor descriptive of the patient and other prognostic variables relate more to disease biology, multiple types of "high-risk" groups may exist, necessitating different post-induction strategies.

Continued Therapy

Consolidation and Maintenance Therapy

Post-induction chemotherapy in children with ALL has been demonstrated in randomized controlled trials to prolong remission duration and survival and to be an essential component of curative therapy. The use of more intensive post-induction therapy in "high-risk" children appears to be of added benefit. These observations have resulted in multiagent consolidation (or intensification) and maintenance therapies becoming a standard part of protocols for treatment of adult ALL. Adequate testing of these principles in randomized trials has not been completed in adult patients. Thus, optimal agents, schedule, and duration of treatment for this phase of treatment remain uncertain.

Most reported case series employ a phase of consolidation therapy in which multiple drugs are administered in a dose and schedule that induce significant marrow aplasia. Commonly used drugs include an anthracycline, a corticosteroid, cytarabine, and an antimetabolite such as methotrexate or 6-thioguanine. Subsequent maintenance therapy, in which a lesser degree of pancytopenia is induced, is usually continued for 30 to 36 months. Maintenance treatment usually consists of oral methotrexate and 6-mercaptopurine as administered in children. Multiple other agents are used in some protocols.

Again, the specifics of various consolidation and maintenance schemes are complex, and protocol specifics should be reviewed in original publications. Drugs used in the post-induction therapy of recent reports are indicated in Table 3. As previously indicated, these case series cannot be directly compared.

Central Nervous System Therapy

As with other aspects of therapy in adult patients, measures to prevent recurrence of leukemia in the central nervous system (CNS) have been patterned after practices developed in children. The need for CNS prophylaxis has been clearly demonstrated in childhood ALL. Components of treatment may include methotrexate, given intrathecally and in "intermediate" or "high" intravenous doses, and radiation. In adults, analyses of case series and cohort studies suggest that these therapies decrease the incidence of CNS relapse and improve relapse-free and overall survival rates. However, unlike results observed in children, unequivocal benefit has not been demonstrated in randomized controlled trials. Prophylactic treatment with intrathecal methotrexate and cranial radiation has been shown in one randomized trial to result in significantly fewer CNS relapses, but number of total relapses, remission duration, and survival were not altered.

Despite the lack of evidence from randomized trials, prophylactic CNS therapy continues to be regarded as a standard component of adult regimens. As treatment objectives are curative rather than palliative, available data would support this practice. The fact that unequivocal benefits have not yet been observed underscores the difficulties that persist in the treatment of ALL in adults. Current methods of CNS prophylaxis are indicated in Table 4. Incidence of risk factors for CNS relapse, including CNS leukemia at presentation and FAB L3 morphology or B cell immunophenotype, vary between these case series. This precludes comparison of these case series; optimal modalities, dose, timing, and schedule of CNS prophylaxis are yet to be determined.

Bone Marrow Transplantation

The role of allogeneic marrow transplantation for adult patients in first remission remains controversial. Most reports of this modality are case series rather than comparative trials. No randomized controlled trials have been conducted. As multiple patient and disease factors may determine prognosis, outcome differences observed between case series cannot be confidently attributed to treatment choice.

Two trials comparing "standard" consolidation and maintenance therapy to transplantation in first remission have been reported. A policy of maintenance therapy only was compared with allogeneic or autologous marrow transplantation in a prospective cohort study reported by Proctor. The combined transplantation groups appeared to have a superior 3-year disease-free survival (40 percent versus 20 percent), but small patient numbers precluded achievement of statistical significance. The pooled outcomes of two multicenter German trials employing consolidation and maintenance therapy were compared with results of transplantation in first remission in patients reported to the International Bone Marrow Transplant Registry. Regression techniques were used to adjust for prognostic characteristics. No difference in leukemia-free survival was observed, with 35 to 40 percent of patients alive and free of leukemia at 5 years in both groups. As treatment choices were not determined by random allocation in either of these studies, it is not possible to form definitive conclusions regarding a policy of transplantation in first remission.

Case series reporting results of allogeneic transplantation in first remission in which the proportion of adult patients can be determined are indicated in Table 5. Disease-free survival appears to be at least similar to that observed in more recent trials employing consolidation and maintenance therapies. Treatment failures are more

Table 3 Clinical Trials of Therapy: Post-induction Therapy

Author	Consolidation Drugs	Maintenance Drugs	CCR Duration*
Schauer et al, J Clin Oncol, 1983	Cytarabine + Thioguanine Cytarabine + Methotrexate Vincristine + Prednisone + Cyclophosphamide + L-asparaginase	Vincristine Prednisone Doxorubicin Cyclophosphamide BCNU Mercaptopurine Methotrexate Actinomycin D	66% at 30 months
Hussein et al, Blood, 1989	Cytarabine + Thioguanine Cytarabine + Methotrexate Vincristine + Prednisone + Cyclophosphamide + L-asparaginase	Vincristine Prednisone Doxorubicin Cyclophosphamide BCNU Mercaptopurine Methotrexate Actinomycin D	50% at 23 months
Hoelzer et al, Blood, 1984	Vincristine + Doxorubicin + Dexamethasone Cytarabine + Thioguanine + Cyclphosphamide	Methotrexate Mercaptopurine	50% at 24 months
Linker et al, Blood, 1987	Vincristine + Prednisone + Daunorubicin + L-asparaginase Cytarabine + Teniposide Methotrexate + Leucovorin	Methotrexate Mercaptopurine	53% at 36 months
Radford et al, J Clin Oncol, 1989	None	Vincristine Prednisone Doxorubicin Cyclophosphamide BCNU Mercaptopurine Methotrexate Actinomycin D	53% at 36 months

*Continuous complete remission (patients not achieving remission have been excluded).

commonly due to transplant-related complications than to relapse of leukemia; disease relapse does, however, appear more frequent than in comparable patients with acute nonlymphocytic leukemia. Prognostic variables influencing outcome in transplant series largely relate to measures used to prevent graft versus host (GVH) disease. Specifically, the use of corticosteroids has been associated with improvements in leukemia-free survival. Whether this is a surrogate marker for lesser degrees of GVH and an associated graft versus leukemia effect cannot be determined. Patient age appears to remain a prognostic variable, with younger patients continuing to have superior outcomes. Pretreatment disease variables have been less consistently shown to impact on outcome in transplant series.

In summary, whether adult patients in first remission should undergo marrow transplantation remains uncertain. Allogeneic transplantation does appear to be a reasonable option for patients with adverse disease-related prognostic factors such as high pretreatment leukocyte count, null phenotype, presence of Philadelphia chromosome, and prolonged time to remission. The usefulness of autologous marrow transplant in first remission has not been adequately described and remains investigational. Properly stratified randomized trials remain necessary to determine optimal strategies of post-induction therapy.

MANAGEMENT OF LONG-TERM COMPLICATIONS

Relapse of leukemia remains the major long-term risk to the health of most patients. However, significant

Table 4 Clinical Trials of Therapy: CNS Prophylaxis

Author	*Methods of Prophylaxis*	*Percent CNS Relapses*	
		Isolated	*CNS + Marrow*
Schauer et al, J Clin Oncol, 1983*	Methotrexate (intrathecal or intraventricular) given during phases of induction, consolidation, and maintenance	3.2	4.9
Hussein et al, Blood, 1989	Methotrexate (intrathecal or intraventricular) given during phases of induction, consolidation, and maintenance	6.9	4.3
Hoelzer et al, Blood, 1988†	Intrathecal methotrexate and cranial radiation (24 Gy) given after induction	6.3	1.4
Linker et al, Blood, 1987†	Intrathecal methotrexate and cranial radiation (18 Gy) given after induction; intermediate-dose methotrexate given during consolidation	0	1.5
Radford et al, J Clin Oncol, 1989	Intrathecal methotrexate and cranial radiation (24 Gy) given after induction	9.1	Not indicated

*Includes results of L 10 and L 10 M protocols.
†Additional therapy given to patients with CNS involvement at time of diagnosis.

Table 5 Bone Marrow Transplant in First Remission: Case Series

Author/Reference	*Number of Patients*	*% Adults*	*% Disease-Free Survival*	*Relapses (%)*	*Toxic Deaths (%)*
Vernant, J Clin Oncol, 1988	27	100	59 at 3 years	11	30
Blume, Transplantation, 1987	39	97	63 at 3 years	10	26
McCarthy, Bone Marrow Trans, 1988	32	72	50 at 4 years	22	22
Wingard et al, J Clin Oncol, 1990	18	94	42 at 5 years	11	44

physiologic and psychological problems may occur in patients who are apparently cured. These problems result from complications of both the underlying leukemia and treatment modalities. Careful attention to these long-term issues is required to ensure a return to an optimal quality of life for patients and their families.

Common post-treatment problems include issues related to fertility, the risk of second malignancies, neurologic disorders, and potential cardiac dysfunction. The incidence of infertility and second malignancies appears to be less than in patients, such as those with Hodgkin's and non-Hodgkin's lymphoma, who have treatment regimens that include high cumulative doses of alkylating agents. However, fertility may be compromised, particularly in women who are over the age of 27 to 30 years or receive craniospinal (or abdominal) irradiation and men who receive testicular irradiation. These risks are thus most significant in patients who undergo marrow transplantation and receive total body irradiation. An increased risk of developing secondary myelodysplasia and acute nonlymphocytic leukemia has been reported in children and can be assumed to be present in adults.

Neurologic problems include persisting peripheral neuropathy secondary to vincristine, visual disturbances secondary to cataract formation, and leukoencephalopathy. Peripheral neuropathy associated with vincristine administration will usually resolve completely although wrist or foot drop may only partially improve. The most devastating neurologic complication is that of leukoencephalopathy. This syndrome typically presents with alterations in intellect and most frequently occurs in patients receiving combined modality therapy with intrathecal and high-dose intravenous methotrexate plus cranial radiation. Treatment for both of the above mentioned disorders consists largely of rehabilitative and supportive measures. Cardiac dysfunction secondary to anthracycline use is most common in patients who have pre-existing heart disease or relapse and thus receive further chemotherapy with "second-line" protocols. Monitoring of left ventricular ejection fraction values during therapy is necessary if continued administration of an anthracycline agent is planned for these patients.

Psychological difficulties are extremely common and may be neglected in many patients. Problems include fear of relapse, change in self image, loss of confidence as contact with the treatment team diminishes, adjustments to any persisting physical disorders (including infertility), and isolation from family, friends, and colleagues. Return to "normal" social and employment activities may be compromised by any number of these factors. Attention to such potential difficulties with arrangements for appropriate counseling, including involvement with support groups, should be considered.

MANAGEMENT OF RELAPSED LEUKEMIA

Recurrence of ALL in adults carries an ominous prognosis and is associated with survival of 1 to 2 years in less than 10 percent in nontransplanted patients. Treatment objectives should thus be directed at achieving remission and proceeding to marrow transplantation in patients in whom curative intent remains reasonable and effectively palliating symptoms for patients in whom intensive treatment is not feasible. Optimal treatment regimens have not been determined for these patients; entry into trials testing investigational agents and new combinations of drugs should be considered.

The major prognostic variable associated with success of re-induction treatment is the duration of first remission. Patients with brief first remissions, particularly those who relapse while on continued therapy, have the poorest outlooks. These patients should be treated with regimens similar to those used to induce remission in patients with acute nonlymphocytic leukemia. Commonly described regimens include standard or high-dose cytarabine combined with an additional agent such as daunorubicin, idarubicin, mitoxantrone, m-AMSA, or teniposide. Remission rates as high as 50 to 70 percent have been observed. In patients who relapse after more prolonged first remissions, comparable remission proportions can be achieved with protocols used in initial induction treatment. Such treatment is usually associated with less toxicity.

Optimal treatment of patients achieving a second remission is with marrow transplantation. Options include allogeneic transplantation from an HLA-matched sibling or matched unrelated donor and autologous marrow reinfusion after intensive chemotherapy. Allogeneic transplantation is usually available only for patients younger than 50 years and is limited by the availability of a donor. The largest body of data exists for patients receiving a matched sibling transplant. Five-year actuarial leukemia-free survival rates of 25 to 45 percent have been observed in combined populations of adults and children in second remission. Superior results appear to be achieved in series that include a larger proportion of children. In comparison with transplants performed in first remission, relapse, seen in approximately 50 percent of cases, is the most common cause of treatment failure.

For patients in whom a sibling donor is not available, transplantation from an unrelated matched donor can be considered. Problems related to this treatment option include difficulty obtaining an HLA-matched donor during the time period in which a second remission can be maintained and the apparent increased incidence of GVH. This approach should currently be regarded as investigational; long-term results remain unknown.

Autologous marrow transplantation is similarly investigational. This option includes the theoretical advantage of greater availability and avoidance of GVH. Most reported series include in vitro purging of harvested marrow with either chemotherapeutic agents, monoclonal antibodies, or immunotoxins. A cohort series comparing autologous with matched sibling allogeneic transplantation in adults and children demonstrated comparable 4-year relapse-free survival rates of 20 and 27 percent, respectively. Autologous transplantation was less toxic with more rapid marrow engraftment, shorter initial hospitalizations, and fewer treatment-related deaths. Relapse rate was increased, however: 79 percent in the group undergoing autologous transplantation compared with 56 percent with allogeneic transplantation.

The optimal type of transplant remains uncertain. Chances for prolonged disease-free survival may be best with a matched sibling allogeneic transplant given that a continuous rate of relapse may be observed with autologous transplantation. Therefore, patients with an HLA-matched sibling should be first considered for allogeneic transplantation. Choices for patients without such donors are less certain.

The management of adult patients who experience an isolated CNS relapse also remains uncertain because reports of therapy are limited to case series that include small numbers of patients. The prognosis of these patients appears to parallel those with marrow relapse. Therefore, in addition to treatment directed at the CNS, re-introduction of systemic therapy is recommended. Components of CNS treatment can include intrathecal or intraventricular methotrexate and cytarabine, high-dose intravenous methotrexate, and cranial or craniospinal irradiation. Decisions regarding the specifics of CNS treatment should be integrated with long-term treatment plans, including marrow transplantation. One approach to therapy is to administer systemic and CNS therapy concurrently with intrathecal or intraventricular methotrexate and cytarabine and high-dose intravenous methotrexate. Other systemic agents may include doxorubicin, cyclophosphamide, and vincristine. Subsequent radiation treatment should be administered, but dose and timing will depend on the feasibility of marrow transplantation.

FUTURE DEVELOPMENTS

Advances in treatment are expected over the next decade. Further developments in the understanding of the molecular biology of ALL should lead to an improved ability to detect minimal residual disease and thus more accurately determine remission status. Such investigations include studies of gene rearrangement and oncogene expression, which will be facilitated with techniques such as the polymerase chain reaction.

The use of hematologic growth factors may allow testing of the role of chemotherapy dose while reducing treatment toxicity. Biologic response modifiers may play a role in achieving or maintaining remission. The use of interferon has been demonstrated to prolong remission status following marrow transplantation, although an effect on survival was not observed. Formal testing of interferon, other biologic agents, and the therapeutic use of monoclonal antibodies may lead to important advances.

Developments in transplantation biology may include improvements in techniques to prevent fatal GVH and to purge autologous marrow. These measures may then allow marrow transplantation to be a more feasible option because of an increase in the donor pool, a reduction in transplant-related toxicity with unrelated donors, and a reduced risk of relapse following autologous marrow reinfusion.

SUGGESTED READING

Barrett AJ, Horowitz MM, Gale RP, et al. Marrow transplantation for acute lymphoblastic leukemia: Factors affecting relapse and survival. Blood 1989; 74:862–871.

Hoelzer D, Thiel E, Loffler H, et al. Intensified therapy in acute lymphoblastic and acute undifferentiated leukemia in adults. Blood 1984; 64:38–47.

Hoelzer D, Thiel E, Loffler H, et al. Prognostic factors in a multicenter study for treatment of acute lymphoblastic leukemia in adults. Blood 1988; 71:123–131.

Hussein KK, Dahlberg S, Head D, et al. Treatment of acute lymphoblastic leukemia in adults with intensive induction, consolidation, and maintenance chemotherapy. Blood 1989; 73:57–63.

Kersey JH, Weisdorf D, Nesbit ME, et al. Comparison of autologous and allogeneic bone marrow transplantation for treatment of refractory high-risk acute lymphoblastic leukemia. N Engl J Med 1987; 317:461–467.

Linker CA, Levitt LJ, O'Donnell M, et al. Improved results of treatment of adult acute lymphoblastic leukemia. Blood 1987; 69:1242–1248.

Radford JE Jr, Burns CP, Jones MP, et al. Adult acute lymphoblastic leukemia: Results of the Iowa HOP-L protocol. J Clin Oncol 1989; 7:58–66.

Schauer P, Arlin ZA, Mertelsmann R, et al. Treatment of acute lymphoblastic leukemia in adults: Results of the L-10 and L-10M protocols. J Clin Oncol 1983; 1:462–470.

Wingard JR, Piantadosi S, Santos GW, et al. Allogeneic bone marrow transplantation for patients with high-risk acute lymphoblastic leukemia. J Clin Oncol 1990; 8:820–830.

ACUTE MYELOID LEUKEMIA

RICHARD M. STONE, M.D.
ROBERT J. MAYER, M.D.

Acute myeloid leukemia (AML) represents a clonal malignancy of hematopoietic stem cells. With an annual incidence in the United States of approximately 11,000 new cases, this disorder is uncommon, accounting for only 1 to 2 percent of all malignancies. Although AML is the third leading cause of cancer in young adults (ages 18 to 30 years), it appears most often in older patients, having a median age at the time of diagnosis of about 60 years. AML has been the object of intense study for two major reasons: (1) recent advances in antineoplastic therapy and supportive care have made the disease treatable in most patients and curable in many, and (2) the presence of easily obtainable malignant tissue in blood and bone marrow has allowed in-depth investigations into the nature of human leukemic cells.

After outlining etiologic associations, classification, and presenting features, this brief review will focus on contemporary management strategies for the treatment of adults with AML. Such strategies, particularly those relating to the use and timing of bone marrow transplantation, remain controversial.

ETIOLOGY

The vast majority of patients with AML have no clearly definable predisposing condition. The risk for the development of AML is increased if chromosomal aberrancies occur through environmental, neoplastic, or congenital mechanisms. The use of cytotoxic drugs, most notably alkylating agents when given as anticancer therapy in the treatment of Hodgkin's disease, ovarian cancer, and non-Hodgkin's lymphoma, or as immunosuppressive treatment in the management of so-called collagen-vascular disorders, can lead to bone marrow damage and the emergence of "secondary" AML 4 to 8 years after exposure. Such alkylating agents, including nitrogen mustard, busulfan, chlorambucil, and cyclophosphamide, bind to DNA, resulting in mutagenesis and the occasional emergence of a leukemic clone of hematopoietic stem cells. Prior exposure to ionizing radiation or benzene also has been associated with an increased incidence of AML, presumably through a similar mechanism of DNA damage, although it is generally difficult to define a specific causative link in any given patient. Certain chronic bone marrow diseases, especially if presumed to be caused by abnormalities in the pluripotent stem cell, may evolve into a clinical syndrome consistent with AML. Such disorders include the myeloproliferative syndromes (agnogenic myeloid metaplasia, essential thrombocythemia, polycythemia vera, and chronic granulocytic leukemia), the myelodysplastic syndromes (refractory anemias with or without excess bone marrow myeloblasts), and paroxysmal nocturnal hemoglobinuria. Congenital diseases characterized by chromosomal abnormalities, such as Down's syndrome (trisomy 21), Fanconi's anemia, Bloom's syndrome, and perhaps Turner's (XO) and Kleinfelter's syndromes (XXY), predispose to the development of AML. Despite evidence that leukemia in lower primates may be caused by retroviral infection, there are no data in humans to suggest that AML is induced by viruses.

As with most cancers, AML is believed to represent a clonal disorder in which the malignant cells originate from a single cell. The AML progenitor cell is thought to be derived from a hematopoietic stem cell, normally engaged both in self-replication and in differentiation. Such processes ultimately lead to the production of mature circulating blood cells. A perturbation in the normal replication/differentiation balance in favor of replication may result in AML. This so-called block in differentiation may occur as a result of oncogene activation, a loss of tumor suppressor genes, or both. The specific stage in the hematopoietic hierarchy at which such a block occurs determines the clinical phenotype of AML.

Although it has generally been accepted that chemotherapy must ablate the leukemic clone for normal hematopoiesis to resume and as a prerequisite for long-term disease eradication, the results of recent provocative studies imply that unique markers of leukemic cells may be found in granulocytes during clinical remission, suggesting the ability of malignant blasts to differentiate. This evidence for the existence of abnormal hematopoiesis during apparent remission may provide a partial explanation for the disturbingly high rate of subsequent relapse.

PRESENTATION

Patients with AML generally seek medical attention because of the bleeding, infection, and weakness that result from replacement of normal bone marrow by leukemic blast forms (myelophthisis), leading to thrombocytopenia, neutropenia, and anemia.

DIAGNOSIS

Morphology

The diagnosis of AML is based on morphologic, cytochemical, immunophenotypic, and cytogenetic studies performed on cells recovered from circulating blood or bone marrow aspiration, as well as the histologic appearance of a bone marrow biopsy specimen. The minimum criterion for the diagnosis of AML is the finding of more than 30 percent replacement of the bone marrow with myeloblasts. Myeloblasts are large, irregularly shaped cells with pale blue, often granular, cytoplasm, and a nucleus having coarsely clumped chromatin and discrete nucleoli. The cytoplasmic granules may coalesce to form oblong inclusion forms known as Auer rods (or Auer bodies). Myeloblasts usually can be distinguished morphologically from lymphoblasts (found in acute lymphoblastic leukemia), which display a sparse non-granulated cytoplasm and a more centrally located nucleus (Table 1). Cytochemical studies, when applied to myeloblasts, generally reveal avid staining for peroxidase or nonspecific esterase (in the case of monocytic or myelomonocytic leukemias); in contrast, lymphoblasts tend to exhibit avidity to the periodic acid-Schiff (PAS) reagent. The combination of morphologic and cytochemical analysis can be used to place AML cells into one of seven subtypes as defined by the French-American-British (FAB) classification system. These entities include acute myeloid leukemia (without [M-1] or with [M-2] maturation), acute promyelocytic leukemia (M-3), acute myelomonocytic leukemia, (M-4), acute monocytic leukemia (M-5), erytholeukemia (M-6), and megakaryoblastic leukemia (M-7).

Immunophenotype

The use of monoclonal antibodies directed against cell surface antigens that characterize various stages of cellular differentiation has permitted further refinement in the definition of leukemic cells as being of myeloid (AML), lymphoid (ALL), or both myeloid and lymphoid (biphenotypic) origin. Such an effort frequently serves to confirm the diagnostic impression made on morphologic grounds alone, but not uncommonly clarifies an otherwise ambiguous situation, thereby defining therapy. Approximately 10 percent of adult patients presenting with acute leukemia will have either no lineage-specific markers or evidence of both lymphoid and myeloid origin on their leukemic blast cells. It is hypothesized that in such cases the leukemic clone has arisen from a relatively primitive cell in the hematopoietic hierarchy. The prognosis for these patients is generally considered

Table 1 Distinguishing Features between ALL and AML

	ALL	AML
Morphology		
Shape	Round	Irregular
Cytoplasm	Dark blue rim	Pale blue
Nucleus	Central	Eccentric
Nuclear chromatin	Homogeneous	Coarse clumps
Auer bodies (rods)	Absent	Present in 50% of cases
Histochemistry		
Periodic acid-Schiff	+	−
Peroxidase	−	+
Esterase	−	±
Enzymology		
Terminal transferase (TdT)	+	−

worse than that for other patients with AML, perhaps because the more primitive cells may be more resistant to chemotherapy.

The enzymatic marker terminal transferase (TdT), present in the leukemic cells of 95 percent of ALL patients and absent from the cells of 95 percent of AML patients, may provide confirmation of leukemic classification. This unique DNA polymerase apparently acts as a ligase for rearranged gene fragments of immunoglobulin (B cells) or surface receptor (T cells) proteins during lymphoid maturation and, therefore, serves as a marker of lymphoid lineage.

Cytogenetics

With the availability of quinacrine banding techniques, a nonrandom karyotypic abnormality has been identified in approximately 50 percent of patients with AML. Chromosomal changes may reflect modal loss (e.g., monosomy 7) or gain (e.g., trisomy 8), translocations from one chromosome to another [t(8:21) associated with M-2 histology, t(15:17) associated with M-3 subtype], or rearrangements of material within a given chromosome (inversion of chromosome 16 in cases of M-4 associated with bone marrow eosinophilia). In addition to adding precision to diagnostic power, cytogenetic analysis has proved highly useful as a predictor of clinical outcome because most of the defined chromosomal changes have been shown to have prognostic significance.

UNUSUAL FEATURES

The clinician must be aware of special clinical situations arising during the early management of patients with AML that call for specific intervention.

Leukostasis

Thrombi caused by clumping of myeloblasts may occur when the peripheral leukemic cell count exceeds 100,000 cells/μl. This phenomenon, known as leukostasis, is unique to myeloblasts. It can cause reversible pulmonary infiltrates; more ominously, the phenomenon may lead to neurologic dysfunction and potentially irreversible cerebral damage due to thrombosis, infarction, and intracranial swelling. The presence of a circulating myeloblast count in excess of 100,000 cells/μl at the time of diagnosis mandates the rapid initiation of intravenous hydration (200 to 250 mL/hour) to expand the intravascular volume and dilute the myeloblast concentration. Some physicians experienced in the management of patients with AML also favor the use of leukapheresis, whereas others prefer to administer oral hydroxyurea (50 mg/kg) as additional means of reducing the peripheral blast count. Cranial radiation therapy to destroy leukemic thrombi also has been proposed if neurologic abnormalities suggestive of cerebral damage develop.

Myeloblastoma

Localized extramedullary deposits of myeloblasts, known as myeloblastomas, granulocytic sarcomas, or chloromas, can lead to subcutaneous nodules, pleural effusions or intestinal obstruction. Although localized radiation therapy is indicated if such a mass were to cause significant localized symptoms, the prompt initiation of systemic chemotherapy is generally considered to be the preferred therapeutic approach.

Coagulopathy

Acute promyelocytic leukemia (M-3) is characterized by the presence of dysplastic, granule-laden promyelocytes in the peripheral blood and bone marrow. A consumptive coagulopathy often develops as these thromboplastin-containing granules are released, either because of spontaneous cell death or the effects of chemotherapy. The use of low doses of heparin has been proposed as a means of counteracting this potential cause of hemorrhage. The role of such heparin therapy remains uncertain, however, because similarly high rates of remission have been observed in the presence or absence of anticoagulation, as long as management includes the administration of fresh-frozen plasma and platelet concentrates.

Extramedullary Infiltrations

A unique feature of acute monoblastic leukemia (M-5), and to a lesser extent, acute myelomonocytic leukemia (M-4) is the tendency of the leukemic blasts to infiltrate the gingiva and buccal mucosa, resulting in painful, swollen gums. Such infiltration may also involve the skin (leukemia cutis). Interestingly, spread to the meninges (leukemic meningitis) appears far less commonly in patients with AML than in those with ALL.

METABOLIC ABNORMALITIES

Urate nephropathy, occurring as a result of spontaneous or therapy-induced leukemic cell death in patients with high tumor cell burdens, was formerly a frequent cause of mortality. This life-threatening complication can nearly always be prevented through the aggressive intravenous administration of saline (200 to 250 mL per hour) and the administration of allopurinol (300 to 600 mg per day) prior to the administration of antileukemic chemotherapy. If the urine remains acidic (pH less than 6.0) despite adequate hydration, sodium bicarbonate should be administered to alkalinize the urine and make urate deposits more soluble. A less common metabolic abnormality that may be observed at the time of diagnosis in patients with AML or ALL when elevated circulating white blood cell counts are excessive is renal loss of potassium leading to hypokalemia. The cause of this finding is uncertain.

The prognosis for patients with AML has improved during the past 10 to 20 years for several reasons besides

Table 2 Induction Regimen for AML

Initial treatment	
Daunorubicin	45 mg/m^2/d × 3 days
Ara-C	+
	100–200 mg/m^2/d × 7 days continuous IV infusion
Day 14 marrow examination	
Hypoplasia: await remission, then begin intensification	
Residual leukemia: proceed to second induction	
Second induction	
Daunorubicin	45 mg/m^2 × 2 days
Ara-C	100–200 mg/m^2/d × 5 days continuous IV infusion

the appreciation of these metabolic complications. Although effective chemotherapeutic strategies have been devised (see below), improvements in supportive care such as the widespread availability of platelet transfusions and the development of potent, broad-spectrum antibiotics have permitted far better tolerance of profound myelosuppression. The administration of blood products, antimicrobials, and chemotherapy also has been enhanced by the use of indwelling central venous devices such as Hickman and Broviac catheters.

REMISSION-INDUCTION THERAPY

When the diagnosis of AML has been made, patients generally should be stabilized metabolically with 12 to 24 hours of parenteral hydration and given necessary blood products prior to the initiation of chemotherapy. Because of the continuous need for large quantities of intravenous products, including chemotherapeutic agents, antibiotics, blood transfusions, and fluids, the placement of an indwelling intravenous access device (e.g., Hickman catheter) into the subclavian vein via a subcutaneous tunnel is highly desirable. Antibiotic therapy should be instituted in the presence of persistent fever or clinical evidence of infection. Despite the use of such antimicrobial agents, the absence of functional neutrophils may prevent the control of infections. Attempts at eradicating infections in newly diagnosed patients with AML through the prolonged use of antibiotics most often prove fruitless. Hence, the initiation of definitive antileukemic therapy should not be delayed for more than 48 hours.

Perhaps the most frequently used remission-induction regimen combines daunorubicin (45 mg per m^2 per day by intravenous push daily for 3 days) with cytarabine (ara-C) (100 to 200 mg per m^2 per day given by continuous intravenous infusion for 7 days) (Table 2). The use of this so-called 3 + 7 treatment program has been associated with a 65 percent overall complete response rate in patients with *de novo* AML and a 35 percent complete response rate in those patients with a history of a prior hematologic disorder (i.e., secondary AML). Complete response rates are clearly age dependent, being 70 to 80 percent in *de novo* AML patients under 60 years of age but only 50 percent in older individuals. The addition of 6-thioguanine to daunorubicin and ara-C (TAD regimen) has not proved to be more effective than the use of 3 + 7 alone. Although the substitution of a newer anthracycline, idarubicin, for daunorubicin, has resulted in encouraging preliminary data, daunorubicin probably should still be considered the anthracycline of choice in AML induction programs.

A bone marrow examination is generally performed 14 days after the initiation of induction therapy to assess the effect of treatment. If persistent leukemic blasts are present or if the cellularity is in excess of 15 to 20 percent, a second course of treatment using an attenuated dose schedule (2 days of daunorubicin [45 mg per m^2 per day] and 5 days of continuous infusion ara-C [100 to 200 mg per m^2 per day]) is recommended (see Table 2). Such a second induction course, required in about 30 percent of patients with AML, delays the time to marrow recovery from 21 days to 35 days but does not appear to affect the outcome adversely if remission is achieved. Conversely, if the bone marrow examination performed 14 days after the start of therapy is devoid of blasts and reveals hypocellularity, no further therapy is needed. The bone marrow examination should be repeated weekly until the qualitative pattern of the recovering marrow (i.e., remission "vs" leukemia) can be determined. Once marrow remission has been documented, a lumbar puncture should be performed to rule out the occult presence of leukemic blasts in the cerebrospinal fluid.

POST-REMISSION STRATEGIES

The most controversial issue regarding the management of patients with AML deals with the design of optimal post-remission treatment (Table 3). It is clear that post-remission treatment is necessary because virtually all patients will relapse if no further chemotherapy is administered. It seems apparent, therefore, that a clinically undetectable leukemic cell burden remains after the achievement of remission and the restoration of normal hematopoietic function. How best to eradicate this residual leukemic burden is the focus of ongoing clinical studies.

Various post-remission treatment strategies have been advanced, ranging from the prolonged use of additional chemotherapy at doses less than those used during induction (maintenance), repeating the induction regimen in an identical dose schedule (consolidation), increasing the intensity of the dose schedule compared to that given during induction (intensification), or offering marrow ablative treatment followed by stem cell rescue either from an histocompatible sibling (allogeneic bone marrow transplant) or the patient himself (autologous bone marrow transplant).

The use of consolidation or maintenance treatment

Table 3 Post-Remission Management Alternatives in AML

Intensive chemotherapy
Allogeneic bone marrow transplantation
Autologous bone marrow transplantation

in patients with AML who have achieved complete response results in an increase in the median duration of remission from 4 to 8 months to 10 to 15 months, with 17 to 33 percent of such individuals projected to remain free of their disease for at least 4 years. Most randomized studies have demonstrated that chemotherapy administered for more than 8 to 16 months after the achievement of remission results in little or no additional benefit.

Recent clinical investigations have focused on methods of intensifying treatment during the post-remission period for patients with AML. Such efforts at intensification take advantage of the steep dose-response curve for ara-C, which has been shown in experimental tumors and short-term cultures of human leukemic cells. Several uncontrolled studies involving the use of high-dose ara-C (1 to 3 g per m^2 for 6 to 12 doses) have been associated with a projected 45 to 55 percent likelihood of continued complete remission after 24 months in patients under 40 years of age. Preliminary results from a study conducted by the Eastern Cooperative Oncology Group indicate that the probability of continued remission in patients who received one course of intensive post-remission therapy containing ara-C when administered in such a high-dose fashion was 50 percent greater than that of a similar cohort who received 2 years of low-dose maintenance treatment. Unfortunately, the administration of high-dose ara-C is poorly tolerated in elderly patients, leading to irreversible cerebellar dysfunction in about 10 percent of individuals older than 60 years of age.

Bone marrow transplantation from an histocompatible donor following myeloablative chemotherapy either with or without radiation therapy is an alternative approach to post-remission intensification for patients with AML. Allogeneic transplantation is associated with a reduction in the rate of leukemic relapse from 55 to 75 percent following chemotherapy to 15 to 25 percent. However, life-threatening toxicities associated with allogeneic transplantation, such as graft-versus-host disease (GVHD) and interstitial pneumonitis, reduce the long-term survival of transplanted patients to 45 to 50 percent. The complication rate of allogeneic transplantation is much lower in those patients under 30 years of age, and eligibility for this procedure is ordinarily restricted to those patients under age 45 years. Although the incidence of potentially fatal GVHD can be reduced by purging the donor bone marrow of T-lymphocytes, which are thought to mediate this complication, such attempts have thus far failed to demonstrate improvement in survival owing to a higher incidence of graft rejection and leukemic relapse. Based on the higher leukemic relapse rate in patients receiving marrow from an identical twin (syngeneic transplant), in whom GVHD does not occur, as well as the reduced relapse

rate in those with clinically significant GVHD who survive, it has been postulated that some of the lymphoid cells responsible for GVHD also may possess antileukemic activity (graft-versus-leukemia phenomenon).

Allogeneic bone marrow transplantation has been compared prospectively to post-remission chemotherapy in at least four clinical trials; three of these studies reported statistical superiority for the allograft in terms of disease-free survival, whereas the outcome of the other study suggested that the two approaches are equivalent. The lack of comparability between the transplant and chemotherapy cohorts in these studies with regard to treatment intensity and compliance in the chemotherapy groups as well as the potential selection biases with regard to age, percentage of patients with histocompatible donors, and referral patterns make the results of these trials inconclusive. A comparison of the outcomes from the largest and most mature transplant series with more preliminary data from similar (albeit slightly older) individuals who received short courses of intensive chemotherapy, usually including high doses of ara-C, demonstrates a similar probability of disease-free survival after 3 years. Allogeneic bone marrow transplantation represents the only therapeutic modality with curative potential in adults with AML in first relapse or second remission. The results from intensive chemotherapy in first remission and transplantation appear to overlap; therefore, some investigations have suggested that allogeneic transplantation be deferred and offered as a salvage procedure for those eligible patients who develop a recurrence.

Because the median age of AML is approximately 60 years and only 30 to 35 percent of patients may be expected to have an HLA-identical donor, only a small proportion of individuals with AML will be eligible for allogeneic transplantation, and alternative approaches are required. One such approach is autologous bone marrow transplantation. Bone marrow is harvested and cryopreserved while the patient is in remission. Because of the potential that the harvested marrow may harbor residual leukemic cells, treatment of the marrow with chemotherapeutic agents or monoclonal antibodies and complement is often attempted; however, the efficacy of such purging remains unproved. The patient subsequently receives similar marrow ablative treatment as administered in the allogeneic setting, the stored marrow is thawed, and then reinfused. Preliminary data suggest a 35 to 45 percent likelihood of disease-free survival after 3 years following autografting in adults with AML in first remission, an outcome similar to that associated with intensive chemotherapy or allogeneic bone marrow transplantation. Whether autografting will merely prove to be equivalent to intensive chemotherapy or serve as an effective means of "late intensification" remains to be determined.

Given the absence of new chemotherapeutic agents of significant promise, novel approaches for the treatment of patients with AML are required to improve on current cure rates. Several such approaches are currently under study. The use of hematopoietic growth factors, either to allow added tolerance for high-dose therapy or to synchronize leukemic cells kinetically, is being examined by several groups of investigators. The administration of immunotoxins (a drug or cell poison chemically linked to a leukemia-specific monoclonal antibody) has been associated with promising results in eradicating minimal residual disease in animal models. Finally, attempts at harnessing the "graft-versus-leukemia" effect without the eligibility restrictions and toxicities associated with allografting through the use of lymphokines that enhance natural killer cell activity also have proved to be effective in preclinical trials.

SUGGESTED READING

International bone marrow transplant registry. Transplant or chemotherapy in acute myelogenous leukaemia. Lancet 1989; 1:1119–1122.

Lowenberg B, Verdonck LJ, Dekker AW, et al. Autologous bone marrow transplantation in acute myeloid leukemia in first remission: Results of the Dutch prospective study. J Clin Oncol 1990; 8:287–294.

Mayer RJ. Current chemotherapeutic treatment approaches to the management of previously untreated adults with *de novo* acute myelogenous leukemia. Semin Oncol 1987; 14:384–386.

Mayer RJ. Allogeneic transplantation versus intensive chemotherapy in first-remission acute leukemia: Is there a "best choice"? J Clin Oncol 1988; 6:1532–1536.

ACUTE LEUKEMIA IN CHILDHOOD

STEPHEN E. SALLAN, M.D.
AMY LOUISE BILLETT, M.D.

ACUTE LYMPHOBLASTIC LEUKEMIA

Acute lymphoblastic leukemia (ALL), the most common childhood malignancy, accounts for 75 percent of the 2,000 to 2,500 new cases of acute leukemia diagnosed each year in children in the United States under the age of 15 (Table 1). In the 1950s, almost all children diagnosed with ALL died of their disease within months. In the 1990s, we expect that 65 percent to 70 percent of patients will be cured (Fig. 1).

General Principles of Therapy

The treatment of ALL includes multiple-drug systemic and intrathecal chemotherapy for all patients and cranial irradiation for some. Treatment is usually divided into four phases, beginning with intensive *remission-induction* chemotherapy, which is designed to eradicate all measurable disease. With modern-era chemotherapy, 95 percent of children will achieve complete remission with restoration of normal bone marrow function and no detectable leukemia on bone marrow examination. There is, however, still unmeasurable residual disease at this time.

Table 1 Acute Leukemia in Children

Type	FAB Classification*	Frequency (%)	Cases/Year (US children < age 15)
Acute Lymphoblastic Leukemia (ALL)			1,500–2,000
	L1	85	
	L2	14	
	L3	1	
Acute Myelogenous Leukemia (AML)			400–500
AML—acute myelogenous leukemia	M1	20	
AML—acute myelogenous leukemia with differentiation	M2	20	
APML—acute promyelocytic leukemia	M3	3	
AMMol—acute myelomonocytic leukemia	M4	25	
AMOL—acute monocytic leukemia	M5	26	
Erythroid leukemia	M6	4	
Acute megakaryocytic leukemia	M7	2	

*French–American–British.

The next two phases of therapy, *central nervous system (CNS) therapy* and systemic *intensification*, are often administered concurrently. All children have leukemic invasion of the meninges at diagnosis, although only 3 percent have measurable CNS disease by examination of the cerebrospinal fluid (CSF). Because most systemic chemotherapy does not penetrate into the CNS, specific CNS therapy must be given. Radiation therapy to the cranium and intrathecal chemotherapy have been the mainstay of CNS treatment to date. In an attempt to avoid late effects, however, many investigators are omitting radiation in some patients. Concurrent with specific CNS therapy, it is important to treat intensively the residual systemic disease. *Intensification* therapy with multiple, non–cross-resistant drugs to prevent the emergence of drug-resistant leukemia is given for 1 to 6 months.

The final phase of treatment, *continuation* (or *maintenance*) chemotherapy, consists of less intensive therapy administered to eliminate any residual leukemia cells. Although mercaptopurine and methotrexate have been the mainstay of this phase of therapy, we recommend the addition of prednisone and vincristine. Parenteral therapy is used when possible to obviate problems with poor compliance and drug absorption. We continue treatment for a total of 2 years of continuous complete remission.

Treatment Factors

It is important to identify factors at the time of diagnosis that can guide treatment decisions. Once called *prognostic factors*, we believe that it is more appropriate to call them *treatment factors*, because intensive therapy can change outcome. The most important adverse factors that indicate the need for more intensive therapy include high initial white blood cell count (greater than 20,000 per cubic millimeter); age less than 2 years or greater than 9 years; T-cell immunophenotype; and CNS disease at diagnosis. Still more intensive therapy may be indicated for patients with an initial white blood cell count greater than 100,000 per cubic millimeter, age less than 1 year, or certain chromosomal translocations such as t(9;22) in all patients and t(4;11) in infants. Identification of treatment factors allows the use of the most intensive therapy for the patients at highest risk of relapse.

Presentation

Children with ALL usually present with the signs and symptoms of bone marrow replacement with or without extramedullary invasion. Pallor, fatigue, bleeding, fever, and bone pain are typical manifestations of bone marrow replacement. Extramedullary disease findings include adenopathy, arthralgias, and hepatosplenomegaly.

Diagnosis

The diagnosis of ALL is established by examination of the bone marrow, including morphology, cytochemical

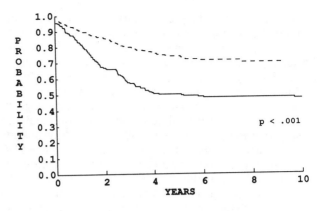

legend:

——— 210 children treated 1973-1979 (DFCI protocols 73-01 and 77-01)

- - - - - 550 children treated 1980-1987 (DFCI 80-01, 81-01, 85-01)

An event was defined as induction-failure, death from any cause, or relapse of leukemia. Patients were censored at time of last known follow-up or when taken off study, other than for failure.

Figure 1 Event-free survival in children with acute lymphoblastic leukemia (ALL) (Dana-Farber Cancer Institute Protocols). An event was defined as induction-failure, death from any cause, or relapse of leukemia. Patients were censored at time of last known follow-up or when taken off study, other than for failure.

stains, immunologic cell surface markers, and cytogenetics. These latter two studies are critical to identify treatment factors at the time of diagnosis, although initial treatment plans can often be developed on the basis of morphology and cytochemical stains alone. Once the diagnosis of leukemia is suspected or established, all patients should be referred to a center staffed by pediatric oncologists familiar with the many aspects of this disease and its treatment. Specific therapy should not be instituted until the diagnosis has been established, except in the rare instance in which a patient is in imminent danger. Because ALL is a rare disease and each patient can contribute to the development of more effective, less morbid future treatments, we always recommend therapy on a research protocol.

Support Care at Diagnosis

Initial management and supportive care to stabilize the patient must be carried out before the institution of specific antileukemia therapy. A chest radiograph can identify the presence of an anterior mediastinal mass. When neurologic assessment reveals a specific deficit, CNS imaging studies are indicated. Somnolence, seizures, stroke, tachypnea, or hypoxemia can be manifestations of leukostasis, which is best treated with leukophoresis or exchange transfusions. Initial metabolic assessment includes measurements of electrolytes, creatinine, uric acid, calcium, phosphate, and magnesium. All patients need twice-maintenance hydration with sodium bicarbonate to maintain high urine output and to alkalinize the urine to prevent urate crystal precipitation within the renal tubules. Immediate institution of allopurinol will help prevent further urate formation. Metabolic parameters must be followed carefully over time, as abnormalities may worsen when specific therapy is instituted and cell lysis occurs. Symptomatic anemia or a hematocrit less than 25 percent requires transfusion with packed red blood cells. All transfused blood products should be irradiated to prevent possible graft-versus-host disease; a white blood cell filter should be used to prevent cytomegalovirus (CMV) transmission and reduce the risk of alloimmunization; and CMV-negative blood should be used if no white blood cell filter is available and the patient is not known to be CMV-positive. Thrombocytopenia is common, and platelet transfusions are indicated for any platelet count less than 20,000 per cubic millimeter if there is any active bleeding. Transfused platelets should be CMV-negative, irradiated, and obtained from a single donor, if possible.

Fever present at the time of diagnosis or at any time during remission-induction chemotherapy requires a thorough physical examination with inspection of all possible sites of disease such as paronychia, perirectal abscess, bone marrow aspiration sites, and all mucocutaneous surfaces. The usual signs of infection, including pus, may be minimal or absent in neutropenic patients. Cultures should be obtained from blood and urine, and CSF if indicated. Antibiotics to treat both gram-positive and gram-negative infections should be instituted immediately in febrile patients. Initial antibiotic choices should be governed by each institution's usual pathogens and patterns of antibiotic resistance. We usually use a combination of mezlocillin and gentamicin.

Remission-Induction Chemotherapy

Remission-induction chemotherapy at our institution includes the use of prednisone daily for 21 days, vincristine weekly for four doses, doxorubicin, methotrexate, and asparaginase at the initiation of therapy, and two doses of intrathecal drug over the course of the first month (Table 2). We use the same regimen for all patients regardless of treatment factors because we believe that initial eradication of disease is crucial. Previous studies have shown improved survival in the setting of four-agent induction and more intensive consolidation and maintenance chemotherapy. Improvements in supportive care have reduced the occurrence of toxic deaths during induction to approximately 3 percent. Most patients require hospitalization throughout remission-induction chemotherapy.

At the end of induction, a bone marrow aspiration should be performed to assess if complete remission, less than 5 percent blasts in the bone marrow and normal peripheral blood counts, has been achieved. If a cytogenetic marker was present in leukemia cells at the time of diagnosis, repeat bone marrow cytogenetic studies should be obtained to document cytogenetic as well as morphologic remission. Although there are currently no reliable molecular techniques to measure minimal residual disease, this will be important in the future management of ALL.

Supportive Care After Induction

Supportive care after the attainment of complete remission includes trimethoprim-sulfamethoxazole administered three consecutive days per week to prevent *Pneumocystis carinii* and other bacterial infections. Varicella zoster virus (VZV) titers should be measured at diagnosis, and patients at risk of disease should receive varicella zoster immune globulin within 96 hours of a known exposure to prevent or ameliorate disease. When VZV vaccine becomes available, it will be indicated for all patients with negative VZV titers. Acyclovir should be given to any child with an active VZV infection to prevent severe, systemic disease.

Central Nervous System Treatment

We initiate CNS therapy during remission-induction chemotherapy with several doses of intrathecal cytarabine. Once complete remission has been obtained, definitive therapy should be instituted. Intrathecal drug

Table 2 Drugs Used for Remission Induction in Acute Lymphoblastic Leukemia
(Dana-Farber Cancer Institute)

Drug	Usual Dosage	Route	Principal Side Effects
Prednisone	40 mg/m^2 daily for 21 days, divided in three doses	PO	Hypertension, hyperglycemia, edema, immunosuppression, obesity, mood changes
Vincristine	1.5 mg/m^2 weekly for three doses (2.0 mg maximum)	IV	Peripheral neuropathy, constipation, alopecia
Doxorubicin	30 mg/m^2 daily for two doses	IV	Mucositis, emesis, myelosuppression, alopecia, cardiac damage, tissue necrosis if extravasation
Methotrexate	40 mg/m^2, one dose	IV	Mucositis, myelosuppression, hepatitis
Asparaginase	20,000 IU/m^2, one dose	IM	Coagulopathy, pancreatitis, allergic reactions, encephalopathy, hepatitis

should also be administered on a regular basis throughout all subsequent treatment. Significant, long-term CNS sequelae related to irradiation and intrathecal drug include growth failure, neuropsychiatric sequelae, and second malignant neoplasms such as brain tumors. We recommend 1,800 cGy to the cranium with concurrent administration of four doses of intrathecal methotrexate and cytarabine for high-risk patients, and we treat others with intrathecal chemotherapy alone. For those rare patients who present with CNS leukemia at diagnosis, we give intrathecal drugs twice weekly until the CSF is clear of blasts and then institute cranial radiation therapy with concurrent intrathecal therapy after complete hematologic remission has been obtained.

Intensification and Continuation Therapy

Once complete remission has been obtained, we institute intensive chemotherapy concurrent with specific CNS therapy (Table 3). Patients between ages 2 and 9 years, with white blood counts less than 20,000 per cubic milliliter, and with no other adverse factors at diagnosis, receive 20 weekly doses of intramuscular asparaginase (25,000 IU per square meter). Approximately 30 percent of patients develop a mild allergic response to *Escherichia coli* asparaginase, such as local tenderness and erythema or mild systemic urticaria. Two-thirds of these patients will tolerate *Erwinia* asparaginase.

Concurrent with the intensive use of asparaginase, patients receive regular chemotherapy that includes a 5-day course of prednisone (40 mg per square meter per day) every 3 weeks, intravenous vincristine (2 mg per square meter) every 3 weeks, a 14-day course of oral mercaptopurine (50 mg per square meter per day) every 3 weeks, and intramuscular methotrexate (40 mg per square meter) weekly 1 day after asparaginase. Once 20 doses of asparaginase have been completed, patients continue to receive the other four drugs until a total of 2 years of continuous complete remission has been obtained. We also give intrathecal methotrexate and cytarabine every 18 weeks throughout the course of therapy.

Patients with high-risk features such as white blood cell count over 20,000 per cubic millimeter, age less than 2 years or greater than 9 years, CNS disease, anterior mediastinal mass, or T-cell disease at diagnosis receive more intensive therapy with 6 to 9 months of asparaginase and doxorubicin. Doxorubicin is administered at 30 mg per square meter every 3 weeks to a cumulative total dose of 360 mg per square meter. Weekly intramuscular asparaginase is given concurrently with doxorubicin. During this time period, vincristine, prednisone, and mercaptopurine are administered as described previously. Methotrexate then replaces doxorubicin and asparaginase, and all patients continue to receive systemic and intrathecal chemotherapy until they have been in continuous complete remission for a total of 2 years.

Because modern chemotherapy results in cure for approximately two-thirds of children with ALL, we do not recommend bone marrow transplantation in first remission except for patients with the Philadelphia translocation, t(9;22). The natural history of mature

Table 3 Drugs Used for Intensification and Continuation Therapy in Acute Lymphoblastic Leukemia (Dana-Farber Cancer Institute)

Drug	Usual Dosage	Route	Principal Side Effects
Asparaginase*	20,000 IU/m² weekly for 5–9 months	IM	Coagulopathy, pancreatitis, allergic reactions, encephalopathy, hepatitis
Prednisone	40 mg/m² in three divided doses daily for 5 days every 3 weeks	PO	Hypertension, hyperglycemia, edema, immunosuppression, obesity, mood changes
Vincristine	2 mg/m² every 3 weeks (2 mg maximum)	IV	Peripheral neuropathy, constipation, alopecia
Methotrexate†	30 mg/m² weekly	IM or IV	Mucositis, myelosuppression, hepatitis
6–Mercaptopurine	50 mg/m² daily for 14 consecutive days every 3 weeks	PO	Myelosuppression, mucositis, hepatitis
Doxorubicin‡	30 mg/m² every 3 weeks until cumulative dose is 360 mg/m²	IV	Mucositis, emesis, myelosuppression, alopecia, cardiac damage, tissue necrosis if extravasation

*Asparaginase is given weekly for 20 doses in patients with no high-risk treatment factors and concurrent with doxorubicin in all other patients.

†Methotrexate is started as soon as patient is in remission if there are no high-risk treatment factors and at completion of doxorubicin if there are any high-risk treatment factors.

‡Doxorubicin is given to patients with any high-risk treatment factor.

B-cell ALL with surface immunoglobulin and L3 morphology mimics that of advanced Burkitt's lymphoma. We therefore treat these patients with a 2-month, very intensive regimen with cyclophosphamide, cytarabine, and methotrexate. We do not have a separate treatment program for patients with T-cell ALL, but we treat them as we do other children with high-risk treatment factors.

Relapsed Acute Lymphoblastic Leukemia

Relapsed ALL is currently the sixth most common childhood malignancy in the United States, and outcome is usually dismal. Adverse prognostic factors at the time of relapse include a short duration of initial remission, bone marrow involvement, and intensive initial therapy. Reinduction therapy should include the use of multiple drugs such as vincristine, prednisone, asparaginase, and an anthracycline. As primary therapy has become more intensive, second complete remission rates have dropped from above 90 percent to less than 75 percent.

If complete remission is obtained, intensive chemotherapy to eradicate minimal residual disease is indicated. Continuation chemotherapy, however, cures less than 30 percent of patients in most reported series. Because survival after matched, allogeneic transplantation in second remission is 30 percent to 70 percent in different studies, we recommend transplantation for all patients who achieve a second remission. For the 80 percent of patients without a potential allogeneic donor, we recommend purged, autologous transplantation when feasible. Survival at 2 years is approximately 30 percent with this treatment. The efficacy of matched unrelated donor transplantation or mismatched transplantation for relapsed ALL is currently under investigation.

For patients without a bone marrow transplantation option, intensive chemotherapy is indicated, although overall prognosis is poor. In the setting of multiply relapsed ALL, experimental treatment such as innovative chemotherapy, matched unrelated donor transplantation, mismatched transplantation, or immunotherapy may be indicated.

ACUTE MYELOGENOUS LEUKEMIA

Acute myelogenous leukemia (AML) represents approximately 15 percent to 20 percent of all childhood leukemia. Advances in therapy in the past 20 years have resulted in complete remission rates of approximately 80 percent, with 65 percent of patients remaining in continuous complete remission.

Although many of the treatment concepts in AML are similar to those in ALL, there are some important differences. In theory, much more myelosuppressive therapy with different drugs is required to treat AML than ALL because AML is a stem-cell disease. If complete remission is achieved, allogeneic bone marrow transplantation is recommended because such therapy has resulted in more long-term cures. Whether or not autologous bone marrow transplantation will be superior to chemotherapy is currently under active investigation. If bone marrow transplantation is not performed, chemotherapy while the patient is in remission is indicated.

Presentation

The presentation of AML is very similar to that of ALL, with certain exceptions. In general, children with AML are sicker at the time of diagnosis than children with ALL. Leukostasis is more common in AML, and disseminated intravascular coagulation is often seen in association with acute promyelocytic leukemia (M3). Infants with AML may present with hepatosplenomegaly, leukemia cutis, CNS disease, very high initial white counts, and monocytic leukemia (M5). Chloromas or myeloblastomas may occur in any soft-tissue location.

Diagnosis

The differential diagnosis of a child who presents with AML includes ALL, chronic myeloproliferative disorders, myelodysplastic syndromes, aplastic anemia, and overwhelming infection. In infants with trisomy 21, a transient myeloproliferative syndrome must be excluded. The diagnosis of AML is established by morphologic and cytochemical stains of the bone marrow and further characterized by studies of immunologic cell surface markers and cytogenetics.

Supportive Care

Initial management and supportive care do not differ significantly between AML and ALL, although hyperleukocytosis and leukostasis are more common in AML. Specific therapy for AML should be instituted as soon as a patient is stable and the diagnosis is unequivocal. We always recommend treatment on a research protocol at an institution familiar with the diagnosis and treatment of children with this disease.

Induction

The goal of induction therapy is to reduce the leukemia cell burden to undetectable levels by both clinical and hematologic parameters. A combination of daunorubicin and cytarabine form the basis of most successful induction regimens. Thioguanine or etoposide are often used in conjunction with these agents. Because single-arm studies suggest that the use of a third agent may increase the complete remission rate in pediatric AML, we currently use a three-drug regimen including cytarabine (100 mg per square meter per day) administered as a 7-day continuous infusion, daunorubicin (45 mg per square meter per day) administered as three consecutive bolus doses, and thioguanine (100 mg per square meter per day) administered for a total of 1 week.

Induction therapy requires careful attention to the

issues of toxicity of therapy and supportive care. Five to ten percent of the patients die from complications such as infection or hemorrhage. Chemotherapy-induced mucosal damage and concurrent severe myelosuppression frequently cause gastrointestinal problems. Patients are at high risk of infection, and enterocolitis or typhlitis is relatively common.

Central Nervous System Therapy

Central nervous system disease at the time of diagnosis occurs in approximately 20 percent of patients but is not an adverse prognostic factor. Historical data have shown that without specific CNS therapy, CNS relapse will occur in approximately 20 percent of patients in hematologic complete remission. Intrathecal drugs such as cytarabine and methotrexate and radiation therapy are all effective agents to prevent CNS relapse. We currently use intrathecal cytarabine alone.

Continuation Chemotherapy

As in ALL, there is presumed residual disease at the end of induction chemotherapy; thus, continuation therapy is indicated. There are no data to support the use of more than 1 year of treatment in remission. With less intensive regimens, approximately 30 percent of patients remained in continuous complete remission for 2 or more years from diagnosis. The most intensive chemotherapy regimens have provided long-term continuous complete remission rates of 45 percent.

Bone Marrow Transplantation

Because chemotherapy is curative in less than 50 percent of patients with AML, allogeneic bone marrow transplantation in first complete remission has become the treatment of choice. Leukemia-free survival can be expected in 60 percent of children with AML after allogeneic bone marrow transplantation in first remission. The major causes of death are graft-versus-host disease and interstitial pneumonitis, although toxicity is usually less severe in children than in adults. In contrast, most failures after transplantation for ALL result from recurrent leukemia.

Because only 20 percent of patients have an allogeneic donor, the role of autologous bone marrow transplantation is under active investigation. Current protocols randomize children who do not have a donor to receive either a short course of chemotherapy or an autologous bone marrow transplant with in vitro purging of the marrow. Results of such studies are too early to evaluate.

Relapsed Acute Myelogenous Leukemia

When children with AML have a relapse, reinduction is extremely difficult, and fewer than 50 percent of such children achieve a second complete remission. If second remission is obtained, its duration is usually short, despite ongoing chemotherapy. Allogeneic or autologous bone marrow transplantation, either in early relapse or in second complete remission, is recommended. For those few patients who relapse after initial chemotherapy, achieve second complete remission, and undergo bone marrow transplantation, survival ranges from 30 percent to 40 percent.

SUGGESTED READING

Brochstein JA, Kernan NA, Groshen S, et al. Allogeneic bone marrow transplantation after hyperfractionated total-body irradiation and cyclophosphamide in children with acute leukemia. N Engl J Med 1987; 317:1,618–1,624.
Clavell LA, Gelber RD, Cohen HJ, et al. Four-agent induction and intensive asparaginase therapy for treatment of childhood acute lymphoblastic leukemia. N Engl J Med 1986; 315:657–663.
Lampkin BC, Masterson M, Sambrano JE, et al. Current chemotherapeutic strategies in childhood acute nonlymphocytic leukemia. Semin Oncol 1987; 14:397.
Riehm H, Gadner H, Henze G, et al. Results and significance of randomized trials in four consecutive ALL-BFM studies. In: Buchner T, Shellong G, Hiddemann W, et al, eds. Haematology and blood transfusion 33: Acute leukemias II. Berlin: Springer-Verlag, 1990:439–450.
Rivera GK, Santana V, Mahmoud H, et al. Acute lymphocytic leukemia of childhood: The problem of relapses. Bone Marrow Transplant 1989; 4 (Suppl 1):80–85.

HAIRY CELL LEUKEMIA

LEONIDAS C. PLATANIAS, M.D.
MARK J. RATAIN, M.D.

Hairy cell leukemia is a rare lymphoproliferative disease, usually of B-cell origin. The disease has a chronic course characterized by splenomegaly, pancytopenia, and the appearance of the characteristic "hairy cells" in the peripheral blood and bone marrow. Even though this disease compares favorably in terms of prognosis to other lymphoproliferative disorders, it still has a progressive course and is usually complicated by severe cytopenias and life-threatening infections, requiring therapeutic intervention. Over the last few years, significant progress has been made in the understanding of its biology and treatment. The use of interferon and pentostatin has led to a dramatic improvement in the prognosis of patients with hairy cell leukemia. The therapeutic options for the physician are clearly better than they were in the recent past. Before deciding the appropriate therapy for each individual patient, a careful diagnostic evaluation to confirm the diagnosis, and a precise assessment of the disease status must be performed.

DIAGNOSIS

The diagnosis of hairy cell leukemia can be established by the clinical presentation, the peripheral blood smear, and the bone marrow biopsy. Patients may present with symptoms related to pancytopenia such as fatigue secondary to severe anemia, bleeding secondary to thrombocytopenia, and bacterial or opportunistic infections associated with neutropenia or the underlying immune deficiency. Splenomegaly is usually the most prominent physical finding, and in some patients it can cause pain and easy satiety. Fifty percent of the patients are pancytopenic at the time of diagnosis. Approximately 20 percent of the patients present during the leukemic phase of the disease and have a white blood cell count higher than 10,000 per μl, with more than 50 percent hairy cells in the peripheral blood smear. A bone marrow biopsy is required to establish the diagnosis of hairy cell leukemia definitively. The bone marrow is usually hypercellular with diffuse infiltration by hairy cells. The staining for tartrate-resistant acid phosphatase (TRAP) is almost always positive, but this finding is not pathognomonic and can be found in other lymphoproliferative disorders. In atypical cases in which a diagnostic dilemma exists, electron microscopy is sometimes useful by demonstrating the characteristic morphology of hairy cells. Immunocytochemistry can also be useful in difficult cases. Staining of the bone marrow with monoclonal antibodies against antigens expressed by hairy cells, such as CD11c, CD22, and CD25, may be helpful in the differential diagnosis of lymphoproliferative disorders.

INDICATIONS FOR TREATMENT

Approximately 10 percent of patients with hairy cell leukemia have a long-term survival of more than 10 years without receiving any form of therapy. Therefore, it is important before instituting any form of therapy to establish an absolute indication for treatment. Table 1 lists the criteria used to decide which patients require treatment. It is not uncommon to see asymptomatic

Table 1 Criteria for Institution of Treatment

Hemoglobin <10 g/dl
Platelet count <100,000/μl
Granulocyte count <1,000/μl
Recurrent bacterial or opportunistic infections
Symptomatic splenomegaly
Leukemic phase (WBC >20,000/μl)
Tissue infiltration (i.e., bony lesions)
Autoimmune complications

patients with mild pancytopenias who were diagnosed with hairy cell leukemia subsequent to a routine blood count. Many of them require only observation and careful follow-up of their disease status until evidence of disease progression.

SPLENECTOMY

Despite the significant advances in the management of hairy cell leukemia over the last few years, splenectomy remains the treatment of choice for many newly diagnosed patients. The aim of splenectomy in these patients is not cure, but rather palliation of symptoms and temporary control of the manifestations of the disease. In patients with hairy cell leukemia the spleen is almost always involved, but the degree of splenomegaly varies. Hypersplenism contributes significantly in the development of pancytopenia in these patients. Therefore, splenectomy is a logical approach for the control of cytopenias in patients who present with significant splenomegaly but only minimal or moderate bone marrow involvement. The size of the spleen has not been found to correlate with response to splenectomy, and the factor that determines the response to surgery is the degree of bone marrow cellularity and/or leukemic infiltration. Patients with a bone marrow cellularity of less than 85 percent seem to have good and prolonged responses to splenectomy, and unless other indications for systemic therapy are present, should be considered candidates for surgery. Approximately 50 percent of the patients who undergo splenectomy will show a partial response with a return of their blood counts to normal values. Another 40 percent will have a minor response with a rise of one or two hematologic parameters. Despite the dramatic effects of splenectomy in carefully selected patients, most patients will relapse within 5 to 10 years and will require systemic therapy.

The preoperative care of a patient with hairy cell leukemia who is to undergo splenectomy is not different from other hematologic diseases where splenectomy is indicated. A vaccine for pneumococcal infection should be administered preoperatively, and special attention should be undertaken in the immediate diagnosis and treatment of infectious complications, especially in neutropenic patients. The procedure is usually not problematic for experienced surgeons despite the very large spleen size. The postoperative recovery of the patients is similar to that of other patients who undergo abdominal surgery. The first sign of hematologic recovery is a rise in the platelet count that occurs within days or weeks. The neutrophil count and the hemoglobin follow subsequently.

As mentioned earlier, splenectomy has an important role in the management of many patients with hairy cell leukemia. In rare instances in which the diagnosis cannot be established despite the routine diagnostic work-up, splenectomy can be useful diagnostically. There are occasional patients who present with splenomegaly and pancytopenia, without circulating hairy cells in the peripheral blood, and with an atypical bone marrow morphology. In these cases the diagnosis of hairy cell leukemia versus other low-grade lymphoproliferative malignancies can be very difficult. Splenectomy may be indicated in such patients both for its therapeutic role in restoring blood counts, and to provide ample material for pathologic examination.

INTERFERON-ALPHA

Interferon-alpha was first reported to have activity in hairy cell leukemia in 1984. Its activity was confirmed in multicenter trials in the United States, and the drug is now approved by the FDA for use in this disease. Interferon-alpha is a biologic response modifier that also has shown activity in other hematologic diseases such as nodular lymphomas, multiple myeloma, and chronic myelogenous leukemia. Hairy cell leukemia is the disease in which interferon-alpha seems to be most effective. Its mechanism of action is not well understood. Possible mechanisms for its effect, supported by in vitro experimental data, include induction of differentiation of hairy cells, activation of natural killer cells with subsequent killing of the malignant cells, and induction of class II major histocompatibility antigens on the surface of hairy cells. Other studies have shown that interferon inhibits the release of growth factors for hairy cells such as tumor necrosis factor (TNF), and low-molecular–weight B-cell growth factor (BCGF), postulating that its action may be by disruption of autocrine loops. Finally, interferon-alpha may have a direct action on the in vitro differentiation of multilineage lympho-myeloid stem cells and enhance the formation of normal hematopoietic elements.

Two types of recombinant interferon-alpha have been used extensively in clinical trials in hairy cell leukemia: Interferon alpha-2a (Hoffmann-LaRoche), and interferon alpha-2b (Schering-Plough). Both of these products have shown similar activity in the induction of remission, but the incidence of neutralizing antibodies subsequent to use of interferon alpha-2a appears to be higher, as discussed later. Interferon-alpha has activity both in previously splenectomized patients with disease progression and in patients who never underwent splenectomy. Its use is clearly indicated in patients who have a relapse after initial remission with splenectomy, as well as in patients who do not show a significant response to splenectomy.

As shown in Figure 1 there is a group of patients who may best benefit by initial treatment with interferon. Patients with a very hypercellular bone marrow (cellularity >85 percent), patients in the leukemic phase of the disease, and patients with tissue involvement such as

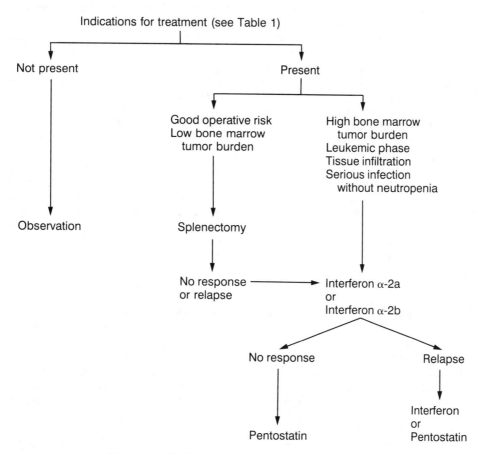

Figure 1 Guide for treatment in hairy cell leukemia.

bony lesions or large lymphadenopathy are better candidates for initial interferon induction therapy. A small number of patients present with opportunistic infections without neutropenia. These patients have a serious underlying cellular immunodeficiency and will benefit more by the use of interferon-alpha. Patients with indications for splenectomy who refuse surgery should also be offered interferon treatment.

The usual dose of interferon alpha-2b is 2×10^6 per square meter units three times a week administered subcutaneously. The treatment should be continued for 12 months. Prolongation of treatment to 18 months delays the relapse rate while the treatment continues, but does not extend the length of remission duration after treatment is discontinued. Therefore, treatment beyond 12 months should be considered only if there are no significant side effects and the treatment is well tolerated. However, this is not the case in most patients who continue treatment for more than 12 months, as they develop a chronic fatigue syndrome necessitating discontinuation of treatment. Studies using a lower dose regimen (2×10^5 units/m^2 given three times per week) have shown inferior results to the standard regimen (2×10^6 u/m^2 three times per week), and this low-dose regimen is not recommended in the treatment of hairy cell leukemia. It is possible that chronic maintenance treatment with lower doses may be useful in maintaining remission induced with standard doses, although this use is clearly investigational. Interferon alpha-2a is usually administered at a dose of 3 million units daily for 6 months. It is not clear which dose, product, and schedule is better, but the treatment three times weekly with interferon alpha-2b allows easier evaluation of patients who develop fever during treatment in distinguishing infections from interferon toxicity.

The side effects of treatment are usually well tolerated. During the first week of treatment patients develop a flu-like syndrome that resolves after 2 to 4 weeks. The fever that these patients develop can be controlled with acetaminophen. Other side effects include fatigue, dry mouth, and discomfort at the site of injection. A significant percentage of patients may experience toxicities such as transient skin rashes and gastrointestinal disorders. Only rare patients develop central nervous system toxicity or peripheral neuropathy that requires discontinuation of treatment. Myelosuppression, including a decrease in both neutrophil and platelet counts, occurs in many patients within the first month of treatment. These decreases are transient, and the treatment should be continued despite the decreases.

The assessment of therapeutic response in pancytopenic patients receiving interferon therapy should be primarily based on hematologic parameters. A rise in the platelet count is often the first evidence of response, and usually normalizes within 2 months. The hemoglobin and neutrophil counts usually normalize over the subsequent 1 to 8 months of therapy. In patients with the leukemic phase of the disease the white blood cell count should decrease within 2 weeks and normalize by 8 weeks. In nonsplenectomized patients, the spleen size decreases slowly. Similarly the bone marrow biopsy in these patients shows gradual reduction in the number of infiltrating hairy cells. The immunologic abnormalities also correct with interferon therapy, and the initially decreased monocyte and natural killer cell counts will improve after about 3 months of treatment. With the normalization of the neutrophil count and the correction of the immunologic abnormalities, the number of infectious episodes decreases dramatically. Neutrophil alkaline phosphatase (NAP) and the serum soluble interleukin-2 receptor are two markers that have been shown to correlate with disease activity. With interferon treatment the levels of both of these decrease gradually and have been shown to correlate with the response to treatment. Serial follow-up of these markers may be useful to assess response and possibly predict future relapse.

As has been previously reported in a large multicenter trial, approximately 80 percent of patients have a partial response with normalization of all three cell lines and associated decrease of bone marrow involvement, and 7 percent have a minor response with improvement of at least one blood count. Other studies have demonstrated similar results, confirming the therapeutic efficacy of interferon in this disease. From the follow-up of the patients who were treated with interferon-alpha in large clinical trials it seems that approximately 50 percent of them relapse within 2 years after cessation of therapy. These patients may again develop anemia, thrombocytopenia, neutropenia, hyperleukocytosis, or tissue infiltration, and almost all patients will require further treatment. However, most patients will respond to a second course of interferon and obtain second remissions.

It is not clearly defined which patients should be retreated with interferon or receive 2'-deoxycoformycin at the first relapse. It seems that the treatment of relapsed patients should be individualized based on the previous tolerance to interferon treatment and the duration and quality of response. For instance, a patient who obtained a remission with previous interferon therapy and presents with a relapse after a long period of remission (i.e., 2 to 4 years), should be retreated with interferon. On the other hand, a patient who relapsed only a few months after obtaining a partial remission with interferon should probably receive pentostatin treatment, as discussed in the following section.

Recently, it has been recognized that some patients can develop resistance to interferon associated with the development of neutralizing antibodies during treatment. Both neutralizing and non-neutralizing antibodies to interferon alpha-2a develop in approximately 60 percent of patients receiving this treatment. Half of these patients develop neutralizing antibodies and one-third of them become resistant to treatment. Whether these antibodies are of clinical significance is still questionable, and further studies to evaluate their association with failure to response are required. In contrast to interferon alpha-2a, development of antibodies to interferon-alpha-2b is very rare, and in our institution we observed only one case in 69 treated patients.

2'-DEOXYCOFORMYCIN (PENTOSTATIN)

Pentostatin is still an experimental drug, currently used in clinical trials in the United States. The drug has shown significant activity in this disease, inducing complete remission in approximately 50 to 80 percent of patients with hairy cell leukemia and partial remissions in the remainder. The drug is a purine analogue with potent inhibitory activity against adenosine deaminase (ADA), and thus has selective toxicity against lymphocytes. Adenosine deaminase is an enzyme that regulates intracellular adenosine levels through deamination of adenosine and deoxyadenosine. Normal T and B lymphocytes have high levels of this enzyme, but most leukemic cells have much higher levels. There is evidence to suggest that pentostatin, by inhibiting adenosine deaminase, can cause single-strand DNA breaks, deplete NAD levels, and inhibit transcellular methylation reactions and intracellular ATP levels. It is of interest that hairy cells have lower levels of ADA than other malignant and normal lymphoid cells, and this could explain their extreme sensitivity to pentostatin. This agent has activity in many lymphoproliferative diseases, including chronic lymphocytic leukemia, prolymphocytic leukemia, acute T-cell leukemia, mycosis fungoides, and hairy cell leukemia. Responses in hairy cell leukemia can be obtained with relatively low, less toxic, doses of the drug, in contrast to the other malignancies that require high doses with subsequent serious toxicities.

As mentioned earlier, pentostatin is still an experimental agent, and its activity and safety are still being tested in patients with resistance to interferon as well as in previously untreated patients. The high number of complete responses that has been obtained in preliminary clinical trials strongly suggests that the drug will have a major role in the routine management of hairy cell leukemia. So far, almost all of the complete responses are durable (with a median follow-up of 2 years), in contrast to those obtained with interferon treatment. It is possible that pentostatin may be curative in hairy cell leukemia, although longer follow-up is necessary to determine if this drug will keep its clinical promise.

The drug is administered intravenously at a dose of 4 to 5 mg per square meter every 14 to 28 days. The most important toxicities are nausea, vomiting, conjunctivitis, skin rash, and myelosuppression. At the dose levels used in hairy cell leukemia, renal insufficiency is rare and reversible after discontinuation of the drug. The major concern for the use of pentostatin is its immunosuppressive effects and the potential for long-term immunosuppression. Studies have shown that pentostatin induces lymphopenia and a decrease of natural killer cell function, in contrast to interferon therapy, which has an opposite immunostimulatory effect. The pentostatin-induced immunosuppression has been reported to last at least 6 months after discontinuation of therapy. The clinical consequences of this phenomenon are unclear, however, because affected patients do not develop increased incidence of opportunistic infections in short-term follow-up, although sporadic cases of opportunistic infections have been reported.

The response to pentostatin is rapid with a platelet count rise seen within the first 2 weeks of treatment. The hemoglobin and neutrophil count improve within the first 2 months, and clearance of the hairy cells from the bone marrow is seen within 6 months. The size of the spleen decreases rapidly, and the levels of NAP and serum-soluble interleukin 2 receptor also decrease rapidly, reflecting the rapid decrease of hairy cell tumor burden.

Until this drug is better studied and obtains FDA approval, our recommendation is that only patients in whom interferon therapy has failed or in whom relapse occurs after initial response to interferon be treated with pentostatin. Patients can receive pentostatin by participating in the ongoing clinical trials or by obtaining the drug from the National Cancer Institute through the special exception mechanism. This mechanism gives clinicians the opportunity to obtain pentostatin for individual patients by applying to the Division of Cancer Treatment of the NCI.

Interferon and pentostatin are compared in Table 2.

CHEMOTHERAPY

The use of chemotherapeutic agents other than pentostatin has thus far been of limited success. Chlorambucil as a single agent was used prior to the institution of interferon treatment, and has been shown to induce partial remissions in some patients. High-dose methotrexate with leucovorin rescue has also given partial responses in patients refractory to splenectomy, but the experience with this treatment has been limited. It seems that with the current advances in the treatment of this disease with interferon and pentostatin other traditional chemotherapeutic agents have little place in its management.

SUPPORTIVE THERAPY

Infections

Infection is the major cause of morbidity and mortality in hairy cell leukemia. Bacterial infections in neutropenic patients with hairy cell leukemia should be managed promptly with rapid institution of broad-spectrum antibiotics. Life-threatening infections in these patients also have been reported in the absence of absolute neutropenia. Special attention should be given to neutropenic patients receiving pentostatin, because the drug is myelosuppressive and causes further decrease of the neutrophil count early in its course. In neutropenic patients with fever, antibiotic therapy

Table 2 Interferon and Pentostatin in the Treatment of Hairy Cell Leukemia

Drug	Mechanism of Action	Complete Remissions	Partial Remissions	Adverse Effects
Interferon-alpha	Unknown	< 5 %	80%	Fever Flu-like syndrome CNS toxicity GI toxicity Chronic fatigue syndrome Myelosuppression Development of antibodies
Pentostatin	ADA inhibitor	60–90 %	10–40 %	Nausea Vomiting Skin rash Myelosuppression Renal toxicity Immunosuppression

should be continued for 2 weeks even in the absence of an infectious source. Most of the patients with neutropenia and fever will respond to treatment within the first 3 to 4 days. If the fever persists, antifungal therapy with amphotericin B should be instituted.

Recently it has been reported that neutropenic patients with hairy cell leukemia can respond to granulocyte-colony stimulating factor (G-CSF) with a significant rise of the neutrophil count. It is possible that the administration of this agent in neutropenic patients with serious infection could have an impact in clinical outcome.

Because of the underlying cellular immunodeficiency, patients with hairy cell leukemia are susceptible to infections with a variety of opportunistic organisms, including atypical mycobacteria, *Pneumocystis carinii,* cytomegalovirus and *Toxoplasma gondii.* Increased suspicion for the diagnosis and prompt institution of the appropriate therapy are required to avoid possible catastrophic sequences from these infections. Patients with hairy cell leukemia who present with fever, respiratory symptoms, and a diffuse interstitial infiltrate should undergo bronchoscopy to establish the diagnosis of opportunistic infection. Cultures for *Mycobacterium tuberculosis* and atypical mycobacteria should be sent to the laboratory. Acid-fast stain and Giemsa or Gomori methenamine silver stains should be obtained. The diagnosis of cytomegalovirus or *Toxoplasma* can be established accurately by demonstrating intranuclear and cytoplasmic inclusion bodies and trophozoites, respectively, in the tissue obtained from the lung biopsy. If the material obtained by the bronchoscopy is not sufficient to establish the diagnosis, an open lung biopsy should be undertaken. In our institution, patients with hairy cell leukemia who present with *Mycobacterium avium-intracellulare* (MAI) infection are treated with a five-drug regimen that includes rifampicin, ethambutol, streptomycin, cycloserine, and ethionamide. Although the efficacy of this regimen is still under investigation, we recommend this aggressive antibiotic regimen, concomitantly with interferon treatment for hairy cell leukemia if indicated, because this infection can be successfully treated in those patients who show a response to interferon.

Bleeding

Life-threatening bleeding is rarely a problem in patients with hairy cell leukemia, even in the presence of serious thrombocytopenia. When necessary, platelet transfusions should be given. With the rapid increase of the platelet count in patients undergoing splenectomy or receiving systemic therapy one should not expect serious problems for prolonged periods of time. In the rare instances in which patients present with severe thrombocytopenia and bleeding, emergency splenectomy should be considered. The patients should receive enough platelet transfusions to make the surgery feasible.

FUTURE THERAPIES

One agent that may be clinically useful is 2-chlorodeoxyadenosine, an adenosine deaminase–resistant purine analogue that selectively accumulates in cells rich in deoxycytidine kinase and has high specificity for malignant cells. In a preliminary trial the drug has been shown to induce complete remissions in five of six patients treated, with virtually no toxicity. These remissions have lasted as long as 2 years. This drug is very promising because of the lack of toxicity and its probable high therapeutic efficacy, and in the future may prove to be better than interferon and pentostatin.

Future therapies may focus on agents that would interrupt the autocrine loops required for leukemic cell growth. Tumor necrosis factor has been shown to be an autocrine growth factor for leukemic hairy cells. It is possible that TNF antagonists or monoclonal antibodies to TNF may have activity in hairy cell leukemia. Laboratory studies are now underway to better define this phenomenon, and these may lead to new, efficient, and more specific ways of treating this rare disease.

SUGGESTED READING

Golomb HM, Jacobs A, Fefer A, et al. Alpha-2 interferon therapy of hairy-cell leukemia: A multicenter study of 64 patients. J Clin Oncol 1986; 4:900–905.

Ratain MJ, Golomb HM, Vardiman JW, et al. Relapse after interferon alpha-2b therapy for hairy cell leukemia: analysis of prognostic variables. J Clin Oncol 1988; 6:1714–1721.

Ratain MJ, Vardiman JW, Barker CM, et al. Prognostic variables in hairy cell leukemia after splenectomy as initial therapy. Cancer 1988; 62:2420–2424.

Spiers ASD, Moore D, Cassileth PA, et al. Remissions in hairy-cell leukemia with pentostatin (2'-deoxycoformycin). N Engl J Med 1987; 316:825–830.

ALLOGENEIC BONE MARROW TRANSPLANTATION

HANS A. MESSNER, M.D., Ph.D., FRCPC

Allogeneic bone marrow transplants (BMT) are performed with curative intent in a wide variety of hemopoietic disorders. These include severe aplastic anemia, immune deficiency disorders, acute leukemia, chronic myeloid leukemia, and other hemopoietic malignancies, as well as a number of genetic defects. The commonly used preparative regimens usually combine high-dose chemotherapy with total body irradiation (TBI). The purpose of these pretreatment schedules is to suppress the immune system of the host to induce graft tolerance and to eliminate malignant cell populations in recipients with hemopoietic neoplasms. Chemotherapy and TBI are delivered at maximum dose as determined by the toxic influence on the next most sensitive organ or organ system. Complications of BMT may relate to toxicity of the preparative regimen or its failure to control immunologically active, or residual malignant cell populations of the host. The transplant procedure also may be associated with poor engraftment, slow reconstitution of the immune system, or the development of graft-versus-host disease.

PREPARATIVE REGIMENS

The majority of transplant centers have used regimens that combine one or more chemotherapeutic agents with TBI. Some centers have explored the use of high-dose single or combination chemotherapy without radiation for various indications.

Total Body Irradiation

The classic regimen for hemopoietic malignancies combined cyclophosphamide (CTX) at a dose of 60 mg per kilogram per day for 2 days with 1,000 cGy TBI. At the different centers, TBI was delivered either by cobalt sources or linear accelerators at dose rates that varied from 2 to 85 cGy per minute. This schedule resulted in sustained engraftment and prolonged disease-free and relapse-free survival. However, it was also associated with radiation-induced interstitial pneumonitis in a significant proportion of recipients when radiation was delivered in dose rates that exceeded 5 to 8 cGy per minute. Two changes in the delivery of radiation have nearly eliminated radiation-induced interstitial pneumonitis:

The majority of transplant teams adopted fractionated total body irradiation (FTBI), where a cumulative dose of 1,200 to 1,350 cGy is given in six fractions at dose rates up to 30 cGy per minute.

Based on a large experience with palliative, wide-field radiation, our own institution elected to reduce TBI to a single dose of 500 cGy delivered at 50 to 85 cGy per minute by a single cobalt source.

Both schedules appear to result in comparable disease-free survival rates as a measurement of their biologic effect on malignant cell populations.

Chemotherapy

Many centers have continued to use CTX as previously described. Other groups have added additional chemotherapeutic agents such as cytosine arabinoside at various doses, dimethylmyleran, doxorubicin (Adriamycin), melphalan, and others. In some studies, particularly those of high-risk patients, CTX was replaced by VP-16, high-dose cytosine arabinoside, or high-dose cytosine arabinoside combined with mitoxantrone. None of these variations have improved disease-free survival significantly, although the regimen combining VP-16 with FTBI shows some promise.

The combined use of high-dose busulfan and CTX and the omission of TBI represents an alternative approach to the above mentioned regimens with similar long-term, disease-free survival in comparable patient populations.

CLINICAL RESULTS

Leukemia

Single-institution studies and BMT registry reviews have identified a number of recipient-related risk factors that contribute to the clinical outcome of BMT. These include recipient age, disease status at BMT, and history of exposure to cytomegalovirus (CMV). The observed clinical results in various analyses are generally in agreement. Patients transplanted in first remission acute myeloid leukemia (AML), acute lymphoblastic leukemia (ALL), or chronic phase chronic myeloid leukemia (CML) have a 50 to 65 percent long-term, disease-free and relapse-free survival. The results are less favorable when the procedure is performed in patients who have more advanced disease. The survival rates may vary from as low as 10 to 35 percent. The difference in long-term survival of both patient groups is related to an increased relapse rate in patients transplanted with more advanced disease.

Other Hemopoietic Malignancies

The benefit of BMT for other hemopoietic malignancies is less well defined. For instance, patients with myeloma and malignant lymphoma appear to have a very high relapse rate, and only 20 to 30 percent of transplant recipients demonstrate long-term, disease-free survival.

Aplastic Anemia

Until very recently, BMT was the treatment of choice for patients with severe aplastic anemia. A cure rate that exceeded 80 percent was observed for patients who were untransfused before receiving the transplant. The recent use of methotrexate (MTX) and cyclosporine as prophylaxis for graft-versus-host disease (GVHD) appears to approach these results for previously transfused patients. However, developments such as the availability of antithymocyte globulin (ATG), the effectiveness of cyclosporine in the treatment of severe aplastic anemia, and the future use of recombinant hemopoietic growth factors such as erythropoietin and GM-CSF, G-CSF or IL3 may require re-evaluation of BMT for this disease. Currently, the advantage of BMT is related to a more complete re-establishment of hemopoiesis. Disadvantages include graft rejection and transplant-related complications such as GVHD and CMV pneumonitis. Patients treated with ATG or cyclosporine respond slowly and often incompletely; however, they do not develop transplant-related complications. This therapeutic approach may be preferable for older patients with severe aplastic anemia.

As an adult transplant center, our center has performed a pilot study to test whether patients with severe aplastic anemia in whom ATG has failed can subsequently receive a successful bone marrow transplant. All patients with severe aplastic anemia presented to our institution were initially treated with ATG. Seventeen of these 21 are alive with improved or re-established normal bone marrow function. The patient population included six patients with HLA identical donors. Four of these recovered with ATG therapy. Two failed to respond to ATG treatment and subsequently received a BMT. Both patients had no difficulties with engraftment and have re-established normal hemopoietic parameters.

Metabolic Disorders

The use of BMT in genetically determined metabolic disorders has been successful in approximately 36 reported indications with reversal of the disease causing enzyme defects.

FAILURE ANALYSIS AND THERAPEUTIC APPROACHES

Failure to achieve long-term, disease-free survival after BMT may relate to multiple problems. The three most commonly encountered problems are related to life-threatening infections, the development of GVHD, and relapse of the underlying hemopoietic malignancy.

SELECTED INFECTIOUS COMPLICATIONS

BMT recipients remain severely immunocompromised for weeks and months and may be exposed to a series of life-threatening infections of various causes. A number of prophylactic and therapeutic approaches have shown promise in successfully controlling some of the problems.

Bacterial Infections

Bacterial infections are common during the neutropenic early post-BMT period. The majority of these infections can be controlled with aggressive antibiotic therapy. Patients who have undergone a splenectomy or who are functionally asplenic are at risk of developing rapidly progressive diplococcal septicemia. Early therapy with penicillin or erythromycin is essential. In spite of timely administration of these antibiotics, patients may succumb to this infectious complication. The role of a pneumococcal vaccine has not been fully evaluated. However, its use appears to be of limited effectiveness. Alternatively, patients may carry a supply of penicillin or erythromycin and initiate therapy at the earliest sign of an infection.

Pneumocystis carinii

The prophylactic use of trimethoprim-sulfamethoxazole during the early post-transplant period may prevent some of the gram-negative infections. However, attention should be drawn to the fact that its use may lead to the development of trimethoprim-sulfamethoxazole–resistant indole-negative *Escherichia coli*–related infections.

Trimethoprim-sulfamethoxazole is also effective in preventing *Pneumocystis carinii*–related pneumonias. For this purpose, it is sufficient to administer the drug on three consecutive days per week at a dose of two tablets orally every 12 hours. Therapy should likely be continued for 1 year.

The therapy of *Pneumocystis carinii*–related pneumonia may present a problem because it usually occurs in BMT recipients who have developed a hypersensitivity to trimethoprim-sulfamethoxazole and therefore had the drug stopped or in whom the drug had been discontinued because of low peripheral blood values and decreased bone marrow cellularity. The typical therapeutic dose for *Pneumocystis carinii* infection is four ampules administered every 6 hours through a peripheral intravenous access; the drug has to be diluted in a large volume, for instance 500 ml of 5 percent dextrose in water. If administered through a central venous catheter, the drug can be given safely in smaller volumes. A full course requires therapy for 3 weeks. If no response is observed after 1 week, trimethoprim-sulfamethoxazole may be replaced by pentamidine, to be administered at a dose of 4 mg per kilogram per day intramuscularly or intravenously. The treatment should be maintained for 14 to 21 days.

Herpes Simplex and Zoster

The advent of antiviral agents such as acyclovir has changed the clinical course of herpes infections in BMT recipients. Herpes simplex, a common problem during the early post-BMT period, can almost be eliminated if acyclovir is used prophylactically at a dose of 200 mg orally every 8 hours. Discontinuation of the drug, however, may rapidly lead to viral shedding and development of virally induced lesions. The disadvantage of a post-BMT course of acyclovir is delayed engraftment.

Herpes zoster infections, a common occurrence even in BMT recipients with normal peripheral blood counts, also respond to therapy with acyclovir. Intravenous therapy at a dose of 10 mg per kilogram every 8 hours is recommended for patients with normal renal function when more than two dermatomes are involved or if dissemination has occurred. The therapy should be continued until the lesions have dried. Acyclovir may prevent further spreading and may reduce posthepetic neuralgia. The role of oral acyclovir in herpes zoster is not established. We have investigated its use in patients with lesions that are limited to one or two dermatomes. The examined patients did not demonstrate further spreading. However, further study is necessary.

Cytomegalovirus-Induced Disease

The development of CMV-related disease, in particular CMV-induced pneumonitis, represents a life-threatening and often fatal complication of BMT. CMV disease may result from reactivation of CMV residing in the BMT recipient or by transmission through CMV-containing blood products. Approaches to improve the clinical outcome focus on prevention as well as on the exploration of new therapeutic modalities.

Preventive measures include the administration of immunoglobulin preparations with high antiCMV titer. A series of studies suggest that symptomatic cytomegalovirus infections and interstitial pneumonia occur with lower frequency in patients who receive prophylactic immunoglobulins.

The exclusive use of CMV-negative blood products for CMV-negative recipients also was associated with a significantly reduced frequency of CMV disease. It will be necessary to combine both approaches and to evaluate critically if the influence of immunoglobulin is upheld when only CMV-negative blood products are given to all patients.

The availability of acyclovir and 9-(1,3 dihydroxy-2-propoxymethyl) guanine (DHPG) have added further opportunities to develop new prophylactic and therapeutic strategies. Caution with the use of these antiviral agents has to be applied, since both are toxic to bone marrow and may impair renal function.

It is difficult to influence the clinical course of established CMV disease, particularly CMV pneumonitis. Although both acyclovir and DHPG may have been effective in individual cases, larger studies do not show a significant improvement in survival when these drugs are used. DHPG was found to be effective in reducing or eliminating shedding of CMV in patients with biopsy-proved, CMV-induced disease when used at the recommended dose of 5 mg per kilogram every 12 hours for a total of 10 mg per kilogram per day. Unfortunately, if DHPG is introduced late into the treatment schedule, tissue damage may have progressed to an irreversible state. This appears to be of particular importance when CMV-induced lung disease is treated.

Therefore, the use of DHPG early in the clinical course may be more effective. It will be necessary to conduct studies in which patients are treated with DHPG at the moment when shedding of CMV is documented, without the development of CMV-related disease. Under these conditions, it also may be feasible to reduce the usually administered dose of DHPG and to reduce the toxic effect on the newly established graft. In addition to the administration of DHPG alone, the drug may also be combined with immunoglobulins that contain high antiCMV titers. Preliminary studies show some promise.

GRAFT-VERSUS-HOST DISEASE

Prophylaxis and Treatment of Acute Graft-Versus-Host Disease

Acute and chronic graft-versus-host disease have plagued the prognosis of BMT recipients. The incidence of GVHD is age dependent and may vary from 50 to 75 percent in adults. Severe GVHD (grades II to IV) may occur in 25 to 50 percent of all patients. This frequency was similar when MTX or cyclosporine was used prophylactically. More recently, the combination of MTX and cyclosporine appears to have reduced the incidence and severity of GVHD. Patients that develop GVHD in spite of MTX and cyclosporine prophylaxis may benefit from steroid medications in a conventional dose of 40 mg per meter squared per day. This dose may be escalated in nonresponders. However, combined administration of cyclosporine and high-dose steroids may cause central nervous system (CNS) side effects, including seizures.

Alternative methods to prevent GVHD include the use of procedures that eliminate or reduce the frequency of donor-derived T lymphocytes in the BMT inoculum. Centers that have performed these studies report a very low incidence of GVHD and a severity that usually does not exceed grade II. Unfortunately, the use of T cell–depleted transplant inocula has resulted in graft rejections in 10 to 20 percent of recipients and is associated with a significantly increased relapse rate in patients with hemopoietic malignancies. The increased relapse rate may relate to the absence of a beneficial graft anti-leukemic effect observed in patients that display some GVHD. In particular, recent studies in chronic myeloid leukemia show a relapse rate that significantly exceeds the previous experience. The observation of increased relapse rates is not confirmed by all BMT teams that use T cell depleted bone marrows. Further studies will be necessary to determine whether the higher relapse rate and poor engraftment may be linked to the use of specific antibodies, to the completeness of T-cell removal, or to the additional use of other medications such as cyclosporine.

Chronic GVHD

Chronic GVHD may result in syndromes that are reminiscent of rheumatoid disorders such as the sicca syndrome and progressive systemic sclerosis. Occasionally, prolonged liver dysfunction and jaundice can be observed. These disorders require intensive management with immunosuppressive agents. The disease process gradually decreases in some patients. However, other patients demonstrate a failure to thrive that is associated with progressive worsening of the symptoms and that may eventually lead to their death. Treatment approaches with steroids, azathioprine, CTX, and cyclosporine, either alone or in combination, have shown some benefits. Thalidomide is also being explored.

RELAPSE OF HEMOPOIETIC MALIGNANCIES

Unfortunately, a certain proportion of BMT recipients relapse with their underlying disease. The frequency of relapse varies from study to study and ranges from 10 to 40 percent for patients transplanted with AML in first remission. Recent experience in acute leukemia and CML has clearly demonstrated that this relapse rate may relate to the manipulation of the BMT inoculum prior to infusion.

A significantly higher relapse rate is universally observed for patients transplanted with more advanced disease. A study replacing the more conventionally used CTX and TBI with VP-16 (60 mg per kilogram total dose) and FTBI (1,350 cGy total dose) shows some promise and results in a 48 percent disease-free survival rate at 2 years. It will therefore be mandatory to develop novel approaches to eliminate the malignant disease in the host prior to transplantation and to consider further interventions after the transplant. The latter approach was examined for patients with previous CNS leukemia. Continuing intrathecal therapy with MTX after transplantation has lowered the CNS relapse rate. In addition to the administration of chemotherapy post-transplantation, one may consider the use of biologic response modifiers such as interferon as alternative interventions.

FUTURE DIRECTIONS

Some of the problems discussed earlier may relate to the fact that BMT recipients usually do not demonstrate a complete normalization of hemopoiesis when bone marrow function is assessed by the frequency of hemopoietic precursors. The reduced numbers suggest incomplete engraftment and a poor reserve. The availability of hemopoietic growth factors obtained by recombinant technology may provide additional means to increase the rate of engraftment and to enhance the probability of re-establishing a more complete reserve. Various hemopoietic growth factors may either be used to stimulate clonogenic precursors in the transplant inoculum or to be administered directly to the patient. The safety of these maneuvers may have to take into account that some malignant precursors may be receptors for the same growth factors.

In summary, BMT is a form of therapy that facilitates the increase of chemotherapy and radiation beyond the level of bone marrow tolerance. It allows us to determine whether or not escalated dose schedules are able to control proliferation of malignant hemopoietic cells. At the moment, it is not clear whether transplantation of allogeneic cells contributes to the disease control as suggested by the graft-versus-leukemia effect and by the increased relapse rate in T-cell–depleted transplant patients. The putative benefit of these interactions between donor-derived cell populations and residual malignant cell populations in the host has to be further explored. The use of hemopoietic growth factors may facilitate the administration of intensive courses of chemotherapy without the requirement for a bone marrow transplant. This approach may allow a direct comparison of the clinical outcome in patients receiving the same aggressive treatment protocol with and without transplantation.

SUGGESTED READING

Appelbaum FR, Barrall J, Storb R, et al. Bone marrow transplantation for patients with myelodysplasia: Pretreatment variables and outcome. Ann Intern Med 1990; 112:590–597.

Appelbaum FR, Fisher LD, Thomas ED, et al. Chemotherapy v. marrow transplantation for adults with acute nonlymphocytic leukemia: A five-year follow up. Blood 1988; 72:179–184.

Blaise D, Gaspard MH, Stopp AM, et al. Allogeneic or autologous bone marrow transplantation for acute lymphoblastic leukemia in first complete remission. Bone Marrow Transplantation 1990; 5:7–12.

Cassileth PA, McGlave PB, Harrington DP, et al. Comparison of post remission therapy in AML: Maintenance versus intensive consolidation therapy versus allogeneic bone marrow transplantation. Proc Am Soc Clin Oncol 1989; 8:197.

Champlin R, Jansen J, Ho W, et al. Retention of graft-versus-leukemia using selective depletion of CD8-positive T-lymphocytes for prevention of graft-versus-host disease following bone marrow transplantation for chronic myelogeneous leukemia. Transplant Proc 1991; 23:1695–1696.

Conde E, Iriondo A, Rayon C, et al. Allogeneic bone marrow transplantation versus intensification chemotherapy for acute myelogenous leukemia in first remission: a prospective controlled trial. Br J Haematol 1988; 68:219–226.

Emanuel D, Cunningham I, Jules-Elysee K, et al. Cytomegalovirus pneumonia after bone marrow transplantation successfully treated with the combination of ganciclovir and high dose intravenous immune globulin. Ann Intern Med 1988; 109:777–782.

Goldman JM, Gale RP, Horowitz MM, et al. Bone marrow transplantation for chronic myelogeneous leukemia in chronic phase. Ann Int Med 1988; 108:806:814.

Hermans J, Suciu S, Stijnen TH, et al. Treatment of acute myelogenous leukemia: An EBMT-EORTC retrospective analysis of chemotherapy versus allogeneic or autologous bone marrow transplantation. Eur J Cancer Clin Oncol 1989; 25:545–550.

Lomen PL and the XOMA BMT Study Group. Anti CD-5 immunoconjugate in acute GVHD. In: Champlin RE, Gale RP eds. New strategies in bone marrow transplantation. New York: Wiley-Liss, 1991; 137:285–293.

Löwenberg B, Verdonck LJ, Dekker AW, et al. Autologous bone marrow transplantation in acute myeloid leukemia in first remission: Results of a Dutch prospective study. J Clin Oncol 1990; 8:287–294.

McGlave PB, Beatty P, Ash R, Hows JM. Therapy for chronic myelogeneous leukemia with unrelated donor bone marrow transplantation: Results in 102 cases. Blood 1990; 75:1728–1732.

Meyers JD, Reed EC, Shepp DH, et al. Acyclovir for prevention of cytomegalovirus infection and disease after allogeneic marrow transplantation. N Engl J Med 1988; 318:70–75.

Reed EC, Bowden RA, Dandliker PS, et al. Treatment of cytomegalovirus pneumonia with ganciclovir and intravenous cytomegalovirus immunoglobulin in patients with bone marrow transplants. Ann Intern Med 1988; 109:783–788

Reiffers J, Gaspard MH, Maraninchi D, et al. Comparison of allogeneic or autologous bone marrow transplantation and chemotherapy in patients with acute myeloid leukaemia in first remission: A prospective controlled trial. Br J Haematol 1989; 72:57–63.

Thomas ED, Clift RA. Indications for marrow transplantation in chronic myelogenous leukemia. Blood 1989; 73:861–864.

AUTOLOGOUS BONE MARROW TRANSPLANTATION

MICHAEL J. BARNETT, B.M.
GORDON L. PHILLIPS, M.D.

Extensive laboratory studies have shown that malignant cells generally exhibit a steep dose-response curve to both radiation and chemotherapeutic agents. In humans, the cure of Hodgkin's disease with radiation and the cure of Burkitt's lymphoma with cyclophosphamide represent prime examples of how this principle has been successfully applied in clinical practice. Although such dose escalation results in a greater antitumor effect, it also causes increased toxicity to normal tissues. Indeed, toxicity to the marrow is frequently dose-limiting.

Intravenous infusion (i.e., transplantation) of hematopoietic stem cells after intensive therapy for malignant disease allows the administration of chemotherapy or chemoradiotherapy in doses that would otherwise result in prolonged or permanent myelosuppression. The stem cells are obtained from marrow donated by a compatible family member or unrelated volunteer (allogeneic) or an identical twin (syngeneic) or from the patient (autologous).

The present interest in the treatment of malignant disease with intensive therapy and autologous marrow transplantation began some 15 years ago. It was then based, in large part, on the results of earlier studies in which patients with leukemia had been treated with high-dose cyclophosphamide and total-body irradiation made possible by transplantation of marrow from a sibling sharing the same human leukocyte antigen (HLA) type. These studies showed that a proportion (albeit small) of patients with otherwise refractory acute leukemia could be cured. However, the approach was clearly of limited applicability owing to the lack of suitable donors for the majority of patients and the immunologic consequences, notably graft-versus-host disease (GVHD), which necessitated that an age limit of 45 to 50 years be imposed. It was appreciated that the use of autologous rather than allogeneic marrow transplantation might allow intensive and potentially curative therapy to be offered to considerably more patients. Furthermore, in the absence of GVHD, autologous marrow transplantation would be safer and might therefore be utilized in older patients, thereby further increasing its applicability.

It has subsequently become apparent that the cure of leukemia by treatments utilizing allogeneic marrow transplantation is due not only to the intensive therapy but also to an action of the allograft, the so-called graft-versus-leukemia effect, which is a consequence of histocompatibility differences between the graft and the leukemia cells. This has relevance to autografting, in which an antileukemic effect of the graft might not be expected. In this regard, the results of syngeneic marrow transplantation (in a sense, the ideal autograft) are informative. Although relapse rates are higher when compared .with allografts, cures of leukemia can be achieved with syngeneic marrow transplantation, indicating that the intensive therapy alone has the capacity to eradicate the leukemic clone in some patients. Thus, the success of syngeneic marrow transplantation has provided a strong impetus for the use of autologous marrow transplantation.

There are, however, a number of unique problems related to the use of autologous hematopoietic cells to support intensive therapy. One is that prior to harvesting the autograft, normal stem cell function may have been compromised by previous chemotherapy, leading to delayed, incomplete, or unsustained hematologic recovery after infusion. This is particularly likely for diseases in which the conventional chemotherapy used to induce remission is especially myelosuppressive, notably acute myelogenous leukemia. Another is that despite harvest of marrow during morphologic remission, occult malignant stem cells may contaminate the autograft. Obviously, this is of greater concern for the hematologic malignancies, in which marrow contamination is an intrinsic feature, rather than for other malignancies such as germ cell tumors and ovarian cancer, in which it is not. Finally, at present, the origin of recurring malignant cells after treatments involving autografting cannot be established. Thus, it is not possible to determine whether relapse in any individual patient was due to an inability of the intensive therapy to eradicate the disease or to the transplantation of undetected but viable malignant stem cells in the autograft.

Recent surveys carried out in North America and Europe indicate that an increasing number of autografts are being undertaken for both hematologic malignancies and solid tumors (Fig. 1). Nevertheless, various aspects of this treatment modality remain controversial, and it cannot, as yet, be considered standard therapy. It is against this background that the subject is discussed in broad terms and with a tendency toward expression of personal views rather than those of the consensus.

COMPONENTS OF AUTOGRAFTING

Patient

Age, performance status, previous therapy, and function of the major organs are all important factors when considering a patient for intensive therapy and autografting. As previously mentioned, allogeneic marrow transplantation is generally restricted to patients aged less than 45 to 50 years, primarily because of the high incidence of fatal complications (e.g., GVHD and interstitial pneumonitis) in those older than this. The use of autologous marrow avoids GVHD and associated fatalities and potentially raises the age limit by a decade, (i.e., to 60 years).

The performance status of the patient is an important factor because those in whom this is low suffer more therapy-related toxicities. In addition, low performance status correlates with advanced disease, which in turn predicts for poor outcome.

The details of previous therapy and function of the major organs also require consideration. For example,

patients with abnormal liver function (e.g., after transfusion-related hepatitis) or those who have previously received radiation to the chest may, after intensive therapy and autografting, be at increased risk of developing veno-occlusive disease of the liver or interstitial pneumonitis, respectively. A case can be made for performing a liver biopsy on those patients with abnormal liver function in addition to the routine pretransplant tests of cardiac, pulmonary, and renal function.

Disease

Diseases selected for intensive therapy and autografting should be responsive to standard-dose therapy, which is amenable to dose escalation. In addition, to minimize the risk of infusing malignant stem cells in the autograft, it is generally felt that the marrow must be at least microscopically free of disease at procurement.

Cure of some acute leukemias with chemotherapy and some lymphomas with chemotherapy and radiation, coupled with the successes of allogeneic and syngeneic marrow transplantation in the treatment of refractory hematologic malignancy, serve as a rationale for the use of autografts to extend the benefits of intensive therapy to more patients with these diseases. Other diseases for which autografting would be a reasonable option include neuroblastoma, Ewing's sarcoma, germ cell tumors, and multiple myeloma as well as breast, ovarian, and small-cell lung cancers.

Intensive Therapy

The components of intensive therapy regimens should ideally have established efficacy at conventional dose, exhibit a steep dose-response relationship, have myelosuppression as the dose-limiting toxicity, and allow substantial dose escalation before the development of significant nonhematologic toxicity. The most commonly used agents are busulfan, carboplatin, carmustine (BCNU), cyclophosphamide, cytosine arabinoside, etoposide, melphalan, and total-body irradiation (TBI). Some combinations are more widely employed than others, specifically cyclophosphamide and TBI, busulfan and cyclophosphamide, and cyclophosphamide, BCNU, and etoposide.

In terms of efficacy, the superiority of any one regimen over another for a particular malignancy has yet to be proven. Nevertheless, in the setting of autografting in which there is no need for pretransplant immunosuppression, the treatment regimen can be chosen solely on the basis of antitumor activity. For example, in the treatment of ovarian cancer and germ cell tumors, high-dose carboplatin (a weak immunosuppressive) may be selected as the major component of the regimen. Previous treatment may also influence the choice of intensive therapy. An example of this is Hodgkin's disease, for which a number of patients have received prior mediastinal radiation and for whom an all-chemotherapy regimen (e.g., cyclophosphamide, BCNU, and etoposide) carries less risk of fatal interstitial pneumonitis than a TBI-containing regimen.

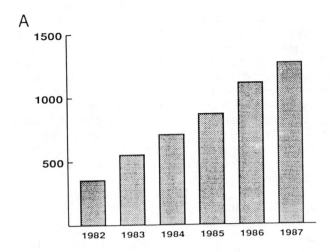

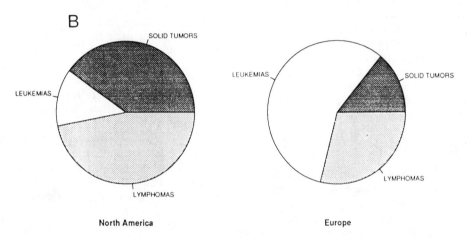

Figure 1 Survey of 112 centers worldwide. *A*, Annual number of autotransplants, 1982 to 1987. *B*, Indications for autotransplants in North America and Europe. (From Gorin NC, Gale RP, Armitage JO. The Advisory Committee of the International Autologous Bone Marrow Transplant Registry. Autologous bone marrow transplants: Different indications in Europe and North America. Lancet 1989; 2:317-318.)

In view of the inevitable morbidity and mortality (5 percent to 25 percent) associated with intensive therapy and autografting, a uniform system for grading regimen-related toxicity is important. Such a system has been proposed by the Seattle group and will no doubt be employed by others.

Hematopoietic Stem Cells

Not infrequently, a clear indication for the use of intensive therapy may exist, but a choice has to be made concerning the source of hematopoietic stem cells for transplantation (i.e., autologous versus allogeneic). Which method is preferable depends on the age of the patient, disease under consideration, likelihood of marrow involvement, adverse effects of GVHD, and the possibility of a graft-versus-tumor effect.

In certain circumstances, the potential advantages of the transplantation of allogeneic marrow, namely the more predictable hematologic recovery, the absolute certainty of avoiding the infusion of malignant stem cells, and the likelihood of a graft-versus-tumor effect, hold sway. It can be reasoned that such would be the case for many patients in remission of acute myelogenous leukemia who are aged less than 45 to 50 years and have an HLA-identical sibling to act as a donor.

Conversely, for Hodgkin's disease, the routine use of autologous marrow is favored in order to avoid the consequences of GVHD. This decision is based on the observation that marrow involvement with Hodgkin's disease is unusual at presentation (approximately 5 percent of cases) and is even less common at progression or first relapse. It is therefore assumed that for most patients the probability of infusing malignant stem cells in an autograft will be low and the anticipated problems due to GVHD would outweigh any possible benefits of an allograft.

Blood may be used instead of marrow as a source of

hematopoietic stem cells. It has been shown that such cells, after being obtained by multiple leukapheresis collections (usually approximately eight), can rescue patients given intensive therapy. The major advantage of this approach is that it can be employed when harvesting of the marrow is impossible (e.g., after pelvic irradiation) or when the marrow is overly contaminated with malignant cells. There is, however, the disadvantage of increased demands on labor, with each leukapheresis collection requiring individual cryopreservation and storage. The decision to use peripheral blood stem cells routinely is, therefore, usually based on local interests and available resources.

Finally, another possibility exists. This pertains to the fact that, with the exception of cyclophosphamide and TBI or busulfan and cyclophosphamide, most intensive therapy regimens are not myeloablative. Indeed, the BACT regimen (BCNU, cytosine arabinoside, cyclophosphamide, and 6-thioguanine), developed at National Institutes of Health many years ago and a prototype for other regimens, can clearly be given without the support of an autograft with satisfactory hematologic recovery, albeit after a prolonged period of myelosuppression. It may therefore be reasonable to consider the use of such intensive therapy without an autograft but in conjunction with hematopoietic cytokines to stimulate hematologic recovery from endogenous hematopoietic stem cells.

In Vitro Treatment of the Autograft

A concern regarding the use of autologous marrow in transplant protocols is the possibility that malignant stem cells may contaminate the autograft and be a potential source of disease recurrence. Obviously, the type of malignancy and its propensity to involve the marrow will dictate the likelihood of this (e.g., the subtypes of non-Hodgkin's lymphoma, in which marrow involvement is likely in lymphoblastic but not in large-cell disease).

Over the last decade, much effort has gone into the development of various physical, immunologic, chemical, biologic, and photodynamic methods to rid ("purge") the autograft of malignant stem cells. A prerequisite of these so-called negative-selection methods is that the potential of the remaining normal stem cells in the autograft to reconstitute the hematopoietic system should not be significantly compromised. Furthermore, theoretically, all malignant stem cells have to be removed by negative selection if the autograft is not to carry the potential for disease recurrence. A logical and perhaps better strategy may be to isolate (i.e., positively select) normal stem cells, relatively few of which may be required to restore hematopoiesis. Clinical studies using the latter approach are now underway.

Unfortunately, at present it is very difficult to assess the efficacy of any in vitro treatment technique because the source of disease recurrence cannot be determined. Furthermore, in the clinical setting, a trial designed specifically to evaluate the effect of a given in vitro treatment method by comparing the relapse rates in patients receiving untreated versus in vitro treated marrows would only be informative if the intensive therapy regimen were sufficiently effective to produce a low intrinsic relapse rate. Such trials would also require large numbers of patients, which is impractical in most situations.

It should be stressed that until such time as the antitumor effect of intensive therapy and autografting is significantly improved, contamination of the graft will continue to be an infrequent cause of treatment failure.

TIMING OF AUTOGRAFTING

It may be argued that the optimal time for the use of intensive therapy and autografting is during an initial remission induced by primary chemotherapy. This is based on the assumption that eradication of such "minimal residual disease" would be more likely and cumulative organ toxicity would be at a minimum. However, because intensive therapy and autografting is generally more toxic than conventional treatment, this policy could only be justified if patients at high risk of relapse could be identified. The following examples illustrate the problem and reflect our current practice.

At present, for certain malignancies it is difficult to identify reliably, either at diagnosis or in an initial remission, patients at high risk or relapse. Such is the case in Hodgkin's disease, in which the response to optimal primary chemotherapy (regimens comprising seven or eight drugs) does, however, correlate well with outcome. Thus, patients in whom an initial complete remission is not achieved or in whom disease recurs have a sufficiently poor prognosis to justify the toxicities of intensive therapy and autografting. This strategy of prompt autografting at the first sign of failure of standard therapy would improve efficacy and diminish overall toxicity by limiting the use of autografting in Hodgkin's disease to the minority of patients who actually require it. A similar approach may be adopted with other malignancies that also usually carry a good prognosis with standard therapy (e.g., large-cell lymphoma and germ cell tumors).

For other diseases, it may be possible to identify a subgroup of patients at presentation in whom remissions are unlikely to be durable. Examples of this situation are acute leukemia with high white cell count, advanced small noncleaved cell lymphoma, lymphoblastic lymphoma with marrow involvement, and ovarian cancer with significant residual disease at the completion of primary laparotomy. In these circumstances, patients may well benefit from intensive therapy and autografting during an initial remission induced by primary chemotherapy.

TECHNICAL ASPECTS

The techniques employed for the various stages of autologous marrow transplantation are, in general, well established and will not be discussed. Mention will, however, be made of a few recent developments.

When the marrow is harvested, an attempt is usually made to procure a minimum of 1.0×10^8 nucleated cells per kilogram of patient weight. The actual number of hematopoietic stem cells (i.e., those capable of self-renewal) required is, of course, much smaller. Unfortunately, at present, an assay that measures directly and exclusively hematopoietic stem cells with in vivo reconstituting potential does not exist. Based on experiments in the mouse, it seems likely, however, that the cells capable of initiating hematopoiesis in the long-term culture system may be representative of those able to reconstitute the hematopoietic system in vivo. Based on this premise, a new quantitative assay for a very primitive hematopoietic cell has been developed in Vancouver. In brief, test cells are seeded onto pre-established, irradiated human marrow adherent cells, which eliminates the requirement for an adequate supportive population to be generated from the marrow sample being evaluated for its stem cell content. The endpoint of the assay is the total hematopoietic colony-forming cell (progenitor) content (adherent plus nonadherent) of the resultant cultures harvested 5 weeks later. Studies are now underway to correlate the results of this long-term culture initiating cell assay with in vivo reconstituting potential after autografting.

Attempts to isolate normal stem cells from the autograft (i.e., positive selection) depend on the ability to distinguish such cells from their malignant counterparts. In this regard, the CD34 antigen, present on virtually all normal hematopoietic progenitor cells, has clinical relevance. Highly enriched populations of CD34-positive cells have been isolated using monoclonal antibodies and column separation. Preliminary experiments indicate the approach is feasible on a large scale (i.e., for the treatment of an autograft), and clinical studies are underway.

When the intensive therapy takes only a few days to administer, it is possible to store the marrow at 4°C and then infuse with resultant satisfactory restoration of hematopoiesis. In most cases, however, the duration of the intensive therapy is longer or the marrow is to be used in the future, and it must then be frozen to maintain hematopoietic stem cell viability. The standard method for the cryopreservation of marrow involves use of the cryoprotectant dimethylsulfoxide (DMSO), freezing at a controlled rate, and storage in liquid nitrogen. Recently, storage of prepared marrow in a freezer at a higher temperature has been suggested to be a more convenient and economical alternative, at least for short periods of time (which is usually all that is required).

CURRENT PRACTICE AND RESULTS

Lymphomas

A steadily increasing number of autografts are being carried out for Hodgkin's disease. The most frequently employed intensive therapy has been the CBV (cyclophosphamide, BCNU, and etoposide [VP–16–213]) regimen supported by an untreated autograft. Recent reports suggest that if this approach is applied at the first sign of failure of conventional chemotherapy, 40 percent to 50 percent disease-free survival may be a possible projection.

The non-Hodgkin's lymphomas (NHL) are the diseases for which the most autografts have been done. Studies to date have mainly involved patients with intermediate-grade and high-grade NHL, for whom recurrence after initial therapy carries a dismal prognosis. A variety of treatment regimens have been used, and some groups have treated the autograft in vitro. For patients in so-called "sensitive relapse" (i.e., disease responsive to chemotherapy), disease-free survival of approximately 40 percent can be achieved. In contrast, those with primarily resistant disease or with "resistant relapse" (i.e., disease unresponsive to chemotherapy) are unlikely to benefit from this approach. It would also appear that patients with recurrent large-cell lymphoma after more effective primary therapy (e.g., the so-called third-generation regimens) are less likely to be cured by autografting than those who have previously received less intensive chemotherapy. Unfortunately, patients with large-cell lymphoma who have the most to gain from autografting (i.e., those in an initial remission but at high risk of relapse) are difficult to identify.

Studies of autografting for myeloma and low-grade lymphoma are also now underway. The indolent nature of low-grade lymphoma will, however, require a long follow-up to evaluate these efforts.

Leukemias

Considerable interest has been shown in autografting for acute myelogenous leukemia (AML), particularly in Europe. Both TBI-containing and all-chemotherapy regimens have been supported by an untreated autograft or one treated in vitro (typically with a derivative of cyclophosphamide). Results of 40 percent to 60 percent disease-free survival after autografting for AML in first remission have been used to support the superiority of this approach over postremission chemotherapy. These results should, however, be interpreted with caution, because in most series, the median duration of remission prior to autografting is approximately 6 months, and time-censoring becomes an important factor. Thus, patients who relapse before receiving an autograft are obviously excluded from the autografting results but not from the chemotherapy results with which the former are compared. The subject would perhaps be best addressed in a trial in which patients in first remission of AML are randomized to receive conventional chemotherapy or intensive therapy and an autograft.

Most autografts to date for acute lymphoblastic leukemia (ALL) have been carried out in patients with disease in second or subsequent remission. Typically, TBI-containing regimens have been used and an immunologic method has been employed to treat the autograft in vitro. With this approach, disease-free survival has been reported in 20 percent to 30 percent of patients, which is not dissimilar to the results achieved with allogeneic marrow transplantation (the increased relapse rate in the former being balanced by the higher procedure-related mortality in the latter).

Previous efforts to treat chronic myeloid leukemia (CML) using autografting have involved the infusion of blood or marrow cells (taken and cryopreserved during chronic phase) after intensive therapy for blast-phase disease. Not surprisingly, this has at best allowed reestablishment of another limited period of chronic-phase disease. Recently, a new strategy has been developed in Vancouver that may allow autografting for CML to be given with curative rather than palliative intent. This is discussed further later.

Solid Tumors

Intensive therapy and autografting for patients with advanced solid tumors has produced few cures. Nevertheless, diseases have been identified for which this approach might successfully be employed at an earlier stage. Such studies are now underway employing a variety of treatment regimens supported by an untreated autograft. For neuroblastoma and Ewing's sarcoma, this appears to be an effective strategy. In addition, results of these efforts in other malignancies such as germ cell tumors and cancers of the breast and ovary, although preliminary, are sufficiently encouraging to warrant guarded optimism.

NEW DIRECTIONS AND FUTURE PROSPECTS

Enhancing the Antitumor Effect of Autografting

It seems unlikely that further dose escalation of existing agents will be of overall benefit, as any improvement in efficacy will be offset by increased toxicity to normal tissues. One approach is to link radioisotopes to monoclonal antibodies, thereby targeting radiotherapy to the tumor. In this way, a higher dose of radiation can be delivered to sites of disease (e.g., the marrow) while sparing normal tissues.

Another strategy to increase the efficacy of intensive therapy and autografting is to evoke a graft-versus-tumor effect. To this end, the Baltimore group is evaluating the use of cyclosporine after autograft to induce GVHD. The possible antitumor activity of lymphokine-activated killer (LAK) cells generated by interleukin-2 is also being investigated in the autograft setting in several centers.

Isolation of Normal Hematopoietic Stem Cells

New approaches to the isolation of normal hematopoietic stem cells may allow the administration of intensive therapy to patients with diseases hitherto considered incurable by autografting. Experiments carried out in Vancouver a number of years ago demonstrated that when marrow from patients with CML is set up in long-term culture, malignant (Philadelphia chromosome [Ph^1]-positive) stem cells are often not maintained, whereas any coexisting normal (Ph^1-negative) stem cells are. The use of autologous marrow maintained in culture is now being evaluated for its ability to allow the administration of intensive and potentially curative therapy to patients with CML.

It has also recently been reported that sufficient hematopoietic stem cells might be obtained from the umbilical cord blood of a newborn to serve as an autograft. Although this has been a disturbing concept to some, it could be possible to cryopreserve a person's cord blood at birth against the eventuality of their developing a malignancy in the future.

Hematopoietic Cytokines

In the last few years, clinical experience has been gained with the use of several hematopoietic cytokines. Granulocyte colony-stimulating factor (G-CSF) and granulocyte-macrophage colony-stimulating factor (GM-CSF) have been given after autografting for malignant disease. The ability of these CSFs to stimulate myeloid leukemic stem cells has restricted such studies to patients with lymphomas, ALL, and solid tumors. Results to date suggest that for patients who have not been heavily pretreated, the period of neutropenia after autograft may be shortened by 5 to 7 days. Administration of GM-CSF has also been used to allow the collection of peripheral blood cells, which in combination with autologous marrow appear to enhance hematologic recovery after intensive therapy. In the future, it is likely that an array of hematopoietic cytokines will form an important part of the oncologist's armamentarium.

Gene Transfer

Long-stem stable gene transfer to hematopoietic stem cells now appears feasible using recombinant retroviruses. Applied to autografting, this may allow the progeny of such genetically marked cells to be followed in the recipient and, in the event of disease recurrence, the origin of malignant cells to be determined. Furthermore, and potentially of great importance, such techniques may eventually usher in the era of gene therapy for malignant disease.

Acknowledgements. Some of the work discussed was supported by grants from the National Cancer Institute of Canada and the British Columbia Health Care Research Foundation. We also thank Sandra Bonner for typing, Linda Williams for editing, and Connie Eaves and Joseph Connors for critical review of the manuscript.

SUGGESTED READING

Armitage JO. Bone marrow transplantation in the treatment of patients with lymphoma. Blood 1989; 73:1,749–1,758.

Cheson BD, Lacerna L, Leyland-Jones B, et al. Autologous bone marrow transplantation: Current status and future directions. Ann Intern Med 1989; 110:51–65.

Gale RP, Butturini A. Autotransplants in leukaemia. Lancet 1989; 2:315–317.

Herzig GP. Autologous marrow transplantation in cancer therapy. Prog Hematol 1981; 12:1–23.

Treleaven JG, Kemshead JT. Removal of tumor cells from bone marrow: An evaluation of the available techniques. Hematol Oncol 1985; 3:65–75.

MULTIPLE MYELOMA AND RELATED MONOCLONAL GAMMOPATHIES

ANN M. BENGER, M.D., FRCPC
WILLIAM E. C. WILSON, M.D., C.M., FRCPC, F.A.C.P.

Individuals proved to have myeloma come to medical attention for a variety of reasons. Patients with overt disease present with symptoms that generally involve one or more of three pathogenetic mechanisms: skeletal destruction, bone marrow failure, and synthesis of an abnormal protein. The symptomatic consequences of cortical bone destruction may be bone pain, hypercalcemia, pathologic fracture, and spinal cord compression. Bone marrow failure may manifest itself with the symptoms of anemia, susceptibility to infection related to leukopenia, or a hemorrhagic diathesis consequent to thrombocytopenia. The dysproteinemia of multiple myeloma may become symptomatic as a consequence of renal failure, hyperviscosity, amyloid deposition, coagulation disturbance, and/or impaired humoral immunity. Finally, nonspecific symptoms of malignancy may accompany those related to these three pathogenetic mechanisms.

At the other extreme, a patient destined to die from myeloma may first be recognized by the presence of a small monoclonal protein identified during the investigation of an unrelated problem.

The challenge presented to the clinician by this range of immunoproliferative disease is to identify those patients whose prognosis is sufficiently poor to warrant the risks attendant upon any therapy. For those who do require treatment, the physician must devise a therapeutic strategy that provides the best chance for active productivity for the patient's remaining limited life.

ASSESSMENT OF PROGNOSIS

When a diagnosis of myeloma is established, several clinical and laboratory parameters have an adverse effect on prognosis. These are renal failure, hypercalcemia, anemia, leukopenia, thrombocytopenia, light chain disease, and poor performance status. The marked reduction in median survival associated with Bence Jones proteinuria, complicating IgG and IgA myeloma, is due to a strong association with uremia. For a given amount of paraprotein, patients with IgA myeloma fare worse than those whose tumor cells secrete IgG. It is clear that several of these factors relate well to tumor load.

In addition to clinical staging, more specialized laboratory techniques may assist in assessing prognosis. The tritiated thymidine labeling index of plasma cells is low in patients with indolent or smoldering myeloma. In patients who are not azotemic, the beta-2 microglobulin level correlates well with the tumor burden.

Current studies are exploring methods by which patients with a very poor prognosis might be identified for participation in trials of more radical therapy. Heavy marrow infiltration with malignant plasma cells is negatively associated with prognosis in patients with IgG and light chain myeloma. Immature morphology of tumor cells predicts a poor prognosis and is accompanied by preB cell phenotype and chromosomal abnormality. In vitro assays for melphalan sensitivity have demonstrated that these cells are drug resistant. In another study, determination of the RNA content of myeloma cells by flow cytometry revealed that a low level of RNA was associated with greater resistance to initial and salvage chemotherapy.

GENERAL PLANS OF MANAGEMENT

Monoclonal Gammopathy of Undetermined Significance

Because the term benign monoclonal gammopathy can only be used retrospectively with any certainty, a patient who presents with a small monoclonal protein that is identified incidentally must be considered a potential myeloma candidate. A history and physical examination to exclude the other causes of dysproteinemia should be recorded.

In the absence of contraindicating illness or infirmity, the initial investigation should include a bone marrow aspiration and biopsy, determination of the parameters of bone marrow function, evaluation of renal function, a serum calcium level, estimation of the serum levels of the three major classes of immune globulin, serum immunoelectrophoresis, a 24-hour urine collection for total protein measurement and electrophoresis, and a skeletal x-ray survey.

The individual least likely to develop overt myeloma is older and has no further abnormalities identified by the additional investigation.

A repeat serum protein electrophoresis should be obtained after 3 months. If the abnormality is stable, the interval may safely be increased to 6 months.

Indolent or Smoldering Myeloma

Not all patients with multiple myeloma have an overtly progressive malignancy. When a patient presents with multiple myeloma (more than 10 percent plasma cells in the bone marrow and an MCP in excess of 30 g per liter), who is asymptomatic and lacks hematologic, biochemical, and radiologic evidence of overt myeloma, it is reasonable to withhold chemotherapy. Many patients of this type remain stable, and, therefore, are best protected from the complications that attend chemotherapy.

The interval for initial reassessment should be 2 months. If the protein abnormality remains stable, the follow-up interval can be lengthened progressively to 6 months. For patients in this group, treatment should be considered if the abnormal protein level increases by 50 percent or if the symptoms of complications become evident.

Overt Multiple Myeloma

Generally, patients with overt multiple myeloma have symptoms related to skeletal damage, renal failure, or compromised bone marrow function, and have a progressive disease. Historical data indicate a median survival of 7 months without treatment. Melphalan and prednisone therapy has extended the median survival to 30 months.

Whether initial therapy with intensive multidrug chemotherapy can improve the outlook for most patients with multiple myeloma remains controversial. Until this controversy is resolved, it is generally reasonable to institute therapy with melphalan, 9 mg per meter squared per day for 4 days, orally on an empty stomach every 4 weeks. The dose should be increased to 12 mg per meter squared for 4 days if the granulocyte nadir is over 500.

If the patient does not respond with a fall of MCP, the dose should be increased progressively to 15 mg per meter squared per day for 4 days, 18 mg per meter squared per day for 4 days, etc., until clear evidence of hematologic toxicity is observed, thereby indicating adequate absorption of melphalan. Prednisone, 100 mg orally, should accompany each day of melphalan.

An expected 70 percent of patients demonstrate a drop in the MCP to 50 percent of the pretreatment value. A slow, progressive diminution in the level of abnormal protein signifies a better prognosis than a rapid fall.

The duration of chemotherapy is controversial. Cessation results in earlier relapse, but not necessarily a shortening of median survival. Continued therapy might increase the likelihood of refractory anemia and acute leukemia. Until more data are available, it is reasonable to discontinue therapy at 2 years in those patients who have had a good response.

A trial is currently underway to determine if the addition of alpha interferon might increase the duration of remissions induced with melphalan and prednisone.

Cyclophosphamide is a reasonable substitute for patients who are allergic to melphalan or are intolerant to melphalan in other ways.

Advanced Myeloma

Some patients present with manifestations of disease that warrant aggressive therapeutic intervention if major morbidity or immediate mortality are to be avoided. Examples of this include patients with serious hypercalcemia and those with critical neurologic complications. For those in this category who seem otherwise fit, consideration should be given to one of the multiagent regimens. In an uncontrolled study of 46 previously untreated patients, the M-2 protocol produced objective responses in 87 percent. Other multiagent regimens may be superior to melphalan and prednisone in this setting.

SPECIFIC CLINICAL PROBLEMS

Solitary Myeloma

An occasional patient presents with an apparently isolated bone lesion. This is generally symptomatic. After the diagnosis is established by biopsy, the initial assessment parameters outlined previously should be obtained. If these reveal no abnormality or only a small monoclonal protein peak, the patient may have a localized malignancy and may possibly be cured by intense radiotherapy. Most patients who present with apparently localized disease manifest progressive disease within 2 years. If a monoclonal protein is present and does not disappear with radiation, overt multiple myeloma can be anticipated.

Extramedullary Plasmacytoma

Plasma cell tumors presenting outside bone are generally found within the respiratory tract. The lymph nodes and the gastrointestinal tract are less frequent sites. They are generally single, but may be multiple. Therapy has included resection and/or radiation, depending on location. Although local recurrence or metastases to soft tissues (lymph nodes) or bone can be anticipated, the prognosis is generally better than that of overt multiple myeloma.

Nonsecretory Myeloma

Fewer than 5 percent of patients with multiple myeloma have tumor cells that do not secrete clinically measurable amounts of abnormal protein into the serum or urine. Nonsecretory tumors generally are identified because of bone lesions. The tumor cell mass tends to be less and the levels of hemoglobin and normal immune globulin tend to be preserved. The prognosis of these patients is better than that seen in patients with overt multiple myeloma.

Pathologic Fractures

Pathologic fracture is a frequently presenting manifestation of overt disease. In non–weight-bearing areas, therapy for the systemic disease is generally followed by relief from the local symptoms. When fracture of a major long bone occurs, internal fixation followed by local irradiation is recommended.

Patients with a pathologic vertebral collapse must be immediately assessed with respect to spinal cord compression. If no evidence of cord compromise is present, urgent local radiotherapy should be initiated and be accompanied by high-dose dexamethasone therapy. The patient must be reassessed during the first few days of radiotherapy for signs of spinal cord compression. Patients with evidence of compromised spinal cord function should be considered for immediate decompression laminectomy followed by local radiotherapy. Because the ultimate outlook for the patient depends on their tolerance for chemotherapy, the volume of active bone marrow irradiated should be as conservative as is reasonable.

Spinal Cord Compression

Spinal cord compression that is identified and treated early because of an accompanying pathologic fracture generally has a good prognosis. Occasional patients with myeloma have spinal cord compression from an extradural deposit that is not associated with overt bone destruction. These patients are often not diagnosed until major impairment of spinal cord function has been present for some time. The tumor is usually identified by the neurosurgeon. Once the diagnosis is established, the patient should receive local radiation while being assessed for systemic chemotherapy. As permanent neurologic sequelae are all too frequent, active rehabilitation therapy should be instituted as soon as the postoperative state allows.

Renal Failure

The most common renal lesion to complicate multiple myeloma is tubular atrophy and degeneration. Dimers of light chains filtered by the glomerulus are reabsorbed and catabolized in the tubular cells. Patients who excrete light chains are more likely to have impaired renal function.

Other possible mechanisms of deterioration in renal function include interstitial tumor cell infiltration, dehydration, hypercalcemic nephropathy, pyelonephritis, and amyloid deposition in the glomeruli.

Management of the renal failure should include prompt correction of any recognized complicating factors (i.e., hypercalcemia, dehydration, and infection) and aggressive treatment of the myeloma. The patient may require the support of dialysis. Acute renal failure may reverse with forced alkaline diuresis and dialysis. Occasional reports suggest an added benefit from plasmapheresis.

Bone Marrow Failure

Some manifestation of impaired bone marrow function can be anticipated in most patients being treated for multiple myeloma. The degree of marrow failure usually worsens temporarily with initiation of treatment, and the patient may require transfusions.

Disproportionate neutropenia often complicates chemotherapy in patients with advanced myeloma. When this is associated with major marrow infiltration, chemotherapy sometimes has to be cautiously continued in the hope that a reduction of the tumor burden will be followed by increased granulopoiesis.

Plasma cell leukemia is a rare and particularly malignant form of marrow failure. Affected patients typically have a high tumor burden, disproportionate tissue and organ involvement, and a median survival of 2 months in one series.

Acute leukemia, often preceded by a period of refractory anemia, is a recognized complication of melphalan therapy. In one series, the incidence of acute leukemia in patients with multiple myeloma after alkylator therapy was 1.9 percent (actuarial 2.8 percent at 5 years, 10.1 percent at 10 years). When a refractory anemia develops, alkylating therapy should be stopped. Patients who develop acute myeloid leukemia and who are otherwise fit may respond to intense chemotherapy.

Hyperviscosity

The hyperviscosity syndrome is not a common manifestation of multiple myeloma, since it is more frequently found in Waldenström's macroglobulinemia. However, certain IgA proteins and some monoclonal IgG molecules of the IgG 1 and IgG 3 subclasses may aggregate in vivo, thereby resulting in increased serum viscosity. Prompt reversal of the manifestations of the hyperviscosity syndrome can be anticipated from plasmapheresis. Long-term control, however, depends on response to chemotherapy.

Hypercalcemia

Hypercalcemia is present at the time of diagnosis in 30 percent of patients with multiple myeloma. It is generally not severe and responds to treatment of the underlying malignancy. Symptomatic hypercalcemia can usually be ameliorated temporarily by hydration and diuretic administration while the chemotherapy exerts its effect. Occasional severe cases may benefit from mithramycin, calcitonin, or oral phosphate solutions.

Amyloid Deposition

Myeloma patients with significant amyloid deposition in vital organs have a dismal prognosis, with a median survival of 5 months in one series. In the absence of cardiac amyloid, some patients respond to chemotherapy. The responsive patients have a median survival in excess of 2 years.

Myeloma in the Elderly

The incidence of multiple myeloma rises with age from 7 per 100,000 at age 50 to more than 20 per 100,000 at age 80. Because of increased longevity, elderly patients are coming more frequently to medical attention for treatment of myeloma. In a large, multi-institutional study of myeloma therapy, patients over 80 years seemed to be underrepresented when compared with a broader epidemiologic survey. This possibly reflected referral bias and investigator bias with exclusion of those considered too frail or otherwise unable to tolerate chemotherapy. However, for those elderly patients who were included in the study group, the prognostic risk factor representation was the same as that of younger patients. The older patients had responses and survival rates equivalent to the younger patients. Hematologic toxicity was no greater in the older group. The older patients did experience greater gastrointestinal toxicity in the treatment arm employing melphalan and prednisone. The authors conclude that myeloma treated without bone marrow ablation has a similar outcome when young patients were compared to the elderly.

RELAPSED OR RESISTANT MYELOMA

If treatment is discontinued, myeloma relapses in patients who have responded well to therapy with melphalan and prednisone. Relapse in this setting is best treated by reinstitution of melphalan and prednisone.

The outlook is poor for most patients when their disease progresses despite therapy with melphalan and prednisone. In addition to the manifestations of advancing disease, which may include impaired mobility related to bone pain and/or pathologic fractures, the clinical problem is often complicated by impaired tolerance to chemotherapy because of previous treatment and recurrent infection. For the subset of patients judged to be preterminal, the judicious but liberal use of narcotics may constitute the best therapy. Prednisone pulse therapy may provide some palliation for patients unable to tolerate more toxic regimens.

Four-day infusions of vincristine and doxorubicin combined with dexamethasone pulse therapy has produced a 70 percent response rate in patients whose myeloma was resistant to alkylating therapy. This observation requires confirmation in a larger group of patients. The regimen involves an indwelling catheter, the need for hospitalization for the chemotherapy infusion each month, and admission for treatment of the infectious complications.

Bone marrow transplantation is currently under investigation. When the donor is an identical twin, response is seen, but progression of the myeloma generally supervenes. The results of allogeneic transplantation have not been encouraging. Autologous bone marrow transplantation studies demonstrate that dosage escalation can overcome drug resistance to some extent. The clinical benefits observed to date have been disappointing, perhaps because the patients were in a state of advanced disease and marrow purging had not been carried out.

The treatment of patients with plasma cell dyscrasias has been improved by the recognition that chemotherapy can be safely withheld from some.

A combination of melphalan and prednisone is the mainstay of therapy for overt disease. For those whose disease becomes progressive and requires therapy, most die of multiple myeloma within 3 or 4 years of initial diagnosis.

Physicians who accept responsibility for the care of patients with myeloma should attempt to align themselves with a myeloma study group in the hope that expanded clinical research will improve the results of therapy.

SUGGESTED READING

Alexanian R. Localized indolent myeloma. Blood 1980; 56:521.

Barlogie B, Smith L, Alexanian R. Effective treatment of advanced multiple myeloma refractory to akylating agents. N Engl J Med 1984; 310:1353.

Corwin J, Lindberg RD. Solitary plasmacytoma and their relationship to multiple myeloma. Cancer 1979; 43:1007.

Durie BGM, Salmon SE. A clinical staging system for multiple myeloma: correlation of measured myeloma cell mass with presenting clinical features, response to treatment, and survival. Cancer 1975; 36:842.

Durie BGM, Salmon SE. The current status and future prospects of treatment for multiple myeloma. Clin Haematol 1982; 11:181.

Greipp PR, Kyle RAP. Clinical, morphological, and cell kinetic differences among multiple myeloma, monoclonal gammopathy of undetermined significance and smouldering multiple myeloma. Blood 1983; 62:166.

THE HEMOPHILIAS

JEANNE M. LUSHER, M.D.

DIAGNOSIS AND CLINICAL MANIFESTATIONS

Hemophilia A (factor VIII deficiency) and hemophilia B (factor IX deficiency) are clinically indistinguishable. Both are inherited as X-linked traits and thus affect men almost exclusively. Both are characterized by bleeding into joints and soft tissues. If one performs the usual coagulation screening tests, the activated partial thromboplastin time (APTT) will be quite prolonged, whereas the prothrombin time (PT), thrombin (TT), and bleeding time will be normal. In order to distinguish between the two disorders, one must perform factor VIII and factor IX assays.

Because neither factor VIII nor factor IX cross the placenta, the diagnosis can be made from a cord blood sample. Thus, if a woman who is a known or possible "carrier" is pregnant and does not desire in utero diagnosis, arrangements should be made in advance for her obstetrician to collect a cord blood sample (from a vessel in the fetal side of the placenta) for factor VIII or factor IX assay. Blood should be collected into a standard "blue-top" (liquid citrate) tube and transported to the laboratory immediately.

Carrier Detection and Prenatal Diagnosis

If a woman is a possible carrier of hemophilia A or B, one can assay her factor VIII or factor IX coagulant level, and if it is below the lower limits of normal (the normal range in most labs being 0.60 to 1.50 factor VIII U per milliliter), she would be classified as a carrier of the gene for hemophilia A or B. However, many known carriers have factor VIII or factor IX levels within the normal range (because of the random inactivation of the X chromosome in somatic cells of women). In order to improve the probability of carrier detection for hemophilia A, one can measure factor VIII-related antigen (factor VIII R:Ag) along with factor VIII coagulant activity and determine the ratio of the two. If she has more factor VIII R:Ag than factor VIII coagulant activity (indicating that she is producing some nonfunctional factor VIII), a ratio of less than 0.6 can be equated with a 90 percent likelihood of her being a carrier.

The underlying molecular pathology of the hemophilias is quite heterogeneous. In a minority of families with hemophilia, the precise DNA mutation can be determined. In such families, carrier detection and pre-natal diagnosis can be made with certainty. In most families, however, one must rely on indirect gene-linkage testing with restriction fragment length polymorphisms (RFLPs). An affected male in the family as well as other appropriate family members, must be available for study, in order to have informative linkage data. With currently available intragenic polymorphisms for the factor VIII gene, approximately two-thirds of kindreds will be heterozygous and thus informative in linkage studies.

Similarly, in hemophilia B, more precise determination of carrier status is possible using polymorphic DNA markers. Combined analysis with the available intragenic RFLPs will be informative in approximately 80 percent of families.

Limitations of RFLP testing include the fact that one must be able to test many family members (in order for useful linkage data to be produced). Also, if there is only one hemophiliac in a family (sporadic hemophilia), frequently one cannot identify the mutation. Here, RFLP linkage studies can only be used for exclusions of inheritance of the hemophilic X chromosome.

For those who desire diagnosis in the first trimester of pregnancy, prenatal diagnosis can be accomplished by direct fetal blood sampling or, in certain families (as discussed previously), by RFLP analysis. Analysis of RFLP can be performed on chorionic villus samples (CVS) obtained between 8 and 11 weeks' gestation, or on amniocytes obtained by amniocentesis between 14 to 16 weeks. Fetal blood can be obtained by fetoscopy at 17 to 18 weeks' gestation; the fetal blood can be used for coagulation and DNA studies. Among the technical difficulties associated with these diagnostic techniques is the fact that amniocytes usually require in vitro culturing for 10 to 14 days to achieve sufficient numbers of cells for DNA extraction. Following extraction of DNA, the development of an interpretable autoradiograph takes 1 to 2 weeks. Newer techniques, such as the polymerase chain reaction, have speeded up the process considerably.

There is a high mutation rate for both factor VIII and factor IX deficiency. In approximately one-third of newly diagnosed cases, there is no family history of hemophilia.

Bleeding Manifestations in Infancy

Although cephalohematomas or occasionally intracranial hemorrhage can occur in hemophiliac neonates during vaginal delivery (especially if the mother is a primigravida who has a long, difficult labor), infants with hemophilia rarely have bleeding episodes requiring treatment unless subjected to surgery or unusual trauma. In general, tongue and mouth bleeding and bleeding into joints or soft tissues begin in toddlers who are learning to walk and have frequent falls and bumps. From that time on, persons with hemophilia have repeated episodes of joint and soft-tissue bleeding.

MANAGEMENT: GENERAL PRINCIPLES

Musculoskeletal Bleeding

Bleeding into joints or muscles should be treated immediately! An acute hemarthrosis should be considered a medical emergency, with prompt infusion of the missing clotting factor. If joint bleeding is not treated immediately, a destructive cycle of events is set in motion: blood in the synovial space serves as an irritant and results in synovial proliferation and increased vascularity. The highly vascular synovium then protrudes into the joint space, where it can be easily traumatized with walking or other normal activities. Thus, rebleeding occurs, and a vicious cycle of repetitive bleeding leads to chronic synovitis and eventual erosion of the cartilage and underlying bony surface. Crippling deformities ensue.

One of the many benefits of home treatment (self-infusion, or infusion of a child by a parent) is prompt treatment of joint bleeding. Treatment consists of intravenous infusion of factor VIII or factor IX (see Tables 1 and 2 for recommended dosage), and a period of non–weight bearing for the particular joint involved. If an acute hemarthrosis is treated early, often a single dose of clotting factor will suffice. On the other hand, if the joint has already become swollen and painful (indicating a more extensive hemorrhage), two or three larger doses may be required.

Intramuscular bleeding generally requires several doses of clotting factor. This is particularly true for extensive intramuscular hemorrhages involving large muscle masses (e.g., iliopsoas or thigh bleeding). Although the iliopsoas muscle is not visible on physical examination, one should suspect an iliopsoas hemorrhage if the patient has pain on extension of the thigh, prefers to keep his thigh flexed at the hip, and has numbness or paresthesias around the inguinal region. Radiologic studies (radiography, ultrasound) will confirm the suspected diagnosis and will convey the extent of the hemorrhage. Large iliopsoas bleeds should be managed by bed rest and several days of treatment with clotting factor concentrates given every 12 hours.

Tongue and Mouth Lacerations

These generally occur in toddlers who have bitten their tongue or have fallen, with or without a toy or other object in their mouth. Although infusion of clotting factor will stop the bleeding, rebleeding almost invariably occurs. Thus, most pediatric hematologists routinely admit toddlers with tongue or mouth lacerations. The child is given nothing by mouth (NPO) except for an

Table 1 Hemophilia A: Recommended Dosages of Factor VIII*

Type of Bleeding	Initial Dose (Factor VIII U/kg)	Repeat Dose (Factor VIII U/kg)	Other Treatment
Acute hemarthrosis			
Early	10	Seldom necessary	Ice packs, non-weight-bearing
Late	20	20 q12h	sling, or lightweight splint may be helpful; rarely, joint aspiration is helpful
Intramuscular hemorrhage†	20–30	20 q12h (often several days of treatment)	Non-weight-bearing support; complete bed rest for iliopsoas hemorrhage
Life-threatening situations‡	50	25–30 q8–12h or (preferably) as a continuous infusion (3–4 U/kg/hr)	
Intracranial hemorrhage			
Major surgery			
Major trauma			
Tongue or neck bleeding with potential airway obstruction			
Severe abdominal pain‡	20–40	20–25 q12h	
Tongue and mouth lacerations‡	20	20 q12h	An antifibrinolytic agent (tranexamic acid or ACA), sedation, NPO in small child; local application or oradhesive gauze may be beneficial for gum bleeding
Extractions of permanent teeth	20	20 q12h; however, often not necessary in uncomplicated extractions	Antifibrinolytic agent beginning 1 day preop; continue 7–10 days
Painless spontaneous gross hematuria	None		Increased PO fluids. Corticosteroids or Factor VIII used by some

*Refers to viral-attenuated Factor VIII.
†In individuals who have mild hemophilia A, DDAVP (desmopressin) is the treatment of choice rather than Factor VIII concentrates.
‡These situations should be treated in a comprehensive hemophilia center. If first seen in another hospital, the hemophilia center should be contacted and the patient transferred after emergency treatment is given at the local hospital.
(Adapted from Lusher JM. Management of hemophilia. In: Westphal RG, Smith DM eds. Treatment of hemophilia and von Willebrand's disease. New developments. Arlington, VA: American Association of Blood Banks, 1989.)

antifibrinolytic agent (Amicar or Cyclokapron syrup) and is kept heavily sedated; factor VIII or factor IX and intravenous fluids are administered. Poorly formed, friable clots should be removed. Topical thrombin may be used, but one should avoid cauterization and should also avoid sutures unless absolutely necessary. The use of an oradhesive gauze may be helpful in protecting a laceration or oozing surface other than the tongue.

Dental Extractions

Although important for everyone, good dental hygiene is particularly important for persons with hemophilia in order to avoid gum bleeding and the need for extractions of permanent teeth. However, if the latter must be done, an antifibrinolytic agent should be given starting the evening before the procedure, and it should be continued for 7 to 10 days following extraction. (Because the tissues of the oral mucosa are rich in fibrinolytic material, fibrin clots are rapidly lysed unless an antifibrinolytic agent is given.) Novocaine blocks by deep injection (e.g., mandibular block) should be avoided. Nitrous oxide or a short-acting anesthetic may be used. The oral surgeon should be experienced in the care of persons with hemophilia. If good local care is used, often only one dose of factor VIII (or factor IX) given pre-extraction is required.

Central Nervous System Bleeding

Head trauma should be cause for immediate alarm and immediate treatment. Unless judged trivial, any closed head injury should be regarded as a medical emergency. If the patient is on home treatment and he, or someone, can mix and infuse factor VIII (or factor IX) quickly, this should be done before he is taken to the medical facility for evaluation. One should obtain a pertinent medical history and physical assessment, as well as a computed tomography (CT) scan. Depending on the nature and extent of intracranial hemorrhage (ICH), if present, appropriate medical and neurosurgical management can be instituted. In general, one should aim for a factor VIII level of greater than 50 percent in the case of ICH; such levels should be continuously maintained by continuous infusion (rather than bolus doses) of factor VIII. This regimen should be maintained for approximately 3 weeks. If the patient's condition is then stable, prophylaxis (with a bolus dose of factor VIII given every other day) should begin and should be continued for 6 to 12 months, as the rate of spontaneous recurrence of ICH is high.

In small children in whom venous access is a problem, one can arrange for a central venous catheter (e.g., Broviac catheter) or Port-a-Cath. Although these devices may result in local bleeding or infection, one must weigh these risks against the risk of recurrent ICH.

Table 2 Hemophilia B: Recommended Dosage Schedule

Type of Bleeding	Initial Dose and Source of Factor IX* (Factor IX U/kg)	Repeat Dose and Source of Factor IX* (Factor IX U/kg)	Other Treatment
Acute hemarthrosis† In individual with mild hemophilia B	15 ml (FFP)	None	
Early, in severe hemophilia B	20 (PCC)	None	Seldom necessary
Late (pain, swelling, limitation of motion), in severe hemophilia B	30 (PCC)	20–25 (PCC) q12h	Ice packs, non-weight-bearing support, and a sling may be useful; rarely, joint aspiration is helpful
Intramuscular hemorrhage‡ In individual with mild hemophilia B	15 ml (FFP)	10–15 ml (FFP) q12h	
In severe hemophilia B	30–40 (PCC)	30 (PCC) q12h	Non-weight-bearing support; complete bed rest for iliopsoas hemorrhage
Life-threatening situations‡ Intracranial hemorrhage Major trauma Tongue or neck bleeding with potential airway obstruction	50 (PCC)	20–25 (PCC) q12h or as a continuous infusion	AT III concentrate of 1 unit FFP source of AT III; add heparin to reconstituted PCC (see text)
Severe abdominal pain‡ In mild hemophilia B	15 (FFP)	10 (FFP) q12h	
In severe hemophilia B	40 (PCC)	20 (PCC) q12h	

*PCC refers to heat-treated or otherwise viral-attenuated PCC. As soon as a nonthrombogenic factor IX concentrate is licensed and available, it would become the preferred product for most of the situations cited in the table.

†In infants and children under 4 years of age, some still prefer to use FFP rather than PCC, even in those with moderate or severe hemophilia B.

‡These situations should be treated in a comprehensive hemophilia center. If first seen in another hospital, the hemophilia center should be contacted and the patient transferred after emergency treatment is given at the local hospital.

Abbreviation: FFP = fresh frozen plasma.

(Adapted from Lusher JM. Management of hemophilia. In: Westphal RG, Smith DM eds. Treatment of hemophilia and von Willebrand's disease. New developments. Arlington, VA: American Association of Blood Banks, 1989.)

Surgical Procedures

If surgery is judged necessary in a person with hemophilia, there must be close cooperation and communication between medical and surgical personnel. Unless the surgery is of an emergency nature, one should screen the patient for an unexpected inhibitor antibody to factor VIII (or factor IX). Assuming that no inhibitor is found, the hematologist can calculate the dose of factor VIII (or factor IX) required to achieve the desired factor VIII levels (see dosage calculation later). In general, the initial bolus dose of factor VIII (or factor IX) is given 30 to 45 minutes preoperatively. This should then be followed by a continuous infusion of factor VIII, which can be maintained throughout the postoperative period.

In the case of persons with hemophilia B given prothrombin complex concentrates (PCCs), one must be aware of the potential for disseminated intravascular coagulation (DIC) and thromboembolism (see section on factor IX concentrates). This risk is particularly great in persons who undergo orthopedic surgical procedures involving the lower extremities, in which thromboplastic materials may enter the circulation and the patient is immobile. However, thrombotic complications associated with the use of PCCs may occur in *other* situations as well. Although PCCs contain some clotting factors in an activated form, other new, purer forms of factor IX appear to be much less thrombogenic and should be used for any person with hemophilia B who requires hemostasis for a period of time (as for surgery).

Hematuria

Painless, spontaneous gross hematuria occurs not infrequently in persons with hemophilia. Although one should make sure that the patient does not have another condition, such as acute glomerulonephritis, flank trauma, renal calculus, or severe thrombocytopenia, most often there *is* no apparent cause for the bleeding and it is painless. Some physicians use corticosteroids or factor VIII (or factor IX) concentrates and prescribe bed rest. For many years, however, it has been our policy to use no treatment and to allow the patient to go about his usual activities. In general, gross hematuria will stop within a few days.

Avoidance of Drugs Causing Platelet Dysfunction

Persons with hemophilia (or any other underlying coagulation disorder) should avoid aspirin and all aspirin-containing compounds, as these cause platelet dysfunction, which can enhance bleeding once it begins. Certain other drugs, including nonsteroidal antiinflammatory agents, antihistamines, and certain antibiotics in high dosage, can also interfere with platelet function. Acetaminophen is a useful alternative to aspirin for relief of pain or fever.

Dosage Consideration

In calculating factor VIII dosage, one can assume that a dose of one factor VIII unit (U) per kilogram body weight will raise the recipient's factor VIII level by 0.02 U per milliliter (2 percent). In contrast to factor VIII, factor IX is a much smaller molecule and thus diffuses into the tissues rather than remaining intravascular. One factor IX U per kilogram will raise the recipient's factor IX level by only 0.01 U per milliliter (1 percent). Thus, if one wishes to raise the factor VIII level to 0.50 U per milliliter in a person whose baseline value is less than 0.01 U per milliliter, a dosage of 25 U per kilogram should be given, whereas in a person with severe factor IX deficiency, a dosage of 50 U per kilogram would be required to achieve this same level.

ADMINISTRATION: INTERMITTENT VERSUS CONTINUOUS INFUSION

For most purposes, a single bolus dose or intermittent bolus doses of factor VIII or factor IX are used. In certain situations, however, one would prefer to have a steady-state level of factor VIII, rather than peaks and troughs. Most physicians who treat hemophilia recommend continous intravenous infusions for surgery (particularly in the postoperative period) and for central nervous system hemorrhage. Advantages of continuous infusions in such situations include the ability to obtain a meaningful factor VIII assay value at any time point and the avoidance of delayed bolus doses, which might result in very low factor VIII levels and rebleeding. In using continuous infusions of factor VIII, an initial bolus dose of 40 to 50 U per kilogram should be given. Then a dosage of 3 U per kilogram per hour will usually maintain a factor VIII level of 0.50 U per milliliter; 4 U per kilogram per hour will usually maintain a level of 0.75 U per milliliter. One should not merely assume these levels, however, but should obtain a daily factor VIII assay to see if the desired level is being maintained.

AVAILABLE PRODUCTS

Products for Persons with Hemophilia A

A variety of products are now available for persons with hemophilia A. These include DDAVP (1-deamino-8-D-arginine vasopressin; desmopressin), for those with mild or moderate factor VIII deficiency; cryoprecipitate; plasma-derived factor VIII concentrates; and recombinant factor VIII.

DDAVP

The synthetic agent DDAVP is regarded as the treatment of choice for persons with mild or moderate hemophilia A, whenever an approximate threefold increase in factor VIII will suffice for control or prevention of bleeding. This agent, which was first used in persons with mild hemophilia A and von Willebrand's disease in the late 1970s, effects a rapid release of factor VIII and von Willebrand factor (vWF) from storage sites. In severe hemophilia A, there is nothing to be released and, thus, the drug is ineffective. In those with mild or moderate hemophilia A with baseline factor VIII values of 0.05 to 0.10 U per milliliter (5 percent to 10 percent), however, intravenous infusion of DDAVP will result in a very rapid increase of 2- to 15-fold (average, 3-fold) over baseline values. The magnitude of the response is usually consistent in the same individual over time, as long as doses are not given in rapid succession. The recommended dose for hemostatic purposes (in contrast to its use for diabetes insipidus) is 0.3 µg per kilogram per dose. It is usually given intravenously, although it can be given subcutaneously or intranasally. The formulation currently licensed in the United States is too dilute for hemostatic use; however, a more highly concentrated intravenous spray form is available in Europe and is being used as an investigational drug in at least two hemophilia centers in the United States at present.

If one plans to use DDAVP for surgical coverage, one must be aware that many (but not all) recipients will exhibit tachyphylaxis (diminishing response with repeated doses), to reflect transient depletion of storage sites. The drug is remarkably free of side effects. If DDAVP is given to small children or surgical patients with no attention to fluids and electrolytes, however, hyponatremia and water intoxication may result. Such complications can be avoided by limiting fluids or monitoring fluids and electrolytes following administration of DDAVP.

Cryoprecipitates

Cryoprecipitates are an excellent source of factor VIII, as well as vWF and fibrinogen. Cryoprecipitates are still preferred by some, especially if they are prepared from plasma donated by one or a small number of repeatedly tested donors. However, most patients and physicians prefer factor VIII concentrates, as they are easier to store, reconstitute, and administer: they are labeled with the number of factor VIII units contained (whereas most bags of cryoprecipitate vary considerably in factor VIII content); and, perhaps most importantly, they can be subjected to pasteurization or other methods of viral attenuation.

Commercially Prepared Factor VIII Concentrates

Lyophilized, commercially prepared factor VIII concentrates have been the mainstay of treatment since their introduction two decades ago. Throughout the 1970s, these products were not subjected to viral attenuation processes, because it was thought that too much (heat-labile) factor VIII would be destroyed in the process. By the mid-1970s, however, it had become apparent that most hemophiliacs receiving commercially prepared clotting factor concentrates had hepatitis, many had persisting elevations of alanine amino transferase (ALT), and some had progressed to chronic hepatitis or even cirrhosis. In an attempt to produce a hepatitis-safe factor VIII concentrate, Hyland Laboratories began dry-heat treating their concentrate; in 1981, it introduced Hemofil-T, a factor VIII concentrate heated in the dry state at 60°C for 30 hours. Although

studies in chimpanzees suggested that this product was hepatitis-safe, 85 percent of human hemophiliac children who received only Hemofil-T developed evidence of a non-A, non-B hepatitis (NANBH). It was thus apparent that this method of dry heating was not effectively destroying hepatitis virus; however, when the agent causing the acquired immunodeficiency syndrome (AIDS) was identified in early 1985, it became apparent that this agent (now called human immunodeficiency virus, HIV) was uniquely heat-sensitive. There is no doubt that some hemophiliacs who had been switched to Hemofil-T in the very early 1980s were probably spared from HIV infection.

In the early 1980s, with AIDS becoming an increasing concern, all manufacturers of factor VIII concentrates attempted to develop better viral attenuation methods. By 1987, factor VIII products produced and treated by a variety of methods were becoming available, although the dry-heat–treated concentrates had become the mainstay at most hemophilia centers. However, a flurry of reports of seroconversions to HIV in persons who had received only dry-heat–treated concentrates (most being associated with one method of dry heating) resulted in a dramatic change in product availability in early 1988. Without warning, dry-heat–treated factor VIII concentrate almost disappeared from the US marketplace, whereas factor VIII concentrates prepared by newer purification and viral attenuation methodologies were not yet available in sufficient quantity. Thus, throughout much of 1988, the question of how one should choose among products became "What can we get?" By late 1988, the factor VIII shortage seemed to have abated, although the only readily available products in many parts of the country were the monoclonal antibody purified factor VIII concentrates. These were (and still are) much more costly than the "old" dry-heat–treated concentrates (Table 3); to date, however, the monoclonal antibody purified concentrates have had an excellent track record in terms of viral safety. Produced and distributed by three US companies, the so-called "monoclonal products" are now being used by the majority of hemophiliacs in the United States. Several logs of virus are lost in the purification process; dry heating, pasteurization, or solvent-detergent treatment are used as an additional safeguard. Intermediate purity viral attenuated factor VIII concentrates available in the United States include those that are pasteurized, solvent-detergent–treated, or heated in the wet state in n-heptane. All of these appear to be safe in terms of HIV transmission, with no case of seroconversion to HIV being attributable to any currently marketed factor VIII concentrates.

Hepatitis safety is more difficult to document with any new product, as hepatitis safety trials must be conducted in previously untreated human subjects. The numbers of such subjects are small, and most are infants. Nonetheless, in order to establish the hepatitis safety of new products, one must follow the rather stringent guidelines that were established by the International Committee on Thrombosis and Haemostasis in 1984, and reaffirmed in 1988. Data concerning

Table 3 Wholesale Prices and Availability of Factor VIII Concentrates*

	Price/unit (cents)		
Process	Fall 1987	Spring 1988	Winter 1989
Dry heat†	6–9	12	20
Heated in n-heptane	14	25	38
Solvent and detergent	14	28	28
Heated in solution	42–45	42–45	42–45
Immunoaffinity purified	55	55–60	43–65

*Pricing data and the number of total available units of factor VIII concentrate manufactured were obtained by polling 33 randomly selected treatment centers and all clotting factor manufacturers. In 1987, 591 million units were consumed in the total US market. In 1988, 475 million units were available. In 1989, it is estimated that 475 million untis will be available. Many variables will have an impact on the estimate, including approvals by the Food and Drug Administration of new products, the final disposition of the withdrawn American Red Cross product under review by the Food and Drug Administration, and the potential for increasing the yield of factor VIII during production.

†The demand for dry-heated product in 1988 was more than double the available supply of 125 to 175 million units.

From Pierce GF, Lusher JM, Brownstein AP, et al. The use of purified clotting factor concentrates in hemophilia. Influence of viral safety, cost and supply on therapy. JAMA, 1989; 261:3434–3438.

the hepatitis safety of most new products thus come from relatively small numbers of subjects. To date, hepatitis safety trials with Armour's Monoclate, Hyland's Hemofil-M, Behringwerke's Humate-P, and the New York Blood Center's solvent-detergent–treated factor VIII concentrate indicate that these products did not transmit NANBH (or HIV) to any of the study subjects.

Recombinant Factor VIII

In 1984, two groups simultaneously announced the successful cloning of the factor VIII gene and the in vitro expression of its product. This remarkable feat led to the development of factor VIII concentrates prepared by recombinant DNA technology. Although not yet licensed, two companies' recombinant factor VIII concentrates have been in multicenter prelicensure clinical trials for some time. Both Hyland's and Cutter's recombinant factor VIII appear to be identical to human plasma-derived factor VIII, and to be hemostatically effective and safe. The recombinant factor VIII developed by scientists at Genetics Institute and produced by Hyland Laboratories was first infused into an adult with hemophilia in 1986; numerous patients have now received this product. To date, 95 human subjects have been infused with the recombinant factor VIII developed by Genentech and produced by Cutter Biological, Miles, Inc. In studies with both of these products, recombinant factor VIII has been well tolerated. Once licensed in the United States, recombinant factor VIII may well become the treatment of choice for persons with factor VIII deficiency.

Products for Hemophilia B

The development of purer, safer products for hemophilia B has lagged behind, presumably because of the smaller market. Thus, at present, the only products for hemophilia B that are licensed in the United States are the intermediate purity prothrombin complex concentrates (PCCs), which contain factors II, VII, IX, and X, proteins C and S, and some partially activated clotting factors as well. As noted earlier, PCCs have been associated with additional complications—not only transmission of blood-borne viruses but thrombotic complications as well. The risk of DIC and thromboembolism is greatest in persons with hemophilia B who are immobile after orthopedic surgical procedures or who have sustained crush injuries. However, those with severe hepatocellular dysfunction are also at risk, as clotting factor intermediates are not readily cleared from the circulation, and such patients may have low antithrombin III (AT III) levels.

One must be aware of such complications whenever prescribing PCCs. Large repetitive doses should be avoided, and if one must use PCCs for the "high-risk" situations described previously, it is wise to provide a source of AT III and to closely monitor the patient for evidence of DIC or deep venous thrombosis.

Several US companies have developed purer factor IX products that, in prelicensure clinical trials, appear to be less thrombogenic; however, none of these are licensed as of April, 1990.

Products for Patients with Inhibitor Antibodies to Factor VIII or Factor IX

Approximately 15 percent of persons with severe hemophilia A develop inhibitor antibodies to factor VIII; 1 percent to 2 percent of those with severe hemophilia B develop factor IX inhibitors. Although the presence of an inhibitor does not increase the frequency of bleeding, it does make treatment of bleeding difficult. Those who form antibody only in low concentration following factor VIII stimulus (the so-called "low responders") can generally be treated with human factor VIII in a somewhat higher dosage. On the other hand, those who have a brisk anamnestic response following any exposure to human factor VIII (so-called "high responders") generally cannot. It is the latter group who are particularly difficult to manage.

PCCs and Activated PCCs

Over the past two decades, PCCs have been the mainstay of treatment for hemophiliacs with inhibitors. For this purpose, a larger dose of PCCs is required. Most use 50 to 75 factor IX U per kilogram per dose. Although PCCs appear to "bypass" the need for factor VIII (or factor IX) in the clotting sequence, the precise mechanism by which this occurs is still not known. This therapy leaves something to be desired, as PCCs are not predictably effective in controlling bleeding in inhibitor patients, and often several doses are required. Such large, repetitive doses are not without risk. A number of cases of myocardial infarction (several fatal) have been reported in young hemophiliacs with inhibitors who received PCCs. In using large repeated doses of PCCs, this risk should be kept in mind. If the patient's bleeding fails to respond to two or three doses of PCCs, it is unlikely that additional doses will be effective.

Two purposely activated (A) PCCs, Hyland's Autoplex and Immuno's FEIBA, were developed in the late 1970s specifically for use in inhibitor patients. These products contain more activated clotting factor than do "standard" PCCs, and should never be used in noninhibitor patients! As is the case with "standard" PCCs, the APCCs cannot always be relied upon. Even in the same patient, APCCs may be effective on some occasions but not at all on other occasions. Recommended dosage for APCCs is 50 to 75 U per kilogram per dose. Although controlled double-blind studies conducted in the late 1970s and early 1980s showed little or no advantage of APCCs over "standard" PCCs in controlling joint bleeding, many hemophilia treaters are now using one of the APCCs, feeling that they are more likely to be effective. In fact, most of the authors' inhibitor patients receive APCCs as first-line treatment for bleeding episodes.

Polyelectrolyte Porcine Factor VIII

Because most factor VIII inhibitors have some degree of species specificity, human factor VIII inhibitors generally destroy human factor VIII to a much greater extent than other species' factor VIII. Speywood Laboratories in the United Kingdom produce a highly purified, polyelectrolyte porcine factor VIII, Hyate:C. This product has been licensed in the United States since 1986 for use in life- or limb-threatening bleeding episodes and has proved life-saving in a number of instances. (The author has successfully used Hyate:C for two instances of ICH, four surgical procedures, and one instance of massive intra-abdominal hemorrhage.) Although it is recommended that one obtain an antiporcine inhibitor level to see if a particular patient's inhibitor is likely to destroy infused Hyate:C, most subjects whose human factor VIII inhibitor level is less than 50 Bethesda Units will have a favorable response to Hyate:C. Recommended starting dosage is 50 to 100 U per kilogram, with subsequent dosage being determined by assaying the recipient's factor VIII level. The main advantage of this product (in addition to its effectiveness) is that one can objectively measure the recipient's factor VIII level. Disadvantages include the risk of allergic reactions (as it is a foreign species protein) and development of antibodies to porcine factor VIII. However, many patients have neither of these complications. Thrombocytopenia, which was common with older porcine factor VIII preparations used in the 1950s, is quite uncommon with Hyate:C. This agent has been a very useful addition to one's therapeutic armamentarium for factor VIII inhibitor patients.

Other Bypassing Approaches

Other agents that are not licensed for use in humans but are currently undergoing clinical trials in humans or animals include recombinant factor VIIa, Xa-phospholipid, and recombinant nonlipidated tissue factor. NOVO's recombinant factor VIIa is the only one of these that has been tried in humans. Recombinant factor VIIa has been used successfully in major surgery and in life-threatening bleeding episodes in several hemophiliacs with inhibitors in Europe and the United States. This agent is now undergoing phase 2 trials in the United States and abroad. The author is involved in these trials with recombinant factor VIIa and has been impressed with this agent's efficacy and safety. However, the number of patients treated to date is still relatively small. The other two investigational agents have been used in Giles' hemophiliac dogs in Canada, but they have not yet been infused into human subjects.

Transient Removal of Inhibitors

Nilsson and colleagues in Sweden developed immunoabsorption columns in the early 1980s and were able to remove factor VIII (or factor IX) inhibitors (as well as other IgG antibodies) transiently by extracorporeal circulation through these columns, which contained sepharose coupled to staphylococcal protein A. A similar system has been developed by the Dupont Company; the Dupont immunoabsorption columns are undergoing clinical trial at a few US hemophilia centers. Because other IgG antibodies are also removed, Nilsson and colleagues began adding intravenous IG at the end of the procedure. They found that this delayed reappearance of the inhibitor. These investigators now use a combination of intravenous IG, cyclophosphamide, and human factor VIII (immediately following the immunoabsorption procedure) in an attempt to achieve immune tolerance. The author has not had personal experience with this approach, however.

Attempts to Eradicate Inhibitors

A variety of approaches have been used in an attempt to suppress or eradicate inhibitors. During the 1980s, a number of investigators developed and used less costly and less demanding modifications of Brackmann's original "Bonn protocol." However, even these modified immune tolerance regimens are expensive, require good venous access, good patient compliance, and a considerable amount of factor VIII. Although such modified regimens have appeared to suppress completely inhibitors in many patients, enthusiasm for *any* attempts to achieve immune tolerance waned in 1988 owing to the shortage of factor VIII, plus the fact that the majority of US hemophiliacs were infected with HIV and had declining cellular immunity. Thus, many were concerned that immune tolerance regimens, particularly those that used immunosuppressive drugs, might hasten progression of HIV disease.

THE ROLE OF COMPREHENSIVE CARE AND THE IMPACT OF HIV/AIDS

It is beyond the scope of this chapter to describe the many benefits of comprehensive care. The regional comprehensive hemophilia centers that were established in the late 1970s evolved out of the recognized need for a multifaceted approach to hemophilia and its many complications—not only for the person with hemophilia but for his family members as well. The comprehensive care teams generally consist of one or more hemophilia nurses, social worker(s), physical therapist, orthopedic surgeon, dentist, genetic counselor, and pediatric and adult hematologist(s). Home treatment training programs are provided. Counseling, vocational guidance, and education concerning various aspects of hemophilia and its treatment are provided. At each patient's semiannual comprehensive clinic visit, he is seen and evaluated by each team member, a blood sample is assayed for such things as inhibitors, liver enzymes, and often for cellular immunity as well, and a set of recommendations are formulated for his care. Obviously, patients' needs differ, and the comprehensive hemophilia team tailors its approach to the individual. Over the past 5 years, concerns about HIV/AIDS have overshadowed other more basic hemophilia-related concerns, but the latter must not be ignored. Nonetheless, concerns about HIV/AIDS—the need for confiden-tial testing, education, counseling, screening sexual partners and offspring, risk-reduction strategies, drug trials (as with AZT), management of HIV-related illnesses, and death of patients we have known so well—have required an enormous amount of time and effort on the part of hemophilia team members, and have been quite emotionally draining for many.

SUGGESTED READING

Hilgartner MW, Pochedly C, eds. Hemophilia in the child and adult. 2nd ed. New York: Raven Press, 1989.

Kasper CK, ed. Recent advances in hemophilia care. New York: Alan R. Liss, 1990.

Lusher JM: Management of hemophilia. In: Pizzo P, Wilfert C, eds. Pediatric AIDS (in press).

Lusher JM: Etiology, natural history and management of Factor VIII inhibitors. Ann NY Acad Sci 1987; 509:89–102.

Pierce GF, Lusher JM, Brownstein AP, et al. The use of purified clotting factor concentrates in hemophilia. Influence of viral safety, cost and supply on therapy. JAMA 1989; 261:3434–3438.

Wesphal RG, Smith DM Jr, eds. Treatment of hemophilia and von Willebrand's disease: New developments. Arlington, VA: American Association of Blood Banks, 1989.

VON WILLEBRAND DISEASE

ZAVERIO M. RUGGERI, M.D.
THEODORE S. ZIMMERMAN, M.D.

PATHOGENESIS AND CLASSIFICATION

Von Willebrand disease is a congenital bleeding disorder characterized by a complex hemostatic defect. Abnormal platelet function, expressed by prolonged bleeding time, is a consistent finding and may be accompanied by decreased factor VIII procoagulant activity. The pathogenesis of von Willebrand disease is based on quantitative and/or qualitative abnormalities of von Willebrand factor, a large multimeric glycoprotein that circulates in plasma complexed with the factor VIII procoagulant protein. These two proteins form the factor VIII–von Willebrand factor complex. When present, the decreased factor VIII procoagulant activity is secondary to the reduced concentration of von Willebrand factor. The von Willebrand factor, but not the factor VIII procoagulant protein, is present in endothelial cells, the subendothelium, platelets, and megakaryocytes, as well as plasma.

Different forms of von Willebrand disease can be identified by their patterns of genetic transmission as well as by von Willebrand factor abnormalities in plasma and the cellular compartment. The distinction of various von Willebrand disease subtypes is important for correct therapy. These include the following.

Autosomal Dominant Inheritance

Type I. These patients may represent over 70 percent of all cases. Concentrations of factor VIII procoagulant and von Willebrand factor in plasma are decreased, usually to the same relative degree. Concentration of von Willebrand factor in the cellular compartment is normal in the majority of patients, although cases have been reported with low platelet content of the protein. All sizes of von Willebrand factor multimers are present, although there may be a relative decrease in the largest multimers and the structure of individual multimers may be altered. The characteristic hemostatic and laboratory abnormalities result from reduced plasma concentrations of the factor VIII–von Willebrand factor complex.

Type II. Concentrations of factor VIII procoagulant activity and von Willebrand factor may be decreased or normal in plasma. Von Willebrand factor concentration is usually normal in the cellular compartment. Plasma lacks large multimeric forms of von Willebrand factor. Several type II variants have been described based on altered structure and function of von Willebrand factor. With the exception of type IIB variants, ristocetin-induced platelet–von Willebrand factor interaction is decreased.

In type IIB, there is heightened ristocetin-induced platelet–von Willebrand factor interaction resulting from an increased affinity of the abnormal von Willebrand factor for the platelet glycoprotein Ib receptor. In some families, this heightened interaction results in chronic thrombocytopenia and the presence of platelet aggregates in the circulation.

Platelet type or so-called pseudo von Willebrand disease is similar in many respects to type IIB von Willebrand disease. However, the defect lies in the platelet receptor for von Willebrand factor, which has an increased affinity for the protein.

Autosomal Recessive Inheritance

Type III. Patients with type III disease are homozygous or double heterozygous for abnormal gene(s) inherited from both parents, who are usually clinically normal. Factor VIII procoagulant activity is markedly decreased. Von Willebrand factor is undetectable or present in trace amounts both in plasma and in the cellular compartment. These patients are clinically the most severely affected. A subset of patients with complete homozygous deletion of the von Willebrand factor gene is prone to develop antibodies to von Willebrand factor after repeated infusions of concentrates containing the protein.

GENERAL PRINCIPLES OF THERAPY

The aim of therapy in von Willebrand disease is to correct the prolonged bleeding time and, if present, the abnormality of blood coagulation. To achieve this, both von Willebrand factor and factor VIII procoagulant activity must be raised to normal levels in plasma. A normal concentration of a *functionally normal* von Willebrand factor must be achieved in patients with qualitative abnormalities of the protein.

Most patients with the more common autosomal dominant form of von Willebrand disease have a relatively mild bleeding tendency. In children, mucosal bleeding, particularly epistaxis and gingival bleeding, are common symptoms. Excessive blood loss following dental extraction, tonsillectomy, or other common surgical procedures is also frequent, as are cutaneous bleeding and easy bruising. Gastrointestinal bleeding is not infrequent and can be without identifiable cause. In females, menorrhagia is not uncommon, particularly after the first menses and in adolescent girls in general. Excess postpartum bleeding can also occur. However, spontaneous joint and muscular bleeding are exceptional.

Bleeding symptoms may be present in patients with normal plasma levels of factor VIII procoagulant activity. Therefore, it is not surprising that effective therapy requires correction of the quantitative and/or qualitative von Willebrand factor defect. If this is not achieved, poor control of bleeding will be observed even if concentrations of factor VIII procoagulant activity are raised to normal or above.

The clinical picture of the recessive form of von Willebrand disease is more severe. Mucosal and cutaneous bleeding, as well as hemorrhages from the female genital tract, occur more frequently and are of greater severity. Excessive bleeding after dental extractions or surgery can be controlled only by replacement therapy. Hemarthroses and muscular hematomata are not uncommon, and permanent disability may ensue in some cases. In these patients, correction of both the von Willebrand factor and factor VIII procoagulant defect is mandatory. In nonmucosal bleeding, particularly in cases of joint or muscle hemorrhage, raising the factor VIII procoagulant levels may be sufficient for effective hemostasis even when the bleeding time is not normalized. This is fortunate because individuals with homozygous von Willebrand factor gene deletion may develop antibodies to von Willebrand factor, which may render von Willebrand factor replacement therapy ineffective.

There are two main approaches to the therapy of von Willebrand disease. One is replacement therapy, i.e., the infusion of exogenous factor VIII–von Willebrand factor derived from normal plasma. The second is to induce release of endogenous factor VIII–von Willebrand factor from tissue stores using 1-deamino-[8-D-arginine]vasopressin (DDAVP). Replacement therapy is the only possibility in patients with severe (type III) von Willebrand disease who have markedly reduced levels of the factor VIII–von Willebrand factor related activities in both plasma and tissue stores. Infusion of DDAVP may release cellular factor VIII–von Willebrand factor into the circulation and increase its concentration to adequate levels in patients with the dominant form of von Willebrand disease who have normal tissue stores of von Willebrand factor. Occasional patients with type I and a larger percentage of those with type II variants do not respond to this drug.

DDAVP is contraindicated in both type IIB and platelet type (pseudo) von Willebrand disease because raising the endogenous von Willebrand factor in either of these disorders results in thrombocytopenia.

REPLACEMENT THERAPY AND BLOOD DERIVATIVES

Replacement therapy is performed by infusing plasma fractions enriched in the factor VIII–von Willebrand factor complex. Infusion of blood derivatives in patients with von Willebrand disease promotes a delayed increase in factor VIII procoagulant activity that is disproportionate to the amount administered. After the peak reached at the end of the infusion, factor VIII procoagulant activity continues to rise for 12 to 24 hours. On the contrary, von Willebrand factor starts to decrease immediately after the end of the infusion. Therefore, a discrepancy between factor VIII procoagulant activity and von Willebrand factor is found between 12 to 48 hours after treatment. Correction of the bleeding time defect is even shorter than that of the von Willebrand factor plasma levels. The delayed rise of factor VIII procoagulant activity is characteristically observed in all forms of von Willebrand disease, with the exception of the recessive form in patients who have developed an inhibitor antibody to factor VIII–von Willebrand factor (see below).

Of the available sources of factor VIII–von Willebrand factor, only single-donor cryoprecipitate appears to correct both von Willebrand factor (bleeding time) and factor VIII procoagulant activity. Commercial concentrates of factor VIII–von Willebrand factor prepared from large pools of plasma are effective in raising the factor VIII procoagulant levels, but usually fail to correct the bleeding time, even when they bring the ristocetin cofactor activity up to normal levels. Single-donor cryoprecipitate contains the larger von Willebrand factor multimers that are necessary for shortening bleeding time. Most commercial concentrates of factor VIII–von Willebrand factor have lacked these larger multimers. Correction of both the bleeding time and procoagulant activity is important to achieve normal hemostasis in von Willebrand disease patients. Correction of the former is particularly important in the case of mucosal bleeding or whenever platelet adhesion to the subendothelium plays a major role in stopping hemorrhage. In most surgical procedures, when primary hemostasis can be bypassed by surgical hemostasis, correcting the factor VIII procoagulant abnormality becomes most important.

In severe bleeding episodes, a dose of cryoprecipitate between 30 and 50 U per kilogram is recommended. This dosage should raise factor VIII procoagulant activity and correct the bleeding time if the material contains the larger von Willebrand factor multimers. This effect on bleeding time, however, is transient and lasts less than 12 hours, probably because the larger forms of von Willebrand factor are rapidly cleared from the circulation. Therefore, cryoprecipitate should be administered twice a day if hemostasis must be kept normal at all times.

Replacement therapy with human blood derivatives, particularly those obtained from large plasma pools, carries a relatively high risk of transmitting viral hepatitis. This is particularly true in patients who have had no or limited exposure to factor VIII-von Willebrand factor concentrates. Single-donor cryoprecipitate is preferred for this reason as well as for its ability to correct the bleeding time and factor VIII-procoagulant activity levels. However, there is a risk of transmitting the human immunodeficiency virus with cryoprecipitate. Although all donors are screened for antibodies to the virus, single-donor cryoprecipitate is not heat treated.

THE USE OF DDAVP

DDAVP (0.3 µg per kilogram) is the treatment of choice because of the virtual absence of serious side effects. However, it is not equally efficacious in all forms of the disorder. It is not effective in the severe recessive form (type III), in which tissue stores of von Willebrand factor are markedly reduced or absent. On the other hand, most patients with type I von Willebrand disease will have a complete correction of their

hemostatic abnormality lasting for 4 to 6 hours provided that von Willebrand factor concentration in plasma reaches normal levels. In type II disease, the bleeding time may not be corrected even though von Willebrand factor levels are increased to well within normal ranges. This ineffectiveness is due to the fact that the multimeric structure of plasma von Willebrand factor will not be normalized in these patients. However, factor VIII procoagulant levels will be restored to normal, and this may be sufficient for some surgical procedures in which primary hemostasis can be achieved by suturing or cautery. Where this is not possible (as in tooth extraction, gastrointestinal bleeding, or childbirth), normalization of factor VIII procoagulant activity without correction of the bleeding time will usually not secure hemostasis. Cryoprecipitate should be used in type II von Willebrand disease whenever primary hemostasis must be assured. It also should be used in type I patients who do not obtain an adequate response to DDAVP.

Because DDAVP causes thrombocytopenia in type IIB and platelet type (pseudo) von Willebrand disease, its use should not be attempted in these disorders. Cryoprecipitate is usually effective in type IIB. Cryoprecipitate should be used sparingly in platelet type von Willebrand disease because large amounts can cause thrombocytopenia.

PREGNANCY AND CHILDBIRTH

During pregnancy, factor VIII–von Willebrand factor levels tend to rise. In many individuals, particularly those with type I von Willebrand disease, this will be sufficient to restore hemostasis to normal. However, complete correction will not occur in patients with severe von Willebrand disease (type III) or those producing abnormal von Willebrand factor (type II). It is therefore recommended that the *bleeding time* be followed during pregnancy and, if it has not been corrected, that replacement therapy be given at the time of delivery.

INHIBITOR ANTIBODY DEVELOPMENT AFTER REPLACEMENT THERAPY

In a subset of patients with severe (type III) von Willebrand disease, replacement therapy will induce the appearance of antibodies directed toward the factor VIII–von Willebrand factor complex. The individuals so affected have a homozygous deletion of the von Willebrand factor gene. These inhibitors may complicate the treatment of bleeding episodes, and correcting the abnormal hemostasis may be impossible when the inhibitor titer is too high. Since antibodies in these cases are specifically directed against von Willebrand factor, inactivation of factor VIII procoagulant activity probably occurs as a result of steric hindrance. Correcting the bleeding time abnormality is therefore more difficult than correcting the coagulation abnormality. This contrasts with the inhibitors seen in hemophilia A, which are directed at the factor VIII procoagulant protein and do not characteristically affect the bleeding time.

From the clinical point of view, management of soft tissue or joint hemorrhages in the presence of von Willebrand factor inhibitors may be satisfactory if plasma factor VIII procoagulant activity is raised. On the other hand, the inability of replacement therapy to shorten the bleeding time is associated with poor control of mucosal bleeding. Reactions have been described in patients with these inhibitors who are infused with factor VIII–von Willebrand factor concentrates. Most of these reactions are probably due to the precipitating nature of the antibodies, with formation of circulating antigen–antibody complexes. Infusion of factor VIII–von Willebrand factor concentrates into these patients will inevitably cause an amnestic rise of the inhibitor titer. Avoiding replacement therapy, on the contrary, may lead to disappearance of the antibody. To choose the correct dosage, antibody titers should be measured before replacement therapy is administered. Plasma factor VIII procoagulant activity and ristocetin cofactor activity should be tested in vitro to evaluate in vivo recovery of infused factor VIII-von Willebrand factor and to determine the successive dosage of replacement therapy often required. Post-transfusional antibody titers should also be monitored at periodic intervals.

ACQUIRED VON WILLEBRAND DISEASE

A bleeding diathesis similar to inherited von Willebrand disease is occasionally seen on an acquired basis. This syndrome has been reported in association with lupus erythematosus, monoclonal gammopathy, hypernephroma, lymphoproliferative disorders, and angiodysplastic lesions. Antibodies to von Willebrand factor have been detected in a minority of these cases. However, von Willebrand factor is usually decreased in plasma, often to an impressive degree. The principles of replacement therapy outlined above apply to these patients. When antibodies have been detected, they should be monitored before and after replacement therapy.

SUGGESTED READING

Fujimura Y, Ruggeri ZM, Zimmerman TS. Structure and function of human von Willebrand factor. In: Zimmerman TS, Ruggeri ZM, eds. Coagulation and bleeding disorders. The role of factor VIII and von Willebrand factor. New York: Marcel Dekker, 1988.
Berkowitz SD, Ruggeri ZM, Zimmerman TS. von Willebrand disease. In: Zimmerman TS, Ruggeri ZM, eds. Coagulation and bleeding disorders. The role of factor VIII and von Willebrand factor. New York: Marcel Dekker, 1988.
Ruggeri ZM, Zimmerman TS. von Willebrand factor and von Willebrand disease. Blood 1987; 70:895–904.

DEFICIENCIES OF THE VITAMIN K DEPENDENT CLOTTING FACTORS

HAROLD R. ROBERTS, M.D.
VIRGIL L. ROSE, M.D.

Prothrombin, factors VII, IX, and X, and proteins C and S are synthesized in the liver, and vitamin K is required for their complete synthesis. Within the hepatocyte, precursor proteins of these factors undergo postribosomal modification by vitamin K–dependent hepatic carboxylase, resulting in the addition of a carboxyl group to 10 to 12 glutamyl residues on the amino terminal ends of these molecules. This results in the formation of gammacarboxyglutamyl (GLA) residues, which are necessary for calcium-dependent phospholipid interactions. The number of GLA residues on the vitamin K–dependent clotting factors is variably reduced in the presence of warfarin drugs, vitamin K

deficiency, liver disease, and some rare congenital bleeding disorders.

Proteins C and S are discussed in Chapter 29, and hereditary deficiency of factor IX (hemophilia B) is discussed in the chapter "The Hemophilias."

DIAGNOSIS OF DEFICIENCIES OF THE VITAMIN K–DEPENDENT FACTORS

The diagnosis of these coagulation factor deficiencies is made in patients with a history of bleeding and laboratory tests that document low levels of one or more of the aforementioned clotting factors. Usually screening tests of coagulation function, i.e., the prothrombin time (PT) and activated partial thromboplastin time (APTT), are prolonged in the presence of low levels of clotting factors. Accurate diagnosis rests upon specific assays for individual clotting factors.

Clotting factor deficiencies may be congenital or acquired, as shown in Table 1. Usually only a single clotting factor is deficient in hereditary disorders, whereas in acquired disorders multiple clotting factors are usually affected.

Table 1 Causes of Deficiencies of the Vitamin K-Dependent Factors

Congenital Deficiencies
  Prothrombin: Hypoprothrombinemia, Dysprothrombinemia
  Factor VII deficiency
  Factor IX deficiency (Hemophilia B)
  Factor X deficiency
  Combined deficiencies: factors, II, VII, IX, and X

Acquired deficiencies
  Hemorrhagic disease of the newborn
  Warfarin ingestion: Therapeutic, toxic, surreptitious
  Superwarfarin ingestion
  Antibiotic administration
  Other drugs: Cholestyramine, vitamins A and E, mineral oil, hydantoins, and salicylates
  Dietary deficiency
  Liver disease: Hepatitis, cirrhosis, malignancy
  Malabsorption: Pancreatic disease, small bowel disease, biliary tract obstruction
  Other causes: Amyloidosis, nephrotic syndrome, acquired inhibitors to clotting factors

CONGENITAL FACTOR DEFICIENCIES

Prothrombin

Prothrombin (factor II) deficiency is inherited as an autosomal recessive disorder. Approximately 30 cases have been described. Homozygotes for true hypoprothrombinemia may have prothrombin levels of 2 percent to 25 percent of normal. These patients may experience significant hemorrhage. Patients heterozygous for hypoprothrombinemia are asymptomatic. Dysprothrombinemias are characterized by structural abnormalities in the prothrombin molecule. Patients with dysprothrombinemia may be symptomatic in the heterozygous state. Affected patients exhibit easy bruising, epistaxis, menorrhagia, postpartum hemorrhage, and postsurgical hemorrhage. Both the PT and APTT are prolonged, and functional prothrombin levels are low when measured by specific assay.

The biologic half-life of prothrombin is approximately 72 hours. To achieve normal hemostasis, the level of functional prothrombin should be raised to about 25 percent or higher. Prothrombin levels are followed to judge the frequency of infusions, but cessation of hemorrhage is the best guide to the efficacy of therapy. The preferred treatment for bleeding episodes in patients with either hypo- or dysprothrombinemia is fresh frozen plasma in a loading dose of 10 to 15 ml per kilogram of body weight, followed by maintenance infusions of 3 to 6 ml per kilogram of body weight every 24 hours if necessary. Usually single doses suffice for isolated bleeding events, but in the case of surgery or sustained bleeding, replacement therapy may need to be continued for 5 to 10 days.

Commercially available prothrombin complex concentrates (PCCs) have been used for treatment of bleeding episodes (Table 2). Currently available PCCs are produced from pooled human plasma and may transmit hepatitis B and C. These concentrates have also been associated with thromboembolic events (Table 3). For treatment of severe hemorrhagic episodes, however, PCCs may be indicated and can be infused at a dose of 40 U per kilogram of body weight, followed by 15 U per kilogram of body weight every 24 to 36 hours.

Factor VII

Factor VII deficiency is a rare disorder; it is inherited as an autosomal recessive characteristic that occurs in about 1 in 500,000 persons. It is the only hereditary clotting factor deficiency characterized by a prolonged PT and a normal APTT. Severely affected individuals (factor VII levels < 1 percent) have hemorrhagic episodes beginning in childhood, including umbilical cord hemorrhage, epistaxis, intracranial bleeding, menorrhagia, and hemarthroses. In severely affected factor VII–deficient patients, hemorrhage is as severe as that seen in classic hemophilia. Mild and moderate forms of factor VII deficiency also occur, but the severity of bleeding with trauma or surgery varies to a surprising degree. At times, no bleeding occurs in mildly affected patients, even after major surgery.

Plasma replacement therapy is the current treatment of choice for bleeding episodes. Major surgery can be carried out under coverage of normal plasma. In severely affected patients, factor levels of 10 percent to 20 percent are considered effective for hemostasis. Plasma in a loading dose of 10 to 15 ml per kilogram of body weight is usually effective in single doses for hemarthroses, dental procedures, or other limited bleeding events. Prophylactic plasma replacement is given for dental procedures to prevent bleeding. For surgery, loading doses of plasma, as noted previously, should be followed by maintenance doses given every 6 to 12 hours for 5 to 10 days depending on the type of surgery. In some severely affected patients, it has been suggested that major bleeding episodes may require treatment with PCCs every 6 to 12 hours. As shown in Table 2, one must be certain that the PCCs contain factor VII. The dosage is calculated as 0.5 U (factor VII) × body weight (kg) × desired increase (percent of normal). We have had little experience in the treatment of factor VII–deficient patients, but our preference is to use plasma replacement therapy rather than PCCs if possible. Plasma is generally safer than currently available PCCs, but it has the risks listed in Table 4.

Highly purified recombinant factor VIIa, free of infectious agents, has been prepared by Novo Laboratories and could conceivably be used to treat factor VII–deficient patients, although it has not yet been used for this purpose. Rather, recombinant factor VIIa is currently undergoing clinical trials in patients with classic hemophilia and Christmas disease complicated by circulating antibodies to factors VIII and IX, respectively.

Factor IX

Factor IX deficiency (hemophilia B) is discussed in the chapter "The Hemophilias."

Table 2 Commercially Available Prothrombin Complex Concentrates

Name	Factors (units/100 U of factor IX)*			
Prothrombin complex concentrates	**II**	**VII**	**IX**	**X**
Proplex T† (Baxter Hyland)	(50)	(400)	(100)	(50)
Konyne-HT (Cutter)	(100)	(20)	(100)	(140)
Profilnine Heat-Treated (Alpha Therapeutic)	(148)	(11)	(100)	(64)
Activated prothrombin complex concentrates‡				
Autoplex T† (Baxter Hyland)	II, VII, IX, X, and variable amounts of VIIa, IXa, and Xa			
FEIBA VH Immuno (Immuno)	II, VII, IX, X, and variable amounts of VIIa, IXa, and Xa			

*Prothrombin complex concentrates are usually labeled in units of factor IX per vial and come in sizes ranging from approximately 250 to 1,000 U.

†It contains heparin, 1 to 2 units per milliliter of reconstituted material.

‡Activated PCCs are used to treat patients with hemophilia A and B with inhibitors to factors VIII and IX, respectively. They contain more activated factors than unactivated PCCs and presumably possess materials that "bypass" inhibitors.

Table 3 Adverse Effects Associated with the Use of Prothrombin Complex Concentrates

Viral infections (hepatitis C and B)
Thrombosis
    Thromboembolism
    Disseminated intravascular coagulation (especially in the presence of liver disease)
Chronic hepatitis (secondary to viral hepatitis, 50% of transfusion-related infections become chronic)
    Chronic persistent hepatitis
    Chronic lobular hepatitis
    Chronic active hepatitis
    Cirrhosis (occurs in approximately 10% of chronically infected patients)
Allergic reactions (including anaphylaxis)

Table 4 Adverse Effects of Plasma Replacement Therapy

Type of adverse effect	Risk*
Viral infections	
Hepatitis B virus	1/1000
Hepatitis C virus	1–2/100
Human immunodeficiency virus	1/36,000–150,000
Cytomegalovirus	1/10-12
Hepatitis delta virus	1/3,000
Epstein-Barr virus	1/200
Human T-cell lymphotropic viruses	rare
Allergic reaction	1/1,000
Anaphylaxis	1/150,000
Hemolysis	1/2,500-5,000
Hypervolemia	Variable

*The risk of an adverse reaction is listed per unit of transfused plasma. Risks cited are approximate and will vary according to the donor population in a particular region. Allergic or anaphylactic reactions usually do not occur without previous exposure to blood products.

Factor X

Factor X deficiency is a rare disorder (approximately 1 per million of the population) and is inherited as an autosomal recessive characteristic. It is often heralded by umbilical cord bleeding. As with other clotting factor deficiencies, genetic heterogeneity is characteristic of the disorder, and several point mutations in the factor X gene have been reported. Depending upon the genetic abnormality, bleeding in factor X deficiency may be mild, moderate, or severe. The hemorrhagic tendency in factor X deficiency ranges from easy bruisability, epistaxis, and menorrhagia in mildly or moderately affected patients, to spontaneous hemorrhages in severely affected patients.

Treatment of factor X deficiency is determined by the severity of the hemorrhage. In mild bleeding episodes, the treatment of choice is fresh frozen plasma, which is given in doses sufficient to raise the factor X level to 20 percent to 30 percent of normal. The half-life of transfused factor X is 24 to 48 hours (mean, 40 hours) so that plasma infusions every 12 to 24 hours usually result in a gradual rise in levels of factor X. A loading dose of plasma (10 to 15 ml per kilogram of body weight) is followed by 3 to 6 ml per kilogram of body weight every 12 hours when one dose will not suffice to control bleeding. In severe hemorrhagic episodes or with major surgical procedures, PCCs that are known to contain factor X (see Table 2) may be given in a dose of 50 U per kilogram every 12 to 24 hours. Prothrombin complex concentrates should be used only if the deficiency is profound or if fluid overload from large amounts of plasma is a concern.

Combined Deficiencies of Vitamin K–Dependent Factors

Rare combined congenital deficiencies of factors II, VII, IX, and X have been reported. These patients exhibit defective gammacarboxylation of glutamyl residues in all the vitamin K–dependent factors. Antigenic levels of the vitamin K–dependent factors are near normal, but functional activities may be markedly decreased. Large doses of oral vitamin K should be tried in these patients because it has resulted in an increase in functional levels of vitamin K–dependent factors in some of them.

General Comments

Patients with hereditary deficiencies of vitamin K–dependent clotting factors should receive comprehensive care. From the time of diagnosis, every attempt should be made to prevent long-term complications. Whenever possible, fresh frozen plasma is selected over PCCs because the risk of hepatitis B and C is much greater with PCCs. Thromboembolism, including disseminated intravascular coagulation (DIC), may occur with all preparations of PCCs. When plasma is not acceptable, whether owing to volume overload or severity of bleeding, several PCCs are available. Prothrombin complex concentrates are usually labeled in units of factor IX per bottle. Proplex T lists the number of units of both factors VII and IX. An approximation of the content of factors II, VII, and X per 100 U of factor IX in PCCs is provided in Table 2. The main advantage of PCCs is that factor levels of 50 percent or greater can be achieved without volume overload. In addition, PCCs can be stored in the lyophilized form at 4°C for prolonged periods of time and are easy to reconstitute. Therefore, they can be used for home therapy in patients with frequent bleeding episodes.

The major disadvantage of PCCs has proved to be transmission of viral diseases (see Table 3). Currently available PCCs are now heat-treated in the lyophilized state. This procedure inactivates human immunodeficiency virus (HIV) but does not reliably eradicate the hepatitis viruses. A recently developed enzyme-linked immunoassay for detection of hepatitis C (non-A, non-B hepatitis), which presumably will be available in the near future, should exclude source plasma contaminated with hepatitis C. All patients not previously exposed to hepatitis B should be appropriately immunized. There is a real need for PCCs free of viral contamination. When such concentrates will be available is not known.

Most severely affected patients with hereditary hemorrhagic disorders who received blood products before 1985 are seropositive for the HIV antibody. Patients infected with HIV are best managed in conjunction with an infectious disease specialist. It is particularly important to counsel these patients about safe sexual practices so that sexual partners are protected.

Home therapy, using either plasma or PCCs, is important in the management of patients with severe deficiencies of any of the blood clotting factors. Patients are taught self-infusion techniques for treatment at the earliest sign of bleeding. With hemarthroses, prompt administration of deficient factor may limit joint destruction.

Dental care is a critical part of the overall management of patients with congenital clotting factor deficiencies. Patients should receive dental cleaning every 6 months and other appropriate prophylaxis for dental problems.

Progesterone or one of the oral contraceptives should be given to affected women with menorrhagia.

ACQUIRED DEFICIENCIES OF VITAMIN K–DEPENDENT FACTORS

Hemorrhagic Disease of the Newborn

Hemorrhagic disease of the newborn is an acquired deficiency of vitamin K due to poor transport of the vitamin to the fetus from the placenta, the lack of intestinal bacterial flora in the fetus, and immaturity of the fetal liver. Premature infants are at greater risk for developing vitamin K deficiency and bleeding than are term infants. Even in term infants, levels of vitamin K–dependent factors may decrease significantly on the second and third days after delivery. Human milk is a poor source of vitamin K, resulting in a greater tendency for breastfed infants to develop bleeding. The preferred prophylaxis for hemorrhagic disease of the newborn is intramuscular administration of vitamin K_1 in a dose of 0.5 to 1.0 mg as soon after delivery as possible.

Warfarin Therapy

One of the most common causes of decreased availability of functional levels of vitamin K in the hepatocyte is warfarin therapy. Warfarin decreases carboxylation of glutamyl residues of prothrombin and factors VII, IX, and X by inhibition of vitamin K reductase. This results in unavailability of reduced vitamin K for carboxylase activity. The most sensitive indicator of warfarin effect is a decrease in factor VII, which results in a prolonged PT. Other vitamin K–dependent factors are eventually decreased as well, resulting in a prolongation of the aPTT.

The most common complication of warfarin therapy is hemorrhage. The effects of warfarin can be reversed within 4 to 12 hours by vitamin K_1 administration. In patients who are taking warfarin for therapeutic purposes, however, vitamin K should not be given unless clearly indicated, because the patient will be rendered resistant to warfarin for several days thereafter. In nonbleeding patients, overdosage of warfarin can be managed by discontinuing the drug and allowing clotting factors to increase gradually to more desirable levels. If emergent correction is necessary, fresh frozen plasma, 10 to 15 ml per kilogram of body weight, should be administered rapidly and repeated in a dose of 5 ml per kilogram of body weight every 6 to 12 hours if necessary. When temporary reversal of warfarin effect is desired, fresh frozen plasma is the treatment of choice because resumption of warfarin therapy can be initiated in the usual dose. Plasma therapy has the risks listed in Table 4.

Surreptitious Warfarin Ingestion

Surreptitious ingestion of warfarin, often by medical or paramedical personnel, must be considered in an acquired deficiency of the vitamin K–dependent factors in bleeding patients without a previous history of disease. Overdoses of warfarin have been taken in attempted suicides but are more commonly ingested for secondary gain. The treatment of choice is vitamin K$_1$ at a dose of 1 to 2 mg intravenously or 5 to 10 mg subcutaneously. Repeated doses of vitamin K may be required for overdoses of warfarin. If patients are bleeding in vital areas, fresh frozen plasma should be used.

Superwarfarin

Superwarfarins, such as brodifacoum or difenacoum, which were developed as rodenticides, have a very long duration of action. An ingestion of one of the superwarfarins taken for secondary gain, attempted suicide, or accidentally by a child may effectively inhibit vitamin K reductase for 50 days or more. Superwarfarins cause a marked and prolonged reduction of the vitamin K–dependent factors. Repeated large doses of vitamin K are required to control the effects of a superwarfarin. Therapy with high doses of vitamin K, e.g., 50 to 100 mg per day orally or parenterally, may be required for weeks to months. In addition, fresh frozen plasma is often necessary to control bleeding.

Antibiotic Administration

Vitamin K–dependent clotting factor deficiencies may occur as a complication of the use of certain broad-spectrum antibiotics. It is widely held that the vitamin K deficiency resulting therefrom is due to eradication of vitamin K–producing gut bacteria. Although this has not been disproved, recent evidence suggests that antibiotics containing a methyltetrazolethiol (MTT) group, such as cefamandole and cefoperazone, interfere with intrahepatic metabolism of vitamin K to cause these clotting factor deficiencies. Iatrogenic "deficiency" of vitamin K secondary to antibiotic administration is best reversed with parenteral vitamin K at a dose of 5 to 10 mg per day for 3 to 5 days. A slow response to therapy may occur if the offending antibiotic is continued, in which case longer supplementation with the vitamin is necessary.

Other Drugs

There are other drugs that interfere with vitamin K and result in clotting factor deficiencies. Cholestyramine, which binds bile acids, prevents absorption of fat-soluble vitamins, including vitamin K. Ingestion of excessive quantities of mineral oil has a similar effect. Excessive doses of vitamin A or vitamin E interfere with vitamin K absorption and possibly the metabolism of vitamin K. Salicylates and hydantoins antagonize vitamin K metabolism. In these instances, withdrawal of the offending drug or supplementation with vitamin K at a dose of 5 to 10 mg daily for 3 to 5 days is the treatment of choice.

Dietary Deficiency

Dietary deficiency of vitamin K generally occurs in debilitated patients who are not eating well or who avoid eating green vegetables. Chronically ill patients on parenteral nutrition without vitamin K supplementation are especially prone to vitamin K deficiency. Dietary deficiency of vitamin K is often overlooked until bleeding occurs or the PT is noted to be prolonged. Vitamin K in doses of 5 to 10 mg corrects the defect. Green leafy vegetables, cheeses, and vegetable oils are excellent sources of the vitamin and should be added to the diet when possible.

Protein-calorie malnutrition (marasmus, kwashiorkor) may cause hypoprothombinemia by amino acid deprivation, a condition not responsive to vitamin K administration. If bleeding occurs in these conditions, fresh frozen plasma is the treatment of choice.

Hepatocellular Disease

In hepatocellular disease, reduction in vitamin K–dependent factors results from abnormal metabolism of vitamin K or from an overall decrease in protein synthesis. Deficiencies of vitamin K–dependent factors are frequently seen in patients with hepatitis, cirrhosis, hepatic malignancies, or other types of liver disease. Usually multiple clotting factors are decreased, as shown in Table 5. Vitamin K may be given to patients with liver disease, but it is usually not effective. As a general rule, the coagulopathy of liver disease requires no treatment unless the patient experiences significant hemorrhage. In this event, the treatment of choice is fresh frozen plasma, which contains all of the coagulation factors. Currently available PCCs are generally not given to correct the coagulopathy of liver disease because of the danger of infecting patients with viral hepatitis superimposed on a compromised liver. In addition, there is the danger of thromboembolic events induced by PCCs, especially in the presence of liver dysfunction. Fresh frozen plasma in a loading dose of 10 ml per kilogram of body weight may be given, followed by maintenance doses of 3 ml per kilogram of body weight every 8 to 12 hours if necessary. With plasma therapy, there is always the danger of hypervolemia, which may contribute to increased bleeding in some patients (see Table 4). Deamino-arginine vasopressin (DDAVP) may be of value in the treatment of bleeding resulting from liver disease. DDAVP is given intravenously or subcutaneously in doses of 0.3 µg per kilogram of body weight. Side effects are few, but they do occur and include nausea, vomiting, severe headache, and hyponatremia.

Table 5 Coagulopathy of Liver Disease

Mild liver failure: Reduction in Vitamin K-dependent factors VII, X, II, and IX

Moderate liver failure: Reduction in above as well as factors V and fibrinogen

Severe liver failure: Reduction in all factors, including factor VIII

Malabsorption

Malabsorption may occur in a variety of conditions affecting the gastrointestinal tract. Biliary obstruction interferes with absorption of fats and fat-soluble vitamins A, D, E, and K, by blocking bile acid secretion. If the obstruction has been present for several days, vitamin K should be given by intramuscular or subcutaneous injection (10 mg) prior to any surgical attempt to relieve the blockage. Small bowel disease such as regional ileitis, short bowel syndrome, or "overgrowth" by intestinal bacterial flora may cause a decrease in vitamin K–dependent factors. Pancreatic insufficiency, with malabsorption and steatorrhea, is another etiology of fat-soluble vitamin deficiency. In these cases, parenteral administration of vitamin K (10 to 25 mg) should correct the defect. In patients with chronic disorders, intermittent repeated doses of vitamin K may be necessary.

Acquired Deficiencies of Single Factors

Single factor deficiencies may be acquired in a variety of conditions. Isolated acquired deficiency of prothrombin is rare but has been reported in lupus erythematosus due to an antiprothrombin antibody. Occasionally, prothrombin levels are extremely low, probably because the prothrombin-antibody complex is rapidly cleared from the circulation. Treatment with steroids may be of benefit in this condition.

Acquired factor VII deficiency has been described in homocystinuria and reportedly responds to a low-methionine diet. Factor IX levels may drop due to urinary loss in nephrotic syndrome. Acquired inhibitors to vitamin K–dependent factors are extremely rare. When they do occur, immunosuppressive therapy may be of benefit.

Amyloidosis, usually of the primary type, is occasionally associated with an isolated factor X deficiency. This deficiency is characterized by a short biologic half-life of factor X, presumably because of absorption of factor X from the plasma onto amyloid fibrils. Because production of factor X is not impaired in amyloidosis, vitamin K administration is not effective. In addition, fresh frozen plasma is ineffective because of the short in vivo half-life of factor X in the presence of amyloid. Prothrombin complex concentrates containing factor X may be necessary for profound bleeding, but the risk of hepatitis should be weighed against the possible benefit. Splenectomy, by removing a source of the amyloid deposits, has been associated with improvement in some patients.

SUGGESTED READING

Alperin JB. Coagulopathy caused by vitamin K deficiency in critically ill, hospitalized patients. JAMA 1987; 258(14):1916–1919.

Lipsky JJ. Antibiotic-associated hypoprothrombinaemia: Review. J Antimicrob Chem 1988; 21:281–300.

Menache D. New concentrates of factors VII, IX and X. In: Kasper C, ed. Recent advances in hemophilia care. New York: Alan R. Liss, 1990; 177–187.

Olson RE. Vitamin K. In: Colman RW, Hirsh J, Marder VJ, eds. Hemostasis and thrombosis. Philadelphia: JB Lippincott, 1987: 846–860.

Roberts HR, Foster PA. Inherited disorders of prothrombin conversion. In: Colman RW, Hirsh J, Marder VJ, eds. Hemostasis and thrombosis. Philadelphia; JB Lippincott, 1987:162–181.

ACQUIRED ANTICOAGULANTS

SANDOR S. SHAPIRO, M.D.

Acquired anticoagulants are generally antibodies directed against specific coagulation factors or against negatively charged phospholipids (so-called lupus anticoagulants). Antibodies in the former category usually are associated with an increased risk of hemorrhage; the most common of these antibodies are directed against factor VIII or factor IX. Antibodies in the latter category, to the contrary, appear to be associated with a high risk of thrombosis. Therapeutic considerations in these two classes are therefore quite different, and the two classes will be discussed separately.

CIRCULATING INHIBITORS (ANTICOAGULANTS) TO SPECIFIC COAGULATION FACTORS

Although antibodies have been described against nearly all coagulation factors, the vast majority are directed against FVIII or, to a lesser extent, FIX. The present discussion will be limited to FVIII and FIX antibodies. For a more general discussion, the reader should consult one of the references at the end of this chapter.

Antibodies to FVIII occur in 10 to 20 percent of treated patients with moderate or severe hemophilia A as a consequence of exposure to exogenous FVIII. The prevalence of FIX antibodies in severe hemophilia B is somewhat lower. When they occur, antibodies usually do not cause a worsening of the hemorrhagic diathesis, but may severely complicate treatment of bleeding episodes. About 20 percent of patients with antibodies are "weak responders," whose antibody levels do not exceed 2 to 5 Bethesda U per milliliter despite repeated exposure to FVIII or FIX. The remaining 80 percent behave in the manner expected for most antibodies: anamnestic responses occur 4 to 10 days after antigenic challenge, while withholding antigen results in a gradual fall in titer. Occasionally, patients with mild hemophilia A develop FVIII antibodies after treatment with FVIII. Generally, such antibodies are transient, but while present, they often increase the severity of the patient's hemophilia. Individuals who are not suffering from genetic coagulation factor deficiencies may also develop inhibitors, most frequently against FVIII, which induce a hemorrhagic disorder; usually there is no antecedent history of exposure to blood products.

Acute Treatment

Proper treatment requires adequate laboratory facilities including, as a minimum, accurate quantitative assays for the coagulation factor in question and for the coagulation inhibitor. For the latter purpose, the Bethesda assay is highly recommended. Because inhibitors occur with some frequency in treated hemophiliacs, it is important to measure coagulation factor and inhibitor levels on a regular basis, including an assessment of in vivo yield after infusion of coagulation factor concentrates. Any patient whose clinical response to infusion seems suboptimal should be checked for the presence of an inhibitor.

Inhibitor patients who are "weak responders" can generally continue treatment with FVIII or FIX, although at higher doses than usual. Dose can be calculated by estimating the FVIII or FIX needed to neutralize the inhibitor and adding to that the amount needed to achieve hemostasis in the specific clinical situation. For example, a 50-kg youngster with hemophilia A and an elbow hemorrhage, whose FVIII antibody is 2 BU per milliliter, would require approximately 2,000 U of FVIII to neutralize the antibody — 2 BU per milliliter × 40 ml per kilogram plasma volume × 0.5 (the definition of the Bethesda unit is that concentration of antibody neutralizing 50 percent of the FVIII in an equal volume of normal plasma) — plus 700 U to treat the hemarthrosis (14 U per kilogram is a dose sufficient to treat a hemarthrosis in an uncomplicated hemophiliac), or a total of 2,700 U FVIII. "Weak responder" antibody patients can be placed on home therapy and respond well to treatment.

The situation with strong responders is much more complex. Once antibody levels exceed 10 BU per milliliter it is impractical to give replacement therapy with FVIII or FIX. In addition, treatment can be expected to result in a substantial increase in antibody titer. Thus replacement therapy with concentrate is generally reserved for life-threatening situations. An alternative form of treatment is the use of prothrombin complex concentrates (PCCs), either the nonactivated varieties (such as Konyne or Proplex) or the activated types (such as Autoplex or FEIBA). Although the active principle "bypassing" the inhibitor has not been identified, control studies have demonstrated that single infusions of nonactivated PCCs at a dose of 75 FIX U per kilogram are effective in treating hemarthroses in 50 percent of cases (vs. a success rate of 25 percent for placebo). Activated PCCs (at a dose of 75 bypassing units per kilogram) may be slightly more effective (55 to 60 percent). Uncontrolled studies suggest that effectiveness may be increased with 2 to 3 doses (6 to 8 hours apart). PCCs can be used in hemophilia A patients with FVIII inhibitors and also in hemophilia B patients with FIX inhibitors. Since PCCs induce a mild prothrombotic state, care must be taken to avoid their use in patients with serious liver dysfunction and to refrain from using EACA concomitantly. Since variable amounts of FVIII antigen are present in PCCs, some patients show rises in FVIII antibody levels after treatment, although rarely to more than two to three times pretreatment levels. Treatment should almost always be initiated with nonactivated PCCs, in view of the small difference in efficacy and the large difference in cost. Activated PCCs should be used only after failure of the nonactivated variety. The only exception is serious cranial hemorrhage, where the slight advantage of activated PCCs, as well as the need for immediate treatment, outweigh the cost factor.

Since FVIII therapy is, by definition, the treatment of choice in hemophilia A, several approaches have been taken to circumvent high antibody titers and produce circulating levels of FVIII. Plasmapheresis has been used, but has not been uniformly successful. Although, theoretically, 60 to 85 percent of the plasma antibody can be removed with a 3- to 4-liter plasmapheresis, this goal is rarely achieved and is, in any event, insufficient in the face of a high-titer antibody. Almost all FVIII and FIX antibodies are IgG, whose distribution is only 45 percent intravascular. Furthermore, antibody production appears to be stimulated by the procedure, since pre-plasmapheresis antibody levels are frequently reattained within 48 hours. Thus it may be necessary to perform daily plasmapheresis for 2 to 3 days before antibody levels are reduced by 75 percent. At that point, massive doses of concentrate may neutralize the inhibitor and achieve hemostatic levels of FVIII. Until the last plasmapheresis, replacement should probably be with 5 percent albumin in normal saline, because hemodynamic, metabolic, and immunologic complications have occasionally occurred when plasma has been used for volume replacement.

Because of the species specificity of many FVIII antibodies, another approach to replacement therapy is the use of FVIII concentrates of animal origin. Prior experience with porcine and bovine concentrates had been complicated by the frequent occurrence of allergic reactions and thrombocytopenia. Recently, a polyelectrolyte-fractionated porcine FVIII has been prepared (Hyate C, Speywood Laboratories, Irvine, CA) that is largely free of these side effects. Allergic reactions, when they occur, are generally mild and easily controlled with antihistamines and/or steroids. If the use of porcine FVIII is contemplated, inhibitor titers must be measured against the porcine product and calculations of replacement quantities made on this basis. Usually a patient's antibody will react much less, or not at all, against the porcine material, so that hemostatic levels of FVIII can be achieved after infusion. Because it is a foreign protein and can induce antibody formation, efficacy of porcine FVIII may decrease with repeated use, and the risk of allergic reactions may increase. Thus this product should be reserved for life-threatening situations. In anticipation of its use, and to prevent problems in emergencies, all inhibitor patients should have antiporcine FVIII levels determined, and a small stock of porcine FVIII should be available wherever inhibitor patients are treated.

Several maneuvers have been proposed to blunt the anamnestic response when FVIII or FIX is used in patients with hemophilia A or B and inhibitors. Immunosuppressive agents, such as cyclophosphamide, have been administered intravenously (in single doses of 10 to 20 mg per kilogram) at the initiation of infusion therapy, but results have not been convincing. Immunosuppressive therapy also has been used in attempts to eradicate inhibitors (to be discussed). Recently intravenous IgG (IVIgG) has been used as an adjunct to treatment. IVIgG, made from large pools of normal plasma, has been shown to contain anti-idiotypic antibodies capable of neutralizing many patients' inhibitors in vitro and in vivo; responses may vary from patient to patient and, in a given patient, from lot to lot of IVIgG. The usual dose is 0.3 to 0.4 g per kilogram, and infusions have been given daily for as long as 8 days. When a response is seen, a substantial fall in inhibitor occurs, which may last 4 to 12 weeks. Current data would suggest that in vitro testing is a good predictor of in vivo results. Thus inability of IVIgG to neutralize the inhibitor when admixed with patient plasma argues against its in vivo use.

In inhibitor patients who are capable of synthesizing FVIII to some extent (mild hemophiliacs) or normally (nonhemophiliacs), treatment with DDAVP (1-deamino-8-D-arginine vasopressin) may play a role. This drug stimulates the release of von Willebrand factor from endothelial cell stores and, indirectly, raises the level of FVIII. It has been used in place of FVIII or PCCs as preparation for dental extraction, for example; however, it is unlikely to be effective unless the inhibitor level is low. The drug is administered as an intravenous dose of 0.3 μg per kilogram in 50 ml normal saline over about 15 minutes. Rarely, recipients have mild vasopressin-like side effects, but usually the drug is well tolerated, with only occasional flushing or tachycardia. Antifibrinolytic therapy should be given at the same time (oral EACA, 20 g daily in four divided doses), because DDAVP also releases tissue plasminogen activator from endothelial cells, leading to an increase in blood fibrinolytic activity. DDAVP is ineffective in hemophilia B patients with FIX antibodies.

EACA alone has been used with moderate success as an adjunct to therapy in dental extractions in inhibitor and noninhibitor patients. Its use is based on the concept that the small degree of hemostasis achieved by the patient is aided by temporarily shutting off the normal fibrinolytic response at the site of extraction. EACA is given orally, 20 g per day in four divided doses, for 4 to 5 days, starting a few hours before the dental surgery. EACA should be avoided in patients with hematuria. Finally, dental extraction is much more successful in well-relaxed patients, and training patients in relaxation techniques, including hypnosis, has proved useful.

Eradication of Antibodies

A number of approaches have been taken in attempts to eradicate antibodies. Cyclophosphamide and azathioprine, with or without steroids, have been used at the time of antigenic challenge with blood products, but success has been rare except, perhaps, when treatment has been given at the time of appearance of the inhibitor. Greater success has been achieved with nonhemophilic inhibitors, using long-term oral treatment. A typical regimen would be 150 mg cyclophosphamide and 30 to 50 mg prednisone daily. Antibody titers fall slowly, and treatment frequently must be continued for many months.

Induction of specific tolerance has been attempted as well. Patients with hemophilia A and inhibitors have been treated with massive daily doses of FVIII—the so-called Bonn regimen—for months to years, with disappearance of antibodies, without recurrence when the regimen was stopped, and FVIII therapy on a need basis was reinstituted. This regimen is enormously expensive and psychologically trying, especially for young patients, and has not found much favor. However, less stringent administration schedules may achieve similar ends. It is the general impression that patients on home treatment, receiving infusion once or twice weekly, do not form antibodies at the expected rate, perhaps owing to this phenomenon.

The most recent attempts at inducing tolerance have involved the use of IVIgG, together with immunosuppressives and concentrates. However, a larger experience and longer patient follow-up will be necessary before this approach can be evaluated.

In summary, hemophiliacs with "strong responder" inhibitors pose a serious therapeutic challenge. The usual type of hemorrhagic events can be treated fairly successfully with PCCs. Life-threatening hemorrhage, or operative procedures requiring coverage for 7 to 10 days, require other approaches. Plasmapheresis may play a useful role in lowering high antibody levels so as to make replacement therapy more effective. Porcine FVIII may be useful in these circumstances. IVIgG may be useful in some patients for similar reasons. Inhibitors in mild hemophiliacs and in nonhemophiliacs may fall after DDAVP infusion (always given together with EACA), and this approach may be useful for dental extractions. Eradication of inhibitors probably involves induction of tolerance. Although not yet perfected, several promising approaches are currently under investigation.

LUPUS ANTICOAGULANTS

Lupus anticoagulants are a frequent cause of a prolonged PTT. Less frequently, they may be associated with a prolongation of the PT as well. A variety of coagulation tests have been used for their detection, none of which is absolutely specific. Of these, the dilute Russell viper venom time (RVVT) is probably the simplest and the most specific. Lupus anticoagulants interfere, to a greater or lesser extent, with all phospholipid-dependent coagulation tests. These "anticoagulants," in and of themselves, are rarely, if ever, a cause of bleeding. To the contrary, patients with lupus anticoagulants have a 25 to 30 percent prevalence of thromboembolic disorders. In addition, women with histories of repeated abortion frequently have lupus anticoagulants. In almost all cases, patients with lupus anticoagulants have elevated levels of anticardiolipin antibodies, but the dilute RVVT seems to be a better indicator of thrombotic risk.

Nonpregnant patients with lupus anticoagulants and a documented history of thrombosis should be placed on oral anticoagulant therapy. Control of therapy can usually be achieved by following the prothrombin time, which is rarely prolonged. Mild prolongations do not interfere with treatment, which should aim for a PT ratio of 1.3 to 1.5.

Elimination of the lupus anticoagulant can frequently be achieved with steroids, but the antibody tends to recur after cessation of steroids. Steroids have also been used to carry spontaneous aborters to term, and the rate of fetal salvage is high. However, side effects are also significant, and alternative treatments are currently being investigated. In both situations, reduction of lupus anticoagulant levels may not be accompanied by diminution in the titer of anticardiolipin antibodies.

SUGGESTED READING

Harris EN. Antiphospholipid antibodies. Br J Haematol 1990; 74:1–9.
Kasper CK, Aledort LM, Counts RB, et al. A more uniform measurement of factor VIII inhibitors. Thromb Diath Haemorrh 1975; 34:869–872.
Love PE, Santoro SA. Antiphospholipid antibodies: Anticardiolipin and the lupus anticoagulant in systemic lupus erythematosus (SLE) and in non-SLE disorders. Ann Int Med 1990; 112:682–698.
Shapiro SS, Siegel JE. Hemorrhage disorders associated with circulating inhibitors. In: Ratnoff OD, Forbes CD, eds. Disorders of hemostasis. Philadelphia: WB Saunders, 1991:245.
Triplett DA, Brandt J. Laboratory identification of the lupus anticoagulant. Br J Haematol 1989; 73:139–142.

THALASSEMIA

MELVIN H. FREEDMAN, M.D., F.R.C.P.C.

Thalassemia is an inherited disorder characterized by a decreased rate of synthesis of one or more globin chains. This quantitative abnormality leads to imbalanced globin chain synthesis, defective hemoglobin production, and shortened red cell survival. The various forms of thalassemia are shown in Table 1.

It is conservatively estimated that there are 180 million heterozygote carriers for the various types of thalassemia throughout Asia, North Africa, and Europe. This high gene frequency results in a significant annual number of births of homozygote and compound heterozygote states that pose clinical problems.

At the molecular level, most of the α-thalassemias are due to deletions of one or more genes from the α-globin complex located on the short arm of chromosome 16. Currently, 20 such deletional mutants have been described. In contrast, most β-thalassemias are nondeletional mutations in or near the β-globin gene cluster on chromosome II that affect the transcription of β–globin messenger RNA. There are more than 90 different mutations that account for the β-thalassemias.

Table 1 Classification of the Thalassemias

α-Thalassemia syndromes
  "Silent carrier" state
  α-Thalassemia trait
  Hb H disease
  Hydrops fetalis with Hb Bart's
  Hb Constant Spring syndromes
  α-Thalassemia + β-thalassemia
  Hb S or Hb SS/α thalassemia

β-Thalassemia syndromes
  β-Thalassemia minor
  Thalassemia intermedia
  β-Thalassemia major

Rare thalassemias
  γ-Thalassemia
  δ-Thalassemia
  γδβ-Thalassemia

Thalassemias with other hemoglobinopathies
  sickle/β-thalassemia
  Hb C/β-thalassemia
  Hb E/β-thalassemia
  Hb Q/α-thalassemia
  Hb G/α-thalassemia

Hereditary persistence of fetal hemoglobin
  Pancellular
  Heterocellular

Despite this striking biologic diversity in molecular pathology of the α- and β-thalassemias, the clinical phenotypes are remarkably similar for most patients, and all of the examples shown in Table 1 can be resolved into a small number of simplified, generic categories:

- Silent. The thalassemia gene is present but is "masked" because the hematology is normal or minimally abnormal and the blood smear is unremarkable. Examples are the "silent carrier" state for α-thalassemia (one gene deletion), heterozygous Hb Constant Spring trait, and "silent" expression of β^+-thalassemia minor.
- Mild. The hemoglobin level is normal or mildly reduced and remains stable. Red cells are hypochromic and microcytic disproportionately when compared to the hemoglobin level. Classical examples are α-thalassemia trait (two gene deletion), and the various clinical types of heterozygous β-thalassemia minor, which include the high Hb A_2 variety, δβ-thalassemia, the form with normal Hb A_2 and Hb F, and Hb Lepore trait.
- Moderate. The hemoglobin level is moderately reduced, but regular blood transfusions are not required. There may be symptoms related to anemia. There are almost always abnormal physical findings, including skeletal changes, splenomegaly, and cardiomegaly. This category encompasses a number of disorders termed β-thalassemia "intermedia." The three main explanations for this syndrome are (1) the co-inheritance of α-thalassemia, (2) the presence of a milder molecular defect of β-chain production, or (3) unusually effective synthesis of γ-chains of Hb F.
- Severe. The hemoglobin level falls progressively late in the first year of life or shortly thereafter, and there is a requirement for regular life-long blood transfusions. In the untransfused or inadequately transfused state, the disease is severe, debilitating, and ultimately lethal. This category includes homozygous β-thalassemia (thalassemia major or Cooley's anemia), and the compound heterozygous interactions of β-thalassemia minor with structurally abnormal hemoglobins such as Hb E/β°-thalassemia.
- Hemolytic anemia. The features of this category are chronic hemolysis with a stable anemia of variable severity, reticulocytosis, and splenomegaly. Regular blood transfusions are usually not necessary. Examples are Hb H disease (3-gene deletion), interactions of α-thalassemia trait and Hb Constant Spring trait, and homozygous Hb Constant Spring.
- Lethal. Affected fetuses are stillborn or die shortly after birth as a result of profound intrauterine anemia. The infants have marked anasarca and extreme extramedullary hematopoiesis with massive hepatosplenomegaly. Fetal hydrops syndrome with Hb Bart's (4-gene deletion) is the outstanding example.

SILENT AND MILD FORMS

Genetic Counseling, Education, and Prevention

Because thalassemias are inherited, all individuals and couples at risk for bearing affected offspring need information and support through genetic counseling. Effective counseling depends on the counselor's depth of knowledge, experience, and communicative skills. The goal is to provide precise and complete information on thalassemia in an atmosphere of strict confidentiality that will help affected individuals understand the disorder and formulate decisions.

Most experience with prevention has been with β-thalassemia. One approach is by prospective screening whereby total school-age populations are tested and carriers are warned about the risks of having offspring with another carrier. The success of such a large-scale program has not been determined.

The other approach is by prenatal diagnosis. This entails screening mothers at their first prenatal visit, screening fathers in cases in which the mother is a thalassemia carrier, and offering the couple the possibility of prenatal diagnosis and therapeutic abortion if they are both carriers of a gene for a severe form of thalassemia. Prenatal diagnosis is also offered to parents who have already had an affected child. Currently, these programs are used mainly for prenatal diagnosis of the severe transfusion-dependent forms of homozygous thalassemia. Some experience has also been gained in prenatal diagnosis of mothers at risk of having a fetus with the Hb Bart's hydrops syndrome.

The technology for prenatal diagnosis of thalassemia is still changing. Fetal blood sampling with globin-chain synthesis analysis has been supplanted by direct analysis of fetal DNA. The DNA can be obtained from fetal cells in amniotic fluid relatively late in pregnancy, but also from a chorionic villus biopsy as early as the ninth week of gestation. Depending on the nature of the molecular pathology involved, the diagnosis can be established by one or more of the following: Southern blot analysis of fetal DNA in disorders associated with major deletions; "cutting" fetal DNA with restriction endonucleases and mapping the gene for syndromes with point mutations that alter restriction enzyme sites; oligonucleotide probing when the mutation is known; and, in cases in which the mutation is not known, restriction fragment length polymorphism analysis of parental chromosomes to determine if the fetus has received both affected chromosomes from parents.

Advances in DNA technology will greatly facilitate the development of prenatal diagnosis programs. An important new technique is the polymerase chain reaction (PCR), which allows small amounts of DNA to be amplified rapidly. Using PCR together with oligonucleotide probes and nonradioactive labeling techniques, it is possible to develop a simple "dot-blot" analysis to determine rapidly whether a fetus has inherited a severe form of thalassemia.

Treatment

The mild forms of thalassemia, such as α-thalassemia trait and β-thalassemia minor, do not require therapy. Indeed, no form of treatment is effective in raising the hemoglobin level in these conditions. Iron supplementation is never given unless a patient has proven iron deficiency. Unfortunately, many individuals are mistakenly diagnosed as having iron deficiency and are given long-term iron therapy without benefit. There is a theoretical possibility that such inappropriate and prolonged iron treatment may gradually produce significant hemosiderosis. There is also no role for folate or vitamin B_{12} supplements or other "hematinics" in the management of uncomplicated thalassemia.

In women with β-thalassemia minor, a decline in hemoglobin can occur during pregnancy in the face of normal iron, folate, and vitamin B_{12} stores. Occasionally, the anemia may be severe enough to require blood transfusion. The falling hemoglobin level may be aggravated by an iron or folate deficiency state related to pregnancy, and iron stores and folate status must always be assessed in these cases so that the appropriate management can be planned.

MODERATE FORMS

The moderate forms of thalassemia comprising the thalassemia "intermedia" disorders pose a variety of clinical problems, some of which are difficult to manage. Almost all of these problems can be resolved by maintaining the hemoglobin in the normal range using a regular, life-long transfusion program. However, because of the penalty of transfusion-induced iron overload and the necessity for a concurrent iron chelation program (see section on severe thalassemia), determined efforts should always be made to refrain from transfusing these patients if possible.

Hypersplenism

If a regular transfusion program is being considered for a patient with thalassemia "intermedia," the role of the spleen size in the production of the anemia should be carefully evaluated beforehand. Exacerbation of anemia due to splenomegaly is a common feature and may be due to splenic red cell pooling, increased red cell destruction, or both. Clinical experience has generally shown that a palpable spleen more than 6 to 8 cm below the costal margin is associated with shortened red cell survival. This can result in a sustained, modest decline in annual mean hemoglobin levels and produce slowing of growth in children, complaints of fatigue and weakness, and increasing skeletal changes such as thalassemia facies, osteoporosis, bone pain, and pathologic fractures. In this clinical setting, splenectomy generally restores the hemoglobin to its highest previous level, ameliorates the signs and symptoms to a degree, and removes the need for regular transfusions.

If splenectomy is planned, an ultrasound of the gallbladder should always be performed before surgery. Because of sustained hyperbilirubinemia in thalassemia "intermedia," pigment stones are common and cholecystectomy is often necessary. If stones are identified, a strong argument can be made for removing the gallbladder at the time of splenectomy, even if the gallstones are not causing a clinical problem. This may spare the patient a second operation at a later date.

Prior to splenectomy, polyvalent pneumococcal vaccine should be given to all patients of all ages; in addition, *Haemophilus influenzae* type b vaccine should be given to pediatric patients. Since the introduction of these vaccines, the need for long-term antibiotic prophylaxis has not been determined, but most workers in the field still prescribe an appropriate agent following splenectomy that "covers" pneumococci and *Haemophilus influenzae*. Compliance with long-term antibiotic administration can be a problem, however, and in the event of unexplained fever in a splenectomized patient, immediate blood cultures must be taken and broad-spectrum antibiotics started.

Folate Deficiency

An increased demand for folic acid to sustain the heightened degree of marrow erythropoiesis in thalassemia "intermedia" can result in biochemical and hematologic evidence of a folate deficiency state. This is especially true in ethnic groups that enjoy folate-poor diets. Because of the morphologic abnormalities associated with thalassemia, the bone marrow may not always show typical features of megaloblastic erythropoiesis. An extremely low hemoglobin level at presentation or a progressive decline in hemoglobin with time should prompt consideration of folate deficiency. Long-term folate supplements (5 mg per day) will correct the deficiency and induce an increase in hemoglobin level.

Special Problems

Increased gut absorption of dietary iron may occur in thalassemia "intermedia" and, if sustained over many years, can lead to hemosiderosis. The iron overload can be detected by a serum ferritin measurement of greater than 1000 μg per liter, and a high serum iron with a fully saturated iron-binding capacity. A liver biopsy for histology and for quantitative iron estimation is also a good measure of iron overload, but it is invasive and usually not performed routinely. To determine if iron chelation therapy is needed, a test dose of deferoxamine (Desferal, DFO), 500 mg IM, is administered, and urine is then collected for 24 hours. Urinary iron excretion of more than 2.5 mg per 24 hours in a vitamin C–replete patient indicates moderate iron loading and justifies starting iron chelation treatment with DFO.

Leg ulcers can be very troublesome and cannot be cured with the usual variety of topical ointments or with oral zinc sulfate supplements. The only totally effective treatment is an intensive transfusion program to keep the hemoglobin level in a sustained, normal range until healing is complete. Occasionally, skin grafting is needed, but it will fail unless it is coupled with the transfusion program.

Pregnancy with thalassemia "intermedia" is associated with a fetal loss rate of about 50 percent. A regular transfusion program to maintain a high hemoglobin level throughout the gestation, coupled with folate supplements, completely corrects the high risk of fetal wastage.

HEMOLYTIC ANEMIA

Hb H disease is the main example of this form of thalassemia. In Hb H disease, there is decreased synthesis of α-globin chains and a two- to fivefold excess of β-chains. "Hb" H is not a real hemoglobin but consists of aggregates of β-chain tetramers. Red cells containing Hb H are sensitive to oxidative stress, and the hemolytic anemia may be aggravated by drugs that induce oxidant injury. Thus, the same family of drugs that induces hemolysis in patients with G6PD deficiency should also be avoided in patients with Hb H disease, especially sulfonamides.

Several problems observed in patients with thalassemia "intermedia" are also seen in patients with Hb H disease. Probably the most common complication is severe splenomegaly with associated hypersplenism. A declining hemoglobin level, especially with leukopenia and thrombocytopenia, or development of a transfusion requirement in a previously stable patient constitutes strong evidence for the existence of hypersplenism. Red cell survival with splenic scanning by ^{51}Cr-labeled red cells is not useful and may even be misleading because the label binds selectively to β-chains and may, by selective removal of Hb H inclusions from erythrocytes in the spleen, give a falsely high index of splenic destruction. Most patients with Hb H disease who undergo splenectomy have a mean rise of hemoglobin of 20 to 30 g per liter after the procedure. Thus, splenectomy is justified in patients with evidence of hypersplenism.

General therapy for Hb H disease includes prescription of folic acid supplements, avoidance of iron supplements (as well as oxidant drugs), prompt attention and treatment of infection, and judicious use of transfusions. Transfusion may be needed during pregnancy because the anemia usually becomes worse.

SEVERE FORMS

Beta-thalassemia major requires life-long medical supervision and is best directed by a comprehensive care clinic skilled in the disease. The minimal requirements for a thalassemia clinic are a dedicated, experienced medical director, a motivated nurse, and an effective social worker. Also essential is a good blood banking facility, a biochemistry laboratory capable of measuring serum and urinary iron levels and serum ferritin concentrations, and a solid infrastructure of consultants in cardiology, endocrinology, ophthalmology, audiology, and radiology. The successful management of thalassemia requires commitment as well as the highest standards of medical care.

At time of presentation, thalassemia major must be distinguished from the various thalassemia "intermedia" syndromes because regular, intensive transfusions combined with iron chelation therapy may not really be necessary. Thalassemia major can usually be distinguished by routine bloodwork and hemoglobin electrophoresis on the patient and family members, but globin-chain synthesis rates and DNA analysis may be necessary in some cases.

Timing of Transfusions

When the diagnosis is confirmed, a decision has to be made regarding the start of the transfusion program. Some useful guidelines regarding the timing and initiation of transfusions are as follows: (1) children presenting with symptoms before 1 year of age should be started on regular transfusions; (2) patients presenting in their second year should be started on transfusions if they do not thrive clinically; and (3) children who thrive without transfusion into their third year have a milder form of disease and may not require transfusions. The hemoglobin level can also be used as the indication for starting transfusions, which are usually instituted when the hemoglobin level falls and remains below 70 g per liter because of the deleterious effects on growth and bone at this degree of anemia.

Prior to the first blood transfusion, a complete red cell phenotype should be performed on the patient's cells. This will be the last chance to obtain an accurate red cell profile before the transfusion program is initiated. The data can be used for phenotype-specific cross-matches, although this tends to be more costly than standard group-specific cross-matching. If phenotype-specific cross-matches are not performed, one can expect isoimmunization and red cell antigen antibody formation in about one-third of thalassemia patients, usually anti-K_1 and anti-E.

Hepatitis B vaccine should be given to patients who are negative for antibody against the virus before or shortly after the transfusion program begins to prevent the transmission of the disease by blood. The dose is 0.5 ml for children and 1.0 ml for adults given intramuscularly according to the following schedule: first dose at an elected date, second dose 1 month later, and third dose as a booster 6 months after the first dose.

Once the transfusion program is started, the hemoglobin level should be measured just prior to each transfusion. This will provide a guide to the volume of transfused blood needed and the frequency of transfusions that will maintain the hemoglobin at a desired level (see section on choice of transfusion regimen). Alternately, the pre- and post-transfusion hemoglobins can be measured, which allows a calculation of the mean hemoglobin maintained by transfusion. To prolong the interval between transfusions, the mean hemoglobin level must be raised to a higher level; however, raising it excessively may result in deleterious expansion of blood volume with increased viscosity. Moreover, changing the transfusion interval may significantly affect the overall iron accumulation; e.g., a transfusion interval of 5 weeks to maintain a given hemoglobin value results in a 20 percent greater iron intake per year compared to a 3-week interval. Thus, one should aim for an interval of 3 to 4 weeks after having established a satisfactory mean hemoglobin level.

Choice of Transfusion Regimen

The ideal pretransfusion hemoglobin level that confers maximum clinical benefits is not known. Two transfusion formats have been proposed, each with strong advocates. The "hypertransfusion" program is designed to maintain the pretransfusion hemoglobin above 100 g per liter, and the "supertransfusion" regimen, above 120 g per liter. Compared to the era of sporadic transfusions, patients with thalassemia receiving either hypertransfusion or supertransfusion are taller, have less hepatosplenomegaly, have milder skeletal changes, and are healthier. There are claims that supertransfusion has three further advantages over hypertransfusion via a mechanism of suppressed marrow erythropoiesis: reduced gastrointestinal iron absorption, less bone demineralization, and prevention of hypersplenism. Some of these claims are supported by clear-cut data and some are not, and it is important for the physician who supervises the program to know which benefits are speculative, which are proven, and which are of clinical importance.

In general, a modified hypertransfusion program is currently the preferred and most widely used format in which the pretransfusion hemoglobin level is maintained above 115 g per liter. This entails the transfusion of 15 ml per kilogram of packed red cells every 3 to 4 weeks.

Blood Products

If whole blood or concentrated red cell preparations are used, most patients develop febrile, nonhemolytic transfusion reactions with or without urticaria. These reactions are due to prior sensitization to donor plasma protein antigens or, more importantly, to the in vivo destruction of transfused white cells, usually neutrophils but sometimes lymphocytes and platelets. Thus, whole blood and concentrated red cell preparations are unsuitable products for transfusion therapy of thalassemia major, and their use should be avoided. Instead, leukocyte-poor red cells for transfusion of these patients should always be requested from the blood bank. The three main techniques for depleting white cells from red cells are by filtration, by an automated red cell wash in a blood cell processor, and by a freeze-thaw-wash procedure.

Experimental programs using apheresis and cell-separation techniques allow the infusion of blood enriched with young erythrocytes, termed *neocytes*, which have the longest survival time following transfusion. Such efforts are designed to reduce total transfusion requirements by extending the circulation time of transfused cells. The transfusional iron burden is also reduced owing to the removal of aged erythrocytes from the preparation, which have a short survival following transfusion. These programs remain largely experimental but are being utilized in centers treating large numbers of patients.

If febrile, nonhemolytic reactions occur, acetaminophen should be given in a dose of 10 to 15 mg per kilogram PO for children, and 650 to 1,000 mg total dose PO for adults. For urticaria, diphenhydramine hydrochloride (Benadryl) is usually effective in a dose of 1.5 mg per kilogram PO or IV for children and 25 to 50 mg total dose PO or IV for adults.

Splenectomy

The incidence of marked splenomegaly and hypersplenism has significantly declined since the introduction of hypertransfusion and supertransfusion programs. One should still be alert to this possibility, however, and, in general, an increasing transfusion requirement in the absence of antibody-mediated red cell destruction is suggestive of hypersplenism. Although neither sequestration of ^{51}Cr-labeled red cells nor size of the spleen reliably reflect the degree of hypersplenism, splenomegaly of more than 6 cm below the costal margin is nearly always associated with increased transfusion requirements. A clinically enlarged spleen even in the absence of overt hypersplenism accounts for a large volume of total circulating blood, and its removal often leads to a marked immediate, although transient, reduction in transfusion requirements. Any degree of physical discomfort from an enlarged spleen is also an indication for splenectomy.

As a practical guideline for the need for splenectomy, one can use the total annual transfusion volume. When yearly requirements exceed 200 to 250 ml per kilogram to maintain the desired pretransfusion hemoglobin, splenectomy is recommended. Most patients with annual transfusion requirements exceeding 200 ml per kilogram before splenectomy achieve a moderate but significant reduction in red cell requirements to the desired value of 200 ml per kilogram per year after splenectomy.

The preventative precautions regarding splenectomy described previously apply equally to patients with thalassemia major (see section on hypersplenism under moderate forms).

Iron Chelation

The major consequence of regular transfusions is iron overload. If untreated, the progressive accumulation of body iron causes considerable morbidity and, ultimately, a cardiac demise in most patients. Hence, a modern, aggressive transfusion regimen must be coupled with an iron chelation program; currently, DFO is the most effective and widely used chelator available for treatment of transfusional hemosiderosis in man.

If started early in the transfusion program and if used conscientiously, DFO almost always establishes a negative iron balance, which means that the rate of iron excretion in urine and stool exceeds that of iron accumulation. In the first few months of chelation therapy, serum ferritin levels often fall rapidly, probably reflecting improved hepatocellular function as well as diminished iron stores. With continued DFO therapy, serum ferritin levels reach normal or near-normal levels, reflecting the removal of excessively stored iron.

Deferoxamine is minimally effective when given orally, and slow parenteral infusions are more effective than bolus administration. Thus, the current standard technique consists of a daily subcutaneous infusion of DFO by means of a battery-operated syringe pump attached to a narrow-gauge butterfly needle inserted under the skin of the anterior abdominal wall, legs, and arms in daily rotation. In practice, the infusions are administered overnight to minimize inconvenience to the patient, and the dose of the drug varies with the age of the patient and the degree of iron overload. When given in a standard dose of 50 mg per kilogram per day by subcutaneous infusion, most patients older than 3 years attain a negative iron balance. Pruritus, swelling, and pain at the injection site can jeopardize the chance of long-term compliance with the program. This can be prevented in many cases by adding 0.1 mg of hydrocortisone to each milliliter of DFO at the time of infusion. Use of cold towels can also reduce the discomfort once the local reaction has developed.

When vitamin C supplements are given to iron-overloaded thalassemia patients concurrently with DFO therapy, urinary iron excretion increases two- to tenfold, and stool excretion remains the same or increases. Therefore, ascorbic acid supplements, 100 mg per day, will benefit thalassemia patients who show enhanced DFO-induced urinary iron excretion. Patients with cardiac disease are not suitable candidates for ascorbic acid supplements, especially in large doses (500 mg per day), because of possible cardiac decompensation coincident with their administration during DFO therapy.

The exact age to initiate chelation for maximal benefit is not clear. Patients must accumulate about 3 to 4 g of iron, equivalent to a serum ferritin of more than 500 μg per liter, before DFO infusions induce a substantial urinary iron output; in some patients, this may take months to years of regular transfusions. Nevertheless, some investigators have recommended starting chelation very early anyway, and in our clinic, we infuse intravenous DFO at the time of each transfusion, starting with the third or fourth exposure, and start a subcutaneous DFO program when the serum ferritin reaches upper normal limits. The ultimate benefits and safety of this early approach have not been proven, but the data are very promising because young patients have been kept continually in a negative iron balance. There may be a risk in very young patients, however, of DFO-induced bony changes and growth failure.

Not all patients can be treated successfully with subcutaneous infusions of DFO. Older individuals with large iron stores or those with iron-induced cardiac dysfunction may progress to failure or death before sufficient iron can be removed by this method. Other patients, especially teenagers, may not comply with subcutaneous chelation therapy. For these patients, daily intravenous infusions of high doses of DFO (5 to 12 g per 24 hours) through an externalized catheter, such as a Hickman or Broviac type, or through a subcutaneous port may be a successful alternative. Intravenous therapy reduces the discomfort of subcutaneous administration and improves compliance. This method also increases the amount of DFO that can be given with each infusion, which improves iron excretion. Daily, high-dose, intravenous therapy with DFO can reduce high serum ferritin levels to normal within 12 to 24 months. Some patients treated by this method have dramatic reversal of cardiac disease, including arrhythmias and heart failure. However, iron-induced endocrine disorders such as hypoparathyroidism and diabetes mellitus do not improve despite the reduction in body iron stores.

There are major neurotoxic side effects of DFO that result in impairment of vision, hearing, or both in some patients. The visual abnormalities include reduced acuity, impaired color vision, poor dark adaptation, and central scotomata. The auditory abnormalities range from a subclinical, high-frequency sensorineural hearing loss detected only by an audiogram, to a severe low- to high-frequency deficit with clinical deafness requiring hearing aids. Patients with neurotoxicity tend to be younger, have lower ferritin levels, and administer higher DFO doses than those who are unaffected. This suggests that the toxicity of DFO develops when there is a disproportionate amount of available chelator relative to the degree of iron overload.

The early recognition of visual impairment and reduction of the DFO dose or temporary cessation of chelation therapy will result in clinical improvement. The auditory problems are more difficult to manage and require serial monitoring with audiograms. The following guidelines allow effective yet safe administration of DFO. A dose of 50 mg per kilogram by subcutaneous infusion is recommended in those without audiogram abnormalities. With mild toxicity, a reduction to 30 or 40 mg per kilogram per dose should result in a reversal of the abnormal results to normal within 4 weeks. Moderate abnormalities require a reduction of DFO to 25 mg per kilogram per dose with careful monitoring. In those with symptoms of hearing loss, the drug should be stopped for 4 weeks, and when the audiogram is stable or improved, therapy should be restarted at 10 to 25 mg per kilogram per dose. Serial audiograms should be performed every 6 months in those without problems and more frequently in young patients with normal serum ferritin values and in those with auditory dysfunction. Similarly, every patient should have a yearly ophthalmology assessment if asymptomatic, but an assessment should be done immediately and more frequently if problems arise.

Oral Iron Chelators

An inexpensive, safe, and orally effective iron chelator is highly desirable. Two agents are currently in human trials, and a few others are being studied in animals that have potential. If any of these oral agents are shown to work as well as or better than DFO, DFO will probably be phased out as the agent of choice.

The hydroxypyridones represent a potentially useful class of oral iron chelators. One of these compounds, 1,2-dimethyl-3-hydroxypyrid-4-one (L1) induces urinary iron excretion at a rate comparable to that obtained with DFO in iron-overloaded patients with thalassemia. The stool excretion of iron with L1 varies but is usually much less than the urinary elimination. In initial clinical trials with a small group of patients, daily L1 therapy did not induce a consistent fall in serum ferritin levels after several months of treatment. However, longer trials of treatment with L1 are underway with detailed monitoring of iron stores by liver biopsy and imaging techniques. These trials should determine the agent's full potential. L1 has had few side effects when used in animal and human studies. The safety and efficacy of other hydroxypyridones are currently being evaluated.

Pyridoxine isonicotinoyl hydrazone (PIH) is another oral chelator composed of pyridoxine and isoniazid, both of which have been used for treatment of other disorders without major toxicity. In the rat, PIH removes iron from both parenchymal and reticuloendothelial cells. However, total iron excretion in short-term clinical trials is less than that seen with conventional doses of DFO given by subcutaneous infusion. Thus, PIH is unlikely to be useful for treating transfusional iron overload but may be effective in preventing the more slowly progressive iron overload due to increased iron absorption in patients with thalassemia "intermedia."

Other potentially useful oral agents have not been tested in humans yet. However, one of these, N,N'-bis (o-hydroxybenzoyl) ethylenediamine N,N'-diacetic acid, (HBED) appears to be the most promising. In animal studies, HBED is comparable to DFO in its ability to remove iron. Detailed chronic toxicity studies have shown that the agent is very safe. A dimethyl ester derivative of HBED also appears to be very effective and significantly exceeds DFO in promotion of iron excretion; however, it is difficult to synthesize. Clinical evaluation of HBED is currently in the planning stages.

Major Problems of Iron Overload

If iron chelation is started too late, e.g., after 10 years of regular transfusions, or if compliance with DFO is poor, the inevitable problems of iron overload ensue. The three target tissues that suffer the most serious damage are cardiac, hepatic, and endocrine. Although most patients load iron in a similar manner in the three target tissues, magnetic resonance imaging (MRI) has disclosed that some patients load iron in the heart but not in the liver, and some load iron in the liver but not in the heart. Thus, there may be biologic differences in iron loading that should be taken into account in assessing patients.

Cardiac

Iron-induced heart disease due to deposition of iron in the pericardium and myocardium evolves slowly but progressively over several years. Echocardiography and radionuclide cineangiography provide functional information on the evolution of cardiac siderosis. Diastolic dysfunction is the first abnormality to be detected and occurs early in the illness at a time when systolic function is preserved. By the time systolic dysfunction develops, heart disease is well advanced. Clinically, pericarditis is a frequent and early syndrome and is sometimes accompanied by atrial arrhythmias. Within months to years of the onset of pericarditis, patients develop ventricular ectopy as well as ventricular tachyarrhythmias. Heart failure ensues and leads to a cardiac demise at an unpredictable future date.

Treatment of pericarditis includes bed rest, acetylsalicylic acid, other analgesia for chest pain if needed, and anti-inflammatory drugs such as indomethacin. Atrial arrhythmias have been suppressed in the past with digoxin, propanolol (a class II antiarrhythmic agent), or calcium channel-blocking drugs (class IV), but there is a current trend to use class IC agents such as propafenone hydrochloride. Ventricular arrhythmias may be more difficult to manage. If they are asymptomatic, they probably do not require therapy unless there is evidence of hemodynamic compromise. A portable Holter device can be helpful in monitoring the severity of ventricular arrhythmias. If therapy is instituted, the current direction is to give class III or class IA agents such as amioderone hydrochloride or disopyramide phosphate, respectively. Combinations of quinidine, propanolol, and digoxin may also be needed.

The onset of congestive heart failure requires aggressive management. The conventional approach of salt restriction, diuretics, and digoxin is currently being supplanted by intensive diuresis coupled with vasodilatory agents used individually, such as captopril, or in combinations, like hydralazine plus isosorbide dinitrate.

Hepatic

In patients receiving regular transfusions but without adequate chelation, hepatomegaly occurs as a result of progressive engorgement of hepatic parenchymal and phagocytic cells with hemosiderin. Further increases in hepatic iron deposition can induce intralobular fibrosis. End-stage cirrhosis may ensue, but this is an infrequent cause of death compared to heart disease. The only proven way to halt irrevocable liver disease induced by iron is by aggressive, regular chelation with DFO.

Hepatic enzymes may be mildly elevated chronically in some patients. This may be due to hepatocellular destruction induced by iron, chronic, smoldering type B hepatitis in those not previously protected by vaccination, or type C (non-A, non-B) hepatitis. Claims of efficacy of interferon in ameliorating type C hepatitis require substantiation.

Endocrine

Growth retardation becomes obvious after 10 years of age in less than one-half of patients. Even in well-transfused patients, there is a decrease in growth rate in late childhood and an absent or greatly diminished pubertal growth spurt. The basis for this growth retardation is not known. There is no evidence of growth hormone deficiency, but there is speculation that somatomedin (insulin-like growth factor) deficiency may play a role. No therapy is currently recommended.

Failure of sexual development occurs in the majority of patients with iron overload and, in general, is related to hypothalamic-pituitary dysfunction with lack of luteinizing hormone (LH) and follicle-stimulating hormone (FSH) production rather than to primary end-organ unresponsiveness. For those with delayed puberty but who otherwise have reasonable general health, satisfactory nutrition, and an adequate transfusion program, conventional treatment involves testosterone or estrogen supplementation after 15 years of age.

Diabetes mellitus occurs in less than 10 percent of patients and is due to both pancreatic hypoproduction and, in some cases, insulin resistance. When glucose tolerance tests are performed, as many as 50 percent of thalassemic patients have "chemical diabetes," and most of these have normal or elevated circulating insulin levels. Subsequently, when the diabetes becomes symptomatic, insulin output decreases, as is the case in most patients with juvenile diabetes, and insulin supplementation is required.

Hypoparathyroidism also occurs in a small fraction of patients and can present with classic tetany, hypocalcemia, and hyperphosphatemia. Emergency treatment for tetany consists of an intravenous infusion of calcium gluconate coupled with oral vitamin D_3 (1,25-dihydroxycholecalciferal, calcitriol). Once normocalcemia has been achieved, therapy can be continued with vitamin D_3, or with vitamin D_2 which is less costly. An adequate calcium intake should be ensured with supplements, if necessary.

Iron deposition in thyroid parenchymal tissue is often extensive, but dysfunction is usually limited to primary subclinical hypothyroidism. Similarly, early iron deposition in the adrenals is limited primarily to the zona glomerulosa, the site of mineralcorticoid production, although mineralcorticoid regulation is seldom impaired.

Bone Marrow Transplantation

Bone marrow transplantation (BMT) can cure thalassemia major, but patients and families must be willing to accept the risk that the patient may die from the procedure. They must also understand that survivors of BMT may have considerable morbidity from graft-versus-host disease, especially during the first year following BMT.

The aim of BMT for thalassemia is to improve the quality of life and survival in transfusion-dependent patients. Disease-free survival cannot be obtained with any other form of therapy for this disease. Because BMT for thalassemia is still not conventional treatment, the only appropriate candidates for the procedure are those with family member donors who are HLA-matched and mixed-leukocyte culture unresponsive. The best results from BMT are seen in well-chelated patients under 16 years of age who do not have either hepatomegaly or portal fibrosis on liver biopsy. The chance for cure of thalassemia by BMT in this group is 94 percent.

Genetic Therapy

Successful treatment of thalassemia major might be accomplished by reactivation of γ-globin gene function or by substitution of normal β-globin genes for the defective genes. Reactivation of γ-gene function could ameliorate the imbalanced globin-chain synthesis, resulting in a reduction of the ineffective erythropoiesis and hemolytic anemia of the disease. Introduction of normal β-genes into hematopoietic stem cells would allow them to function normally and would correct the β-globin deficit.

In utero, active γ-genes are hypomethylated, but after birth they become methylated when deactivation occurs. The drug 5-azacytidine induces hypomethylation of γ-genes, increases γ-chain synthesis, and has been shown to produce an increase in hemoglobin level in a limited clinical trial in β-thalassemia "intermedia." The agent has not been used widely, however, because of concerns regarding its oncogenic potential. Hydroxyurea is a second drug that induces an increase in fetal hemoglobin but probably by the mechanism of recruitment of Hb F–producing BFU-E erythroid progenitors. It is generally felt that hydroxyurea does not have the same oncogenic risk as 5-azacytidine and is a safer drug for long-term use. Brief trials with both hydroxyurea and 5-azacytidine have been reported in small numbers of patients with thalassemia or sickle cell disease without evidence of long-term clinical benefit. This therapy should be considered experimental and only used in qualified and authorized centers.

Despite dedicated research, the possibility of successful gene replacement in thalassemia is unlikely in the immediate future. Techniques for isolating specific human genes and inserting them into the DNA of other cells have been accomplished and have raised the hopes for cure of many genetic diseases. However, major problems are involved in placing new genes into a human and ensuring their sustained, active expression. At this time, attempts to perform such experiments in humans with thalassemia are premature.

SUGGESTED READING

Cohen A. Treatment of transfusional iron overload. Am J Pediatr Hematol Oncol 1990; 12:4–8.

Freedman MH. Management of beta-thalassemia major using transfusions and iron chelation with deferoxamine. Transfusion Med Rev 1988; 2:161–175.

Modell B, Berdoukas V. The clinical approach to thalassemia. London: Grune & Stratton, 1984.

Weatherall DJ. The thalassemias. In: Hematology. 4th ed. Williams WJ, Beutler E, Erslev AJ, et al, eds. New York: McGraw-Hill, 1990: 510–539.

DISSEMINATED INTRAVASCULAR COAGULATION

ANTHONY J. BLEYER, M.D.
WILLIAM R. BELL, M.D.

The hemostatic mechanism results from a delicate balance between activators, inhibitors, and clearance of activated factors. This system functions optimally when there is a localized stimulus for hemostasis. Endothelial damage causes activation of factor XII to factor XII_a, and the intrinsic pathway commences. Fibrin monomers join to preserve the integrity of the intravascular compartment and promote wound healing. At the same time, plasminogen is transformed to plasmin, which acts as a scavenger for the degradation of fibrin strands and activated clotting factors. In this way, fibrin and activated coagulation proteins that were not utilized in clot formation are inactivated. The final result is formation of a localized hemostatic plug while avoiding fibrin deposition throughout the body.

In disseminated intravascular coagulation (DIC), there is persistent, overwhelming, and often diffuse activation of the coagulation cascade. Fibrin is formed throughout the circulation instead of just at the site of injury. Plasminogen is extensively converted to plasmin, with degradation of factors throughout the circulatory system. The body is no longer able to maintain hemostasis for new wounds, as the orderly mechanism of fibrin deposition is lost. This disorganized activation and degradation may result in either a predominance of bleeding or thrombosis. Usually there is clinical evidence of hemorrhage, and laboratory tests may reveal organ systems affected by fibrin deposition.

Many different clinical processes result in this disturbance. Entrance into the circulation of a procoagulant, a thromboplastic substance from damaged, hypoxic, or infarcted tissue, will induce activation of the coagulation and fibrinolytic systems and cause aggregation of platelets. Malignant neoplasms and amniotic fluid have high tissue thromboplastin activity. When released into the circulation, they can cause overwhelming activation of the coagulation cascade. Endotoxin converts factor XII to factor XII_a, lyses white blood cells, and activates platelets. Trauma may result in the release of large amounts of tissue thromboplastin. Concurrent hypoxia and acidosis in the damaged tissue can further aggravate the situation.

Under the influence of these diverse clinical problems, there is formation of fibrin diffusely through the circulation. Unlike normal hemostasis, fibrin is not deposited at a single site, but rather small fibrin aggregates precipitate in arterioles, venules, and capillaries throughout the circulation. Although occasionally manifested as venous thrombosis, this is recognized clinically as an elevation in hepatic enzymes or a decrease in glomerular filtration rate.

The conversion of plasminogen to plasmin is stimulated by factor XII_a. Plasmin circulates and dissolves exposed arginyl-lysyl bonds. Fibrin is degraded, resulting in dissolution of hemostatic plugs throughout the body. Fibrinogen is also lysed into fragments X, Y, D, and E, of which Y, D, and E cannot polymerize. Protein C, antithrombin III, and many clotting factors are also degraded by plasmin.

Disseminated intravascular coagulation also results in activation of the prekallikrein-kallikrein system and the complement system, further amplifying the coagulopathy. Factor XII_a transforms prekallikrein to kallikrein, with the eventual formation of kinin. This agent causes vasodilation and increased vascular permeability. Plasmin activates the complement system, which results in red cell and platelet lysis.

The blood-forming elements are quantitatively decreased and qualitatively altered. Platelets are directly damaged and attach to fibrin mesh throughout the circulation, resulting in a decrease in platelet number. Fibrin degradation products also bind to the platelet surface, resulting in a qualitative loss of platelet function. Red blood cells are damaged as they pass through vessels occluded with fibrin, forming a variety of schistocytes. They are also lysed by the complement system.

In summary, diffuse activation of thrombus-forming and plasminolytic mechanisms results in thrombosis and hemorrhage, with qualitative and quantitative destruction of platelets, coagulation factors, and red blood cells.

DIAGNOSIS

Diagnosis of DIC usually results from suspicion in a patient with evidence of bleeding or in a patient with an appropriate underlying clinical syndrome.

Frequently, DIC presents as bleeding or a tendency to bleed in a patient who is severely ill or has been suffering from a chronic illness. Often the patient is on multiple medications and is in the intensive care unit. There may be oozing from venipuncture sites or hematomas resulting from minimal trauma. Stools may test positive for occult blood or be frankly bloody. Blood-tinged fluid may be draining from the nasogastric tube or Foley catheter. A careful fundoscopic and neurologic exam may identify additional sites of bleeding. Occasionally, the patient may only have a tendency to bleed despite severe DIC. A routinely drawn prothrombin time (PT) or activated partial thromboplastin time (APTT) may show unexpected prolongation. Of the two tests, the APTT is the more sensitive.

Almost any medical disorder can cause DIC; however, certain conditions are frequently associated with DIC, and screening for defects in coagulation will alert the physician to their presence. For instance, promyelocytic leukemia is frequently associated with DIC, and a possible diagnosis of DIC should be confirmed before induction chemotherapy. The cirrhotic patient who has recently undergone placement of a LeVeen shunt must be observed for the development of DIC. The pregnant patient with toxemia, abruptio placenta, or retained dead fetus in utero must be followed for DIC, as this may prompt immediate evacuation of the uterus. The patient with DIC from a head injury should be identified preoperatively. In these situations, the presence of DIC may alter therapy or the timing of certain therapeutic maneuvers.

Thrombosis is an uncommon presentation of DIC except in Trousseau's syndrome and septic thrombophlebitis. However, laboratory data may raise the question of pulmonary, hepatic, or renal damage secondary to thrombus formation.

LABORATORY DIAGNOSIS

Diagnosis depends on laboratory tests that show evidence of both coagulation and fibrinolysis. Associated platelet and erythrocyte pathology may aid in confirming the diagnosis. No single laboratory test is pathognomonic of DIC, and as will be pointed out, test results that are consistent with DIC may reflect underlying conditions.

The first diagnostic procedure is examination of the peripheral blood smear, which should be prepared directly from finger puncture. A striking reduction in platelet number will occur in over 85 percent of patients. Erythrocyte fragmentation will occur in approximately one-half of patients. A condition in which extensive red blood cell fragmentation, thrombocytopenia, and DIC occur is thrombotic thrombocytopenic purpura–hemolytic uremic syndrome (TTP-HUS). A platelet count should be performed. In many cases, the platelet count will be between 40,000 and 70,000 per cubic millimeter. Other causes of thrombocytopenia must be considered, such as heparin, H_2 receptor antagonists, and hypersplenism.

Clot formation in a glass tube should be observed. One milliliter of freshly drawn blood should be placed in a clean glass tube and tilted every 30 seconds. Clot formation should occur within 10 minutes. If the clot that is formed is approximately the volume of the blood placed in the tube, the fibrinogen level is at least 100 mg per 100 ml. The clot should then be observed at 30-minute intervals for evidence of retraction. If adequate platelets are present, clot should begin to retract within 1 hour. If the clot forms quickly and retracts within 1 hour, it is unlikely that the patient has DIC.

In DIC, clot formation usually takes place, but owing to decreased fibrinogen, thrombocytopenia, and excessive fibrinolysis, the clot will not retract and instead a lumpy liquid forms. Sometimes it is difficult to see any clot formation. In this situation, the blood should be placed in a shallow dish and observed for formation of very small fibrin aggregates.

A variation of this test is Page's test, in which 0.1 ml of bovine thrombin is added to 1 ml of freshly drawn blood in a clean glass tube. The thrombin accelerates clot formation. The tube is then observed as previously detailed. A prolonged PT or APPT frequently leads to consideration of the diagnosis of DIC. However, these tests are not routinely helpful in establishing the diagnosis of DIC. These tests are quite variable through the course of DIC, and their predictive value is low. The APTT and the thrombin time are more sensitive than the PT.

The most useful tests when considering DIC are the fibrinogen level and the presence of elevated quantities of fibrinogen-fibrin degradation products (FDP-fdp). The fibrinogen level is usually low in DIC, although it may be high in Trousseau's syndrome or at the time of onset of DIC. It is important how the fibrinogen level is measured, as FDP-fdp may seriously interfere with several different methods of assay for fibrinogen. A non–rate-dependent thrombin coagulable protein assay must be utilized. Rate-dependent and salting-out techniques frequently provide erroneous results. In severe DIC, the fibrinogen concentration is usually between 10 and 50 mg per 100 ml.

Fibrinogen levels may be low in patients with compromised synthetic function who do not have DIC. Also, fibrinogen levels and platelet count may be normal in early DIC. For this reason, it is important to measure FDP-fdp. Degradation of fibrinogen and fibrin occurs only through the fibrinolytic system, and the presence of FDP-fdp must raise high suspicion of DIC. As with the fibrinogen level, there are many assays for FDP-fdp. The most sensitive and specific test is the immunologic tanned red cell hemagglutination immunoinhibition assay.

Many other tests have been suggested in order to "confirm" the diagnosis of DIC. These tests include the euglobulin lysis test and measurement of D-dimer. These tests have not been found to be distinctly helpful, as there have been many false-positive and false-negative tests in our experience. These tests only add confusion, and they are not needed if good assay techniques of fibrinogen and FDP-fdp are used. Other tests precipitate fibrin monomer and soluble fibrinogen-fibrin complexes. Ethanol and protamine are frequently used to elicit precipitation, but these reagents also precipitate many other proteins. These tests also do not aid in diagnosing DIC.

In summary, the peripheral smear, platelet count, whole blood clotting time, fibrinogen level, and FDP-fdp assays constitute the cornerstone in making the diagnosis of DIC. None of these tests alone can accurately diagnose DIC, as many conditions produce abnormalities in one or several of these tests in the absence of DIC. It is important that other causes of laboratory abnormalities be investigated, as different etiologies mandate different therapies. A prolonged PT may respond to vitamin K, and thrombocytopenia may respond to discontinuation of an H$_2$ receptor blocker.

TREATMENT

The first step in therapy is identification of the underlying illness. Often this condition is obvious, as in promyelocytic leukemia or trauma. When the underlying illness cannot be found, occult sepsis must be considered, especially in the immunodeficient or chronically ill. Broad-spectrum antibiotics should be considered if there are other signs of infection. Other silent underlying conditions include neoplasm and aneurysm.

Nowhere in medicine is the paradigm "treat the underlying cause" as important as in DIC. The more quickly the primary condition is corrected, the faster DIC will resolve. In association with incurable illness such as terminal cancer, DIC may be one of the final mechanisms leading to death. Moreover, studies of various therapeutic interventions show that the awareness of underlying disease is more important than the therapy provided.

Associated metabolic problems must also be treated, as they may aggravate the coagulopathy. Aggressive correction of hypotension, acidosis, hypoxia, and electrolyte imbalance is of paramount importance. The patient should be kept at relative bed rest and precautions should be taken against falls and bleeding. Phlebotomies should be performed with the smallest possible needles, withdrawing only absolutely necessary minimal amounts of blood. The patient should have his or her blood typed by the blood bank in case of hemorrhage.

A daily physical examination should be performed to check for new bleeding or thrombosis. Neurologic and mental status examinations should be performed frequently, and the extremities should be examined for cords, swelling, and absent pulses.

The specific treatment of DIC with heparin, antithrombin III, or gabexate (a serine synthetic protease inhibitor of thrombin) is an issue of significant controversy. Although there is general consensus that heparin should be used to treat Trousseau's syndrome and septic thrombophlebitis, specific treatment of DIC in other circumstances is an unresolved issue.

Heparin is a polysaccharide that binds to antithrombin III in such a way as to greatly increase its antagonism of clotting factors. Antithrombin III combines with all factors except VII and irreversibly inactivates them. By inactivating clotting factors, heparin should help decrease the overreactivation of the clotting cascade. The result of this should be decreased formation of fibrin and thrombus. There should also be decreased activation of the fibrinolytic system. Although it would appear that heparin should be an ideal therapy for DIC, there are no double-blind case-controlled studies that show heparin improves survival in DIC.

It is very difficult to carry out such a trial. First, DIC is not a common disorder, and a multicenter study would be needed to recruit enough patients. Second, it is very difficult to control these trials for the type of illness, its severity, and the underlying health of the patient involved. Until such a trial is performed, it is impossible to say whether heparin is of benefit in DIC for a given medical condition. It has been shown that heparin may normalize laboratory measurements in patients with DIC. However, whether this results in clinical improvement remains to be seen.

Despite the lack of hard evidence, many clinicians claim anecdotal improvement from heparin and routinely prescribe it for patients with DIC. We, however, do not routinely use heparin in the management of this condition and have had excellent results with conservative therapeutic management but very aggressive diagnostic pursuit of the underlying illness. The patient who has had no response to conservative therapy and who is actively deteriorating, should not be denied a trial of heparin. A low dose of heparin (5 to 10 U per kilogram per hour) should be tried, and the patient should be observed closely for a change in his condition.

An alternative treatment that has been suggested is antithrombin III concentrate. In many instances of DIC, the level of antithrombin III may be low. Some investigators believe heparin is ineffective in these situations because there is not enough substrate (antithrombin III) present. Other studies have failed to identify significant reduction of antithrombin III in the blood. Future studies may show an improvement in survival with this agent. At this time, it may be prudent to use fresh frozen plasma instead of cryoprecipitate if repletion of plasma proteins is needed, as this will provide antithrombin III.

There have been some attempts to use both heparin and antithrombin III concentrate. The combination of these agents may result in increased hemorrhage and should be avoided.

Gabexate mesilate ([ethyl p-(guanidinohexanoylaxy) benzoate] methane sulfonate) is a synthetic serine proteinase inhibitor of thrombin, factor X_a, plasmin, and kallikrein. It is marketed in Japan under the commercial name FOY, although it has not been approved for administration in North America. Gabexate does not require antithrombin III and is therefore of theoretic benefit. Its efficacy is currently being evaluated and at present is unknown.

The following sections consider specific clinical situations in which DIC may be encountered.

Trousseau's Syndrome

The patient who presents with recurrent migratory arterial and/or venous thrombosis has Trousseau's syndrome. These patients usually have an elevated fibrinogen level with no other evidence of a hypercoagulable state. There is an exquisite response to heparin, and the abrupt recurrence of thrombosis after discontinuation of heparin is almost pathognomonic of Trousseau's syndrome.

Disseminated intravascular coagulation may be a prominent manifestation of this condition. An example is a patient who presented with recurrent thrombosis that responded to heparin. The patient was placed on a therapeutic regimen of warfarin, and heparin was discontinued. Twenty-four hours after stopping heparin, the PT was 75 seconds, the APTT was 180 seconds, the FDP-fdp titer was 1:2048, and the fibrinogen level was 28 mg per deciliter, and thrombosis recurred. Heparin was resumed at 30 hours after discontinuation, and 2 days later the PT, APTT, fibrinogen level, and FDP-fdp titer were normal. The patient was discharged on heparin, 5,000 U SC every 8 hours. The patient underwent an extensive workup for malignancy, including several computed axial tomographic studies of the abdomen and chest. No malignancy could be detected. Ten months later, the patient died from cerebrovascular accident. Autopsy revealed a poorly differentiated neoplasm, 2 to 3 cm in diameter, in the submucosa of the left main-stem bronchus. Hilar nodes contained metastatic tumor.

This case demonstrates the severity of DIC that may be present with Trousseau's syndrome. These patients should undergo a very extensive search for a neoplasm. Adenocarcinomas are the most common primary neoplasms, although any neoplasm can cause DIC. These patients must remain on heparin and can often be maintained on subcutaneous administration as outpatients.

Leukemia

Leukemias have long been associated with bleeding, and one-half of all leukemias in the past were associated with death from hemorrhage. With the institution of more effective chemotherapy and blood product support, death from hemorrhage became significantly less common.

Although all leukemias may cause DIC, promyelocytic leukemia is most often linked to DIC. It has been shown that all leukemic cells have a high tissue thromboplastin activity. Also, these cells contain enzymes such as elastase that can digest clotting factors. Why promyelocytic leukemia is more frequently associated with DIC is unknown. The cause of DIC is believed to be within the promyelocytes. Thus, chemotherapy, which results in cell lysis, may initiate or augment DIC.

Many investigators believe that heparin therapy has resulted in a decreased mortality in promyelocytic leukemia. However, no randomized, well-controlled, double-blinded studies have been performed. Recently, the use of heparin has been questioned. It does not appear that heparin has an effect on survival or induction of remission. The clinical benefit that was previously ascribed to heparin was possibly due to improved chemotherapy.

Appropriate chemotherapy and induction of remission is the most important therapy for DIC in leukemia. We do not routinely use heparin as therapy in this disorder. It is important to note that the thrombocytopenia in these patients may not be the result of DIC, and platelet transfusions should be attempted if thrombocytopenia is severe. If the patient obtains an increment from platelet transfusion, the therapy should be continued as needed. Patients with promyelocytic leukemia should not be treated with heparin if DIC cannot be identified.

Obstetrics

Several conditions in pregnancy may result in DIC. Abruptio placenta, which occurs in approximately 1 percent of all births, may cause DIC. Characteristically, the abruption is severe, and the baby is almost always in severe distress or dead if DIC is present. The amount of vaginal bleeding does not necessarily correlate with the true blood loss, as the retroplacental bleeding may not be continuous with the vagina. If DIC has occurred, the amount of blood loss is usually great, with estimates of usually 4 or more units. Therefore, the patient should immediately be cross-matched, and the hematocrit value followed closely. FDP-fdp are known to slow uterine contractions, and, given the concomitant fetal distress, the patient usually requires an immediate cesarean section. After evacuation of the uterus, DIC should resolve, and the patient should be given fresh frozen plasma as needed postoperatively.

Intrauterine fetal demise is another condition that has been associated with DIC. Usually DIC develops several weeks after fetal demise, and not immediately. Delivery of the dead fetus usually occurs at less than 2 weeks following onset of death, so that coagulopathy is not always an associated problem.

When intrauterine death of a twin occurs, there is a possibility of development of DIC in the viable fetus. If the twins are monozygotic with monochorionic placentas, there are frequently vascular anastomoses that result in transfer of agents that could cause DIC. Although it has been reported, heparin should not help the viable fetus because heparin cannot cross the placenta. In this situation, ultrasound should be performed to determine if the placentas are monochorionic and whether or not there are vascular anastomoses. In the event that a monochorionic placenta is present, early delivery is encouraged, because coagulopathy frequently results in hemorrhage in the viable fetus.

One of the most feared complications of pregnancy is amniotic fluid embolism. During strenuous labor, after rupture of membranes, there may be infusion of amniotic fluid into the maternal circulation. This material has very high tissue thromboplastin activity and can cause severe DIC. The acute respiratory distress syndrome frequently results, and the mortality of this condition is high. Treatment is supportive. There are experts who recommend high-dose heparin, intermediate-dose heparin, or no heparin. We do not use heparin in treating this disorder.

Aneurysm

Disseminated intravascular coagulation is not uncommon in aortic dissection with aneurysm formation, and patients may actually present with petechiae and purpura without any evidence of chest pain. Fisher and colleagues prospectively studied 76 patients presenting with aneurysm. Fibrin degradation products were elevated preoperatively in most patients, and the presence of FDP-fdp did not correlate with intraoperative bleeding. However, patients who presented with petechiae and low platelet counts required significantly more blood intraoperatively.

Patients with aneurysm formation with DIC must be carefully monitored, but they still may undergo surgery for correction. Indeed, surgery is required to correct the coagulopathy. These patients are likely to develop serious hemorrhage from femoral puncture sites for arteriography. These sites must be watched closely for 48 hours following the procedure. Four or more liters of blood loss intraoperatively should be anticipated, and a large supply of blood, as well as a high-speed autotransfuser, should be available.

Once surgery has been accomplished, coagulation studies will quickly return to baseline. These authors did not use heparin preoperatively in their patients.

Liver Disease

Consumptive coagulopathy is common in patients with liver disease of any type because of decreased coagulation factor production and decreased removal of FDP-fdp by the reticuloendothelial system.

A specific problem is DIC after placement of a LeVeen shunt. In these patients, other causes of DIC, such as sepsis, should be carefully excluded. If the coagulopathy is not severe, these patients may be observed for several weeks to months with improvement. If there is no resolution of the DIC, the LeVeen shunt should be taken down.

SUGGESTED READING

Bell WR. Disseminated intravascular coagulation. Johns Hopkins Med J 1980; 146:289–299.
Bell WR, Starksen NF, Tong S, et al. Trousseau's syndrome. Am J Med 1985; 79:423–430.
Feinstein DI. Treatment of disseminated intravascular coagulation. Semin Thromb Hemost 1988; 14:351–362.
Finley BE. Acute coagulopathy in pregnancy. Med Clin North Am 1989; 43:723–743.
Fisher DF, Yawn DH, Crawford ES: Preoperative DIC associated with aortic aneurysms. Arch Surg 1983; 118:1,252–1,255.

ANTITHROMBIN III, PROTEIN C, AND PROTEIN S DEFICIENCY

MORRIS A. BLAJCHMAN, M.D., FRCPC
PHIL WELLS, M.D., FRCPC

The presence of activated clotting factors in the circulation would result in intravascular clot or thrombus formation if such activity were unopposed. Thus, an integral part of the complex series of reactions known as the clotting or coagulation cascade is the presence of inhibitors that can act at various steps in the cascade. The purpose of these critical inhibitors of coagulation is to prevent the occurrence of uncontrolled intravascular coagulation. Antithrombin III, protein C, and protein S are three of the key inhibitors of coagulation. A deficiency of any of these can result in life-threatening disease, manifested by the increased incidence of thromboembolic events. In this chapter we try to provide

insights into the nature of these proteins; an understanding of their concomitant deficiency states; and guidelines for the treatment of patients with such deficiency disorders.

HUMAN ANTITHROMBIN III AND ITS DEFICIENCY STATES

Antithrombin III (AT-III) is a single-chain glycoprotein with a molecular weight of approximately 60,000 daltons. It has a half-life in the circulation of approximately 65 hours. Antithrombin-III is synthesized predominantly in the liver but is also reported to be manufactured in vascular endothelial cells. It is a member of the Serpin super family of serine protease inhibitory proteins, a group of inhibitors that evolved from a common ancestral gene approximately 500 million years ago. In addition to AT-III, the proteins of the Serpin family include α_1-antiplasmin, α_1-antitrypsin, the protein C inhibitor (PCI), and the plasminogen activator inhibitor (PAI). Thus, in addition to inhibiting the activated serine proteases of the coagulation system, they also inhibit the activated serine protease of the complement system and the fibrinolytic cascade. Antithrombin-III inhibits several activated clotting proteins, including factors IX_a, X_a, XI_a, and XII_a, but the main actions are to inhibit thrombin and factor X_a. This is accomplished through the formation of a covalent complex between inhibitor and protease, which is rapidly removed from the circulation. An irreversible reaction occurs when the serine protease lyses AT-III at its reactive center, ser393-arg394, to form a 1:1 stoichiometric covalent complex. The formation of this complex results in both the inactivation of the enzyme and its rapid removal from the circulation. This is accomplished by an as yet undefined receptor associated with the liver. The half-life, in the circulation, of the protease–AT-III complex is approximately 5 minutes. The inactivation of thrombin, and other serine proteases, by AT-III is greatly enhanced by the mucopolysaccharide heparin sulphate. The exact mode of heparin action is somewhat controversial. It appears that the binding of heparin to AT-III enhances its reactivity with thrombin by altering the conformation of the inhibitor in a way that promotes attack by the protease. At least two heparin-binding domains on AT-III have been identified: amino acid residues 41 to 49 comprise heparin-binding region I and amino acid residues 107 to 156 comprise heparin-binding region II. Heparin enhances the rate of thrombin inhibition by AT-III at least 1,000-fold and factor X_a inhibition by approximately 100-fold. In addition to causing a conformation change in AT-III, heparin also interacts with thrombin, a further possible mechanism enabling heparin to enhance the interaction between thrombin and AT-III. Heparin is not normally found in the circulation, but a closely related naturally occurring vessel wall glycosaminoglycan, heparan sulfate, probably provides the in vivo cofactor activity.

The Classification of Inherited Antithrombin III Deficiency

Antithrombin-III activity can be measured in the clinical laboratory using three types of assay: one measures the antigen level; the second, heparin cofactor activity; and the third, progressive antithrombin III activity in the absence of heparin. The classification of patients with congenital deficiency of AT-III is based upon these three parameters. There are four types of AT-III deficiency (Table 1), with type 1 being, by far, the most common. Type 1 AT-III deficiency is a quantitative abnormality of AT-III, with all three AT-III assays being decreased equally to approximately 50 percent of normal. This is due to the absence of an AT-III translation product from one of the two autosomal AT-III alleles, which are located on the long arm of chromosome 1. Type 2 AT-III deficiency is a qualitative defect in AT-III characterized by a point mutation in the gene causing an amino acid substitution in the part of the protein that interacts with the serine protease. In an individual with such a mutation, the AT-III antigen level

Table 1 Classification of Inherited Human Antithrombin III Deficiency

Type 1	Absence of an AT-III protein translation product from one of the two AT-III alleles
Type 2	The presence of abnormal AT-III protein in the circulation due to a mutation in the thrombin-binding region of gene
Type 3	The presence of abnormal AT-III protein due to a mutation in the heparin-binding region of the gene
Type 4	The presence of mutant AT-III protein due to a mutation affecting a site in the gene not included in any of the above

is normal (100 percent), whereas progressive AT-III functional activity or heparin cofactor activity is 50 percent of normal. Type 3 AT-III deficiency is also a qualitative defect characterized by abnormalities in heparin cofactor activity. Again, AT-III antigen level is normal (100 percent), whereas heparin cofactor activity is 50 percent of normal. Individuals with type 3 AT-III deficiency have thromboembolic problems primarily when homozygous, whereas individuals with type 1 and type 2 AT-III deficiency have evidence of thromboembolic disease, even when heterozygous. One consanguineous kindred with two children with homozygous type 1 AT-III deficiency has recently been reported. Both affected infants died within 3 weeks of birth, with evidence of disseminated thrombi in small and large vessels associated with tissue necrosis. Homozygous AT-III deficiency of types 1 and 2 are thus probably incompatible with life. A fourth type of AT-III deficiency has been described in at least three kindreds. All three kindreds manifested impaired heparin cofactor activity without clinical evidence of an increased incidence of thromboembolic events.

The precise prevalence of AT-III deficiency in the general population is unclear, as appropriately designed studies have not yet been done. Nonetheless, the prevalence of congenital AT-III deficiency can be looked at from three perspectives. The first is the prevalence of AT-III deficiency in the general population. Available limited information suggests that AT-III deficiency occurs in asymptomatic individuals with a frequency of 1 in 2,000 to 1 in 20,000. The second perspective is the prevalence of AT-III deficiency in patients who have a known thromboembolic history. In unselected individuals with thromboembolic events, less than 1 percent have congenital AT-III deficiency. However, in patients with a history of thromboembolic events diagnosed before they reach the age of 45 years, approximately 5 percent have inherited AT-III deficiency (usually type 1). Indeed, in patients less than 45 years of age, several recent studies suggest that up to 20 percent will be found to be deficient in either AT-III, protein C, or protein S, with the prevalence of each approximately equal.

A third way of looking at the prevalence of AT-III deficiency is to examine the prevalence of thromboembolic events in patients with known AT-III deficiency. It appears that 50 percent to 60 percent of patients with heterozygous type 1 or type 2 AT-III deficiency will have at least one thromboembolic event sometime during their lifetime. In contrast, the incidence of thromboembolic events in individuals with heterozygous type 3 AT-III deficiency has been estimated to be only 6 percent. Thus, the overall risk in patients with type 1 or 2 AT-III deficiency of having a thromboembolic event is approximately 1 percent per year. This risk generally increases with age, but it also increases during events known to increase the risk of thrombosis in the general population (i.e., trauma, surgery, pregnancy, prolonged immobilization, and chronic inflammatory disease).

It is important to keep in mind the clinical situations in which to suspect AT-III deficiency. These include (1) a thromboembolic event that occurs before the age of 45, particularly in pregnant women; (2) a thromboembolic event occurring when there is a family history of thromboembolism; (3) patients with recurrent thromboembolic events; (4) a thromboembolic event that occurs in a patient at an unusual site (i.e., inferior vena cava, mesenteric, renal, or cerebral veins); (5) a thromboembolic event in a patient associated with documented heparin resistance; and (6) neonates with arterial or venous thrombosis. In all these situations, one should also think about the possibility of protein C and protein S deficiency.

The Treatment of Patients with Inherited Antithrombin III Deficiency

The clinical setting usually dictates the form of therapy required. We consider only the treatment of patients with heterozygous type 1 and type 2 AT-III deficiency, as individuals with type 3 AT-III deficiency appear not to be at risk unless they are homozygous. At this time, the treatment of patients with AT-III deficiency involves primarily the use of heparin and the vitamin K antagonist oral anticoagulants. However, the recent availability of AT-III concentrates will allow an evaluation of this new modality in the treatment of patients deficient in AT-III.

Antithrombin-III concentrates are prepared from plasma by affinity elution from heparin-Sepharose beads or gels. The resulting product is then pasteurized by heating at 60°C for 10 hours to inactivate any viruses that may be present. Although there is some loss of activity with such treatment, the administration of 1 U per kilogram body weight, in an average adult, will increase the plasma AT-III level by 1.8 percent. Recovery is reduced to 1 percent or less in patients with shock or disseminated intravascular coagulation (DIC). The half-life of infused AT-III in such patients can be as short as 5 hours.

The first clinical setting to consider is the healthy asymptomatic individual with known heterozygous type 1 or type 2 inherited AT-III deficiency. Although no study has formally addressed the question as to whether anticoagulation is required in such individuals, it is our opinion that they be anticoagulated with a small dose of oral anticoagulants to prolong the INR to 1.5 to 2.0, but only during high-risk periods. Prophylaxis with AT-III

concentrates may be used, if available, but, as indicated previously, the precise place of AT-III concentrates in the treatment of AT-III deficiency remains to be established. An important fact to remember is that individuals with asymptomatic AT-III deficiency should be counseled about the increased thromboembolic risk associated with pregnancy, surgery, and trauma. In particular, women should be advised against the use of oral contraceptives, especially if no prophylactic measures are taken to prevent thromboembolic events.

The second clinical setting to consider is that of a patient with an established deep venous thrombosis (DVT). Full intravenous heparin anticoagulation is generally indicated in such patients. This is usually accomplished with a 5,000 U bolus, followed by heparin infusion at a rate of 1,200 U per hour, in order to prolong the activated partial thromboplastin time (APTT) to twice the normal value. In these patients, it is important to keep in mind four important points: (1) reach therapeutic heparin levels within the first 24 hours to prevent recurrence; (2) individuals with inherited AT-III deficiency may be difficult to heparinize; one way to deal with this eventuality is to initiate oral anticoagulant therapy early, usually within a few days of initiating heparin therapy; (3) consider the use of AT-III concentrates if heparin resistance occurs; and (4) consider the use of long-term oral anticoagulation.

Pregnancy is the third clinical setting we would like to address. It is important, first of all, to counsel all women with AT-III deficiency about the increased risk of thromboembolism during pregnancy. Another risk, for those on oral anticoagulants, is the increased risk of fetal developmental abnormalities due to the oral anticoagulants. While planning a pregnancy, a patient who is on oral anticoagulants should have pregnancy tests done frequently. Once the pregnancy begins, the switch to heparin should occur by approximately the eighth week of conception. Once a pregnancy starts, women deficient in AT-III should be anticoagulated because of the increased risk of thrombosis during the pregnancy. Heparin should be given subcutaneously every 12 hours using a dose to mildly prolong the APTT by 5 to 10 seconds. Such a regimen has been reported to be effective when compared to historical controls.

Heparin should be used throughout the pregnancy. If this is not possible, then oral anticoagulants ought to be used, but only during the second and third trimester, as oral anticoagulant embryopathy occurs primarily during the first trimester. At the start of labor, the heparin should be discontinued and AT-III concentrates used, if available, to raise the AT-III levels to 100 percent. This usually requires 50 U of AT-III per kilogram body weight daily. This should be continued until either the heparin or the oral anticoagulant has been restarted and is established in the therapeutic range. If oral anticoagulants are not going to be used on a long-term basis, then heparin should be started within 24 hours of delivery and continued into the postpartum period, for at least 2 weeks. The newborn will need to be evaluated for AT-III deficiency, but in the absence of complications, this should be delayed for at least 6 months, at which point adult levels of AT-III are attained. Neonatal AT-III levels are approximately 50 percent that seen in adults.

Surgery is the last clinical setting that we will address. For minor surgical procedures (i.e., lymph node biopsies, excisions under local anesthesia, and so forth), asymptomatic patients probably require no intervention. If oral anticoagulants have been used, reversal with vitamin K just prior to the procedure is usually sufficient, and oral anticoagulant therapy should be restarted a few days later. For major surgery, the use of low-dose heparin (8,000 U twice daily) is indicated, followed by oral anticoagulation for up to a month postoperatively. If AT-III concentrates are available, AT-III concentrates should be used at a dose of 50 U per kilogram per day in combination with the reversal of the oral anticoagulants. Antithrombin-III levels should be monitored to be sure that the administered AT-III brings the level to within the normal plasma range. The AT-III concentrates should be continued until the risk of bleeding is small. This may require 3 to 4 weeks of therapy in the case of neurosurgical or cardiovascular procedures. Please note that these recommendations for AT-III replacement are based on theoretical considerations only. Antithrombin-III replacement represents a logical consideration in this setting; however, at the time of writing, there are insufficient data available to demonstrate the real value of AT-III replacement in patients with AT-III deficiency.

Acquired Antithrombin III Deficiency

A mild to moderate reduction in AT-III level is common following surgery. This is thought not to have major clinical significance. Clinically significant acquired AT-III deficiency is known to occur in patients with nephrotic syndrome, in which the protein is excreted in the urine; protein-losing enteropathy due to inflammatory bowel disease and loss of AT-III in the bowel contents; severe liver disease, in which there is decreased production; and DIC states, in which there is increased catabolism of AT-III. The small drop in AT-III concentration that occurs postoperatively and during the postpartum period does not appear to predispose to thrombosis. The AT-III deficiency that can develop in patients with nephrotic syndrome, severe liver disease, or protein-losing enteropathy may predispose to thrombotic events if the AT-III level goes below 50 percent. Therapy with AT-III concentrates or anticoagulation cannot be recommended routinely for such patients at this time, although this may prove to be a useful intervention in the foreseeable future. In the setting of patients with DIC, preliminary data indicate that AT-III concentrates, particularly when AT-III levels are low, prevent the continuation of the DIC. The available data, however, are preliminary, and the routine use of AT-III replacement in such patients cannot be recommended until adequate randomized studies are published indicating utility.

PROTEIN C DEFICIENCY

Protein C is a plasma glycoprotein with an approximate molecular weight of 62,000 daltons that is present in the circulation in a double-chain form. It is a vitamin K–dependent zymogen that becomes a serine protease when activated by thrombin. Activated protein C (APC) regulates blood coagulation by inactivating thrombin-activated factor V and factor VIII. The congenital deficiency of protein C has been associated with a high incidence of thromboembolic events in affected individuals. The molecular basis of protein C deficiency is largely unknown, but several point mutations have recently been identified. Both type 1 (concordant reduction in antigenic and functional activity) and type 2 (normal antigen level with reduced functional activity) inherited protein C deficiency have been described. Both types may have similar clinical manifestations (See Table 2).

The current concepts explaining the anticoagulant effect of protein C are as follows: Thrombin, when formed, binds tightly to an endothelial receptor called thrombomodulin. This 1:1 binding to thrombomodulin induces a conformational change in the thrombin molecule so that it is capable only of activating protein C. Formation of the thrombomodulin-thrombin complex therefore directly inhibits the capacity of thrombin to clot fibrinogen; to activate platelets; to activate factor XIII; and to activate factors V and VIII. When

Table 2 Classification of Inherited Protein C and Protein S Deficiency and Their Clinical Effects

Deficiency	Clinical Effect
Protein C Deficiency	
Heterozygous	Increased frequency of thromboembolic events
	Oral anticoagulant-induced skin necrosis
Homozygous (or doubly heterozygous)	Purpura fulminans in the neonate
Protein S Deficiency	
Heterozygous	
Homozygous (or doubly heterozygous)	Increased frequency of thromboembolic events

complexed to thrombomodulin, thrombin activation of protein C to form APC is enhanced by at least three orders of magnitude. The APC then complexes with protein S (see later) on the surface of the endothelium and in this form can cleave activated factor VIII and activated factor V, eliminating their procoagulant cofactor ability. This results in the decreased generation of factor X_a and thrombin. Activated protein C has been shown also to accelerate fibrinolysis, a topic beyond the scope of this chapter.

Congenital Protein C Deficiency

Congenital protein C deficiency is inherited as an autosomal dominant trait. The protein C gene has been isolated and has been determined to reside on chromosome 2. The heterozygous state has been reported to occur in as many as 1 in 300 individuals (blood donors). Functional and immunologic assays for protein C exist, but these must be carefully standardized within individual laboratories. Prevalence of thromboembolic events suggests that as few as 1 in 70 of these protein C heterozygotes is at risk of thrombosis. Currently, there is no laboratory test that can predict which of these individuals is at risk. The best predictor of thrombosis risk is whether there is a family history of thromboembolic events associated with heterozygous protein C deficiency. In some kindreds, there is a very strong thrombotic tendency and the risk of thromboembolic events, before the age of 45 years, may be as high as 65 percent. The documentation of protein C deficiency in an individual presenting with a thrombotic event can be attributed to the protein C deficiency primarily where there is a coexisting positive family history of thrombosis. In such instances, one should probably consider that individual to be at risk for recurrent DVT.

Patients with protein C deficiency also appear to be at risk for the phenomenon of oral anticoagulant–induced skin necrosis. This event is due to thromboses occurring in the small vessels of the skin on the second to fifth day following the initiation of the oral anticoagulant therapy. The skin necrosis tends to occur primarily in the skin over the breasts and flanks. The occurrence of skin necrosis has been attributed to the production, by the oral anticoagulants, of a temporary hypercoagulable state as the result of the very short plasma half-life of protein C. It is postulated that the rapid decrease in the protein C level induced by the oral anticoagulant quickly exceeds that of the procoagulant vitamin K–dependent factors, thus inducing thrombosis. Why only the skin is involved in such instances is unclear.

Protein C deficiency is autosomally inherited; thus, the homozygous (or double heterozygous) state can and does occur. Protein C deficiency appears to be a very heterozygous disorder; thus, most patients who inherit two abnormal protein C genes will most likely be doubly heterozygous, rather than homozygous. However, until this issue is clarified, patients with two-allele protein C deficiency will generally be referred to as homozygous. Homozygous protein C deficiency has been estimated to

occur in 1 in 500,000 live births. Some cerebral and ophthalmic thrombotic complications occur in most instances. This can lead to hydrocephalus, mental retardation, seizures, and blindness. Within 2 to 5 days of birth, purpura and DIC occur in the majority of patients so affected. There are occasional documented cases that the DIC appears only when the child was several months or even several years of age. The purpura occurs in two phases, the first being reversible, if the neonate is treated with plasma or protein C concentrate. In the second phase, the skin necrosis is irreversible and may often need surgical debridement. It may be difficult to diagnose homozygous protein C deficiency because protein C levels are usually very low in most "sick" infants. Furthermore, neonates with DIC usually have very low levels of protein C, even when the protein C deficiency is not inherited. The diagnosis of protein C deficiency can usually be established by the presence of the typical skin lesions and often by a family history of such events having been observed in previous children born within that family.

Management of Protein C Deficiency

Prophylactic therapy of asymptomatic protein C deficient heterozygous individuals is not recommended at this time. In patients with acute thromboembolic events, heparin is indicated. It is probably wise not to begin oral anticoagulant therapy with a loading dose because of the risk of oral anticoagulant–induced skin necrosis. For the same reason, full anticoagulation with heparin is indicated before beginning oral anticoagulant therapy. The optimal length of treatment required for these patients is controversial; however, if there is evidence of recurring thromboembolic events, or a strong family history, then lifelong anticoagulation with oral anticoagulants should be recommended even with the first thrombotic event. Similarly, in asymptomatic heterozygotes, if there is a strong family history of thrombosis associated with documented heterozygous protein C deficiency, lifelong anticoagulation should be considered. If there is no family history of thrombosis, the decision to anticoagulate the heterozygous protein C–deficient patient is more difficult. It is our opinion that heterozygous protein C–deficient individuals should probably not be committed to lifelong anticoagulant therapy except when there is a strong family history or there is evidence that a thrombotic event developed spontaneously, without the concomitant presence of known risk factors.

There are also special situations to examine, such as pregnancy and surgery. Without prophylaxis, 26 percent of heterozygous protein C–deficient patients will develop a thrombotic event in such situations, with most occurring in the early postpartum period in pregnant women. During pregnancy, therefore, one should start heparin during the second trimester; it should be continued during the remainder of the pregnancy and for 2 to 3 weeks into the postpartum period. Postoperatively and in other situations of prolonged immobilization, such as following an accident, subcutaneous heparin is probably indicated.

The treatment of the oral anticoagulant–induced skin necrosis is difficult. This generally consists of the discontinuation of the oral anticoagulants and the administration of vitamin K and fresh frozen plasma. Extensive surgical debridement of the necrotic areas may also be necessary. A highly pure and safe protein C concentrate has recently been developed. When this product becomes licensed and readily available, it will likely be a useful adjunct in the management of oral anticoagulant–induced skin necrosis as well as in the prophylaxis of pregnant and surgical patients with heterozygous protein C deficiency. It is also very likely that recombinant human protein C preparations will become available within the next few years.

The treatment of patients with homozygous (or doubly heterozygous) protein C deficiency is limited at this time to the use of fresh frozen plasma. Fresh frozen plasma should be used at a dose of 8 to 12 cc per kilogram every 12 hours for 4 to 8 weeks or until the skin lesions have healed. At this initial treatment, slow oral anticoagulation may be instituted. Factor IX concentrates (which contain some protein C) have also been used in such patients at a dose of 200 U per kilogram to achieve a 100 percent protein C plasma level. This can be administered every 48 hours, but care should be taken to initiate such therapy only after adequate heparinization has been achieved. Such an approach has been used successfully in several infants, for over a 2-year period, to prevent the complications of this dreaded disease. Patients with homozygous protein C deficiency will benefit enormously with the availability of protein C concentrates, whether obtained from recombinant DNA technology or purified from plasma.

Protein C deficiency states can also be acquired. This can occur in patients with liver disease given oral anticoagulants; in patients with DIC; in association with hemodialysis therapy in patients with chronic renal failure, and in patients undergoing plasma exchange. Protein C levels are also often decreased in patients taking high-estrogen birth control pills, in patients with nephrotic syndrome, and in diabetic patients with diabetic complications. The clinical significance of these acquired states is unknown at this time.

PROTEIN S DEFICIENCY

Protein S is also a vitamin K–dependent protein, but it is unique among them in that it is not a zymogen, but a cofactor. Protein S interacts with the phospholipid on the endothelial cell surface, in the presence of calcium, to increase by one order of magnitude the activity of APC. Protein S exists in plasma in both the free form (averaging 35 percent to 40 percent of the total) and the bound form. In the bound form, protein S is found complexed with the C4b binding protein. It appears that only the free form of protein S is coagulantly active. Protein S is synthesized in the liver, but the decrease in protein S induced by oral anticoagulants is proportionately less than that of the other vitamin K–dependent factors. This has led investigators to postulate that there may be extrahepatic synthesis sites for protein S, but these sites have yet to be identified. Functional assays for protein S are not very good at this time. Several immunologic assays are available using the ELISA technique. These assays, however, frequently underestimate the amount of free protein S in the circulation. Liver disease will decrease the level of free protein S, as will pregnancy and acute illness. The latter is likely the result of the fact that the C4b binding protein is an acute-phase reactant whose concentration increases during acute illnesses. This means that during pregnancy or in patients with an inflammatory state, the C4b binding protein level goes up, leading to a decrease in free protein S level.

Congenital deficiency of protein S can be divided into two types: type 1 and type 2 (Table 2). In type 1 deficiency, the free protein S level is greatly decreased and most of the protein present is detected in the bound form. This form of protein S deficiency is the most common. Type 2 protein S deficiency is rare. Type 2 patients have decreased levels of both free and bound protein S. The prevalence of protein S deficiency in patients under the age of 45 years with diagnosed thrombotic events may be as high as 5 percent to 8 percent. Thromboembolic risk during pregnancy appears to be slightly less than with the other deficiency syndromes discussed, but it is still increased compared to nondeficient individuals. The prevalence of asymptomatic protein S deficiency is unknown, as is the risk of a thrombotic event in individuals with protein S deficiency. Individuals with known heterozygous protein S deficiency and a family history of thromboembolic events appear to be at high risk. Sixty percent of such individuals will have thromboembolic events before the age of 40; this is similar to the findings in individuals with AT-III and protein C deficiency. The approach to therapy is the same as outlined for individuals with heterozygous protein C deficiency, except for the use of protein C concentrates. Protein S concentrate preparations are not yet available, but these are likely to be developed within the next 5 years.

SUGGESTED READING

Esmon CT. The roles of protein C and thrombomodulin in the regulation of blood coagulation. J Biol Chem 1989; 264:4,743–4,746.

Gallus AS. Replacement therapy in antithrombin III deficiency. Transfusion Med Rev 1989; 4:253–263.

Mann KG, Jenny RJ, Krishnaswamy S. Cofactor proteins in the assembly and expression of blood clotting enzyme complexes. Ann Rev Biochem 1988; 57:915–956.

Manson HE, Austin RC, Fernandez-Rachubinski F, et al. The molecular pathology of inherited human antithrombin III deficiency. Transfusion Med Rev 1989; 4:264–281.

IMMUNE THROMBOCYTOPENIA

RICHARD H. ASTER, M.D.

ACUTE IDIOPATHIC THROMBOCYTOPENIC PURPURA

Acute idiopathic thrombocytopenic purpura (ITP) is a relatively common childhood disorder characterized by a sudden reduction in platelet levels and hemorrhagic manifestations. About one-half of the cases are preceded by an upper respiratory infection or, less commonly, by specific viral infections such as measles or chicken pox. Platelet destruction in acute ITP is thought to be mediated by autoantibodies or immune complexes somehow triggered by exposure to viral antigens, but its exact pathogenesis is not understood. Serologic tests capable of diagnosing acute ITP with precision are not yet available. Accordingly, the diagnosis is made on the basis of clinical and nonspecific laboratory findings and exclusion of other causes of thrombocytopenia.

Therapeutic Approach

Passive Management

Acute ITP is usually self-limited and untreated cases recover spontaneously, often within a week or two, occasionally after 4 to 6 months. Watchful waiting while avoiding trauma is an acceptable form of therapy, especially in mild cases.

Corticosteroids

Carefully conducted clinical trials provide evidence that platelet levels increase more rapidly in children given corticosteroids than in untreated children. Other trials fail to demonstrate this distinction. Considering the relatively minor side effects associated with corticosteroid administration for a few weeks in children, it is reasonable to prescribe prednisone, 2 mg per kilogram daily, for a maximum of 2 or 3 weeks, to symptomatic patients pending resolution of this controversy. Higher doses of prednisone or intravenous prednisolone are recommended for children with profoundly reduced platelet counts (less than 5,000 per microliter) and severe hemorrhagic symptoms. After a few days of treatment, bleeding symptoms often diminish in severity, reflected by clearing of purpuric lesions in the skin and buccal mucosa. At this point, the dose of prednisone can be reduced to 0.5 to 1 mg per kilogram even if the platelet count has not yet risen. Children receiving corticosteroids are subject to th same side effects as adults, i.e., fluid retention, cushingoid changes, psychiatric abnormalities, and increased susceptibility to infection, and they should be followed closely. The medication can be tapered and then discontinued as soon as the platelet count exceeds 50,000 per microliter.

Intravenous Gamma Globulin

Intravenous gamma globulin provides a therapeutic alternative to corticosteroids in patients with severe hemorrhagic symptoms. The dose currently recommended is 0.4 g per kilogram body weight daily for 5 days. About 80 percent of children so treated experience signifi-cant elevations in platelet counts, often to normal levels. In approximately half of these cases, the elevation is sustained. In the others, thrombocytopenia recurs, but may respond again to intravenous gamma globu-lin infusion. Intravenous gamma globulin is thought to impair the ability of macrophages to clear immuno-globulin-coated platelets, but other mechanisms of action are also possible. At the recommended doses, the side effects of intravenous gamma globulin are minor, consisting mainly of fever and headache. There is no evidence that any one of the various commercial preparations available is superior to the others.

Management of Intracranial Hemorrhage

Less than 1 percent of children with acute ITP present with intracranial hemorrhage or develop this complication soon after diagnosis. Such cases require aggressive treatment with high-dose corticosteroids, intravenous gamma globulin, and platelet transfusions. Surgical evacuation of subdural or epidural hematoma is sometimes required. It is reasonable to perform a splenectomy in patients capable of tolerating surgery, although the effectiveness of this procedure is not fully established. Exchange transfusion has been employed in a few cases.

Platelet Transfusions

Transfused platelets are rapidly destroyed in children with acute ITP and, except in patients with intracranial hemorrhage, or other severe bleeding symptoms, are contraindicated because of potential infectious complications.

Refractory Cases

Children who remain thrombocytopenic after 4 to 6 months of observation rarely recover spontaneously thereafter. Such patients generally have a different form of autoimmune thrombocytopenia – chronic ITP. Splenectomy is the mainstay of treatment for this disorder (see below). Repeated courses of intravenous gamma globulin are sometimes effective in symptomatic children. Removal of the spleen in young children results in increased susceptibility to postsplenectomy sepsis. Children undergoing splenectomy should be immunized with pneumococcal and *Haemophilus influenzae* vaccine, and their parents should be cautioned to seek medical consultation at the first sign of infection. If splenectomy must be performed in a child younger than 5 to 6 years of age, consideration should be given to prophylactic antibiotic therapy.

CHRONIC IDIOPATHIC (AUTOIMMUNE) THROMBOCYTOPENIC PURPURA

Chronic ITP is generally more insidious in onset than acute ITP of childhood, although the degree of thrombocytopenia and severity of bleeding symptoms vary widely from patient to patient. Women are affected about four times as often as men. The disorder appears to be a true autoimmune condition in which certain glycoproteins on the surface of platelets are the target autoantigens. The underlying cause of chronic ITP is almost certainly a failure of immunoregulation, but the exact basis for this abnormality is unknown. Chronic ITP usually occurs in isolation, but develops in association with a number of other conditions, including Hodgkin's and non-Hodgkin's lymphoma, systemic lupus erythematosus, hyperthyroidism, and infection with HIV-I. The diagnosis is made on the basis of clinical and nonspecific laboratory findings that exclude other causes of thrombocytopenia. Serologic methods for detecting and characterizing platelet reactive autoantibodies are becoming more precise, and specific serologic diagnosis may soon be possible.

Therapeutic Approach

Passive Management

Occasional patients with mild thrombocytopenia and minimal hemorrhagic symptoms can be followed without specific therapy, sometimes for many months or even years.

Corticosteroids

Corticosteroids are the primary therapy for patients with more severe thrombocytopenia as well as purpuric lesions. A distinction is often made between patients with wet purpura and those with dry purpura. In the former group, hemorrhagic bullae and generalized oozing from mucosal surfaces is seen, and the risk of intracranial hemorrhage appears to be greater. Such patients should be hospitalized for their initial treatment. The conventional initial dose of prednisone is 1 mg per kilogram per day. Doses two or three times higher are indicated in patients with extensive wet purpura and profound thrombocytopenia (platelets less than 5,000 per microliter). In many patients, there is clearing of purpura before the platelet count rises.

The exact mechanism of corticosteroid action is not known, but they are thought to act by inhibiting the capacity of macrophages to remove antibody-coated platelets from the circulation and, perhaps, by suppressing autoantibody production. Most patients respond with a rise in platelet count within 1 or 2 weeks of the time treatment is initiated. As soon as purpura clears and the platelet count exceeds 100,000 per microliter, the medication can be tapered gradually. A reasonable schedule is to reduce the dose of prednisone by 10 mg per week initially and 5 mg per week after the dose reaches 0.5 mg per kilogram. Platelet counts should be determined weekly and the regimen modified if thrombocytopenia recurs. All patients receiving long-term corticosteroids should be observed for side effects, which include fluid retention, cushingoid features, hypertension, aggravation of diabetes, gastric complications, and psychosis.

Splenectomy

In nearly all patients with chronic ITP, thrombocytopenia recurs as the dosage of corticosteroids is reduced. Some patients can be managed for long periods of time on doses of prednisone sufficiently low to minimize side effects. Others require splenectomy if there is no contraindication to surgery. The benefit of splenectomy derives from removing the major site in which antibody-coated platelets are destroyed and removing a major site of autoantibody production. About 75 percent of patients achieve a permanent remission after surgery. The response rate is higher in younger patients than in persons older than 50 years. Patients who fail to achieve a complete remission can often be managed on low doses of prednisone.

Recurrent Thrombocytopenia

Thrombocytopenia sometimes recurs many years after a splenectomy-induced remission. In most cases, this is a consequence of increased autoantibody production and destruction of platelets in extrasplenic sites. In a minority of cases, the recurrence results from hypertrophy of an accessory spleen, which can be detected by spleen scan. Surgical removal of the accessory splenic tissue is often curative.

Refractoriness to Prednisone and Splenectomy

A number of second line therapies are available for patients who fail to respond initially even to high-dose prednisone or in whom splenectomy is ineffective.

Intravenous Gamma Globulin

More than half of patients with chronic ITP achieve an increase in platelet levels following administration of intravenous gamma globulin, 0.4 g per kilogram body weight daily for 5 days. Intravenous gamma globulin appears to act by impairing the ability of macrophages to clear antibody-coated platelets from the circulation, but other mechanisms are also possible. Several commercial preparations of intravenous gamma globulin are available; none has been shown to be clearly superior to the others. The duration of the response to gamma globulin is variable. Some patients have only a modest elevation in platelets for a few days. In others, the platelet count is normalized for several weeks, and sometimes for months. In the majority of cases, thrombocytopenia recurs, but occasional patients develop a sustained remission for reasons not currently understood. Side effects of intravenous gamma globulin are limited to headache and occasional fever, but the current treatment is expensive and should be reserved for patients who fail to respond to prednisone and splenectomy.

Immunosuppression

Several immunosuppressive regimens have been used to treat patients who fail to respond to standard therapy or who are not candidates for splenectomy. The highest response rate appears to have been achieved with vincristine, 1 to 2 mg intravenously every 7 days for 3 to 4 weeks. Some patients achieve a sustained remission, but thrombocytopenia recurs within weeks or months in most. Patients receiving repeated doses of vincristine should be monitored for the development of peripheral neuropathy. It has been suggested that vincristine is more effective if infused slowly over a 6-hour period than when it is given as a bolus injection.

Cyclophosphamide, in doses ranging from 50 to 200 mg per day orally with prednisone, produces at least a transient elevation in platelet levels after 3 to 8 weeks of treatment in about one-third of cases. A minority of responders develop permanent, unmaintained remissions. Patients receiving cyclophosphamide should take large amounts of fluid daily to prevent cystitis and should have blood counts performed at least weekly. Azathioprine, in doses of 100 to 300 mg per day with prednisone, leads to platelet elevations in about 25 percent of cases, sometimes after 6 to 9 months of treatment. Side effects of this regimen are minimal, but blood counts should be monitored periodically.

Colchicine

Colchicine, in doses ranging from 0.6 to 1.2 mg four times daily, has been reported to raise platelet levels in some refractory patients. Its mechanism of action is unknown, but inhibition of macrophage function has been suggested. Gastrointestinal side effects may limit therapy in individual patients. Up to 4 to 6 weeks may be required for a therapeutic effect.

Danazol

Danazol is a nonvirilizing, modified androgen found empirically to raise platelet levels in some patients with refractory ITP when given with prednisone. In some series, about one-half of treated patients have achieved significant benefit.

Platelet Transfusions

Platelets transfused to patients with chronic ITP are usually destroyed rapidly and produce little therapeutic benefit. Their use should be limited to patients with severe, life-threatening bleeding, in whom they may be of transient benefit. It may be necessary to give platelet concentrates every few hours to maintain a hemostatic effect in such cases. Platelets can be given preoperatively to patients undergoing splenectomy, but surgery is often tolerated without transfusion. A more sustained elevation in platelet count is achieved if platelets are given after the splenic pedicle is clamped. Alternatively, the transfusion can be given after a single dose of intravenous gamma globulin, 0.4 g per kilogram.

Plasma Exchange

Machine-assisted, therapeutic plasma exchange has been advocated for patients with life-threatening bleeding in an attempt to lower circulating levels of autoantibody. This approach is worthy of trial in critically ill patients, but often is without beneficial effect.

Idiopathic Thrombocytopenic Purpura in Pregnancy

Special therapeutic considerations apply in pregnant women with ITP because of the potential effects of treatment on the fetus and the risk of neonatal thrombocytopenia resulting from transplacental passage of autoantibody. Most women can be managed during pregnancy with modest doses of prednisone. In rare instances, splenectomy has been performed successfully in the second or third trimester. Intravenous gamma globulin can also be utilized and is not known to be harmful to the fetus. In general, the severity of thrombocytopenia in the newborn is proportional to the severity of the disease in the mother, but there are many exceptions. Infants with severe thrombocytopenia have been born to women previously splenectomized and who have normal platelet counts. Currently, it is not possible to predict by serologic testing whether an infant will be born thrombocytopenic. There is some evidence that administration of prednisone, 0.5 to 1.0 mg per kilogram, to the mother during the last 2 or 3 weeks of pregnancy reduces the severity of thrombocytopenia in the newborn. Opinions differ as to whether caesarean section should be performed to reduce the chance of intracranial hemorrhage in the infant. When labor is routine, even thrombocytopenic infants generally do well with vaginal delivery. Sometimes, a scalp vein platelet count is performed shortly after rupture of the membranes, and vaginal delivery proceeds if the infant's platelet count is greater than 50,000 per microliter. In infants with lower counts, caesarean section is performed. Probably, a platelet count done on fetal blood obtained by percutaneous sampling of the umbilical vein provides a better index of fetal platelet levels. In affected infants, thrombocytopenia sometimes persists for several months and can usually be managed with prednisone, 1 to 2 mg per kilogram per day. Intravenous gamma globulin, 0.4 g per kilogram per day for 5 days, can also be utilized. With further experience, this may become the treatment of choice. Exchange transfusion is indicated only in severely affected infants who fail to respond to these therapies.

It must be kept in mind that most women who develop mild thrombocytopenia during pregnancy do not have ITP. "Gestational thrombocytopenia" occurs in 5 to 7 percent of normal pregnancies and does not require specific treatment.

SUGGESTED READING

Aster RH. "Gestational" thrombocytopenia. A plea for conservative management. N Engl J Med 1990; 323:264–265.
Aster RH, George JN. Thrombocytopenia due to enhanced platelet destruction by immunologic mechanisms. In: Williams WJ, Beutler E, Erslev AJ, Lichtman MA, eds. Hematology, 4th Ed. New York: McGraw-Hill, 1990:1370.
Berchtold P, McMillan R. Therapy of chronic idiopathic thrombocytopenic purpura in adults. Blood 1989; 74:2309–2317.
Chessells J. Chronic idiopathic thrombocytopenic purpura: Primum non nocere. Arch Dis Child 1989; 64:1326.
Warkentin TE, Kelton JG. Current concepts in the treatment of immune thrombocytopenia. Drugs 1990; 40:531–542.

THROMBOTIC THROMBOCYTOPENIC PURPURA

JOEL L. MOAKE, M.D.

PATHOGENESIS

Thrombotic thrombocytopenic purpura (TTP) is an extraordinary example of the thrombotic process in the arterial circulation. It is a combination of thrombocytopenia, microangiopathic hemolytic anemia (i.e., intravascular hemolysis with schistocytes on peripheral blood films), and fluctuating ischemic vascular signs (Table 1). Ischemia can affect any organ, but must include the central nervous system. The formation of platelet occlusive lesions occurs in arterioles and capillaries throughout the microcirculation. The intravascular platelet thrombi probably form and disperse repeatedly, causing the characteristic intermittent symptoms and signs of ischemia in many organs.

Most patients with TTP have no other known disorder. Sometimes, however, TTP is associated with infections, immunologic abnormalities (including systemic lupus erythematosus and acquired immunodeficiency syndrome [AIDS]), drugs (including mitomycin C and cyclosporin A), or pregnancy. About two-thirds of patients with TTP have a single episode that never recurs after successful treatment. An intermittent form of TTP, characterized by subsequent occasional infrequent relapses, ensues in about one-third of patients. It has been possible to recognize this intermittent type of TTP because many patients now survive their initial TTP episodes. Chronic relapsing TTP, characterized by episodes of varying severity about every 3 weeks that require prophylactic plasma infusion, is the rarest type of the disorder (Table 2).

It has been suggested that episodes of TTP may be caused by (1) inadequate endothelial cell production of PGI_2, or excessive lability of PGI_2, due to a deficiency of either an endothelial cell stimulating or stabilizing factor present in normal plasma; (2) deficient plasminogen activator production by endothelial cells and, consequently, inadequate fibrinolysis; (3) deficient production of IgG molecules that may normally interfere with platelet aggregation, perhaps by combining with an as yet unidentified microbe (or microbial product) capable of aggregating platelets; or (4) presence in the circulation of a substance or substances capable of inducing intravascular platelet aggregation. The first three hypotheses are unlikely explanations for TTP because infusions of PGI_2, streptokinase, urokinase, or concentrated IgG have not been consistently demonstrated to be effective modes of therapy. The fourth explanation is most likely. The aggregating substances in the bloodstream have been reported by different investigators to include one of several small proteins in the 40- to 60-kD

Table 1 Diagnosis of Thrombotic Thrombocytopenic Purpura

Intravascular platelet aggregation
  Thrombocytopenia
  Ischemic vascular signs (including neurologic)
Microangiopathic hemolytic anemia (schistocytosis and elevated LDH level)
  ± Fever
  ± Acute renal failure

Table 2 Types of Thrombotic Thrombocytopenic Purpura

Single episode
  Idiopathic
  Secondary
Intermittent (occasional, infrequent, irregular relapses)
Chronic relapsing (frequent, regular, periodic relapses)

range, a cysteine protease, or unusually large (UL) von Willebrand factor (vWF) multimeric forms. These UL-vWF multimers are derived from endothelial cells that may be injured or intensely stimulated to secrete their contents of Weibel-Palade bodies (containing ULvWF forms) during a single episode of TTP. In the intermittent or chronic relapsing types of TTP, autoantibodies may inactivate a "depolymerase" activity in normal plasma responsible for converting ULvWF forms from endothelial cells to the somewhat smaller vWF forms normally in circulation. Unusually large vWF multimers have been demonstrated to be present between episodes in patients with both the intermittent and chronic relapsing types of TTP and to disappear along with platelets during TTP relapses. These findings indicate that both ULvWF multimers and some as yet unidentified cofactor are involved in the pathogenesis of TTP episodes. The intravascular thrombi formed during episodes of TTP stain strongly for vWF antigen but only weakly for fibrinogen. (In contrast, the opposite immunohistochemical results have been obtained on thrombi in patients with disseminated intravascular coagulation.) These observations provide additional evidence for the involvement of vWF in the pathogenesis of TTP episodes.

The extent of intravascular clumping during TTP episodes is related to the degree of thrombocytopenia. Platelet counts are often less than 10,000 per microliter. Erythrocyte fragmentation has been presumed to occur because red blood cells are injured and partially disrupted as they move through partially occluded arterioles and capillaries. Recently, however, young red cells have been found to have surface receptors for unusually large vWF multimers. These young red cells adhere to endothelial cells via ULvWF multimeric forms on subendothelial cell surfaces and may be susceptible to disruption by shear forces in areas of rapid blood flow. The result may be the microangiopathic hemolytic anemia and elevated serum lactate dehydrogenase (LDH) levels characteristic of TTP episodes.

In TTP, ischemic arterial signs and symptoms can involve any organ; however, for the diagnosis to be made, ischemia must involve the central nervous system. Clinical manifestations range from behavioral changes to sensory-motor dysfunction to coma. Renal failure and fever may or may not be present (see Table 1).

Thrombotic thrombocytopenic purpura is a clinical diagnosis. Tissues obtained from biopsy of bone marrow or gingiva may not capture the evanescent arterial thrombi and are not considered necessary (or even, in some circumstances, safe) to acquire.

TREATMENT

In about 50 to 75 percent of patients, TTP episodes can be reversed by intensive plasma manipulation. This is best done by plasma exchange (i.e., the combination of plasmapheresis and plasma infusion; 3 to 4 L per day) using normal fresh frozen platelet-poor plasma. It is presumed that platelet aggregating substances (ULvWF multimers plus some other cofactor?) are being removed by plasmapheresis and that normal plasma is providing some antiaggregating agent that is present in patient plasma in inadequate amounts (unusually large vWF "depolymerase"?).

Immediately after diagnosis, infusion of normal fresh frozen plasma at the rate of about 30 ml per kilogram per day can be initiated until plasmapheresis and plasma exchange can be arranged. (This should be within 24 to 48 hours in most circumstances.) Patients with TTP and coma, cardiac failure, or renal dysfunction should receive exchange plasmapheresis commencing immediately after diagnosis, if possible (Table 3).

Relapses in some chronic relapsing patients with TTP may respond to, or be prevented by, transfusion of normal fresh frozen plasma alone (in quantities varying from one to several units) without the need for concurrent plasmapheresis.

Some patients have recovered from TTP episodes without receiving glucocorticoids, and a few have recovered in association with glucocorticoid therapy only. The majority of reported patients who have recovered from initial TTP episodes have, however, received glucocorticoids. This is the basis for their frequent use in TTP.

In some patients, the apparent effectiveness of glucocorticoids may be related to an underlying autoimmune pathogenesis (production by the patient of endothelial cell autoantibodies in single-episode TTP; or of autoantibodies against the ULvWF "depolymerase," or against endothelial cell attachment sites for the plasma ULvWF "depolymerase," in the intermittent or chronic relapsing types of TTP?). It is probably advisable for methylprednisolone to be started immediately following diagnosis in a dosage of about 0.75 mg per kilogram IV every 12 hours, and continued until the patient recovers.

Depending on the hemoglobin level and intensity of hemolysis, red blood cell transfusions may be required. If the platelet count is very low and bleeding is a primary problem, or if intracranial bleeding is demonstrated by computed tomography (CT) or magnetic resonance imaging (MRI), then platelet transfusions are necessary. In a few patients, however, the transfusion of platelets has been temporally associated with exacerbation of the microcirculatory thrombotic process in the cerebrovascular or coronary circulation.

Plasma exchange should be continued until responding patients attain a normal neurologic status, a platelet count greater than 150,000 per microliter, a rising hemoglobin level, and a normal serum LDH value.

Table 3 Treatment of Thrombotic Thrombocytopenic Purpura

Immediate infusion of fresh frozen plasma (30 ml/kg/day)
Exchange transfusion with fresh frozen plasma (3–4 L/day) to
  commence as soon as possible
Red cell transfusions as needed
Platelet transfusions only for intracerebral (or other life-
  threatening) hemorrhage

Plasma exchange should then be done for 2 to 3 additional days in order to minimize the possibility of immediate relapse. If this occurs, the same treatment protocol should be repeated. In patients who achieve a partial response without deterioration in clinical condition, plasma exchange should be continued for a period of a few to many additional days in an effort to achieve a complete remission.

If a patient does not respond within the first 5 days of therapy, or deteriorates within the first 3 days, other forms of therapy should be tried (Table 4). Options include addition of vincristine (1.4 mg per square meter, but not exceeding 2 mg total dosage, given by intravenous push on day 1, followed by 1 mg on days 4, 7, and 10); substitution in the plasma-exchange procedures of cryosupernatant (plasma depleted of the cryoprecipitate fraction that contains the largest plasma vWF multimeric forms, as well as fibrinogen and fibronectin) for fresh frozen plasma; splenectomy (removal of cells producing vWF cofactor, or immunologic cells producing autoantibodies against endothelial cells or the ULvWF "depolymerase"?), and addition of other immunosuppressive agents (e.g., azathioprine or cyclophosphamide) to suppress autoantibody formation.

The use of aspirin and dipyridamole is controversial. Aspirin may exacerbate hemorrhagic complications in TTP patients with severe thrombocytopenia. Neither drug has been unequivocally demonstrated to be useful. The same comments pertain to intravenous prostacyclin (PGI_2), dextran, and fibrinolytic agents. Heparin in therapeutic dosages is contraindicated. Transfusions or exchange transfusions with fluids other than plasma or its cryosupernatant fraction (e.g., albumin, gammaglobulin) are almost always ineffective.

When a patient achieves remission and the plasma exchanges (or infusions) have been discontinued, the platelet count should be monitored regularly. Patients with a protracted initial episode who have not achieved a complete remission, as well as patients with the chronic relapsing form of TTP, usually relapse within a few weeks of discontinuation of therapy. In the intermittent

Table 4 Treatment of Refractory Thrombotic Thrombocytopenic Purpura

Vincristine
Cryosupernatant (plasma minus vWF-rich cyroprecipitate)
Splenectomy
Azathioprine (Imuran) or cyclophosphamide (Cytoxan)

type of TTP, the disorder may not recur for months (or, occasionally, years). Detection of ULvWF multimers in the EDTA-plasma of patients after recovery from an initial episode of TTP has proved to be a reliable indication of the propensity for recurrence.

SUGGESTED READING

Bukowski RM, Hewlett JS, Reimer RR, et al. Therapy of thrombotic thrombocytopenic purpura: An overview. Semin Thromb Hemost 1981; 7:1–8.

Byrnes JJ, Moake JL. Thrombotic thrombocytopenic purpura and the hemolytic-uremic syndrome: Evolving concepts of pathogenesis and therapy. Clin Haematol 1986; 15:413–442.

Byrnes JJ, Moake JL, Panpit K, et al. Effectiveness of the cryosupernatant fraction of plasma in the treatment of refractory thrombotic thrombocytopenic purpura. Am J Hematol 1990; 34:169–174.

del Zoppo GJ. Antiplatelet therapy in thrombotic thrombocytopenic purpura. Semin Hematol 1987; 24:130–139.

Gordon LI, Kwaan HC, Rossi EC. Deleterious effects of platelet transfusions and recovery thrombocytosis in patients with thrombotic microangiopathy. Semin Hematol 1987; 24:194–201.

Gutterman LA, Stevenson TD. Treatment of thrombotic thrombocytopenic purpura with vincristine. JAMA 1982; 247:1433–1436.

Moake JL, Rudy CK, Troll JH, et al. Therapy of chronic relapsing thrombotic thrombocytopenic purpura with prednisone and azathioprine. Am J Hematol 1985; 20:73–79.

Moake JL, McPherson PD. Abnormalities of von Willebrand factor multimers in thrombotic thrombocytopenic purpura and the hemolytic-uremic syndrome. Am J Med 1989; 87:3-9N–3-15N.

Rosove MH, Ho WG, Goldfinger D. Ineffectiveness of aspirin and dipyridamole in the treatment of thrombotic thrombocytopenic purpura. Ann Intern Med 1982; 96:27–33.

Shepard KV, Bukowski RM. The treatment of thrombotic thrombocytopenic purpura with exchange transfusions, plasma infusions, and plasma exchange. Semin Hematol 1987; 24:178–193.

IMMEDIATE AND DELAYED ADVERSE REACTIONS TO TRANSFUSIONS

J. A. MCBRIDE, M.D., F.R.C.P.(Edin), FRCPC, F.R.C.P.
PAMELA A. O'HOSKI, A.R.T.

Blood transfusion in the 1990s is still a relatively safe procedure despite valid concerns about the transmission of disease. Nevertheless, in a small number of patients who receive transfusion, complications do occur. Although these complications are generally not serious, they are uncomfortable for the patient. In rare cases, these reactions can be serious and have a morbidity of their own and may even lead to the death of the patient. Serious life-threatening reactions to transfusion are discussed first and less serious but more common reactions later. Finally, the possible consequences of contamination of blood products are also discussed.

LIFE-THREATENING TRANSFUSION REACTIONS

Immediate Immune Hemolysis

Red cell lysis occurs when potent antibodies that are invariably present in the patient's serum react with transfused red cells. Severe hemolysis may be seen after as little as 50 to 100 ml of incompatible red cells have been transfused. For this reason, it is wise to run the first portion of blood into a patient slowly. The patient should be closely monitored during this time. Hemolysis is usually immediate and occurs both intravascularly and extravascularly. The patient frequently complains of pain at the site of injection of the blood, severe crushing chest pain, and pain in the lumbar region that occasionally radiates into the limbs. Fever and chills are common. Tachycardia occurs, and severe shock with hypotension and circulatory failure may develop. Occasionally, the patient develops a hemorrhagic state.

Patients who receive incompatible transfusion while under general anesthesia may not show any of these signs, and indeed, a generalized bleeding tendency may be the first and only sign of a transfusion reaction.

Management

1. Stop the transfusion but maintain an intravenous access with normal saline to ensure a urine flow of at least 100 ml/hr.
2. Recheck the identity of the blood and the identity of the patient.
3. Obtain post-transfusion recipient blood samples from the arm opposite the site of transfusion.

Both a serum and an ethylenediaminetetraacetic acid (EDTA) sample are required.
4. Ensure the return of the appropriate samples and the suspect blood unit, together with its giving set and filter, to the Blood Bank.
5. Collect the first sample of urine passed by the patient after the incident.
6. Maintain an accurate record of fluid intake and urinary output.

When a major transfusion reaction is suspected, the Blood Bank must be informed immediately. A major ABO-incompatible transfusion reaction is almost always the result of a clerical error or the misidentification of a patient or a unit of blood for transfusion. Under these circumstances, there is always the possibility of a second error, and every attempt should be made to detect this error and prevent a second transfusion reaction in another patient.

A very uncommon cause of an immediate transfusion reaction is interdonor incompatibility. This is when a unit of blood, the plasma of which contains an antibody, is given to a patient who either possesses the antigen on his own cells, or has previously been transfused a unit of antigen-positive blood. The antibody involved is usually within the Kell blood group system, and the reaction is less severe than an ABO mismatch.

Treatment

After the immediate acute phase of hemolysis, the patient usually develops hemoglobinuria that may be transient, and jaundice develops in about 6 to 12 hours. The jaundice is usually mild but may persist for several days. Treatment of this phase of a transfusion reaction is the same as the treatment for shock. The patient's blood volume and urinary output must be maintained, and this can be done by the administration of normal saline. Diuresis can be encouraged by the use of a diuretic such as furosemide or ethacrynic acid. The aim is to maintain a urinary output of about 100 ml per hour. Mannitol-induced diuresis has been described in much of the older transfusion literature, but there is little experimental evidence to support its use. Vasopressive drugs that restrict blood flow through the kidneys should not be used. If the patient develops a generalized hemorrhagic tendency, treatment consists of replacement of the coagulation factors by cryoprecipitate or fresh-frozen plasma. Thrombocytopenia can be corrected by the use of platelet concentrates. In the event that a patient requires further transfusion of red cells, he or she should be transfused with group O cells and if necessary given group AB plasma. Oliguria and rising creatinine and urea levels are the first signs of renal failure, and the clinical picture soon becomes that of acute tubular necrosis. The mortality from acute hemolytic transfusion reaction is estimated to be between 10 and 25 percent.

Anaphylactic Reactions to Blood

Approximately 1 in 500 of the population is totally deficient in IgA protein. Such patients recognize all subgroups of IgA as foreign, and can, when stimulated, produce complement-binding IgG class–specific antibodies. When patients who are IgA deficient have become sensitized, either by previous transfusion or by pregnancy, they can have an anaphylactic reaction to plasma products. Traditionally, the transfusion reaction has been fast and starts almost immediately on beginning the transfusion. Plasma or a plasma product is the usual culprit. Red cell concentrates do contain enough plasma to provoke anaphylaxis. Gamma globulin or Rhesus immunoglobulin, if given intravenously, can also provoke this severe reaction. If a patient has had such a reaction in the past and requires further transfusion, IgA can be removed either by washing donor red cells or by the use of frozen red cells that are washed during processing. If IgA-deficient donors of the appropriate group are available, plasma from such donors may be used with considerable safety. Perhaps the best method for avoiding such a serious side effect, if there is time, is the use of autologous blood for transfusion.

Infected Blood Product

The transfusion of a blood product contaminated by live bacteria or bacterial toxin fortunately is extremely uncommon. The annual incidence of positive bacterial cultures in red cells or in platelets, as recently tested by the Canadian Red Cross over a 10-year period from 1980 to 1989, has been reviewed. Approximately 31 percent of red cell products and 42 percent of platelet products were found to be positive on microbiologic culture. These figures are not thought to be significantly different from those obtained in other large transfusion organizations.

Despite these data, the number of clinically significant episodes of bacterial sepsis reported is very low. Most bacteria do not grow in the cold, but recently bacteremia caused by *Yersinia enterocolitica* has been described in seven patients who had received a transfusion of packed red cells that had been stored at 4° C for up to 42 days. This has led to some concern by regulatory authorities who are reconsidering the recommended storage shelf life of red cells. The modern tendency to store platelets at room temperature at least increases the possibility for bacterial growth. Small amounts of infected blood products, for example, the volume of a platelet transfusion, can result in immediate, severe shock and peripheral circulatory failure, and the rapid death of the patient. The organisms responsible are usually Gram negative and may be organisms that in other circumstances are not usually regarded as pathogenic (e.g., *Serratia marcesens*). The most commonly isolated organisms from platelet concentrates are *Staphylococcus epidermidis*, the diptheroids, and *Staphylococcus aureus*. The diagnosis is suggested by the clinical picture of shock, peripheral failure, high fevers and rigors, hypotension, tachycardia, and frequently vomiting. As in all transfusion reactions, the patient may complain of pain in the arm or in the general area of the vein in which the blood product is being infused. Treatment, which is frequently unsuccessful, consists of aggressive measures to combat shock—the use of plasma volume expanders, steroids, pressor agents, and broad-spectrum antibiotics. It is important that when this complication is suspected, blood samples be taken from the patient for cultures. The blood product bag and any closed segments on the bag should be returned to the Blood Bank for microbiologic culture. It is necessary to inform the supplier of this blood product immediately, because other blood products derived from the same donor unit may be similarly contaminated.

Some plasma products that are thawed in a water bath may become contaminated either through microscopic flaws in the plastic of the bag or by droplet infection at the time of entry for infusion. It is also important when these plasma products are thawed that the temperature during thawing be strictly controlled. The transfusion of overheated blood products that contain coagulated proteins may activate complement, which can produce a pulmonary hypersensitivity transfusion reaction.

LESS SERIOUS TRANSFUSION REACTIONS

Delayed Hemolytic Transfusion Reactions

Delayed hemolytic transfusion reaction is much milder than the direct reaction described above and occurs from 2 to 14 days after the administration of blood that appears to be cross-match compatible. Following transfusion, the patient is immunized either by an antigen present on the transfused cells to which he or she has never been exposed, or there is a secondary immune response with the renewed production of a previously stimulated antibody. Symptoms are usually mild; the only manifestation of a delayed transfusion reaction may be unexpected failure to maintain the patient's hemoglobin value after transfusion or the development of mild jaundice. There is no real treatment. The incidence of delayed transfusion reaction has been the subject of much controversy, but a recent prospective study of over 2,700 patients in Hamilton, Ontario, Canada showed that a delayed hemolytic reaction occurred in 1.5 percent of patients. The major challenge to the physician is the prevention of further delayed transfusion reactions if the patient requires repeated blood transfusions. Prevention depends on the use of accurate records kept by the Blood Bank, in the physician's office, or by the patient. The knowledge that an antibody had at one time been detected in the patient's serum allows the infusion of red cells negative for that particular antigen in the future if transfusion is required. About 15 to 20 percent of patients are good antibody formers and tend to produce multiple antibodies following transfusion. Patients who develop multiple antibodies and still require transfusion are a difficult ongoing clinical problem. The Blood Bank should be informed as far in advance of an intended transfusion as possible in order to allow for extensive search either by computer or by manual screening for suitable antigen-negative, cross-matched compatible red cells. If widespread screening is unsuccessful, suitable blood might be found among the patient's immediate blood relatives. If the patient's clinical condition improves to the point that transfusion is no longer required, he or she should be encouraged to donate red cells to be frozen in the Rare Donor Bank. If the patient requires elective surgery, autologous transfusion should be considered.

Apparent delayed transfusion reactions have been seen following the passive infusion of antibody contained in intravenous immune globulin, immune serum globulin, and preparations of antitetanus immune antiglobulin.

Febrile Reactions Following Transfusion of Blood Product

Febrile reactions are common in patients receiving multiple transfusions. In general terms, the frequency and severity of febrile reactions become greater as the number of transfusions increases. This type of reaction is probably attributable to the development in the patient's plasma of antibodies directed against human leukocyte antigens (HLA) carried on leukocytes. These antibodies react in turn with leukocytes in the transfused blood. Fever occurs toward the end of the transfusion. The patient's temperature characteristically falls once the transfusion has stopped. It is necessary to stop the transfusion and initiate a transfusion reaction investigation (Table 1). Characteristically, the patient's temperature falls once the transfusion has stopped. The reason for stopping the transfusion is that an initial febrile reaction may conceal a more serious transfusion reaction. In patients who are in a chronic transfusion program and experience febrile reactions, it is often advisable to transfuse leukocyte-poor blood. This may be accomplished by centrifugation of the blood and removal of the identifiable buffy coat, or by the use of 40 micron millipore filters that will remove about 95 percent of the leucocytes present, or by a fiber-filled filter that can remove more than 99 percent of the white cells present. Similar filters have been developed for the removal of white cells from platelet concentrates.

Allergic Reactions

Allergic reactions to blood products are relatively common. They usually consist of hives or a wheal and flare reaction. This may occur at any time during the course of the transfusion. It is not usually necessary to stop the transfusion when the allergic reaction is mild, but the person performing the transfusion must be aware that the earliest sign of an anti-IgA potentially anaphylactic reaction is the appearance of a red

Table 1 Laboratory Tests Performed at Time of Suspected Hemolytic Transfusion Reaction

1. Find the pretransfusion sample, and compare the patient identification data with the post-transfusion sample
2. Spin and check blood for visual evidence of hemolysis (pretransfusion sample acts as a control)
3. Repeat the ABO group, the Rhesus type, and perform a direct antiglobulin test on pre- and post-transfusion samples side by side
4. Repeat the cross-match and antibody screen on both samples
5. In the event that all of these investigations prove negative, consider retesting the donor bag for ABO, Rhesus type, and perform an antibody screen on the plasma

rash on the skin. Edema of the face and the larynx is uncommon, but laryngeal edema is an important potential complication of any allergic reaction. The transfusion should be slowed, and an antihistamine drug such as diphenhydramine (Benadryl or Clortripolon) given. Alternatively, the patient may be given hydrocortisone intravenously. This usually brings the reaction under control, the patient becomes much more comfortable, and the transfusion can continue. Premedication with these same drugs should precede future transfusions.

Noncardiogenic Pulmonary Edema Syndrome

This increasingly recognized complication is an example of transfusion-associated adult respiratory distress syndrome. This syndrome is also known as transfusion-related acute lung injury (TRALI). The patient usually develops chills and fever within a relatively short time after transfusion starts. The temperature may be persistently raised for up to about 48 hours, and changes of so-called allergic pneumonitis appear on x-ray films within a few hours after the transfusion. Clinical examination of the chest may be negative or may reveal diffuse, fine, basal crepitations. This syndrome is probably caused by an HLA antibody present in the donor plasma. Even when traditional packed cells are used, the packed cell preparation contains up to 80 ml of plasma, which is sufficient to produce this syndrome. The syndrome is usually self-limiting, and all the changes generally clear within 72 hours. Treatment should be expectant, with strict control of transfusion requirements and fluid balance and the vigorous use of diuretics. Steroids may be helpful if the dyspnea and cyanosis are persistent or severe. In the most severe cases, treatment with a respirator may be necessary. Multiparous women have been identified as the donors of the blood that produces these reactions. Implicated donors should be removed from the donor registry.

Pulmonary overload also can occur when patients who are chronically anemic are transfused too rapidly and are given too much volume. The first step is to recognize that the patient has an expanded blood volume and has pulmonary edema. Treatment entails the production of a forced diuresis and strict control of fluid balance. Patients who have an expanded blood volume should be transfused very slowly with well-packed red cells.

Graft-Versus-Host Reaction

This disease was probably originally described as postoperative erythroderma (POE) in patients who were tranfused fresh blood following heart surgery in Japan. It is now recognized to be acute graft-versus-host disease. Graft-versus-host disease occurs following the transfusion of blood products that contain immunologically competent lymphocytes. Patient groups at risk include neonates, persons with congenital immune deficiencies, recipients of both allogeneic and autologous marrow transplants, and patients recovering from intensive chemotherapy or radiotherapy. There is also some controversy about the danger of exposing patients with untreated Hodgkin's disease to graft-versus-host disease associated with transfusion. At the time of this writing, no case of graft-versus-host disease has been attributed to transfusion in a patient with acquired immunodeficiency syndrome (AIDS).

Irradiation of blood and blood products destroys the ability of lymphocytes to produce this complication. The American Association of Blood Banks has recommended that blood from closely related, directed donors should be irradiated to prevent this syndrome. The dose of radiation required is not clear, but most authorities in the literature suggest that between 2,500 to 5,000 cGy is required.

Delayed Post-Transfusion Purpura

Delayed post-transfusion purpura is a rare syndrome that occurs in multiparous women 5 to 7 days after a blood transfusion. Characteristically, the patient develops a profound thrombocytopenia that may persist for 4 to 6 weeks. Patients generally respond to plasma exchange and may respond to administration of intravenous gamma globulin. The syndrome is caused by the existence of an alloantibody in the serum of a recipient previously immunized to a platelet antigen (usually anti-Pl^{a1}). If patients who develop this syndrome require future transfusion, it may be prudent to consider the use of washed red cells to remove contaminating platelets.

Citrate Toxicity

Patients may develop citrate toxicity as a result of ultramassive transfusions of blood or plasma during prolonged surgical procedures or following trauma.

The monitoring of ionized calcium seems to be the optimal although impractical way to manage this complication. Replacement of ionized calcium can be accomplished by the administration of calcium chloride or calcium gluconate.

Mild tetany is not uncommon during rapid plasma exchange, as for example during therapeutic plasmapheresis. Management is to slow the infusion rate. Calcium replacement is seldom necessary in these circumstances.

Situations That May Mimic Transfusion Reactions

Occasionally the transfusionist is asked to see a patient who appears to be having a transfusion reaction. This is particularly prone to occur when an underlying event takes place at the same time that the patient is receiving a transfusion for another reason.

1. Such reactions are seen in patients with glucose-6-phosphate dehydrogenase deficiency who have been exposed to an oxidant drug at the same time as they are receiving red blood cells for another reason. In this case it is the patient's own cells that are being lysed, not the transfused cells.
2. Blood that has been handled poorly, e.g., damaged in an inappropriate condition of storage, may lyse rapidly when transfused into a patient. This produces hemoglobinemia and hemoglobinuria, which may resemble a transfusion reaction.
3. After transurethral resection of the prostate, bladder lavage is occasionally carried out with sterile, distilled water. Some of the perfusate finds its way into the venous system and may cause significant intravascular hemolysis and hyponatremia. This is less of a hazard now that most surgeons use a glycine solution or normal saline for this purpose.
4. *Clostridium welchii* septicemia, for example following gallbladder surgery, can produce fulminant intravascular hemolysis that may be mistaken for a transfusion reaction if the patient has received a transfusion in the course of the surgery.
5. Almost any cause of intravascular hemolysis, however rare (e.g., paroxysmal nocturnal hemoglobinuria), may superficially appear to be a transfusion reaction when, in fact, the patient's own cells are being lysed.
6. The use of intravenous dimethylsulfoxide has been associated with a reaction that mimics a severe direct transfusion reaction.

TRANSMISSION OF DISEASE

Any blood transfusion carries with it a risk, although a small one, of transmitting disease. Two diseases, syphilis and hepatitis B, are routinely tested for. The transmission of syphilis and hepatitis B by blood transfusion is now a rarity. However, transmission of non-A, non-B hepatitis continues unabated. The causative virus has recently been identified, and the disease is now called hepatitis C. Routine screening for hepatitis C in donors is underway at most major blood centers. The current form of testing is thought to identify approximately 85 percent of carriers, but the impact of testing on the incidence of non-A, non-B hepatitis cannot yet be assessed. It may be necessary to continue the already existing surrogate testing to identify donors who have other forms of viral hepatitis. Delta-agent hepatitis continues to be a small but troublesome problem.

Much has been said about the transmission of the human immunodeficiency virus and its relationship to transfusion. It is now quite clear that in donors who have been exposed to this virus, antibodies can be tested for, and confirmation of the exposure by the use of a Western blot technique should eliminate the majority of potentially infected donors. Other retroviruses, such as human T-cell leukemia virus type 1 (HTLV-1), can also be transmitted by transfusion. The antibody to this virus will soon be routinely tested for by transfusion services. The donor who has recently been exposed to either virus and who has not yet formed antibodies will continue to be a hazard.

Infectious mononucleosis and cytomegalovirus can be transmitted by blood transfusion; however, the risk of transmission of the latter is thought to be reduced by the elimination of donor lymphocytes by the use of a suitable filter.

Transmission of malaria by blood transfusion is well documented. There have been reports of transmission of other protozoal infections in temperate climates by the transfusion of blood from donors who are either suffering from a protozoal disease or who are chronic carriers of it.

Chagas disease (*Trypanosoma cruzi*) has occurred following the transfusion of blood from South American donors. Babesiosis (*Babesia microti*), which is endemic in some North Eastern and Central states, has been transmitted to at least seven patients by blood transfusion. Indeed, the screening of donors for Babesia antibodies has been considered in the states where the parasite is endemic because the range of its vectors appears to be increasing.

The culture of *Borrelia burgdorferi* and the demonstration that the parasite can persist in blood stored under transfusion conditions, makes it likely that Lyme disease will be the next disease associated with transfusion. These diseases, although uncommon, must be considered in any patient who has a persistent fever following transfusion.

The recent war in the Persian Gulf may lead to the exclusion of a significant number of otherwise healthy blood donors. This is because many of the diseases endemic in the Persian Gulf are capable of being transmitted by transfusion. These diseases include malaria (*Plasmodium vivax* and *Plasmodium falciparum*), Congo-Crimean hemorrhagic fever, hepatitis A and B, and Leishmaniasis. The major blood collecting agencies are preparing guidelines for screening such donors.

SUGGESTED READING

Aber RC. Transfusion-associated *Yersinia* enterocolitica. Transfusion 1990; 30:193–195.

Anderson KC, Weinstein HJ. Transfusion-associated graft-versus-host disease. N Engl J Med 1990; 323:315–321.

Cohen ND, Munoz A, Reitz BA, et al. Transmission of retroviruses by transfusion of screened blood in patients undergoing cardiac surgery. N Engl J Med 1989; 320:1172–1176.

deGraan-Hentzen YCE, Gratama JW, Mudde GC, et al. Prevention of primary cytomegalovirus infection in patients with hematologic malignancies by intensive white cell depletion of blood products. Transfusion 1989; 29:757–760.

Dzik WH, Kirkley SA. Citrate toxicity during massive blood transfusion. Transfusion Med Rev 1988; 2:76–94.

Gasser RA, Magill AJ, Oster CN, Tramont EC. The threat of infectious disease in Americans returning from Operation Desert Storm. N Engl J Med 1991; 324:859–864.

Goldman M, Blajchman MA. Blood product-associated bacterial sepsis. Transfusion Med Rev 1991; 5:73–83.

Grant IH, Gold JWM, Wittner M, et al. Transfusion-associated acute Chagas' disease acquired in the United States. Ann Intern Med 1989; 111:849–851.

Heddle NM, O'Hoski PL, McBride JA, et al. A prospective study to determine the frequency and clinical significance of delayed transfusion reactions. (Unpublished data)

Issitt PD. Transfusion reactions. In: Issitt PD, ed. Applied blood group serology. 3rd ed. Miami: Montgomery Scientific, 1985:498.

Laschinger CA, Naylor DG. Anti-IgA antibodies and transfusion reactions in Canada. Can Med Assoc J 1983; 1281:381–382.

Leitman SF, Holland PV. Irradiation of blood products. Transfusion 1985; 25:293.

Levy GJ, Shabot MM, Hart ME, et al. Transfusion-associated noncardiogenic pulmonary edema. Transfusion 1986; 26:278–281.

Nickerson P, Orr P, Schroeder ML. Transfusion-associated *Trypanosoma cruzi* infection in a non-endemic area. Ann Intern Med 1989; 111:851–853.

Popovsky MA. Transfusion-transmitted babesiosis. Transfusion 1991; 31:296–297.

Popovsky MA. Immune mediated transfusion reactions. In: Nance SF, ed. Immune destruction of red blood cells. Arlington, VA: American Association of Blood Banks, 1989.

Yersinia enterocolitica bacteremia and endotoxin shock associated with red blood cell transfusion—United States, 1987–1988. MMWR 1988; 37:577–578.

Zuck TF, Sherwood WC, Bove JR. A review of recent events related to surrogate testing of blood to prevent non-A, non-B post-transfusion hepatitis. Transfusion 1987; 27:203–206.

PLASMA EXCHANGE AND INTRAVENOUS IMMUNE GLOBULIN

GAIL ROCK, Ph.D., M.D.

The concept of therapeutic benefit from removal of blood with release of various "humors" originated in the Renaissance period and has now become the basis for the modern medical discipline of plasma exchange. In 1909, Fleig first reported on the benefits of selective removal of plasma; then in 1913 and 1914, Able described plasmapheresis as "a method by which the blood . . . may be submitted to dialysis outside the body, and again returned to the natural circulation." One of the papers concludes that "it appears probable . . . that a considerably greater prolongation of life by this method will be obtained in future experiments, when the limits of the procedure and the details of the most advantageous technique have been developed." Today, we are well on our way to an understanding of the limits of these procedures and an understanding of some of the disorders in which plasma removal can be of benefit; however, there is, as yet, very little detail determining the most advantageous technique for plasma removal.

For more than three decades, it has been accepted that removal of plasma (plasmapheresis) is of benefit to patients with Waldenström's macroglobulinemia and manifestations of hyperviscosity. Manual plasmapheresis with collection of whole blood, ex vivo separation of the cells from the plasma, and return of the cells to the patient with disposal of the plasma became routine therapy in this disorder. Subsequently, it was recognized that other diseases might benefit from plasma removal; however, the relatively large amounts of plasma that must be removed to effect benefit in the majority of cases greatly limited clinical application of plasmapheresis. The subsequent development of highly automated machines that permit online separation of blood components and selective removal of any of the blood fractions made it possible to apply plasma removal clinically on a wide basis.

These automated cell separators separate blood components through centrifugation, filtration, or a combination of both principles to remove selectively any one of the blood components and return the other components to the patient or donor. The cell separator was originally developed in order to collect large numbers of granulocytes for transfusion to septic patients; however, it was quickly realized that the ability to obtain good separation of the various components would permit collection of large numbers of platelets or plasma, and these applications now account for the majority of the apheresis procedures.

The general term *apheresis* is used to describe the group of procedures in which one or several of the various blood components are selectively removed. Plasmapheresis involves the removal of plasma in volumes generally not exceeding 5 to 600 ml. Replacement fluid is usually not given. Plasma exchange, on the other hand, involves removal of large volumes of plasma (normally 3 to 5 L or between 1 to 1.5 plasma volumes) and replacement of the plasma with crystalloids, colloids, or plasma. Therapeutic plateletpheresis procedures are used to remove platelets in disorders such as thrombocythemia. Similarly, granulocytes may be removed for therapeutic reasons when the elevated white cell count causes problems related to viscosity and blood flow. Granulocytes are also removed in patients with acute myelogenous leukemia (AML) of the M3 variety, in which the large numbers of promyelocytes contribute to disseminated intravascular coagulation (DIC).

The rationale for the use of plasma exchange is the removal of an abnormal plasma constituent or the replacement of a deficient, normal plasma constituent, as summarized in Table 1. In many cases, the proposed mechanism of action has not been established as truly causative but rather is implied from what is currently known about the disease. Depending on the nature of the toxic compound and its distribution in the body (i.e., if there is tissue distribution), one calculates the plasma volume to be removed.

CURRENT ACTIVITIES IN THERAPEUTIC PLASMA EXCHANGE

Several countries have organized national registries in order to determine the activity in plasma exchange and to help plan randomized prospective clinical trials to resolve the many unanswered questions regarding appropriate application. At the present time (1990), Canada and France appear to have the most comprehensive reporting system. Efforts are being made by the American Society for Apheresis (ASFA) and the European Society for Haemapheresis (ESH) to gather similar information. Since the Canadian Apheresis Study Group was founded in 1980, it has established and maintained records on the majority of exchange procedures carried out in Canada; these records probably represent the most comprehensive basis on which to assess the field of apheresis at the present time.

In 1989, with a population of approximately 25

Table 1 Possible Mechanisms of Action of Therapeutic Plasma Exchange

Mechanism of Action	Disorder
Removal of autoantibody	Myasthenia gravis
Removal of alloantibody	Rh alloimmunization in pregnancy
Removal of immune complexes	Systemic lupus erythematosus
Removal of monoclonal protein	Hyperviscosity syndrome
Removal of toxin	Mushroom poisoning
Replenishment of specific plasma factor	Thrombotic thrombocytopenic purpura
Placebo effect	Rheumatoid arthritis

million people in Canada, 5,793 plasma-exchange procedures were carried out (Fig. 1) on 706 patients who were treated an average of 8.2 times each. The diseases for which plasma exchange was carried out are shown in Table 2. By broadly classifying diseases as neurologic, hematologic, collagen-vascular, and nephrologic, it is apparent that most of the procedures were carried out for neurologic disorders (Fig. 2). This current emphasis on the treatment of neurologic disorders is seen in most other countries. Of the neurologic disorders, which represent 51 percent of the total procedures in Canada, the majority were for acute Guillain-Barré syndrome, followed by chronic Guillain-Barré syndrome and myasthenia gravis (Fig. 3).

PE IN CANADA

TOTAL PROCEDURES

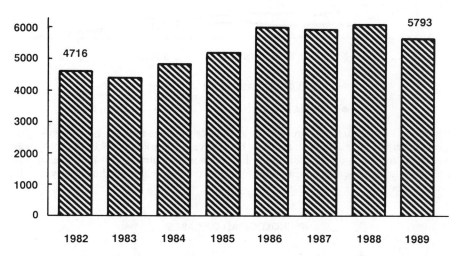

Figure 1 Total number of plasma-exchange procedures performed in Canada. The CASG has reports on the majority of plasma-exchange procedures carried out in Canada since 1982. As shown, the number of procedures increased from 4,716 in 1982, leveled off at slightly over 6,000 per year between 1986 and 1988, and then decreased to 5,793 in 1989.

Table 2 Diseases Treated by Plasma Exchange*

ABO incompatible bone marrow	Lupus
Agranulocytosis	Macroglobulinemia
Alveolar hemorrhage	Miscellaneous inhibitors
Amyloid neuropathy	Multiple sclerosis
Autoimmune hemolytic anemia	Myasthenia gravis
Behçet's syndrome	Myeloma
Biliary cirrhosis	Paraneoplastic syndrome
Breast cancer	Peripheral neuropathy
Convulsions	Polycythemia
Cryoglobulinemia	Polymyasitis
Dermatitis herpetiform	Primary biliary stenosis
Dermatomyositis	Raynaud's disease
Eton-Lambert syndrome	Red cell aplasia
Fabry's disease	Renal calculi
Factro VIII antibodies	Rh disease
Glomerulonephritis	Rheumatoid arthritis
Goodpasture's syndrome	Scleroderma
Grave's disease	Severe exopthalmos
Guillain-Barré syndrome	Sjögren's syndrome
Hemolytic-uremic syndrome	Systemic lupus erythematosus
Henoch-Schönlein	Thrombocythemia
Hypercholesterolemia	Thombotic thrombocytopenic purpura
Hyperviscosity	Transplant rejection
Immune thrombocytopenic purpura	Unspecified nephritis
Leukemia	Vasculitis
Light-chain disease	

*Other diseases have also been treated by plasma exchange; however, this list represents the most common applications.

PE PROCEDURES BY DISEASE CATEGORIES

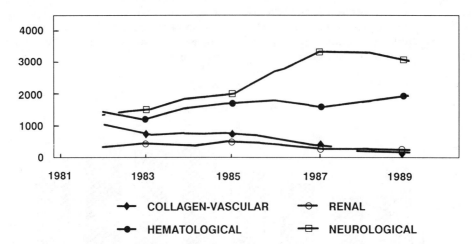

Figure 2 Plasma-exchange procedures in Canada organized by disease category. The level of activity in neurologic diseases has increased markedly since 1982, whereas treatment for hematologic indications has remained relatively constant. Renal and collagen-vascular diseases now account for approximately 500 procedures per year.

NEUROLOGICAL DISEASES*

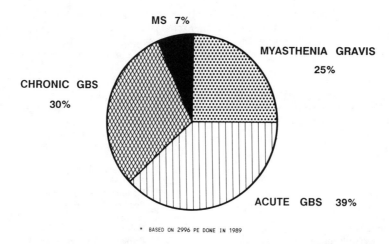

Figure 3 Plasma-exchange procedures done in Canada for neurologic diseases: (based on 2,996 plasma-exchange procedures done in 1989). Treatment of Guillain-Barré syndrome (GBS) by plasma-exchange accounted for almost 60 percent of the total procedures performed within the neurology category.

In 1989, hematologic disorders accounted for 1,922 procedures, collagen-vascular for 200, and renal for 244. This distribution of activity has changed considerably since 1984 (see Fig. 2) and likely represents results from randomized prospective clinical trials that showed considerable advantage to plasma exchange in acute Guillain-Barré syndrome and little benefit in rheumatoid arthritis.

EQUIPMENT

Plasma exchange generally utilizes a two-arm technique in which the blood is removed from the patient via a needle in one arm and returned to the other; this procedure is considerably faster than those involving a single-needle procedure. A variety of centrifugation devices are available, and although all operate on the same basic principle of separation of blood components via centrifugation, there are relative differences in the devices that allow for varying levels of cross-cellular contamination in the plasma or removal of platelets with varying number of white cells. Because white cell contamination affects both platelet storage and immunization, current trends are toward use of the most leukocyte poor platelet preparations.

Membrane devices operate using either hollow fiber filtration or flat sheet filtration to separate plasma and plasma proteins from the cells. Complement activation has been a concern in the development and operation of some of the membrane devices. With today's improved technology, however, this is not a problem in most procedures.

REPLACEMENT FLUID

In the early days of plasma exchange, replacement was often carried out using fresh frozen plasma. Because of the advent of acquired immunodeficiency syndrome (AIDS), a switch to albumin or crystalloids was made, and in most centers, fresh frozen plasma is currently used only for the treatment of thrombotic thrombocytopenic purpura (TTP).

There has been considerable debate about the effects of removing large volumes of plasma on hemostasis. Although many of the proteins do decrease in concentration, the effect has been transient and generally not found to be problematic.

Similarly, many investigators have concern for the problem of citrate toxicity due to the anticoagulant used to collect the blood. Supplementation with calcium gluconate is routine in some centers and never carried out in others.

Interesting progress has been made in several immunologic diseases in which efforts have been directed to immune suppression by the use of intravenous IgG in conjunction with plasma exchange. It appears that the presence of an anti-idiotype antibody in the intravenous IgG may have an immunosuppressive effect. Thus, intravenous IgG has been used with plasma exchange in the treatment of Rh disease, idiopathic thrombocytopenic purpura, and refractory TTP, in which benefit has been reported in several cases.

CURRENT STATUS

Randomized prospective clinical trials have shown the benefit of plasma exchange in TTP, multiple sclerosis, and acute Guillain-Barré syndrome. An international trial of plasma exchange and cyclophosphamide for the treatment of systemic lupus erythematosus has just begun and should help to assess effect in that disorder. Historically, a great deal of anecdotal evidence exists to show benefit in myasthenia gravis (particularly in respirator-dependent patients) and in Goodpasture's syndrome such that it is likely impossible to carry out

prospective randomized trials in these disorders. Plasma exchange is also generally considered as appropriate therapy in patients with severe Rh disease, in which small-volume plasma exchange on a biweekly schedule has been seen to be of benefit in reducing antibody titer.

SELECTIVE ABSORPTION OF PLASMA CONSTITUENTS

A natural progression in the application of therapeutic plasma exchange has been the selective removal of toxic materials from plasma and the subsequent return of the patient's own depleted plasma. This is accomplished by a variety of methods, including plasma filtration, with exclusion of macromolecules such as cryoglobulins by using an appropriate pore size on the filter, and immunoabsorption, with affinity column removal of selected antigens. The latter approach has been used with great success in the treatment of hypercholesterolemia. Homozygous patients have undergone repeat plasma perfusion over columns containing monoclonal antibody to low-density lipoproteins (LDLs), with subsequent decrease in the level of LDLs, increase in high-density lipoproteins (HDLs), and resolution, in some reports, of atheromatous plaques. Although very encouraging, the labor-intensive nature of this approach and the relatively few homozygous patients have limited application. However, should benefit be found in the heterozygous population, widespread use may occur. Such studies are currently underway in Germany and in the United States.

The selective removal of antibody or immune complexes by the use of staphylococcal A columns has similarly intrigued investigators. Early reports indicated that there was reduction in size or complete resolution of some solid tumors following plasma perfusion over the columns. Subsequently, removal of IgG and immune complexes from plasma has been found to benefit patients with thrombocytopenia and AIDS, with removal of antiplatelet antibodies corresponding to an increase in platelet count. Staphylococcal A columns have also been successfully used to remove IgG from hemophiliacs with factor VIII inhibitors.

The costs of these staphylococcal A columns and the fact that, to date, many of the mechanisms involved in their use are not well understood, have limited their use. However, as more is learned and the columns become reusable and, therefore, less expensive, more widespread use will undoubtedly ensue.

REACTIONS TO PLASMA EXCHANGE

Although the majority of procedures are carried out without any difficulty, side effects to plasma exchange do occur. In 1989, the CASG reported on 5,235 plasma exchange procedures in which reactions occurred 612 times. These were classed as mild (72 percent; transient in nature, responded quickly to simple measures, with little or no clinical significance), moderate (24 percent; caused considerable discomfort to the patient, who did not respond quickly to treatment but, in general, didn't require termination of the procedure), and severe (4 percent; patient clinically unstable and required vigorous resuscitative measures; these reactions usually required termination of the procedure).

Similar data have been reported from the French National Registry. Plasma exchange has been associated with death in most countries; therefore, it cannot be considered an innocuous procedure. Careful attention to fluid balance and to citrate reactions is a necessity, as is a thorough understanding of the pathophysiology of the underlying disease that is being treated in order to avoid the various problems that can arise.

SUGGESTED READING

McKhann GM, et al. Role of therapeutic plasmapheresis in the acute Guillain-Barré syndrome. J Neuroimmunol 1988; 20(2–3):297–300.

Pineda AA. Selective extraction of plasma constituents [editorial]. Transfusion 1989; 29(4):283–284.

Rock G, ed. Apheresis. Proceedings of the 2nd Congress of the World Apheresis Association. New York: Alan R. Liss Publishing, 1990.

Shumak KH, Rock GA. Therapeutic plasma exchange. N Engl J Med 1984; 310:762.

Selective removal of plasma components to achieve immune modulation. Semin Hematol 1989; 26(2, Suppl 1):1–51.

IRON CHELATION THERAPY

GEORGE J. KONTOGHIORGHES, PH.D.
A. VICTOR HOFFBRAND, D.M., F.R.C.P., F.R.C.PATH.

Iron chelation is life saving for many thousands of patients with thalassaemia major and other severe chronic refractory anemias who require regular blood transfusions. Current therapy with subcutaneous desferrioxamine (Desferal) is limited to only a small portion of these patients worldwide because of its high cost and the difficulty of administration, which cause poor compliance. A cheap and safe orally active chelator is, therefore, needed. We review here the present status of treatment with subcutaneous desferrioxamine and with the most clinically advanced chelator 1,2-dimethyl-3-hydroxypyrid-4-one (L_1).

IRON AND CHELATION

Iron is an important trace element, and it is required by many proteins involved in metabolic pathways essential for growth and development in humans. Body iron levels are regulated by the gut through absorption; there is no regulatory mechanism for iron excretion. In transfusional iron overload, as the body iron burden increases from the multiple red cell transfusions, the concentration of the iron storage proteins, and of hemosiderin in particular, increases many fold. Transferrin iron saturation also increases, and in most patients is over 100 percent. In such situations, nontransferrin iron also may be present in plasma. All these iron pools and an intracellular low molecular weight iron pool are thought to be in equilibrium. Iron toxicity may arise mainly from the incapacity of cells to store excess iron with lysosomal rupture and also from the catalytic formation of oxygen-activated products such as lipid peroxides by low molecular weight iron.

Chelators are molecules that can use two or more of their ligands to bind to a metal. Ligands such as $-PO_3$, $-SH$, $-COOH$, $-OH$, and $-NH_2$ are naturally occurring and widely distributed in biomolecules such as proteins and lipids. Naturally occurring low molecular weight chelators such as citrate and ATP and high molecular weight chelators such as transferrin and lactoferrin bind to iron under physiologic conditions and compete with exogenous chelators. An iron chelator that reduces the iron burden and also inhibits the catalytic activity of the low molecular weight iron pool will reduce the toxicity of iron in transfusional iron overload. Effective iron removal by exogenous chelators depends on their ability to reach the iron pools, mobilize iron from the iron pools, compete effectively with naturally occurring chelators, and form an iron complex that is nontoxic and can be excreted.

IRON OVERLOAD

Each unit of blood contains 200 to 250 mg of iron, and the average daily intake of iron as hemoglobin in adult transfusion-dependent patients is approximately 25 to 30 mg. The body is unable to excrete this iron, and it accumulates stored intracellulary in the proteins haemosiderin and ferritin in the reticuloendothelial system, in parenchymal cells of the liver, in endocrine and other tissues and, most importantly, in the heart. Damage to these organs is clinically apparent following the transfusion of about 50 to 100 units of blood, but may occur much earlier, especially in children. In patients with thalassaemia major, without iron chelation therapy, death usually occurs in the second or third decade of life from cardiac arrythmia or congestive heart failure.

CHELATION WITH SUBCUTANEOUS DESFERRIOXAMINE

The mainstay of iron chelation therapy currently is desferrioxamine (DF) given by subcutaneous infusion. The drug is inactive by mouth, and it has a short plasma half-life of less than 5 minutes; slow infusion is therefore needed to maintain effective plasma levels and achieve substantial iron excretion. In practice, this is given as a 10 to 20 mL infusion by a battery-driven pump into the subcutaneous tissues of the abdomen or thighs. The amount of iron excreted in any patient varies not only with the dose of drug and length of infusion but also with the patient's iron load, vitamin C status, and state of erythropoiesis.

Iron excretion in response to DF occurs largely in the urine. The exact proportion lost by the fecal route is variable, but it has been assumed to be up to one-third that in the urine, fecal loss being proportionately increased by a high hemoglobin level (with consequent inhibited erythropoiesis) and lower body iron content. In most patients, infusions of 40 to 50 mg per kg body weight for 5 to 6 nights each week over a 10- to 12-hour period with additional intravenous DF infusion of 2 g with each unit of blood transfused are sufficient to maintain body iron stores at around 5 to 10 times normal and, in compliant patients, to prevent serious cardiomyopathy.

The mortality rate from cardiac complications of thalassaemia major before the age of 15 years in a large multicenter Italian study has been reduced from 13.8 percent in those born between 1960 and 1964 to 5 percent in those born between 1970 and 1979, coinciding with the introduction of subcutaneous DF therapy. Although other aspects of management also may have improved in these years, it is likely that the introduction of effective iron chelation therapy in 1976–1977 has made the major impact.

Side-effects

Desferrioxamine has proved a remarkably safe drug in view of the large doses that have been administered daily to many thousands of patients worldwide during the last 14 years. Nevertheless, some side-effects have emerged. These include damage to the retina (with increased pigmentation, loss of visual acuity, and night blindness), an optic neuropathy with central scotomata, auditory dysfunction (resulting particularly in high tone deafness), reduced growth in infants and children, and bone abnormalities. The exact mechanisms for these toxicities are unclear, although they seem to relate to high peak levels of DF in the face of relatively low iron stores and low serum ferritin levels. In addition, DF may exacerbate potentially fatal *Yersinia enterocolitica* infection by making iron available to this organism.

Compliance and Costs

Compliance with subcutaneous DF therapy is a major problem, especially in teenagers. A number of studies have documented increased cardiac disease and mortality in noncompliant patients. Increased use of DF can reverse cardiac damage in some of these patients. In-dwelling intravenous catheters (Port-a-Cath or Hickman) have been inserted into some patients to allow continuous chelation in the hope of reversing cardiac damage. The main problem worldwide with DF, however, is the high cost of the drug, pump, infusion needles, and tubing, which makes the drug unavailable to the majority of patients with thalassaemia major and other transfusion-dependent anemias. Many thousands of patients die annually for this reason.

ORALLY ACTIVE CHELATORS

Searching for an Oral Iron Chelator

Of the many hundreds of chelators tested in animals only few have shown potential for clinical use (Table 1). Of those tested in humans only one 1,2-dimethyl-3-hydroxypyrid-4-one (L_1) appears to be promising so far. Several other α-ketohydroxypyridines also appear to be good candidates for clinical trials on the basis of results of animal studies and will probably be tested soon in patients (see Table 1). A major consideration in the search for an oral iron chelating drug is safety because high doses will be needed long-term to maintain iron stores near normal in the face of continuing blood transfusions. Moreover, as the body iron stores decrease, the amount of iron excreted per given dose of chelator will also decrease and, as found for DF, the potential toxicity of a chelator will increase. There is, therefore, a requirement for an effective chelator with a high margin of safety during long-term administration both for patients with heavy iron loads and for near-normal iron loads.

Several other considerations have to be included in the requirements of an oral iron chelator that are not relevant to subcutaneous DF. Examples of these are (1) stability of the chelator in the acidic environment of the stomach, (2) the effect of dietary constituents on the absorption of the chelator, (3) the possibility of increasing or decreasing the absorption of iron and of other metal ions, e.g., aluminum or copper, from the gut, and (4) reabsorption of the chelator and its iron complex

Table 1 Promising Oral Iron Chelators with Clinical Potential for Replacing Subcutaneous Desferrioxamine

α-ketohydroxypyridines:
  1-(methyl-, ethyl-,2'-methoxyethyl-, 3'-ethoxypropyl- and allyl)
    2-methyl or 2-ethyl, 3-hydroxypyrid-4-one
  1,4-dihydroxy-pyrid-2-one
Phenolic ethylene diamines (e.g., HBED)
Pyridoxal isonicotinoyl hydrazones (PIH)
Desferrithiocin
Desferrioxamine derivatives and polymeric hydroxamates

Table 2 Major advantages of L₁ over Desferrioxamine

L₁	*DF*
High compliance	Low compliance
Daily and repeated oral administration	10–12 hours/day, 5 days/week subcutaneous administration
Solid/solution easy to carry	Injections/pump uncomfortable
Cheap	Expensive

Table 3 Properties of L₁ in Animals and In Vitro

Stability in acid (pH 1.0) and base (pH 12)
Iron removal from ferritin, hemosiderin, and transferrin
Inhibition of iron-containing proteins, e.g., cyclooxygenase, lipoxygenase, ribonucleotide reductase
Inhibition of free-radical formation
Inhibition of iron uptake by red cells and mobilization of iron from macrophages and hepatocytes
Increase of iron and aluminum excretion in animals when administered intragastrically or parenterally
Median lethal dose in rats is 600–700 mg/kg (intraperitoneal) and 2–3 g/kg (intragastric)
Chronic administration of 200 mg/kg has been reported to cause a decrease of the white cells in rats and mice, hyperplasia of the adrenals, increases in cholesterol level, and hypersalivation

following biliary excretion. On the other hand, compliance will not be a major problem with an oral chelator unless it is not well tolerated because it causes gastric disturbances or because a need for frequent administration separate from food interferes with the dietary habits of the patient.

Of the compounds that have undergone clinical trials 2,3-dihydroxybenzoic acid was abandoned because of ineffectiveness. Cholylhydroxamic acid was tried in humans but abandoned because of unacceptable diarrhea at therapeutic doses. Pyridoxal isonicotinoyl hydrazone (PIH) is nontoxic but not sufficiently effective to cause negative iron balance in regularly transfused patients. It is currently undergoing clinical trials in patients with thalassaemia intermedia. Related compounds such as pyridoxal benzoyl hydrazone and pyridoxal-2-pyrimidinyl-ethoxycarbonyl metholramide (PPEM) are also effective in animals but require further preclinical studies before being given to humans. Diethylenetriamine pentacetic acid (DTPA), a cheap but not orally active chelator, is effective in removing iron from patients, but because of the removal of other trace metals such as zinc cannot be widely used safely in transfusional iron overload.

The most promising group of oral iron chelators are the α-ketohydroxypyridines, which include L₁. L₁ (MW 139) forms a 3:1 chelator:iron complex at physiologic pH. It has a higher binding constant for iron (log β3 = 36) than that of DF (log β3 = 31), and L₁ is capable of removing iron not only from hemosiderin and ferritin but also from transferrin. It is very hydrophilic with a partition coefficient (K_{par}) between the lipid and aqueous phases of 0.19. This ensures low accumulation in lipids and therefore low potential toxicity to cell membranes. The median lethal single dose in rats is 600 to 700 mg/kg with an intraperitoneal injection and over 2 g/kg by intragastric administration.

The major criteria for replacing DF with L₁ or any other chelator in the treatment of transfusional iron overload are cost, effectiveness, and safety (Table 2). A new one-step synthesis of L₁ and several of its analogs from maltol and ethyl maltol will result in much lower costs of production than is the current situation with DF. With regard to effectiveness, L₁ given several times daily appears to cause sufficient iron excretion to bring heavily iron loaded patients to negative iron balance.

The first clinical trials showed that L₁ was effective at increasing excretion of iron but not of calcium, zinc, copper, or magnesium in multitransfused patients with myelodysplasia. Subsequent studies in patients with

thalassaemia major confirmed the effectiveness of L₁ and showed that doses of up to 100 mg/kg divided into two or three doses daily could lead to excretion of more than 30 mg of iron (and in some patients more than 100 mg) in 24 hours in thalassaemia major patients, thus achieving negative iron balance, and this level of excretion could be maintained for many months. In studies performed for 1 to 15 months in patients in London, Bombay, and Berne, a drop in serum ferritin has been observed in some but not all the patients. Follow-up studies with adequate doses of L₁ to maintain negative iron balance for prolonged periods in more patients are needed to confirm that L₁ can maintain iron stores in these patients as low as those that can be achieved in some patients with subcutaneous DF. The results so far in over 50 thalassaemia major patients worldwide who have taken L₁ for more than 1 year are very encouraging. The properties of L₁ in animals and in vitro are listed in Table 3.

Pharmacology of L₁

Pharmacokinetic studies in humans have indicated that L₁ is rapidly absorbed from the stomach and appears in the blood within minutes of ingestion. It is then mostly metabolized to a glucuronide. Eighty to ninety percent of L₁ is cleared from plasma within 5 to 6 hours of administration, and it is almost totally excreted in the urine within 24 hours in the form of a glucuronide but also as free drug and as an iron complex (Table 4). Fecal iron excretion does not appear to be increased by L₁. Neither is the drug–iron complex absorbed. Variations in the metabolism and rate of clearance of L₁ have been noted in the eight individuals studied so far. These differences in the pharmacokinetics and metabolism of L₁ may have implications not only for the effectiveness of the drug in increasing iron excretion but also for its toxicity. It may, therefore, be appropriate to assess the pharmacokinetic profile and metabolism of L₁ in each patient, especially those who are likely to embark on intensive and prolonged chelation therapy. A further potential advantage of L₁ and other α-ketohydroxypyridines over DF is their lack of promotion of growth of *Yersinia enterocolitica*. In contrast to the case with DF, the organism cannot use the

Table 4 Pharmacology of L_1 in Humans

Absorption through the stomach within minutes
Appearance in the blood within 5–10 minutes and entry into organs, e.g., liver
Metabolism proceeds mainly through conjugation with glucuronic acid
Excretion is almost completely in the urine, mainly as a glucuronide metabolite and to a lesser extent as an iron complex or unchanged molecule
Half-life of plasma elimination is 47–134 minutes and maximum plasma clearance of 85–90% is within 5–6 hours

---

L_1–iron complex, and L_1 inhibits rather than promotes the growth of *Yersinia*.

The major outstanding hurdle for introducing L_1 to all transfusional iron overloaded patients is the requirement for completing long-term toxicity studies in animals and more long-term clinical trials in patients at effective doses.

Adverse Effects Observed During Trials with L_1

The drug, made up in 0.5-g gelatin capsules, has been well-tolerated without gastrointestinal symptoms. Over 160 patients have received the drug for periods of a few weeks up to 24 months. No skin rashes or changes in cardiac, renal, or liver function have been noted. No neurologic effects have been observed clinically, and no changes in visual or auditory function have been detected on sensitive testing.

The following adverse effects have been observed during the trials with L_1 (Table 5). Mild joint or muscle pains developed in patients in two centers, London and Bombay. Among 13 patients treated at the Royal Free Hospital four complained of joint pains after starting L_1 therapy. In one effusions occurred, which subsided coinciding with discontinuing the drug, whereas in two, transient pains disappeared despite continuation of the drug. In the fourth patient, pain occurred from knees affected by previously symptomless osteoarthritis, but this did not require discontinuation of the drug. Among 34 patients treated in Bombay, two developed joint effusions, which subsided on stopping the drug but reappeared when therapy was restarted. In another five patients, mild joint or muscle pains occurred that subsided spontaneously and did not require discontinuation of the drug. Among patients studied by groups in Canada, Switzerland, Holland, and Italy no joint or

Table 5 Adverse Observations with L_1 in Humans

Transient joint pains and musculoskeletal pains in 11 of 150 iron-loaded patients
Increased titer of the rheumatoid factor in 2 patients
Transient L_w antibody and agranulocytosis in a Blackfan-Diamond patient
Agranulocytosis in a thalassemia major patient

---

muscle pains have been reported. Whether this is because of a difference in the patient population or a difference in the dose protocol is uncertain.

One patient with Blackfan-Diamond anemia developed a rare red cell antibody, L_w, that made cross-matching blood difficult. She was given steroid therapy and transfused Rhesus negative blood, which showed normal survival. The antibody disappeared when L_1 was stopped and did not reappear in the 6 weeks when L_1 was given again after a 3-month interval without L_1 therapy. Six weeks after restarting L_1, this same patient developed agranulocytosis and thrombocytopenia, which recovered 3 weeks after the drug was stopped. One female thalassemia major patient developed a granulocytosis lasting 7 weeks, 6 weeks after commencing L_1 104 mg per kg daily. This recovered spontaneously. No other patient has been reported to develop a fall in white cell or platelet count while receiving L_1, however, and indeed in one patient with myelodysplasia with severe pancytopenia before starting L_1, no further falls occurred in neutrophil or platelet levels during a year of receiving the drug and no infections or spontaneous bleeding developed.

SUGGESTED READING

Bartlett AN, Hoffbrand AV, Kontoghiorghes GJ. Long-term trial with the oral iron chelator 1,2-dimethyl-3-hydroxypyrid-4-one (L_1). II. Clinical observations. Br J Haematol 1990; 76:301–304.

Kontoghiorghes GJ, Bartlett AN, Hoffbrand AV, et al. Long-term trial with oral iron chelator 1,2-dimethyl-3-hydroxypyrid-4-one (L_1). I. Iron chelation and metabolic studies. Br J Haematol 1990; 76: 295–300.

Kontoghiorghes GJ, Hoffbrand AV. Prospects for effective and oral chelation in transfusional iron overload. Rec Adv Haematol 1988 5:75–98.

Modell B, Berdoukas V. The clinical approach to thalassaemia. London: Croane and Strutton, 1984.

Nathan DG Ed. Oral iron chelators. Semin Haematol 1990; 27: 83–85.

BLOOD COMPONENT THERAPY IN PLATELET DISORDERS

RICHARD S. EISENSTAEDT, M.D.

Platelet disorders are classified into those caused by thrombocytopenia (arising from either inadequate marrow production, excessive peripheral destruction, or both) and qualitative defects (where platelets, though normal in numbers, fail to function properly to prevent and control bleeding). The latter is most often caused by ingested drugs such as aspirin or by underlying diseases such as uremia or von Willebrand's disease.

Platelet disorders are optimally managed by diagnosing and treating the specific cause of the underlying quantitative or qualitative defect. However, the primary cause may be unknown, or if known, may not be amenable to specific therapy that is reliably effective. Furthermore, the patient may be acutely bleeding or otherwise emergently ill so that waiting for specific treatment to work may be hazardous. In such instances, the nonspecific transfusion of platelets or plasma components is appropriate.

RANDOM DONOR PLATELET TRANSFUSION

Platelets are most often available for transfusion as a pooled product concentrated from randomly donated units of whole blood following centrifugation procedures to limit red blood cell (RBC) contamination and reduce plasma volume. One unit of whole blood will usually yield 5 to 10×10^{10} platelets. Alternatively, 5 to 10 units from a single donor may be prepared by plateletpheresis using automated cell separators. Platelets are stored in vitro for up to 5 days at 20 to 24° C. Gas permeable plastic bags and constant agitation help maintain physiologic pH, but in vivo viability is still reduced 25 to 50 percent after storage as compared to fresh platelets.

Transfused platelets from one unit of whole blood will raise the platelet count of a normal 70 kg recipient by approximately 10,000 per microliter. Such knowledge may provide a rough guideline in selecting the number of units of platelets for transfusion, but must be tempered by the insight that platelet recipients are virtually never "normal" and commonly have problems that shorten platelet survival and thus reduce the theoretical response. Problems such as infection, bleeding, hypersplenism, and disseminated intravascular coagulation often contribute to the need for platelet transfusion in the first place. Obtaining a platelet count immediately after transfusion is the only way to assess reliably the adequacy of therapy.

The decision to transfuse platelets is based most directly on the presence of bleeding complications to which underlying thrombocytopenia or, less often, qualitative defects are contributing. In patients with severe thrombocytopenia (platelet counts less than 30,000 per microliter), such a contribution can be confidently assumed. Bleeding in patients whose platelet count is mildly depressed (between 80,000 to 150,000 per microliter) should *not* be attributed to underlying thrombocytopenia, and a more relevant cause such as disruption of the vasculature or defects elsewhere in the hemostatic defense should be pursued. Platelet transfusion per se is not apt to help much in controlling such bleeding. Patients with intermediate degrees of thrombocytopenia usually have other important problems to account for their bleeding, but some will benefit from platelet support.

Several other factors may help in the decision to transfuse platelets. First, an abrupt fall in platelet count is usually more symptomatic than a gradual decline to the same low level. Thrombocytopenia caused mainly by excessive peripheral destruction leads to enhanced marrow production of platelets that tend to be younger and better functioning than a similar number of more aged platelets seen in the thrombocytopenia of inadequate marrow production. The same disorders that cause thrombocytopenia also may produce qualitative defects that may create a greater hemostatic defect than one might estimate from platelet count alone. Finally, recognizing the specific cause of thrombocytopenia and knowing its treatment or its inherently self-limited nature may obviate the need for platelet transfusion.

Patients requiring platelet support should receive six to eight units pooled from random blood donors. The post-transfusion platelet count and impact on bleeding will dictate additional transfusion requirements. Platelets for transfusion need not be selected for donor–recipient red cell compatibility, as major ABO and Rh antigens are not well expressed on platelets and the number of contaminating red cells is too small to incite serious immunological transfusion reaction. However, since the RBC count may be sufficient to sensitize recipients, Rh-negative women of childbearing age should always receive Rh negative products. Donor antibodies in the suspending plasma may passively bind to recipient red cells and produce positive antiglobulin tests that may be confusing or, more rarely, may actually precipitate hemolysis.

COMPLICATIONS

The transmission of hepatitis (most often due to hepatitis C virus) is the major risk of platelet transfusion, as in the case for other cell and plasma components. The incidence of post-transfusion hepatitis (PTH) in red cell recipients is probably 1 to 2 percent, the average recipient receiving blood from three different donors. Although the relationship between increased donor exposure and increased hepatitis risk has not been clearcut in some studies, it nonetheless seems logical that it exists and that hepatitis would develop in a higher percentage of patients receiving pooled products from at least six to eight donors.

PTH may rarely lead to fulminant hepatocellular necrosis and death from liver failure. More often, the acute illness is mild, and in fact is often unrecognized. However, of concern is the fact that 50 percent of patients with PTH continue to have fluctuating transaminase elevations and histological evidence of chronic hepatitis years after their transfusion. Whether these patients will ultimately develop morbidity and mortality from evolving cirrhosis is not yet known.

Other infections may be spread through platelet transfusion. Human immunodeficiency virus (HIV) can be transmitted in platelet concentrates, though deferring high-risk groups from donating and testing those that do for antibody to the acquired immunodeficiency syndrome (AIDS) virus has markedly reduced that likelihood. There is no evidence that blood provided by donors designated for a specific recipient is any safer than that provided by the community-at-large, and good moral, ethical, and financial arguments exist for discouraging such "designated donation." Other retroviruses, such as HTLV-1, that are linked to human lymphoma and leukemia theoretically can be transmitted by platelet transfusion. Stored at room temperature for up to 5 days, platelets provide a potentially fertile medium for bacterial growth and are more likely than other blood components to transmit such infection, although its occurrence remains rare. Patients who develop high fever and other signs of sepsis while receiving platelets should, following appropriate cultures, be treated with broad-spectrum antibiotics.

Cytomegalovirus and more exotic diseases such as malaria and babesiosis may also be transmitted by platelet transfusion.

About half of patients exposed to allogeneic platelets form antiplatelet antibodies. These antibodies, occurring typically 4 to 6 weeks after initial exposure, are most often directed against HLA antigens and result in rapid destruction of transfused platelets, negating the expected clinical benefit of transfusion. A platelet count measured 1 hour after transfusion is specific in distinguishing alloimmunization from other nonimmunological factors that shorten platelet survival. Those patients who become sensitized to random-donor platelets should be HLA typed and subsequently transfused with single-donor HLA compatible products.

A small percentage will remain refractory. A variety of platelet cross-matching techniques have been described that may aid in selecting compatible donors, although none has emerged as specific, reproducible, and simple enough for routine use in hospital transfusion centers. Intravenous gamma globulin, given at 400 mg per kilogram per day over 5 days, may reduce platelet destruction in alloimmunized recipients previously refractory to even HLA-matched donors, although clinical experience with this therapy is scant and therapy failures are reported.

Platelet transfusions may elicit other immunologic reactions, most often characterized by fever and occasionally accompanied by an urticarial rash. These symptoms usually resolve spontaneously, or may be treated with acetaminophen, 650 mg, plus diphenhydramine, 25 mg intravenously or 50 mg orally. Anaphylactic reactions with bronchospasm, hypotension, and disseminated intravascular coagulation are rare.

Platelet products contain immunocompetent white cells capable of causing graft-versus-host disease in susceptible recipients. In such cases, platelet units should be irradiated prior to transfusion.

CARDIOVASCULAR SURGERY

Patients undergoing open heart surgery commonly develop thrombocytopenia and, in addition, acquire a qualitative platelet defect during cardiopulmonary bypass. Although platelet transfusions are often given to these patients, their routine use will not decrease blood loss. Instead, platelet transfusions should be reserved for heart surgery patients whose thrombocytopenia and prolonged bleeding time are accompanied by untoward bleeding. It should be kept in mind that bleeding may be more related to defective surgical hemostasis than abnormal platelet function.

IMMUNOLOGICAL THROMBOCYTOPENIC PURPURA

Platelet transfusions may be useful in treating emergent bleeding in patients with ITP. Survival of transfused platelets will clearly be shortened but may nonetheless increase platelet counts for an adequate duration to help patients who are exsanguinating or bleeding into the central nervous system. High-dose corticosteroids, i.e., methylprednisolone, 120 mg intravenously, should be given and intravenous gamma globulin, 400 mg per kilogram per day for 5 days, should be started simultaneously. Platelet transfusions should be avoided in the absence of life-threatening bleeding. In general, prophylactic transfusion is contraindicated, and may not be needed even for thrombocytopenic patients undergoing therapeutic splenectomy.

SINGLE-DONOR PLATELET TRANSFUSION

There are theoretic advantages to using single-donor platelets for transfusion routinely. Decreased donor exposure will reduce the incidence and delay the onset of platelet alloimmunization and possibly decrease the incidence of post-transfusion hepatitis. These theoretical advantages, however, are either unproved or of marginal clinical utility in controlled investigation. Furthermore, the time, expense, and limited donor base available for plateletpheresis prohibit uniform reliance on single-donor products.

Single-donor HLA-matched platelets are indicated

for sensitized recipients who are refractory to random-donor platelets. Single-donor non-HLA–matched platelets may be optimal for patients with aplastic anemia awaiting bone marrow transplantation.

PROPHYLACTIC TRANSFUSION

Prophylactic platelet transfusion should be given to patients when the severity and duration of thrombocytopenia suggest that bleeding is likely to occur. Marrow injury in patients being treated for acute leukemia results in severe and sustained thrombocytopenia. Infection and additional nonhematologic chemotherapy toxicity heighten bleeding risk. Although controlled studies of prophylactic platelet transfusion have produced inconsistent results, prophylactic administration of six to eight units of platelets to leukemic patients whose platelet count is less than 20,000 per microliter seems prudent. Similar guidelines are appropriate for patients with lymphoma or other solid tumors, although their drug-induced marrow toxicity is usually more rapidly reversible. The threshold for prophylactic transfusion should be higher in patients with chronic aplastic anemia. First, these patients may tolerate lower platelet counts without bleeding during periods when they are not infected and not being treated with drugs or antithymocyte globulin. Second, their indefinite need for support entails repetitive exposure to the toxicity of transfusion.

Surgical patients should be prophylactically transfused in the perioperative and immediate postoperative period for platelet counts below 50,000 per deciliter. For delicate eye or neurosurgery, prophylaxis should be considered for modest thrombocytopenia. Thrombocytopenic patients scheduled for invasive procedures such as subclavian vein catheter insertion, lumbar puncture, or liver biopsy should also receive prophylactic transfusion. Several factors should be considered in this decision: (1) thrombocytopenia should be interpreted first and foremost as a risk factor for bleeding following such procedures that may or may not be palliated or prevented by platelet transfusion. The need for the procedure and the existence of safer alternatives (i.e., antecubital vein cut-down versus central venous catheter insertion) should be re-assessed. (2) A bleeding time may help in evaluating the qualitative impact of intermediate degrees of thrombocytopenia and, if normal, may obviate the need for prophylaxis. (3) Delaying an emergency procedure while awaiting platelet transfusion (i.e., lumbar puncture in a patient with suspected meningitis) is unacceptable even if thrombocytopenia is severe.

The bleeding time may be useful for evaluating patients with a suspected bleeding disorder; however, abnormalities of this test when used to screen otherwise asymptomatic patients preoperatively do not predict excessive surgical bleeding and does not mandate prophylactic platelet transfusion.

PLASMA COMPONENTS

Thrombotic Thrombocytopenic Purpura

Thrombotic thrombocytopenic purpura is a heterogeneous syndrome with diverse pathophysiology and inconsistency in response to therapy. Although corticosteroids and inhibitors of platelet function are often used, plasma therapy is likely of greater importance. A blood volume plasma exchange should be performed using fresh-frozen plasma for replacement fluid. Although improvement may be dramatic, exchange transfusion should be continued, four to five times per week for 2 to 3 weeks, in less responsive patients. Some patients clearly respond to plasma administration rather than to plasmapheresis. These patients may be treated with infusion of fresh-frozen plasma, 2 to 4 units per day, though intravascular volume overload may require plasma exchange for these patients as well.

Post-transfusion Purpura

Post-transfusion purpura occurs when patients who lack the PLA-I antigen are transfused with PLA-I positive blood products and develop autoimmune thrombocytopenia 7 to 14 days later. Platelet administration often causes serious transfusion reactions in this condition. Patients with significant bleeding should receive plasma exchange transfusion.

von Willebrand's Disease (vWD)

Qualitative platelet defects in this disease occur because of an abnormality of von Willebrand factor (vWF), a plasma factor required for normal platelet adhesion. An increasing number of vWD subtypes have been identified with differing vWF deficiencies. Patients with severe type I and most patients with type II von Willebrand's disease should be treated with cryoprecipitate, 0.1 to 0.15 units per kilogram. The need for subsequent treatment depends on correction of bleeding time and impact on clinical bleeding.

Uremia

The qualitative platelet defect in uremia should initially be treated with hemodialysis. Patients whose defect persists may also respond to cryoprecipitate transfusion. Improved platelet function is, however, inconsistent. Desmopressin infusion may be equally effective and safer in avoiding the infectious risk of blood components. The bleeding time and perhaps bleeding risk in anemic patients will improve if the hematocrit is corrected to 30 percent.

SUGGESTED READING

Castillo R, Monteagudo J, Escolar G, et al. Hemostatic effect of normal platelet transfusion in severe von Willebrand disease patients. Blood 1991; 177:1901–1905.

Lind SE. The bleeding time does not predict surgical bleeding. Blood 1991; 77:2547–2552.

Menitove JE: The decreasing risk of transfusion associated AIDS. N Engl J Med 1989; 321:966–968.

Murphy S. Guidelines for platelet tranfusion. J Am Med Assoc 1988; 259:2453–2454.

Platelet transfusion therapy, consensus conference. J Am Med Assoc 1987; 257:1777–1780.

Tremolada F, Casarin C, Tagger A, et al. Antibody to hepatitis C virus in post-transfusion hepatitis. Ann Int Med 1991; 114:277–281.

DIAGNOSTIC, PROGNOSTIC, AND THERAPEUTIC SIGNIFICANCE OF IMMUNE MARKERS IN ACUTE LEUKEMIA

PETER B. NEAME, M.D., FRCPC, FACP, FRC Path
PRANITI SOAMBOONSRUP, BSc. MT(ASCP)SH

The diagnosis of acute leukemia requires the morphologic examination of peripheral blood and bone marrow. Distinction between acute lymphoblastic and acute nonlymphoblastic or myeloid leukemias is important in view of the different therapeutic regimens and patient outcome. The most widely accepted classification system of acute leukemia has been the French-American-British (FAB). The production of immunologic reagents, first heteroantisera and then monoclonal antibodies, has supplied an alternative method to classify acute leukemia. Two major techniques are frequently used, either (1) immunoenzymatic staining (usually alkaline phosphatase-antialkaline phosphatase, or APAAP) of peripheral blood and bone marrow smears or (2) immunofluorescence staining of a blood or marrow cell suspension followed by fluorescence microscopy or flow cytometry.

DIAGNOSTIC SIGNIFICANCE OF IMMUNE MARKER EXPRESSION IN ACUTE LEUKEMIA

Use of an Immunophenotypic Panel in Diagnosis

Immune marker expression on leukemic cells can be used to classify acute leukemia. Immune antibodies can react with surface (e.g., CD33, CD19, CD2), cytoplasmic (e.g., c-CD3, c-CD22, Cμ), or nuclear (e.g., TdT) antigens. Table 1 shows an example of a panel of immunologic reagents that is employed to categorize acute leukemia cases using a flow cytometer. It was developed to obtain the maximum of information using the smallest number of tests. It is performed in sequence so that the most useful information is likely to be derived from specimens that contain an insufficient number of cells for complete analysis. The first-line screen is used to distinguish acute myeloid (AML) from acute lym-

phoid leukemia (ALL) and to separate acute granulocytic (nonmonocytic) from monocytic leukemia and B-lineage ALL (B-ALL) from T-lineage ALL (T-ALL). The second-line panel is used to further subtype AML and ALL and to distinguish a rare case not recognized by the first panel. The third panel recognizes the less common erythroid and megakaryocytic types of AML and further discriminates subtypes of ALL. Similar panels are used by other investigators using commercial or locally prepared reagents.

Specificity and Sensitivity of the First-Line Panel

Table 2 shows the sensitivity, specificity, and predictive values of our first-line panel in identifying AML. Using My7 and My9 positivity alone to identify AML in 191 patients, the sensitivity is 98 percent and the specificity is 75 percent, the latter because 25 percent of ALL patient's cells were also positive with My7 or My9 or with both monoclonal antibodies indicative of biphenotypic expression. When negativity with lymphoid antibodies (B4, Tll/Leul) was included in the analysis, the specificity increased to 99 percent, but the sensitivity dropped slightly from 98 percent to 90 percent. The percentage drop was related to the biphenotypic AML patients (AML with B4$^+$ or Tll/Leul$^+$) who were not detected.

Table 3 shows the sensitivity, specificity, and predictive values of our first-line panel in identifying ALL in 100 patients. When B4 or Tll/Leul positivity alone was used, good specificity (89 percent) and sensitivity (85 percent) were achieved. When negativity with myeloid antibodies (My7, My9) was included in the analysis, the specificity was 100 percent; however, the sensitivity dropped to 77 percent owing to the elimination of the biphenotypic ALL patients.

In summary, the vast majority of acute leukemia cases can be assigned to their major classes when using the first-line panel. Twelve percent of the cases showed biphenotypic expression. These cases could be further discriminated according to the results of the second-line panel.

Comparison of Immunophenotyping with the FAB Classification

Immunophenotyping has certain advantages over the FAB classification. It will supply information not obtainable from the FAB classification, which is also prone to error because of its subjective interpretation.

Table 1 Immunophenotyping Panel for Classifying Acute Leukemia (Using Flow Cytometry)

Panel	Acute Nonlymphocytic Leukemia			Acute Lymphocytic Leukemia		
First Line						
Strategy	Nonmonocytic	vs	monocytic	T-lineage ALL	vs	B-lineage ALL
Antibodies	CD13(My7)* + CD33(My9)		CD14(My4)	CD2(T11) + CD5(Leu1)		CD19(B4)
Second Line						
i Strategy	Stage of differentiation and maturity			Subclassification of ALL		
Antibodies	CD15(LeuM1), HLA-DR(Ia), CD34(My10)			CD3(T3), CD1(T6), CD71(T9)		TdT, HLA-DR, CD10(J5), Cμ†, SIgκ.λ
ii Strategy	Identification of rare cases not differentiated by first line					
Antibodies	My8, CD11 (MO1), above second-line antibodies			CD7(Leu 9) CD3†		cCD22†
Third Line						
Strategy	Identification of erythroid and megakaryocytic AML variants			Further subclassification of ALL		
Antibodies	GpA, GpC CD41(IIb/IIIa), PLT1, CD42 a + b, Factor VIIIR			(CD8)T8, CD4(T4), Delta 1, WT31		CD20 (B1) CD21 (B2)

*Cluster differentiation number established by the 1st to 4th International Workshop on Human Leukocyte Differentiation Antigens in order to identify clusters of similar monoclonal antibodies.
†Cytoplasmic antigens recognized by flourescent microscopy.

Table 2 Sensitivity, Specificity, and Predictive Value of First-Line Panel (AML versus Non-AML)

Antigen Expression*	AML	ANML (ALL)	SENS (%)	SPEC (%)	PPV (%)	NPV (%)
My7$^+$, My9$^+$ or My7/9$^+$ CD13$^+$, CD33$^+$ or CD13/33$^+$	187/191	24/96	98	75	89	95
B4$^-$, T11/Leu1$^-$, My7$^+$ or My9$^+$ or My7/9$^+$ CD19$^-$, CD2/5$^-$, CD13$^+$ or CD33$^+$ or CD13/CD33$^+$	157/174	1/92	90	99	99	84

*Positive reaction is defined as 20 percent of leukemic cells more fluorescent than the control.
Abbreviations: NPV = negative predictive value, PPV = positive predictive value, SENS = sensitivity, SPEC = specificity.

Table 3 Sensitivity, Specificity, and Predictive Value of First-Line Panel (ALL versus Non-ALL)

Antigen Expression*	ALL	ANLL (AML)	SENS (%)	SPEC (%)	PPV (%)	NPV (%)
B4$^+$ or T11/Leu1$^+$ CD19$^+$ or CD2/CD5$^+$	85/100	21/189	85	89	80	92
B4$^+$ or T11/Leu1$^+$, My7$^-$, My9$^-$ CD19$^+$ or CD2/CD5$^+$, CD13$^-$, CD33$^-$	72/94	0/190	77	100	100	90

*Positive reaction is defined as 20 percent of leukemic cells more fluorescent than the control.
Abbreviations: NPV = negative predictive value, PPV = positive predictive value, SENS = sensitivity, SPEC = specificity.

Immunophenotyping (1) allows the reproducible discrimination of AML from ALL and T-ALL from B-ALL; (2) recognizes cases undifferentiated by morphology and cytochemistry; (3) identifies cases of acute mixed leukemia usually not demonstrated by morphology and cytochemistry; (4) identifies heterogeneous ALL subgroups not recognized by the FAB classification; and (5) demonstrates only myeloid antigens in some cases diagnosed by conventional FAB criteria as typical ALL.

The immunophenotypic classification of acute leukemia can be performed independently of the FAB morphologic-cytochemical classification. Although the ALL immunophenotypic subtypes usually do not correspond with the FAB classification, there is correlation in many instances between the AML subtype morphology and a composite immunophenotype. As has been previously suggested, the composite immunophenotype probably reflects a related but somewhat different view of the status of cell differentiation and maturation than obtained by morphologic-cytochemical analysis. For the classification of AML, immune marker analysis can be made together with morphologic-cytochemical analysis, as each technique complements the information supplied by the other.

Identification of Residual Disease or Early Relapse

A major limitation in the therapy of acute leukemia has been the inability to detect minimal residual disease or early relapse in the bone marrow. Several techniques, e.g., the use of clonal gene rearrangements together with the polymerase chain reaction, have been proposed but require evaluation. The use of immunophenotypic markers as indicators of residual disease or early relapse has not, in most instances, been proven to be of value because a specific tumor antigen has not been identified. However, early identification of leukemic cells in the cerebrospinal fluid may be detected by identifying cells with an indicative immune marker(s). The APAAP method is a useful technique in this respect. More sensitive laboratory techniques than are currently available are required to detect residual leukemic cells in the bone marrow.

PROGNOSTIC SIGNIFICANCE OF IMMUNE MARKER EXPRESSION IN ACUTE LEUKEMIA

The FAB classification has only been minimally successful in recognizing groups of clinical relevance. In theory, immunophenotyping may identify subgroups of ALL and AML patients with different response rates to standard therapy. The prognostic impact of the immunophenotype may also differ with age.

Immune Marker Expression and Patient Outcome in Childhood ALL

Initial studies suggested a relationship between the immunophenotype in childhood ALL and patient outcome. In these studies, remission reduction rate and remission duration were observed to be lowest in T-ALL, better in null-ALL, and highest in c-ALL (see Table 4). A subsequent study showed that pre-B-ALL responded poorly to treatment.

The predictive value of the clinical and biologic features that have prognostic significance in childhood ALL can vary with the efficacy of the treatment delivered. Recent use of intensive chemotherapy in high-risk patients (e.g., Dana-Farber Institute or Berlin-Frankfurt Munster Group Protocols) has resulted in prolonged continuous complete remission in 60 percent to 80 percent of the children with T-ALL. B-ALL (SIg$^+$), often represented morphologically as FAB L3, has a poor prognosis, although improvement has again been reported with recent treatment regimens. It seems that only the elevation of the leukocyte count (>20 to 50 × 10.9 per liter), age (<2 or >9 years), and chromosomal abnormality have consistently been shown as independent indicators of patient outcome. In a number of studies, the blast cell immunophenotype has emerged as an independently significant prognostic factor, but

Table 4 Relationship of Immunophenotype to Patient Outcome in ALL*

	Childhood ALL†	Adult ALL
Worse prognosis	c-ALL	T-ALL
↓	T-ALL	c-ALL
	null-ALL	null-ALL
	pre-B-ALL	B-ALL
	B-ALL	

*Patient outcome must be evaluated in the context of the therapy administered. Age, white count, and chromosomal abnormality are important independent prognostic factors.
†c-ALL = CD19$^+$, CD10$^+$, Cμ$^-$, SIg$^-$; T-ALL = CD2$^+$, CD5$^+$ or CD7$^+$; null-ALL = CD19$^+$, CD10$^-$, Cμ$^-$, SIg$^-$; pre-B-ALL = CD19$^+$, CD10$^{+/-}$, Cμ$^+$, SIg$^-$; B-ALL = CD19$^+$, CD10$^{+/-}$, Cμ$^+$, SIg$^+$.

with more effective therapy, its contribution to patient outcome in childhood ALL has been reduced. Nevertheless, in order to assign the patients, using a number of specific criteria, to standard or high-risk protocols, it is necessary to determine the immunophenotype.

Immune Marker Expression and Patient Outcome in Adult ALL

Adult ALL has a worse prognosis than childhood ALL. In contrast to childhood ALL, a number of studies have now shown the best prognosis in adults with T-ALL who were receiving intensive therapy. In a German prospective multicenter study of 368 adult ALL patients, the probability of being in continuous complete remission (CCR) at 5 years or greater was 0.55 for T-ALL, 0.34 for c-ALL, and 0.24 for null-ALL. Other prognostic factors unfavorable for remission duration included time to complete remission (CR) of more than 4 weeks, a leukocyte count greater than 30×10^9 per liter, and age older than 35 years. In contrast to c-ALL or T-ALL, the outcome in null-ALL was only slightly worsened when the other adverse factors were present. Table 4 shows the relationship of the immunophenotype to patient outcome in ALL.

Immune Marker Expression and Patient Outcome in Adult ANLL

Table 5 shows results of relating immune marker expression to patient outcome in adult acute nonlymphoblastic leukemia (ANLL). It will be seen that patients whose leukemic cells have some of the same antigens have shown different response rates to therapy. On the available evidence, it seems premature to attribute prognostic significance to immune markers in ANLL. Further study of a large number of cases is required to assess the relationship of marker expression to patient outcome. It may be possible in the future to select patients for alternate therapy if certain antigens or groups of antigens, expressed on ANLL cells, reveal a subgroup of patients with different response rates to standard therapy.

Table 5 Relationship of Antigen Expression to Patient Outcome in Adult ANLL

Investigators	No. Patients Analyzed	Therapy	Overall Complete Remission Rate (%)	Patient Outcome
Holowiecki et al. Acta Haematol 1986; 76:16–19	242	Daunorubicin + Ara-C or TAD	51	CD15+ (VIM-D5) of ANLL cells predicted ability to achieve CR
Griffin et al. Blood 1986; 68:1232–1241.	161	Standard Ara-C daunorubicin	65	My7+ (CD13) and My4+ (CD14) predicted low CR rate, [My4⁻My7⁻] phenotype a high CR rate. Ia+, My8+, or M01+(CD11) associated with decreased CCR. My8+ predicted short survival. MCS–1 (CD15) showed no relationship to CR rate, CR, or survival
Borowitz et al. Am J Clin Pathol 1989;91:265–270.	75	High- or low-dose induction therapy	52	Patients with CD34 (My10)-positive leukemia were less likely to enter a CR even when receiving a high-dose induction-type chemotherapy. No difference in CR rate between CD13+ and CD13⁻ patients
Ward et al. Blood 1989; 74:238a.	103	Standard Ara-C anthracycline or high-dose Ara-C	60	Patients with cells (+) for My7(CD13), My4(CD14), and My10(CD34) did not have lower CR rate than those whose cells did not express those antigens ($P = 0.58, 0.74$ and 0.75 resp.). No difference in CR between CD15+ and CD15⁻ patients
Gayathri et al. Blood 1989; 74:357a.	59	Standard therapy	52	Analysis of response indicated that no marker, including CD13(My7), CD14(My4), and HLA-DR, predicted remission rates
van der Schoot et al. Blood 1989; 74:371a.	127	—	—	Expression of CD13 was significantly related to CR induction ($P = 0.00027$). Patients with CD13-negative blasts had higher chance to reach CR (77% vs 38%)
Schwarzinger et al. J Clin Oncol 1990; 8:423–430.	145	Modified 3 + 7 daunorubicin + cytarabine	65	Reactivity of My7 was predictive for CR: My7+, 59%, vs My7⁻, 91% ($P < .003$). Probability of significantly lower survival rate My7+, ($P < .03$). VIM-D5 (CD15) was significantly associated with a higher probability of CCR ($P < .01$)

CR = complete remission, CCR = continuous complete remission.

Immune Marker Expression and Patient Outcome in Childhood ANLL

Because ANLL in childhood is a less common disease than ALL, there are few data on the relationship between the immunophenotype and patient outcome. Adolescent patients who have the FAB criteria for ANLL but express the CD2 antigen have been shown to have a poor response to induction therapy. These cases will be included in the following section on acute leukemia with biphenotypic expression.

Biphenotypic Expression in Acute Leukemia and Patient Outcome

Acute leukemia with biphenotypic expression (mixed-lineage phenotype) is found in about 12 percent to 15 percent of patients with acute leukemia. It is more commonly found in ALL cases, as defined by FAB morphologic-cytochemical criteria, being observed in about 15 percent to 25 percent of adult or childhood patients. It is noted in about 8 percent to 12 percent of AML cases.

A number of terms have been applied to the condition. These have included *biphenotypic, hybrid, chimeric,* and *mixed.* The terms *biclonal* and *bilineal* have been used to describe the rare case of acute leukemia with separate populations of lymphoblasts and myeloblasts. Mirro and Kitchingman of St. Jude Children's Research Hospital in Memphis have used the term *acute mixed-lineage leukemia* when the leukemic blasts have coexpressed lymphoid and myeloid characteristics. They have proposed certain criteria to define the condition so that comparisons can be made between investigators and institutions. The criteria have included immunophenotypic, cytochemical, molecular, and karyotypic characteristics, which were assigned a relative weight according to the considered lineage specificity of the marker. Of the papers previously published on acute leukemia with biphenotypic expression, few would qualify as acute mixed-lineage leukemia by the proposed criteria.

Although preliminary data suggested that childhood ALL patients expressing myeloid-associated antigens had inferior outcome on standard induction therapy, investigation of a larger group of patients showed that the CR rate was the same for childhood ALL patients with or without myeloid markers. Another study in adult

Table 6 Biphenotypic Acute Leukemia and Patient Outcome

Investigators	Number Studied	Age Group	Therapy	FAB	Biphenotypic Marker Expression	Positive Patient (%)	Patient Outcome
ALL + My⁺ Marker							
Sobel et al. N Engl J Med 1987; 316:1111–1117	76	>14 yr	Standard anthracycline, vincristine, prednisone	ALL	MCS2(CD13), My9(CD33)	33	My$^+$ patients had fewer CRs than My$^-$ patients (35% vs 76%, $P<0.01$). My$^+$ identifies a high-risk group of patients with adult ALL
Pui et al. Blood 1989; 74:160a.	267	Childhood	Intensive combination therapy	ALL	CD11b, CD13, CD33, CD36, CD15, CD14, CD12	16.4	All children achieved CR. At a median follow-up of 2.5 yr, event-free survival did not differ significantly between My$^+$ and My$^-$ patients. My$^+$ in ALL of childhood lacks prognostic value in context of intensive chemotherapy
AML + L⁺ Marker							
Cross et al. Blood 1988; 72:257–587.	94	Mostly adolescent	Intensive multiagent therapy	AML	CD2	9.5	Patients with CD2$^+$ AML had poorer responses to remission induction therapy (50% vs 80% entered complete remission, $P = .05$)
Benedetto et al. J Clin Oncol 1986; 4:489–495.	133	Adult	L-14 and L-14M protocols	AML	TdT	22	Remission-induction rates were higher for the Tdt$^-$ patients, with 68% vs 48% for the TdT$^+$ patients ($P = .05$) TdT$^-$ patients also experienced longer remission ($P = .003$) than TdT$^+$ patients
Swirsky et al. Br J Haematol 1988; 70:193–198.	304	Adult and childhood	DAT 1 + 5	AML	TdT	8.1	There were no significant correlations between TdT$^+$ in AML and CR rate, duration of remission, or survival
Schwarzinger et al. J Clin Oncol 1990; 8:423–430.	123	>14 yr	Modified 3 + 7 daunorubicin and cytarabine	AML	TdT	15	Reactivity of TdT was predictive for CR (TdT$^+$, 28% vs TdT$^-$, 71% ($P<.001$). Probability of lower survival in TdT$^+$ cases ($P<.001$)

patients showed a lower CR for ALL patients in whom blast cells expressed myeloid antigens. Follow-up studies of this group have not yet been published. Further evaluation is required.

Following investigation of 10 AML patients in childhood that expressed the CD2 antigen, it was suggested that AML with CD2$^+$ may be indicative of a poor response to induction therapy; however, most patients in the CD2$^+$ AML subgroups were adolescents. Further investigation of a larger group using multivariant analysis to identify independent prognostic indicators is necessary. The presence of TdT$^+$ on AML blasts was initially associated with a poor remission induction rate, but a larger multicenter trial failed to confirm it. In a recent report, TdT$^+$ AML patients had a lower RR rate and a significantly lower survival rate. Reports on

the outcome of patients with acute leukemia with biphenotypic expression are shown in Table 6.

THERAPEUTIC USE OF MONOCLONAL ANTIBODIES IN ACUTE LEUKEMIA

Monoclonal antibodies have been used to purge the bone marrow of malignant leukemic cells or T cells in autologous or allogeneic bone marrow transplantation or in vivo as immunophenotype specific therapy (serotherapy).

Marrow Purging

Purging of bone marrow of malignant cells in autologous bone marrow transplantation or deleting the marrow of T cells in allogeneic bone marrow transplantation has been recently investigated.

Autologous bone marrow transplants have been performed for patients with acute lymphocytic and acute nonlymphocytic leukemia. A major concern with autologous marrow transplantation is the strong possibility of residual leukemia cells in the cryopreserved remission bone marrow. It may be possible to eliminate the leukemic cells in vitro using cytotoxic monoclonal antibodies reactive against differentiation antigens present on the leukemic cells but unreactive with antigens on pluripotential stem cells. Following the use of monoclonal antibodies AML-2-23 and PM-81 in ANLL or monoclonal antibodies or antisera reactive against B- or T-lymphocyte differentiation antigens in ALL, attempts to eliminate antibody-labeled cells have been performed with complement and by the use of immunotoxins or by other techniques. The clinical consequences of this in vitro preparation of bone marrow requires further evaluation.

In *allogeneic* bone marrow transplantation of patients with acute leukemia, attempts to prevent acute graft-versus-host disease (GVHD) by depleting T-lymphocytes from the donor marrow using an anti–T-cell monoclonal antibody and complement have reduced the incidence and severity of acute GVHD. However, T-cell depletion has been associated with an increased risk of graft failure and leukemic recurrence. Prevention of the higher risk of graft failure by additional pretransplant immunosuppression and of increased leukemic relapse by intensification of the conditioning regimen is under investigation. Further evaluation of the ex vivo elimination of T-lymphocytes is required. Apart from antibody elimination of T-cells, other physical methods, such as counterflow centrifugation, have been used.

Immunophenotype Specific Therapy (Serotherapy)

The therapeutic use of monoclonal antibodies in cancer therapy has recently been investigated. An immunophenotype-specific monoclonal antibody can be administered intravenously to locate on the tumor cell membrane, giving support to the concept that it may be useful therapeutically in targeting tumor-specific antigens. Nevertheless, it is not yet clear whether truly tumor-specific antigens exist on tumor cells. It seems possible that there may be quantitative differences in antigen expression between leukemic and normal cells. These differences might be exploited in antibody-mediated therapy. Investigation into the use of immunoconjugates suggests monoclonal antibodies can be used to carry drugs, toxins, and radioisotopes to malignant cells. However, serotherapy is still in an early phase of investigation and requires further evaluation.

SUGGESTED READING

Ball ED, Mills LE, Cornwell GG, et al. Autologous bone marrow transplantation for acute myeloid leukemia using monoclonal antibody-purged bone marrow. Blood 1990; 75:1199–1206.

Champlin R, Gale RP. Acute lymphoblastic leukemia: Recent advances in biology and therapy. Blood 1989; 73:2051–2066.

Drexler HG, Gignac SM, Minowada J. Routine immunophenotyping of acute leukemias. Blut 1988; 57:327–339.

Greaves MF, Janossy G, Peto J, et al. Immunologically defined subclasses of acute lymphoblastic leukemia in children: Their relationship to presentation features and prognosis. Br J Haematol 1981; 48:179–197.

Griffin JD, Davis R, Nelson DA, et al. Use of surface marker analysis to predict outcome of adult acute myeloblastic leukemia. Blood 1986; 68:1232–1241.

Hoezler D, Thiel E, Löffler H, et al. Prognostic factors in a multicenter study for treatment of acute lymphoblastic leukemia in adults. Blood 1988; 71:123–131.

Mirro J, Kitchingman GR. The morphology, cytochemistry, molecular characteristics and clinical significance of acute mixed-lineage leukemia. In: Scott CS, ed. Leukaemia cytochemistry: Principles and practice. Chichester, England: Ellis Horwood Ltd, 1989:155.

Neame PB, Soamboonsrup P, Browman GP, et al. Classifying acute leukemia by immunophenotyping: A combined FAB-immunologic classification of AML. Blood 1986; 68:1355–1362.

Oldham RK, Thurman GB, Talmadge JE, et al. Lymphokines, monoclonal antibodies, and other biological response modifiers in the treatment of cancer. Cancer 1984; 54:2795–2806.

Pui C-H, Crist WM. High-risk lymphoblastic leukemia in children: Prognostic factors and management. Blood Rev 1987; 1:25–33.

Santos GW. Marrow transplantation in acute nonlymphocytic leukemia. Blood 1989; 74:901–908.

AIDS: MANAGEMENT OF THE HEMATOLOGIC MANIFESTATIONS

RALPH ZALUSKY, M.D.

Over the past decade, the acquired immunodeficiency syndrome (AIDS) has gained major prominence as a significant disease entity with a high rate of morbidity and mortality. A retrovirus, designated the human immunodeficiency virus (HIV), has been shown to be the etiologic agent, with tropism for $CD4^+$ T lymphocytes. Transmission has been highest in homosexual men, intravenous drug abusers, infants born of infected mothers, hemophiliacs, and other recipients of transfused blood products. Since antibody testing for HIV became available in 1985, donors of blood products for the latter two groups have largely been screened from the pool. The Centers for Disease Control has established criteria for different stages of the infection, whose major manifestations include a variety of opportunistic infections and neoplastic diseases. The latter will be discussed in a separate chapter of this book. In this chapter, the hematologic manifestations and their management are considered.

No organ system has been spared the devastation wrought by HIV, and a variety of clinical manifestations have been observed. The hematologist has frequently been consulted for effects of the virus, or that of therapy, on the blood-forming tissues. Early on in the epidemic, a syndrome of persistent generalized lymphadenopathy was described in which lymph node biopsy demonstrated a picture of florid reactive hyperplasia, distinguishing this entity from malignant lymphoma. Leukopenia, thrombocytopenia, and anemia, either singly or in combination, have been frequently observed. Bone marrow studies in these situations are generally not revealing, but they have occasionally yielded diagnostic information when granuloma formation, such as infection with *Mycobacterium avium intracellulare*, is present. In addition, the bone marrow is frequently normocellular to hypercellular, and shows excessive plasma cells, lymphoid aggregates, and reticulin fibrosis. Direct involvement of marrow progenitor cells by HIV has been postulated and may partially account for the peripheral blood findings.

Ultimately, the therapy for these hematologic manifestations will be obviated by the prevention (vaccine) or specific therapy of the retrovirus. At the present time, the major antiviral agent in general use is Zidovudine (azidothymidine, or AZT); other dideoxynucleosides, such as 2', 3'dideoxyinosine (ddI), are undergoing clinical trials. Azidothymidine carries its own hematologic toxicity.

HIV-ASSOCIATED THROMBOCYTOPENIA

Early on in the epidemic, reports of significant thrombocytopenia began to appear, not infrequently as the sole manifestation of HIV infection. Because thrombocytopenia appeared in patients who were otherwise asymptomatic, drug-induced causes were unlikely, even in former intravenous drug abusers who had refrained from recent use of these agents. Clinically, the thrombocytopenia had all the features of immune-mediated peripheral destruction, with large platelets on peripheral smear, normal to increased megakaryocytes in the bone marrow, and the absence of splenomegaly. Furthermore, studies showed that the platelets from these patients were excessively coated with immunoglobulin but differed from classical autoimmune thrombocytopenia in that a higher proportion of patients showed immune complexes as opposed to 7S IgG antiplatelet antibodies.

Our therapeutic approach to the management of HIV-associated thrombocytopenia takes into account the clinical status of the patient and the presence or absence of bleeding manifestations. In the absence of the latter, no therapy has been recommended if the platelet count is greater than 30,000 per cubic millimeter. However, this approach is being modified based on early reports that AZT given orally may ameliorate the thrombocytopenia after several weeks of therapy. It should be pointed out that there is a 10 percent to 20 percent spontaneous remission rate, so that conservative management is appropriate in the asymptomatic patient. Furthermore, when the asymptomatic thrombocytopenic patient develops infection, a rise in platelet numbers has occasionally been observed.

For individuals with platelet counts below 30,000 per cubic millimeter, and especially if evidence of abnormal bleeding is present, more active intervention is indicated. Recognizing that these patients are already immunosuppressed, we begin with a regimen of prednisone. 40 to 60 mg PO per day for 2 weeks, and then taper this rapidly to a maintenance dose of 10 to 15 mg per day. A majority of patients will respond with platelet counts exceeding 50,000 per cubic millimeter, but generally relapse when corticosteroid therapy is discontinued. Next, depending on the overall clinical status of the patient, i.e., those not debilitated by advanced AIDS, splenectomy should be considered. Results from this procedure generally bring the platelet count to normal levels in more than 70 percent of patients.

Concern has been expressed that corticosteroids or splenectomy may accelerate the progression to full-blown AIDS in these compromised patients. However, it would appear that this progression is determined more by HIV positivity than the occurrence of thrombocytopenia in the asymptomatic state.

In classical autoimmune thrombocytopenia, additional modalities of therapy have been applied, and these also have roles in HIV associated thrombocytopenia. High-dose intravenous gamma globulin, 0.4 g per kilogram daily for 5 days, has been shown to be very effective in raising the platelet count to acceptable levels in more than 80 percent of patients. Because the effect is transient for this expensive therapy, we have reserved its use for patients who are actively bleeding or who are scheduled for operative procedures. Also, in hemophilia patients with severe thrombocytopenia, an especially disastrous combination, the initial use of high-dose intravenous gamma globulin is warranted. Recently, the use of anti-Rh(D), probably working by a similar mechanism of reticuloendothelial system blockade, has been shown to have efficacy, and at a much reduced cost. However, it is too early to make recommendations for this modality, which is still in the investigative stage.

When a patient's clinical condition disallows consideration for splenectomy, or when low-dose corticosteroids fail to maintain a platelet count above 30,000 per cubic millimeter, vincristine, 2 mg IV weekly, has been tried. If there is no response by the fourth injection, it is unlikely that this agent will be beneficial. In those who do respond, however, and do not develop untoward neurologic toxicity, intermittent injections separated by intervals of 2 to 3 weeks off therapy may be tried.

Although a few instances of responses to Danazol, 200 mg PO four times a day, have been reported, we have had little success with this agent.

HIV-ASSOCIATED ANEMIA

Anemia in HIV-positive individuals tends to be related to the stage of the disease. Asymptomatic individuals with $CD4^+$ lymphocyte counts greater than 500 per cubic millimeter have a low incidence, but as the disease progresses to AIDS, anemia becomes very common. In most respects, the anemia can be characterized as the anemia of chronic disease: normochromic, normocytic indices, low reticulocyte response, and decreased serum iron and iron-binding capacity with normal to elevated serum ferritin levels. Adding to the complexity of the etiology, these patients are frequently infected and are on a variety of drugs.

In 1986, a clinical trial with AZT for the treatment of HIV disease was begun. Because the double-blind placebo-controlled study showed a survival benefit in patients with AIDS by 24 weeks, it was felt to be unethical to continue the placebo arm. These patients were treated with 200 mg of AZT PO every 4 hours. Anemia resulted in approximately one-third of these patients; two-thirds of these patients required transfusion. It was of some interest that leukopenia also frequently occurred but the platelets were spared. The anemia was macrocytic in most instances, although normochromic, normocytic anemia and, rarely, red cell aplasia were also observed. Because of the frequency of anemia, an interinstitutional study on the effect of recombinant human erythropoietin (rHuEPO) was undertaken. The results from the double-blind placebo-controlled portion of this study demonstrated a modest effect on reducing the red cell transfusion requirements of those on rHuEPO. The dose was 100 U per kilogram

IV three times per week. In retrospect, it was shown that patients with baseline endogenous serum EPO levels of 500 mIU per milliliter or less accounted for most of the responders, whereas those with levels greater than 500 mIU per milliliter showed no response. Whether this growth factor will be more widely used will have to await the results of studies in which rHuEPO is being administered in doses up to 500 U per kilogram three times a week, and in which the subcutaneous route has been found to be as efficacious as the intravenous route. The role for rHuEPO will have to be reassessed in the future, because a large-scale study of asymptomatic HIV-positive individuals with $CD4^+$ counts of less than 500 per cubic millimeter showed a survival advantage with a total daily dose of 500 mg of AZT. At this dosage, hematologic toxicity, anemia, and neutropenia were minimal. It would appear that the hematologic toxicity is related to AZT dose, and the lowest dose that will still show anti-HIV efficacy needs to be established. In patients with advanced AIDS, however, even a dose as low as 500 mg per day may still induce significant anemia.

Other causes of anemia in these patients should not be overlooked. Iron deficiency, though uncommon, needs to be considered in patients with excessive blood loss. Considering the poor nutritional intake of many of these patients, folic acid and vitamin B_{12} status can be easily ascertained from serum levels of the vitamin, and replacement can be given as indicated. There is some evidence that defects in cobalamin transport may be operative and, thus, blunt response to vitamin B_{12} therapy.

HIV-ASSOCIATED LEUKOPENIA

As an overall manifestation of defective bone marrow function, leukopenia is a common occurrence in HIV-positive patients. Superimposed on the evidence for direct HIV involvement of marrow progenitors is the added insult of drugs directed against the virus, such as AZT, as well as agents used to treat the infectious complications, such as ganciclovir (DHPG), pentamidine, trimethoprim-sulfamethoxazole, pyrimethamine-sulfadiazine, and acyclovir. When confronted with this array of myelotoxic agents, the hematologist must balance the benefit of these agents against the problems of the underlying disease. Maintenance of an absolute neutrophil count greater than 500 per cubic millimeter requires judicious juggling.

Early trials utilizing hematopoietic growth factors have shown promise in treating the neutropenia associated with HIV disease. Patients with AIDS or AIDS-related complex (ARC) responded to intravenous recombinant granulocyte-macrophage colony-stimulating factor (GM-CSF) in a dose-dependent manner. Cessation of therapy resulted in a return to baseline white blood cell counts within a period of 3 to 9 days. Daily subcutaneous injections have similarly been given for extended periods of time, and refractoriness to this agent has not been shown. Side effects have been minimal, consisting of myalgias, fever, nausea, and mild transient liver function abnormalities. Even in the presence of AZT, itself a myelotoxic agent, GM-CSF has been shown to improve the neutropenia. Concern was expressed that proliferation of the monocyte-macrophage pool would increase the reservoir of the retrovirus, but in vitro studies have shown that the inhibition of HIV replication by AZT in the presence of GM-CSF is augmented. Granulocyte colony-stimulating factor (G-CSF) shows similarly good responses in HIV-positive patients with neutropenia. In this rapidly emerging field, it is likely that interleukin-3 (IL-3), which acts at an earlier progenitor stage, will undergo clinical testing as well.

At the present time, specific recommendations on the use of these factors, or combinations thereof, must await their availability after data from current studies are completed.

HIV-ASSOCIATED COAGULATION ABNORMALITIES

In our own experience, and that of several others, antiphospholipid antibodies of the lupus anticoagulant type have been demonstrated frequently in patients with HIV disease. In a group of 52 patients with AIDS, 26 were found to have a prolonged activated partial thromboplastin time (APTT) that was not corrected by the addition of normal plasma in vitro. The majority of these patients had active *Pneumocystis carinii* pneumonia at the time. In other series, however, a correlation between the presence of the anticoagulant and active opportunistic infection was not seen. Analysis of the anticoagulant indicated that most belonged to the IgM subclass, unlike the characteristic IgG subclass seen in association with other diseases. A further distinction is the relative rarity of associated thrombotic complications. Although no specific therapy is indicated for this finding, it is important to recognize, because the hematologist is frequently called upon to assess these patients for biopsy and other surgical procedures.

SUGGESTED READING

Castella A, Croxson TS, Mildvan D, et al. The bone marrow in AIDS: A histologic, hematologic, and microbiologic study. Am J Clin Pathol 1985; 84:425–432.

Karpatkin S. Immunologic thrombocytopenic purpura in HIV-seropositive homosexuals, narcotic addicts and hemophiliacs. Semin Hematol 1988; 25:219–229.

Scadden DT, Zon LI, Groopman JE. Pathophysiology and management of HIV-associated hematologic disorders. Blood 1989; 74: 1455–1463.

DIAGNOSTIC AND THERAPEUTIC IMPLICATIONS OF THE GROWTH OF HEMATOPOIETIC PROGENITOR CELLS IN VITRO

ALLEN C. EAVES, M.D., Ph.D., FRCP(C)
CONNIE J. EAVES, Ph.D.

The diagnostic use of in vitro colony assays for the detection of hematopoietic progenitors is becoming increasingly important in a number of hematologic disorders. These include the myeloproliferative syndromes (MPS), myelodysplastic syndromes (MDS), aplastic states, and myeloid leukemias. In general, culture conditions have been optimized most successfully for progenitors giving rise to colonies of red cells, megakaryocytes, granulocytes and macrophages, or combinations of these cell types. Considerable progress has also been made in the definition of semisolid culture systems that support lymphoid cell proliferation, resulting in the formation of T cells, B cells, and myeloma or lymphoma cells. However, the reproducibility and clin-ical usefulness of these latter culture procedures have not been well established. Moreover, even though experience with the diagnostic use of in vitro colony assays for myeloid progenitors is more advanced, considerable variability in findings due to the lack of standardized culture media has hampered interlaboratory comparisons for many years, and this problem is compounded even further by the subjectivity of colony scoring.

Hematopoietic progenitors have been utilized for some time for therapeutic purposes, primarily in cancer patients requiring hematopoietic rescue following administration of otherwise lethal doses of chemoradiotherapy to obtain a better antitumor effect. Hematopoietic rescue is usually achieved by the transplantation of an allogeneic (genetically nonidentical) or autologous (the patient's own) marrow transplant, although peripheral blood, which also contains primitive hematopoietic cells, has also been used for this purpose. Most often, unmanipulated marrow or blood cell suspensions are transplanted; however, more recently, in vitro cell separation ("purging") procedures to remove potentially contaminating neoplastic cells from autologous marrow harvests (to reduce the risk of relapse) or to remove T cells from allogeneic transplants (to reduce graft-versus-host disease) are being introduced. Strategies focused on the positive selection of normal hematopoietic stem cells or the use of cell culture procedures to increase the number or growth potential of primitive hematopoietic cells in a transplant are now also being explored as alternative therapeutic possibilities. Initiatives in this latter direction are based largely on the development of a liquid "long-term" culture system that allows the sustained production and differentiation of primitive hematopoietic progenitors in vitro for many weeks.

The long-term culture system is quite different from the semisolid culture systems used for colony assays. In the latter, optimal concentrations of soluble stimulatory factors are incorporated into the medium to achieve maximal plating efficiency (detection) of the clonogenic progenitors present in the test cell suspension and the cells are diluted in a semisolid medium at a sufficiently low cell concentration to allow the colonies that subsequently form to be visualized individually. In contrast, long-term cultures are initiated by placing cells at relatively high cell concentrations in a liquid medium to which no exogenous growth factors are added. Maintenance of hematopoietic cell production under these conditions is dependent on the presence of a supportive layer of mesenchymal "stromal" cells that appear when these cultures are initiated with bone marrow cells. This adherent layer appears to mimic the in vivo function of the marrow stroma by providing various positive and negative regulatory factors via close-range interactions with adjacent hematopoietic cells that are also found in this fraction of the culture. For reasons not yet well understood, conditions established in long-term cultures set up with unseparated marrow appear to allow expression of the hematopoietic potential of a very primitive type of cell, more primitive than cells detectable in conventional clonogenic assays. The long-term culture system has provided an approach both to quantitating the most primitive human hematopoietic progenitors known and to analyzing the mechanisms by which the marrow stroma regulate their differentiation into mature blood cells.

Recent studies have shown that leukemic progenitors may be selectively removed from the patient's marrow by relatively short incubation periods (10 days) of marrow under long-term culture conditions. Although the mechanism underlying this phenomenon is still a mystery, the therapeutic potential of cultured autologous marrow to support intensive treatment of leukemia is now being evaluated. Improvements in the culture media and procedures used to establish and maintain long-term cultures in combination with further developments in gene transfer technology will also facilitate the future use of genetically engineered autologous hematopoietic progenitors for the correction of a variety of inherited genetic disorders by transplantation into affected recipients.

TYPES OF PROGENITORS

The first colony assay for a hematopoietic progenitor cell was the spleen colony assay described in 1961. In this report, the appearance of myeloid colonies in the spleens of lethally irradiated mice 10 days following the intravenous injection of small numbers of normal marrow cells from a syngeneic donor (i.e., from the same inbred strain of mouse) was noted and the term *colony-forming unit-spleen* (CFU-S) was proposed to designate the cell, or cells, responsible for giving rise to each of these colonies. Each spleen colony was subsequently formally shown to represent the progeny of a single cell. However, the operational term *CFU* persisted to accommodate the fact that some cells with the potential to form a colony may not do so. For example, only 10 percent of the cells in normal marrow with spleen colony-forming potential are thought to express this potential following their injection into irradiated recipients, the remainder being undetected primarily because they home to other organs, both hematopoietic and nonhematopoietic. Some of the spleen colonies generated in this way, and most that are visible 12 to 14 days after injection, contain combinations of daughter red cells, megakaryocytes, and granulocytes or their precursors, demonstrating that the original cells from which such colonies derive have the potential to differentiate along multiple lineages. Most such colonies can also be shown to contain daughter cells with the capacity for generating secondary multilineage spleen colonies, indicating that the original cell from which the primary colonies arise also undergo some self-renewal during their first divisions.

Conditions suitable for obtaining hematopoietic colony growth in vitro from both mouse and human progenitors began to be defined a few years later. Eventually, appropriate cocktails of nutrients and growth factors for generating colonies containing many different types of mature progeny, both singly and in combination, were identified. Accordingly, terminology was developed that reflected both the generic clonogenic ability and the specific lineage potentialities of the progenitors of these different types of colonies. Subsequent comparisons of the characteristics of their progenitors and, finally, the ability to separate them physically showed that different types of colonies are derived from distinct progenitor populations representing specific stages of differentiation along each of the various hematopoietic lineages. The interrelationships of these primitive hematopoietic cells are now considered well established, and the resultant hierarchical scheme of progenitor cell differentiation that they define is shown in Figure 1. Although this scheme includes both multipotent and lineage-restricted colony-forming progenitor types, most clinically useful colony assay data are at present derived from measurements of the number or properties of progenitors committed to either the erythroid or ganulocyte-macrophage lineages. Therefore, the following discussions are focused on the use of these particular types of assays. Note that the scheme shown in Figure 1 does not preclude the existence of other transitions. However, based on available data, such transitions, if they occur, are normally relatively uncommon. One should note also that the scheme shown in Figure 1 does not attempt to portray how commitment of pluripotent cells to any single differentiation pathway is

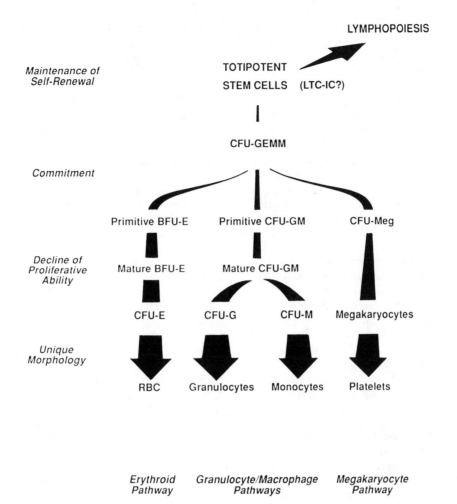

Figure 1 Schematic representation of the various stages of hemopoietic cell differentiation identified by in vitro assays for clonogenic cells (colony-forming units, or CFU) and long-term culture-initiating cells (LTC-IC).

brought about. In fact, very little is known about this process except that it does not appear to involve a well-ordered sequence of lineage-restricting events nor does it appear to be readily manipulated by extrinsic factors.

The most primitive progenitors in the hematopoietic hierarchy are responsible for the long-term maintenance of all hematopoietic lineages and are capable of regenerating and sustaining these lineages after transplantation into receptive and immunologically compatible recipients. The ability of single cells in normal adult mouse marrow to repopulate the entire immuno-hematologic system of irradiated recipients has now been well established from retroviral marking experiments, and in human marrow transplant recipients, analysis of X-linked methylation-sensitive restriction fragment length polymorphisms (RFLPs) has provided evidence of occasional monoclonal (single cell origin) hematopoiesis of normal (allogeneic) donor origin, suggesting the existence of a similar primitive totipotent repopulating cell population in adult human marrow also. Recent purification studies have suggested that

long-term repopulating cells in the marrow of mice include a very minor subset of CFU-S or may not even be detectable by this assay and, similarly, may not be detectable by current in vitro colony assay methodology. On the other hand, we now know that murine lympho-myeloid stem cells with long-term in vivo repopulating potential can proliferate in the long-term marrow culture system. Therefore it should be possible to use this culture system to develop a quantitative assay for repopulating cells (discussed later).

CULTURE METHODS

A complex mixture of different types of hematopoietic cells is found in both blood and marrow, and in both cases the progenitors are present at relatively low frequencies ($< 1/1,000$ cells). The presence of red cells at the concentrations at which they are normally present in samples of human blood or marrow would usually preclude colony recognition if such samples were plated directly in colony assays. Therefore, some preliminary preparation is undertaken to reduce the red cell content and sometimes to obtain additional progenitor enrichment. Because each manipulation of the blood or marrow sample inevitably results in some progenitor cell loss, the method chosen represents a balance between the need for red cell removal, the need for progenitor enrichment to facilitate scoring (and increase plating efficiency), and the disadvantage of reduced progenitor recovery. In our experience, the simplest and most reproducible method for preparing marrow samples is simply to lyse the red cells by brief exposure to a buffered ammonium chloride solution. For blood, granulocytes and red cells are usually removed by density centrifugation on Ficoll-Hypaque or Percoll using solution densities standardized for isolating lymphocytes and monocytes.

Because of how blood and marrow samples are obtained, progenitor quantitation in each also is different. Progenitors in the marrow can only be expressed relative to the number of other cells present (e.g., per 2×10^5 nucleated marrow cells), not absolutely (e.g., as "n" progenitors per kilogram body weight or per unit of marrow volume), as would be ideal and is possible in mice. Thus, any change in the number of marrow cells that do not form colonies in the assay being performed (e.g., lymphoblast infiltrates in acute lymphocytic leukemia [ALL]) will distort the measured relative frequency of myeloid progenitors, even if the absolute number of these present is normal. In contrast, progenitors in the circulation can be expressed as absolute concentrations (per milliliter of blood) as well as on relative basis (e.g., per 4×10^5 light-density nucleated blood cells). Absolute values for circulating progenitor numbers may not, however, always reflect the total body content of progenitors, as a variety of factors (e.g., myelofibrosis) may independently influence the proportion of progenitors that are in the circulation.

One of the greatest problems with in vitro hematopoietic colony assays has been a lack of standardization of culture conditions, particularly between different laboratories. This has been due in part to the fact that all culture requirements are still not molecularly defined. To obtain conditions of optimal plating efficiency, it is therefore necessary to search, by empirically testing, for "optimal" batches of fetal calf serum (FCS), bovine serum albumin (BSA), and methyl cellulose (or other gelling agent). Consistency of culture conditions can then be achieved by sequential screening of all reagents used, and if these are purchased in bulk, most individual components can be held constant for several years. Even with standardized culture reagents and cell-preparation procedures, significant variation in colony morphology is observed, particularly with human samples, even those from different normal individuals. Thus, close attention needs to be paid to the criteria used for colony recognition and scoring, and inclusion of internal controls (e.g., cultures without added growth factors) may be important. In our experience, it requires several months of training in colony scoring before staff acquire the experience to be able to evaluate reliably the diversity of clinical material for which colony assay data are likely to be solicited.

Colony Assay Procedures

Progenitor cells are detected by virtue of their ability to generate mature, recognizable blood cell progeny that remain associated as individual colonies because of the presence of a gelling agent in the media that greatly decreases cell movement. The colonies that are produced are relatively easy to see because the more mature cells that make up the majority of the cells in either blood or marrow usually lyse within a few days after being placed in culture to leave the intervening media clear. Methyl cellulose is now widely used as a gelling agent because it allows better support of erythroid colony growth than other types of semisolid support systems while also allowing optimal granulopoietic colony formation so that both types of progenitors can be assayed in the same cultures. In addition, methyl cellulose increases the viscosity of the medium without converting it to a solid. Thus, the colonies produced in methyl cellulose cultures can be readily removed either in bulk or individually, and the cells can then be washed and resuspended for morphologic or cytogenetic analysis. To ensure a reasonable space between colonies, cells are usually plated at a concentration anticipated to give not more than 100 to 200 colonies per milliliter of medium, e.g. 2×10^5 nucleated normal marrow cells. Thus, only 1 million nucleated cells are required to ensure obtaining useful data from most marrow samples, assuming two replicate 35-mm diameter petri dishes are plated, each with 2×10^5 nucleated cells in approximately 1 ml of complete culture medium.

In our laboratory, granulocyte-macrophage colonies are scored after 2½ to 3 weeks of incubation, when virtually all colonies have matured. A somewhat arbitrary minimum of 20 cells per colony is used as the lower cut-off. However, this varies between laboratories. Many use somewhat higher cut-offs of 40 or 50 cells. Granulocyte-macrophage colonies can also be subdivided into those containing more, or less, than 500 cells. This is done because the progenitors (CFU-GM) in normal marrow from which the larger (> 500 cell) colonies arise display three features of very primitive hematopoietic cells: (1) they are normally noncycling (i.e., they belong to a normally quiescent compartment); (2) they have a high proliferative potential (> 8 to 9 cell divisions); and (3) they are relatively sensitive to inhibition by TGF-β. TGF-β is a reversible negative regulator of hematopoietic cells that has greater effects on more primitive cells than more mature myelopoietic cells. CFU-GMs that give rise to colonies of more than 500 cells are thus referred to as primitive CFU-GM. Similarly, CFU-GM that give rise to colonies of more than 20 but less than 500 cells are referred to as "mature CFU-GM. Groupings of less than 20 to 50 cells, but more than 4 to 5 cells, are often referred to as clusters. Because of their very small size, granulocyte-macrophage clusters are extremely labor-intensive to score. In general, granulocyte-macrophage cluster data have not been found to add much information to that provided by CFU-GM counts and therefore are not widely reported. An important exception to this, however, is in the assessment of patients with acute myelogenous leukemia (AML) or myelodysplasia (MDS) where the generation of blast clusters has diagnostic usefulness (discussed later).

Erythroid colonies need to be scored at two different times. The smaller erythroid colonies are best scored after 10 to 12 days because they tend to lyse and become difficult to detect at later times. Erythroid progenitors with greater proliferative capacity give rise to groups of CFU-E–derived colonies. Because differentiation is semisynchronous, hemoglobinization begins in a rather sudden fashion after an initial period of growth when the erythroid nature of the developing colony is not yet obvious. For this reason, such large erythroid colonies were first called *bursts*, and the term *burst-forming unit-erythroid* (BFU-E) was assigned to their progenitors. Colonies containing what appear as three to eight CFU-E–derived colonies are considered to have originated from "mature" BFU-E; larger groupings are said to be derived from "primitive" BFU-E. This latter distinction in erythroid colony size is used to separate BFU-E into "primitive" and "mature" subpopulations that show distinct properties analogous to those that distinguish primitive and mature CFU-GM.

Assays Using Long-Term Cultures

When marrow cells are placed in liquid cultures containing horse serum and corticosteroid (but without added agar or methyl cellulose), at cell densities greater than approximately 5×10^5 cells per milliliter, the cells settle to the bottom of the culture dish and an adherent layer of fibroblasts, fat cells, and other mesenchymal cell types forms. Within 2 to 3 weeks, this adherent layer becomes quite extensive but can be disrupted with trypsin and a cell suspension obtained. These adherent layer cells can then be plated in secondary methyl cellulose cultures that show that most of the more "primitive" hematopoietic progenitors in the entire culture are present in this adherent layer. The overlying nonadherent layer of the primary cultures consists mainly of terminally differentiating granulocytic cells, macrophages, some mature CFU-GM, and an occasional BFU-E. With weekly changes of the media in these cultures, hematopoiesis may be maintained for several months, hence the name *long-term culture*. Both the survival and the proliferative behavior of the primitive hematopoietic progenitors in the adherent layer are regulated by the nonhematopoietic cells with which they are closely associated. In the absence of the nonhematopoietic cell feeder, the primitive cells proliferate continuously but are not maintained and rapidly disappear. In contrast, in the presence of such a feeder, the primitive cells are sustained but held in a quiescent state at least in part by the endogenous production of TGF-β. However, appropriate perturbation of the nonhemato-

poietic cells by agents such as horse serum, interleukin-1, or platelet-derived growth factor leads to the activation of adjacent primitive hematopoietic cells that then enter S-phase, divide, and differentiate. The amplified progeny produced as a result are then released into the nonadherent fraction, where some (e.g., the erythroid progenitors) die owing to an absence of the factors required for their support and further differentiation, but others (e.g., the granulopoietic progenitors) mature further.

Recent studies indicate that the initial marrow contains a distinct population of very primitive cells that may not be capable of forming colonies in standard methyl cellulose assays but that are the progenitors of the clonogenic cells detectable in long-term cultures that have been maintained for periods of several weeks. For human cells, assessment of the number of clonogenic cells present in 5-week-old long-term cultures has been found to provide a useful endpoint to quantitate these very primitive cells (long-term culture–initiating cells), because this measure of clonogenic cell output is a linear function of the number of cells originally added (providing that the required supportive stromal cells are present at nonlimiting numbers). Although this assay is very lengthy (5 weeks for the long-term culture, plus 3 weeks for the secondary methyl cellulose colony assays) and the need for pre-established, irradiated long-term culture adherent feeder layers must be anticipated 2 to 3 weeks before initiating the assay, this approach may prove extremely important for the quantitation and characterization of the human progenitor cell that may be responsible for engraftment after BMT.

Assessment of Progenitor Proliferative Status

Hematopoietic progenitors normally represent rare members of the cell suspensions in which they are found and cannot be uniquely identified. Therefore, to determine their proliferative state, standard kinetic methods such as determination of labeling indices following exposure to ^{3}H-thymidine or assessment of DNA distributions by flow cytometry cannot be used. Instead, a method referred to as the thymidine suicide assay is used. This assay is based on the selective uptake by S-phase cells of high specific activity ^{3}H-thymidine (or hydroxyurea) during a short exposure period, resulting in the subsequent selective inactivation of these cells only when they are stimulated to proliferate. The number of colonies obtained from cells exposed to ^{3}H-thymidine by comparison to controls (similarly handled but exposed to no or cold thymidine) thus provides a measure of the proportion of progenitors in the original suspension that were in S-phase. A significant reduction in colony formation (approximately 50 percent) is observed if most of the colony-forming progenitors are actively proliferating. Conversely, if most of the progenitors are in a G_0 resting state, exposure to ^{3}H-thymidine will have no effect on their clonogenic capacity.

Early studies of the proliferative state of murine

progenitors showed that the majority of the most primitive progenitors in the marrow are not normally actively cycling, but rather are in a G_o state indicative of a very slow rate of turnover of the population. Accordingly, it was anticipated that analogous progenitor populations in the human hematopoietic hierarchy would display similar kinetic features under steady-state conditions. Subsequent studies verified this prediction. Both primitive BFU-E and CFU-GM as well as CFU-GEMM (i.e., the progenitors of multilineage colonies), have been found to be quiescent populations in normal adult human marrow, whereas more mature clonogenic progenitor types are actively proliferating. Interestingly, all circulating myeloid progenitors, including those considered to be more mature (some of which are also present in the blood, although at decreased numbers relative to marrow), are normally found to be quiescent. Although the presence of cycling progenitors in the circulation or of primitive populations in the marrow is not normally seen, this situation can change following gross perturbation of hematopoiesis, e.g., as occurs during regeneration of the system following treatment of individuals with myeloablative therapy and bone marrow transplantation. In the unperturbed individual, however, quiescence of primitive cells is a very stable feature and thus has diagnostic usefulness.

DIAGNOSTIC AND PROGNOSTIC USES

Polycythemia Vera

The diagnosis of polycythemia vera has become greatly simplified by the discovery in 1974 by Prchal and Axelrad that these patients have erythroid progenitors that can differentiate into mature red cell colonies in vitro in the absence of erythropoietin. Subsequent studies by a number of groups showed that virtually all patients meeting the diagnostic criteria of the Polycythemia Vera Study Group (PVSG) will show this feature of erythropoietin independence. Because this abnormality persists, even after years of treatment, erythropoietin independence is useful in establishing the correct diagnosis in all patients with polycythemia vera, including those with a normal hematocrit as a result of previous treatment, bleeding, iron deficiency, and so forth or because they are in the "burnt out" phase or progressing to myelofibrosis. Because erythropoietin independence is an intrinsical abnormal property of the neoplastic erythroid progenitor, it is manifested regardless of whether such cells are obtained from blood or marrow. The ability to make the diagnosis by assessment of blood progenitors has the advantage of avoiding the need for a marrow aspirate. However, marrow cultures are useful, not only because they allow independent confirmation of the diagnosis but because they sometimes may reveal the presence of erythropoietin-independent cells that were missed in peripheral blood assays. This is due to the fact that the proportion of erythroid progenitors that are erythropoietin-

independent is lowest in the most primitive erythroid progenitor compartments (BFU-E) and highest in the most mature erythroid progenitor compartments (CFU-E). Because the latter are more prevalent in the marrow, erythropoietin-independent cells are readily detected in marrow assays.

Detection of erythropoietin-independent progenitors requires the use of culture conditions that give zero background. False-positive results can occur, even with normal marrow, if the fetal calf serum used in the cultures has not been carefully selected to be low in erythropoietin content. Similarly, the cells tested must be carefully washed prior to placing them in culture to prevent carry over of any serum erythropoietin, especially in patients with secondary erythrocytosis who may have significantly elevated serum erythropoietin levels.

Although the presence of readily detectable numbers (usually > 10 percent) CFU-E or BFU-E showing erythropoietin independence appears to be diagnostic of polycythemia vera, the proportion present in a given patient has not shown obvious prognostic importance. In polycythemia vera, the percentage of erythropoietin-independent progenitors in individual patients does not appear to increase significantly with time from diagnosis. In retrospect, this should not be viewed as surprising, because by the time of diagnosis, most of the hematopoietic progenitors seen in patients with polycythemia vera are members of the neoplastic clone, but only a proportion of these exhibit erythropoietin independence. Thus, the extent to which the neoplastic cells show erythropoietin independence may be more a unique feature of individual polycythemia vera clones, perhaps reflecting some heterogeneity in the genetic abnormalities that may result in this disease phenotype.

As mentioned previously, all patients with myeloproliferative disorders thus far studied have shown deregulation of their hematopoietic progenitors such that no quiescent populations are found in these individuals. (This does not exclude their presence, however, because this method detects only the behavior that is exhibited by the majority of the cells.) Thus, thymidine suicide studies can, like erythropoietin independence measurements, distinguish between patients with polycythemia vera and patients who have an erythrocytosis that is secondary to some other cause. Interestingly, the heightened proliferation characteristic of the neoplastic progenitors in polycythemia vera does not lead to a marked increase in their numbers, which appear to remain within normal limits. It can therefore be inferred that the increased progenitor proliferation observed may be associated with an increased rate of progenitor cell death. Only at the terminal stages of erythropoiesis and, to a minor extent, in other lineages in some patients is there an increased output of mature progeny.

Essential Thrombocytosis

Erythropoietin-independent erythroid growth in culture is also commonly seen in patients with a clinical diagnosis of essential thrombocytosis. The percentage of abnormal progenitors is often lower than that seen in polycythemia vera, although it is usually greater than 10 percent. Also, the extent of hemoglobinization of the erythroid colonies that mature in the absence of erythropoietin may be less than that seen in corresponding polycythemia vera cultures. As in patients with polycythemia vera, however, exhibition of erythropoietin independence in vitro appears constant with time, being detectable even many years following the initial diagnosis. This is consistent with the sustained presence of a dominant neoplastic clone that is thought to take over the marrow in these patients. Patients with essential thrombocytosis who show erythropoietin independence also show deregulated cycling control of all primitive progenitor types.

Myelofibrosis

Myelofibrosis as a primary diagnosis is often associated with the presence of erythropoietin-independent erythroid progenitors. In this case, erythropoietin independence is again demonstrable in both blood and marrow assays, and, once seen, it is usually evident on subsequent cultures. Myelofibrosis is often seen to develop in patients with a previously established diagnosis of polycythemia vera or essential thrombocytosis (or chronic myelogenous leukemia [CML]). In all cases, increased numbers of circulating myeloid progenitors (measured as the number of CFU-E, BFU-E, CFU-GM, and CFU-GEMM per milliliter of blood) are often seen. This increase in progenitors can be many times above the upper limit of the normal range. Because of these similarities, it is possible that even primary myelofibrosis patients simply represent examples of individuals with a preceding asymptomatic history of polycythemia vera or essential thrombocytosis, analogous to CML patients presenting in blast crisis as ALLs or AMLs. Further work at the molecular and genetic level will clearly be required to develop more definitive classifications of these various disease entities.

Chronic Myelogenous Leukemia

A marked increase in the number of progenitors per milliliter of blood is typical of CML. In fact, the number of circulating progenitors increases as an exponential function of the white blood cell count, regardless of treatment. Thus, when the clone is smaller or reduced by therapy, the number of circulating progenitors may lie within the normal range, whereas when the white blood cell count increases to 10- to 50-fold normal values, the circulating progenitors may be increased several hundred to a thousand-fold. Curiously, this is true with respect to all progenitor types, including erythroid progenitors (CFU-E and BFU-E) and megakaryocyte progenitors (CFU-MK) as well as granulocyte-macrophage progenitors (CFU-GM). Even though the marrow is very cellular in CML and there may be a significant absolute increase in the number of he-

matopoietic progenitors in the marrow, this cannot be appreciated from marrow culture results, because these can only be expressed on a per-marrow-cell basis (as discussed previously).

Erythropoietin-independent erythroid colony growth is frequently seen in assays of blood or marrow from CML patients. However, the colonies produced in the absence of erythropoietin rarely become fully hemoglobinized. This is similar to the situation frequently seen in essential thrombocytosis assays, but it is in contrast to the erythropoietin-independent erythroid colonies seen in polycythemia vera cultures, which tend to complete their maturation more successfully. Cells of CML differ from those of essential thrombocytosis and polycythemia vera in that expression of erythropoietin independence in vitro is less consistent even in individual patients and is thus not always seen in sequential samples. On the other hand, abnormal cycling of CML progenitors is seen in all patients and persists throughout the course of the disease.

The development of an accelerated phase or blast crisis in CML is not usually heralded by unique changes in numbers of progenitors, except those predicted by an uncontrolled increase in the white blood cell count, nor does the detection of frequency of erythropoietin-independent erythroid progenitors change significantly. However, the development of numerous, small, poorly differentiated "blast colonies" may occasionally be seen. The presence of such colonies or clusters then helps to confirm the existence of a more aggressive subclone. Because of the rapid growth of these "blast" colonies, although typically only to a small size (<20 to 50 cells) and their tendency to lyse soon afterwards, it is difficult to document their presence reliably unless they are produced in large numbers. In the latter situation, normal granulocyte-macrophage colonies are rarely seen, although erythroid colonies typical of those present in assays of chronic phase CML patients' samples may still differentiate apparently normally. Sometimes, it appears that the erythroid lineage is also involved in the blast-phase subclone, in which case very abnormal appearing colonies showing some degree of hemoglobinization may be seen, either as the only type of erythroid colony present or together with normal erythroid colonies generated from coexisting chronic-phase progenitors.

Myelodysplastic Syndromes

The diagnosis of MDS requires a marrow examination in order to meet the French-American-British (FAB) criteria and for subclassification. Direct cytogenetics is also useful because this provides additional objective evidence of a clonal abnormality in approximately 40 percent of MDS patients meeting FAB diagnostic criteria. In vitro colony assays show reduced numbers of progenitors in most patients, with blast colony formation in approximately 25 percent. The presence of blast colonies may be particularly useful in establishing the diagnosis of MDS in those patients who have a cytopenia but who do not meet FAB criteria or do not have a chromosomal abnormality.

The prognostic significance of reduced progenitors or blast colony formation needs further study. In general, blast colony formation appears to be associated with higher numbers of marrow blasts and, hence, a poorer prognosis of FAB criteria (i.e., refractory anemia with excess blasts [RAEB] or RAEB in transformation [RAEBIT]). However, very reduced numbers of progenitors (in the absence of blast cell colonies), or no in vitro growth at all, has also been associated with short survival in some studies.

Acute Myelogenous Leukemia

The majority of patients presenting with acute myelogenous leukemia (AML) show numerous blast cell colonies when either blood or marrow is cultured. Most of the remaining patients show reduced or absent progenitors. From a diagnostic perspective, the presence of blast cell colonies confirms a diagnosis of either AML or MDS, as in vitro growth patterns alone do not allow a distinction to be made between these two diagnoses. Decreased numbers of marrow progenitors, without blast cell colonies, is also not particularly discriminating, as it is consistent with either AML, MDS, a hypoplastic state, or an infiltrate. The prognostic significance of in vitro growth patterns in AML at presentation has remained controversial. This is likely due to the considerable heterogeneity in the biology and response to treatment of the neoplastic clones that develop in different individuals, all of whom are classified under this common disease heading. Heterogeneity at the cytogenetic and molecular level in both AML and MDS is now widely appreciated; however, at least to date this has not facilitated the clinical exploitation of culture data. Complex, multifactorial analysis of the response of blast colony progenitors to particular cytokines in liquid and semisolid culture systems are now being explored, but it also already appears unlikely that this will provide simple procedures for planning therapy.

THERAPEUTIC IMPLICATIONS

It is now known that in man (as in mice) the hematopoietic system of a single individual can be repopulated and maintained by a single or small number of transplanted stem cells. An in vitro assay that allows these cells to be identified and quantitated has not yet been clearly established. However, it seems likely that such cells either do not form colonies in conventional semisolid culture systems or, if they do, the colonies they generate are not distinguishable from those derived from primitive BFU-E, CFU-GM, and CFU-GEMM. An alternative approach has been to adapt the long-term culture system to allow quantitation of cells that can give rise to primitive clonogenic progenitors in vitro for at least 5 weeks (as described previously). Because these cells are precursors of clonogenic progenitors, they must,

by definition, be more primitive. Moreover, results of studies of murine long-term cultures have shown that totipotent murine repopulating cells not only persist but also proliferate under these conditions, making it very likely that a similar situation will eventually be shown to prevail in long-term cultures initiated with human marrow given the numerous other similar features they are known to share.

The availability of an assay for repopulating cells would allow definitive measurements to be made regarding the response of these cells to various drugs (or radiation) and to evaluate suspensions to be used for bone marrow rescue and the subsequent rate of recovery in the recipients' hematopoietic tissues. Such an assay is also key to stem cell purification strategies. These have now progressed to the point where monitoring clonogenic cell populations is no longer predictive of the cell of interest. Besides providing additional and critical assay methodology, the availability of a culture system that supports human stem cells in vitro has several other therapeutic implications. These pertain to situations in which manipulation of stem cells in vitro prior to transplantation in vivo is required. One example now under investigation is the use of "culture purging" to remove leukemic cells from patients' marrows and hence allow the development of protocols involving autologous marrow transplants. A second example, still at the preclinical stage, is the area of gene transfer. Finally, there exists the possibility of using stem cell cultures as in vitro "factories" to amplify stem cells from small innocula or to generate therapeutically useful quantities of mature blood cell progeny. Although both of these may appear rather futuristic at the present time, the clinical pay-offs would be enormous and there are many centers now working towards these goals.

Culture Purging

The long-term culture system has been used extensively to analyze the process of stromal cell-mediated regulation of growth and differentiation of both normal and neoplastic hematopoietic progenitors. In the course of studies of cultures initiated with marrow from patients with CML, it was found that the Ph^1-positive clonogenic progenitors decreased rapidly in the first few weeks of culture so that they were usually undetectable 6 to 8 weeks later. Nevertheless, in some cultures, some hematopoiesis persisted and cytogenetic studies revealed that this was due to the sustained production of normal (Ph^1-negative) progenitors. The simplest interpretation of these findings is that leukemic and coexisting normal hematopoietic cells are differentially affected by the conditions prevailing in these cultures, the former being selected against, the latter being favored. Accordingly, this suggested that the culture procedure itself might be used as a method of purging. Similar results were also obtained with cultures from a proportion of AML patients. This approach is now being tested in clinical trials in both Vancouver, Canada, and Manchester, Great Britain. Preliminary results suggest that marrow held in culture for 10 days can be used to transplant nonleukemic hematopoiesis, thereby allowing patients who are ineligible for allogeneic bone marrow transplantation to be given intensive and potentially curative treatment. Although these findings are encouraging, assessment of the duration of engraftment and long-term disease-free survival will clearly require additional patients and several more years of follow-up.

Gene Therapy

Genes can be efficiently transferred into hematopoietic cells using amphotropic retroviral vectors, although electroporation and microinjection may also prove eventually to be competitive procedures with advantages in terms of the amount of new genetic material that can be readily transferred. Exposure of the target cells to growth factors that have stimulatory effects on them in vitro appears important to obtaining maximal levels of gene transfer using retroviruses and is also likely to be important if additional in vitro selection procedures are used prior to transplantation in vivo. The potential of microinjection to achieve gene transfer to human marrow cells is based at present on extrapolation from experimental studies with cell lines. Analogous work with human marrow has had to await the development of procedures for obtaining pure, or close to pure, progenitor populations, and for fixing them reversibly and viably to a solid matrix support to allow them to be microinjected. Although considerably more must still be learned about the cellular and molecular biology of gene transfer to hematopoietic stem cells, results from animal models over the last several years have shown that high levels of transfer to even purified stem cell populations is achievable and long-term expression is feasible. Gene transfer for marking human T-cell populations is already a clinical reality, and similar applications in bone marrow transplantation are a likely prelude to gene therapy of congenital diseases within the next few years.

THE FUTURE

Continued progress in the use of in vitro colony assays to facilitate the diagnosis and choice of treatment of various hematopoietic disorders will depend primarily on the further characterization of the most primitive types of hematopoietic cells, their growth factor requirements, and identification of conditions that will allow their rapid stimulation and differentiation in vitro. One exciting possibility is the extension of phenotype analysis using modern flow cytometric instrumentation to enable the characterization and, hence, quantitation of subsets of primitive cells currently identifiable only by assays that detect their growth potential. Such an approach offers the obvious appeal of providing information immediately, thus allowing its direct incorporation into therapeutic planning. The main use of hematopoietic cultures might then well become focused on applications in which stem cell maintenance, amplification, selection, or differentiation is desired.

Acknowledgements. Some of the work summarized in this review was funded by operating grants from the National Cancer Institute of Canada, which also supports C.J. Eaves as a Terry Fox Cancer Research Scientist. The authors also wish to thank Ms. Laurie Trarup for expert secretarial assistance.

SUGGESTED READING

Barnett MJ, Eaves CJ, Phillips GL, et al. Successful autografting in chronic myeloid leukaemia after maintenance of marrow in culture. Bone Marrow Transplant 1989; 4:345.

Eaves AC, Cashman JD, Gaboury LA, et al. Clinical significance of long-term cultures of myeloid blood cells. CRC Crit Rev Oncol Hematol 1987; 7:125.

Eaves AC, Eaves CJ. Erythropoiesis in culture. Haematol 1984; 13:371.

Eaves AC, Krystal G, Cashman JD, et al. Polycythemia vera: In vitro analysis of regulatory defects. In: Zanjani ED, Tavassoli M, Ascensao JL, eds. Regulation of erythropoiesis. New York: PMA Publishing Corp, 1988:523.

Eaves CJ, Eaves AC. Erythropoiesis. In: Golde DW, Takaku F, eds. Hematopoietic stem cells. New York: Marcel Dekker 1985:19.

Hughes PFD, Eaves CJ, Hogge DE, et al. High-efficiency gene transfer to human hematopoietic cells maintained in long-term marrow culture. Blood 1989; 74:1,915.

Metcalf D. Hemopoietic colonies: In vitro cloning of normal and leukemic cells. In: Recent results in cancer research. New York: Springer-Verlag, 1977.

Prchal JF, Axelrod AA. Bone marrow responses in polycythemia vera. (Letter). N Engl J Med 1974; 290:1382.

Raskind WH, Fialkow PJ. The use of cell markers in the study of human hemopoietic neoplasia. Adv Cancer Res 1987; 49:127–167.

Sutherland HJ, Lansdorp PM, Henkelman DH, et al. Functional characterization of individual human hemopoietic stem cells cultured at limiting dilution on supportive marrow stromal layers. Proc Natl Acad Sci USA, 1990; 87:3,584.

Szilvassy SJ, Fraser CC, Eaves CJ, et al. Retrovirus-mediated gene transfer to purified hemopoietic stem cells with long-term lympho-myelopoietic repopulating ability. Proc Natl Acad Sci USA 1989; 86:8,798.

Turhan AG, Humphries RK, Phillips GL, et al. Clonal hematopoiesis demonstrated by X-linked DNA polymorphisms after allogeneic bone marrow transplantation. N Engl J Med 1989; 320:1,655.

THROMBOCYTOSIS

ANDREW I. SCHAFER, M.D.

The finding of thrombocytosis (generally considered when the platelet count is >450,000 per microliter) has greatly increased since the advent of automated platelet counting. A wide variety of conditions can cause either transient or longstanding thrombocytosis. The critical differential diagnosis in patients with thrombocytosis is to distinguish between essential thrombocythemia (ET) and secondary (reactive) causes of thrombocytosis. An elevated platelet count per se may be dangerous only in ET; however, secondary thrombocytosis is important to recognize because it is often the manifestation of a potentially dangerous underlying disease.

Essential thrombocythemia is one of the myeloproliferative disorders, which constitute a group of related disorders of the pluripotent hematopoietic stem cell that also includes polycythemia vera (PV), chronic myelogenous leukemia (CML), and myeloid metaplasia with or without myelofibrosis (MMM). The other myeloproliferative disorders, which may also be associated with thrombocytosis, are generally characterized by diagnostic markers: an elevated red cell mass in PV, the presence of a Philadelphia chromosome in CML, the pathologic finding of marrow fibrosis in MMM. In contrast, ET usually remains a diagnosis of exclusion. As is the case with other myeloproliferative disorders, ET may transform to acute leukemia, and the risk of this conversion is markedly increased by treatment with alkylating agents. The major causes of morbidity and mortality in ET are bleeding and thrombosis. Bleeding complications are typically those encountered in patients with platelet disorders, i.e., superficial hemorrhage into skin and mucous membranes. Thrombotic complications are most frequently deep vein thrombosis and pulmonary embolism. However, other more characteristic thrombotic problems may arise in ET. Cerebrovascular and digital ischemia syndromes, presumably caused by predominantly platelet occlusions of blood vessels, are particularly common.

DIFFERENTIAL DIAGNOSIS

The Polycythemia Vera Study Group (PVSG) has established stringent diagnostic criteria for ET, as outlined in Table 1. Most of these criteria were designed to exclude patients who have thrombocytosis associated with one of the other myeloproliferative disorders. As noted previously, these distinctions are occasionally difficult in clinical practice. The last criterion listed by the PVSG is to rule out other possible causes of nonmyeloproliferative, reactive thrombocytosis.

Acute hemorrhage is associated with transient thrombocytosis. Reactive thrombocytosis caused by

Table 1 Diagnostic Criteria for Essential Thrombocythemia*

Platelet count >600,000/μl.
Hemoglobin ≤ 13 g/100 ml/dl or normal red cell mass (men <36 ml/kg, women <32 ml/kg)
Stainable iron in marrow or failure of iron trial (<1 g/100 ml/dl rise in hemoglobin after 1 mo of iron therapy)
No Philadelphia chromosome
Collagen fibrosis of marrow
  Absent, or
    < 1/3 biopsy area without both splenomegaly and leukoerythroblastic reaction
No known cause for reactive thrombocytosis

*As determined by the Polycythemia Vera Study Group.

chronic iron deficiency is reversible within 7 to 10 days of repletion of iron stores. Chronic inflammatory diseases (most strikingly inflammatory bowel disease), various malignancies, and chronic bacterial or fungal infections are frequently associated with elevated platelet counts that only rarely exceed 1,000,000 per microliter. Finally, splenectomy for any reason is characteristically followed by thrombocytosis that usually resolves within weeks to months, but may persist for years in some cases.

INITIAL EVALUATION

Because the diagnosis of ET is often one of exclusion, causes of secondary thrombocytosis should be sought first. Iron deficiency should be evaluated by blood tests for the status of iron stores. Chronic inflammatory or infectious diseases causing reactive thrombocytosis are usually clinically apparent, but approaching the possibility of occult malignancy is more troublesome and should be guided by simple screening tests (e.g., pursuit of abnormalities in the physical examination, stools for occult blood, chest radiograph). Bone marrow aspirate and biopsy characteristically reveal megakaryocytic hyperplasia in both ET and secondary thrombocytosis. However, bone marrow megakaryocytes in ET are more often dysplastic and occur in large clusters, associated with masses of platelet debris (referred to as "platelet drifts"). Furthermore, the bone marrow sample can be analyzed by cytogenetics to exclude Philadelphia chromosome-positive CML with thrombocytosis. Coagulation tests are generally unhelpful. The bleeding time is usually normal, and prolongations do not correlate with bleeding risk in ET. Platelet aggregation studies may show a variety of nonspecific abnormalities; however, the finding of an isolated and complete loss of platelet responsiveness to epinephrine is a very strong indication that the patient has ET rather than a reactive thrombocytosis.

CYTOREDUCTION

The first and most critical decision in the treatment of patients with thrombocytosis is to determine the need

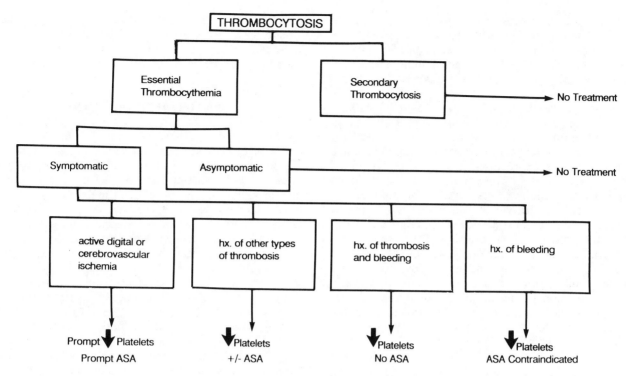

Figure 1 Algorithm for treatment of thrombocytosis.

for suppressing the high platelet count (cytoreduction). In patients with secondary thrombocytosis, the elevated platelet count per se generally poses no threat and should not be reduced. In contrast, the issue of platelet cytoreduction in thrombocytosis caused by ET or other myeloproliferative disorders is the subject of considerable controversy. In general, the weight of evidence in the literature fails to demonstrate a clear correlation between the platelet count, however high, and the risk of either bleeding or thrombosis in ET. Although no controlled, prospective studies are available, it presently appears that the risk of treatment outweighs any potential benefit of chronic cytoreductive therapy in *asymptomatic* patients with ET. However, such treatment should be considered for patients with ET who have had bleeding or thrombotic complications, because largely anecdotal experience suggests that lowering the platelet count in such cases may prevent further hemostatic problems. Platelet cytoreduction is particularly indicated in patients with cerebrovascular or digital ischemia symptoms.

Plateletpheresis

Lowering the platelet count by plateletpheresis has been reported to abrogate active clinical complications. This approach is of value primarily in the acute setting (e.g., cerebrovascular or digital ischemia), in which rapid reduction in the platelet count may be required. Up to about a 50 percent reduction in platelet count can be achieved with plateletpheresis. It is at best a temporary measure, which may be followed within a few days by an even higher "rebound" thrombocytosis.

Alkylating Agents

Melphalan, busulfan, thiotepa, uracil mustard, and chlorambucil have all been successfully used to suppress the platelet count in patients with ET and other myeloproliferative disorders. Although clearly effective, these alkylating agents are associated with a prohibitive leukemogenic risk. Except in rare cases in which other treatments (vide infra) cannot be used, alkylating agents have now been abandoned in the management of patients with myeloproliferative disorders.

Hydroxyurea

Hydroxyurea, a simple derivative of urea, is an S-phase–specific drug that inhibits ribonucleotide reductase. When administered orally, it is readily and rapidly absorbed from the gastrointestinal tract. Peak plasma concentrations are attained in 1 to 2 hours, and the drug disappears from plasma within 24 hours after a single oral dose.

Because of its ease of use and remarkable lack of serious toxicity, hydroxyurea has now become the chemotherapeutic agent of first choice to suppress blood counts in the myeloproliferative disorders. It is first-line chemotherapy not only to reduce the platelet count in ET but also to reduce the white blood count in CML or red cell count in PV. The only significant toxicity of hydroxyurea is myelosuppression, particularly leukopenia. Because it is not an alkylating agent, the development of acute leukemia has not been considered to be a risk; nevertheless, its leukemogenic potential will have to be excluded by more long-term experience with the drug.

Hydroxyurea acts rapidly, with a nadir of platelet cytoreduction expected within about 3 days. The nadir of white cell counts occurs 6 to 7 days after an oral dose, with rapid subsequent recovery. Frequent blood counts (at least weekly) are required initially after beginning therapy. Because the effects of the drug are rapid in onset and are readily reversible, the chronic maintenance dose of hydroxyurea, which may vary greatly among different patients, can be titrated relatively easily. When indicated for the suppression of thrombocytosis, hydroxyurea is administered orally at a dose of generally 0.5 ot 3.0 g daily. Although the proper dose of the drug can be readily regulated in most patients, protracted myelosuppression is inexplicably encountered in rare patients; therefore, some caution is required to avoid too cavalier an approach to monitoring of blood counts during chronic maintenance therapy.

Interferon

Based on the efficacy of recombinant α-interferon in the treatment of CML, this cytokine has been recently explored in ET. In three initial clinical trials, platelet cytoreduction has been achieved quite rapidly in all cases, with a greater than 50 percent decrease in platelet counts within 4 weeks, at a dose of 3 million units daily administered subcutaneously. Furthermore, clinical symptoms attributable to ET have been found to resolve promptly in all cases. The cytoreductive actions of α-interferon in ET have been relatively selective for platelets, with a lesser decrease in white cell counts and little, if any, decrease in hemoglobin observed in most patients.

The major adverse effects of interferon are the almost invariable influenza-like symptoms. Despite the use of acetaminophen, these symptoms can be sufficiently incapacitating to necessitate discontinuation of treatment. Therefore, although this promising therapeutic modality offers predictable and relatively rapid platelet cytoreduction in ET in short-term studies, its role in chronic therapy and its long-term efficacy have yet to be determined.

Anagrelide

Anagrelide is an orally administered, nonmutagenic drug that has been found to cause a selective lowering of the platelet count in ET. Its cytoreductive mechanism of action probably involves suppression of megakaryocytopoiesis. Platelet counts drop to normal within 12 days of starting the drug in most patients with ET. In addition to its thrombocytopenic effect, anagrelide also has potent antiplatelet activity. Although the initial study did not find serious bleeding complications, this remains a potential risk of this drug in patients with ET who may already have a pre-existing functional platelet defect. Long-term results and toxicity with this experimental drug have not yet been reported.

ANTIPLATELET AGENTS

Most of the experience with antiplatelet drugs in ET has involved the use of aspirin. However, consideration should be given in the future to newer agents that interfere with platelet function, such as ticlopidine, monoclonal antibodies to platelet membrane glycoproteins, and omega-3 fatty acid–containing fish oils. Guidelines for the use of aspirin and other antiplatelet drugs in ET have not been clearly established; therefore, recommendations must be based on largely anecdotal experience in the literature.

As in the case for cytoreductive agents (vide supra), there is no rationale for the use of aspirin in patients with secondary or reactive thrombocytosis. In ET, the decision to use antiplatelet therapy must be strictly individualized and based on clinical history. Laboratory tests (e.g., bleeding time, platelet aggregation studies) have been generally unreliable in predicting the risk of bleeding or thrombosis and are therefore at best of marginal ancillary value in making treatment decisions. Furthermore, the degree of thrombocytosis, however extreme, should not be used to dictate the use of aspirin. When the PVSG conducted a prospective, randomized trial of antiplatelet therapy in PV, it found that a regimen of aspirin (300 mg three times daily) plus persantine (75 mg three times daily) not only failed to prevent thromboembolic complications but actually caused an increased incidence of serious gastrointestinal bleeding. In patients with ET or other myeloproliferative disorders, aspirin can cause an exaggerated prolongation of the bleeding time.

Some general guidelines for the use of aspirin in ET can be proposed based on fragmentary information in the medical literature. Patients with ET with recurrent bleeding problems should be instructed to avoid aspirin. Asymptomatic patients or patients with a mixed history of both bleeding and thrombotic complications probably should not receive aspirin; when its use is found to be necessary in these cases, it should be administered with caution. In contrast, aspirin can be recommended for patients with ET with a history of only thrombosis. Finally, patients with ET who have had either cerebrovascular, coronary, or digital ischemia syndromes should take aspirin regularly. The optimal dose is unknown, but one tablet (300 mg) daily should be adequate, and an enteric-coated preparation can be substituted if there is gastrointestinal intolerance.

It can be concluded that the indiscriminate use of aspirin in ET, even with extreme thrombocytosis, is potentially hazardous. The decision to treat patients with aspirin should be individualized, based primarily on the clinical situation, and reassessed periodically in each case.

SUGGESTED READING

Mitus AJ, Schafer AI. Thrombocytosis and thrombocythemia. Hematol Oncol Clin North Am 1990; 4:157–178.

Murphy S, Iland H, Rosenthal D, et al. Essential thrombocythemia: An interim report from the polycythemia vera study group. Semin Hematol 1986; 23:177–182.

Schafer AI. Bleeding and thrombosis in the myeloproliferative disorders. Blood 1984; 64:1–12.

Schafer AI. Essential thrombocythemia. In: Coller BS, ed. Progress in Hemostasis and Thrombosis. Vol. 10 (in press).

DIAGNOSTIC AND THERAPEUTIC SIGNIFICANCE OF ALTERED GENES IN HEMATOLOGIC MALIGNANCIES

MARK MINDEN, M.D., Ph.D., FRCPC

A variety of recurrent genetic changes have been identified in hematologic malignancies. In some cases the changes are associated with the development of the disease (disease-specific changes), whereas in other instances the changes are related to lineage-specific processes that occur both in normal and malignant cells (disease-associated changes). In clinical medicine, the identification of these genetic events makes it possible to add to diagnostic accuracy and to monitor the presence and progression of the disease; it may also be useful in the choice of therapy. In this chapter I review the methods used to detect genetic changes occurring in hematologic malignancies, illustrate the uses of these techniques in chronic myelogenous leukemia (CML) and acute leukemias, and briefly discuss the application of these methods to the detection of minimal residual disease.

Genetic abnormalities were first detected in hematologic malignancies using metaphase chromosome analysis; the cytogenetic changes include balanced chromosome translocations, loss or addition of specific chromosomes, interstitial deletions, formation of iso chromosomes, and evidence of gene amplification by the presence of marker chromosomes, double minutes and homogenously staining regions. The detection of chromosome abnormalities depends on the availability of fresh cells that are proliferating; the co-existence of normal proliferating bone marrow cells with tumor cells may mask the genetic abnormalities present in the malignant cell population. The abnormality has to be large enough that it can be seen through a microscope. In the case of chromosome translocations, the abnormality must produce different sizes of chromosomes or an altered banding pattern of a chromosome. For interstitial deletions to be observed it is necessary to delete an entire band from a chromosome; an individual band has been estimated to contain a minimum of 10^6

base pairs (bp). Technical problems such as poor metaphase spreads and differential sensitivities of the cells in the sample to hypotonic lysis also can limit the detection of chromosomal alterations. These limitations require that a large number of metaphases be analyzed to maximize the chance of detecting an abnormal metaphase. Despite these problems, cytogenetics has been valuable in directing research aimed at identifying specific genes that are altered in malignant cells using the techniques of modern molecular biology.

The molecular biology methods that are currently employed make it possible to study DNA, RNA, and protein from malignant cells. In the following section the techniques used to study DNA, RNA, and protein in a clinical setting are reviewed and their advantages and limitations discussed. Specific abnormalities and the methods used to detect them are listed in Tables 1 and 2.

EVALUATION OF DNA

One of the most frequently used techniques used to study DNA is Southern blot analysis. In this technique, DNA is digested with specific restriction enzymes, size fractionated by gel electrophoresis, transferred to a solid support, probed with a fragment of the gene of interest, and visualized by autoradiography. Alterations of the mobility of a fragment indicate either point mutation, insertion or deletion of a piece of DNA, or gene rearrangement. To obtain enough DNA for analysis one needs 10^5 to 10^6 cells; unlike cytogenetics, the cells do not need to be proliferating. Although it is possible to obtain DNA from fixed specimens, it is preferable that the DNA be from fresh or frozen cells. The Southern blot technique is relatively insensitive such that in 5 μg of DNA (this is the amount of DNA that can be extracted from approximately 5×10^5 cells) 0.5 to 1 percent of the cells must contain the same new fragment of DNA in order to be detected. Also, the new fragment must be significantly different in size from the normal fragment so that it can be detected. Thus, the Southern blot technique is useful in cases in which a significant proportion of the sample is made up of tumor cells and a relatively large sample is available. The Southern blot technique is most useful for detecting gene rearrangement, insertion or deletion, and point mutation; for the latter the technique is relatively insensitive.

A second more sensitive method is the polymerase

Table 1 Microscopic Chromosomal Abnormalities

Abnormality	Genes Involved and Consequence of Change	Method of Detection
Acute Myeloblastic Leukemia		
t15;17	Retinoic acid receptor α on chromosome 17 and MYL on chromosome 15 forms a fusion protein	C, S, N, P
t8;21	Unknown	C
t9;22	BCR and ABL form a fusion protein	C, S, N, P, F
t1;3	Evi-1 on chromosome 3, dysregulation of transcription	C, S, N, I
Acute Lymphoblastic Leukemia		
t1;19	PBX1 on chromosome 1 and E2a on chromosome 19 form a fusion protein	C, S, N, P
t1;14	Tal-1 on chromosome 1 and TCR δ on chromosome 14, dysregulation of transcription	C, S
t10;14	Tcl-3 on chromosome 10 and TCR δ on chromosome 14	C, S, P
t8;14	c-MYC on chromosome 8 and Ig heavy chain or TCR α on chromosome 14, dysregulation of transcription	C, S
t9;22	BCR and ABL form a fusion protein	C, S, P, F
Chronic Myelogenous Leukemia		
t9;22	BCR and ABL form a fusion protein	C, S, N, P, F
trisomy 8	Unknown	C
iso 17q	Probably abnormal remaining p53	C
Non-Hodgkin's Lymphoma		
t8;14	c-MYC and Ig heavy chain or TCR α	C, S
t2;8	Ig κ light chain and c-MYC, dysregulation of transcription	C, S
t8;22	Ig λ light chain and c-MYC, dysregulation of transcription	C, S
t11;14	Bcl-1 on chromosome 11 and Ig heavy chain on chromosome 14	C, S
t14;18	Bcl-2 on chromosome 18 and Ig heavy chain on chromosome 14, dysregulation of transcription	C, S, P

C = cytogenetics; S = Southern blot; N = Northern blot; P = PCR with sequencing; F = fluorescent in situ hybridization to interphase nuclei; I = immunohistochemistry or immunoprecipitation.

Table 2 Sub-microscopic Chromosomal Abnormalities

Abnormality	Genes Involved and Consequence of Change	Method of Detection
Acute Myelogenous Leukemia		
Point mutation	p53 mutant protein	S, P, I
Point mutation	FMS mutant protein	P
Point mutation	N-RAS or K-RAS mutant protein	P, O
Acute Lymphoblastic Leukemia		
Deletion	5′ of Tal-1 gene dysregulation of transcription	P
Point mutation	p53 mutant protein	P
Chronic Myelogenous Leukemia		
Rearrangement	p53 no protein made or mutant protein	S, P, I
Point mutation	N-RAS mutant protein	P, O

C = cytogenetics; S = Southern blot; N = Northern blot; P = PCR with sequencing; F = fluorescent in situ hybridization to interphase nuclei; I = immunohistochemistry or immunoprecipitation; O = probing with oligonucleotides specific for a point mutation.

chain reaction (PCR). In this technique oligonucleotide primers complementary to opposite strands of DNA and spanning the region of interest are annealed to denatured single-stranded DNA and, in the presence of DNA polymerase, new DNA is produced. By repeating the process of denaturation, annealing of primers, and DNA replication, it is possible to amplify the sequences between the primers 10^6 times in several hours. Point mutations may be detected in the PCR product in a number of ways including (1) direct sequencing; (2) RNase protection; (3) single-strand separation electrophoresis; and (4) probing the PCR product with specific oligonucleotides; with oligonucleotide probes it is possible to detect 1 in 10 cells carrying a specific point mutation. PCR also may be used to detect consistent insertions, deletions, or rearrangements with the ability to identify one tumor cell carrying a specific rearrangement in 10^5 to 10^6 cells. One of the major limitations of PCR is the likelihood of contamination. Because the technique is so sensitive, if even one molecule of cloned DNA gets into a sample, it will be detected. For this reason special precautions must be taken when using PCR; these include having separate sets of pipettes for set up and analysis and using separate rooms for set up and analysis and negative controls in each experiment. Another limitation is the size of the DNA fragment that can be amplified; in general, it is preferable to amplify fragments less than 1 kb in length, although it is possible to amplify fragments up to 4 kb in length.

ANALYSIS OF RNA

Northern blot analysis is used to study the steady state level of expression and size of a specific mRNA. RNA is extracted from 10^6 fresh or frozen cells, separated according to size by gel electrophoresis, transferred to a solid support, and probed for the gene of interest. The presence of a specific RNA may also be determined by in situ hybridization, RNase protection, or PCR. In order to detect an RNA by PCR it is first necessary to convert the RNA template to a DNA template using reverse transcriptase. Once this has been done, the DNA is amplified in the manner described previously. The advantage of the in situ hybridization technique is that it is carried out at a single cell level; however, it is not possible to determine if the RNA is of normal size or sequence with this method. Mutations present in RNA may be detected either by RNase protection or analysis of the PCR product as described earlier. The disadvantage of Northern blot analysis is that it requires relatively large numbers of cells. The disadvantages of PCR are similar to those discussed previously.

ANALYSIS OF PROTEIN

The size and presence of a specific protein may be determined by immunoprecipitation of radiolabeled cellular proteins or by Western blotting. Both of these techniques require a relatively large number of cells. The presence of a specific protein that is relatively abundant can be determined by immunohistochemistry. Although this technique does not give any indication about the size of the protein, it is possible to generate antibodies that are specific to the mutated but not the normal form of a protein. The advantage of this is illustrated in the following section.

SPECIFIC GENETIC ABNORMALITIES OCCURRING IN HEMATOPOIETIC CELLS

Chronic Myelogenous Leukemia

In CML, the Philadelphia chromosome or a variant of it can be found in the leukemic cells of more than 95 percent of patients. The Philadelphia chromosome is part of a balanced translocation involving chromosome 9q34 and 22q11. At a molecular level, the BCR gene on chromosome 22 is joined to the ABL oncogene on chromosome 22, such that the resulting mRNA contains either exon 13 or 14 of BCR adjacent to exon 2 of ABL. A fusion protein of 210 kd with enhanced tyrosine kinase activity and predominantly cytoplasmic localization is produced by this RNA. At the genomic level, the breakpoint in the ABL gene can occur over a span of greater than 100 kb; however, the breakpoints in the BCR gene are clustered over a distance of approximately 4 kb, which is referred to as the major breakpoint cluster region (M-BCR). Using probes derived from the M-BCR and appropriate restriction enzymes, it is possible to detect evidence of the rearrangement by the appearance of a new band on a Southern blot in almost all cases of Philadelphia chromosome–positive CML. Rearrangement of the BCR locus and production of the BCR-ABL fusion protein also are seen in cases with complex three-way translocations that involve chromosomes 9, 22, and another chromosome; also, in some cases in which there is no apparent involvement of chromosomes 9 or 22, there is rearrangement of the BCR and ABL genes. These latter cases with "masked" Philadelphia chromosomes have a clinical course that is similar to that in individuals with Philadelphia chromosome–positive disease. The ease with which one can detect evidence of the Philadelphia chromosome by Southern blot analysis has resulted in the use of this test in the diagnosis and follow up of patients with CML.

The use of interferon and allogeneic or autologous bone marrow transplant can reproducibly result in the disappearance of the Philadelphia chromosome from the bone marrow and the establishment of hemopoiesis from cytogenetically normal cells. We have found that it is convenient, reliable, and cost effective to use Southern blot analysis rather than cytogenetics to monitor the proportion of Philadelphia chromosome–positive cells in CML patients after treatment with interferon or bone marrow transplantation.

The Philadelphia chromosome becomes undetectable in the bone marrow in approximately 20 to 30 percent of patients treated with interferon, with the loss of the Philadelphia chromosome occurring over several months to years. It has been our experience that bone marrow samples from patients on interferon frequently yield no or too few metaphases to assess accurately the percentage of Philadelphia chromosome positive and negative metaphases. Because of this, we have set up a semiquantitative Southern blot analysis to follow patients with CML being treated with interferon. On each gel there is a standard set of samples containing a mixture of DNA from normal bone marrow cells and CML cells in which the amount of CML DNA varies from 0, 1, 5, 10, 20, 50, 75, to 100 percent. By using scanning densitometry and comparing the intensity of the normal BCR germline band to the intensity of the rearranged BCR band it is possible to determine the relative concentration of Philadelphia chromosome positive and negative cells in the patient's sample. The same method can be used to follow the disappearance or the re-emergence of CML cells following bone marrow transplant. However, the loss of the rearranged band does not indicate eradication of CML as Southern blot analysis cannot detect fewer than 0.5 percent leukemic cells. To improve on this result, it is possible to use PCR analysis, which can detect as few as 1 in 10^5 to 10^6 leukemic cells in a sample.

The breakpoint in the ABL gene can occur over a large distance, thus it is not possible to easily apply PCR to the study of genomic DNA; however, the fusion RNA contains either BCR exon 13 or 14 joined to ABL exon 2 and so it is possible to use PCR of RNA to detect the presence of CML cells. This technique has been applied to the study of patients treated with interferon or bone marrow transplantation. In most cases of CML treated with interferon in which the bone marrow has become negative for the Philadelphia chromosome by cytogenetics or Southern blot analysis, the CML clone can still be detected by PCR. Despite this, patients may remain clinically disease free; further study is required to determine the significance and nature of these residual cells. For example, the residual cells may be long-lived B cells that are unlikely to be involved in leukemic relapse. In patients who have had a bone marrow transplant it is not unusual to detect the CML clone by PCR following the transplant for up to 1 year; the presence of CML cells detected by PCR after this time or evidence of increasing numbers of CML cells as detected by PCR does suggest leukemic relapse. Great care against false-positive results caused by contamination must be taken when using the PCR technique for detecting BCR-ABL transcripts.

Over time, the chronic phase of CML gives way to blast crisis. This change is associated with the acquisition of new chromosomal abnormalities including an extra Philadelphia chromosome, trisomy of chromosome 8, and an iso-chromosome 17q. Periodic chromosome evaluation is useful in predicting the development of a blast crisis. Using molecular techniques it has been found that the p53 gene on the short arm of chromosome 17 is frequently rearranged in the leukemic cells of patients with a myeloid blast crisis.

The p53 gene is a nuclear phosphoprotein that has growth suppressing activity and is postulated to be a tumor suppressor gene. The p53 gene product may be rendered inactive by deletion (the p53 gene is deleted from one chromosome by the formation of an iso-17q chromosome), gene rearrangement, which disrupts the gene, and point mutations, which alter the immunophenotype of the protein and its ability to interact with viral antigens such as the large T antigen of SV40. Alterations of p53 may be detected by Southern blot analysis, PCR, and immunohistochemistry. Southern blot analysis will demonstrate only gross rearrangements of the gene and not point mutations. To detect point mutations investigators have used PCR to amplify specific exons from genomic DNA or the coding region of RNA. The PCR product is then sequenced to detect point mutations. Recently a monoclonal antibody has been developed that reacts with mutant forms of the protein but not the native protein. This antibody can be used to detect mutant forms of p53 either by immunoprecipitation or on fixed cells. It will be interesting to determine if the emergence of mutant p53 cells, as detected by flow cytometry, will predict impending myeloid blast crisis. If this proves to be the case, it may be possible to screen for such cells on a routine basis and when they first appear either give high-dose conventional chemotherapy or proceed to bone marrow transplantation with the aim of eradicating the mutant p53 clone.

The previous discussion illustrates the means by which it is possible to use molecular techniques to diagnose a certain disease, to detect small numbers of malignant cells, and to identify progression of the disease. Similar approaches can be used to identify and use other genetic abnormalities that have been characterized at the molecular level (see Table 1). The abnormalities discussed earlier represent disease-specific changes. It is also possible to evaluate malignant cells using disease-associated genetic changes.

Examples of disease-associated molecular changes are the rearrangements of the immunoglobulin (Ig) and T cell antigen receptor genes (TCR). During normal development of B cells and T cells their antigen recognition genes must undergo somatic rearrangement before a functional protein can be produced. Through this process of rearrangement one of a number of variable or V genes is juxtaposed to a diversity (D) or joining (J) segment; the joining is imprecise, and a variable number of extra nucleotides are added (this is N region diversity and is unique for each rearrangement). In a clonal population of cells it is possible to detect rearranged genes by Southern blot analysis. In a polyclonal population, however, because of the large number of possible rearrangements and hence a great variation in the size of the resulting rearranged fragment, one observes a smear rather than a discrete band. In order to see a discrete band a clone of cells possessing the same rearrangement pattern must constitute more than 0.5 percent of cells. This can then be used to advantage to study malignant populations of cells, which by their nature are clonal proliferations.

In clinical practice it is occasionally difficult to determine whether the expansion of hemopoietic cells is clonal and whether they belong to the B cell, T cell, or myeloid lineage. Some light can be shed on this problem by performing Southern blot analysis using probes to the Ig heavy and light chain loci and to the TCR β, γ, and δ loci. The finding of a rearranged band using any one of these probes indicates that one is dealing with a clonal expansion of cells; some caution must be used in interpreting results of TCR γ as there is a limited number of possible rearrangements; in general, this probe should not be used as the sole indicator of clonality.

During B cell development the Ig heavy chain gene rearranges before the κ light chain gene, which rearranges before the λ light chain genes. The finding of both Ig heavy and light chain gene rearrangements indicates that the tumor is of the B cell lineage. However, only Ig heavy chain gene rearrangements have been found in a significant number of cases of acute myeloid leukemia. In the case in which there is only Ig heavy chain rearrangement, the assignment of lineage must take into account other information such as cell morphology, cell surface phenotype, and the expression of lineage-specific genes.

During T cell development the TCR genes undergo rearrangement. From studies of the thymus it appears that the order of rearrangement is TCR δ before γ, before β, before α. Owing to the dispersal of the Jα segments over approximately 85 kb, it is not convenient to study rearrangements of TCR α. Rearrangements of the TCR genes occur in T cell malignancies but also are seen in B cell tumors and acute myeloid leukemia. It is not unusual to see TCR and Ig rearrangements in B cell malignancies, although the converse, that is TCR and Ig rearrangements in T cell malignancies, is uncommon. TCR gene rearrangements are a convenient means for detecting clonality, and the finding of a rearranged TCR gene suggests that the malignancy is of T cell origin; however, because of the finding of TCR gene rearrangements in non-T cell malignancies, the assignment of lineage must take into account all of the available information including other gene rearrangements and cell surface markers. It has been suggested that the best marker of the T cell lineage is CD3 either on the cell surface or in the cytoplasm.

For routine clinical samples it is convenient to use the Southern blot technique. This technique is relatively insensitive, however, and is not useful for detecting minimal residual disease; the sensitivity of detecting small numbers of residual leukemic cells can be increased by using PCR that has been adapted to identify either Ig heavy chain or TCR γ gene rearrangements. To detect Ig heavy chain gene rearrangements that are specific to the leukemic clone it is necessary to identify the sequence generated by the joining of V, D, and J segments and the intervening N regions. With this knowledge, a patient-specific primer can be made. By using the patient-specific primer and a second primer that is found in all J regions, it is possible to distinguish gene rearrangement that occurred in the leukemic cells from gene rearrangements that occurred in contaminating normal B cells. As mentioned above, it is necessary to avoid contamination of any of the reagents used for PCR because contamination may give a false-positive result.

Minimal Residual Disease

Following chemotherapy of leukemia and lymphoma it is possible to obtain complete remissions, defined by the disappearance of masses and in the case of leukemia fewer than 5 percent blast cells in the bone marrow. Unfortunately, disease frequently recurs, indicating that the definition of remission is optimistic. As illustrated above, it is possible to improve the detection of residual leukemia or lymphoma cells. In addition to the PCR-based methods described, immunohistochemical methods based on the aberrant expression of proteins can detect one tumor cell in 10^4 cells. Although classic cytogenetics is an insensitive technique for detecting residual leukemic cells, in situ hybridization can be used to detect specific chromosomal abnormalities in interphase nuclei. For example, if the leukemic cells have a specific translocation, cells containing the translocation can be detected by using probes to either side of the breakpoint; depending on the number of cells screened, it is possible to detect very infrequent tumor cells.

The significance of finding residual leukemic cells is not clear. In one study in which residual AML cells were detected by aberrant expression of cell surface markers, patients who had residual disease relapsed at a faster rate than patients whose bone marrow was negative in the assay; however, relapses did occur in both groups. In the case of CML following bone marrow transplantation, the presence of BCR-ABL–positive cells can persist for up to 1 year and not indicate impending relapse. On the other hand, the appearance of BCR-ABL–positive cells in patients who were previously negative does predict relapse.

At our center we have followed patients with CML after bone marrow transplantation with Southern blot analysis. Patients who show re-emergence of the CML clone have been treated with interferon with subsequent reversion to the negative state. We are in the process of carrying out PCR analysis of the bone marrow of these patients to see if the negative state is due to the reduction of the Philadelphia chromosome–positive cells to a level below the sensitivity of the Southern blot assay or the eradication of the leukemic clone.

As the techniques for detecting residual leukemic cells become easier to apply it will be possible to test the value of early intervention in diseases such as AML, ALL, and lymphoma.

SUGGESTED READING

Brisco MJ, Tan LW, Orsborn AM, et al. Development of a highly sensitive assay, based on the polymerase chain reaction, for rare B-lymphocyte clones in a polyclonal population. Br J Haematol 1990; 75:163–167.

Campana D, Coustan-Smith E, Janossy G. The immunologic detection of minimal residual disease in acute leukemia. Blood 1990; 76:163–171.

Deane M, Norton JD. Immunoglobulin gene "fingerprinting": An approach to analysis of B lymphoid clonality in lymphoproliferative disorders. Br J Haematol 1991; 77:274–281.

Gorska-Flipot I, Norman C, Addy L, et al. Molecular pathology of chronic myelogenous leukemia. Tumor Biology 1990; 11(Suppl 1):25–43.

Hughes TP, Morgan GJ, Martiat P, et al. Detection of residual leukemia after bone marrow transplantation for chronic myeloge-nous leukemia: Role of polymerase chain reaction in predicting relapse. Blood 1991; 77:874–878.

Lane DP, Benchimol S. p53: Oncogene or anti-oncogene? Genes and Development 1990; 4:1–8.

Tkachuk DC, Westbrook CA, Andreeff M, et al. Detection of bcr-abl fusion in chronic myelogenous leukemia by in situ hybridization. Science 1990; 250:559–562.

PREVENTION AND TREATMENT OF INFECTIONS IN NEUTROPENIC HOSTS

COLEMAN ROTSTEIN, M.D., FRCPC

Infections are a significant cause of morbidity and mortality in neutropenic patients with malignant disorders despite the remarkable progress that has been made in their prevention, recognition, and therapy. Infection has been identified as the cause of death in 60, 65, and 40 percent of patients with leukemia, lymphoma, and solid tumors, respectively. The armamentarium of antineoplastic chemotherapy and radiation continues to improve survival, but simultaneously has rendered those exposed more susceptible to opportunistic pathogens. In addition, supportive care measures such as the use of implanted venous access devices although facilitating patient care and enhancing survival have also predisposed patients to an increased risk of infection.

Compromised host defenses and their interrelationship with endogenous and exogenous microflora play key roles in determining the types of infection seen in cancer patients. Neutrophils are the most important cellular defense against infection. Neutropenia, if present, is the overriding host defense defect predisposing patients with cancer to infection. Other important factors interacting with neutropenia and predisposing neutropenic patients to infection are a breakdown in host physical defense barriers (i.e., the integumentary system and mucous membranes), colonizing microflora, and the microflora present in the patient's immediate environment. It is well known that a breakdown in host physical defense barriers such as a mucositis secondary to chemotherapy provides an excellent portal of entry for microorganisms. In fact, the bacteria that have colonized various surfaces and orifices of the body become pathogens. Similarly, in the case of aspergillosis, organisms acquired from the host's immediate environment and usually acting as colonizers of the lung become virulent pathogens.

The most common microorganisms causing infections in neutropenic patients are bacteria, fungi, and viruses. Parasites such as *Pneumocystis carinii* and *Toxoplasma gondii* are unusual pathogens in neutropenic patients. *Pneumocystis carinii* infections most often occur after neutrophil recovery in patients with an underlying T-cell defect such as those with lymphoma or acute lymphocytic leukemia.

Bacterial isolates predominate among pathogens in neutropenic patients and account for approximately 60 percent of documented infections. Although previously gram-negative bacilli were the most common pathogens isolated, currently gram-positive isolates have superceded them whether or not patients are receiving antibacterial prophylaxis. This may be related to the upsurge in the use of central venous access devices. Initial bacterial isolates include coagulase-negative staphylococci, *Staphylococcus aureus*, viridans streptococci, *Enterobacteriaceae*, and *Pseudomonas aeruginosa* (Table 1). Bacterial infections occurring later in the course of chemotherapy are caused by more resistant organisms such as *Corynebacterium jeikeium*, *Xanthomonas maltophilia*, and anaerobes. It should be noted that the incidence and severity of bacterial infections are inversely proportional to the absolute neutrophil count and the duration of neutropenia. The most common sites of bacterial infection in neutropenic patients are the bloodstream, lungs, skin, oral pharynx, and perianal area. In general, the organism producing infection in these areas is the organism that previously colonized these areas.

Invasive fungal infections are frequent in patients rendered neutropenic by antineoplastic chemotherapy. Autopsy studies have revealed that 30 to 50 percent of the patients with hematologic malignancies have histopathologically documented invasive fungal infections. Candidiasis and aspergillosis are the most common fungal infections observed in neutropenic cancer patients. Candidiasis may present early in the course of neutropenia, whereas aspergillosis usually manifests itself after approximately 3 weeks of profound neutropenia (neutrophil count $< 0.5 \times 10^9$ per L). Hepatosplenic candidiasis, which occurs later in the clinical course, is a particularly difficult problem both diagnostically and therapeutically.

Owing to our inability to diagnose viral infections, the full extent of these infections is still unrecognized in neutropenic cancer patients. Reactivated herpes simplex and varicella-zoster infections account for the bulk of

Table 1 Organisms Causing Infections in Neutropenic Cancer Patients

Bacteria	Fungi	Viruses	Parasites
Early	Early	Herpes Simplex	*Pneumocystis carinii*
Gram positive	*Candida*	Cytomegalovirus	*Toxoplasma gondii*
Coagulase-negative staphylococci		Varicella-Zoster	
Staphylococcus aureus			
Streptococcus viridans			
Gram negative			
Enterobacteriaceae			
Pseudomonas aeruginosa			
Late	Late		
Gram positive	*Aspergillus*		
Corynebacterium jeikeium	*Zygomycetes*		
Gram negative	*Trichosporon*		
Xanthomonas maltophilia	*Fusarium*		
Multiply resistant species			
Anaerobes			

these infections. The contribution of cytomegalovirus (whether primary or reactivated disease) to febrile episodes in neutropenic patients is undergoing investigation. Viral infections may occur at any time during the neutropenic period and may produce more severe illness in neutropenic hosts than in immunocompetent hosts.

PREVENTION OF INFECTION IN NEUTROPENIC HOSTS

Infectious complications expose patients to potentially toxic antimicrobial agents and increase the costs of cancer treatment. Moreover, infectious complications may precipitate modifications in the dose intensity of antineoplastic therapy, potentially compromising successful treatment of the malignancy. Considerable effort has, therefore, been directed toward reducing infectious morbidity.

Infections in neutropenic patients arise predominantly from endogenous sources through either colonization of mucosal surfaces and skin or reactivation of a latent infection. In addition, another mode of infection transmission may be from environmental sources including foods (*Pseudomonas* can be found on fresh fruit and vegetables), air *(Aspergillus),* and contact with medical personnel who do not practice good hand washing technique. As a result, investigators have endeavored to interrupt these mechanisms of transmission with prophylactic nontoxic antimicrobial agents and environmental controls (Fig. 1). These attempts, however, have met with mixed results.

Prevention of Bacterial Infections

Environmental Control Measures

Total protective isolation (TPI) was conceived as a means of preventing the neutropenic host from acquiring pathogenic bacteria from the environment. A sterile environment is achieved by cleaning the patient's immediate area using high-efficiency particulate air (HEPA) filters and disinfection of all physical surfaces. Food and water are prepared to lower their microbial burden. In conjunction with TPI, rigorous washing of the skin and the use of oral nonabsorbable antimicrobials (gentamicin, vancomycin, nystatin, colistin, bacitracin, and neomycin) are employed to suppress endogenous microflora.

The frequency of bacterial infectious complications in neutropenic patients housed in TPI and using oral nonabsorbable antibiotics was significantly lower than the frequency noted for controls in a number of controlled clinical trials. Also, when TPI was compared with conventional ward care, fewer bacterial infections were observed. Although TPI lowered the incidence of bacterial infection, it had no impact on the survival of neutropenic hosts. With the more potent parenteral antibacterial agents available today, the potential attraction of TPI leading to fewer bacterial infections without prolonged survival has faded. The high costs of TPI and problems with compliance have placed this method of infection prevention in disfavor.

Reverse isolation, that is, isolation without HEPA filtration, is costly and poses a psychological burden for patients. This type of isolation may actually impede care by health care personnel while offering no additional protection for the patient. Reverse isolation has no advantage over a strict hand washing policy.

Oral Nonabsorbable Antibiotics

To eliminate the need for isolation, oral nonabsorbable antibiotics have been administered to reduce bacterial infections. These antibiotics have successfully suppressed the gastrointestinal tract reservoir of bacteria in clinical trials, but have no impact on microorganisms colonizing other body sites. As a result, infections still occurred at other sites. Moreover, owing to the drawbacks of cost, compliance, and the emergence of resistance, oral nonabsorbable antibiotics should not play a major role in attempts to prevent infectious complications in neutropenic cancer patients.

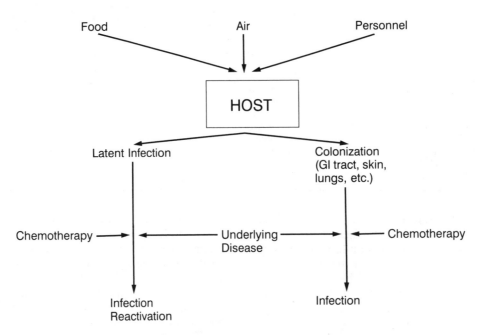

Figure 1 Pathogenesis of infection.

Oral Absorbable Antibiotics

The rationale for using oral absorbable antibiotics is to achieve therapeutic blood levels of the drugs in an effort to prevent bacterial infection. Activity against both gram-positive and gram-negative bacteria is necessary because these are common pathogens in neutropenic cancer patients. Drugs that have been employed for this purpose include nalidixic acid, trimethoprim-sulfamethoxazole (TMP-S), and the quinolones, norfloxacin and ciprofloxacin. Of the aforementioned antimicrobials, resistance emerged quickly to nalidixic acid.

Besides having activity against gram-positive and gram-negative bacteria, TMP-S has the additional attribute of protecting against *Pneumocystis carinii* pneumonia. This is of particular benefit to neutropenic patients with T-cell dysfunction such as those with lymphoma and acute lymphocytic leukemia. The initial enthusiasm for TMP-S prophylaxis has diminished. The cumulative results from a number of trials have shown that TMP-S does not decrease the number of febrile days or the need for parenteral antibiotics, or increase survival. Nevertheless, TMP-S does decrease the incidence of microbiologically documented infections, particularly gram-negative bacteremia and concomitant septic shock. TMP-S is superior to trimethoprim alone for the prevention of infectious complications in neutropenic patients. One must also be cognizant of the emergence of resistant organisms and fungi with the use of TMP-S and the prolonged neutrophil recovery that has been reported.

The quinolones, norfloxacin and particularly cipro-floxacin, are currently the best candidates for the prevention of bacterial infections in neutropenic hosts. Both agents have been demonstrated to be effective in reducing the incidence of both gram-positive and gram-negative bacterial infections in controlled clinical trials. In fact, ciprofloxacin's efficacy in preventing infection surpassed that of TMP-S plus colistin. One must be cautious though about the emergence of resistant gram-positive organisms such as viridans streptococci as major pathogens in patients taking quinolone prophylaxis.

The role that selective decontamination plays in preventing bacterial infection in neutropenic patients is unclear. The rationale for selective decontamination is the preservation of anaerobic flora of the gastrointestinal tract making it more difficult for newly acquired organisms such as aerobic gram-negative bacilli to gain a foothold. Both nonabsorbable (colistin, polymyxin) and absorbable oral antibiotics (TMP-S, quinolones) suppress aerobic pathogens and preserve colonization resistance; however, clinical studies have demonstrated the emergence of resistant gram-negative bacilli even though colonization resistance has been achieved. Moreover, the systemic absorption of drugs such as TMP-S and ciprofloxacin casts serious doubt on the fact that one is merely observing the effect of colonization resistance.

Prevention of Fungal Infections

Invasive fungal infections are a major infectious complication among neutropenic patients with cancer.

Although bacterial infections are most likely to occur during the first week of profound neutropenia, the prospect of developing an invasive fungal infection increases dramatically beyond the initial week of profound neutropenia. Fungal infections are often life-threatening, as evidenced by their prevalence in autopsy studies. In addition, these infections pose a number of problems for clinicians. First, it may be difficult for a clinician to make an early diagnosis of invasive fungal infection. Second, few agents effective for the treatment of these infections are available, and those that are effective in vitro often are not as effective in human infections. This observation underscores the lack of adequate standardized in vitro susceptibility testing for fungi. Third, even if a diagnosis is made and effective therapy is available, we often do not know when to stop therapy. As a result, prevention of fungal infections is imperative.

The most common invasive fungal infections in neutropenic hosts are candidiasis, aspergillosis, zygomycosis, and trichosporosis. By far, candidiasis is the most frequent, followed by aspergillosis; however, the pathogenesis of these invasive fungal infections is quite disparate. It is generally accepted that the gastrointestinal tract constitutes a major reservoir for *Candida* sp., although *Candida* also may be isolated from the skin. Exogenous sources for *Candida* such as food, intravenous catheters, and fluid are far less frequent.

Aspergillosis, on the other hand, is mainly an air-borne disease, and outbreaks among neutropenic patients are usually due to heavy air contamination.

Owing to the different pathogenesis of the most common fungal infections, prevention of invasive fungal infections among neutropenic patients has focused on environmental control measures and chemoprophylaxis.

Environmental Control Measures

Simple hygienic measures such as careful hand washing are effective in reducing the interpersonal transmission of *Candida* organisms. Restricting the patient's diet to cooked foods also may be beneficial. To prevent aspergillosis, plants and flowers must be prohibited in the neutropenic patient's environment. Vigilant surveillance of the environment and patients during both interior and exterior construction may be predictive of the development of invasive aspergillosis in these predisposed hosts.

More specifically, TPI has been employed to reduce the incidence of invasive fungal infections in neutropenic hosts. TPI in combination with nystatin was effective in reducing the incidence of both disseminated and localized candidiasis. Moreover, as *Aspergillus* conidia are ubiquitous in the environment, TPI with HEPA filters has been demonstrated to reduce the incidence of aspergillosis among neutropenic hosts in medical centers where this infection is a problem. The removal of conidia from the air by HEPA filtration drastically reduces the morbidity and mortality due to aspergillosis. However, such units are very expensive. TPI with HEPA filters should only be advocated to protect patients in situations in which a high incidence of aspergillosis exists among neutropenic patients with cancer. Otherwise, housing neutropenic patients in private rooms, provided that the ambient hospital air meets present day engineering standards, and enforcing a strict hand washing policy are sufficient and more cost-effective.

Chemoprophylaxis

Oral chemoprophylaxis is a cost effective means of preventing invasive fungal infections in neutropenic patients, but it has not met expectations. Most of the available oral antifungal agents have been evaluated for the prevention of candidiasis. Whether a specific regimen is effective in reducing the incidence of disseminated disease remains controversial. Among orally administered polyenes (nystatin and amphotericin B), nystatin has been proved to be ineffective, and trials of oral amphotericin B have produced divergent results. Despite a reduction in yeast colonization, inconsistent results were seen for invasive candidiasis.

Because of its ease of administration, ketoconazole has been most extensively studied among the imidazoles. Ketoconazole at a dose of 400 mg per day had a beneficial effect in neutropenic cancer patients. Concerns about its absorption, hepatic side effects, and the emergence of fungal resistance (*Candida glabrata* and *Aspergillus*) remain. Recently developed triazoles such as fluconazole and itraconazole also have been employed prophylactically. Early findings have noted that fluconazole in particular has reduced the frequency of invasive candidiasis in neutropenic cancer patients. Fluconazole may, in fact, be the drug of choice for fungal prophylaxis. Further studies are underway with other triazoles.

Although intravenous miconazole has been used for the prevention of fungal sepsis, it did not reduce the need for empiric parenteral amphotericin B in febrile neutropenic patients. Topical clotrimazole troches were ineffective in preventing invasive fungal infection in neutropenic patients.

Orally administered antifungal agents have been of no benefit in preventing aspergillosis, which is an airborne infection. Clinical investigations assessing the potential value of fluconazole and itraconazole for the prevention of aspergillosis are yet to be completed. There are some preliminary findings that indicate that intranasally inhaled amphotericin B may be of benefit in preventing invasive pulmonary aspergillosis. Once the diagnosis of invasive aspergillosis has been made in a neutropenic host, the prophylactic administration of intravenous amphotericin B for subsequent chemotherapy-induced neutropenic episodes has been shown to be effective.

Prevention of Viral Infections

Reactivated herpes simplex virus infections are a significant cause of morbidity in immunocompromised patients. These reactivated infections occur in more than 50 percent of adult patients receiving timed sequential chemotherapy for acute leukemia who had pretreatment complement fixation titers 1:16 or higher. Acyclovir has been found to be an effective inhibitor of herpes simplex virus. Acyclovir at a dosage of 250 mg/m^2 every 8 hours intravenously, beginning 3 days after the first day of chemotherapy and continuing for a total of 32 days or less if the patient is discharged, is effective in preventing herpes simplex virus infection in patients with acute leukemia. Oral acyclovir at a dosage of 400 mg five times a day has also been effective prophylaxis in bone marrow transplant recipients. Both oral and intravenous acyclovir are recommended for prophylaxis in patients with malignancy and anticipated chemotherapy-induced neutropenia if pretreatment antibody titers are 1:16 or higher.

In summary, a number of issues have been raised relating to antibacterial, antifungal, and antiviral prophylaxis in neutropenic cancer patients (Table 2). A number of questions remain to be answered. Clearly, most neutropenic patients can be cared for in a private room; strict hand washing technique should be adhered to to prevent the transmission of pathogens from personnel and the environment if the ambient hospital air attains present day engineering standards. TPI would be useful only if one knows that a significant incidence of airborne infections such as aspergillosis exists. Patients with anticipated neutrophil counts of less than 0.5 × 10^9 per L for 7 days or longer do benefit from antibacterial and antifungal prophylaxis. The prophylaxis should be initiated within 24 hours of starting antineoplastic chemotherapy and continued until neutrophil recovery or parenteral antibacterial and antifungal therapeutic agents, respectively, are initiated. For patients with acute nonlymphocytic leukemia and autologous bone marrow transplantation, ciprofloxacin 500 mg given orally twice per day should be the antibacterial prophylactic agent of choice combined with fluconazole, 200 to 400 mg per day orally, as antifungal prophylaxis. For patients with acute lymphocytic leukemia and lymphoma, TMP-S (160 mg trimethoprim twice a day), which provides additional protection against *Pneumocystis carinii* pneumonia, should be employed in combination with fluconazole. If a patient with a solid tumor is anticipated to have a neutrophil count of less than 0.5 × 10^9 per L for 7 days or longer after receiving intensive chemotherapy, ciprofloxacin in conjunction with fluconazole is appropriate. Acyclovir prophylaxis may be employed for all patients receiving chemotherapy with anticipated

neutropenia if their prechemotherapy herpes simplex antibody titers are 1:16 or higher.

Future Prospects for Preventing Bacterial and Fungal Infections in Neutropenic Patients

Trials are currently underway evaluating the effects of granulocyte-macrophage colony-stimulating factor (GM-CSF) on neutropenia. Recombinant GM-CSF has been observed to reduce the time of significant neutropenia associated with chemotherapy in solid tumors and lymphomas. Its effectiveness in neutropenia related to antileukemic therapy remains to be evaluated. The role of immunotherapy in preventing infection in neutropenic patients is under investigation.

TREATMENT OF INFECTIONS IN NEUTROPENIC HOSTS

Despite intensive infection prevention programs, the clinical course of patients with neutropenia continues to be complicated by fever and infection. The development of infection is significantly influenced by the level of neutropenia (significant neutropenia being defined as less than 1.0 × 10^9 per L neutrophils), the duration of neutropenia, and the rate of decline in neutrophil count. Fever (defined by a single temperature of 38.3° C or higher or 38° C or higher over at least 1 hour) is invariably present as an early sign of infection. Sixty percent of such febrile episodes have been reported to represent microbiologically or clinically documented infections. As mentioned previously, bacterial isolates account for the majority of infections in neutropenic patients and are usually the cause of initial infections. However, the incidence of invasive fungal infections is rising. Infections in neutropenic hosts still remain difficult to diagnose and are frequently refractory to standard modalities. Failure to initiate therapy early in the course of the infection is a cause for significant morbidity and mortality among these patients.

Treatment of Bacterial Infections

Gram-positive isolates such as coagulase-negative staphylococci, *Staphylococcus aureus,* and streptococci are now responsible for the majority of bacterial infections in neutropenic patients. Nevertheless, gram-

Table 2 Summary of Prophylaxis in Neutropenic Cancer Patients

	Acute nonlymphocytic leukemia; Autologous bone marrow transplants	Acute lymphocytic leukemia, Lymphoma	Solid tumors
Antibacterial	Ciprofloxacin	TMP-S	Ciprofloxacin
Antifungal	Fluconazole	Fluconazole	Fluconazole
Antiviral-Herpes Simplex	Acyclovir	Acyclovir	Acyclovir

negative isolates are still common. *Escherichia coli, Klebsiella* sp., and *Pseudomonas aeruginosa* comprise the majority of initial gram-negative pathogens.

Empiric therapy with broad-spectrum antibiotics administered with the development of fever or the first sign of infection is now a universally accepted principle. The use of antimicrobial agents active against gram-negative pathogens is mandatory because of the rapid clinical deterioration that can occur when a neutropenic patient develops a gram-negative bacillary infection. However, the specific composition of the empiric antibiotic therapy remains controversial.

In choosing the initial antibiotic regimen, one should consider the type, incidence, and antibiotic susceptibility of bacterial isolates usually seen in neutropenic patients. Issues also to be taken into consideration include penicillin allergy; renal or hepatic dysfunction; and the co-administration of nephrotoxic drugs such as cisplatin, amphotericin B, vancomycin, and aminoglycosides. Recommended therapeutic options are a combination of an aminoglycoside with an antipseudomonal beta-lactam, the combination of two broad-spectrum antipseudomonal beta-lactam antibiotics, monotherapy with a single broad-spectrum antipseudomonal beta-lactam antibiotic, or vancomycin with a combination of an antipseudomonal beta-lactam and an aminoglycoside.

The use of a broad-spectrum antipseudomonal beta-lactam (ticarcillin [with or without clavulanic acid], mezlocillin, piperacillin, azlocillin, cefoperazone, ceftazidime, or imipenem-cilastatin) plus an aminoglycoside (gentamicin, tobramycin, or amikacin) has been extensively evaluated in clinical trials. The advantages of combination antibacterial therapy are potential synergistic effects against gram-negative bacilli and minimal emergence of resistance. The disadvantages are the lack of activity of these combinations against resistant gram-positive isolates and the nephrotoxicity and ototoxicity associated with aminoglycosides. A variation on this approach with beta-lactams such as ceftazidime and imipenem-cilastatin, is the concept of "front-loading" with an aminoglycoside. Although the aminoglycoside and ceftazidime or imipenem-cilastatin combination is commenced initially, the aminoglycoside is stopped after 72 hours if no microbiologically or clinically documented infection is present. Thereafter, only the broad-spectrum beta-lactam is continued.

The double beta-lactam regimen (e.g., cefoperazone-mezlocillin or piperacillin, ceftazidime-piperacillin, etc.) is a less toxic but still synergistic combination. There are the disadvantages of high cost, the emergence of resistant organisms, and possible antagonism of the beta-lactams with certain bacterial infections.

Ceftazidime or imipenem-cilastatin alone have been employed successfully as empiric therapy in febrile neutropenic patients with cancer. This type of "monotherapy" is useful in patients with pre-existing renal dysfunction. However, concerns remain regarding the development of resistant organisms.

In centers where methicillin-resistant coagulase-negative staphylococci, methicillin-resistant *S. aureus,* and *Corynebacterium* sp. are frequent pathogens in febrile neutropenic patients, vancomycin may be included in the initial regimen; however, this remains controversial. Such regimens include vancomycin plus an aminoglycoside and an antipseudomonal beta-lactam, or vancomycin in combination with ceftazidime or imipenem-cilastatin. The mortality rate associated with gram-positive infections is drastically lower than that which occurs with gram-negative infections, whereas the cost and potential toxicity of vancomycin are considerable; however, one must balance this with the fact that in two clinical trials the inclusion of vancomycin resulted in more rapid resolution of the first infection fever, fewer days of bacteremia, and fewer instances of treatment failure. An approach to this issue may be the use of a combination of an antipseudomonal beta-lactam with an aminoglycoside initially because of the likelihood of gram-negative infections in those neutropenic patients not on antibacterial prophylaxis, with the option of adding vancomycin later. As for those febrile neutropenic patients taking an antibacterial prophylactic agent such as ciprofloxacin or TMP-S who have a low probability of developing gram-negative infection but may have a resistant gram-positive infection, vancomycin with ceftazidime or imipenem-cilastatin is a reasonable alternative as initial therapy. Vancomycin should be included in the initial antibiotic regimen if evidence of a central venous access device infection such as a cellulitis exists.

For microbiologically or clinically documented infections and fevers of unknown origin that respond to the initial antibiotic regimen, antibiotic therapy should be continued for a minimum of 7 days and until the neutrophil count rises to higher than 0.5×10^9 per L for longer than 48 hours (Fig. 2). Should resistant bacteria be isolated, adjustment of the initial regimen to cover these microorganisms is necessary. In the case of a fever of unknown origin, if the patient remains febrile beyond the initial 72 hours, one may consider adding vancomycin intravenously to the empiric regimen. Another option in such a febrile patient would include the initiation of antianaerobic coverage (metronidazole or clindamycin) if the patient's clinical course suggests evidence of mucositis or an infection of gastrointestinal origin.

A fever persisting for 5 days in a profoundly neutropenic patient with a microbiologically or clinically documented infection or fever of unknown origin mandates a meticulous reassessment of the patient. If no focus of infection is determined, there is strong support for the addition of empiric parenteral amphotericin B by day 5 to 7 of antibiotic therapy. The use of amphotericin B in febrile neutropenic patients will be discussed further below. If the neutrophil count rises higher than 0.5×10^9 per L for longer than 48 hours and no infection is evident in a continuously febrile patient, one may consider stopping antibiotic therapy and watching expectantly.

The duration of antibiotic therapy in febrile neu-

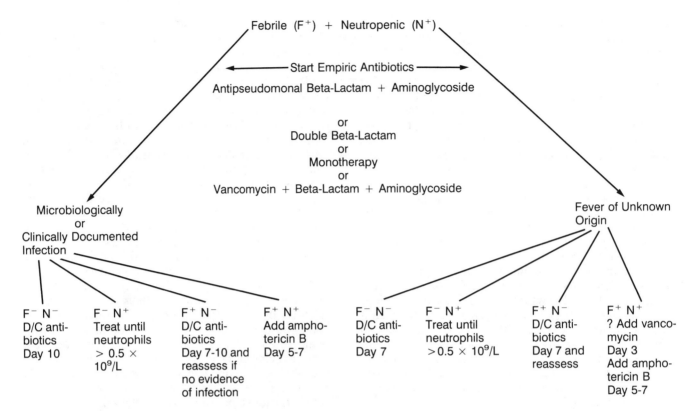

Figure 2 Approach to empiric antibiotic and antifungal therapy in febrile neutropenic patients.

tropenic patients is not well defined. The single most important determinant of the duration of therapy is the neutrophil count. Once the neutrophil count surpasses 0.5×10^9 per L, the likelihood of the persistence or recrudescence of infection or fever is greatly diminished, and antibiotics may be discontinued providing no focus of infection exists. When neutropenia persists, antibiotic therapy should be maintained until the neutrophil count exceeds 0.5×10^9 per L for more than 48 hours.

Treatment of Fungal Infections

As mentioned previously, fungal infections are well-documented sequelae of chemotherapy-induced neutropenia and a cause of significant mortality in neutropenic cancer patients. These infections are usually manifested beyond the first week of profound neutropenia with candidiasis appearing early in the neutropenic course. Other fungal infections such as aspergillosis, zygomycosis, and trichosporosis are caused by more resistant pathogens that emerge later. The increasing prevalence of fungal infections centers around enhanced survival during the early phases of marrow aplasia owing to advances in the treatment of bacterial infection and other supportive care modalities such as blood product support and the management of the tumor lysis syndrome. Although these measures have prolonged survival, they have rendered the patient more immunosuppressed and more susceptible to fungal

infection. In addition, the prolonged use of antibacterial agents has enhanced fungal overgrowth in the gastrointestinal tract, the primary focus of these fungal pathogens. Indeed, most *Candida* infections are of endogenous origin, whereas infections such as aspergillosis are acquired exogenously.

Antifungal therapy may be subdivided into therapy for documented fungal infections and empiric therapy. At present, therapy for documented fungal infections accounts for a smaller proportion of antifungal therapeutic courses than empiric therapy. Therapy for documented fungal infections is directed against fungemias, pneumonias, and cellulitis often caused by resistant organisms. The agent of choice is currently amphotericin B at a dose of 0.6 to 1.0 mg per kg per day. At times, 5-fluorocytosine has to be added. Imidazoles have produced inconsistent results for such infections in neutropenic patients.

It is well known that the majority of fungal infections in febrile neutropenic patients are occult. In the past, these infections were not diagnosed until autopsy. The lack of inflammatory effector cells in these patients mutes localizing tissue-specific physical signs, making clinical findings characteristically nonspecific early in the course of infection. Invasive procedures are often contraindicated because of marrow aplasia, and fungal antigen or antibody detection systems have provided inconclusive results. As a result, the empiric use of antifungal therapy after 5 to 7 days of refractory fever has gained support because of the observed clinical response. Here also, amphotericin B (0.6 mg per kg per day intravenously) is the agent of choice. The empiric use of the new triazoles for this indication is under investigation.

Indications for empiric amphotericin B include the following clinical scenarios: the failure of a neutropenic patient with a microbiologically or clinically documented bacterial infection (that is not related to central venous catheter placement) to respond to 5 to 7 days of appropriate antibacterial therapy with no new evidence of bacterial infection present but colonization with the same species of fungus at two body sites; the failure of a neutropenic patient with a fever of unknown origin to respond to 5 to 7 days of appropriate antibacterial therapy; the recurrence of fever with no obvious focus of infection in a neutropenic patient who initially responded to antibacterial therapy and was afebrile for at least 4 days but now is colonized with the same species of fungus at two body sites; and a neutropenic patient with a focal pulmonary infiltrate unresponsive to 5 to 7 days of antibacterial therapy.

Although amphotericin B therapy is associated with toxicity, its benefits far outweigh its drawbacks when employed for both empiric and documented fungal infections in neutropenic patients.

Treatment of Viral Infections

The treatment of viral infections in neutropenic patients is still in its infancy. Acyclovir is the mainstay of therapy for both herpes simplex and varicella-zoster infections. Oral acyclovir (200 mg five times a day for 7 to 10 days) is effective treatment for mild herpes simplex mucositis. The intravenous form (5 mg per kg every 8 hours) used for moderate to severe infections and those patients who cannot tolerate the oral form. For patients with varicella-zoster infections, intravenous acyclovir (500 mg per M^2 every 8 hours for 7 days) is employed.

Recently, ganciclovir has been approved for the treatment of cytomegalovirus infections. Responses are generally favorable at a dosage of 5 mg per kg every 12 hours intravenously for 14 to 21 days.

Acknowledgement. The author wishes to thank Mrs. Donna Erwood for her assistance in the preparation of this manuscript.

SUGGESTED READING

Bodey G. Antibiotics in patients with neutropenia. Arch Intern Med 1984; 144:1845–1851.
Hermann F, Schulz G, Wieser M, et al. Effect of granulocyte-macrophage colony-stimulating factor in neutropenia and related morbidity induced by myelotoxic chemotherapy. Am J Med 1990; 88:619–624.
Hughes WT, Armstrong D, Bodey G, et al. Guidelines for the use of antimicrobial agents in neutropenic patients with unexplained fever. J Infect Dis 1990; 161:381–396.
Meunier F. Prevention of mycoses in immunocompromised patients. Rev Infect Dis 1987; 9:408–416.
Pizzo PA. Considerations for the prevention of infectious complications in patients with cancer. Rev Infect Dis 1989; 11:S1551–S1563.
Pizzo PA, Robichaud KJ, Gill FA, Witebsky FG. Empiric antibiotic and antifungal therapy for cancer patients with prolonged fever and granulocytopenia. Am J Med 1982; 72:101–111.

VENOUS THROMBOSIS AND PULMONARY EMBOLISM

CHRISTINE DEMERS, M.D. FRCP
JEFFREY S. GINSBERG, M.D. FRCPC

Deep venous thrombosis (DVT) and pulmonary embolism (PE) are common problems. These two entities are closely related and frequently both are present in the same patient. In fact, half of patients with venographically proven proximal DVT have PE, whereas 70 percent of patients with objectively proven PE have DVT that can be demonstrated venographically. Because effective therapy is available and the diagnosis of DVT and PE on clinical grounds is unreliable, early diagnosis with validated objective tests is mandatory.

DIAGNOSIS

Deep Venous Thrombosis

The clinical diagnosis of DVT is nonspecific and should always be confirmed by objective testing. In fact, over one-half of patients who present with clinically suspected DVT have no evidence of DVT on venography. The validated objective tests for the diagnosis of DVT include contrast venography, impedance plethysmography (IPG), radioactive fibrinogen uptake scanning (RFUS), duplex ultrasonography, and Doppler ultrasonography.

Contrast venography is the gold standard, and, when adequately performed, a normal test excludes DVT. Unfortunately, venography is invasive, expensive, and occasionally associated with chemical phlebitis, allergic reactions, and volume overload. Furthermore, in 10 to 15 percent of patients, venography is technically inadequate. For these reasons, several noninvasive techniques have been validated over the last few years.

Impedance plethysmography is sensitive (92 to 95 percent) and specific (96 percent) for proximal DVT (thrombus in the popliteal or more proximal veins). Because IPG is insensitive for calf vein thrombosis, serial testing should be performed for 7 to 10 days in patients whose initial IPG is normal, to exclude the possibility of calf vein thrombosis extending into the proximal veins. The safety of withholding anticoagulant therapy in patients with negative serial IPG has been demonstrated in several large prospective trials.

Radioactive fibrinogen uptake scanning is sensitive and specific for calf vein thrombosis but relatively insensitive to proximal DVT, and a result is not obtained for at least 24 hours. Therefore, leg scanning alone should never be used in patients with clinically suspected DVT. The combination of RFUS and IPG is a good alternative to venography, and the safety of withholding anticoagulant therapy in patients with normal IPG and RFUS has been demonstrated.

Duplex ultrasonography is the combination of real-time B-mode ultrasound imaging and Doppler ultrasonography. In patients presenting with clinically suspected DVT, duplex ultrasonography is sensitive and specific for proximal DVT, but not calf DVT. The major limitations of duplex ultrasonography are the subjectivity and the requirement for considerable experience and skill to obtain reliable results.

Doppler ultrasonography is a noninvasive, inexpensive test that is sensitive and specific for proximal, but not calf, DVT. The major limitations are its subjectivity and dependence upon the skill of the examiner. The safety of withholding anticoagulant therapy in patients whose Doppler ultrasound is normal has not been demonstrated.

To summarize, for patients with clinically suspected DVT, three diagnostic approaches have been validated in large prospective trials, as described in Figure 1: contrast venography, serial IPG, and the combination of IPG and RFUS. It is likely that the approach of serial duplex ultrasonography is valid and is a reasonable alternative to the options listed first.

Recurrent Deep Venous Thrombosis

The diagnosis of recurrent DVT is a challenge because symptoms in patients with previous DVT can be caused by the postphlebitic syndrome and venography may be difficult to interpret in patients with previous disease. An approach that has been validated in patients with suspected recurrent DVT is described in Figure 2. Withholding anticoagulant therapy, if IPG and RFUS remain negative, is associated with a low risk of thromboembolic events on follow-up and is therefore a safe approach.

Pulmonary Embolism

It is mandatory to perform objective testing in patients with clinically suspected PE because the clinical diagnosis of PE is inaccurate. Pulmonary angiography is the gold standard for the diagnosis of PE, but it is invasive and associated with a mortality rate of 0.25 percent and a morbidity rate of 1.5 percent. Perfusion and ventilation (V/Q) lung scanning are the most useful noninvasive tests in patients with clinically suspected PE. It is widely accepted that a normal lung scan excludes PE and that a high-probability lung scan (defined as a segmental or greater perfusion defect with normal ventilation) indicates PE in the vast majority of cases. Unfortunately, 40 to 60 percent of patients with suspected PE have neither a high-probability lung scan nor a normal lung scan. This lung scan pattern, which is sometimes referred to as non-high probability, and sometimes low or indeterminate probability, includes segmental perfusion defects with matched ventilation defects, subsegmental perfusion defects with or without ventilation defects, and perfusion defects with corresponding abnormalities on chest radiograph. In this group, the prevalence of PE is 21 to 40 percent. The clinical management of this group of patients is problematic because treating them all means exposing at least 60 percent of patients without PE to the risks of anticoagulant therapy, whereas leaving them all untreated will be disastrous in a substantial number of

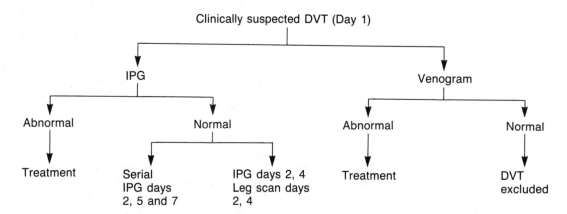

Figure 1 Diagnostic approaches to a patient with clinically suspected deep venous thrombosis (DVT). IPG = impedance plethysmography.

patients with PE. Our approach to patients with non–high-probability scans is to determine whether concomitant DVT is demonstrable by IPG or venography. If IPG or venography is abnormal, the patient should be treated with anticoagulants, whereas if these tests are normal, PE cannot be excluded because about one-half of patients with PE have normal IPG and 30 percent have normal venography. In this case, a reasonable option is to perform pulmonary angiography to exclude or confirm PE. In a subgroup of patients with non–high-probability lung scans and good cardiopulmonary reserve, an approach that has been validated is follow-up with serial IPG. The rationale for this approach is that in the absence of proximal vein thrombosis, clinically evident recurrent venous thromboembolism is rare, even though PE may be present at presentation. A recent cohort study in which anticoagulant therapy was withheld in patients with good cardiopulmonary reserve, non–high-probability scans and normal serial IPG demonstrated a low rate (2.7 percent) of new thromboembolic events. The approach to patients with clinically suspected PE is summarized in Figure 3.

PROPHYLAXIS OF THROMBOEMBOLISM

Risk factors for venous thromboembolism include recent surgery, increasing age, previous venous thromboembolism, cancer, obesity, estrogen consumption, congestive heart failure, stroke, and pregnancy. Patients can be classified as low, moderate, and high risk for venous thromboembolism according to the presence of risk factors (Table 1).

Primary Prophylaxis

Standard heparin given subcutaneously in doses of 5,000 U every 8 to 12 hours is effective in preventing proximal DVT and fatal PE in patients undergoing general, urologic, and orthopedic surgery. Because there may be a slight increase in bleeding with standard heparin, heparin is often avoided in patients undergoing neurosurgery and urologic surgery.

Adjusted-dose standard heparin given as 3,500 U subcutaneously every 8 hours and adjusted to prolong a 6 hours postinjection activated partial thromboplastin time (APTT) to 31.5 to 36 seconds has been shown to be effective and safe prophylaxis in patients undergoing elective hip surgery.

Low-molecular-weight heparin is effective in reducing DVT in patients undergoing elective hip surgery and general surgery and involves a minimal bleeding risk. Several ongoing studies are evaluating the efficacy and safety of low-molecular-weight heparin in patients undergoing other types of orthopedic surgery and neurosurgery.

Warfarin therapy started preoperatively, for patients undergoing elective hip surgery or knee surgery, and postoperatively, in patients undergoing fractured hip surgery, is effective in preventing venous thromboembolism.

Dextran is effective in reducing DVT in patients undergoing general and hip surgery, but frequent side effects, such as volume overload and hypersensitivity, may occur.

Graduated compression stockings are effective in reducing the incidence of thromboembolism in patients undergoing general surgery; however, they should not be used alone in moderate-risk or high-risk patients.

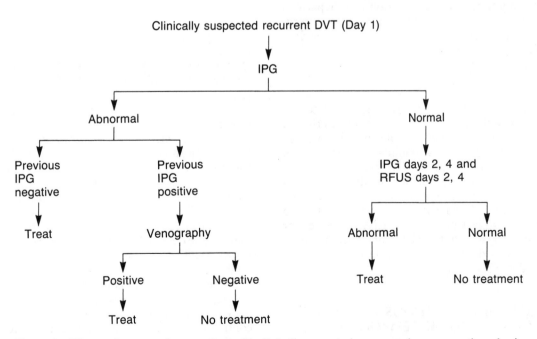

Figure 2 Diagnostic approach to a patient with clinically suspected recurrent deep venous thrombosis (DVT). IPG = impedance plethysmography.

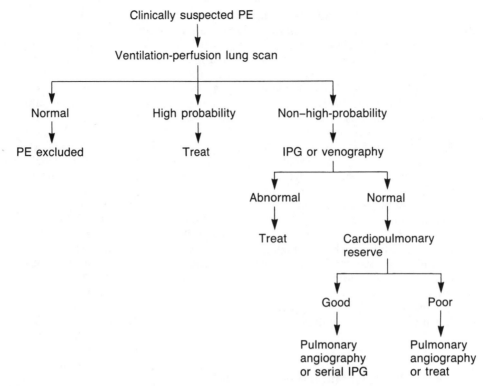

Figure 3 Diagnostic approach to a patient with clinically suspected pulmonary embolism (PE). IPG = impedance plethysmography.

Intermittent pneumatic leg compression is effective in reducing DVT in patients undergoing neurosurgery, major knee surgery, and urologic surgery, and it is the prophylaxis of choice when anticoagulants are contraindicated.

Dihydroergotamine in combination with heparin is more effective than heparin alone in preventing thromboembolism in patients undergoing general surgery or orthopedic surgery.

Surveillance

Surveillance techniques with RFUS, IPG, and duplex ultrasonography can be used either as an alternative to, or in addition to primary prophylaxis in high-risk patients. Unfortunately, these noninvasive tests are not as sensitive for screening the high-risk postoperative patient as they are in symptomatic outpatients. For this reason, these tests should not replace primary prophylaxis and should only be used alone in patients who cannot receive primary prophylaxis. Risk categories for DVT, proximal DVT, and fatal PE and recommendations for prophylaxis in low-, moderate-, and high-risk groups are described in Table 1.

TREATMENT OF DEEP VENOUS THROMBOSIS AND PULMONARY EMBOLISM

Anticoagulant therapy with heparin followed by oral anticoagulants is effective in preventing fatal PE, non-fatal PE, and recurrence in patients with DVT and PE. The pharmacology and side effects of the drugs used in the treatment of DVT and PE are reviewed briefly, and then the treatment approach will be summarized.

Drugs

Heparin is a glycosaminoglycan with a molecular weight range of 10,000 to 16,000 daltons. Heparin for clinical use is extracted from beef lung or porcine gut mucosa. The antithrombotic effect of heparin is mainly related to the potentiation of antithrombin III, which inhibits factors II_a, X_a, IX_a, and XI_a. Heparin also causes in vitro aggregation of platelets and can cause prolongation of the bleeding time. Heparin can be administered intravenously or subcutaneously, with mean half-lives of 60 to 90 minutes and 6 to 10 hours, respectively.

The effects of administered heparin are usually monitored with in vitro coagulation assays such as the APTT, which is the most widely used test. Monitoring of the heparin level is indicated when the APTT is not therapeutic despite high doses of heparin and in patients whose APTT is prolonged owing to a nonspecific inhibitor.

The side effects of heparin include bleeding, thrombocytopenia, and osteoporosis. The frequency of bleeding with heparin therapy is approximately 5 percent for continuous intravenous infusion and adjusted-dose subcutaneous heparin and significantly higher for intermittent intravenous injection. Because of heparin's short half-life, stopping the heparin infusion is usually suffi-

Table 1 Recommendation for Prophylaxis for Different Risk Groups

	DVT calf	DVT proximal	Fatal PE	
Low-Risk	<10%	<1%	<0.01%	
General surgery <30 min and <40 yr old				Early ambulation +/− compression stockings
Moderate-Risk	10%–40%	2%–10%	0.1%–0.7%	
General surgery >30 min or >40 yr old				Heparin, 5,000 U q12h, or IPC if heparin contraindicated
Neurosurgery				IPC
Prostatic resection				IPC
Myocardial infarct or heart failure				Heparin, 5,000 U q12h
Stroke				Heparin, 5,000 U q12h, or IPC if hemorrhagic
High-Risk	40%–80%	10%–20%	1%–5%	
Recent PE or DVT Pelvic or abdominal surgery for neoplasia				Heparin (adjusted-dose) or warfarin* or heparin, 5,000 U q12h and IPC
Orthopedic Surgery				
Fractured hip				Warfarin* or dextran or low-molecular-weight heparin
Elective hip				Heparin (adjusted-dose) or warfarin* or low-molecular-weight heparin or dextran
Knee surgery				Warfarin* or low-molecular-weight heparin or IPC

*Targeted INR=2.

cient when mild bleeding occurs. If bleeding is severe, heparin can be reversed with a slow infusion of intravenous protamine sulfate (1 mg protamine per 100 U of heparin) given over 10 to 30 minutes. Heparin-induced thrombocytopenia is likely an immunologic phenomenon that is associated with a fall in the platelet count 3 to 15 days after starting heparin. Both arterial and venous thrombosis can occur as a paradoxical complication of this syndrome, which is more common with bovine heparin than porcine heparin. Thus, patients started on heparin therapy should have their platelet count checked regularly (at least 2 to 3 times per week), and consideration should be given to stopping heparin if the platelet count drops by more than 30 percent. Osteoporosis is a rare complication of long-term heparin therapy that manifests as spinal or rib fracture. The risk of osteoporosis is higher with increased duration and daily dose of heparin. It is likely that a subclinical reduction in bone density precedes symptomatic bone fracture. Therefore, patients receiving heparin for more than 3 months in doses of 15,000 U per day or more should have their bone density measured with noninvasive tests.

Vitamin K antagonists exert their antithrombotic effect by inhibiting the vitamin K–dependent gamma carboxylation of factors II, VII, IX, and X and the naturally occurring anticoagulants, protein C and pro-

tein S. The noncarboxylated proteins are nonfunctional because they are unable to bind to calcium and participate in coagulation. Orally administered warfarin (the most widely used vitamin K antagonist) is well absorbed from the gastrointestinal tract, and, in the plasma, 99 percent of warfarin circulates bound to albumin, whereas 1 percent is free; this latter portion is active. The most commonly used laboratory test to monitor warfarin is the prothrombin time (PT). The sensitivity of the PT to decreased vitamin K–dependent factors in patients treated with warfarin depends on the thromboplastin used for the test. The consequence of this variability is a discrepancy between results obtained in different labs and confusion about the optimum intensity of warfarin therapy. In order to standardize PT testing, The World Health Organization (WHO) has developed a reference thromboplastin and has recommended that the PT should be expressed as the International Normalized Ratio (INR). This involves a calculation that incorporates the International Sensitivity Index (ISI) of the individual thromboplastin used with the PT and allows comparison of results obtained in different laboratories.

Side effects of warfarin include bleeding and skin necrosis. There is a well-demonstrated relationship between the risk of bleeding and the degree of prolongation of the INR. Other independent clinical risk factors for bleeding with warfarin therapy include age greater than 65 years, past history of stroke or gastrointestinal bleeding, atrial fibrillation, and the presence of a comorbid condition such as renal failure, recent myocardial infarction, or severe anemia. Patients who develop bleeding while their INR is in the therapeutic range (2 to 3) should be investigated for a remediable lesion, particularly in cases of gastrointestinal or genitourinary bleeding (about one-third of patients who bleed while they are taking warfarin have a remediable cause of bleeding). When mild bleeding occurs, vitamin K, 2.5 to 5 mg SC or PO, should be given to reverse the warfarin effect. If bleeding is more severe, infusion of plasma or a concentrate containing factors II, VII, IX, and X provides a more rapid correction of the INR. Warfarin-induced skin necrosis is a serious, rare complication of warfarin therapy that occurs within the first week of initiation of therapy and is due to a rapid fall in the level of protein C, before levels of the other vitamin K–dependent factors fall. It occurs most frequently in patients with congenital protein C deficiency, but it can occur in any patient started on warfarin. Warfarin should be stopped immediately when this complication occurs.

Drug interactions between warfarin and other drugs are frequent and can alter the absorption, albumin binding, or metabolism of warfarin, producing a prolongation or reduction of the anticoagulant effect. The reader is referred to a more comprehensive review for more details.

Treatment Approaches

Initial Treatment

Heparin is usually initiated with an intravenous bolus of 5,000 U followed by a continuous infusion of 24,000 to 30,000 U per 24 hours in order to prolong the APTT to 1.5 to 2 times control. The maintenance dose can also be given by intermittent intravenous injections with equal effectiveness but with a higher risk of bleeding. Therefore, intermittent intravenous injection should be avoided. Adjusted-dose subcutaneous heparin has been compared to intravenous heparin infusion for the treatment of DVT and PE in randomized trials. In one study, there was a higher recurrence rate with the subcutaneous regimen, but this was probably because early in the course of treatment, the APTT was below the therapeutic range in most of the patients treated with the subcutaneous regimen. Other studies have demonstrated that subcutaneous heparin is comparable to intravenous heparin in both efficacy and safety. At the present time, subcutaneous heparin should be reserved for situations in which intravenous heparin is impossible or impractical. The usual duration of heparin is 7 to 10 days followed by adequate long-term oral anticoagulant therapy. Two recent studies have demonstrated that 4 to 5 days of heparin is adequate, making it possible to discharge patients home sooner.

Subsequent Therapy

When initial heparin therapy is not followed by adequate long-term anticoagulant therapy, a high rate of thromboembolic recurrence occurs. Warfarin, with a targeted INR of 2.0 to 3.0 (PT ratio of 1.3 to 1.5), is associated with a low rate of recurrence (2 percent) and a low bleeding risk (4 percent to 6 percent). There should be at least 4 days of overlap between heparin and warfarin because prolongation of the INR can occur rapidly after warfarin is started, owing to a reduction in factor VII (which has a short half-life) but not factors II, IX, and X (which have longer half-lives). It is likely that the antithrombotic effect of warfarin is not optimal until a reduction in all the vitamin K–dependent clotting factors occurs. Adjusted-dose subcutaneous heparin every 12 hours, in doses to prolong a 6-hour postinjection APTT to 1.5 to 2.0 times control, is a good alternative to warfarin in pregnant women or in cases in which monitoring of warfarin is difficult.

Duration of Treatment

The optimal duration of oral anticoagulant therapy is unknown, but it is reasonable to treat patients with their first episode of proximal DVT or PE for 3 months. The risk of recurrence during the first year after anticoagulants are discontinued is 2 percent to 6 percent. Patients with recurrent DVT or PE should be treated for longer than 3 months because 3 months of therapy is associated with a 20 percent risk of recurrent thromboembolism and a 5 percent risk of fatal PE. There are no randomized trials to provide guidelines, but a reasonable practice is to treat patients for 1 year after a second episode and for the remainder of their lives after a third episode. In symptomatic patients with calf vein thrombosis demonstrated venographically, a reasonable approach is 5 days of intravenous or subcutaneous heparin followed by 6 weeks of oral anticoagulants. Patients with congenital protein C, protein S, or antithrombin III deficiency or with a lupus anticoagulant and one or more thromboembolic events should be considered candidates for long-term anticoagulant therapy. These abnormalities predispose to venous thrombosis, but the prevalence of one of these abnormalities is less than 10 percent in patients with venous thromboembolic disease. It is reasonable to perform assays for the congenital deficiencies in patients with recurrent thromboembolic disease, a family history of venous thromboembolic disorders, thromboembolism before the age of 40, or thrombosis in an unusual site (e.g., superior mesenteric vein, subclavian vein).

Role of Vena Cava Interruption

Interruption of the inferior vena cava by ligation or insertion of an intravascular device such as a Greenfield filter is indicated in patients with acute proximal DVT and (1) an absolute contraindication to anticoagulant therapy (active serious bleeding, recent brain, eye, or spinal cord surgery, recent cerebral hemorrhage or malignant hypertension); (2) bleeding on anticoagulant therapy; or (3) recurrent PE while receiving adequate anticoagulant therapy.

Role of Thrombolytic Therapy

Deep Venous Thrombosis. Thrombolytic therapy causes a more rapid clot lysis than heparin; however, there is still controversy about whether more rapid clot lysis prevents venous valvular damage and subsequent development of the postphlebitic syndrome. At the present time, it would seem reasonable to treat young patients with acute proximal DVT and symptoms for less than 1 week with thrombolytic therapy in order to prevent the postphlebitic syndrome.

Pulmonary Embolism. Several randomized trials have been performed comparing thrombolytic therapy with conventional anticoagulant therapy in PE. Most have reported a more rapid resolution of lung scan abnormalities, pulmonary angiogram, and pulmonary artery pressure abnormalities with thrombolytic therapy compared to heparin. However, no significant differences were observed when the tests were repeated 7 days after therapy, and no improvement in mortality was found. Thus, it is not clear whether rapid clot lysis with thrombolytic therapy reduces long-term morbidity and

justifies the increased bleeding risk of thrombolytic therapy. At the present time, the only clear-cut indication for thrombolytic therapy is for patients in shock with massive PE.

PREGNANCY

Diagnosis

The diagnosis of DVT or PE during pregnancy is problematic because of the fear of exposing the fetus to radiation. On the other hand, because of the inaccuracy of clinical diagnosis of DVT and PE and the potential risks of anticoagulants, a definite diagnosis is highly desirable. The risk of in utero radiation exposure when the different procedures used to diagnose DVT and PE (venography, lung scan, and angiography) are performed has been reviewed recently and appears to be small; there is no increased risk of congenital malformations, but there may be a slight increase in the subsequent risk of childhood cancer.

Our approach to patients with clinically suspected DVT during pregnancy is summarized in Figure 4, and our approach to pregnant patients with clinically suspected PE is summarized in Figure 5.

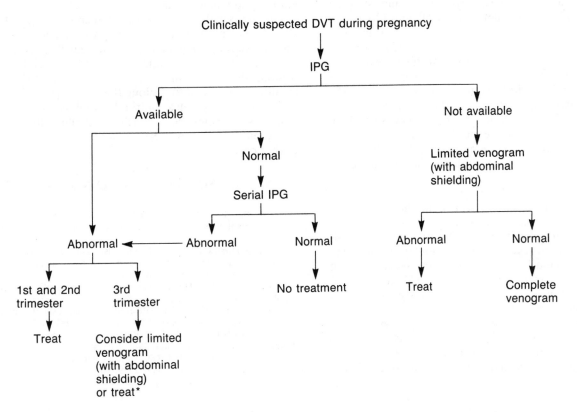

* A false-positive IPG may occasionally occur during the third trimester owing to compression of the pelvic veins by the uterus.

Figure 4 Diagnostic approach to a patient with clinically suspected deep venous thrombosis (DVT) during pregnancy. IPG = impedance plethysmography.

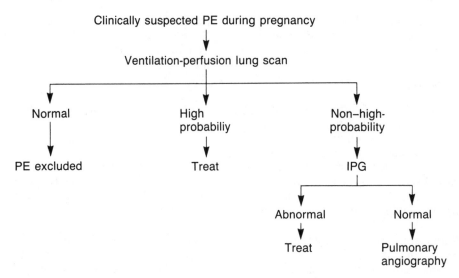

Figure 5 Diagnostic approach to a patient with clinically suspected pulmonary embolism (PE) during pregnancy. IPG = impedance plethysmography.

Anticoagulant Therapy During Pregnancy

Heparin does not cross the placenta and is safe to use during pregnancy. On the other hand, warfarin crosses the placenta and can cause (1) warfarin embryopathy, consisting of nasal hypoplasia and stippled epiphyses with exposure between the 6th and 12th weeks of gestation; (2) central nervous system abnormalities with exposure during any trimester; and (3) abortions and stillbirths. For these reasons, warfarin should be avoided during pregnancy, so heparin is the anticoagulant of choice. Heparin and warfarin are both safe for the breastfed infant when administered to a nursing mother.

Acute DVT or PE during pregnancy should be treated initially with intravenous heparin, as in nonpregnant patients. Intravenous heparin should be followed by adjusted-dose heparin to prolong the 6-hour post-injection APTT to 1.5 to 2 times control throughout pregnancy.

Patients on long-term anticoagulant therapy prior to pregnancy for either recurrent DVT or PE or a prosthetic heart valve should be treated with adjusted-dose subcutaneous heparin throughout pregnancy (as described previously). Two options are available when patients on long-term anticoagulants decide to conceive. The first option is to switch from warfarin to heparin before conception. This ensures that the fetus will not be exposed to warfarin during the early pregnancy but may increase the duration of heparin therapy if conception is delayed. The second option is to continue warfarin and perform frequent pregnancy tests when conception is

attempted. As soon as the pregnancy test becomes positive, warfarin should be discontinued and heparin therapy started. This regimen avoids the critical 6- to 12-week window of exposure during which the warfarin embryopathy may occur.

Patients with a well-documented episode of DVT or PE should be considered for prophylactic heparin therapy during pregnancy. Heparin, 5,000 U every 12 hours, should be given during the first two trimesters, whereas during the third trimester, the dose of heparin should be increased to prolong the 6-hour postinjection APTT to 1.5 to 2 times control. Surveillance with serial noninvasive testing, such as IPG or duplex ultrasonography may be a reasonable alternative to heparin therapy during pregnancy.

SUGGESTED READING

Ginsberg JS, Hirsh J, Turner DC, et al. Risks to the fetus of anticoagulant therapy during pregnancy. Thromb Haemost 1989; 61:197.
Ginsberg JS, Hirsh J, Rainbow AJ, et al. Risk to the fetus of radiologic procedures used in the diagnosis of maternal venous thromboembolic disease. Thromb Haemost 1989; 61:189.
Hull RD, Raskob GE, Hirsh J. The diagnosis of clinically suspected pulmonary embolism. Chest 1986; 89:417S.
Hull RD, Raskob GE, Leclerc JR, et al. The diagnosis of clinically suspected venous thrombosis. Clin Chest Med 1984; 5:439.
Hull RD, Raskob GE, Hirsh J. Prophylaxis of venous thromboembolism: An overview. Chest 1986; 89:374S.
Raskob GE, Carter CJ, Hull RD. Anticoagulant therapy for venous thromboembolism. Prog Hemost 1989; 9:1.

OBSTETRICS AND THROMBOCYTOPENIA

ROBERT F. BURROWS, M.D., FRCSC

Thrombocytopenia is defined as a platelet count less than 150×10^9 per L. With the advent of automated counters, thrombocytopenia has been shown to be a common event in pregnancy, with a prevalence at delivery of approximately 9 percent. Thrombocytopenia occurs in 5 percent of asymptomatic normal pregnant women at term, but it has not been associated with an adverse outcome for the mother or for the fetus (i.e., thrombocytopenia). The remaining patients with low platelet counts have varying causes for their thrombocytopenia. Pre-eclampsia and known immune disorders, systemic lupus erythematosus (SLE) and immune thrombocytopenia purpura (ITP), account for the majority of pathologic thrombocytopenia.

OBSTETRIC CONDITIONS IN WHICH THROMBOCYTOPENIA IS A MAJOR FEATURE

Of the three major causes of thrombocytopenia, reduced production, increased destruction, and sequestration, platelet destruction is by far the most common cause of thrombocytopenia in pregnancy.

Normal Pregnancy

Approximately 5 percent of term pregnancies will have platelet counts less than 150×10^9 per L, a level considered as thrombocytopenic in the nonpregnant woman. In a 1-year study of 1357 consecutive normal patients, we found that the mean platelet count was 225×10^9 per L with the 95th centiles being 109 and 341×10^9 per L. Having continued the study for 4 years, we now consider anyone without a history of immune thrombocytopenia or a medical condition causing low platelets identified incidentally by automation with a platelet count greater than 80×10^9 per L to have incidental thrombocytopenia. In over 400 identified cases of incidental thrombocytopenia in the last 4 years, we have seen only one infant with a cord platelet count less than 100×10^9 per L and this was 98×10^9 per L. The majority of these mothers regained a "normal" platelet count within 5 days postpartum, and none experienced hemostatic incompetence. The thrombocytopenia in normal pregnancy is considered a manifestation of a destructive process and is not just from dilution as evidenced by the mean platelet volume being consistently increased in this condition. Mothers identified with a low platelet count early in pregnancy, only because of automation, are followed serially. If the platelet count is greater than 80×10^9 per L at delivery

no specific interventions are performed, and delivery is conducted based on standard obstetric indications. Even though we have not seen severe neonatal thrombocytopenia, obtaining the fetal cord platelet count is considered part of complete care for this mother and child pair.

Pre-eclampsia

Thrombocytopenia is the most common hemostatic dysfunction seen in pre-eclampsia, a syndrome of hypertension and proteinuria unique to pregnancy, occurring after the 20th week of gestation (Table 1). Clinically significant thrombocytopenia usually occurs in conjunction with evidence of multiorgan dysfunction, and is most common and most severe in patients with preterm pre-eclampsia, occurring in up to 30 percent of patients. Thrombocytopenia that occurs in conjunction with elevated liver enzyme concentrations and hemolysis has been called the HELLP syndrome, although overt evidence of hemolysis is, in our experience, unusual.

The pathophysiology of the thrombocytopenia in pre-eclampsia is unknown but is thought to be either thrombin- or immune-mediated. Overt clinical evidence of thrombin activation is rare, the prothrombin time (PT), partial thromboplastin time (PTT), thrombin clotting time (TCT) and fibrogen levels are usually normal unless there is an associated abruptio placentae.

The ultimate cure of pre-eclampsia and the associated thrombocytopenia is delivery. In-hospital evaluation of the mother and the fetus with aggressive treatment of the hypertension often ameliorates the laboratory abnormalities and improves the clinical state of the mother and fetus enough to allow for a planned and safe delivery. The patient with pre-eclampsia of pregnancy with thrombocytopenia and liver enzyme elevations usually requires delivery within days of presentation. A patient with thrombocytopenia that is associated with persistant alterations in the coagulation profile (PT or PTT) without evidence of abruptio placentae should be delivered within 24 hours of identification.

Neonatal thrombocytopenia in pre-eclampsia is associated with preterm infants manifesting intrauterine growth restriction (IUGR). The neonatologists should be made aware of this infant and the possibility of thrombocytopenia. Extreme neonatal thrombocytopenia, less than 50×10^9 per L is unusual at delivery, and this possibility need not be considered when deciding upon the mode of delivery.

The maternal platelet count often falls postpartum, especially if a cesarean section has been performed. Levels of 20 to 30×10^9 per L can be maintained for days, but these will rise spontaneously by 5 to 7 days after delivery, often with a rebound to excessive counts greater than 500×10^9 per L. This is evidence of the destructive nature of the thrombocytopenia, with reactive thrombocytosis.

We have not routinely used platelet transfusions at cesarean sections regardless of the count, but have platelets available if needed. Platelet transfusions rarely bring about resolution of thrombocytopenia and are not considered immunologically innocuous or completely free from infectious complications. Platelet transfusion may resolve hemostatic concerns at the time of cesarean section, so are not avoidable in all cases.

Thrombotic Thrombocytopenia Purpura

Thrombotic thrombocytopenia purpura (TTP) is a rare disorder, but it has a peak incidence in women of child-bearing age and some features in common with pre-eclampsia–eclampsia (Table 2). There is usually no evidence of activation of the coagulation mechanism, and all clinical findings are explicable on the basis of microvascular occlusion by platelets with secondary red cell and tissue damage. Some patients are acutely ill (Table 3) with a rapidly fatal outcome despite treatment whereas others show a more chronic course. It is the latter that creates confusion with the more common pre-eclampsia syndrome. As there is no evidence that the course of TTP is influenced by delivery, when the platelet count fails to rise in response to delivery, as it will do if the patient is pre-eclamptic, the appropriate diagnosis is made and treatment is instituted. Treatment is by plasma exchange and antiplatelet therapy. The risk to the fetus is determined by the gestation at which it is delivered; the fetus does not develop thrombocytopenia because of the maternal TTP syndrome.

It is difficult to advise a surviving pregnant patient with TTP in regard to future pregnancies because experience is limited and potential exists for relapse.

Table 1 Criteria Defining Pre-eclampsia

Elevation of blood pressure >140/90 for the first time, after 20 gestational weeks of pregnancy with proteinuria >300 mg in a 24 hour urine sample
Variable laboratory abnormalities
  Blood
    Thrombocytopenia
    Microangiopathic hemolytic anemia
  Liver
    Increased enzymes
    Subcapsular hematoma
    Rupture
  Brain
    Visual Disturbances
    Seizures
  Kidney
    Proteinuria
    Oliguria: anuria

Table 2 Diagnostic Criteria of TTP

Thrombocytopenia
Microangiopathic hemolytic anemia
Renal impairment
Neurologic dysfunction
Fever

Similarly, experience with oral contraceptives is limited, and use of these agents is probably ill-advised in the TTP syndrome.

Systemic Lupus Erythematosus

Thrombocytopenia is common in patients with SLE, but rarely is less than 100×10^9 per L. Prognosis for the pregnancy is generally good in patients with SLE without the complications of renal dysfunction and hypertension and in the absence of the lupus anticoagulant and anticardiolipin antibody.

Patients identified with lupus anticoagulant or anticardiolipin antibodies can have poor obstetric histories with thrombosis in the intervillous space leading to increased abortions, stillbirth, early severe pre-eclampsia, and IUGR. As there is lack of standardization of testing for these antibodies, especially the lupus anticoagulant, various treatment protocols have resulted in improved pregnancy outcomes. Our present routine of aspirin, 85 mg daily, and prednisone, 40 mg on alternate days, combined with intense fetal and maternal surveillance has resulted in numerous successful pregnancy outcomes. Those patients presenting with a history of thrombosis or thromboembolism in conjunction with these antibodies are treated with therapeutic doses of heparin in addition to aspirin and prednisone. We have observed no hemorrhagic complications in these pregnancies treated to date.

Immune Thrombocytopenia Purpura

Immune thrombocytopenia purpura (ITP) is a common disorder in reproducing women, and because it is caused by an IgG antibody that readily crosses the placenta, the fetus is also at risk for thrombocytopenia. The management of thrombocytopenia in ITP associated with pregnancy is not unlike that of the patient in the nonpregnant state. No treatment is required for the thrombocytopenia unless it is severe, less than 50×10^9 per L, or associated with evidence of hemostatic incompetence. The pregnant patient with ITP is advised to avoid nonsteroidal anti-inflammatory agents. The mainstay of treatment is prednisone, 1 mg per kg as a starting dose, which is reduced with clinical response, this occurs usually within 1 to 2 weeks. Because of its expense, intravenous immunoglobulin (IV IgG) is not practical for long-term therapy. However, IV IgG has a place for the treatment of hemorrhagic events or for

Table 3 Clinical and Laboratory Features of TTP

Purpura and bleeding with thrombocytopenia
Anemia with red cell fragments and reticulocytosis
Oliguria and uremia
Convulsions and coma
Hemiplegia and dysphasia
Fever
Chest joint and muscle pain
Cardiac arrhythmia

preparing for splenectomy. Splenectomy is best avoided, and is rarely indicated in pregnancy, and avoidance of splenectomy may be the best indication for IV IgG in pregnancy.

The potential risk of thrombocytopenia in the fetus has created controversy in regard to management at delivery. Having recently reviewed our hospital's experience and that of the English literature on pregnancy and ITP it is apparent that (1) the risk to the fetus is overstated, (2) no maternal parameter is totally predictive of fetal thrombocytopenia, (3) a cord platelet count less than 50×10^9 per L occurs in only about 5 percent of the ITP population, and (4) the major risk to the neonate is 24 to 48 hours after delivery and should be preventable with aggressive neonatal therapy.

We reviewed 48 manuscripts published since 1970, comprising reports on 485 liveborn infants. In this group, we found 3 neonatal deaths for a prevalence of death of 6 per 1000 ITP pregnancies. All of these deaths from hemostatic events occurred at least 24 hours after the birth and all were in infants delivered by cesarean section.

We found that maternal platelet count, maternal steroid use, maternal splenectomy, and maternal platelet bound and bindable antibodies were not predictive of fetal thrombocytopenia but only increased or decreased the likelihood of its occurrence. Scalp and cordocentesis data demonstrated a low rate of fetal thrombocytopenia but, more importantly, there was unnecessary morbidity to mother and fetus because of these procedures.

As a consequence of our analysis, we presently manage ITP associated with pregnancy in the following manner (Table 4). The mother is treated in the same manner as the nonpregnant ITP patient and, at term, we allow vaginal delivery in all patients, with cesarean section being performed for obstetric indications only. If the mother is thrombocytopenic, a midline episiotomy is done in preference to a mediolateral one. Cord blood samples are taken for immediate platelet count, and the infant is treated aggressively with IV IgG or steroids in the neonatal period.

Reduced Production

Drugs

In principle, all drugs should be avoided in pregnancy. Table 5 lists those drugs commonly associated with the thrombocytopenia secondary to bone marrow depression. The diagnosis of drug-induced thrombocytopenia is based on the exclusion of other causes and a stoppage of the medication which brings about resolution of the low platelet count. The severity of throm-

Table 4 Management of ITP in Pregnancy

Maternal management same as in the nonpregnant patient
Cesarean delivery only for obstetric indications
Aggressive therapy of the neonate as indicated by the cord platelet count

bocytopenia and the necessity of the drug should determine whether the medication is tolerated, stopped, or changed to a drug less likely to cause a problem. Possible fetal thrombocytopenia should be considered if delivery is imminent, because most medications (except heparin) readily cross the placenta. The prevalence of neonatal thrombocytopenia in maternal drug-induced thrombocytopenia is not documented, so the risk cannot be stated.

Folic Acid Deficiency

Thrombocytopenia secondary to folic acid deficiency is most likely to occur in patients who are economically disadvantaged, in multiparae, in women with twin pregnancies, and in patients with hemolytic anemias. Thrombocytopenia is usually associated with an anemia, which may be characteristically megaloblastic. The anemia and thrombocytopenia usually respond to and are prevented by dietary supplementation with a daily dose of 1 mg of folic acid.

Aplastic anemia, paroxysmal nocturnal hemoglobinuria, and leukemia complicating pregnancy are all rare causes of thrombocytopenia. Because the therapeutic options in these conditions often lead to deterioration of the pregnancy state, the care to these patients must be highly individualized.

Acute Fatty Liver of Pregnancy

Acute fatty liver of pregnancy is stated to be a rare condition. The author, however, disagrees, believing that acute fatty liver of pregnancy is common, often diagnosed as pre-eclampsia and, because delivery effects cure in both, the diagnosis goes unrecognized.

There are several clues to suggest the diagnosis: (1) there is a characteristic history of malaise, nausea, and vomiting for up to a week before presentation; (2) the fetus is usually well grown and late in gestation; (3) thrombocytopenia is more marked than the clinical setting (i.e., if this was pre-eclampsia, the mild increased blood pressure and mild to moderate proteinuria seen usually are not associated with platelet counts this low); and (4) results of coagulation tests (PT, PTT) may be abnormal, this is unusual in pre-eclampsia uncomplicated by abruptio placenta.

The clinical presentation is typically in the last trimester with malaise, nausea, and vomiting. This stage lasts approximately one week with the patient then manifesting liver, renal, and coagulation failure, which progress to coma and death if untreated. Diagnosis is by liver biopsy showing fat in small vacuoles in centrolob-

Table 5 Drugs Associated with Thrombocytopenia

Antibacterial agents, e.g., sulfonamides
Antirheumatic drugs, e.g., indomethacin
Tranquilizers, e.g, chlorpromazine, chlordiazepoxide
Anticonvulsants, e.g., phenytoin, ethosuximide
Miscellaneous, e.g., alcohol, cimetidine, corticosteroids, heparin

ular hepatocytes. As delivery is noted to improve outcome, all pregnancies with this suspected diagnosis are best delivered; the promptness of delivery depends on where the patient is in the evolution of the disorder. Unless the disease is very far progressed, the patient rapidly gets better post-partum. There have been no documented recurrences, and oral contraceptive use appears safe. The risk to the fetus is determined by the gestation at delivery. If the mother is hypoglycemic from liver failure, the fetus also can manifest this problem in the neonatal period.

OBSTETRIC CONDITIONS IN WHICH THROMBOCYTOPENIA IS A MINOR FEATURE

Abruptio Placentae

Premature separation of the placenta, or abruptio placentae, is the most frequent cause of coagulation failure in most obstetric units.

Coagulation failures in abruptio placentae occur only with major placental separation as manifested by fetal distress or fetal death. Fortunately, the majority of coagulation failures are only laboratory findings and are terminated with delivery.

The clotting abnormalities associated with placental abruption are not simply the result of massive extravascular clot formation with component depletion. Activation of the fibrinolytic system and consumption of the soluble components, especially fibrinogen, occur out of proportion to the blood loss.

The coagulation failure should be anticipated when abruptio placentae is associated with fetal death, having a prevalence approaching 40 percent. The platelet count will be variably reduced and the serum fibrinogen concentration will fall, being eventually reflected in a prolongation of the TCT with a rise in fibrin degradation products (FDPs). The mainstay of treatment is to empty the uterus, and in the interim, to support vigorously the intravascular volume with synthetic and human-derived products. Coagulant component therapy administered antepartum is rarely necessary for vaginal delivery. With fetal death, there are already several liters of blood concealed behind the placenta within the uterus and this will not be reflected in the initial hemoglobin/hematocrit. Normal saline and packed red blood cell should be commenced immediately with diagnosis, a urinary catheter placed and coagulation profile obtained. Amniotomy and uterine stimulation should be commenced simultaneously. As the fibrinogen concentration is greatly elevated in pregnancy, the initial TCT may be normal, and serial fibrinogen levels will provide the most useful information of impending coagulation difficulties. When the fibrinogen concentration falls less than 1.5 g per L, the TCT will start to be prolonged. It is now time to consider administration of fibrinogen as cryoprecipitate. Generally, we administer cryoprecipitate in lots of 16 to 20 units. This provides approximately 4 g of fibrinogen, enough to maintain a serum fibrinogen level above 1.5 g per L. It is rarely necessary to replace platelets.

It is essential to maintain circulation volume not only to prevent hypovolemic shock but also to help clearance of FDPs. Fibrin degradation products are potent anticoagulants and are thought to inhibit myometrial activity, which may contribute to a higher prevalence of post-partum hemorrhage associated with abruptio placentae.

Amniotic Fluid Embolism

Amniotic fluid embolism is rare (1:8000 to 1:80,000 deliveries), but it is one of the most devastating complications seen in obstetrics. It is said to occur most commonly in older multiparous patients with large babies at or near term following a short, tumultuous labor associated with the use of uterine stimulants; however, it can occur in a multitude of circumstances. The initial clinical features of amniotic fluid embolism are sudden respiratory distress, cyanosis, and cardiovascular collapse. If the patient is successfully resuscitated from this (the immediate mortality rate can be up to 80 percent) approximately half will experience within 0.5 to 4 hours later a coagulation failure with intractable uterine bleeding. Because of the rarity of the condition, there are no large series using a consistent therapeutic approach on which to rely. Thus, it is impossible to define categorically a treatment plan.

During the initial phase of cardiovascular collapse, treatment is directed toward ventilatory and cardiovascular support. This consists of rapid intubation, mechanical ventilation, and placement of direct central lines to direct cardiovascular support.

It is unclear whether the impending coagulopathy secondary to amniotic fluid embolism can be prevented. Theoretically, the timely administration of heparin might blunt cascade activation and the resulting plasmin activation. In reality, prevention of the coagulopathy is rarely thought of when major resuscitation efforts are in effect.

Because fibrinogenolysis appears to be a dominant feature of amniotic fluid embolism, it may be the only indication for an antifibrinolytic agent in obstetrics, and if the coagulopathy is not controlled with component replacement, this may be considered.

Retention of a Dead Fetus

The association between intrauterine fetal demise and subsequent coagulopathy is well established. The evolution of fetal death syndrome is gradual. The earliest detectable changes occur 3 to 4 weeks after fetal demise; however, approximately 80 percent of women with an intrauterine fetal demise begin spontaneous labor within 2 to 3 weeks. The coagulopathy consists of varying degrees of hypofibrinogenemia decreased plasminogen, decreased antithrombin III (ATIII) activity, increased generation of FDPs, and thrombocytopenia. With the advent of ultrasound examinations and good prenatal care, it is now extremely unusual for an intrauterine death to go undetected for any length of time. When the intrauterine death is diagnosed, it is again unusual that termination has not occurred within the week, because modern methods of induction are now available. This coagulopathy should be an event of the past.

The only circumstance in which the dead fetus may stay in utero is when there is death of one fetus in a set of twins. If maturity is documented, delivery is indicated, but if the surviving fetus is immature, the mother and the other fetus must be considered. The mother should be followed with serial monitoring of fibrinogen levels, knowing that coagulopathy is unusual before 3 to 4 weeks of retention.

The appearance of maternal coagulopathy may necessitate delivery or heparin therapy to correct the coagulopathy before initiating delivery; however, it is unusual for both the coagulopathy to occur and for the pregnancy to continue another 4 to 5 weeks. There is greater risk to the remaining fetus than there is to the mother. The neonatal morbidity associated with an intrauterine death of one twin may be as high as 45 percent in the co-twin. The incidence of neurologic sequelae has been reported to be 20 percent. The risk to the live twin occurs only if there is vascular communication between the twins; therefore, it occurs only in monozygotic twins. Among the first efforts after diagnosis of death of one twin is to determine zygosity, and if possible, to assign risks. Careful scrutiny of the living twin must then occur until delivery is effected.

SUGGESTED READING

Burrows RF, Kelton JG. Thrombocytopenia at delivery: a prospective survey of 6715 deliveries. Am J Obstet Gynecol 1990; 162:731–734.

Hathaway WE, Bonnar J, eds. Hemostatic disorders of the pregnant woman and newborn infant. New York: Elsevier, 1987.

Kitay DZ, ed. Hematologic problems in pregnancy. Oradell, New Jersey. Medical Economics Book, 1987.

Laros RK Jr, ed. Blood disorders in pregnancy. Philadelphia: Lea & Febiger, 1986.

ONCOLOGY

PRINCIPLES OF CANCER MANAGEMENT

PAUL P. CARBONE, M.D., D.Sc. (Hon.), F.A.C.P.

Cancer is not one illness but a spectrum of neoplastic diseases that can arise from and spread to almost every organ and tissue in the body. Each cancer has its unique pattern of presentation and approach to diagnosis, staging, and management. Along with the information in the accompanying chapters on specific cancers, there are principles that will assist the generalist as well as the specialist in the management of their cancer patients. This chapter stresses these overall guidelines of cancer management.

DIAGNOSIS

On presentation, a patient may call attention to a specific mass, but he or she is just as likely to describe vague symptoms such as weakness, weight loss, pain, bleeding per rectum or urethra, an enlarging skin lesion, cough, or change in bowel habits. The physician's index of suspicion of cancer may be high or low depending on the age of the patient, knowledge of personal habits such as smoking or alcohol ingestion, family history, or occupation. However, as a result of regular check-ups and cancer screening procedures such as mammography or lower gastrointestinal endoscopy, more patients are presenting with preneoplastic lesions or very small tumors. These cancers are usually nonpalpable, asymptomatic, and rarely have systemic spread.

A complete physical examination is extremely important. Cancer may be manifested by a specific mass, occult blood in the stool, pleural effusion, or ascites. The physical exam should not only focus on the complaint but should also include careful examination of other areas of the body such as the skin, looking for dysplastic nevi, superficial lymph nodes in the groin, neck and axillary regions, or lumps in the breasts. Every physician also needs to ask the patient about personal smoking habits or the date of the latest mammogram or Pap test, attempting to reinforce good prevention habits.

Laboratory tests must be done with fiscal restraint. No test should be routine, but a sample battery might include a complete blood count, liver enzymes, and a urinalysis. Radiographic procedures are important depending on the degree of suspicion. An ultrasound assessment of the liver or abdomen is often quicker and less expensive to obtain than a computed tomography (CT) scan. Magnetic resonance imaging (MRI) scans and nuclear medicine scans are reserved usually for staging work-up or assessment of specific problems. To diagnose cancer, the CT scan and direct needle biopsies usually provide necessary information that was previously obtained only from a diagnostic laparotomy. Tumor markers such as the CEA, HCG, AFP, and PSA are increasingly able to point to specific diagnoses, however, these are usually most appropriate in situations in which the index of suspicion is very high based on clinical and radiographic findings. At this stage of the work-up, one is trying to determine the possible causes of a complaint and find, if possible, some abnormality that can be safely biopsied.

The diagnosis of cancer has been traditionally based on histologic specimens obtained by excisional or incisional biopsy and aspiration, however, as serum markers become more specific, markedly elevated AFP levels combined with a history of chronic active hepatitis or heavy drinking and ultrasound evidence of liver metastatic deposits indicates, with almost complete assurance, that the patient has a primary liver cancer. Likewise, very elevated HCG levels in a young man or postpartum woman point to a diagnosis of a germ cell or placental neoplasm. Other markers, such as CEA, are not specific and should not be done as screening tests. Markers such as the PSA or CA 125 are beginning to approach some degree of specificity but still should not be used to exclude or diagnose cancer.

Examination of the histologic specimen should be done not only with routine pathologic stains but also with immunochemical or biochemical (estrogen receptors) methods, electron microscope, or flow cytometry, which may aid in defining a specific cancer site as the cause of the malady. In addition to diagnosis, these markers and others serve to add important prognostic information.

STAGING

Once a diagnosis has been established, additional studies are needed to determine the specific stage or extent of the disease. Staging is done to assess extent of the disease, determine therapy, and define prognosis. Treatment today is not only disease-specific but stage- and site-specific. The staging may require additional invasive techniques such as bone marrow, laparotomy, mediastinoscopy, or laparoscopy. The basic strategy is not to assess routinely all possible sites of disease but to tailor the diagnostic testing to the primary treatment approaches planned. Paradoxically, when local modalities are to be used, i.e., surgery or radiotherapy, one needs to be more accurate in order to assess the extent of the disease. If chemotherapy is the planned option, then less invasive staging procedures may be done. In Hodgkin's disease, many physicians are not doing laparotomies if the disease is limited to the mediastinum and is bulky in size. As we know more about the natural history, we also can avoid doing more extensive procedures. For example, a diagnosis of intraductal carcinoma of the breast usually means that axillary dissection is not indicated.

In addition to histologic and clinical procedures designed to assess disease extent, therapy may also be based on molecular biologic and immunologic tests. These include the specific phenotyping of malignant lymphocytes, measurements of receptors, the use of oncogene markers in breast cancer, and cytogenetic aneuploidy and DNA synthesis rates determined by flow cytometry. These latter tests are allowing the oncologist to design specific effective therapy for individual patients. Finally, in assessing disease extent, the physician should define (and measure) those lesions that will be used to assess treatment progress.

THERAPY

Treatment must be directed not only toward cure of the illness and control of potential sites of local recurrences but also to maximizing the quality of life. These objectives entail the use of multidisciplinary approaches and the involvement of several experts. However, this does not mean that each of the specialists performs his or her treatment out of context to what the others are doing, but rather there must be an integration of approaches, with the proposed combined therapy being the least toxic while insuring the best results. The oncologist must also consider whether the patient is eligible to participate in a clinical trial. These trials not only provide the state-of-art therapy for the patient's cancer and specific stage, but they also provide important new data on outcome that advance knowledge and help treat future patients.

Local therapy is being applied not only to improve cure rate but also to meet the patient's perceptions regarding cosmetic outcome. Physicians are obligated to inform patients of therapeutic options that might achieve an equivalent outcome. It is no longer defensible to treat all breast cancers with radical mastectomy when one considers the proven results that can be achieved by minimal surgery and radiation. Likewise, it is also untenable that patients with rectal cancer not receive radiation therapy postoperatively. Many oncologists are offering patients therapies that are not proven, such as preoperative chemotherapy or autologous marrow transplant in breast cancer or combined modality therapy in head and neck cancer. These approaches, advocated by some investigators, are still experimental, and patients receiving these therapies should be part of a clinical trial.

Curative systemic therapy with combination chemotherapy alone is still limited to relatively few diseases such as acute leukemia, Hodgkin's disease, germ cell neoplasms, and large-cell lymphomas. Chemotherapy seems to play a major role as adjuvant therapy to surgery or radiotherapy or to relieve symptoms in advanced disease. Increasingly, biologic therapies such as interferons, lymphokines, monoclonal antibodies, or marrow growth factors are being used either alone or in combination with other modalities. These exciting new treatments are adding significant benefits to cancers such as melanoma, hypernephroma, hairy cell leukemia, and colon cancer.

The management of metastatic disease at specific sites can be characterized as either prophylactic or palliative. In the former, we use prophylactic brain irradiation to prevent central nervous system relapses in small-cell carcinoma of the lung or pelvic radiation in rectal cancer to diminish local recurrences. Symptomatic control of pain, relief of cord compression, and radiation treatment of brain metastasis or bronchial obstruction provides palliation.

Effective symptomatic care is important for those patients who are in pain or suffering emotionally. Besides trying to relieve the specific reason for the problem, such as a pathologic fracture or organ obstruction, pain control can be achieved with the use of effective doses of narcotics. The fear of cancer pain contributes greatly to the psychological horrors of cancer. Likewise, the use of sleeping and antidepressant medications is most helpful to those who have problems resting at night. I would also like to stress the importance of support groups and good old-fashioned listening on the part of the physician. Patients and their families need to feel that the physician is paying attention to them and their questions. Many physicians feel that all their obligations stop after administering the drugs, radiation, or surgery. Continued personal and family counseling is important and may help the patient return to a normal life. Follow-up examinations to assess for metastatic disease and referral to appropriate support groups are important components of total care after the specific therapy has been administered. Rehabilitation service referral after surgery may allow the patient to return to normal activity faster. Increasingly, women are asking about reconstruction surgery after mastectomy, and the effects are very satisfying to them even if it means more surgery. Loss of body parts affects sexuality and family relationships. These needs of the patient assume major proportions as the therapy is completed and patients are in the follow-up phase.

SPECIAL PROBLEMS IN CANCER MANAGEMENT

Cancer is a disease that affects primarily people over 65. More than 50 percent of all deaths occur in that segment of the population over 65 that makes up only 11 percent of our citizens. The elderly are less likely to undergo treatment, be referred to centers, or receive adjunctive treatments. This prejudice against the elderly is hard to appreciate because there is little evidence that cancers are more aggressive or slower growing in that subset of the population. There is also an impression that chemotherapy is more toxic in the elderly. Again most data do not support those concepts. The older individual with or without cancer does have more medical problems, but this does not apply to all of them. Chronologic age is not as important as physiologic age.

Cancer mortality rates in the nonwhite population are often higher for unexplained reasons. These include prostate and breast cancers. For the same stage and histologic type, the outcomes are less favorable in these groups. More research needs to be done to determine the reasons for these differences.

As patients with cancer live longer, the long-term toxicities of chemotherapy or radiation therapy are being recognized. These effects may be manifest as increased second tumors, endocrine organ failure, or changes in mentation. The oncologist and family physician must appreciate the need to continue to follow the patient while recording and observing findings long after the cancer is treated.

BIOLOGIC RESPONSE MODIFIERS

MARK R. ALBERTINI, M.D.
JOAN H. SCHILLER, M.D.

Biologic response modifier (BRM) is a term that was traditionally used for an agent whose antitumor effects were thought to be exerted through modulation of the host's immune system. This is in contrast to the antitumor effects of traditional chemotherapeutic drugs, which kill cancer cells directly. The term, however, has subsequently been applied to a broad range of agents, primarily consisting of human effector cells or their products (cytokines), which have a wide range of effects on both the host and the malignant cell. These effects can be grouped into the following general categories:

1. *Immunologic effects that enhance destruction of the tumor cell.* These activities may be at the level of either the host or the tumor cell and include the following:
   a. *Host.* Augmentation of the host's immune system may be achieved by activating immune effector cells, by enhancing their number, cytotoxicity, or ability to recognize antigens, or by stimulating the production of cytokines.
   b. *Tumor.* Biologic response modifiers may have effects on the tumor cell that make it more susceptible to recognition or killing by immune effector cells or by cytotoxic drugs. For example, enhancement of cell-surface pro- teins or antigens may enhance antigen recog- nition of the tumor cell by effector cells. Alternatively, altering cell membrane charac- teristics may make the tumor cell more sus- ceptible to lysis by cytotoxic agents.
2. *Direct growth-inhibitory effects on the tumor cell.* Although BRMs were first developed for their ability to modify host responses, it is well established that many of these agents also have direct antiproliferative effects.
3. *"Protective" effects on the host from damage to cytotoxic modalities, including chemotherapy and radiation.* Examples of this class of agents include colony-stimulating factors.
4. *Effects on tumor cell biology, including* differenti- ation, angiogenesis, and metastatic ability.

With the exception of alpha-interferon, which is currently approved for the treatment of hairy cell leukemia and Kaposi's sarcoma, no BRMs are currently approved for other than investigational uses in cancer patients. In many cases, the toxicities, therapeutic spectrum, and mechanism of action or biologic activities of these agents are unknown and are undergoing clinical investigation. The objectives of this chapter are to outline the status of the more common BRMs currently under investigation, including possible mechanisms of action, toxicities, and, where known, spectrum of ther- apeutic activity.

INTERFERONS

Interferons (IFNs) are a family of naturally occur- ring proteins produced and secreted by cells in response to virus infection, double-stranded RNA, antigens, or other low-molecular-weight agents. Three different classes (alpha, beta, and gamma) have been identified based on differences in amino acid sequence. Alpha-interferon (IFN-α), which is a family of more than 20 proteins, was the first to be identified, purified, and taken into clinical trials.

Mechanism of Action

Interferons have a broad spectrum of antiviral, immunologic, and antiproliferative properties; which of these is responsible for their antineoplastic effect is unclear. Immunologic properties differ among the three IFN types but include activation of natural killer cells, T cells, killer cells, and macrophages; enhanced secretion of other cytokines; augmentation of antibody-dependent cellular cytotoxicity (ADCC); augmentation of cell-surface protein expression on tumor cells and effector cells, such as histocompatibility class II antigens and tumor-associated antigens; differentiating effects; and effects on oncogenes and angiogenesis. Interferons also induce the synthesis of enzymatic proteins, such as 2,5 oligioadenylate (2,5A) synthetase and protein kinase, which may have important effects on biochemical pathways. Direct antiproliferative effects on tumor cells have generally been considered to be cytostatic, although cytotoxic effects have been reported.

Uncertainties regarding mechanism of action center around the fact that no correlation has been made between enhancement or modulation of any biologic parameter and clinical responses. The role of immunologic mechanisms, however, is supported by murine models in which IFNs have an in vivo antitumor effect despite lack of sensitivity to IFN in vitro. Furthermore, hairy cell leukemia, which is the most sensitive of all malignancies to IFN, is responsive to low doses of IFN. Kaposi's sarcoma, however, requires high doses of IFN to achieve maximal responses. This uncertainty regarding mechanism of activity continues to lead to uncertainties regarding optimal dose to be administered in phase II trials: the maximally tolerated dose (MTD) or the optimal biologic dose (OBD).

Clinical Applications

Two highly purified recombinant IFN-α preparations (IFN-α2a, Hoffmann-LaRoche; and IFN-α2b, Schering-Plough) have been approved by the Food and Drug Administration (FDA) for the treatment of hairy cell leukemia and Kaposi's sarcoma. The clinical activity of these two IFN preparations is nearly identical. The two preparations differ somewhat in the induction of IFN antibodies, although the clinical significance of this antibody induction is unclear. Both IFNs induce clinical responses in approximately 80 percent to 90 percent of patients with hairy cell leukemia, although complete remissions are rare. Partial remissions are associated with a clinical benefit, as evidenced by a decrease in red blood cell and platelet transfusions and a decrease in the incidence of opportunistic infections. Unlike treatment of solid tumors with conventional cytotoxic drugs, remissions may take several months to achieve, may continue for several months following discontinuation of the drugs, and may be reinduced by using the same dose and schedule of IFN therapy. Alpha-interferon may be administered subcutaneously or intramuscularly at low doses (2 million units per square meter three times weekly or 3 million U daily).

Alpha-interferon is effective in patients with acquired immunodeficiency syndrome (AIDS) with Kaposi's sarcoma who have good prognostic parameters: high helper T cell counts (> 400 per cubic millimeter), no B symptoms, and no history of prior opportunistic infections. The response rate decreases from approximately 50 percent to 70 percent in this subset of patients to less than 10 percent in patients with T4 counts less than 100 per cubic millimeter and history of prior opportunistic infections. Unlike hairy cell leukemia, high doses of IFN-α are necessary to achieve maximal response rates (36 million U).

Side Effects

Acute toxicities of IFN consist primarily of an acute influenza-like syndrome, consisting of fevers, chills, rigors, myalgias, headaches, fatigue, malaise, anorexia, arthralgias, and mild nausea. The onset of these symptoms generally occurs between 1 to 3 hours after the administration of IFN and resolves abruptly 2 to 6 hours later. Patients may be premedicated with 650 mg of acetaminophen, and 50 to 75 mg of meperdine may be administered intravenously or intramuscularly for rigors. Because the intensity of these symptoms generally decreases with repeated injections (tachyphylaxis), doses of IFN should generally not be reduced until a sufficient time interval for the tachyphylaxis to occur has passed (usually two to six treatments). Chronic, and often dose-limiting, toxicity consists principally of fatigue, anorexia, and a loss of sense of well-being. Myelosuppression and hepatic toxicity are rarely dose-limiting and usually rapidly reversible. Uncommon central nervous system effects consist of depression, lethargy, and mental slowing, which may progress to stupor and coma.

Beta and gamma-interferons (β-IFN and γ-IFN, respectively) have a different spectrum of in vitro antiproliferative effects and in vivo immunologic activity than IFN-α, and are currently undergoing phase II clinical testing. Their toxicities do not appear to differ substantially from those of IFN-α.

INTERLEUKIN-2 AND CELLULAR IMMUNOTHERAPY

Interleukin-2 (IL-2) is a 15,000 dalton molecular weight glycoprotein that is produced by the helper subclass of T lymphocytes after stimulation by mitogens or specific antigenic stimuli. Production of large quantities of purified recombinant IL-2 became possible after the cloning of the gene for IL-2 in 1983, allowing further evaluation of IL-2 in clinical trials.

Mechanism of Action

Many immunologic changes are induced by in vivo therapy with IL-2, including an increase in the total number of peripheral blood lymphocytes (PBL), an increase in both the number and surface marker intensity of PBLs positive for the CD56 natural killer (NK) cell surface marker, an increase in the proliferative response of PBLs to IL-2, and an increase in the cytotoxic activity of PBLs for NK-resistant targets. Lymphokine-activated killer (LAK) cells result from the in vivo or in vitro exposure of normal lymphocytes to IL-2 and are characterized by their ability to lyse many uncultured, NK-resistant tumor cells. Although NK cells are the primary precursor population for LAK cells, some T cells can also be activated by IL-2 to mediate LAK activity. The generation of LAK effector cells that can mediate cellular cytotoxicity without restriction by the major histocompatibility complex is considered to be the major mechanism for the antitumor effects of in vivo IL-2.

Clinical Applications

Immunotherapeutic trials utilizing IL-2 in various doses and schedules have documented significant immune activation with in vivo IL-2 therapy. Although significant immune responses can be obtained with IL-2 therapy alone and demonstrate an ability to mediate an antitumor effect by the patient's own immune system, these antitumor responses occur infrequently. Preclinical murine models have demonstrated optimal antitumor effects at high and often clinically unachievable doses of IL-2. Clinical trials have evaluated both aggressive, intensive care requiring IL-2 regimens (100,000 U per kilogram, three-times-daily bolus) as well as outpatient regimens of IL-2 therapy (1,000,000 U per square meter per day by continuous infusion). Response rates vary between 4 and 27 percent for patients receiving IL-2 without LAK cells, with most of the higher response rates occurring at the higher doses of IL-2 therapy. The IL-2–mediated toxicity is also clearly greater at the higher IL-2 doses. Diseases that have been most extensively evaluated and have shown the highest response rates include renal cell carcinoma and malignant melanoma.

Many therapeutic protocols are now combining use of a well-characterized IL-2 regimen for immune activation (both bolus and continuous-infusion regimens) along with an additional therapeutic maneuver designed to increase antitumor activity. One strategy has been the combination of exogenously activated LAK cells along with either high-dose or low-dose IL-2 regimens. Renal cell carcinoma and malignant melanoma have been most extensively evaluated and have shown the highest response rates (10 percent to 33 percent). Although it is unclear whether overall response rates and survival have been significantly increased by the addition of LAK-cell infusions to IL-2 therapy, there appears to be a higher percentage of patients who will achieve a complete response with this combined approach. Optimal dose and schedule of IL-2 with LAK-cell infusions are currently being evaluated.

An additional approach has been the isolation and ex vivo IL-2 activation of bulk populations of tumor-infiltrating lymphocytes (TILs), with subsequent adoptive transfer of these IL-2–activated TILs along with IL-2 therapy. Therapy with IL-2–activated TILs has clearly mediated objective tumor responses in some patients, but current approaches have not been significantly improved from IL-2 and LAK cell therapy. Attempts to identify subpopulations of tumor-infiltrating lymphocytes with increased tumor reactivity are now in progress as a means to improve the cellular immunotherapy of human cancers.

Interleukin-2 is also being evaluated in combination with additional cytokines, monoclonal antibodies, and chemotherapy. The selection and scheduling of these therapies with IL-2 will have profound importance both for optimal antitumor responses as well as clinical tolerance.

Side Effects

Subjective clinical toxicities experienced by patients on IL-2 protocols include nausea, vomiting, diarrhea, fatigue, cutaneous reactions, dyspnea, and rigors. Significant clinical toxicities include hypotension requiring pressor support, increased capillary permeability with pulmonary edema and hypoxemia, renal dysfunction due to decreased renal perfusion, cardiac arrhythmias and myocardial infarction, neuropsychiatric complications ranging from disorientation to coma, multiple infectious complications, decreased performance status, weight gain, central venous catheter thromboses, fever, and death. Significant laboratory changes include anemia, neutropenia, eosinophilia with eosinophil counts greater than 10,000 per microliter, thrombocytopenia, increased serum creatinine level, and hyperbilirubinia and increased serum transaminases. Both the frequency and severity of clinical toxicities are greater with the higher-dose IL-2 regimens. Several clinically tolerable IL-2 regimens have been described; however, whether these more tolerable regimens will result in equivalent response rates remains to be determined.

MONOCLONAL ANTIBODIES

The technology to allow fusion of specific antibody-producing B lymphocytes and selected murine myeloma cells was developed by Kohler and Milstein in 1975. These hybrid cells (hybridomas) can produce vast quantities of antibody with defined specificities and can be maintained in culture indefinitely. Monoclonal antibodies have been developed against more than 100 tumor-associated antigens and have tremendous potential applications for tumor diagnosis and monitoring in addition to many potential therapeutic applications.

Mechanism of Action

Monoclonal antibodies can bind to tumor-associated antigens and cause direct tumor cytotoxicity by either complement-mediated or cell-mediated mechanisms. Monoclonal antibodies can also inhibit cell proliferation by binding to growth-factor receptors. Because monoclonal antibodies are foreign proteins, anti-idiotypic monoclonal antibodies can elicit an immune response that may also be directed against the tumor. In addition to unlabeled monoclonal antibodies, antibody immunoconjugates with toxins, cytotoxic drugs, or radionuclides can be formed to "target" therapy to a tumor-associated antigen.

Antibody heteroconjugates, or bispecific antibodies, are a novel means to approximate immune effector lymphocytes and tumor cells in vivo by combining two different Fab fragments in the same monoclonal. Specific binding of the heteroconjugate to the T cell results in T-cell activation. The tumor target is also linked to the antibody heteroconjugate by the antitumor-associated antigen portion of the antibody. The use of chimeric monoclonal antibodies is a different approach that combines murine-derived antigen-binding sites with human constant regions, in an attempt to decrease human antimurine antibody (HAMA) responses. Several chimeric monoclonal antibodies have been able to mediate significant in vitro antibody-dependent, cell-mediated cytotoxicity with human tumor cells, but further in vivo evaluation is needed. Table 1 lists many of the potential therapeutic monoclonal antibodies for human cancers.

Clinical Applications

Most clinical trials with unlabeled monoclonal antibodies have produced only minor clinical responses. Tumors can avoid detection by monoclonal antibodies by antigenic modulation as well as by releasing free antigen into the circulation. Not all cells in a given tumor may express the tumor-associated antigen, and some of the antibodies will have some cross-reactivity with normal tissue. Finally, the inherent lack of significant in vivo cytotoxicity of monoclonal antibodies alone suggests that approaches involving combinations of monoclonal antibodies with other forms of therapy would be necessary to achieve effective antitumor results. Additional studies are also evaluating monoclonal antibodies against growth-factor receptors as well as the use of anti-idiotypic antibodies. Preliminary data suggest potential utility of anti-idiotypic antibodies for human malignant melanoma, and additional clinical trials are now in progress.

"Immunoconjugates" involving monoclonal antibodies linked to toxins, cytotoxic drugs, or radionuclides are also being evaluated. Preliminary data exist for several immunoconjugates, but additional information

Table 1 Potential Therapeutic Monoclonal Antibodies for Human Cancers

Unlabeled Antibodies
　Direct cytotoxicity of monoclonal antibodies
　　Complement-mediated
　　Cell-mediated
　Inhibition of growth-factor receptors
　Induction of specific active immunity with anti-idiotypic
　　monoclonal antibodies

Antibody Immunoconjugates
　Immunoconjugates with toxins
　Immunoconjugates with cytotoxic drugs
　Immunoconjugates with radionuclides

Antibody Heteroconjugates (Bispecific Antibodies)
　Antitumor-associated antigen + anti-CD3
　Antitumor-associated antigen + anti-CD2
　Antitumor-associated antigen + anti-CD16

Chimeric Antibodies
　Murine-derived antigen-binding sites
　Human antibody constant regions

regarding pharmacokinetics, biodistribution, drug dosage, radiation dosimetry, and determination of optimal techniques for immunoconjugation is needed. Polyclonal immunoconjugates, such as polyclonal antiferritin antibodies linked with a radionuclide, are also being evaluated in human hepatocellular carcinoma. Clinical trials will be required to determine the clinical role of antibody heteroconjugates and chimeric antibodies.

Side Effects

Monoclonal antibodies have demonstrated minimal toxicity in most of the clinical trials that have been reported. Significant potential allergic reactions are present if repeated doses of foreign proteins are given. Human antimurine antibodies are seen after therapy with murine monoclonal antibodies and may limit potential effectiveness of these agents. Use of immunoconjugates will likely cause specific toxicities depending on the agent conjugated to the monoclonal antibody.

COLONY-STIMULATING FACTORS

Colony-stimulating factors are growth factors responsible for the survival, proliferation, and maturation of bone marrow stem cells into fully differentiated granulocytes, eosinophils, and monocytes. In addition to their effects on hematopoiesis, colony-stimulating factors (CSFs) are important in stimulating the function of mature cells, such as chemotaxis, phagocytosis, and antibody-dependent cellular cytotoxicity. Although at least five human CSFs have been identified and purified (granulocyte-macrophage colony-stimulating factor [GM-CSF], granulocyte colony-stimulating factor [G-CSF], macrophage colony-stimulating factor [M-CSF], interleukin 5 [eosinophil CSF], and interleukin 3 [multi

CSF]), only two of these (GM-CSF and G-CSF) are currently in phase I and II trials.

Clinical Applications

Clinical trials of CSFs in hematologic and oncologic diseases have centered primarily around two settings: (1) primary bone marrow failure or immunodeficiency states and (2) alleviation of the myelosuppression associated with cytotoxic drugs. In the former setting, CSFs have been used successfully in patients suffering from AIDS and leukopenia, myelodysplastic syndrome and leukopenia, aplastic anemia, idiopathic neutropenia, cyclic neutropenia, chronic severe neutropenia, and cogenital agranulocytosis. Colony-stimulating factors have induced leukocytosis in patients with advanced malignancies and hairy cell leukemia.

Colony-stimulating factors have also been used successfully to stimulate myelopoiesis in patients who are receiving myelosuppressive drugs for malignancies. Randomized, controlled clinical trials have demonstrated either a lesser degree of myelosuppression, a shorter duration of myelosuppression, or both, in patients with transitional cell carcinoma of the bladder, advanced sarcomas, or small-cell carcinomas of the lung who are receiving chemotherapy and CSFs when compared to patients receiving chemotherapy alone. Colony-stimulating factors have also been used successfully in patients receiving autologous bone marrow transplantation to enhance engraftment, reduce the number of febrile days, and recover neutrophil and platelet counts more quickly.

Side Effects

Differences in toxicities between the two CSF preparations that are currently undergoing clinical investigation (GM-CSF and G-CSF) have not been defined. Common side effects include bone pain, skin rash, rigors, local skin reactions, and low-grade fever and chills. Serious adverse reactions at high doses have included pericarditis and pleuritis.

OTHER IMMUNOTHERAPIES

Tumor Vaccines

Another potential use of BRMs is to specifically activate the immune system of the tumor-bearing host against tumor-associated antigens. Both autologous and allogeneic tumor cells, and various preparations derived from them, have been utilized in attempts to generate specific active stimulation of the host's immune system. Although clinical antitumor responses have occasionally been seen with this approach and some patients so immunized subsequently have been able to generate an antigen-specific antibody response, most long-term results have been disappointing. However, some promising results have been seen in patients with malignant melanoma. Clinical trials are now in progress to determine the efficacy of tumor vaccines in the adjuvant setting for patients at high risk of relapse from malignant melanoma. Another approach with tumor vaccines, as discussed previously, is the use of anti-idiotypic antibodies to elicit a specific active stimulation of the host's immune system. This approach is also being evaluated in ongoing clinical trials.

Levamisole

Levamisole is a synthetic antihelminthic drug currently undergoing investigation as an antineoplastic drug because of in vitro and in vivo reports demonstrating immunologic and antitumor effects. The mechanism of action by which levamisole might exert any antineoplastic activity is unknown; however, it has been reported to enhance neutrophil and monocyte chemotaxis, augment cytotoxic T-cell response, and augment monocyte activation. Early clinical reports have shown antitumor activity in metastatic colorectal carcinoma, advanced locoregional breast carcinoma, resectable lung cancer, and multiple myeloma, although these results need to be confirmed. Recently, levamisole plus 5-fluorouracil has been shown to result in improved survival in patients with Duke's C colon cancer in controlled, randomized trials. Levamisole alone was not effective in prolonging survival.

Tumor Necrosis Factor

Tumor necrosis factor (TNF) is a cytokine that was originally identified in the serum of bacillus Calmette Guérin (BCG) sensitized mice injected with endotoxin as the mediator of tumor-necrotizing activity. It has since been found to have cytotoxic and cytostatic activity against a broad range of murine and human carcinoma cell lines, both in vitro and in vivo. It also has been shown to have a wide range of immunomodulatory and biologic properties. Synergistic antitumor effects have been reported when TNF is combined with IFN-γ or IL-2. Phase I trials of recombinant TNF, either as a single agent or in combination with IFN or IL-2, have been completed and phase II trials are underway. Toxicities appear similar to those of other BRMs, consisting primarily of hypotension, fever, rigors and constitutional symptoms.

Bacillus Calmette Guérin

Bacillus Calmette Guérin is an attenuated strain of *Mycobacterium bovis* that is used as a nonspecific immunomodulator, although it also causes delayed-type hypersensitivity to mycobacterial antigens. Although the systemic administration of BCG as an adjuvant treatment following surgery or chemotherapy has been studied extensively in numerous large-scale randomized trials and has not been found to prolong survival, BCG has been shown to be effective as an intravesical agent for the treatment of superficial bladder carcinoma.

Intravesical administration is associated with symptoms of bladder irritation, including dysuria, frequency, urgency, and hematuria, as well as constitutional "flu-like" symptoms similar to those observed with other biologic agents.

FUTURE PROSPECTS FOR IMMUNOTHERAPY

Current BRMs have been largely evaluated in patients with advanced and refractory malignancies. A small, but significant, number of clinical responses have been realized by entirely immunologic therapies. Several potential approaches may help to increase the clinical relevance of BRMs for the majority of patients with cancer. Some improvements may be achieved by adjustments of treatment doses and schedules or by the evaluation of promising BRMs in patients with less advanced disease or in an adjuvant setting. New BRMs will likely be developed. The use of BRMs in a combined immunotherapeutic approach has much theoretical appeal and is now undergoing clinical evaluation. Interleukin-2 can be combined with IFNs, which may increase expression of tumor-associated antigens or synergize with NK-cell activation. Interleukin-2 can be combined with any of the monoclonal antibody approaches described previously and potentially in-

crease either direct cytotoxicity or antibody-dependent cellular cytotoxicity. Effector-cell subpopulations with increased tumor reactivity can be selectively expanded and utilized for adoptive immunotherapy with IL-2 or specific monoclonal antibodies. Finally, the appropriate combination of BRMs with surgery, chemotherapy, or radiation therapy may ultimately produce an effective therapeutic approach for many patients with cancer.

SUGGESTED READING

Borden EC, Sondel PM. Lymphokines and cytokines as cancer treatment. Cancer 1990; 65:800–814.

Foon KA. Biological response modifiers: The new immunotherapy. Cancer Res 1989; 49:1,621–1,639.

Hertler AA, Frankel AE. Immunotoxins: A clinical review of their use in the treatment of malignancies. J Clin Oncol 1989; 7:1,932–1,942.

Margolin KA, Rayner AA, Hawkins MJ, et al. Interleukin-2 and lymphokine-activated killer cell therapy of solid tumors: Analysis of toxicity and management guidelines. J Clin Oncol 1989; 7:486–498.

Moore MAS. Hematopoietic growth factors in cancer. Cancer 1990; 65:836–844.

Schlom J. Basic principles and applications of monoclonal antibodies in the management of carcinomas: The Richard and Hinda Rosenthal Foundation Award Lecture. Cancer Res 1986; 46: 3,225–3,238.

Sosman JA, Hank JA, Sondel PM. In vivo activation of lymphokine-activated killer activity with interleukin-2: Prospects for combination therapies. Sem Oncol 1990; 17:22–30.

CANCER PREVENTION

PETER GREENWALD, M.D., DR.P.H.

The growing prominence of cancer prevention as a means to reduce cancer mortality has arisen from research evidence demonstrating that life-style can affect a person's chances of developing cancer. As much as 90 percent of cancer incidence may be related to life-style and environmental factors, so that, in theory, cancer is largely preventable. Cancer prevention focuses on reducing cancer incidence by avoiding or minimizing exposure to those factors thought to increase cancer occurrence and precancerous progression and encourages the use of cancer prevention practices. A joint effort of physicians and their patients has the potential to improve the nation's cancer statistics and move toward achieving goals for reduced cancer mortality.

Several studies show that physician intervention can exert a powerful influence on patients' adherence to cancer prevention practices. Because the average American aged 45 to 64 years makes 5.1 ambulatory medical visits per year, and those 65 years and older make 6.3 visits per year, there are many encounters during which

physicians can counsel patients about positive behavior changes. In addition, physicians are an authoritative source of health and medical information. Thus, the role of the physician as the primary health care provider is essential in motivating Americans to adhere to preventive habits that may reduce cancer incidence and mortality.

Two factors, tobacco use and diet, are major life-style contributors to cancer mortality, yet they are the most controllable and thus the important focus of cancer prevention strategies. It is estimated that over 30 percent of cancer deaths could be avoided by eliminating tobacco use. The link between tobacco use and cancer at various sites, including the lungs, mouth, and esophagus, is firmly established. Smoking also contributes to cancers of the bladder, pancreas, and kidney.

Because roughly 35 percent of cancer mortality has been estimated to be related to dietary factors, appropriate modification of diet may reduce cancer rates. Although the knowledge of fundamental nutritional mechanisms that affect cancer is incomplete, certain dietary changes are advisable in light of existing evidence. Sufficient laboratory evidence has already accumulated to develop and test several hypotheses in clinical cancer prevention trials with selected nutrient interventions.

In addition to smoking cessation and dietary modification, this chapter discusses chemoprevention, a new area of emphasis in cancer prevention and control. This research, conducted in a series of phases and evaluations, identifies and characterizes chemopreventive agents from natural and synthetic sources that indicate a potential to stop or reverse neoplastic progression. These agents may have the potential to inhibit or arrest genetically initiated cancers or those acquired by exposure to carcinogenic agents in defined risk groups as well as in the general population. With increased understanding of carcinogenic processes, chemopreventive agents may be used to interrupt the development of cancer at one of several different points along its pathway. Fostering lifelong adherence to cancer preventive regimens is a present and future challenge for physicians.

SMOKING PREVENTION AND CESSATION

Although cancer incidence and mortality rates for several cancers in the United States are decreasing, particularly for people under age 65, cancer rates for lung cancer have increased over the past several decades. Lung cancer rates for men have probably peaked, and the latest data indicate a decline consistent with changes in smoking prevalence. However, the lung cancer rates for women continue to increase, and female smoking rates are declining much more slowly than in men. Because lung cancer is almost entirely a result of tobacco use, physicians can effectively intervene by encouraging smoking avoidance and cessation. Evidence from randomized studies shows that physicians informed about smoking cessation techniques can convince 5 percent to 20 percent of their patients not to smoke. The fact that only a small proportion of smokers report that their physician has ever talked to them about cessation indicates the additional impact that physicians could

have if a great number provided smokers with at least brief encouragement to quit. Minimal physician intervention (i.e., physician counseling, educational booklet supplements, and telephone follow-up) was shown to increase quit rates significantly.

Results of Clinical Trials of Smoking Cessation in Physician Practice

Five major intervention trials were sponsored by the National Cancer Institute (NCI) from 1984 through 1989 with the objective of developing brief, structured training and intervention protocols for physicians (and dentists) and their staffs to use in encouraging patients to stop smoking. A profile of the interventions and major trial results are shown in Table 1.

Physician training in smoking cessation produced positive changes in physician-initiated activities, including more time devoted to smoking cessation advice, increased prescription of nicotine gum, increased use of appointments devoted partially or wholly to smoking cessation, more frequent distribution of smoking cessation self-help material, and more frequent establishment of patient quit-smoking dates. Resulting patient smoking cessation rates ranged from 2 percent to 17 percent. Increased success rates were found under three conditions: when comprehensive systems were in place to remind personnel to provide advice; when only patients who were motivated to stop smoking were the focus of the intervention; and when program intensity was increased (e.g., follow-up visits, effective prescription of nicotine gum). Trial results further indicate that the use of intermediary (or community) organizations can increase physician motivation to provide smoking cessation advice. Also, long-term maintenance of simple, office-wide smoking cessation procedures integrated into the reality of medical practice is more effective than a brief, intense program.

Table 1 Profile of Physician (and Dentist) Interventions

Objective	To develop brief, structured training and intervention protocols for physicians and dentists to reduce patient smoking prevalence
Number of trials	5
Methods tested	Nicotine gum use
	Training
	Support and reminder systems
	Relapse prevention
	Self-help
	Protocol compliance
Channels involved	Private practices
	Public clinics
	Health maintenance organizations
	Residency training programs
Number of patients and physicians	107,554 patients
	6,091 physicians and dentists
Primary study period	1984–1989
Major trial results	Consistent patient smoking cessation rates were achieved, ranging from 2% to 17%

Adapted from the Smoking, Tobacco, and Cancer Program 1985–1989 Status Report (in press).

How Best to Advise Your Patient

Within this context, the program elements summarized in Table 2 have been suggested for successful physician intervention in smoking cessation. The physician should identify all patients who smoke, flag their charts, and assess their smoking history and motivation to quit. A personalized discussion of the hazards of smoking and strong recommendation to quit should be given. If possible, a patient's commitment to quit by a certain date should be obtained as part of an individualized plan.

In addition to receiving formal training in smoking cessation, physicians can be more effective if they involve a support team of selected staff members, such as receptionists and nurses, in their smoking cessation procedures, as suggested in Table 2, and systematize the process. Screening patients to determine their level of motivation and focusing on those who are more motivated will result in more efficient use of staff and physician time. To monitor the progress, the staff must ensure that follow-up phone calls or letters and return visits are arranged. One analysis of this approach shows that active follow-up can increase smoking quit rates by 10 percent over rates achieved when follow-up is absent.

Table 2 Essential Elements of a Physician-Guided Smoking Cessation Program

Intake and Screening
Identify smoking status along with vital signs.
Update tobacco use status regularly (6 mo and 12 mo).
Obtain basic data on smoking history and readiness to quit (update regularly if possible).

Physician Actions
Assess motivation and risk profile.
Personalize risk of smoking and benefit of quitting.
Advise to quit.
Obtain quit commitment (set quit date).
Triage (quit plan, including nicotine gum).
Emphasize that progress will be monitored.

Office Staff Actions
Define office resources.
Review quit plan.
Explain nicotine gum use (as necessary).
Explain self-help materials (review special sections).
Facilitate referral to outside resources.
Schedule follow-up contact (link to quit plan).

Follow-up
Conduct rapid follow-up of all patients with plan to change.
Reassess smoking status at next visit.
Triage and recycle relapsers at next visit.

Office Environment
Establish smoke-free office (staff and patients).
Make smoking education materials available.
Publicize smoking cessation program.

From Cullen JW. Principles of cancer prevention: Tobacco. In: DeVita VT Jr, Hillman S, Rosenberg SA, eds. Cancer: Principles and practice of oncology. 3rd ed. Philadelphia: JB Lippincott, 1989: 190; with permission.

Numerous resources are available to help physicians establish and maintain smoking cessation efforts in their offices. The National Cancer Institute has codified physician protocols in a manual entitled *How To Help Your Patients Stop Smoking* (March 1989) and also has other materials available, such as the *Quit for Good* kit for physicians, which contains an information booklet, chart stickers, and copies of self-help and waiting room materials (Office of Cancer Communications, NCI, Bethesda, MD 20892).

Nearly a million deaths were delayed or averted between 1964 and 1985 because millions of Americans decided to quit smoking or refrained from initiating this habit. The 1989 Surgeon General report states that there would be more than 90 million American smokers today instead of some 56 million had the antismoking campaign, begun in 1964, not occurred. Physician efforts in this area can powerfully affect patient motivation and behavior change.

DIETARY MODIFICATION

Although the precise contribution of diet in cancer etiology is not yet determined, existing data provide sufficient evidence for recommending prudent dietary modification that may reduce the risk of some types of cancer. The recent comprehensive National Academy of Sciences' review of diet and cancer is based on the scientific rationale that diet is a controllable risk factor and that cancer incidence could be reduced by dietary modification. The optimal effectiveness of physicians is to provide advice, counseling, and educational materials to assist patients in modifying dietary risks. In many practices, this is viewed as a cooperative process involving nurses, dietitians, and nutritionists.

National Cancer Institute Dietary Guidelines

On the basis of epidemiologic and laboratory evidence showing the cancer promotion or risk reduction of specific dietary components, the NCI has proposed six interim guidelines for increasing the intake of vegetables, fruits, and whole grains (high-fiber foods) while decreasing fat, maintaining desirable weight, and limiting alcohol consumption (Table 3). These guidelines were derived in part from the National Academy of Sciences (NAS) committee report (1982) and were augmented by more recent NCI workshops and a comprehensive review of the data on fiber. These dietary guidelines for cancer prevention undergo periodic reviews based on new research developments. Last reviewed in September 1989, conclusions were that the NCI Guidelines are still timely and appropriate as published.

The National Cancer Institute recommends a reduction in total fat intake from its present level of about 38 percent of calories to below 30 percent. Because diverse populations show a consistent protective effect

Table 3 National Cancer Institute Dietary Guidelines

Reduce fat intake to 30% or less of calories.
Increase fiber intake to 20–30 g/day with an upper limit of 35 g.
Include a variety of vegetables and fruits in the daily diet.
Avoid obesity.
Consume alcoholic beverages in moderation, if at all.
Minimize consumption of salt-cured, salt-pickled, or smoked foods.

From the Division of Cancer Prevention and Control, National Cancer Institute, National Institutes of Health, Bethesda, MD.

associated with dietary fiber intake, NCI recommends that the US adult population increase current dietary fiber intake, from a variety of food sources, to 20 or 30 g from the present average of about 11 g daily. An upper limit of 35 g per day is suggested to avoid any possible adverse effects. Foods high in fiber may also contain other nutritive or nonnutritive substances that reduce cancer risk. Understanding the exact manner in which diet affects tumor incidence and devising and promoting strategies for altering this process are ongoing challenges of nutrition-related cancer prevention research. Until a more specific characterization of the role of dietary factors affecting cancer is developed, the most beneficial course of action is to promote adherence to interim dietary guidelines.

Basis for the Guidelines

Epidemiologic evidence provides consistent support for a relationship between dietary components and the development of certain cancers, including cancers of the gastrointestinal tract and some sex hormone target organs. Vitamins A, C, and E, carotenoids, calcium, selenium, fiber, and a number of nonnutritive components are hypothesized to contribute individually, or in combination, to the apparent cancer-preventive effect of certain food groups. To illustrate the role of primary prevention through intervention, the role of diet in the development of colon cancer is discussed in the following section.

Diet and Colon Cancer

International correlation and migration studies are consistent with the idea that diet is a major factor in the development of colon cancer. These show worldwide use of dietary fiber to be inversely correlated with risk of colon cancer. In westernized countries, the colon cancer rate tends to be substantially higher than in underdeveloped countries, where dietary fiber intake is high. Also of particular interest is Finland, a modern western country with a low colon cancer rate and a high consumption of fiber. Further evidence of the beneficial effects of dietary fiber is seen within country correlations, case-control and cohort epidemiologic studies, and clinical-metabolic studies.

However, not all data are entirely consistent. Differences may exist because dietary fiber from different food sources is a heterogeneous mixture of components,

such as cellulose, hemicelluloses, pectins, gums, and lignin, and therefore may have varying physiologic effects. In addition, fiber components are difficult to quantify accurately in foods, and it has been difficult to separate the effects of fiber from other dietary constituents (e.g., total calories, fats, vitamins, minerals, and nonnutritive components of fruits and vegetables). More information is needed about which specific fiber components are protective.

The other major dietary factor commonly implicated in epidemiologic studies of colorectal cancer is fat. As with breast cancer, the intake of dietary fat is directly related to colon cancer mortality in international correlation settings. Case-control studies on colon cancer and fat are less consistent, probably owing to problems of accurate dietary recall, which tend to bias dietary recall studies in the direction of diminishing true differences.

Studies with animal models of colon cancer indicate a promotional role for dietary fat; both the type of fat consumed and the quantity are important determinants. The results of studies from several laboratories using different carcinogens show that, when the level of dietary fat is increased from 5 percent to 20 or 24 percent, chemically induced colon carcinogenesis is enhanced. Tumor incidence under these conditions increases by 40 percent or 50 percent and occurs when lard, corn oil, or beef fat is used as the fat source.

Recent studies in rodents also demonstrate that dietary fat affects chemically induced colon carcinogenesis, both independently and interactively with fiber. For example, one study shows an enhancing effect of fat on both tumor incidence and tumor multiplicity in rats fed a low-fiber diet, whereas fat had no effect when the fiber content of the diet was high.

Carcinogenesis studies of tumor progression find that fat appears to act during the promotion stage. Feeding high-fat diets to rats before or during treatment with azoxymethane does not enhance tumor yield, whereas the same diet fed after carcinogen administration strongly promotes development of intestinal tumors. One series of experiments suggests that the mechanism of fat promotion in colon carcinogenesis is related to increases in excretion of bile acid, which may act as an intestinal irritant.

Of the micronutrients evaluated for their protective effects on colon cancer, calcium is notable for its activity both in vitro and in vivo. Calcium may have an important role as a fat inactivator in addition to its activity as modulator of epithelial cell differentiation. Limited research testing other types of chemopreventives in colon cancer models has been conducted with selenium and certain antioxidants. These show at least marginal inhibitory activity.

The laboratory effects of macronutrients and certain micronutrients provide strong research leads for developing prevention approaches for colon cancer. Considerable work is under way to better characterize the role of specific types of fat and fiber and the influence of other nutrients, such as calcium, on carcinogenesis.

CHEMOPREVENTION TRIALS

Cancer prevention through the administration of specific chemical regimens is a new area of research with a broad potential for reducing cancer incidence rates. The rationale for chemoprevention is based on strong epidemiologic evidence noting the wide international variations in the occurrence of certain types of cancer and laboratory studies indicating that specific natural and synthetic agents may prevent the initiation or promotion of the neoplastic progress. Chemoprevention research, aided by advancements in understanding the biochemical mechanisms underlying carcinogenesis, has progressed to the point where chemical agents are being identified, characterized, and tested in animal models and clinical trials when a high probability of human efficacy is indicated.

At the NCI, each candidate chemopreventive agent is subjected to an orderly sequence of research phases prior to the initiation of a clinical trial. This preclinical research is designed to identify and test the efficacy, and toxicity, of proposed agents in an in vitro and in vivo screening system. For example, difluoromethylornithine (DFMO) is an irreversible inhibitor of ornithine decarboxylase, the rate-limiting enzyme in polyamine synthesis, whose activity has been implicated in neoplastic cell proliferation. When applied to mouse colon, DFMO appears to act as an antipromotional chemopreventive agent for experimentally induced tumorigenesis. Results such as these, from the preclinical array of tests, may be limited in predicting the effects in humans; thus, clinical intervention trials are necessary to evaluate the efficacy and safety of a promising chemopreventive agent in an actual setting.

Clinical prevention trials require design criteria similar to therapeutic trials such as subject randomization, blinding (when feasible), appropriate controls, dose and treatment schedules, monitoring of subject compliance and accurate data collection and analysis. Chemoprevention trials, however, have some unique features, particularly in regard to the study population and study protocol. The chemoprevention trial selects its study population from healthy subjects, or persons at high risk because of life-style factors, preneoplastic lesions, or a previously treated cancer, whereas the treatment study population consists of cancer patients. The level of toxicity of the chemopreventive agent should be negligible or absent, whereas with therapeutic agents, severe toxicity often is acceptable for malignant disease not otherwise treatable. Both types of trials may require large resource commitments, but generally, prevention studies may require thousands of subjects and may last 10 or more years; thus, they are more expensive. Additionally, subject compliance is easier to maintain with cancer patients than with healthy persons or those at high risk for the development of malignant disease.

As with classical clinical treatment trials, chemoprevention trials pass through an orderly progression of phases. Phase I of the chemoprevention clinical research array involves evaluation of data from preclinical studies as a basis for selection of a safe dose for humans. Pharmacokinetic information can be obtained, including effective blood levels, distribution, metabolism, and elimination of the chemopreventive agent. Phase II trials are essentially screening systems for biologic activity, usually in high-risk populations. After safety and efficacy have been determined in a small population, phase III trials are initiated to administer the agent to many subjects, for extended periods of time. Endpoints in these studies may include overall incidence of cancer, incidence of specific cancers, rate of regression or progression of preneoplastic changes, and changes in cellular or biochemical parameters associated with tumor progression.

Chemoprevention trials supported by the NCI mainly in medical settings are investigating the prevention of cancer at sites such as the colon, breast, lung, cervix, skin, and oral cavity. Selected chemoprevention trials are presented in Table 4. For colon cancer, for example, the targeted risk groups are subjects with adenomatous polyps, and the inhibiting agents under study are fiber, calcium, beta-carotene, vitamins C and E, and the anti-inflammatory antiproliferative drug, piroxicam.

In a recently reported 4-year chemoprevention trial, 58 patients with familial polyposis were treated with either a placebo, with vitamins C (ascorbic acid) and E (alpha-tocopherol), or with these vitamins plus a wheat fiber supplement. When adjusted for patient compliance, the results from the randomized, double-blind trial showed a limited, but statistically significant, inhibition of benign large bowel neoplasia by consumption of dietary fiber supplements of at least 11 g per day. A lesser association was demonstrated between high vitamin C and E intake and the reduction of colon polyps. In a more extensive study, in subjects previously diagnosed with adenomatous polyps, the NCI is further investigating reducing the recurrence of this precancerous lesion by the consumption of a low-fat, high-fiber, and fruit- and vegetable-enriched diet.

The preceding trials are of particular interest because they do not measure cancer incidence as the endpoint but rather assess alterations in precancerous lesions or biochemical, cellular, or molecular indices that may be associated with future malignancy. For example, enhanced colonic epithelial cell proliferation may be a reflection of an increased susceptibility to colon cancer, as low-risk individuals display an epithelium that is more quiescent. In individuals at increased risk for familial colon cancer and those with familial polyposis, supplemental dietary calcium has been shown to decrease colonic cell hyperproliferation, as measured by ^{3}H-thymidine labeling.

Other biologic markers include ornithine decarboxylase inhibition, prostaglandin synthesis inhibition, reversal of abnormal cytology, decreases in fecal mutagens, increased oncogene activation and expression, and inhibition of tumor suppressor genes. To act as successful indicators of future cancer incidence, these markers

Table 4   Selected Current Chemoprevention Intervention Trials*

Target Site	Target/Risk Group	Inhibitory Agents
Breast	Adenocarcinoma	4-HPR
Cervix	Mild/moderate cervical dysplasia	*Trans*-retinoic acid
Cervix	Cervical dysplasia	Folic acid
Colon	Previous colon adenoma	Wheat bran and calcium carbonate
Colon	Previous colon adenoma	Calcium
Colon	High-risk epithelial cell proliferation	Calcium
Colon	Previous adenomatous polyps	Beta-carotene
Colon	Previous adenomatous polyps	Piroxicam
Lung	Chronic smokers	13-*cis*-retinoic acid
Lung	Men, exposed to asbestos	Beta-carotene and retinol
Lung	Cigarette smokers	Beta-carotene and retinoids
Lung	Smoking men	Beta-carotene
Skin	Albinos in Tanzania	Beta-carotene
Skin	Previous basal cell carcinoma	Beta-carotene
Skin	Actinic keratoses patients	Retinol
Skin	Previous basal cell carcinoma	Retinol or 13-*cis*-retinoic acid
Oral cavity	Leukoplakia	13-*cis*-retinoic acid ± beta-carotene
Oral cavity	Leukoplakia	Beta-carotene
All sites	American physicians	Beta-carotene, aspirin

*National Cancer Institute, Division of Cancer Prevention and Control.

must be rigorously validated in large clinical trials and meet strict statistical requirements before researchers can be confident of their predictive value. Biologic markers as predictors of future cancer incidence may have broad clinical applicability in generating additional large-scale intervention trials. These intervention trials have the advantage of requiring less time than a standard prevention trial to achieve comparable statistical power, as well as greatly reduced trial costs.

SUGGESTED READING

Cullen JW. Principles of cancer prevention: Tobacco. In: DeVita VT Jr, Hillman S, Rosenberg SA, eds. Cancer: Principles and practice of oncology. 3rd ed. Philadelphia: JB Lippincott, 1989:181–195.

DeCosse JJ, Miller HH, Lesser ML. Effect of wheat fiber and vitamins C and E on rectal polyps in patients with familial adenomatous polyposis. J Natl Cancer Inst 1989; 81:1,290–1,297.

Greenwald P. Principles of carcinogenesis: Dietary factors. In: DeVita VT Jr, Hillman S, Rosenberg SA, ed. Cancer: Principles and practice of oncology. 3rd ed. Philadelphia: JB Lippincott, 1989:167–180.

Lerman C, Rimer B, Engstrom PF. Reducing avoidable cancer mortality through prevention and early detection regimens. Cancer Res 1989; 49:4,955–4,962.

National Academy of Sciences. National Research Council. Committee on Diet, Nutrition and Cancer. Diet, nutrition, and cancer. Assembly of Life Sciences. Washington, D.C.: National Academy Press, 1982.

National Academy of Sciences. National Research Council. Food and Nutrition Board. Diet and health: Implications for reducing chronic disease risk. Council on Life Sciences. Washington, D.C.: National Academy Press, 1989.

BREAST CANCER: SURGERY

ALONZO P. WALKER, M.D.
WILLIAM L. DONEGAN, M.D.

The management of breast cancer is undergoing substantial change based on new concepts about its biology and natural history. This has had considerable impact upon the surgeon's role in diagnosis and treatment. Currently, the systemic aspect of breast cancer is being addressed even in early stages, and local regional treatment is increasingly conservative. Treatment continues to be a joint effort in which surgery, radiation therapy, and systemic chemohormonal therapy have roles, but the traditional roles are changing, becoming less insular and more integrated into a collaborative overall effort in which patients participate not as a passive recipient but as a decision maker regarding choices of alternative treatments. The disease is also being found more often in its earliest forms through growing use of mammography and regular screening of asymptomatic women. This means that breast cancer is becoming the most frequent cancer of women as well as one of the most curable, and increasingly lends itself to breast-conserving methods of management.

In these circumstances, the surgeon is called upon to adopt new methods of biopsy designed to locate and discretely remove small, nonpalpable lesions found only on mammography. Close collaboration with the radiologist and pathologist is essential to the success of these techniques. Biopsies are now routinely performed without hospital admission or general anesthesia and as a procedure separate from surgical treatment. In the effort to diagnose early, the majority of biopsies do not reveal cancer. As a consequence, morbidity is minimized by emphasis on convenience, cost-effectiveness, and cosmetic considerations. Fine-needle aspiration cytology is replacing core-needle or open biopsy for palpable tumors of the breast because of its convenience and accuracy. Aspirates that show cancer cells can be followed with staging and a decision regarding treatment. An open biopsy designed to identify the occasional false positive can be deferred until the time of treatment.

Beyond issues relevant to biopsy, the most important considerations that define surgical therapy are the histology of the cancer and the stage of disease. This chapter addresses the current role of surgery in the diagnosis of breast cancer, its application to patients with palpable and nonpalpable lesions, and the therapeutic options relevant to histologic type and stage.

DIAGNOSIS OF THE PALPABLE MASS

A palpable mass continues to be the most frequent diagnostic problem relevant to breast disease, and despite the growing use of mammography, most cancers still present as a palpable mass discovered by the patient herself, her husband, or her physician. Fine-needle aspiration of masses serves to distinguish quickly cysts from solid tumors and is widely accepted as the appropriate initial diagnostic maneuver. Careful aspiration rarely causes confusing changes on a subsequent mammogram. With fine-needle aspiration and ultrasound as resources, it is no longer acceptable to perform open biopsies for simple cysts (removal of nonbloody fluid and permanent disappearance of the mass identifies a simple cyst). If no fluid is obtained, the same aspiration conveniently serves to obtain a sample of the tissue for cytologic examination. Identification of cancer cells by this method is rarely an error and bypasses the necessity for separate open biopsy prior to the date of treatment (a two-step procedure). If cytology is unsatisfactory or shows no cancer cells, however, the uncertainty must be resolved with open biopsy, which is now routinely performed as an outpatient procedure under mild sedation and local anesthesia. Malignant tissue found at open biopsy is routinely tested for estrogen and progesterone receptors and more recently for tumor cell ploidy and S-phase fraction with flow cytometry. It must be emphasized that a normal mammogram does not obviate the need to biopsy a mass in the breast, as palpable cancers may fail to be visualized because of dense tissues, a geographic miss, or suboptimal technique. Furthermore, open biopsy with frozen section is still needed immediately preceding treatment to distin-

guish invasive from noninvasive cancers and to identify the occasional false-positive cytology (a one-step procedure).

A modification of biopsy currently used by some physicians, particularly when cancer is strongly suspected, is to excise small masses with a clear margin of normal tissue so that the excisional biopsy serves as a therapeutically acceptable lumpectomy. If the mass indeed proves to be a cancer and all surgical margins are histologically tumor free, there is no need to re-excise the biopsy cavity if the patient decides upon breast-conserving therapy. Re-excision of a biopsy cavity is often an inexact task, necessitating excessive sacrifice of tissue, particularly if another surgeon has performed the initial biopsy, and more so if it was followed by considerable ecchymosis. Needless to say, the best cosmetic result may not be obtained. When this procedure is used, the specimen is oriented with suture tags by the surgeon so that the site of inadequate margins can be precisely identified by the pathologist and additional tissue removed if necessary. To facilitate later examination of margins, the pathologist also paints the specimen with a stain (e.g., India ink) that is visible histologically. With a satisfactory lumpectomy accomplished in this manner, all that remains to complete conservative therapy if the tumor proves invasive is axillary dissection at a subsequent time. Inadequate or indeterminate margins require wider re-excision or mastectomy. It will be appreciated that indiscriminate use of the wide biopsy technique results in unnecessary sacrifice of tissue around many benign lesions (Fig. 1).

NONPALPABLE BREAST LESIONS

Widespread use of mammography for screening has introduced a new dimension to biopsy—the need to determine the nature of nonpalpable lesions in the breasts of asymptomatic women. These subtle mammographic signs of cancer are most often in the form of clustered fine microcalcifications, but also include small stellate masses, architectural distortions, asymmetric densities, and densities containing microcalcifications. Each of these signs is an accepted indication for biopsy; however, the predictive value for malignancy is low, ranging from 9 to 65 percent. Only 20 percent of biopsies for clustered microcalcifications reveal cancer, but when associated with a density, the probability increases to 65 percent. The lowest probability is associated with asymmetric density.

Initially, the entire quadrant of the breast in which the lesion was located was removed to accomplish diagnosis. Currently, "localizing" procedures are in use that permit them to be removed accurately and discretely. Close coordination of surgeon, radiologist, and pathologist is essential for success. The "spot technique" involves injection of a streak of radiocontrast mixed with a visible dye into the lesion with a fine needle under mammographic control. The visible streak of dye leading

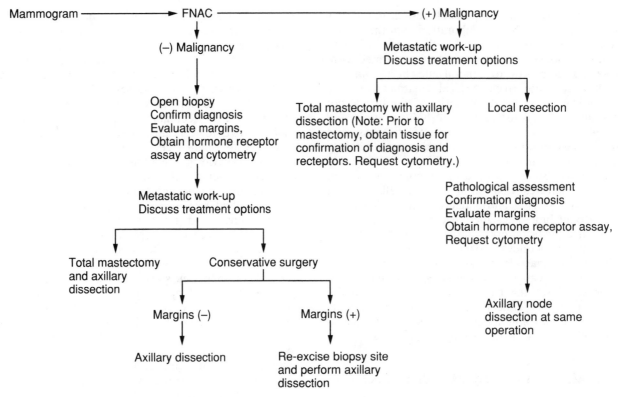

Figure 1 Surgical management of palpable clinical Stage I/II cancers.

(FNAC-Fine needle aspiration cytology)

from the skin to the lesion then serves to guide the surgeon. More widely used are various types of fine sterile wires that are inserted under mammographic guidance to lead the surgeon to the appropriate location in the breast. The biopsy immediately follows localization and is customarily performed with intravenous sedation and under local anesthesia without hospital admission. Accurate removal of microcalcifications and small dense masses can and should be confirmed immediately with a specimen radiograph; the radiologist then locates the precise site of the lesion for the pathologist by placing markers in the specimen. Because the targets are generally small and permit only a limited number of sections for examination, the pathologist often chooses to defer frozen section and save all the tissues for permanent sections. An accurate removal using these techniques can be accomplished in more than 95 percent of cases. When the tissues show no cancer, however, a follow-up mammogram in 2 to 3 months is routine in order to prove that the lesion was in fact removed; if it was not, a repeat biopsy is necessary.

When it is evident on histologic examination that small cancers removed in this fashion have tumor-free margins, the biopsy can provide the basis for breast-conserving treatment without the need for additional surgery on the breast. It is not always feasible to accomplish this at the time of needle-guided biopsy because most of these small cancers are not visible

grossly. Furthermore, the small amount of tumor tissue often does not permit quantitative biochemical determinations of steroid receptors, but they do permit immunocytochemical assay for estrogen receptor protein (ERICA).

In the interval between histologic diagnosis of cancer and treatment, appropriate laboratory and radiographic studies are performed to accomplish accurate staging, primarily to detect distant metastases. A cytologic aspirate consistent with cancer also justifies staging in anticipation of treatment.

THE TNM STAGING SYSTEM

The TNM staging system for breast cancer changed in 1988. The most important changes were that noninvasive carcinomas became stage 0, in keeping with this designation for in situ cancers at most other sites. The previous stage II was divided into two parts, IIA and IIB, the latter to accommodate large, formerly stage IIIA tumors without associated adenopathy and 2- to 5-cm formerly stage II tumors associated with adenopathy. This change served to recognize the relatively benign behavior of large breast cancers without regional spread. Patients with supraclavicular metastases were moved out of stage IIIB and placed into stage IV because of their poor prognosis. The current full staging format is shown in Table 1.

Table 1   1988 Staging System

Definition of TNM

Primary Tumor (T)

Definitions for classifying the primary tumor (T) are the same for clinical and for pathologic classification. The telescoping method of classification can be applied. If the measurement is made by physical examination, the examiner will use the major headings (T1, T2, or T3). If other measurements, such as mammographic or pathologic, are used, the telescoped subsets of T1 can be used.

TX   Primary tumor cannot be assessed

T0   No evidence of primary tumor

Tis*   Carcinoma in situ: Intraductal carcinoma, lobular carcinoma in situ, or Paget's disease of the nipple with no tumor

T1   Tumor 2 cm or smaller in greatest dimension

     T1a   0.5 cm or smaller in greatest dimension

     T1b   Larger than 0.5 cm but not more than 1 cm in greatest dimension

     T1c   Larger than 1 cm but not more than 2 cm in greatest dimension

T2   Tumor larger than 2 cm but not more than 5 cm in greatest dimension

T3   Tumor larger than 5 cm in greatest dimension

T4   Tumor of any size with direct extension of chest wall or skin

     T4a   Extension to chest wall

     T4b   Edema (including peau d'orange) or ulceration of the skin of the breast or satellite skin nodules confined to the same breast

     T4c   Both (T4a and T4b)

     T4d   Inflammatory carcinoma (see definition of inflammatory carcinoma in the introduction)

Regional Lymph Nodes (N)

NX   Regional lymph nodes cannot be assessed (e.g., previously removed)

N0   No regional lymph node metastasis

N1   Metastasis to movable ipsilateral axillary lymph node(s)

N2   Metastasis to ipsilateral axillary lymph node(s)

N3   Metastasis to ipsilateral internal mammary lymph node(s)

Pathologic Classification (pN)

pNX   Regional lymph nodes cannot be assessed (e.g., previously removed or not removed for pathologic study)

pN0   No regional lymph node metastasis

pN1   Metastasis to movable ipsilateral axillary lymph node(s)

     pN1a   Only micrometastasis (none larger than 0.2 cm)

     pNIb   Metastasis to lymph node(s), any larger than 0.2 cm

     pN1bi   Metastasis to one to three lymph nodes, any larger than 0.2 cm and all smaller than 2 cm in greatest dimension

     pN1bii   Metastasis to four or more lymph nodes, any larger than 0.2 cm and all smaller than 2 cm in greatest dimension

     pN1biii   Extension of tumor beyond the capsule of a lymph node metastasis smaller than 2 cm in greatest dimension

     pN1biv   Metastasis to a lymph node 2 cm or larger in greatest dimension

pN2   Metastasis to ipsilateral axillary lymph nodes that are fixed to one another or to other structures

pN3   Metastasis to ipsilateral internal mammary lymph node(s)

Distant Metastasis (M)

MX   Presence of distant metastasis cannot be assessed

M0   No distant metastasis

M1   Distant metastasis (includes metastasis to ipsilateral supraclavicular lymph node(s)

Stage Grouping

Stage 0	Tis	N0	M0
Stage 1	T1	N0	M0
Stage IIA	T0	N1	M0
	T1	N1*	M0
	T2	N0	M0
Stage IIB	T2	N1	M0
	T3	N0	M0
Stage IIIA	T0	N2	M0
	T1	N2	M0
	T2	N2	M0
	T3	N1, N2	M0
Stage IIIB	T4	Any N	M0
	Any T	N3	M0
Stage IV	Any T	Any N	M1

*The prognosis of patients with pN1a is similar to that of patients with pn0.

(From Manual for staging of cancer. 3rd ed. Philadelphia: J.B. Lippincott, 1988.)

NONINVASIVE BREAST CANCER: TNM STAGE 0

Ductal Carcinoma In Situ

Noninvasive breast cancer has two histologic forms, ductal carcinoma in situ (DCIS) and lobular carcinoma in situ (LCIS). The majority of patients with noninvasive cancers have ductal carcinoma in situ, most of which are found as nonpalpable lesions. Ductal carcinoma in situ now accounts for 15 to 20 percent of all cancers found by screening. Compared to 20 years ago, when they were found only because of a palpable mass, nipple discharge, or nipple crusting (Paget's disease), these lesions now are most often clinically silent and found on mammography in association with microcalcifications.

In the recent past, practically all patients with DCIS were treated with total or modified radical mastectomy (Table 2), which in fact achieves excellent local control and 5-year cures that approach 100 percent. However, the demonstration that early invasive carcinomas can be treated successfully with breast-preserving techniques has generated interest in treating DCIS, an even earlier lesion, in similar fashion.

Of concern in this regard are the multifocal nature of DCIS and its occasional association with unsuspected invasive cancer and occult nodal metastases. The likelihood of any of these depends on the size of the DCIS. Those that are smaller than 2.5 cm in size are unlikely to have occult invasion, to be multifocal, or to have lymph node involvement, although the comedo form of DCIS is least predictable in this respect. Uncontrolled studies indicate that complete local excision when possible, nodal removal, and breast irradiation provide survival

Table 2 Operations for Primary Breast Cancer

Operation	Tissues Removed
Radical mastectomy	Large amount of skin, including nipple; breast tissue; pectoralis major and minor muscle; axillary lymph nodes
Modified radical mastectomy (total mastectomy with axillary dissection)	Skin, including nipple; breast tissue; axillary lymph nodes
Total mastectomy	Skin, including nipple; breast tissue
Local resection (segmental mastectomy, lumpectomy, tylectomy, partial mastectomy)	Removal of limited amount of breast tissue containing tumor with tumor-free resection margins
Axillary dissection	Removal of lymph nodes and fatty tissue within the axilla

and local control comparable to modified radical mastectomy. Unsettled issues related to whether axillary dissection is mandatory in view of the small frequency of nodal metastases (1 to 2 percent) and whether breast irradiation is necessary in all cases. It is generally conceded that patients with extensive or multifocal DCIS are best treated by total mastectomy with level 1 axillary lymph node dissection (to remove completely the axillary extension of breast tissue and detect the occasional nodal metastasis). Patients with focal or limited disease that can be completely excised have the option of breast conservation, i.e., a local resection with tumor-free margins, a low axillary dissection, and irradiation of the breast.

In some cases of the most minimal involvement found only by mammography and measuring no more than 2.5 cm in diameter, local excision alone may be adequate treatment if close postoperative observation is possible. Support for this option is based on a small series of carefully selected and closely studied patients. A prospective clinical trial is being conducted by the National Surgical Adjuvant Breast Project (NSABP B-17) to address the issue of whether breast irradiation is necessary after local excision in all cases. Patients are randomized to receive local excision alone (segmental mastectomy) or local excision plus radiotherapy to the breast. Axillary dissection is optional.

Lobular Carcinoma In Situ

The frequency of LCIS is far less than that of DCIS, and its behavior is different, but its management has taken a similar conservative turn. Disagreement continues as to whether LCIS is a preinvasive forerunner of invasive lobular carcinoma or simply a tissue change that indicates an increased risk of developing invasive breast cancer. Those who believe the latter prefer the term *lobular neoplasia*.

Lobular carcinoma in situ is commonly found in premenopausal women, not as a palpable lesion, but microscopically when a biopsy has been performed for

other reasons. It is now appreciated that LCIS is regularly multifocal and dependably bilateral, and its presence indicates that the patient has approximately a 25 percent risk of developing breast cancer in the future, with 11 times the usual risk of dying from it. The problem is that one breast is at no higher risk than the other and that the risk is protracted, with 50 percent of the future cancers occurring after more than 15 years. Interestingly, the LCIS is not always the source of these future cancers; at least half are invasive ductal carcinomas.

In these circumstances, any treatment for one breast would logically apply to the other. Bilateral subcutaneous mastectomy does not remove all breast tissue, is of dubious value for reducing risk, and does not eliminate the need for close observation. Unilateral mastectomy addresses only half the risk, and blind biopsy of the second breast, if negative, still does not reduce the frequency of subsequent cancers in it. Close observation alone is the option being most often recommended for women with LCIS.

Close, frequent follow-up with a physical examination every 6 months, an annual mammogram, and interval monthly breast self-examinations is an accepted method of management for patients with this lesion. Although the risk of an invasive cancer is substantial and affects both breasts, the reality is that the majority of the patients are young and the majority do not develop invasive cancer even after extended observation. Those that do are likely to be diagnosed early and cured. A program of close observation can be expected to entail no more than a 5 percent future risk of dying of breast cancer. These findings support a conservative approach consisting of local resection alone to achieve negative margins and subsequent close follow-up. If an alternative approach is taken, bilateral total mastectomy provides the only complete security and effectively deals with the problems of multicentricity and bilaterality. This procedure should be reserved for patients who, after appropriate counseling, desire not to live with the increased threat of invasive breast cancer or who have a strong family history of breast cancer, with or without severe atypical hyperplasia, or who have diffuse nodular breasts that are difficult to examine either physically or with mammograms. Patients who choose total mastectomies should be offered breast reconstruction to help maintain a positive self-image.

An attempt to further define the natural history of LCIS in prospective fashion is being conducted by the NSABP, which is maintaining a registry of patients with LCIS who undergo local resection alone as primary therapy.

EARLY INVASIVE CARCINOMA: TNM STAGE I AND II

Early invasive stages account for 75 to 80 percent of all cases of breast cancer. Breast conservation for these patients is now solidly supported by the results of several controlled clinical trials that were performed initially in

Europe and now in the United States. Survival and disease-free survival comparable to that after mastectomy have been confirmed for as long as 10 years following treatment, as has acceptable local and regional control of cancer. A review of the history of the events leading to this change is not within the scope of this section; suffice it to say that objection to mastectomy on cosmetic grounds made breast conservation desirable and the ability of high-dose irradiation to control microscopic disease made it feasible. The two surgical options currently available to women with early stages of invasive breast cancer are (1) modified radical mastectomy or (2) breast conservation, with local tumor resection, axillary node dissection, and breast irradiation.

Modified Radical Mastectomy

Modified radical mastectomy is currently the operation most frequently performed for early invasive breast cancer. Also referred to as total mastectomy with axillary node dissection, this operation differs from the Halsted radical mastectomy in preserving the pectoralis major muscle and accomplishing a less complete axillary node dissection. There are no significant differences between the two operations in overall survival, disease-free survival, or rates of local recurrence. The appeal of the modified radical mastectomy is that it provides a more pleasing cosmetic result than the radical procedure and easier breast reconstruction for those who desire it.

Modified mastectomy continues to have the advantages of being universally applicable to stages I and II breast cancers, regardless of tumor size or position, and of sparing the patient the need for irradiation, with its attendant inconvenience and tissue damage. Treatment is also less expensive than breast conservation, unless reconstruction is added. Either because of necessity or patient's choice, this operation is still used in the United States more often than is breast conservation. About 60 percent of cases recently entered into NSABP adjuvant protocols have been treated with this operation either by necessity or by choice.

Breast-Conserving Surgery

For selected cases of stage I or II breast cancer, breast-conserving surgery is a viable alternative to total mastectomy with axillary dissection. In many states, laws now require that patients who are suited for breast conservation be offered this alternative.

A number of terms are used to signify breast-conserving surgery, e.g., lumpectomy, tumorectomy, segmental mastectomy, partial mastectomy, or tylectomy. The best description is a local excision that is sufficiently wide that the tumor is removed with a surgical margin uninvolved with tumor cells. In addition to tumor-free margins, it is necessary that a cosmetic result superior to that achievable with mastectomy plus reconstruction is anticipated. In combination with local excision, an axillary dissection is performed. When

Table 3 Contraindications to Breast-Conservation Surgery and Radiation Therapy

Tumor greater than 5.0 in size
Poorly defined tumor
Large tumor in a small breast
Pregnancy
Previous irradiation in the same site
Multiple tumors within the breast confirmed to be malignant
Mammographically defined diffuse microcalcifications highly suspicious or confirmed malignant
Tumor involving skin or chest wall musculature

healing is complete (approximately 2 weeks), radiation therapy is administered to the remaining breast tissue, ordinarily to a total dose of 5000 cGy. The axilla is not irradiated because recurrence at this site is unusual, and irradiation superimposed on a dissection increases the likelihood of lymphedema.

It should be emphasized that wide local tumor excision without irradiation is associated with a high recurrence rate in the breast when compared to excision and breast radiation. In the NSABP B-06 trial, these frequencies after 5 years were 27.9 percent and 7.7 percent, respectively. Because the objective is to avoid the necessity for a subsequent "salvage" mastectomy, radiation therapy, with or without a "boost" dose to the site of excision, is recommended for all patients treated with local tumor excision.

Patients who desire breast-conserving surgery must be carefully evaluated to be certain it is appropriate for their circumstances. Contraindications are listed in Table 3. Currently, there are no firm contraindications relevant to tumor location, although peripheral locations are most favorable cosmetically. Tumors directly under or close to the nipple may be excised; the nipple may be excised, if necessary, and this may be cosmetically acceptable to some patients. Regardless of location, the primary objective of breast conservation must be to accomplish tumor excision with uninvolved margins and achieve a cosmetic result that will be acceptable to the patient. Axillary dissection remains a part of the conservative treatment of invasive carcinoma because it prevents progression of metastases in the axilla and because it is the only means of determining reliably the presence and extent of axillary metastases. The latter is still the most accurate prognostic indicator of survival.

LOCALLY ADVANCED INVASIVE CARCINOMA: TNM STAGE III

Patients with locally and regionally advanced carcinoma of the breast have a poor prognosis and regularly require multimodal therapy to maximize cure and local tumor control (Fig. 2). The optimal sequence of local-regional and systemic therapy is the subject of most clinical investigations. In the TNM staging system, stage III cancers are subdivided into stages IIIA and IIIB. Stage IIIA cancers are technically resectable, and an operation is feasible as the initial therapy. It is unlikely

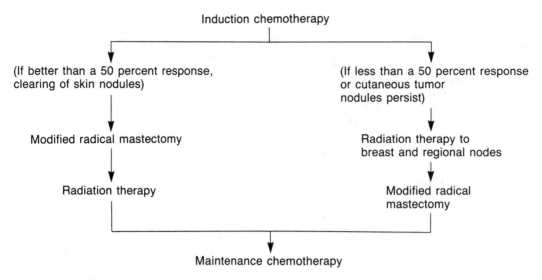

Figure 2 General plan for management of locally advanced breast cancer.

that breast conservation can be safely employed for these large (T3) cancers, regardless of breast size, and the appropriate operation is total mastectomy with axillary dissection. This is often followed by irradiation to the chest wall and residual regional nodes, and regularly by systemic therapy. Initial chemotherapy is employed by many physicians, but whether this is advantageous remains an open question. Even in the event of negative nodes, the high probability of local recurrence and metastases makes adjuvant chemotherapy desirable. Studies seem to indicate that treatment of the breast with surgical removal or with irradiation has little influence on survival provided systemic chemotherapy is effective, but the combination of mastectomy and irradiation achieves local tumor control superior to either alone.

Stage IIIB cancers are not technically resectable and are unsuited for initial surgical therapy. Initial systemic chemotherapy in these cases is appropriate to reduce the extent of tumor involvement as well as to address the distant micrometastases that almost certainly exist. Three to six cycles is standard, but treatment may be continued until an optimum tumor response is obtained. A complete response is followed by total mastectomy with axillary dissection; the axillary dissection should be complete (at least level 2) and should remove all gross disease. After satisfactory wound healing, irradiation is added to improve local control, and patients are placed on maintenance chemotherapy. It is uncertain how long to continue with maintenance chemotherapy; however, the duration is most often not longer than 12 months. When induction chemotherapy produces only an incomplete response, irradiation is a better choice than mastectomy.

Inflammatory carcinoma of the breast customarily presents as stage IIIB disease and receives special attention because of its dramatic features and rapid course. Erythema, edema, warmth, peau d'orange and an ill-defined breast mass, and even pain and tenderness,

are associated with widespread lymphatic permeation of tumor in the parenchyma that often reaches the dermal lymphatics. A high probability of recurrence and dissemination can be expected after local therapy alone, and the same principles of multimodal treatment apply as for other stage IIIB cancers. Induction chemotherapy has been associated with a substantial improvement in the prognosis of these patients, and it is used routinely for initiating treatment. Five-year survival rates between 25 percent and 40 percent are being reported. Until recently, mastectomy was avoided entirely for treatment of inflammatory carcinoma, and irradiation was relied on entirely for local and regional tumor control; however, with operability often restored after treatment with modern chemotherapy and improved prospects for survival, mastectomy has been reintroduced in an effort to further improve control of the tumor on the chest wall and axilla. Induction chemotherapy is followed by radiation therapy or mastectomy depending upon tumor response. A modified radical mastectomy precedes radiation therapy if there is a 50 percent or greater response to chemotherapy and clearing of cutaneous involvement. Otherwise, radiation therapy is employed for further reduction in tumor bulk, and mastectomy is then performed and followed by maintenance chemotherapy.

SUGGESTED READING

American Joint Committee on Cancer. Manual for staging of cancer. 3rd ed. Philadelphia: JB Lippincott, 1988:146–147.

Danforth DN Jr, Lippman ME. Surgical treatment of breast cancer. In: Lippman ME, Lichter AS, Danforth DN Jr, eds. Diagnosis and management of breast cancer. Philadelphia: WB Saunders, 1988: 95–154.

Fisher B. Reappraisal of breast biopsy prompted by the use of lumpectomy: A position paper on surgical strategy. JAMA 1985; 253:3,585–3,588.

Margolese R, Poisson R, Shibata H, et al. The technique of segmental mastectomy (lumpectomy) and axillary dissection: A syllabus from the National Surgical Adjuvant Breast Project Workshops. Surgery 1987; 102:828–834.

Schnitt SJ, Silen W, Sadowski NL, et al. Current concepts: Ductal carcinoma in situ (intra-ductal carcinoma) of the breast. N Engl J Med 1988; 318:898–903.

Spratt JS, Donegan WL. Surgical management. In: Donegan WL, Spratt JS, eds. Cancer of the breast. Philadelphia: WB Saunders, 1988:403–461.

Temple WJ, Jenkins M, Alexander F, et al. Natural history of in situ breast cancer in a defined population. Surgery 1989; 210:653–657.

BREAST CANCER: RADIATION THERAPY

LORI J. PIERCE, M.D.
ROBERT L. GOODMAN, M.D.

Conservative surgery and radiation therapy has become a widely accepted alternative to radical or modified radical mastectomy in the definitive management of stages I and II breast cancer. Retrospective data from single institutions and prospective data from randomized trials have proven the equivalence of radical surgery and conservative management in locoregional control, relapse-free survival, and overall survival. With adequate surgical and radiotherapeutic technique, the conservative approach allows breast preservation with good to excellent cosmesis and minimal complications. Conservative surgery and radiotherapy therefore offers the appropriately selected patient with early-stage breast cancer the opportunity of long-term control with the psychological advantage of organ preservation.

This chapter reviews briefly the randomized trials, discusses criteria for patient selection for conservative management, reviews radiotherapeutic technique with resultant cosmesis and possible complications, and examines locoregional control, patterns of recurrence, and salvage therapy.

RANDOMIZED STUDIES

The World Health Organization (WHO) trial, sponsored primarily by the Institute Gustave-Roussy, randomized 179 patients from October, 1972, through September, 1979, with UICC-AJC T1N0-1 lesions to modified radical mastectomy (MRM) or tumorectomy with a 2-cm margin around gross tumor, low axillary dissection, and radiation to the intact breast. The breast received 45 Gy in 2.5-Gy fractions with Cobalt-60 photons followed by a 15-Gy boost to the tumor bed with either photons or electrons for a total dose of 60 Gy to the excision site. With 10-year mean follow-up, 6/88 locoregional recurrences have been identified in the conservative arm compared to 11/91 who underwent mastectomy. Relapse-free survival (RFS) and overall survival (OS) are essentially identical between the two groups, with 74 percent RFS for conservative therapy and 73 percent for mastectomy, and OS of 79 percent and 80 percent, respectively.

The Cancer Institute of Milan, Italy, compared the classic Halsted mastectomy to quadrantectomy, complete axillary dissection, and breast radiotherapy ("QUART") in 701 patients with clinical T1N0 lesions accrued between June, 1973 and May, 1980. The radiation consisted of 50 Gy in 2-Gy fractions with a 10-Gy boost using photons or electrons. Both the Milan and WHO trials further randomized patients with pathologically positive axillary nodes to regional irradiation and observation and found no survival benefit to nodal irradiation. In addition, patients with positive nodes in the Milan trial received 12 cycles of cytoxan, methotrexate, and 5-fluorouracil. With 13-year median follow-up, 7/349 local recurrences have developed in the mastectomy arm and 11/352 in the QUART arm, with 9 additional patients developing a second ipsilateral breast cancer in the conservative group, resulting in 2 percent and 5.7 percent local failures in the RM and QUART groups respectively. The 10-year overall survival for RM was 76 percent compared to 79 percent for QUART, with RFS curves superimposable for the two groups.

A multi-institutional trial, conducted by the National Surgical Adjuvant Breast and Bowel Project (NSABP-B-06), randomized 1,843 women with clinical stages I and II breast cancers with lesions up to 4 cm to total mastectomy (TM), segmental mastectomy (SM), and SM and breast irradiation. Specimen margins of the SM patients were microscopically negative by protocol design; SM patients with positive margins underwent TM. All patients underwent axillary dissection; those with positive nodes received melphalan and 5-fluorouracil. A dose of 50 Gy was delivered to the intact breast without a boost. However, tissue compensators, which decrease dose inhomogeneity by attenuating the x-ray beam, were not used, resulting in a greater effective dose to the apex of the breast. Eight-year actuarial results showed a significant local benefit in the radiation arm, with 39.4 percent local failures in the SM arm compared to 10.4 percent for SM + XRT (P < 0.001); 8.1 percent locally failed in the TM arm. Relapse-free survivals and OS among all groups were not statistically different.

The National Cancer Institute of the National Institutes of Health began a trial in October, 1979, randomizing patients with clinical stages I and II breast cancer to TM or gross tumor excision with breast irradiation, with all patients undergoing full axillary dissections. The breast received 45 to 50 Gy with a 15- to 20-Gy boost primarily delivered with iridium-192

Table 1 Prospective Randomized Trials

Institution	Clinical Stage	No. of Patients	Definitive Surgery	Conservative Surgery and Radiation	Chemotherapy	Outcome	Results (%) Surgery	XRT
WHO	T_1N_{0-1}	179	MRM	Tumorectomy with 2 cm margin; low axillary dissection; 45 Gy to breast with 15 Gy boost	None	LR DRFS OS	12 73 80	6.8 74 79
							10 year follow-up	
Milan	T_1N_0	701	RM	Quadrantectomy, complete axillary dissection; 50 Gy to breast with 10 Gy boost	Cytoxan Methotrexate 5-Fluorouracil	LR DFS OS	2 76 76	6 77 79
							13 year follow-up	
NCI	T_{1-2},N_{0-1}	224	TM	Gross tumor excision, complete axillary dissection; 45 to 50 Gy to breast with 15 to 20 Gy boost	Cytoxan Adriamycin	LR DFS OS	7 82 85	12 72 89
							5 year follow-up	

Institution	Clinical Stage	No. of Patients	Definitive Surgery	Conservative Surgery and Radiation	Chemotherapy	Outcome	TM	SM	+XRT
NSABP	T_{1-2} up to 4 cm N_{0-1}	1,843	TM	Segmental mastectomy, with negative margins, level I, II dissection; 50 Gy to breast; no boost	5-Fluorouracil Melphalan	LR DFS OS	8 58 71	39 54 71	10 59 76
							8 year follow-up		

DRFS: Distant relapse-free survival, LR: Local relapse, MRM: Modified radical mastectomy, OS: Overall survival, RM: Radical mastectomy, SM: Segmental mastectomy, TM: Total mastectomy, XRT: Irradiation, Surg: Surgery.

implant; regional nodes were irradiated with pathologically positive axillae. All patients with positive nodes received sequential cytoxan and adriamycin. With 68-month follow-up, 5-year actuarial locoregional failure is 12 percent in the conservative group and 7 percent in the mastectomy group; 8-year actuarial results are 20 percent and 11 percent, respectively. Twelve of the 15 local failures among the irradiated group have been successfully salvaged with mastectomy. Relapse-free survival and OS were not significantly different between the two arms (personal communication, K. Straus).

Other randomized trials from Guy's Hospital in London, England, EORTC, and the Danish Breast Cancer Cooperative Group are presently in progress; the results are forthcoming. Retrospective studies have provided longer follow-up of conservatively managed patients, with local control rates of 90 to 95 percent at 5 years and 80 to 90 percent at 10 to 15 years, with DFS and OS comparable to surgical series (Table 2).

PATIENT EVALUATION AND SELECTION

A thorough history is required, including menopausal status, family history of breast cancer, any prior breast malignancies, previous radiation exposure, and medical diseases, including history of connective-tissue disorders. Clinical characteristics of the lesion should be noted, such as date of detection, approximate size, interval growth, associated breast pain or erythema, and nipple discharge. A history of arm pain or swelling, weight loss, new onset of bone pain, or neurologic changes should be elicited. Pertinent features of the physical exam include dimensions of the mass relative to the size of the breast, nipple retraction, skin involvement, tethering or fixation to the chest wall, location relative to the nipple-areolar complex, expression of nipple discharge, and exclusion of separate palpable masses in the remaining ipsilateral breast tissue and contralateral breast. The axillae and supraclavicular fossae are palpated to detect nodal enlargement and to exclude chest wall fixation. A mammogram with adequate compression technique is obtained to characterize the mass fully and to rule out suspicious nonpalpable lesions or calcifications bilaterally. Confirmation of malignancy is established by needle aspiration or open biopsy. Mammographically detected lesions will often require needle localization prior to biopsy. A metastatic evaluation including chest radiograph and liver function tests is obtained, with further evaluation of the liver with abdominal computed tomography scan (CT) or liver scan for abnormal liver enzymes. A bone scan can be

Table 2 Institutional Trials

Physician/ Institution	Clinical Stage	No. of Patients	Conservative Surgery	Radiation	Results (%)	
Solin/University of Pennsylvania	T_{1-2}, N_{0-1}	552	Lumpectomy, level I-II dissection	45-50 Gy to breast with 14-20 Gy boost	LR RFS OS 5-yr follow-up	6 77 94
Recht/Joint Center for Radiotherapy	T_{1-2}, N_{0-1}	607	Gross total excision, level I-II dissection	45-50 Gy with 10-18 Gy boost	LR 5-yr follow-up LR 10-yr follow-up	10 16
Montague/MD Anderson	T_{1-2}, N_{0-1}	311	Gross total excision, level I dissection	45-50 Gy with 10-20 Gy boost	LR DFS 10-year follow-up	5 75
Haffty/Yale	$T_{1-2} N_{0-1}$	278	Gross total excision, axillary dissection	46-50 Gy with 10-20 Gy boost	LR 5-yr follow-up LR 10-yr follow-up	9 20
Kantorowitz/ Rochester	T_{1-2}, N_{0-1}	146	Gross total excision, gross total excision with margin, or quadrantectomy; level I-II dissection	50 Gy with 10–25 Gy boost	LR OS 4.5-yr follow-up	10 82
Bluming/Los Angeles	T_{1-3}, N_{0-1}	145	Gross total excision, complete axillary dissection	45-50 Gy with 15-20 Gy boost	LR DFS OS 8-yr follow-up	12 79 85
Calle/Inst. Curie, France	T_{1-2} to 3 cm, N_0	324	Gross excision with 2 cm margin, level I-II dissection	50 Gy with 10-15 Gy boost	LR DFS 5-yr follow-up	6 90
Clarke/Inst. Gustave Roussy, France	T_{1-2} to 2.5 cm, N_{0-1}	436	Excisional biopsy or quadrantectomy, level I sampling	45 Gy with 15 Gy boost	LR 5-yr follow-up LR 10-yr follow-up	5 7
Delouche/ Charlebourg, France	T_{1-2} to 3.5 cm, N_{0-1}	410	Gross total excision, axillary dissection	50-60 Gy with boost	LR OS 11-yr follow-up	10 63

DFS: Disease-free survival, LR: Local relapse, OS: Overall survival.

obtained as a baseline study because, in the absence of bone pain, the true-positive rate for metastatic disease in early-stage breast cancer is only 1 to 2 percent.

The selection of a patient for conservative surgery and radiation therapy requires close interaction between the surgeon and radiation oncologist in identifying absolute and relative contraindications to the conservative approach. Prior radiation to the breast excludes a patient from further radiotherapy. Diffuse microcalcifications or gross multicentric disease are contraindications for conservative therapy, as studies of mastectomy specimens in patients presenting with multicentric disease or diffuse calcifications have demonstrated an increased tumor burden often involving other quadrants of the breast and multiple axillary nodes. Clinical studies in which multiple excisional biopsies have been performed to remove multicentric disease have resulted in local recurrence rates approaching 40 percent. Candidates for lumpectomy and radiation should have solitary well-defined lesions less than 5 cm or focal microcalcifications that can be easily excised. Pre-existing collagen

vascular diseases, specifically discoid lupus, systemic lupus erythematosus, and scleroderma, may predispose to severe acute and chronic radiation sequelae, including confluent moist desquamation and chest wall necrosis, and should be considered for mastectomy. Relative cosmetic contraindications include retroareolar primaries requiring sacrifice of the nipple-areolar complex to achieve negative tumor margins, a large tumor in a small breast resulting in an unacceptable surgical defect, and breast fibrosis caused by radiation dose inhomogeneity in extremely large, pendulous breasts.

SURGICAL RESECTION

The extent of the surgical resection is a factor contributing to local control in the breast. Incisional biopsies are associated with a three- to four-fold risk of breast recurrence; therefore, at least gross total excision must be obtained. Institutions differ in their surgical objectives, from gross total excision, gross total excision with wide margins, gross excisions with microscopically negative margins, and quadrantectomy. Although extensive resections appear to decrease local failure, cosmesis is often compromised. Our policy has been to excise the gross lesion and a rim of surrounding tissue to obtain grossly and microscopically tumor-free margins, requiring specimen orientation by the surgeon and inking of the margins by the pathologist. If margins are positive, patients undergo re-excision at time of axillary dissection. A retrospective review of 251 patients with early-stage breast cancer from the Hospital of the University of Pennsylvania (HUP) who underwent re-excision owing to uncertainty of the extent of the initial surgery or positive margins demonstrated residual disease in the re-excision specimen in 60 percent of patients with initial positive margins and 49 percent in those with unknown margins. For patients initially presenting with mammographic microcalcifications, a routine postbiopsy mammogram is done to rule out residual radiographically detectable disease. In the HUP study of those patients with residual calcifications on mammogram, 86 percent were found to have residual tumor on re-excision. Our indications for re-excision, therefore, are initial incisional biopsy, positive or unknown margins, and residual calcifications on a postbiopsy mammogram.

An axillary dissection is done for both prognostic and therapeutic indications. Clinical assessment of the axilla is incorrect in 25 to 40 percent of cases when correlated with pathologic results. Axillary dissection provides qualitative evaluation of nodal status for prognostic purposes and identifies patients who may benefit from systemic chemotherapy or hormonal manipulation. Quantitative evaluation of axillary contents also gives prognostic information and has therapeutic implications for long-term regional control. Data from the NSABP-BO4 randomized trial show axillary recurrence as a function of the number of lymph nodes removed; when fewer than 6 axillary nodes were removed, the axillary recurrence rate was 11 percent compared to less than 1 percent recurrence with dissections of greater than 10 nodes. The extent of axillary dissection is variable among surgeons. A node sampling removes only nodes that are clinically suspicious and should be discouraged; a level 1 dissection encompasses nodes located from the lateral border of the latissimus dorsi to the lateral margin of the pectoralis minor muscle; a level 1 to 2 dissection extends to the medial border of the pectoralis minor; and a complete dissection removes the nodes medial to the pectoralis minor muscle. Although a complete axillary dissection provides greatest axillary clearance, it is of limited benefit beyond a level 1 to 2 dissection and appears to increase surgical morbidity, i.e., arm edema. The incidence of skip metastases to level 3 nodes in the absence of positive level 1 and 2 nodes is approximately 2 to 3 percent; thus, the false-negative rate of a level 1 to 2 dissection is low and provides adequate qualitative and quantitative assessment of the axillary contents. Complete axillary dissections are associated with a greater risk of permanent arm edema, especially when followed by regional irradiation. Larson reported a 4 percent incidence of arm edema after radiation alone to the axilla, 8 percent after limited dissection and radiotherapy, and 37 percent after complete axillary dissection and radiotherapy. A complete dissection, therefore, appears to increase significantly the risk of complications and, in the absence of indications such as grossly positive axillary nodes or extracapsular extension, offers little chance of potential gain over a limited dissection.

DEFINITIVE RADIATION THERAPY

Radiation therapy to the breast is generally started within 4 weeks of the last breast surgery and axillary dissection, providing adequate time for wound healing such that the patient may maintain her arm comfortably in the treatment position. Immobilization devices aid in minimizing setup variability. At our institution, styrofoam cradles are made to conform to the contour of each patient prior to the planning session and are used on the treatment machines daily for reproducible patient positioning. Patients receive 46 to 50 Gy over 4 1/2 to 5 weeks to the intact breast using tangent fields with photons from linear accelerators, and wedges are used to reduce dose inhomogeneity throughout the breast. Doses greater than 50 Gy to the entire breast have been shown to result in moderate to severe retraction and breast fibrosis. Good to excellent cosmesis is generally achieved with doses less than or equal to 50 Gy using the skin-sparing effect of megavoltage therapy. A boost with either electrons or implant is delivered to the tumor bed for a total dose of at least 60 Gy to the primary site. In a review of their early data, Harris, at the Joint Center for Radiation Therapy, observed a dose response of the tumor bed, with 4,500 to 5,000 cGy in 5 weeks associated with 12 percent relapse rate, 5,000 to 5,500 cGy in 5 to 6 weeks with 8 percent recurrence, and greater than 60 Gy in 6 to 7 weeks with 0 percent local recurrence. Electrons and iridium implants appear to be equally effective in terms of local control; some reviews, however, suggest a less favorable cosmetic result with the use of larger implants or implants with seeds close to the skin surface. Electrons may be preferred over an implant for parasternal lesions or lesions near to the chest wall because implants may deliver higher doses to the pectoralis muscles and ribs and increase potential complications.

LOCOREGIONAL RECURRENCE

Incisional biopsies and multicentric disease have been shown to increase the risk of locoregional failure following definitive irradiation. Other factors are, however, controversial. In patients with invasive breast cancer, an extensive intraductal component (EIC), defined as the presence of intraductal cancer in 25 percent or more of the tumor mass with intraductal cancer extending beyond the tumor margin into normal breast parenchyma, has been retrospectively identified by the Joint Center to be a risk factor for local recurrence. Patients with EIC had a 33 percent risk of local failure at 10 years compared with 8 percent in patients not found to have an EIC. Extensive intraductal component, as defined previously, has not, however, reproducibly identified patients at higher risk in other institutions. It also has not been shown to be a risk factor in patients with inked margins that are microscopically free of disease. There are no universally accepted pathologic contraindications to conservative surgery and radiation. Young age, in some series, has been associated with a higher breast recurrence, possibly owing to confounding factors such as limited resections without attention to margins. In a review comparing patients 35 years of age and younger to those 36 years and older, Solin found that young patients, when stratified by prognostic factors such as stage, nodal status, receptor status, and negative tumor margins, did not have a statistically increased local recurrence rate at 5 years; longer follow-up, however, is needed.

As demonstrated in Tables 1 and 2, locoregional control obtained with conservative therapy is comparable to that with mastectomy. For those who do experience a locoregional recurrence, failure patterns have differed from mastectomy failures, in whom median time to chest wall failure is 2 years and is associated with synchronous or metachronous metastases in up to 80 percent to 90 percent of patients. In irradiated patients, 75 percent of breast failures occur within the first 5 years, with late failures occurring with longer follow-up. Failures occur primarily at or in the vicinity of the tumor bed; late recurrences occur at greater frequency in other quadrants, which is suggestive of a new primary tumor. For those patients with isolated local recurrences, Fowble noted a 95 percent operability rate, with 92 percent locoregional control after mastectomy, with a 5-year actuarial DFS of 59 percent and an actuarial OS of 84 percent after salvage mastectomy. In general, the survival of patients with an isolated breast recurrence who undergo salvage mastectomy is unchanged from those not experiencing a recurrence.

Although the standard local treatment for isolated breast failures has been mastectomy, trials have been performed in an attempt to select patients who could be considered for limited local re-excision. Kurtz, from Marseille, France, selected 52 patients from a group of 118 patients with an isolated breast recurrence for wedge resection as salvage surgery. Those selected had lesions less than 2 cm without skin changes. With 6-year median follow-up, the actuarial risk of second breast recurrence was 21 percent, with median interval to second locoregional failure of 36 months. Because the success of this approach appears to rely on careful patient selection and the risk of multicentricity exists at time of breast recurrence, until longer follow-up is obtained and the selection criteria are further defined, we continue to advocate mastectomy for an isolated breast recurrence.

Less than 5 percent of patients treated with conservative therapy will develop a regional node failure as first site of relapse; the majority are axillary failures, with less frequent supraclavicular relapses. Internal mammary and infraclavicular failures are rare. A review of nodal failures at the University of Pennsylvania showed that 50 percent of isolated axillary recurrences could be successfully salvaged and are NED; supraclavicular, infraclavicular, and internal mammary recurrences were rarely salvageable and portended a poor overall prognosis.

COMPLICATIONS

Radiation to the breast is generally well tolerated and is associated with minimal major complications. Acute complications include mild edema and erythema of the breast; long-term complications occurring in 5 percent or less of patients include rib fractures, symptomatic pneumonitis, matchline fibrosis, and chest wall pain. Arm edema, related primarily to the extent of axillary dissection, occurs in approximately 10 percent of irradiated patients, with higher estimates reflecting a lower threshold for reportable lymphedema. Contralateral breast tumors and other second malignancies have not been found to be greater in irradiated patients compared with mastectomy patients in the randomized trials.

INTEGRATION OF RADIATION AND CHEMOTHERAPY

Treatment with radiation therapy has not been shown to impede the ability to deliver full-dose chemotherapy. A prospective study by Glick and colleagues, from HUP, of conservatively managed patients who received two concurrent cycles of cytoxan (100 mg per square meter PO) on days 1 through 14 and 5-fluorouracil (600 mg per square meter IV) on days 1 and 8 demonstrated the ability to administer 95 percent of the planned doses of chemotherapy. Six cycles of cytoxan and methotrexate (40 mg per square meter IV) on days 1 and 8 and 5-fluorouracil were then administered at the completion of radiation with no significant differences in mean doses. Lippman, from the National Cancer Institute, looked at the integration of radiation and chemotherapy in patients participating in their randomized trial. The regimen consisted of adriamycin, 30 mg per square meter IV on day 1 and cytoxan, 150 to 200 mg per square meter PO, on days 3 through 6 for irradiated patients and patients undergoing mastectomy. Approximately 85 percent of the irradiated patients received at least 85 percent of the prescribed dose compared to 90 percent of mastectomy patients. Although total white blood cell counts were decreased with therapy, radiation was noted primarily to lower the lymphocyte count; little change was noted in the absolute granulocyte count. Adjustments in chemotherapeutic dosage have since been based upon the absolute granulocyte count.

COSMESIS

The obvious goal of conservative breast treatment is to obtain desirable cosmesis of the intact breast while maintaining locoregional control. Using adequate radiotherapeutic technique, good to excellent cosmesis is obtained in 80 to 90 percent of patients. Rose and Harris reviewed the cosmetic outcome in 593 patients, assigning cosmetic scores based upon detectable radiation and surgical changes, including breast edema and fibrosis, skin retraction, and telangiectasia. The authors found an overall cosmetic score of excellent in 65 percent and good in 25 percent at 5 years of follow-up; at 7 years, 54 percent retained an excellent result and 24 percent were judged as good. In general, breast retraction, telangiectatic changes, and breast edema stabilized after 3 years. Less favorable cosmetic outcomes were associated with the use of adjuvant chemotherapy; 37 percent of patients receiving chemotherapy had an excellent result at 3 years compared to 68 percent without chemotherapy. Other factors affecting cosmesis included tumor size, in which T1 tumors had significantly better cosmesis than T2 lesions owing to less noticeable surgical defects; total dose delivered to the entire breast, with greater risk of skin retraction and fibrosis above 50 Gy; and radiation technique, with improved cosmetic result using megavoltage equipment, wedges to reduce dose inhomogeneity, and no bolus.

INTRADUCTAL CANCER

With the advent of screening mammography and the improvement of mammographic technique, the frequency of detection of nonpalpable intraductal lesions has greatly increased. Historically, intraductal cancer represented 1 to 2 percent of breast malignancies; it now represents 15 to 20 percent of cancers among screened populations. Prior to mammographic surveillance, intraductal lesions frequently presented as clinically palpable masses. Currently, the diagnosis is commonly made from radiographic findings of clustered microcalcifications. The natural history of these two presentations may differ.

Retrospective studies of mastectomy specimens of patients with intraductal cancer have identified multicentric foci in up to 50 percent of cases, with occult invasive cancer in 0 to 21 percent of specimens, dependent upon the degree of pathologic sectioning. The extent of multicentricity and the frequency of occult invasion may reflect tumor size, with larger lesions demonstrating a higher incidence of multicentricity and invasive disease. Reviews by Rosen from Memorial-Sloan Kettering and Page from Vanderbilt of breast biopsies initially interpreted as benign but retrospectively classified as intraductal cancer have demonstrated progression to invasive disease in approximately 33 percent of patients within 10 years of biopsy, usually in the vicinity of the biopsied lesion.

For these reasons, mastectomy has been the standard form of treatment and has been associated with 95 to 100 percent local control and OS. With the growing acceptance of conservative breast therapy for invasive disease, the use of mastectomy for noninvasive disease appeared paradoxical, and trials of local excision and radiotherapy and local excision alone have emerged. The only published randomized data comparing lumpectomy only to lumpectomy and radiation therapy are taken from the NSABP-BO6 trial, in which retrospective pathologic review identified 78 cases initially thought to have invasive disease but were later reclassified as intraductal cancer. Twenty-two patients were treated with local excision alone with negative margins and 29 with excision followed by whole breast radiotherapy. With 39-month mean follow-up, 23 percent recurred in the excision-alone group and 7 percent in the irradiated group. The NSABP-B17 is currently randomizing patients with pure intraductal cancer to lumpectomy with and without radiotherapy and will provide greater insight into the long-term outcome of the two treatments.

Many institutions presently offer lumpectomy and radiation therapy as an alternative to mastectomy for pure intraductal cancer. A review of the literature shows local control in 90 to 95 percent of cases, with up to 11-year median follow-up. Patients selected have presented with palpable lesions or solitary focal calcifications, fully excised with negative margins and negative postbiopsy mammograms prior to radiation. Patients with diffuse or multifocal calcifications are not good candidates for the conservative approach and have been referred for mastectomy.

Excision alone has been used in carefully selected patients, with the largest series reported by Lagios. Seventy-nine patients have been followed after lumpectomy alone; 73 patients were diagnosed by mammographic appearance of microcalcifications, 5 patients by clinical exam, and 1 patient as an incidental finding. The average size of lesions was 6.8 mm. With an average of 48-month follow-up, eight patients (10 percent) have experienced a recurrence, 50 percent as invasive disease and 50 percent as intraductal. All recurrences have been in the same quadrant as the initial disease, generally at the initial biopsy site. All patients with recurrent disease are currently without evidence of disease with either further re-excision or mastectomy. In the absence of long-term follow-up, local excision alone appears to be restricted to patients with solitary lesions less than 1 cm, excised with negative margins, and negative postbiopsy mammograms who are highly motivated for breast conservation with close clinical and mammographic follow-up. At our institution, either lumpectomy and radiation therapy or mastectomy are offered as therapeutic options because of concern of multicentric disease throughout the breast and limited long-term data of local excision alone.

POSTMASTECTOMY RADIOTHERAPY

Selected patients with operable breast cancer who undergo mastectomy have been shown to develop both isolated chest wall failures and local recurrences associated with distant metastases. Haagensen identified positive axillary nodes as a risk factor for chest wall recurrence, with patients having greater than three nodes positive at 20 to 30 percent risk for recurrence. He correlated increasing tumor size with axillary involvement, with lesions 4 to 6 cm having a 40 percent risk of pathologic axillary involvement if clinically node-negative and 80 percent risk if clinically node-positive, placing them at subsequent risk for chest wall recurrence. Because of the complications associated with a chest wall failure, including local pain, infection, tissue necrosis, and bleeding, and the inability to deliver adequate radiation doses to control bulky disease, these patients were referred prophylactically for postoperative chest wall radiotherapy.

Single institutions and multiple randomized trials have compared mastectomy with and without postoperative radiotherapy. Although they have shown a local benefit for radiotherapy, long-term survival has not improved. Many of these trials, however, employed suboptimal radio-therapeutic doses and technique and included patients not at risk for locoregional failure, thus diffusing any discernible survival benefit. Chemotherapy, often administered to address the risk of distant spread, has shown, at best, modest locoregional benefit, with patients with multiple positive nodes and large primary tumors still manifesting a chest wall recurrence. Fowble reviewed the records of 808 women with positive axillary nodes randomized by the Eastern Cooperative Oncology Group to CMF, CMFP (prednisone), CMFPT (prednisone and tamoxifen), if premenopausal, and CMFP, CMFPT, and observation, if postmenopausal, for isolated locoregional failures. She identified four or more positive nodes, tumor size greater than 5 cm, and the presence of tumor necrosis as factors associated with isolated locoregional recurrence. In these patients, the likelihood of an isolated locoregional recurrence paralleled the risk of distant disease, identifying these patients as a subgroup with a potential survival benefit from radiation in addition to chemotherapy.

At the University of Pennsylvania, our indications for postmastectomy radiotherapy are four or more positive nodes, lesions greater than 5 cm, and involved surgical margins. If indications for chemotherapy exist, radiotherapy is given either concurrently or sequentially with drug and has not been shown to impede delivery of full-dose chemotherapy.

SUGGESTED READING

Fisher B, Redmond C, Poisson R, et al. Eight-year results of a randomized clinical trial comparing total mastectomy and lumpectomy with or without irradiation in the treatment of breast cancer. N Engl J Med 1989; 320:822–828.

Fowble B, Gray R, Gilchrist K, et al. Identification of a subgroup of patients with breast cancer and histologically positive axillary nodes receiving adjuvant chemotherapy who may benefit from postoperative radiotherapy. J Clin Oncol 1988; 6:1,107–1,117.

Fowble B, Solin L, Schultz D, et al. Breast recurrence following conservative surgery and radiation: Pattern of failure, prognosis and pathologic findings from mastectomy specimens with implications for treatment. Int J Radiat Oncol Biol Phys 1990; 19:833–842.

Larson D, Weinstein M, Goldbert I, et al. Edema of the arm as a function of the extent of axillary surgery in patients with Stage I-II cancer of the breast treated with primary radiotherapy. Int J Radiat Oncol Biol Phys 1986; 12:1,575–1,582.

Rose M, Olivotto I, Cady B, et al. Conservative surgery and radiation therapy for early breast cancer. Long-term cosmetic results. Arch Surg 1989; 124:153–157.

Sarrazin D, Le M, Arrigada R, et al. Ten-year results of a randomized trial comparing a conservative treatment to mastectomy in early breast cancer. Radiother Oncol 1989; 14:177–184.

Veronesi U, Banfi A, Salvadori B, et al. Breast conservation is the treatment of choice in small breast cancer: Long-term results of a randomized trial. Eur C Cancer 1990; 26:668–670.

BREAST CANCER: SYSTEMIC TREATMENT

CHARLES L. LOPRINZI, M.D.
THEODORE A. BRAICH, M.D.

Breast cancer is the most common malignancy in American women. Despite significant efforts aimed at the prevention or early detection of breast cancer, through means such as life-style modifications and mammography, advanced breast cancer remains a frequent disease. Thus, in addition to locoregional therapies such as surgery and irradiation, systemic drug therapy for this malignancy maintains a prominent role in the practice of oncology.

Systemic antitumor treatment for breast cancer can be subdivided into two major components, hormonal therapy and cytotoxic chemotherapy. Although the concurrent use of chemohormonal therapy continues to be an active research topic, common clinical practice at this time is usually to utilize these two treatment modalities sequentially.

ADJUVANT SYSTEMIC THERAPY

Annually, over 100,000 women present with localized (stage I or II) breast carcinoma in the United States. In addition to questions about locoregional treatment (usually consisting of primary surgery or primary radiation therapy), questions almost always arise regarding the role of adjuvant systemic treatment for these patients. Adjuvant systemic therapy for primary breast cancer is a topic of extensive past and ongoing clinical research. Published results from adjuvant breast cancer trials are frequently at variance with each other and are thus confusing for both medical and lay people.

In September, 1985, the United States National Institute of Health (NIH) sponsored a Consensus Development Conference to address adjuvant systemic breast cancer treatment. Following the presentation of extensive data and considerable discussion, the following conclusions were drawn:

Adjuvant chemotherapy and hormonal therapy are effective treatments for breast cancer patients. While significant advances have been made in the past 5 years, optimal therapy has not been defined for any subset of patients. For this reason, **all patients and their physicians are strongly encouraged to participate in controlled clinical trials**.

Outside the context of a clinical trial and based on the research data presented at the 1985 Consensus Development Conference, the following statements can be made:

For **premenopausal** women with positive nodes, regardless of hormone receptor status, treatment with established combination chemotherapy should become standard care.

For **premenopausal** patients with negative nodes, adjuvant therapy is not generally recommended. For certain high-risk patients in this group, adjuvant chemotherapy should be considered.

For **postmenopausal** women with positive nodes and positive hormone receptor levels, tamoxifen is the treatment of choice.

For **postmenopausal** women with positive nodes and negative hormone receptor levels, chemotherapy may be considered but cannot be recommended as standard practice.

For **postmenopausal** women with negative nodes, regardless of hormone receptor levels, there is no indication for routine adjuvant treatment. For certain high-risk patients in this group, adjuvant therapy may be considered.

Subsequently, these conclusions formed the primary basis for clinical decision making regarding adjuvant breast cancer systemic treatment in the United States.

The next notable historical development occurred in May, 1988, when a Clinical Alert was sent out from the NCI to American clinical oncologists. This communication summarized previously unpublished, preliminary results from three NCI-supported adjuvant therapy trials in women with resected, axillary node-negative breast cancer. Based on the available information from these three studies, this NCI Clinical Alert made the following statements:

Adjuvant hormonal or cytotoxic chemotherapy can have a meaningful impact on the natural history of node negative breast cancer patients.

Outside of a trial setting, the hormonal and chemotherapy treatments described represent credible therapeutic options worthy of careful attention.

This Clinical Alert sparked substantial controversy. In response, several prominent clinical oncologists participated in a roundtable format to discuss clinical and research implications resulting from the NCI communication. These oncologists gave opposing viewpoints when presented with the following question: What do you currently recommend for patients with axillary node-negative primary breast carcinoma who cannot go on a clinical trial? Answers to this query ranged from "... I prefer to treat the majority of node-negative breast cancer patients with chemotherapy, tamoxifen, or both, depending on the individual clinical situation" to "I would prefer not to treat node-negative patients." The three studies described in the NCI Clinical Alert were published the following year in an issue of the New England Journal of Medicine along with three editorials presenting different viewpoints.

Note that another Census Development Conference was scheduled by the United States NIH for June, 1990. This conference was designed to look at treatment issues regarding women with axillary node-negative breast cancer. The conclusions from this conference will probably influence the clinical treatment of such patients in the United States.

Based on the available information and controversy, what practical considerations are appropriate for this topic in clinical medicine? It appears prudent for a medical oncologist, or another informed physician, to discuss adjuvant systemic therapy individually with virtually every newly diagnosed primary breast cancer patient. A reasonable approach is to address each individual case in a stepwise fashion as follows:

1. **Make an estimation of the expected long-term disease-free survival if the patient does not receive any adjuvant systemic treatment**. Patients with positive axillary nodes are at significant risk for relapse, and the risk is proportional to the number of nodes involved. Patients with negative axillary nodes have generally been considered to have a good prognosis. Within this group, however, there are subsets that have risks of relapse as great as 50 percent. Features that help define higher risk groups include negative hormone receptors, larger tumor sizes, higher tumor grades, and high growth fraction tumors.

2. **Estimate, from the available clinical trials information, what survival improvement might be expected with adjuvant systemic therapy.** In premenopausal women, demonstration of a benefit from chemotherapy has been the rule. The evidence is most mature and strongest for node-positive patients. The degree of benefit appears to be greatest for patients with fewer positive nodes. The evidence to support adjuvant chemo-

therapy in node-negative patients is less secure. In a small number of studies with limited follow-up, selected, high-risk patients appear to benefit from chemotherapy.

For postmenopausal patients, adjuvant chemotherapy trials have had variable results. Studies regarding adjuvant hormonal therapy (tamoxifen), however, have demonstrated consistent advantages for prolonged disease-free survival and some evidence for prolonged overall survival. These advantages have generally been numerically small, although statistically significant, and, in the majority of studies, the benefit is restricted to hormone receptor-positive tumors. The benefit appears to be independent of nodal status.

3. **Discuss the preceding two items with the patient along with potential toxicities that may be related to adjuvant systemic treatment.** It is frequently helpful to have family members available for such discussions. The short-term toxicity of chemotherapy can be substantial, although it is generally manageable. Long-term toxicities from limited-term chemotherapy appear to be negligible. Tamoxifen is usually well tolerated, and long-term administration appears safe.

4. **Help the patient make an appropriate decision based on the individual clinical situation.** Age, comorbidity, psychological profile, and social support systems are important variables that need to be considered in this decision-making process.

5. **Document in the patient's medical record a discussion of the preceding issues and the joint decision regarding adjuvant systemic therapy.**

LOCOREGIONAL ADVANCED DISEASE

Locoregional advanced breast cancer is a variably defined term that usually refers to poor prognostic breast cancer involving the breast and the draining lymph node regions, without clinically demonstrable widespread metastatic disease. Included in this category are patients with (1) large primary tumors (>5 cm), (2) cancers invading the skin or chest wall, and (3) characteristics of inflammatory breast cancer. The clinical diagnosis of inflammatory breast cancer calls for the presence of erythema, warmth, and peau d'orange changes involving more than 50 percent of the breast. Histologic evidence of such a diagnosis requires that tumor cells be seen in dermal lymphatic channels. There continues to be disagreement regarding whether the diagnosis of inflammatory breast cancer should require the presence of clinical characteristics, histologic characteristics, or both. Nonetheless, the presence of either characteristic portends a relatively poor prognosis.

Following the diagnosis of inflammatory breast cancer, or locoregional advanced breast cancer that is surgically unresectable, it is generally recommended that patients initially be treated with a doxorubicin-containing combination chemotherapy regimen. Following several cycles of chemotherapy, locoregional therapy (surgery or radiation therapy) is usually employed, frequently followed by further systemic treatment. Utilizing this approach, the majority of patients will be rendered "free of known residual disease," although a majority of them will eventually relapse with metastatic disease. The use of very high doses of chemotherapy with corresponding bone marrow transplantation is actively being studied in these patients. Nonetheless, the use of this approach in a nonresearch setting is not currently recommended.

For patients with resectable locoregional advanced breast cancer, it is also reasonable to initiate treatment with systemic chemotherapy followed by locoregional therapy. However, this treatment approach has not been demonstrated to be superior to treating such patients initially with locoregional therapy followed by systemic chemotherapy.

METASTATIC DISEASE

Patients with breast cancer that has spread outside the bounds of the chest wall and the draining lymph node regions are not considered to be curable with currently available treatment modalities. It is generally recommended that patients with metastatic breast cancer be initially considered for hormonal treatment modalities for two reasons. First, multiple prior randomized trials have not been able to demonstrate improved results from the early use of cytotoxic chemotherapy when compared to initial hormonal therapy in such women. Second, hormonal therapy is generally less toxic than cytotoxic chemotherapy.

A number of factors can be utilized to help predict whether an individual patient is likely to benefit from hormonal treatment. Positive predictive factors for a hormonally sensitive cancer include (1) the presence of positive hormone receptors; (2) a long disease-free interval after primary treatment; (3) no prior systemic treatment; (4) bone or soft-tissue-only metastases; and (5) a longer period of tumor regression with a prior hormone treatment (as opposed to quickly failing a prior hormonal therapy). By using these factors, patients can be placed into groups with high chances of responding to hormone therapy (>80 percent), low chances of responding (<10 percent), or intermediate chances.

Hormonal Treatments

Tamoxifen is the most widely utilized hormonal agent in women with breast cancer. The usual daily dose is two 10-mg tablets. Tamoxifen has a long half-life that allows for once-daily dosing. This drug is well tolerated, with its major toxicity being bothersome hot flashes. In addition, a minority of patients may develop a vaginal discharge. When prescribing tamoxifen, it is wise to alert the patient to the cost of the drug, currently approximately 1 dollar per tablet.

Megestrol acetate is another commonly utilized drug in women with metastatic breast cancer. Its usual daily dose is 160 mg and, like tamoxifen, it is relatively expensive. The major toxicity from megestrol acetate is appetite stimulation with subsequent weight gain. Withdrawal uterine bleeding frequently develops 2 to 3 weeks after stopping megestrol acetate. Alerting postmenopausal women of this phenomenon can prevent frantic phone calls.

Oophorectomy has been a standard hormonal treatment for premenopausal women for all of the twentieth century. In some patients, the antitumor effects from this procedure are not cross-resistant to other hormonal treatments such as tamoxifen. Ablation of ovarian function is usually done by a relatively simple surgical procedure, although irradiation-induced ovarian ablation is occasionally utilized.

High doses of diethylstilbestrol (DES) can be utilized as a hormonal treatment for postmenopausal women. In previously untreated postmenopausal women, DES (15 mg per day) results in similar response rates and response durations as does tamoxifen. Diethylstilbestrol does not cause any untoward toxicities in some women. However, a significant proportion of women will develop prominent side effects from DES, most notably gastrointestinal upset and breast tenderness. One advantage that DES has over many of the other hormonal agents for breast cancer is that it can be purchased at a fraction of their costs.

Fluoxymesterone is an androgenic agent that is frequently used in metastatic breast cancer patients as a secondary or tertiary hormonal therapy. Its usual oral dose is 10 mg twice daily. Not surprisingly, this drug can lead to masculinization, causing appetite stimulation, weight gain, hirsutism, acne, and male-pattern hair loss.

In the not-too-distant past, surgical adrenalectomies were performed as secondary hormonal treatments in women with metastatic breast cancer. This has largely been replaced by aminoglutethimide, a drug that results in a "medical adrenalectomy." Various doses of this drug have been studied with or without the concurrent use of replacement steroids. A relatively standard manner of using aminoglutethimide is to give 250 mg PO twice a day for 2 weeks and then increase the total daily dose to 750 to 1,000 mg per day. Concurrently, hydrocortisone is given at a dose of 100 mg per day (in divided doses) for 2 weeks and then decreased to 40 mg per day. Common toxicities from this drug include lightheadedness, rash (which commonly resolves despite drug continuation), mild gastrointestinal upset, and lethargy. Although the majority of patients will experience some toxicity from this drug, aminoglutethimide-induced toxicity only rarely is severe enough to lead to drug cessation. A cautionary note: Aminoglutethimide occasionally causes severe granulocytopenia or skin desquamation.

Cytotoxic Chemotherapy

As noted previously, hormonal therapy is generally utilized as first-line treatment in patients with metastatic breast cancer. However, cytotoxic chemotherapy eventually has a prominent role to play in the treatment of many such women. Cytotoxic chemotherapy is employed for patients who are believed to have disease that is likely to be resistant to hormonal therapy or for patients with rapidly progressive disease that is considered to be eminently life-threatening. Palliation is the primary goal of chemotherapy in patients with metastatic breast cancer; thus, it is important to weigh potential subjective patient improvements against expected treatment toxicities. A careful balancing of these opposing effects is useful for making appropriate clinical decisions applicable to individual patients. There are approximately eight commonly used cytotoxic drugs for patients with breast cancer. Initial cytotoxic therapy usually consists of a combination of chemotherapy drugs that have differing dose-limiting toxicities. These regimens frequently include cyclophosphamide, 5-fluorouracil, or doxorubicin (Table 1). None of these individual regimens has been demonstrated to be clearly superior to the others.

Chemotherapy-naive patients with measurable metastatic breast cancer can be expected to have a response rate ($\geq$50 percent decrease in cross-sectional diameters) in the 50 to 70 percent range, with complete responses less than 15 to 20 percent of the time. The median time to disease progression in responding patients is in the range of 8 to 10 months from the date of chemotherapy initiation. Patients who have recently received prior adjuvant chemotherapy appear to do more poorly with a lower response rate and shorter response duration.

Historically, patients receiving combination chemotherapy for metastatic breast cancer have had their chemotherapy program continued until they developed disease progression or intolerable toxicity. The use of combination chemotherapy for shorter periods of time has not been well investigated in patients with metastatic breast cancer. In many malignant disease situations, however, the trend has been for giving shorter periods of chemotherapy. Frequently, it is quite reasonable to stop chemotherapy after 5 to 12 months in a stable or responding patient and then observe the patient with or without the use of a hormonal agent. In this situation, one can consider restarting chemotherapy in the event of worsening metastatic disease.

Patients with metastatic disease resistant to an initial combination chemotherapy program can often be treated with an alternative chemotherapy regimen. Single-agent doxorubicin is frequently a reasonable secondary cytotoxic treatment in patients whose initial regimen did not include this drug. Such patients have a response rate of approximately 20 to 30 percent, with a median response duration of 3 to 5 months. Doxorubicin is usually given in total doses of 60 to 80 mg per square meter every 3 to 4 weeks. Divided doses (either given over two to three consecutive days or weekly) may result in similar antitumor activity but less toxicity. Cumulative doses of this drug need to be followed because of an increased risk of cardiac toxicity with high total doxorubicin doses.

Table 1 Frequently Used Combination Chemotherapy Regimens

Acronym	Drugs and Doses	Retreatment Interval
CMF	Cyclophosphamide, 600 mg/m^2 IV, days 1,8 or 100 mg/m^2 PO, days 1–14 Methotrexate, 40 mg/m^2 IV, days 1,8 5-fluorouracil, 600 mg/m^2 IV, days 1,8	4 wk
CFP	Cyclophosphamide, 150 mg/m^2 IV, days 1–5 5-fluorouracil, 300 mg/m^2 IV, days 1–5 Prednisone, 30 mg PO, days 1–7	4–6 wk
CAF	Cyclophosphamide, 100 mg/m^2 PO, days 1–14 Doxorubicin, 30 mg/m^2 IV, days 1,8 5-fluorouracil, 500 mg/m^2 IV, days 1,8	4 wk
FAC	5-fluorouracil, 400–500 mg/m^2 IV, day 1 Doxorubicin, 40–50 mg/m^2 IV, day 1 Cyclophosphamide, 400–500 mg/m^2 IV, day 1	3–4 wk
AV	Doxorubicin, 75 mg/m^2 IV, day 1 Vincristine, 1.4 mg/m^2 IV, days 1,8	3 wk
CMFVP (continuous)	Cyclophosphamide, 60 mg/m^2 PO, qd Methotrexate, 15 mg/m^2 IV, weekly 5-fluorouracil, 300 mg/m^2 IV, weekly Vincristine, 0.625 mg/m^2 IV, weekly ($\times$ 10 wk then stop) Prednisone, 30 mg/m^2 PO, qd on days 1–14; 20 mg/m^2 PO, qd on days 15–28; 10 mg/m^2 PO, qd on days 29–42 then discontinue	

The overall prognosis is generally quite poor in patients who have progressive disease despite second-line chemotherapy. Response rates to tertiary chemotherapy regimens are usually less than 15 percent, and median response durations are quite short. In situations in which it is decided to employ tertiary chemotherapy, mitomycin C, 10 to 20 mg per square meter, can be used with planned retreatment at 4- to 5-week intervals. In addition to usual toxicities associated with cytotoxic drugs, mitomycin C can result in fatal pulmonary toxicity or a commonly fatal hemolytic uremic syndrome.

SUPPORTIVE CARE

As noted in the preceding section, metastatic breast cancer is not currently a curable disease. The vast majority of patients with advanced breast cancer live for many months or years after diagnosis, but eventually die as a result of this disease. As treating physicians, it is our job to provide patients with the best quantity and quality of life. This includes the utilization of antineoplastic systemic therapy as has been outlined. In addition, the primary physician should be well versed in other means of providing supportive care. This includes pain control, treatment of paraneoplastic syndromes such as hypercalcemia, control of nausea and vomiting, treatment of psychological problems, prevention and management of bone fractures, and helping a patient through the dying process.

SUGGESTED READING

Adjuvant chemotherapy for breast cancer. National Institutes of Health Consensus Development Conference Statement. 1985; 5:12.

Adjuvant therapy in node-negative breast cancer. In: Oncology viewpoints, ASCO (American Society of Clinical Oncology), special issue, 1988.

Clinical alert from the National Cancer Institute. May 17, 1988.

Henderson C, Hayes DF, Come S, et al. New agents and new medical treatments for advanced breast cancer. Semin Oncol 1987; 14(1): 34–64.

Ingle JN. Principles of therapy in advanced breast cancer. Hematol Oncol Clin North Am 1989; 3(4):743–763.

ROLE OF DRUGS IN THE TREATMENT OF HEAD AND NECK CANCER

ROBERT L. CAPIZZI, M.D.
DOUGLAS R. WHITE, M.D.

Cancers of the upper aerodigestive tract are malignancies associated with well-identified etiologic agents and precursor lesions (Table 1). Consequently, decreased morbidity and mortality from these neoplasms could stem from vigorous efforts in prevention aimed at modification of behavior and from early detection through screening of high-risk populations. Optimal therapy of advanced disease requires adequate staging and coordinated, prospective, multidisciplinary planning. Historically, surgery and radiation therapy have been the only components of curative therapy and chemotherapy has been used for palliation of advanced locally recurrent or metastatic disease. The demonstration that multidrug chemotherapy programs result in high response rates in previously untreated patients raises the question of the potential role of chemotherapy in initial treatment. The purpose for the incorporation of effective chemotherapy into initial treatment regimens is to increase the local control rate, decrease the morbidity and possibly the mortality from surgery and/or radiation therapy, and increase the overall cure rate through prevention of distant metastasis.

In 1990, it is anticipated that 39,200 new cases of upper aerodigestive tract cancer will be diagnosed and that 11,000 deaths will occur in the United States from these diseases.[1] The overall average 5-year survival for patients diagnosed with head and neck cancer is about 60 percent, and is closely related to location of the primary lesion and stage at diagnosis. Because these cancers usually arise from squamous epithelium, the majority are squamous cell (epidermoid) carcinomas and generally the term head and neck cancer is synonymous with squamous cell carcinoma, both in practice and in the literature.

Table 1 Carcinoma of the Head and Neck

Percentage of total cancers	5%
U.S. Incidence (1986)/Deaths	39,200/11,000
Major risk factors	Tobacco and alcohol abuse
Sex ratio	3–4:1 (M:F)
Premalignant lesions	Leukoplakia
	Erythroplakia
Histology	Squamous cell (epidermoid)
Standard treatment	Surgery and/or radiation
Overall cure rates	60 to 65%
Role of chemotherapy	Palliation
	Investigational in neo-adjuvant and adjuvant setting for cure

Common predisposing factors for the development of squamous cell cancers of the head and neck (SCCHN) in the United States are tobacco use and alcohol consumption. It is estimated that tobacco smokers who do not drink alcohol have two to four times the risk of developing head and neck cancer compared to nonsmokers, and that nonsmoking alcohol consumers are also at increased risk. The risk to smokers who drink may be up to 15 times that of abstainers, suggesting a synergistic rather than simply additive effect. Risk appears to be dose related, both with tobacco and alcohol consumption. Although the majority of reports relating tobacco use to head and neck cancer concern cigarette smokers, an increased incidence of head and neck cancer is also seen in cigar and pipe smokers, and in those who use smokeless tobacco in the form of chewing tobacco and oral snuff.

Oral cancers account for 44 percent of head and neck cancer, and in tobacco smokers are most commonly located in the floor of the mouth, the ventral or lateral tongue, and the soft palate complex. Cancer related to smokeless tobacco use occurs more commonly in sites that are directly exposed to tobacco, such as the buccal mucosa and gingiva. Early lesions in the oral cavity are easily detectable, and these sites should be routinely examined in patients at risk. Early oral cancers are frequently asymptomatic. Although the white patches of leukoplakia are easily observed and have been considered by some to be premalignant, only 2 to 4 percent of leukoplakic lesions are malignant by biopsy. Typically it is the erythroplastic or mixed erythroplastic-leukoplakic lesions that contain carcinoma. Non-neoplastic inflammatory lesions may mimic the changes of early malignancy but usually resolve within 1 or 2 weeks. Lesions that persist for longer than 2 weeks should be biopsied.[2] Laryngeal carcinoma accounts for 32 percent of head and neck cancers. Although more difficult to detect by physical examination, these cancers frequently disclose their presence while still in an early stage by interference with vocal cord functions. Conversely, carcinomas of the oropharynx and nasopharynx, may be difficult to visualize and may remain asymptomatic until far advanced. This, in part, is the reason why pharyngeal carcinomas result in 34 percent of the head and neck cancer deaths while accounting for only 23 percent of the incidence.

Cancer of the head and neck spreads by invasion of contiguous structures and through lymphatics along well-defined pathways. Metastases to lymph nodes are usually ipsilateral in early lateral primaries but are frequently contralateral or bilateral with either advanced or midline primaries. In most cases, death due to head and neck cancer is the result of failure to control local disease rather than the result of systemic metastasis. Clinically detectable systemic metastases ultimately occurs in about 20 percent of head and neck cancer patients, and are reportedly noted in a much higher percent in autopsy series, usually in the setting of incurable locally advanced disease. The most common sites of distant metastasis are lung and lymph nodes.

Staging for primary sites in head and neck cancer utilizes the TNM system, both for individual treatment planning and for outcome comparisons between various treatment regimens and multiple institutions. The staging system is based on clinical rather than pathologic staging. Increasingly sophisticated imaging modalities, particularly MRI scans, may detect occult disease, thereby upstaging patients and making comparison of current studies with older studies impossible. Retrospective reviews reveal that the prognosis of head and neck cancer is related to the primary site, as well as the stage. All stage IV patients do not have an equivalent prognosis, thus primary site must always be considered when evaluating therapeutic outcome. Initial staging of head and neck cancer usually includes panendoscopy, not only to determine the extent of the primary lesion, but also to search for additional synchronous malignancies, because multiple primary lesions in the upper aerodigestive tract occur with sufficient frequency to render this a real possibility. In 5 to 10 percent of patients, one or more additional primary lesions are detected at the time of initial staging and, in about 30 percent of long-term survivors, second primary lesions will occur, especially if high-risk behavior continues. The occurrence of multiple head and neck cancers is believed to result from exposure of multiple areas of squamous epithelium to common risk factors resulting in a field cancerization effect. In addition to defining the extent of local disease by endoscopy, local imaging procedures, including routine x-rays, Panorex views, computed tomography (CT), magnetic resonance imaging (MRI) are routinely used. Computed tomography is superior for delineating bone destruction, while MRI is exquisitely sensitive at detecting soft tissue changes. Generally, a chest x-ray and, in patients with advanced disease, a CT scan of mediastinum is sufficient to exclude systemic metastasis. The presence of abnormal liver function tests, bone pain, or other localizing symptoms should direct attention to these areas prior to initiating "curative" therapy for local disease.

The importance of prospective assessment in a multidisciplinary clinic specializing in head and neck cancer prior to the initiation of therapy cannot be overemphasized. Participants in such a clinic include an otolaryngologist specializing in head and neck malignancies, an experienced radiation oncologist, a medical oncologist, and a dentist. Ancillary personnel such as a speech therapist, a nutritionist, and a social worker should also be available. The purpose of the multidisciplinary head and neck cancer clinic is to allow careful evaluation by multiple observers and to plan a treatment regimen tailored to the individual patient in order to achieve the greatest likelihood of a cure with the least morbidity and the psychosocial well-being of the patient. In a substantial proportion of head and neck cancer patients, treatment options are relatively straightforward, but final decisions may be determined by the geographic availability of suitable radiotherapy facilities or the presence of comorbid medical illnesses such as severe cardiac or pulmonary disease precluding general anesthesia. For some patients with stage II carcinoma of the larynx, laryngectomy may offer a better chance of cure than irradiation, yet for social or psychosocial reasons, the patient may select irradiation in order to preserve normal speech with the future option of some degree of surgical salvage in the event of radiation failure. Thus, social, pyschological, and geographic factors often enter into the selection of appropriate treatment.

Prior to either irradiation or resection, patients must be evaluated by a dentist. The role of the dentist is to determine which teeth are salvageable and to formulate a regimen for their preservation, to extract nonsalvageable teeth and, if required, to plan and construct appropriate intraoral prostheses. Failure to obtain dental consultation prior to initiation of radiation therapy may result in radio-osteonecrosis of the mandible or may increase the difficulty in constructing an adequate intraoral prosthesis postoperatively.

The role of the medical oncologist may include the general medical assessment of the patient, as well as prospective incorporation of chemotherapy into the patient's management. Chemotherapy may be used for palliation of incurable disease or may be incorporated in a multimodality curative program as induction, concomitant, or adjunctive therapy in addition to radiation and/or surgery.

Most patients with advanced localized head and neck cancer require multimodality therapy for cure. Because the majority of deaths are the result of failure to control disease above the clavicle, the focus of primary therapy is local. Traditionally, this has consisted of radical resection followed by external-beam irradiation or high-dose irradiation to unresectable lesions. In general, radiation therapy is not sufficiently effective to achieve permanent control of bulky tumor masses, and results with advanced nonresectable disease are unsatisfactory.

Chemotherapy with either single or multiple drugs has historically been offered to patients who have failed definitive surgery and radiation therapy, or who are incurable because of systemic metastasis. In these situations, the goal of chemotherapy is only palliative, in which case the potential risks and benefits including cost, must be carefully assessed. Although the response rates to a 5-day infusion of cisplatin and 5-fluorouracil may suggest that this is a more effective therapy than oral methotrexate, the inconvenience of hospitalization, and the toxicity and cost of the 5-day infusion may outweigh the benefit of a modest improvement in response rate. Even with improved response rates, an overall improvement in duration of survival is not demonstrable for this group of patients. Palliative effects of chemotherapy include decreased pain and a consequent decrease in the need for narcotic analgesics, which have concomitant side effects; improvement in symptoms secondary to tumor bulk, such as difficulty swallowing; and healing of malodorous ulcerated tumor masses. In some instances, the psychological benefits of "doing something"' outweigh the side effects of therapy, even in nonresponders.

Because responders do benefit from improved symptom control, and patients with more favorable prognostic indicators, especially those with good nutritional and performance status, are likely to respond, these patients should be approached optimistically.

Drugs with therapeutic activity in head and neck cancer are listed in Table 2. Clinical trials evaluating the response of head and neck cancer to various chemotherapy drugs have generally been conducted in patients who have failed prior radiation therapy and/or surgery, and often prior chemotherapy as well. In these patients, responses are usually partial and of short duration. Experience with multiagent regimens (Table 3) has shown significantly higher overall and complete response rates in previously untreated, as compared to previously treated patients, and it is likely that the same is true for single-agent therapy. When using single-agent therapy, the choice of drug may be directed by the presence of significant comorbid disease. Because many head and neck cancer patients have a long-standing history of tobacco abuse, serious lung or heart disease may preclude the use of some drugs.

Methotrexate has been the most extensively evaluated single-agent for the treatment of head and neck cancer. A wide range of doses from 30 to 5,000 mg/m^2 with leucovorin rescue and a variety of schedules and routes of administration have been explored. The summary of all of these investigations is that there does not appear to be a major dose-response effect. The overall response rate is about 30 percent with few complete responses, and the usual duration of response being 3 to 4 months. The optimal dose appears to be 30 to 40 mg/m^2/week administered parenterally (IM, IV, SC). Because methotrexate is excreted in the urine, renal function must be assessed prior to its use. Potential acute toxicities of concern include myelosuppression and stomatitis, which may be particularly severe in patients who have undergone extensive radiation therapy.

Although initial trials using multidrug regimens for the treatment of head and neck cancer failed to demonstrate significantly increased activity as compared with results with single-agents, the evolution of various combinations of cisplatin with 5-fluorouracil appears to hold great promise. When comparing clinical trial results, it is important to note whether patients have received prior chemotherapy or radiation therapy. As shown in Table 3, responses to the same treatment regimen in previously untreated patients may be double those in patients with recurrent disease. Overall, studies that have directly compared single versus multidrug regimens in recurrent or metastatic head and neck cancer have tended to demonstrate a marginal but nonsignificant advantage in response rate and survival for the combination, usually at the cost of increased toxicity. As with single-agent regimens, responders generally survive longer than nonresponders. Because of early reports of efficacy, combinations of 5-fluorouracil with cisplatin have been used in a large number of trials, both as palliative therapy for metastatic or recurrent disease and as induction therapy for locally advanced disease. Response rates in patients with recurrent and metastatic disease range from 11 to 79 percent with complete response rates from 0 to 27 percent and median survival times from 5 to 20 months (Table 4). The causes for this wide range in response rates are multifactorial, including all of the features associated with patient selection as well as differential effectiveness of various permutations of the cisplatin/5-fluorouracil combination (see Table 4). For example, one trial compared bolus administration of cisplatin with 5-fluorouracil to an infusion regimen (Table 4, Kish). In that study, the overall and complete response rates were 72 percent and 22 percent versus 20 percent and 10 percent for the infusion and bolus regimens, respectively.

Induction or neoadjuvant chemotherapy defines the use of chemotherapy prior to local therapy with radiation, surgery, or both. Various rationales have been proposed for the use of induction therapy. Foremost among these is the downstaging of locally advanced

Table 2 Responses to Single Drug Therapy of Recurrent SCCHN

Antimetabolites	Responses*
Methotrexate	30 to 35%
5-fluorouracil	15 to 25%
Ara-C	20%
Natural Products	
Vinblastine	25 to 30%
Vincristine	25 to 30%
Antibiotics	
Doxorubicin	20 to 25%
Bleomycin	15 to 20%
Alkylating Agents	
Cyclophosphamide	30 to 35%
Miscellanoues	
Cisplatin	30 to 35%
Carboplatin	20 to 25%
Hydroxyurea	30 to 35%

*Mostly partial response.

Table 3 Combination Chemotherapy in SCCHN: Previously Treated versus Induction Patients

Drug Combination	Response (%)	
	Treated	Induction
CDDP-BLM	33	70
CDDP-MTX-LCV-BLM	40	80
CDDP-BLM-VBL	45	74
BLM-MTX-VCR	43	71
CDDP-5-FU	50	88

Abbreviations: CDDP = cisplatin, BLM = bleomycin, MTX = methotrexate, LCV = leucovorin, VBL = vinblastine; VCR = vincristine, 5-FU = 5-fluorouracil. (From Erwin TM, Clark JR, Weichselbaum RR. Multidisciplinary treatment of advanced squamous cell carcinomas of the head and neck. Semin Oncol 1985; 12:71–78.)

disease. Secondary considerations include treatment of occult metastases and administration of chemotherapy under conditions advantageous for response such as uninterrupted blood flow to the tumor and improved patient performance status. Published trials with current induction regimens clearly confirm that giving chemotherapy in this setting results in excellent response rates. Overall response rates of up to 94 percent and complete response rates up to 66 percent have been reported. These response rates far exceed those observed with similar treatment regimens in recurrent or metastatic disease because in the induction trials, the response rates have consistently ranged from 73 to 94 percent (Table 5). Emphasis continues to focus on increasing the complete response rate by modification of the basic regimen, which consists of bolus IV administration of cisplatin in conjunction with a 5-day continuous infusion of 5-fluorouracil. Published variations include the addition of oral or intravenous leucovorin as a biochemical modulator of 5-fluorouracil and the administration of cisplatin as a continuous infusion rather than as a bolus injection. In the absence of direct comparison in a Phase III trial, it is difficult to ascertain whether the differences in reported response rates reflect differences in the efficacy of various regimens or are due to patient selection. Published trials suggest that three courses of induction therapy produce optimal response results. In a study of continuous infusion cisplatin/5-fluorouracil and leucovorin, the complete response rate was 26 percent after two cycles of therapy and increased to 66 percent after the third cycle.[3] Although the survival of complete responders is significantly longer than that of nonresponders, the overall survival rate for patients receiving induction chemotherapy is unchanged or perhaps even slightly worse than that for patients treated with standard therapy. A number of reasonable speculations have been proposed to explain the failure of highly effective induction therapy to improve survival. These include the observation that chemotherapy is not particularly effective at eradicating bulky tumor masses; the development of drug resistance; and the possibility that chemotherapy and radiation therapy affect the same tumor cells without additive advantage. Thus, although response to chemotherapy may predict responsiveness to subsequent irradiation, no clinical advantage is achieved by their sequential use. In fact, chemotherapy may worsen the situation in nonresponders by delaying alternative definitive therapy, thereby allowing cancer to progress, selecting out a resistant population of cells, and allowing the overall condition of the patient to deteriorate. Although all of these observations may explain the failure of induction therapy to improve overall survival, it is also reasonable to speculate that induction therapy has not been put to adequate test. To date, no published study has compared optimal induction therapy with conventional therapy alone. The continuous evolution of increasingly effective chemotherapy regimens diminishes the significance of previous trials. Survival has been the only parameter measured but is not the only significant outcome measure. Highly effective induction regimens may obviate the need for extensive resection thereby decreasing morbidity in the absence of a noteworthy effect on mortality. Induction therapy trials provide excellent information regarding the responsiveness of head and neck cancer to various drugs, drug combinations, and their permutations. In the absence of demonstrated benefit, however, and despite high response rates, induction chemotherapy should not be routinely employed as standard therapy. Instead, whenever possible, eligible patients should be entered

Table 4 Studies of Cisplatin/5-Fluorouracil in Patients with Previously Treated Head and Neck Cancers

Investigator	Evaluable Patients (No Prior Treatment)	Overall Response (% CR)	Median Survival Time
Raymond	23 (7)	79% (9)	20 months
Kish	35 (3)	CI 72% (22)	27 weeks
		B 20% (10)	20 weeks
Kish	30 (11)	70% (27)	27.5 weeks
Fosser	30 (9)	67% (20)	–
Rowland	30	60% (17)	CR-14.2 months PR-14 months
Merlano	67	52% (21)	8 months
Khojasteh	23 (8)	52% (4)	–
Amrein	39	46% (18)	5 to 9 months
Mercier	20	35% (5)	6 months
Creagan	30 (4)	25% (0)	7.2 months
Choksi	20	25% (10)	36 weeks
Dasmahaptra	18	11% (0)	–

Abbreviations: CI = 96 hour continuous infusion of 5-fluorouracil and cisplatin, B = Bolus 5-fluorouracil 600 mg/m^2 d 1 and cisplatin, CR = Complete response, PR = Partial response. (From Urba SG, Forastiere AA. Systemic therapy of head and neck cancer: Most effective agents, areas of promise. Oncology 1989; 3:79–88.)

Table 5 Results of Induction Therapy with Cisplatin/5-Fluorouracil in
Advanced Head and Neck Cancer Patients

Investigator	Evaluable Patients	Regimen	Overall Response (CR %)
Kish	26	Cisplatin 100 mg/m^2 5-fluorouracil 1 gm/m^2/day (2 cycles)	88% (19)
Weaver	88	Cisplatin 100 mg/m^2 5-fluorouracil 1 gm/m^2/day (3 cycles)	94% (54)
Thyss	103	Cisplatin 100 mg/m^2 5-fluorouracil 1 gm/m^2/day (3 cycles)	87% (35)
Jacobs C.	30	Cisplatin 100 mg/m^2 5-fluorouracil 1 gm/m^2/day (2 cycles)	83% (43)
Jacobs J.	42	Cisplatin 100 mg/m^2 5-fluorouracil 1 gm/m^2/day (3 cycles)	86% (38)
Amrein	31	Cisplatin 80 mg/m^2 5-fluorouracil 800 mg/m^2/day (2 to 3 cycles)	84% (23)
Clark	53	Cisplatin 20 mg/m^2/day $\times$ 6 5-fluorouracil 1 gm/m^2/day (2 to 4 cycles)	73% (30)

CR = Complete response. (From Urba SG, Forastiere AA. Systemic therapy of head and neck cancer. Most effective agents, areas of promise. Oncology 1989; 3:79–88.)

into clinical trials designed to ascertain the efficacy of induction therapy including evaluation of quality of life.

Some of the objections to induction chemotherapy may be overcome by administering chemotherapy concomitant with definitive irradiation. Incorporation of irradiation into a chemotherapy regimen can be regarded as the addition of another effective agent, the inclusion of which may increase efficacy by circumventing inherent or acquired resistance. Drugs may enhance the effectiveness of radiation therapy by killing cells that are relatively resistant to radiation, by interfering with DNA repair between radiation fractions, or by acting as radiation sensitizers. The incorporation of irradiation into the initial treatment program avoids concerns that the delay of definitive therapy may allow tumor progression or selection of radiation resistant clones by prior induction chemotherapy. Adverse considerations include the likelihood of increased local toxicity, possibly resulting in suboptimal irradiation due to treatment delays. Increased local and systemic toxicity may also interfere with the ability to administer an adequate chemotherapy regimen. On balance, if the toxicity of concomitant therapy is manageable, combining two highly effective therapeutic modalities offers potential advantages for an increased or stable cure rate with decreased long-term morbidity. As anticipated, nonrandomized trials of effective chemotherapeutic regimens, identified in induction programs, when combined with irradiation yield impressive response rates and increased acute toxicity. Complete response rates up to 81 percent are reported with cisplatin/5-fluorouracil/radiation therapy combinations.[4] A number of randomized trials, using single-agent bleomycin, mitomycin-C, or 5-fluorouracil

in conjunction with radiation therapy have reported improved survival.[5] A randomized trial comparing the response rate associated with concurrent chemoradiotherapy to that with similar chemotherapy followed by radiation, reported a significant increase in complete response rate and median survival with the simultaneous therapy.[6] The complete response rate with concurrent therapy was 67 percent versus 32 percent with sequential therapy, and the projected 3-year survival was 68 percent for the concurrent group versus 43 percent for the sequential group. In favorable candidates, there is good reason to anticipate that a combined chemoradiotherapy approach may prove to be a highly effective organ-sparing approach for the control of locally advanced head and neck cancer. The toxicity of combined therapy is formidable, and results from definitive randomized trials are not available.

The role for conventional adjuvant chemotherapy, that is, chemotherapy administered after attainment of a clinical complete response through surgery, radiation, or both is undefined. In view of the high response rates demonstrated in induction trials, it is likely that a majority of patients have cancers that are sensitive to current multidrug regimens. Although distant metastases do not usually present a major problem in the management of head and neck cancer patients, with improved local control, systemic disease may assume significance. The contribution of adjuvant chemotherapy to the control of local disease is more problematic because, despite small numbers, tumor residue after surgery and radiation therapy is likely to be resistant to chemotherapy because of either inherent resistance or local conditions of anoxia or diminished blood flow.

Nevertheless, patients who have achieved clinical complete response have a low tumor burden that should improve the effectiveness of chemotherapy. By definition, most of these patients will have undergone radiation therapy, and tumors responsive to radiation are more likely to respond to chemotherapy. Giving chemotherapy in an adjuvant setting permits earlier institution of definitive radiation and surgery, thereby avoiding the delay associated with induction therapy and the increased toxicity associated with concomitant chemoradiotherapy. Major obstacles to adjuvant chemotherapy have made definitive trials impossible to date. These include refusal of patients who achieve a complete response from local therapy to participate in chemotherapy trials, poor tolerance of chemotherapy, and increased local toxicity after extensive prior radiation and surgery. Although it is likely that some patients would benefit from additional treatment following achievement of a clinical complete response, there has been no evidence of benefit in published trials of classical adjuvant chemotherapy. A published study that does appear to show some survival benefit, administered postoperative or postradiation chemotherapy to patients who had responded to initial induction chemotherapy.[7] In this study, only 46 patients, 63 percent of those eligible, were willing to be randomized, and although the failure-free survival is longer for treated patients than for nontreated patients, it is entirely possible that equivalent results might have been obtained by an additional cycle of induction therapy. Whether to administer adjuvant chemotherapy and, if so, to whom remains an unanswered question. Optimal candidates may be patients who can prospectively be identified as at risk despite early-stage disease.

Although the role of chemotherapy in the definitive management of patients with advanced head and neck cancer has not yet been defined, the high response rates clearly indicate that chemotherapy will be a major factor in decreasing morbidity, mortality, or both.

REFERENCES

Adelstein DJ, Sharan VM, Earle AS. Simultaneous versus sequential combined technique therapy for squamous cell head and neck cancer. Cancer 1990; 65:1685–1691.

Dreyfuss AI, Clark JR, Wright JE. Continuous infusion high-dose leucovorin with 5-fluorouracil and cisplatin for untreated stage IV carcinoma of the head and neck. Ann Intern Med 1990; 112:167–172.

Erwin TM, Clark JR, Weichselbaum RR. Multidisciplinary treatment of advanced squamous cell carcinomas of the head and neck. Semin Oncol 1985; 12:71–78.

Erwin TJ, Clark JR, Weichselbaum RR. An analysis of induction and adjuvant chemotherapy in the multidisciplinary treatment of squamous-cell carcinoma of the head and neck. J Clin Oncol 1987; 5:10–20.

Mashburg A, Samit AM. Early detection, diagnosis, and management of oral and oropharyngeal cancer. Cancer 1989; 39:67–88.

Silverberg E, Boring CC, Squires TS. Cancer statistics 1990. Cancer 1990; 40:9–26.

Urba SG, Forastiere AA. Systemic therapy of head and neck cancer: Most effective agents, areas of promise. Oncology 1989; 3:79–88.

Vokes EE, Weischselbaum RR. Concomitant chemoradiography: Rationale and clinical experience in patients with solid tumors. J Clin Oncol 1990; 8:911–934.

Wendt TA, Hartenstein RC, Wastrow TPU, Lissner J. Cisplatin, fluorouracil with leucovorin calcium enhancement, and synchronous accelerated radiotherapy in the management of locally advanced head and neck cancer: A phase II study. J Clin Oncol 1990; 7:471–476.

ESOPHAGEAL CANCER

BEN SISCHY, M.D., F.A.C.R., D.M.R.T. (EDIN)

Although it is not a common malignancy, squamous cell carcinoma of the thoracic esophagus is an exacting one from the standpoint of patient management and therapy. It is a tumor that has a devastating effect on the host and that presents a great challenge to the treating physician because there is great pessimism regarding a successful therapeutic reponse. In 1990, 10,600 Americans will be diagnosed with cancer of the esophagus and 9,500 patients will die of the disease. Although there is a wide variety of therapeutic options, a standard form of treatment has not yet emerged.

Localized cancer of the esophagus is rarely detected with screening procedures during its asymptomatic phase; however, the diagnosis should be suspected in any patient with dysphagia over the age of 40. The majority of patients at presentation admit to chronic symptoms of 4 to 6 months' duration, and in 80 percent of patients, the disease is advanced to such a degree that survival of more than a year after diagnosis is unusual. By the time the patient presents for an examination due to dysphagia, over 50 percent of the circumference of the esophagus will be involved. By that time, 50 to 90 percent of patients will already have lymph node metastases. Very often the patient reports with aspiration pneumonia, hoarseness, cough, fever, or a choking sensation, all indicative of locally advanced disease. Some patients will already exhibit signs of metastatic disease such as a neck mass or bone pain.

Following the detection of esophageal cancer, it is important to stage the disease as accurately as possible in order to make the optimal therapeutic decisions. Various imaging techniques are available that can assess the extent of the primary lesion and identify the presence of lymph node involvement and metastatic spread. These include chest radiograph, barium esophagram, azygous venography, pneumomediastinography, and computed tomography (CT).

The anatomic features and relations of the esophagus severely limit the curability of malignancy at this site. It is a thin-walled tube surrounded by an inner circular and an outer longitudinal muscularis. There is no fibrous serosa to act as a barrier to the spread of tumor beyond the organ. Distant spread of tumor within the esophagus is not uncommon, and foci of tumor may be observed as far as 4 to 8 cm beyond the margins of the primary tumor.

Approximately 95 percent of esophageal cancers worldwide are squamous cell carcinomas, and the remaining 5 percent are adenocarcinomas. The majority of patients are between 50 and 70 years of age, and men are more frequently affected than women. There are two areas of the world where cancer of the esophagus accounts for a high proportion of cancer deaths, i.e., the Asian Esophageal Cancer Belt, encompassing Iran, Soviet Central Asia, Afghanistan, and the area of Siberia, Mongolia, and China, and Africa (East and South), and France, particularly Normandy. Great Britain, too, has a high frequency of men with the disease. The etiology of esophageal cancer is thought to be multifactorial, but there appears to be a strong indication that chronic ingestion of certain foods and the frequent use of alcoholic beverages increases the risk of developing the disease.

THERAPEUTIC OPTIONS

Surgery

Although Billroth proposed esophageal resections for cure as long ago as 1871, the outcome of any treatment for this disease is extremely poor, and a cure is indeed an unusual event. Earlam and Cunha-Melo, in a review of over 83,000 cases, stated that, following surgery, only 4 percent of patients are alive at 5 years. Resection for squamous cell carcinoma of the esophagus has the highest operative mortality of any routinely performed surgical procedure today. They concluded that neither surgery nor radiotherapy had significant impact on the natural history of the disease and that there was no difference in the 5-year survival figures for either modality. Only 30 to 60 percent of patients are resectable at presentation, and the perioperative mortality rate continues to be relatively high. Approximately 41 percent of surgically resected specimens exhibit lymph node metastases, and 38 percent show tumor extending into the periesophageal tissues.

The possibility of having surgery has increased with the improvement of techniques and anesthesia. Surgery has become more radical. There are advocates for total esophagectomy, which involves splitting the diaphragm and resecting the tail of the pancreas, spleen, and celiac nodes. Reconstruction is performed with a substernal transplant of the right colon, joining the stomach to the cervical esophagus. Another method in lower lesions involves anastomosing the esophagus to the stomach within the chest. However, a corresponding improvement in the results of radical surgery has not followed. The extensive surgery required for resection and reconstruction carries considerable morbidity.

Chemotherapy

Although the role of chemotherapy in the management of this disease has never been a major one, some combinations of drugs have achieved response rates of 18 to 55 percent. Most of these regimens contain cis-platinum, with or without mitomycin C. Single-agent trials have demonstrated that bleomycin, methyl-GAG, vindesine, and cis-platinum have all shown some degree of activity. These agents may be given either definitively or preoperatively. Toxicities may be severe and dose-limiting.

Radiation Therapy

In 1909, there was an initial report from Paris on the use of radium bouginage for esophageal cancer. The use of orthovoltage irradiation followed, which produced severe reactions, chronic side effects, and few cures. Various techniques were introduced in an attempt to alleviate some of the problems, and since then newer technologies have revolutionized both equipment and methods of delivery.

Radiation therapy series are generally comprised of patients who are medically inoperable or who have unresectable disease, and over time this has undoubtedly influenced the results to some extent. It is still a therapeutic dilemma to identify patients for whom curative therapy is appropriate and to determine the preferential palliation for those with advanced disease. This may be due to the fact that no therapy is outstanding in its effectiveness and that every option at this disease site produces morbidities that may be unacceptable in the light of the anticipated prognosis.

The results of radiotherapy are not sufficiently superior to discard all thoughts of surgery, and it appears that currently there are no series comparing irradiation alone with surgery or combined therapy for patients with lesions that are suitable for curative resection.

Definitive Radiation Therapy

Definitive irradiation is commonly used as an alternative to surgery because the number of patients who would benefit from radical surgery is limited. Radiotherapy allows the surrounding structures to be preserved intact while local lateral tumor spread may be encompassed within the target volume. Acute mortality from definitive irradiation is uncommon and is generally confined to the development of a tracheoesophageal fistula or rupture of the aorta; it may be argued that both these events are related to disease rather than therapy.

It becomes difficult to insist on expensive, radical high-risk surgery, which is frequently accompanied by prolonged hospitalizations and chronic morbidity, for a patient population with a characteristic survival of approximately 1 year.

Pearson reported a 5-year survival of 25 percent in a series of 208 patients treated by megavoltage irradiation. Less favorable results have been documented at both the Princess Margaret and Royal Marsden Hospitals. These results approximate those of surgery but with substantially lesser morbidity and mortality.

A report from China on 869 patients who received irradiation doses of 6,000 cGy to 7,900 cGy indicates that patients receiving the higher doses had a 10.8 percent 5-year survival compared to a 1.6 percent for patients at the low end of the dose range.

Preoperative Radiation Therapy

Most series of patients, whether treated by surgery or radiation therapy, demonstrate 5-year survival rates of approximately 5 to 6 percent, and only slightly higher figures are reported when a combination of modalities is used in the management of local disease.

Preoperative irradiation may be advocated in an attempt to convert the tumor to a resectable status. There is an ongoing debate regarding the merits of this modality in the management of esophageal cancer, and there now is an extensive worldwide experience. A vast number of both retrospective and prospective series have been published, and at this time no forerunners in technique or dose schedule appear to be present. Following a review of the literature, one of the possible reasons for the vacillation of opinions regarding therapy becomes evident. It is very difficult to compare the results of many series because there are a number of preselection factors inherent in the patient subgroups. Large trials by different workers all over the world have reported disappointing results without any gain in survival.

Postoperative Radiation Therapy

Some investigators advocate the use of postoperative radiotherapy for those patients with locally advanced disease who have tolerated surgery. Proponents of postoperative irradiation for patients with esophageal cancer argue that following resection, it is possible to direct irradiation to well-defined areas of residual tumor that are accurately identified by the intraoperative placement of radio-opaque clips. It must be recognized, however, that subsequent to colon or stomach interposition, the radiotolerance of these structures in the chest severely limits the dose of irradiation that may be delivered. Some reports indicate an improvement in survival when postoperative irradiation is given as an adjunct to surgery as opposed to when it is deferred to the time of recurrence. In general, however, it appears that its benefit is limited.

Data from Kasai and colleagues concerning the use of postoperative irradiation for esophageal carcinoma indicate that radiation therapy may make a limited but definite impact on survival. When mediastinal and cervical nodes were treated to 6,000 cGy, recurrence at these sites was virtually eliminated. The 5-year survival was improved for patients with no positive nodes at surgery, but nearly two-thirds of these patients developed disseminated disease. Over 90 percent of patients with positive nodes at surgery had recurrence of disease in spite of postoperative irradiation. This would imply that the presence of nodal disease is indicative of systemic disease in most patients.

Brachytherapy

Ever since Guisez reported his use of radium bouginage, intraluminal therapy has been used to some extent in the management of patients with cancer of the esophagus. With the recent availability and increasing role of laser therapy at this disease site, it is likely that there will be a renewed interest in the use of intracavitary irradiation. This, coupled with the current widespread use of afterloading techniques, has led to several articles describing the use of iridium 192 and high-intensity cobalt 60 for boosting primary tumor sites after external-beam therapy.

Innovative Approaches

Therapeutic prospects for squamous cell carcinoma of the esophagus are singularly discouraging, and the overwhelming fact is that the patient's overall chance of survival is poor whether he or she is treated by surgery or radiation therapy. The inability of radiation alone to control local disease reliably is illustrated by a documented tumor sterilization rate of only 30 percent following maximal radiation therapy of 6,600 cGy administered over 7 weeks. There seems to be few prospects of improving either modality beyond their present state without the addition of ancillary agents to augment their effectiveness.

Radiobiologic Modifiers

Neutrons

Esophageal tumors are often ulcerated and necrotic and therefore contain a high percentage of hypoxic cells that are more resistant to the effect of x-rays or gamma irradiation than are well-oxygenated tissues. Several investigators, therefore, have attempted to manage patients with this disease with the use of neutron therapy. Following an initial trial in 1948 that showed disappointing results, the modality was not commonly used for many years. Recently, however, there has been a revival of interest in neutron therapy, and several trials are being initiated in Europe, North America, and Asia. A Radiation Therapy Oncology Group (RTOG) phase I study comparing neutrons alone with mixed-beam therapy for patients with inoperable esophageal cancers showed no difference in survival between the treatment arms.

Alternative Fractionation Schemes

On the premise that several large doses of irradiation produce a greater cell kill than the same total dose given in smaller amounts over the same time period, several investigators have endeavored to gain a survival advantage by using accelerated dose regimens. The results appear to be equivalent to those produced by the use of conventional fractionation schemes.

Another alternative dose schedule that is being used by some radiotherapists is that of hyperfractionation. This is the use of multiple daily fractions of conventional or, more often, smaller size in an attempt to utilize the different rates of cellular repair that are thought to exist between normal and tumor cells. When used for squamous cell carcinomas of the head and neck, the results were encouraging.

Hypoxic Cell Sensitizers

There has been some use of electron affinic, hypoxic cell sensitizer drugs such as misonidazole, but the results do not appear to be better than when radiation therapy is delivered alone.

Chemosensitized Radiation Therapy

There is laboratory evidence in other tumor models that there is an advantage in the use of chemotherapy preoperatively. Theoretically, it appears expedient to use chemotherapy at a time when the metastatic tumor burden is low, as this may diminish the probability of spontaneous drug resistance, and there is evidence of an increased resection rate following neoadjuvant chemotherapy. As a single agent, 5-fluorouracil has a response rate of 17 percent when delivered to patients with carcinoma of the esophagus. Seifert and colleagues documented a greater response rate in patients with colorectal cancer treated with infusional rather than bolus 5-fluorouracil. The established usefulness of 5-fluorouracil in the management of esophageal cancer provides further support for its use in addition to the apparent synergism that occurs when combined with irradiation.

It has been demonstrated both in the laboratory and clinically that when irradiation is combined with 5-fluorouracil, synergistic cell killing takes place. It is also known that the degree of synergism depends on the concentration of cytocidal levels of 5-fluorouracil and the time and method of administration relative to the delivery of the irradiation. Optimal sensitization occurs when the administration of 5-fluorouracil follows irradiation and is in excess of the cell cycle time. It may be that rather than acting as a radiation sensitizer, the radiation may enhance the cytocidal effect of the 5-fluorouracil.

Mitomycin C has also been proven clinically effective in the treatment of esophageal and other gastrointestinal neoplasia. Response rates of 25 percent to 40 percent have been documented in squamous cell carcinoma of the esophagus. Although the cell-killing effect of mitomycin C combined with irradiation appears to be additive and not synergistic, preliminary reports suggest that chronically hypoxic cells may be more sensitive than normal cells. This differential cytoxicity is of potential value because such cells are relatively resistant to radiation and chemotherapy.

Results following the use of preoperative irradiation combined with 5-fluorouracil and mitomycin C for squamous cell carcinoma at other sites, such as the anal canal, have been extremely encouraging and are being reproduced to some degree in the esophagus. Steiger, Franklin, Leichman, and coworkers, from Wayne State University School of Medicine in Detroit, began publishing encouraging reports on the use of chemotherapy combined with radiation therapy and surgery. This created an impetus for this new multidisciplinary approach.

CLINICAL TRIALS

A number of trials have been performed to investigate the role of pre- and postoperative chemotherapy, and the results show that overall the survival rates were not improved over either modality alone, except, predictably, in a subgroup analysis of one trial, patients who responded to chemotherapy had a significantly improved survival when compared to nonresponders or those undergoing surgery alone.

In a selected phase II series, patients received concurrent radiation therapy and chemotherapy followed by surgery. A complete pathologic response was observed in 17 to 27 percent, and the median survival was 12 to 19 months. Other studies have examined the results of radiation therapy combined with chemotherapy as primary treatment, and for the total group (all stages combined), the local control rates were 60 to 79 percent and the median survival was 8 to 24 months.

The Eastern Cooperative Oncology Group sponsored a trial in 1982 that randomized patients to either irradiation alone or irradiation combined with infusional 5-fluorouracil and bolus mitomycin C, with an option of surgery for suitable patients on either arm. Of 119 analyzable patients, 99 (83 percent), have died. The overall median survival is 11.2 months, with a median survival of 9.3 months for the radiotherapy alone arm and 14.8 months for the combined-therapy arm. This difference is significant at $P = 0.02$ after accounting for the factors (stage, performance status, and primary location) used in the randomization procedure. Stage was associated with survival. At 36 months, there was a 28 percent probability of survival for patients with stage I disease treated by combined therapy, versus a 10 percent probability of survival of patients treated by radiation alone. The median survival of patients with stage I disease was 13.7 months and that of patients with stage II was 9.8 months ($P = .03$). Within most subgroups, the pattern of patients doing better with sensitizers was maintained.

PALLIATION

Unfortunately, cancer of the esophagus in the Western world is a disease that is often diagnosed only at a late stage, when any therapy can be expected to fail. This is partly due to the reluctance of some patients to report dysphagia or other symptoms until they become critical and partly because some patients with dysphagia may have normal barium esophograms and endoscopic biopsies.

Many patients present with unresectable disease, characterized by the presence of lymph node metastases or a primary tumor that extends beyond the esophageal wall. This may be recognized clinically by the presence of a tracheoesophageal fistula, obstruction of the superior vena cava, malignant pleural effusion, or paralysis of the recurrent laryngeal nerve. Lymph nodes may often be palpated in the neck or be detected on mediastinoscopy or on CT scan of the thorax.

The philosophy of the best palliation for patients with advanced disease is often personal or institutional. Some prefer to perform a palliative resection or bypass, but this often produces fairly severe sequelae. A gastrostomy tube does not restore the patient's ability to swallow and may not be an option for high-surgical-risk patients.

A nonoperative approach may be the best palliation, and a fairly radical course of irradiation to approximately 5,000 to 6,000 cGy may be advisable. The use of lower doses does not appear to be successful for relief of either pain or dysphagia. Once the tumor mass has regressed, it may be possible to perform periodic esophageal dilatation to relieve dysphagia. If a stricture persists or if a tracheobronchial fistula develops as the tumor shrinks, insertion of a prosthetic tube may be of value. This, however, may be accompanied by a fairly high mortality rate in this patient population.

Symptomatic patients for whom no cure is possible are now being treated endoscopically with a neodymium Yag laser.

ADENOCARCINOMA OF THE ESOPHAGUS

Adenocarcinoma of the esophagus is a rare condition, accounting for approximately 5 to 10 percent of all carcinomas in the lower third of the esophagus. In some situations, it becomes difficult to distinguish a true adenocarcinoma arising in the distal esophagus or esophageal glands, from a lesion in the fundus, cardia, or stomach that has encroached up into the esophagus at the esophagogastric junction. The majority of cases (at least 80 percent) are associated with reflux esophagitis and Barrett's esophagus.

In the United States, there appears to be an increasing number of patients presenting with this histology. A recent article from Boston indicates that 18 percent of esophageal lesions are now adenocarcinomas.

The radiation therapy techniques employed in the management of patients with adenocarcinoma of the esophagus are similar to those used for squamous cell carcinoma of the lower third of the esophagus, i.e., the celiac axis nodes should be irradiated to at least 4,400 cGy.

SUGGESTED READING

DeMeester TR, Levin B, eds. Cancer of the esophagus. Orlando: Grune & Stratton, 1985.

Earlam R, Cunha-Melo JR. Esophageal squamous cell carcinoma: A critical surgical review of surgery. Br J Surg 1980; 67:381–390.

Earlam R, Cunha-Melo JR: Esophageal squamous cell carcinoma: A critical review of radiotherapy. Br J Surg 1980; 67:457–461.

GASTRIC, BILIARY, AND PANCREATIC CANCER: CHEMOTHERAPY

GUILLERMO RAMIREZ, M.D., F.A.C.P.

GASTRIC CARCINOMA

Epidemiology

The incidence of gastric carcinoma has decreased during the last four decades; however, over 23,000 new cases will be diagnosed this year, and an estimated 13,700 patients will die from the disease. The decrease in the death rate cannot be attributed to improvements in either diagnosis or treatment. The prognosis for cancer of the stomach in the western hemisphere continues to be unfavorable. The resectability rate has risen, and the postoperative mortality has declined, but we can meet the challenge of gastric carcinoma only by improving the methods for early diagnosis. The etiology of pancreatic carcinoma remains unknown. Possible etiologic factors commonly cited include pancreatitis, diabetes mellitus, cholelithiasis, industrial exposure, alcohol consumption, and smoking, but there is not conclusive evidence as to the true cause of these tumors.

Diagnosis and Clinical Presentation

The symptoms of gastric carcinoma are usually vague and nonspecific. Pain, anorexia, anemia, or dysphagia often occur when the disease has advanced. The diagnosis is established by upper gastrointestinal radiologic examination, fiberoptic endoscopy, or exfoliative cytology. The use of computed tomography (CT) scanning is useful for staging the patients accurately, but the disease often has spread to the lymph nodes or metastasized to other organs by the time the patients are considered for surgery. Only 18 to 20 percent of the patients have localized disease at the time of diagnosis. Although the 5-year survival for people with localized disease approaches 50 percent, the overall rate is only approximately 12 percent.

Screening is not considered cost-effective in the United States, but for the Japanese, the procedure is almost automated and has enabled them to detect a large number of early cancers. As a result, their 5-year survival for those cases diagnosed in the early stages is around 80 to 90 percent. The technique includes a double-contrast upper gastrointestinal series followed with appropriate endoscopy in the patients with radiologic abnormalities.

Treatment

Surgery remains the treatment of choice when the disease is localized; however, the majority of the patients have a poor prognosis. Because gastric carcinoma extends through the submucosa far beyond to what can be appreciated at the time of surgery, often the patients have more advanced disease, and those with stage III or IV have a worst outlook. The 5-year survival for patients with stage III is less than 15 percent, and, rarely, those with stage IV have a long-term survival. The median survival for patients undergoing "curative" resections of localized stage III/IV lesions is only 8 months; after palliative resection, it is less than 6 months. Although radiation therapy is employed as an adjuvant to surgery, most of the attention is now focused on the use of systemic chemotherapy.

In patients with extensive disease, Lavin and his colleagues have examined pretreatment information to estimate response and survival. Performance status was a major determinant of response and survival. Other factors included more than 5 percent weight loss in 6 months and normal liver chemistries. Response to therapy was associated with an improvement in survival (36 weeks versus 14 weeks) that was above that predicted based on prognostic factors.

Chemotherapy

Chemotherapy with single agents has encountered a limited amount of success. 5-Fluorouracil, doxorubicin, BCNU, methyl-CCNU, mitomycin C, cis-platinum, and etoposide produce a response rate ranging between 15 and 30 percent, but rarely has there been a complete response using a single agent. Several combinations of the aforementioned drugs improve the response rate, but the number of complete responses is low and the gains in survival are not significant. The most commonly used combination of 5-fluorouracil, adriamycin, and mitomycin-C (FAM), first reported by McDonald and colleagues, showed responses of 30 to 35 percent, with a median duration of remission of 6 to 9 months and a median survival of 7 months. The North Central Cancer Treatment Group compared FAM with 5-fluorouracil and adriamycin and 5-fluorouracil alone. They found no difference in survival among the three arms, although the response rate for FAM was higher. Subsequent studies substituting mitomycin C for BCNU (FAB), methyl-CCNU (FAMe), and cis-platinum (FAP) did not yield any better results. Klein and colleagues reported the combination of 5-fluorouracil, adriamycin, and methotrexate as highly effective, with a complete response rate of 10 percent, but their results were not confirmed by other investigators.

Recent reports by Wilke and co-workers, from Hannover, Germany, using a combination of VP-16* 120 mg per square meter IV on days 4,5 and 6, doxorubicin 20 mg per square meter IV on days 1 and 7, and cis-platinum, 40 mg per square meter IV on days 2 and 8 (EAP) or VP-16, 5-fluorouracil, and Leucovorin (ELF), appear quite promising.

In the group receiving EAP, the response rate of 57 percent in 83 of 145 patients with advanced gastric carcinoma included a 15 percent rate of complete responders. Forty nine patients had locally advanced disease, and ninety six had metastatic involvement. The median survival for all patients was 10 months; for those with locally advanced disease, it was 17 months, in contrast to the 8.5 months for patients with metastatic disease and 5 months for the nonresponders. Those patients over 65 years of age or with cardiac risk who could not be treated with anthracyclines were treated with ELF. In this group of 51 patients, the response rate was 53 percent, including 12 percent complete responses. In this group, the median duration of remission was 9.5 months, and the median survival for all patients was 11 months. Katz and colleagues, from a Brazilian group, reported more than 50 percent responses using a modified EAP schedule in patients with advanced disease; 12 percent achieved complete response. The Eastern Cooperative Oncology Group (ECOG), the Dana-Farber Cancer Center, and Memorial Sloan-Kettering are also testing the effectiveness of EAP.

Adjuvant Therapy

Because the results in advanced disease are so discouraging, for many years investigators focused their attention on the use of chemotherapy as an adjuvant to surgery. The Veterans Administration Surgical Group published two studies using thiotepa and 5-fluoxyuridine as single agents. Neither drug proved effective in prolonging survival. Their study of 312 patients using 5-fluorouracil and methyl-CCNU failed to show any benefit. The Eastern Cooperative Oncology Group used the same combination and did not find it to be beneficial. The only positive study using the 5-fluorouracil plus methyl-CCNU combination was reported by the Gastrointestinal Tumor Study Group (GITSG), with a 4-year survival of 44 percent for the surgery-alone group and 59 percent for the group receiving adjuvant chemotherapy. Two other cooperative groups are investigating FAM as an adjuvant to surgery. One study is still in progress, and the other has not made a final report.

Neoadjuvant Therapy

Recently, a major area of interest is the use of neo-adjuvant chemotherapy. The German group reported their results in 35 patients with locally advanced and technically unresectable gastric carcinoma who received preoperative EAP therapy. The response rate was 70 percent (24/35), including 23 percent complete responders (8/35). Twenty of 24 patients with objective response underwent a second-look operation. Six clinical complete responders were pathologically confirmed. After a 19 months' median follow-up, 43 percent of the patients are disease-free. The numbers are too small to draw definitive conclusions, but the data look exciting. The M.D. Anderson Hospital and the Dana-Farber Cancer Center are investigating the usefulness of EAP given preoperatively, and as consolidation following surgery.

PANCREATIC CARCINOMA

Epidemiology

Carcinoma of the pancreas is increasing in frequency in several countries, including the United States. Over 28,000 new cases will be diagnosed this year, and likely 25,000 patients will die from the disease. The high mortality rate of this tumor is in part due to the small number that can be surgically resected. Despite more aggressive surgery and the use of radiation and chemotherapy, overall less than 3 percent of the patients reach a 5-year survival. The majority of the patients die within 1 year from the time of diagnosis.

Diagnosis and Clinical Manifestations

The tumor does not produce specific symptoms in the early stages of the disease, and the diagnosis is difficult with the currently available tests. Most lesions of the body or the tail of the organ are evident only when the disease has spread or metastatic lesions are evident. Asthenia, anorexia, weight loss, and behavioral changes are nondiagnostic, and most of the time they are dismissed by the patients as not important and at times disregarded by their physicians as not related to cancer. Pain is present frequently, with lesions of the body or the tail of the pancreas, but carcinoma is not always the first consideration in the differential diagnosis. Laboratory abnormalities may include anemia, elevated levels of carcinoembryonic antigen (CEA), and hypoalbuminemia, but there is not a panel of tests that will provide an accurate diagnosis. Monoclonal antibodies to pancreatic carcinoma (DU-PAN-2) have shown some preferential binding, but there is some degree of reactivity to normal tissues and other malignant neoplasms. Ultrasound may be useful for localizing a lesion for biopsy and to differentiate cystic lesions, but it does not provide a definitive diagnosis. Radiologic studies are of limited value; if the studies are directed to the upper gastrointestinal tract, there might be some deformities of the duodenal loop, mucosal abnormalities, or displacement of the stomach or the duodenum. The CT scan may offer some help, but on many occasions is not that useful. If a tumor mass is identified by radiographs, percutaneous needle aspiration often provides the diagnosis.

Not uncommonly, the neoplasia is associated with pancreatitis, which makes the diagnosis more difficult because the treatment is directed toward controlling the inflammatory component, thus wasting precious time to make the diagnosis of cancer. The clinical picture, which includes lesions of the head of the pancreas, is somewhat different, for it is not uncommon to see the patient consulting for painless jaundice, when the tumor encroaches the common bile duct. In these cases, the diagnosis may be established by endoscopic retrograde cholangiopancreatography (ERCP), with brushing and exfoliative cytologic examination. The proper staging of the tumor requires surgical assessment. For practical purposes, however, it is only useful if it determines resectability.

Treatment

Surgical resection offers potentially curative treatment for those patients in whom the disease is localized. It may include Whipple procedure, total pancreatectomy, or distal pancreatectomy, depending on the location of the tumor. However, the radical procedures carry a high mortality and morbidity. At times, only a biopsy or a bypass procedure can be performed. The probability of local and regional failures is rather high. In addition, many patients develop distant metastases soon after the surgical intervention. Thus, there is a need to address both the problem of the locoregional control as well as the one of distant metastasis.

Radiation therapy is used as a palliative treatment in pancreatic cancer. The response rate seems directly related to the amount of radiation delivered. Doses of 60 Gy were superior to lower doses, as reported by Haslam and colleagues; however, those results were not confirmed by the GITSG study. In 1969, Moertel and associates reported that radiotherapy appears more effective when combined with 5-fluorouracil. Subsequently, the GITSG confirmed these results, showing that the median survival of the patients receiving the combined treatment of 60 Gy plus 5-fluorouracil was 11.4 months, compared with only 4.3 months for those patients treated with 60 Gy alone. There is renewed interest in the use of radiotherapy given intraoperatively. Peretz and colleagues, from the Memorial Sloan-Kettering Cancer Center, reported the use of intraoperative brachytherapy using iodine-125 implants in 98 patients with unresectable carcinoma of the pancreas. Twenty-seven patients received postoperative external radiation, and 27 patients received chemotherapy. The median survival for the entire group was 7 months. They concluded that in a selected group of patients with adequate implantation, it is possible to achieve high control of the primary tumor and "meaningful long-term palliation of symptoms." A subgroup of patients in their study with T1N0 stage disease who received chemotherapy survived 18.5 months. Another intraoperative technique involving electron-beam irradiation showed encouraging results.

Chemotherapy

The results of chemotherapy in pancreatic carcinoma are disappointing. Single-agent chemotherapy employing 5-fluorouracil, mitomycin C, CCNU, streptozotocin, methyl-CCNU, doxorubicin, *cis*-platinum, methotrexate, dacarbazine, or hydroxyurea yielded responses between 6 percent and 26 percent, but they were short-lasting, and the majority of the patients died within 1 year. Drug combinations, using the aforementioned drugs, produced a higher response rate, but the gains in survival were not significant. The group from Georgetown University reported a response rate of 40 percent using the FAM regimen, but their results were not confirmed by the Cancer and Acute Leukemia Group (CALGB) or the North Central Cancer Treatment Group (NCCTG). There was some enthusiasm with the initial report on the usefulness of the combination of streptozotocin, mitomycin C, and 5-fluorouracil (SMF), but the study by GITSG did not confirm the results.

As pancreatic carcinoma commonly metastasizes to the liver, we thought that including the liver in the initial treatment plan as an adjuvant to surgery would improve the results. We designed a study employing intra-arterial hepatic infusion with 5-fluorouracil, in association with radiation therapy to the liver, pancreas, and regional lymph nodes, following surgery for resectable tumors of the pancreas. The regimen proved rather toxic, and the results were quite disappointing. In patients with resectable tumors, a GITSG study in 43 patients showed that the use of adjuvant external-beam radiation (50 Gy) and 5-fluorouracil improved the overall survival (21 months versus 11 months) and 2-year survival (43 percent versus 18 percent), when compared to surgery (pancreatoduodenectomy) alone.

Because human pancreas contains estrogen and androgen receptors as well as aromatase activity, Lipton and colleagues designed a randomized study in which the patients received FAM or FAM plus aminoglutethimide. The addition of aminoglutethimide did not improve the results obtained with FAM.

TUMORS OF THE ENDOCRINE PANCREAS

Neoplasms of the islet cell can be benign or malignant, and the histologic differentiation is often impossible. This group of diseases comprises two main types of neoplasms: (1) apudomas and (2) carcinoids. Apudomas are derived from cells that are known by their ability to produce polypeptide hormones and to synthesize biogenic amines from amine precursors (amine precursor uptake and decarboxylation = APUD system). These tumors are interesting because approximately 20 percent present clinical pictures associated with excessive endocrine secretions. Commonly, they are associated with hyperplastic or tumoral changes of two or more endocrine glands, and the syndromes of multiple endocrine neoplasia (MEN) have been described as clinically defined entities. The main endocrine tumors of the pancreas are insulinoma, glucagonoma, SRIFoma, VIPoma, PPoma, gastrinoma, and ACTHoma.

Glucagonomas are alpha-cell tumors, commonly located in the tail of the pancreas; over 60 percent are malignant, and the metastases frequently occur in the liver and peripancreatic lymph nodes.

Somastimomas (SRFIomas) were first reported in 1977. They are slow growing and are diagnosed when a tumor mass is detected because they produce little metabolic disturbances and clinical symptoms.

VIPomas, so designated for their production of vasoactive intestinal peptide (VIP), were first described in 1958, when a syndrome of refractory diarrhea and severe hypokalemia was observed in two patients with non–insulin-secreting islet cell tumors. The syndrome was described as pancreatic cholera. The diagnosis is commonly made when symptoms of abdominal colic and pronounced weight loss are not totally explained by diarrhea alone. Potassium levels were below 2.5 mmol per liter, and bicarbonate levels were below 15 mmol per liter in the majority of the patients. Fasting levels of VIP were elevated in all patients, with a range between 48 and 760 pmol per liter (n = 0.5 to 16 pmol per liter).

Gastrinomas, which constitute 20 to 25 percent of endocrine pancreatic tumors are mainly located in the head or the tail of the pancreas. Its association with recurrent peptic ulcers and gastric hypersecretion is known as the Zollinger-Ellison syndrome. Although they grow slowly, 50 to 75 percent have metastases at the time of diagnosis. They are small and difficult to localize; their resection is not possible in 80 to 90 percent of patients because of their location or the presence of metastases.

Insulinomas, or beta cell tumors, are the most commonly diagnosed functioning islet cell tumors, for their classic symptom is hypoglycemia, which frequently occurs in the morning or after vigorous exercise. Early associated symptoms include irritability, flushing, sweating, tachycardia, and nausea, most of them related to sympathetic nervous system irritation. If the hypoglycemia is not treated, central nervous system symptoms appear, including erratic psychiatric behavior, convulsions, and coma. Repeated untreated attacks may cause irreversible brain damage. Diagnosis is made by keeping the patient fasting for at least 24 hours while he or she is kept active. Another diagnostic method is the tolbutamide tolerance test.

Carcinoid tumors are a group of neoplasms derived from the disseminated endocrine cells of the primitive gut and are characterized by the presence of argentaffin granules in their cells, which accounts for the term *argentaffinomas* by which they are also known. They are found in the trachea, bronchial tree or gastrointestinal tract, pancreas, and biliary ducts. They produce 5-hydroxytryptophan, which is broken down and excreted mainly as 5-hydroxyinoleacetic acid (5-HIAA) in the urine, a useful test in making the diagnosis of carcinoid syndrome. They are commonly located in the appendix and are often found incidentally in appendectomies. They may be present in any segment of the intestine.

Their malignancy, as judged by the presence of metastasis, is highest in tumors of the cecum; the tendency to metastasize correlates with their size, and pancreatic carcinoids, because they are discovered late, are almost always considered malignant.

Carcinoid syndrome is frequently associated with carcinoid tumors metastatic to the liver. It is commonly seen in carcinoid tumors of the small intestine, but it could be seen in tumors originated in other locations. Clinically, it is characterized by cutaneous flushing, diarrhea, and asthma-like attacks. Not infrequently, palpitations, tachycardia, hypotension, headaches, nausea, and vomiting are accompanying symptoms. In addition, cardiac valvular damage may occur as a result of the endocardium being covered with a fibrotic layer that may compromise the function of the valves. The flushing can occur spontaneously or be triggered by efforts, a meal, or palpation of the tumor. The mechanisms by which the syndrome occurs are varied, but they are likely associated with the release of histamine, serotonin, bradykinin, or 5-hydroxytryptidine, accounting for elevated urinary excretion of 5-HIAA, which is useful in making the diagnosis.

Treatment

Surgery is the treatment of choice for eradicating endocrine tumors of the pancreas; however, recurrences are frequent. On occasion, because of their location or the presence of metastases, total resection is not possible. When hepatic metastases are present, if they cannot be completely resected, debulking of the lesions may provide symptomatic relief. Embolization of the hepatic artery may be quite effective in controlling the carcinoid syndrome.

Chemotherapy with streptozotocin alone or in combination with 5-fluorouracil is effective and produces long-term remissions. Other drugs used include carmustine, decarbazine, mitomycin C, cyclophosphamide, and doxorubicin. The treatment of Zollinger-Ellison syndrome has been made easier with the use of H_2-receptor antagonists. Symptomatic relief of the symptoms in the carcinoid syndrome can be accomplished by using different drugs. Flushing may be relieved by phenothiazines, pentholamine, or methyldopa. Diarrhea may be treated with opiates and histamine antagonists, like cyproheptadine.

Somatostatin analogues, because of their ability to inhibit the secretion of various pituitary and gastropancreatic regulatory peptides, provide significant symptomatic relief.

TUMORS OF THE HEPATOBILIARY SYSTEM

Neoplasias of the hepatobiliary system represent about 4 percent of the malignant tumors of the gastrointestinal tract. It is estimated that 9,400 new patients will be diagnosed this year and that over 7,000 of them will die from the disease. The high mortality rate and the difficulties in early diagnosis and treatment present a continuous challenge to the oncologists. It is common to group carcinomas of the gallbladder with those of the bile ducts and of the ampulla of Vater, although there are clinical and pathologic differences between those neoplasms. However, because the treatment approaches to these entities, outside of surgery, are similarly limited, we discuss them jointly.

Epidemiology

Carcinomas of the hepatobiliary system are more common in the elderly, being more frequent in the sixth and seventh decades. Gallbladder carcinoma is more common in women (70 percent), whereas cholangiocarcinoma appears more frequently in men (65 percent). Etiologic factors implicated in both tumors include genetic factors, cholelithiasis, inflammatory bowel disease, chemical carcinogens, and typhoid carrier stage. For cholangiocarcinomas, pre-existing conditions like liver fluke infestation, chronic cholangitis, choledochal cysts, Gardner's syndrome, and congenital hepatic fibrosis have been implicated in the cause of these tumors. The most common histology is adenocarcinoma. In the gallbladder, three main subgroups are described: scirrhous (72 percent), papillary (25 percent), and colloid (7 percent). The papillary tumors seem to be less invasive and to have a better prognosis. Carcinomas of the gallbladder and of the biliary tree spread through the lymphatics, the blood stream, intraductally, or intraperitoneally.

Diagnosis and Clinical Manifestations

In the early stages of the disease, the patients are mostly asymptomatic. In gallbladder cancer, the majority of the patients complain of right upper quadrant abdominal pain that often radiates to the back and worsens at night. Weight loss, anorexia, nausea, and jaundice may be present; chills and fever are less common. However, these symptoms are similar to those of benign conditions, and only a change in the pain pattern, from a more sporadic to a steady pain, makes us think of a malignant process. A right upper quadrant mass may be palpable in 50 percent to 70 percent of the cases. Hepatomegaly, jaundice, and ascites usually herald advanced disease. The most common laboratory finding is an elevation of the serum alkaline phosphatase. Radiographic studies like oral cholecystogram are not that helpful, for the nonvisualization does not differentiate between benign disease and malignancy. Ultrasonography may be more useful for visualizing the gallbladder, biliary tree, and surrounding structures and may aid in differentiating obstructive and nonobstructive jaundice. The presence of dilated biliary ducts indicates the need to perform a percutaneous transhepatic cholangiogram, and the study could make the diagnosis of a cholangiocarcinoma. The procedure is useful because, in addition to providing decompression, it allows some brushing on cytologic studies, which could help in the diagnosis of malignancy. Endoscopic retrograde cholangiopancreatography is a useful study, but it does not permit the visualization of the proximal biliary tree.

Treatment

The curative treatment of biliary tract tumors as well as those of the gallbladder rests in the hands of the surgeon. Early diagnosis of gallbladder cancer is an incidental finding at the time of a cholecystectomy for a nonmalignant condition. Not uncommonly, there is direct invasion of the liver by the tumor. A wide resection completely eradicates the tumor.

In carcinomas of the biliary tree, because they frequently produce obstructive jaundice, the diagnosis is made at the time of a decompressing procedure. Unfortunately, quite often the tumors crawl into the hepatic parenchyma, and resection is not possible because the tumor involves an extensive amount of hepatic tissue. The tumors with the best chances of a cure are those of the common duct; these tumors require pancreatoduodenectomy.

Radiation therapy is employed, using either radioactive implants or external-beam radiation. However, the amount of external radiation required to eradicate the tumor is limited by the tolerance of the surrounding organs: liver, duodenum, stomach, and kidney. A report on the use of charged-particle radiation (with helium or neon) showed a 5-year disease-free survival rate of 21 percent. Chemotherapy is used, with a limited amount of success. 5-fluorouracil, 5-fluoxyuridine, BCNU, doxorubicin, and mitomycin C occasionally produce responses, but they are short-lived. FAM therapy has produced responses as high as 31 percent, but the survival advantage is negligible. Combining radiation and chemotherapy, either intra-arterially or systemically, has produced some long-term responders, but the numbers are small.

---

*In patients over 60 years of age, the VP-16 dose was reduced to 100 mg per square meter.

GASTRIC, BILIARY, AND PANCREATIC CANCER: SURGERY AND RADIATION THERAPY

HOLLIS W. MERRICK III, M.D., M.S., F.A.C.S.
RALPH R. DOBELBOWER, M.D., Ph.D., F.A.C.R.

Cancers of the stomach, biliary tree, and pancreas have more in common than anatomic proximity. Adenocarcinomas strongly predominate at each site; the etiology is generally unknown; spread to the liver and peritoneum is extraordinarily common; and although diagnostic evaluation has been revolutionized by the introduction of new technologies in recent decades (flexible endoscopes, computed tomography [CT], magnetic resonance imaging [MRI], and so forth), this has failed to translate into improved survival in most instances. Also, at each site, surgery is the primary treatment modality, and the role of adjuvant therapy is, at present, inadequately defined. Except for early gastric lesions, the ultimate prognosis is almost always death from cancer.

GASTRIC CANCER

Surgery

Surgical resection is the mainstay of therapy for most patients with gastric cancer. The surgical procedure must be tailored to the location and extent of the disease as well as the age and general condition of the host.

Adenocarcinomas extending to the esophagus are best treated by a Lewis (combined abdominal–right thoracic) approach, which permits a thorough mediastinal lymphadenectomy (this is not the case for a left-sided approach) and resection of the esophagus as high as the root of the neck, if necessary, to obtain adequate margins. Lesions of the proximal stomach may be approached by splitting the sternum up to the third intercostal space. This can provide exposure of the esophagus nearly to the level of the inferior pulmonary ligament and is more easily tolerated than a thoracotomy.

Lesions of the distal stomach can be addressed by high distal subtotal gastrectomy, which involves resecting all the stomach except the cardiac region and a portion of the fundus along with the lymphatics of the hepatoduodenal ligament, both omenta, and the first portion of the duodenum. The spleen need not be removed unless the cancer involves the greater curvature or the posterior wall of the body of the stomach; splenectomy may actually have a detrimental effect on survival.

Total gastrectomy customarily involves resection of the entire stomach, the abdominal portion of the esophagus, the first portion of the duodenum, the spleen, both omenta, and the nodes along the left gastric and hepatic arteries. An extended radical total gastrectomy also includes complete resection of the celiac nodes and the body and tail of the pancreas.

The location and extent of disease dictate not only the surgical approach but also, in large measure, the outcome. Cancers of the proximal portion of the stomach carry a much worse prognosis than those of the distal portion of the organ, thus, the outlook after proximal or total gastrectomy is generally bleaker than after distal gastrectomy. The type of resection is at least as important prognostically as the involvement of regional lymph nodes. The prognosis for an exophytic lesion on the greater curvature is much better than that for an ulcerative lesion on the lesser curvature.

Between 40 percent and 70 percent of gastric cancers are resectable. The overall 5-year survival rate is 30 percent to 35 percent following distal gastrectomy and about 20 percent following gastrectomy or proximal gastric resection. For disease limited to the mucosa and submucosa, the 5-year survival rate ranges from 65 percent to 100 percent. Extension to the muscularis drops this figure to 25 percent to 65 percent, and full penetration of the wall decreases it to 12 percent to 25 percent, much the same as lymph node involvement, which confers a prognosis of 2 percent to 24 percent 5-year survival.

Gastric resection may be associated with substantial mortality and morbidity. In addition to hemorrhagic, septic, and pulmonary complications, there is the risk of anastomotic leak, with resultant mediastinitis, peritonitis, shock, and fistula. Long-term effects, including vitamin B_{12} deficiency and dumping syndrome, are seen in most surviving patients.

Radiation Therapy

Radiation therapy for gastric cancer presents a unique set of problems for the radiation oncologist. The adenocarcinoma is only a moderately radioresponsive neoplasm, but the gastric mucosa is very radioresponsive, and the stomach is situated among other critical radioresponsive organs. Furthermore, the organ not only changes in size and shape from minute to minute but may actually lie in different locations within the abdomen from day to day, depending on content and position of the patient.

When irradiating the stomach or the gastric bed, it is important to note that other critical organs may be included in the field of irradiation. It is necessary to establish the anatomic location and functional integrity of the kidney(s) prior to commencing radiation therapy. In patients with normal renal function, up to 50 percent of the total renal parenchyma may be included in the high-dose volume. The spinal cord dose must be kept below 45 Gy in 4½ weeks. The volume of the heart to be irradiated should be minimized, especially when chemotherapy with doxorubicin will be given. It is often necessary to irradiate large portions of the liver, but this usually presents no serious clinical problems if the volume irradiated is less than 70 percent of the total volume of the organ. Significant amounts of costal and vertebral bone marrow may be within the radiation fields. Hematopoietic function will not recover in bones irradiated to doses above 40 Gy, and will be delayed for prolonged periods after doses as low as 20 Gy. It is usually possible to avoid irradiation of large volumes of lung and colon by tailored radiation fields. The same is true to some extent for the pancreas, an organ that can generally tolerate doses above those required for gastric irradiation. Irradiation of the spleen is usually accomplished without clinically significant sequelae.

The importance of field shaping and beam arrangement cannot be overemphasized. One must adhere to the two basic rules of modern radiation therapy: (1) Put the dose on the disease; and (2) spare the normal tissues. Custom field design must incorporate information gained from surgical procedures (preferably with the radiotherapist at the operating table for placement of radiopaque markers), appropriate laboratory studies, imaging studies (radiographs of the upper gastrointestinal tract, intravenous pyelogram, CT, MRI, echography, simulation) and a sound working knowledge of the natural history of the disease and its patterns of recurrence.

Cure of gastric cancer is only rarely accomplished if the gross tumor cannot be removed surgically. Local lymph nodes are involved in as many as 83 percent of patients, and local recurrence occurs in as many as 93 percent. A complete node dissection for gastric cancer is difficult, if not completely impossible, and there is some evidence to suggest that more radical surgery with extended node dissection, splenectomy, and omentectomy does not prevent local recurrence. After "curative" surgery, locoregional recurrence is the most common form of treatment failure. Distant metastases alone are relatively uncommon. Nearly half of peritoneal failures are localized, at least initially, and peritoneal seeding is the most common form of detectable initial tumor dissemination. Intra-abdominal dissemination of disease generally does not occur without recurrence in the upper abdomen. Although microscopic residual disease at the line of resection (usually seen in the submucosal lymphatics) does not guarantee anastomotic recurrence, it does develop more often than not. Therefore, patients with microscopically positive resection margins may particularly benefit from additional local therapy, because this finding most often indicates early recurrence and subsequent death from cancer. Local recurrence of gastric cancer is generally a harbinger of death from disease within 1 year. This points out the importance of local and regional therapy (definitive and adjuvant) in this disease.

Adjuvant Therapy

External-beam radiation therapy is not well tolerated after gastrectomy. This is accentuated by adjuvant

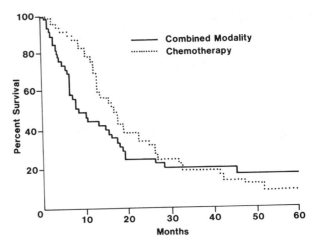

Figure 1 Patient survival, FAMe chemotherapy *vs.* FAMe plus radiation therapy (see text).

chemotherapy. A prospective, randomized study by the Gastrointestinal Tumor Study Group (GITSG) of combination chemotherapy versus radiotherapy plus chemotherapy was closed prematurely when the median survival time was observed to be 35 weeks for the combined modality group compared to 70 weeks for the chemotherapy group. At 3 years, the survival curves crossed, however, and at 5 years, the combined modality group displayed a significantly superior survival rate (18 percent versus 7 percent, Fig. 1). At 10 years, 13 percent of the patients in the combined modality group survived, but all the chemotherapy patients were dead. This underscores not only the potential value of aggressive combined modality therapy for gastric cancer patients with poor prognostic findings but also the toxicity of such therapy and the necessity to provide adequate and often intensive nutritional and general support to patients so treated.

Intraoperative Irradiation

Electron-beam radiation therapy delivered intraoperatively at the time of gastrectomy is not so toxic and appears to be of value. The Japanese have acquired considerable experience with this modality. At Kyoto University Hospital, patients with resected distal tumors without peritoneal or hematogenous dissemination were assigned to treatment by gastrectomy alone (110 patients) or resection plus intraoperative electron-beam therapy (84 patients) on the basis of day of hospital admission. Although this method of "randomization" is open to criticism, the improvement in survival in (Japanese) stages II, III, and IV is impressive (Table 1). The results in stage IV are particularly impressive, as all patients treated with surgery alone died within 2 years, whereas approximately 15 percent of patients treated with adjuvant intraoperative radiotherapy survived 5 years, including 3 of 19 patients with incompletely resected lesions. At our institution, we have adopted this type of approach to the adjuvant therapy of resectable gastric cancer.

Table 1 Intraoperative Electron-Beam Therapy for Resectable Gastric Cancer

	5-Year Survival Rate (%)	
Stage	Gastrectomy	Gastrectomy + IOEBT
I	93	87
II	62	84
III	37	62
IV	0	15

Abe, Kyoto University, Japan.

Palliative Irradiation

The median survival time for patients with untreated, unresectable gastric cancer is approximately 5 months. The operative mortality rate for palliative gastrectomy in such patients is much higher than that for patients with resectable cancers (22 percent and 6 percent, respectively). Moderate-dose external-beam radiation therapy (20 to 40 Gy) effects limited palliation for such patients, but it does not improve survival time. Radiation gastritis is often observed with higher doses. Obstructive symptoms rarely respond to irradiation alone; however, "palliative" irradiation does occasionally result in long-term survival and apparent cure. High-dose external-beam therapy and intraoperative electron-beam therapy have produced a small number of 5-year survivors in selected series.

Gastric Lymphoma

The traditional treatment for gastric lymphoma has been surgical resection, with 5-year survival rates of 25 to 60 percent, but radiation therapy is equally effective in controlling local disease in stage I lesions. For stage II disease, resection combined with radiation therapy seems more effective than either modality alone. The role of radiation therapy is becoming more important, particularly as an adjuvant to resection and as definitive therapy for patients with advanced local disease or disease involving locoregional lymph nodes. Radiation therapy also is an important palliative modality.

With resection alone, the recurrence rate is approximately 50 percent for patients with negative lymph nodes and 75 percent for patients with regional node involvement. Other factors associated with poor prognosis are large primary lesions, deep penetration of the gastric wall, diffuse lesions, multiple lesions, and involvement of adjacent organs. All such patients deserve full benefit of adjuvant or definitive regional radiotherapy. We commonly employ large anterior and posterior upper abdominal fields extending from the diaphragm to the top of the iliac crests to deliver a dose of 25 Gy in 3½ weeks followed by local boost to doses of 40 to 50 Gy, depending on the extent of the disease. Because more than 30 percent of patients, even those with localized gastric lymphoma, subsequently develop distant metastases, adjuvant chemotherapy is probably indicated, but the selection criteria are not clear.

BILIARY CANCER

Surgery

Surgical resection is the treatment of choice for cancer of the biliary tree. The location of the tumor dictates the natural history of the disease and, to some extent, the surgical procedure.

Gallbladder

Lesions of the gallbladder are best treated by radical cholecystectomy, if feasible. Unfortunately, 70 to 80 percent of patients with this disease come to surgical intervention after metastases or local spread of cancer precludes definitive resection. Essentially, the only patients with a good chance of survival are those in whom cholecystectomy is performed because of symptoms of cholecystitis, with the diagnosis having been established only by histopathologic examination of the specimen. In this circumstance, the operative mortality rate is less than 5 percent, whereas it can be as high as 35 percent for aggressive resections of locally advanced disease necessitating partial hepatic resection. Even in patients in whom cancer is not grossly evident, if the microscopic disease penetrates the full thickness of the gallbladder wall (as it does in two-thirds of such patients), all patients will be dead from cancer within 2½ years. If the cancer infiltrates no deeper than the mucosa orsubmucosa, a 5-year survival rate of approximately 65 percent is observed, but such lesions are rare.

Distal Bile Duct

Cancers of the distal portion of the biliary tree are often very difficult to distinguish from carcinoma of the head of the pancreas and are treated in similar fashion with pancreaticoduodenectomy (vide infra) or modifications thereof. The natural history of the disease, the treatment, and the expected outcome are very similar to that of cancer of the head of the pancreas.

Proximal Biliary Tree

Cancers of the proximal biliary tree are usually unresectable because of extension of disease into liver or other adjacent structures. Extended resections involving partial hepatectomy are morbid procedures with operative mortality rates that approach 35 percent. Surgical reconstitution of biliary drainage into the intestinal tract is often a challenge to the skill of the surgeon, if not a factor that limits or precludes complete tumor resection. Bringing jejunum into the hepatic hilus limits the dose of radiation that may be given safely postoperatively.

In spite of all these problems, surgical resection offers the only reasonable hope for cure for tumors of the biliary tree, regardless of location.

Palliative Surgery

The primary symptom of biliary cancer, jaundice—as well as pain, to some extent—may be relieved by a variety of surgical procedures ranging from palliative resection with choledochojejunostomy to simple stent placement. Although the former is generally associated with greater longevity, it also carries the highest morbidity and mortality rates. Biliary stents may be placed at laparotomy, percutaneously or endoscopically. Endoscopic stent placement is more successful and less morbid for lesions of the distal biliary tree, whereas the percutaneous transhepatic approach is more applicable for lesions at or above the hilus. Catheter obstruction with recurring cholangitis and resultant sepsis are common sequelae that may be reduced somewhat by prophylactic catheter replacement every 2 to 4 months. Newer expandable metal stents may obviate this.

Radiation Therapy

In general, the results of surgery for biliary cancer are dismal. An extensive review of 115 reports of surgical series documented only 62 patients who survived for 5 years. Until recent decades, the role of radiation therapy was extremely limited; with the development of new technology, this has begun to change. Clinical experience with the newer modalities is still quite limited, principally because of the relative rarity and adverse natural history of biliary cancer, so it is not known what impact these will have on clinical results.

External-Beam Radiotherapy

With the development of modern megavoltage radiation therapy equipment and the proliferation of radiation therapy simulators and sophisticated computerized treatment planning systems, the radiation oncologist is now able to tailor the radiation dose distribution to the tumor volume as determined by newer imaging modalities such as CT, ultrasound, or MRI. This permits delivery of higher tumor doses with fewer radiation effects in surrounding normal tissues. In spite of these improvements in tumor imaging and dose delivery, which now permit local tumor doses well in excess of 60 Gy, reports of long-term survivors of biliary cancer are still anecdotal, albeit more frequent than in prior decades. Perhaps this reflects the dismal natural history of the disease or, hopefully, simple lack of sufficient clinical experience because of the relative rarity of the disease.

In view of a local recurrence rate that approaches 85 percent, local adjuvant external-beam radiation therapy seems indicated after resection of nearly any biliary cancer. The target volume should be generous, and the dose should be a function of the amount and extent of residual disease as well as the surgical procedure. The external-beam dose to small bowel or anastomoses should not exceed 45 Gy in 4½ to 5 weeks, whereas areas of known residual disease should receive at least 65 Gy. At times, these criteria are incompatible. The radiation field should include, in addition to known tumor and a 2- to 3-cm margin, the hepatic hilus and the celiac node-bearing region. Multiple fields, shrinking fields, and custom blocks are often helpful, as are wedge and rotational treatment plans. Assessment of renal function and location is mandatory at this anatomic site.

External-beam radiation therapy is effective in reducing the pain associated with biliary cancer in as many as 90 percent of patients treated; however, jaundice, the most common symptom, is rarely relieved by radiation therapy alone and should be addressed primarily by other means.

Intraoperative Radiotherapy

At our institution, we are exploring the use of intraoperative electron-beam therapy in the treatment of resectable and unresectable biliary cancer. In both situations, the intraoperative irradiation technique is employed to deliver a single boost dose of 15 to 25 Gy in addition to an external-beam dose of 50 Gy. The total number of reported cases treated by this modality worldwide appears to be fewer than 100 at the time of this writing, with most of the work having been done in Japan. Because of the relative rarity of the disease and the limited availability of intraoperative radiation therapy facilities, several years will be required to evaluate the efficacy of such treatment.

Intraluminal Brachytherapy

If the region of the biliary obstruction can be cannulated by a tube of appropriate internal diameter, the stent may be used as a channel for intraluminal placement of linear sources of radioactivity when the tube provides access to the lumen of the biliary tree without sharp bends. A T-tube is generally not satisfactory for this purpose because of the right-angle bends. The isotope most commonly employed is iridium-192 in the form of wire or seeds. The dose is usually specified at a distance of 0.5 cm from the source(s) and may be given in two or more treatment sessions or in a single application. We use a dose of 30 Gy in a single session, with half-strength sources (0.5 mCi per seed) spaced closely (two seeds per centimeter) as a boost after 50-Gy external-beam therapy, but doses of 10 Gy to 60 Gy have been reported.

The prime advantage of this technique lies in its ability to deliver with accuracy relatively high doses of radiation directly to the site of tumor impingement upon the biliary tract without excessive irradiation of surrounding structures. This is particularly attractive when the radioisotope can be delivered by the nasobiliary route via a catheter placed endoscopically, thus obviating the need for abdominal surgery. When the nasobiliary route is used, the extent of the disease may not be as fully appreciated as at laparotomy. The major disadvantage is the rapid fall-off of dose with distance from the radioactive source(s). Experience with this modality of treatment is still relatively limited, but it appears to be well tolerated.

A major cause of patient attrition after radiation therapy for biliary cancer is sepsis secondary to recurrent cholangitis. This complication should be treated aggressively with antibiotics, change of stent, and general supportive measures, as some patients have expired as a result with no apparent tumor at postmortem examination.

It is still too early to judge the impact on patient survival of the new diagnostic and therapeutic technologies now available.

PANCREATIC CANCER

Surgery

For patients with resectable adenocarcinoma of the pancreas, the treatment of choice is radical surgical excision. The operation should be preceded by upper abdominal CT scan, to search for hepatic metastases and to delineate the primary lesion, and duodenoscopy, to identify and biopsy ampullary and duodenal cancers. Either ERCP or percutaneous transhepatic cholangiopancreatography (PTC) may permit preoperative biliary decompression. Widespread or distant intra-abdominal disease is a contraindication to pancreatic resection.

Exploratory Technique

After the peritoneal cavity is entered, the peritoneum and liver are carefully palpated and inspected. Dimpling or retraction at the base of the mesocolon may represent local extension of cancer. Dilated venous structures may imply obstruction by tumor. Entering the lesser sac permits inspection of the pancreas, whereas a complete Kocher maneuver permits assessment of the distal common duct, the superior mesenteric artery, and the posterior aspect of the pancreatic head. These maneuvers permit detection of most contraindications to resection. Careful examination of the branches of the celiac axis, superior mesenteric vessels, portal vein, and porta hepatis often identifies suspicious lymph nodes that should be biopsied and sent for frozen-section analysis.

If no tumor is encountered to this point, the common bile duct, hepatic artery, and portal vein are dissected and isolated with vascular tapes. The superior mesenteric vessels are identified and the overlying peritoneum is incised over the caudal margin of the pancreas. The anterior aspect of the mesenteric vein is usually free of tributaries, so the surgeon can develop a plane between this structure and the overlying portion of the pancreas and tunnel underneath the gland if invasion of the vein has not occurred. A Penrose drain may be used to elevate the tumor and the gland and to facilitate further retroperitoneal dissection. If no distant metastasis or vascular involvement is found, the lesion may be considered resectable. To this point, the procedure may be terminated without resection, but further steps are generally irreversible.

Resectable Disease

The traditional definitive surgical approach is pancreaticoduodenectomy (Whipple resection) or total pancreatectomy. Debate continues about which is the better procedure. A pylorus-preserving pancreatectomy has been described for use in selected cases. Any resection of the pancreas often lies at the limits of the surgeon's skill (and the patient's endurance); consequently, the procedure should only be undertaken by those who frequently perform this type of surgery. Patients with suspected resectable pancreatic cancer diagnosed by most general surgeons in community hospitals should be decompressed by tube cholecystostomy and transferred to major centers for definitive management. Palliative biliary and gastrointestinal bypass procedures may be indicated at the first operation, but they should be done with cognizance of subsequent surgical procedures so that definitive treatment is not compromised. In general, the patient is better off if he or she is subjected only to a one-stage definitive resection.

Following resection of the cancer, placement of radiopaque clips outlining the tumor bed will greatly facilitate delivery of postoperative radiation therapy. Intraoperative consultation with the radiation oncologist is also of value, allowing him to better appreciate the original location of the tumor and to visualize the anatomic locations of critical anastomoses and of loops of bowel used to construct biliary and gastrointestinal diversions. Intravenous hyperalimentation, adequate ventilatory support, and good intensive nursing care after operation are essential elements of pancreatic surgery.

Unresectable Disease

About 80 percent of patients with pancreatic cancer present with unresectable disease. Approximately half of these have no evidence of metastatic disease, but the tumor is unresectable by virtue of local extension into adjacent structures (portal vein, superior mesenteric vessels, stomach, colon, mesentery, and so forth). Extensive surgical procedures in such patients may do more harm than good, but many patients can be treated with combined radiotherapy and chemotherapy. A few such patients may actually be salvaged. In light of this, it is important to establish the diagnosis histologically at the first laparotomy and to outline the tumor with radiopaque clips to facilitate subsequent radiotherapy. Again, intraoperative consultation with the radiation oncologist is often helpful.

Many surgeons are reluctant to biopsy the pancreas because of the risk of serious complication (fistula). This notion was conceived in the preantibiotic era, but it still persists. Recent experience indicates that with current surgical techniques and appropriate postoperative care, pancreatic biopsy is safe and accurate. Tumors that obstruct the pancreatic duct can produce dilatation of the distal duct system via increased intraluminal pressure. For this reason, pancreatic biopsy should be limited to the tumor itself or performed from the duodenal side of the tumor. Percutaneous or intraoperative needle biopsies are safer (albeit less reliable) than open biopsy. Transduodenal needle biopsy can conceivably avoid the possibility of pancreaticoperitoneal fistula. Associated pancreatitis is often difficult to distinguish from tumor; however, careful palpation can make this determination easier, as can the "feel" of the tissues during needle biopsy.

Obstruction of the gastrointestinal tract is best treated by gastrojejunostomy, whereas biliary obstruction can be treated surgically or, in selected cases, by endoluminal stent, as described previously for biliary cancer. Palliative pancreatic resection is not recommended because the morbidity and mortality outweigh any potential benefit in patients destined to die shortly.

The patient who is asymptomatic after histologic proof of pancreatic cancer and appropriate bypass(es) is best treated expectantly. Quality of life is important. Liberal use of analgesic is the best treatment for selected patients with symptomatic refractory disease. Nutritional support and comfort measures may be the clinician's most important tools in such instances. Diabetes and exocrine insufficiency should be treated when present.

Radiation Therapy

Adjuvant Therapy

Radiation therapy may be administered before, during, or after definitive surgical resection for cancer of the pancreas. Preoperative and intraoperative radiation therapy have been inadequately studied in this setting, but postoperative irradiation does appear to confer a survival advantage. Irradiation should not commence until the patient has recovered from surgery and any postoperative complications have been managed adequately. Pancreatic fistula is only a relative contraindication to irradiation. A dose of 50 Gy is usually well tolerated in daily increments of 1.8 to 2.0-Gy, five fractions weekly.

The radiation fields should be tailored to the tumor bed, excluding from the beams any loops of bowel used for bypass, if feasible. Anastomoses should also be excluded from the fields, except for the pancreaticojejunal anastomosis. Any pancreatic remnant should be included.

Adjuvant 5-fluorouracil can be combined with irradiation during the first and fifth weeks of treatment as a 4-day continuous infusion with a dose of 1,000 mg per square meter per day, not exceeding 1,500 mg per day. Treatment should be interrupted or terminated if reaction is severe. Weekly 5-fluorouracil should follow completion of irradiation. The 5-fluorouracil should be delayed 1 week if the white blood cell count is less than 3,000 or the platelet count is less than 75,000. Nutritional support may be necessary during radiation or drug therapy. Patients should be observed at monthly intervals by the radiation and medical oncologists to assess late toxicity of therapy. Resulting gastritis should be treated by the usual medical means.

Unresectable Disease

Control of unresected pancreatic cancer requires high tumor doses (doses in excess of the radiotolerance of surrounding normal organs). Such doses can be achieved with precision high-dose (PHD) external-beam radiation therapy techniques. This implies accurate three-dimensional localization of the tumor and adjacent normal structures. This is best achieved with CT scanning and radiopaque clips placed at laparotomy to outline gross tumor. Precision high-dose techniques imply good patient immobilization, accurate reproduction of daily treatment set-up, careful simulation with attention to detail, the use of line lasers for daily patient set-up, and transposition from simulator to treatment machine with especially high technologic standards. Beams are angled, blocked, and often extensively custom-shaped to conform the three-dimensional dose profile to that of the tumor and to avoid irradiation of adjacent critical structures as much as possible.

Irradiation should not begin until the patient is well recovered from surgery. Radiation fields should measure no more than 17 cm. Doses of 67 Gy are well tolerated in 1.8-Gy increments if the target volume is closely tailored to the tumor mass. Only high-energy (>4 mV) beams should be used for PHD therapy.

At simulation, the respiratory excursion of the (clipped) mass should be noted and the cephalic and caudal field borders adjusted accordingly. If the excursion is minimal, a margin of 2 cm should suffice. The lateral field margins should be more generous, especially in the regions of the bile duct and the tail of the pancreas, as occult spread of cancer occurs in these directions. A 1.5-cm anterior margin should suffice, as this is the margin of the tumor that is usually most reliably known from surgical exploration, and it is usually covered by peritoneum. The posterior margin is often the most difficult to establish, but in no case should it be less than 1 cm. It is important to include no more than 50 percent of the functional renal parenchyma in the high-dose region. The dose to the remaining renal tissue should be kept below 25 Gy, and the dose to the spinal cord below 45 Gy. After 45 to 55 Gy, the fields may be reduced and reshaped to irradiate only the tumor with "tight" margins.

Adjuvant 5-fluorouracil may be administered concurrently with PHD therapy as a continuous 4-day infusion as described previously or as a daily bolus of 500 mg per square meter for 3 days at the beginning and the end of the course of radiation therapy. Subsequent weekly maintenance therapy is also 5-fluorouracil, 500 mg per square meter. Drug delivery should be delayed 1 week if the white blood cell count is less than 3,000 or if the platelet count is less than 75,000.

If PHD techniques are used meticulously for irradiating pancreatic cancers, fewer and relatively mild complications can be expected. Acute reactions generally consist of mild nausea and vomiting and can be treated with antiemetics or interruption of therapy. Anorexia is more difficult to manage. Delayed reactions (gastritis, gastric bleeding) may be seen in as many as 20 percent of patients 6 to 12 months after treatment. These should be treated medically if possible, but without undue pessimism, as a number of patients with pancreatic cancer who were treated with radiation therapy with curative intent have expired of neglected complications (hemorrhage) or unrelated problems and, at autopsy, have been found free of malignancy.

With aggressive PHD radiation therapy and adjuvant 5-fluorouracil, a median survival time of approximately 1 year may be expected. The occasional patient (5 percent) will survive 5 years. Local tumor control rates in excess of 80 percent can be achieved by the addition of interstitial brachytherapy to the regimen described previously, but this is not recommended. The procedure carries a very high morbidity rate and an operative mortality rate as high as 32 percent, but it adds little, if anything, to patient comfort and survival time. Like pancreatic resection, pancreatic interstitial brachytherapy should only be attempted by skilled, experienced operators who perform the procedure frequently. Intraoperative radiotherapy and treatment with high linear energy transfer beams are currently being evaluated for unresectable pancreatic cancer at specially equipped centers, but no dramatic improvements in clinical results have been seen to date.

Occasionally, the oncologist is presented with a patient with a clinical or surgical diagnosis of unresectable pancreatic cancer. Such patients should not be treated with PHD irradiation or chemotherapy in the absence of histologic confirmation of malignancy (or the appearance of metastases) because myriad diseases, notably pancreatitis, can mimic pancreatic cancer. The risks of chemotherapy and/or high-dose irradiation are not warranted in such situations. Lower doses of radiation may preclude subsequent definitive therapy. In such instances, attempts should be made at histologic confirmation of cancer.

SUGGESTED READING

Dobelbower RR Jr. Gastrointestinal cancer — radiation therapy. Heidelberg, Germany: Springer-Verlag, 1989.

Douglass HO Jr. Gastric cancer. New York: Churchill Livingstone, 1988.

Howard JM, Jordan GJ, Reber HA: Surgical diseases of the pancreas. Philadelphia: Lea & Febiger, 1987.

COLORECTAL CANCER: SURGERY

HERBERT C. HOOVER, Jr., M.D.

Colorectal carcinoma remains second to lung carcinoma as the most common malignancy affecting both men and women in the United States. There are approximately 151,000 new cases and nearly 62,000 deaths each year. As with most human tumors, the cause of colon or rectal cancers remains unknown. Dietary factors, especially the ingestion of saturated fats and a low-fiber diet, tend to be associated with an increased rate of malignant transformation. Addition of fiber to the diet may be a protective factor by increasing the transit time and decreasing the exposure time of the large bowel epithelium to carcinogens.

A number of conditions tend to predispose to malignancies in the large bowel. Among these are chronic ulcerative colitis and familial polyposis. Patients with familial polyposis are felt to have a 100 percent risk of developing carcinoma in the colon or rectum if total colectomy is not performed.

DIAGNOSIS

Screening for colorectal cancer is important because this disease is nearly always curable if detected at an early stage. The commonly utilized screening tests include digital rectal exam, stool test for occult blood, barium enema, rigid or flexible sigmoidoscopy, colonoscopy, and carcinoembryonic antigen (CEA) blood test. Unfortunately, cancers do not always bleed continuously, so occult blood tests are not totally effective in detecting even large cancers. Full colonoscopy is the best screening test, as early lesions are more likely to be detected by direct visualization and biopsy. Shinya and others have shown convincingly that colons kept free of polyps are also kept free of cancer, lending good support to the polyp-to-cancer transition theory. All patients with unexplained large bowel symptoms, guaiac-positive stools, or gross rectal bleeding should be evaluated with a full colonoscopic exam. If symptoms of colonic disease persist after a negative colonoscopy, a barium enema should be performed. Being a large and redundant organ, both radiologic and endoscopic diagnostic procedures can miss significant lesions. Therefore, the two are complementary rather than competitive in their diagnostic potential.

Unfortunately, most patients diagnosed with large bowel cancer present with symptoms representing bowel dysfunction that occurs relatively late in the natural history of this disease. Table 1 shows the symptoms frequently present with rectal, left colon, and right colon cancer. Blood streaking on the stool is the most frequent complaint of patients with rectal cancer, whereas colon cancer patients more frequently complain of pain. Pain in left colon cancer is often colicky, whereas the pain in right colon cancer is usually ill-defined. The differences occur because of the disparities in the caliber of the colon lumen and differences in the character of the stool (solid versus liquid).

Patients found to have colon and rectal cancers

Table 1 Comparison of the Five Most Frequent Symptoms in Rectal, Left Colon, and Right Colon Cancer

Rectum and Rectosigmoid (258 patients)	Left Colon (99 patients)	Right Colon (984 patients)
Melena (85%)	Abdominal pain (72%)	Abdominal pain (74%)
Constipation (46%)	Melena (53%)	Weakness (29%)
Tenesmus (30%)	Constipation (42%)	Melena (27%)
Diarrhea (30%)	Nausea (25%)	Nausea (24%)
Abdominal pain (26%)	Vomiting (23%)	Abdominal mass (23%)

From Postlethwait RW. Malignant tumors of the colon and rectum. Ann Surg 1949; 129: 34–36; with permission.

should have other diagnostic tests prior to operation. Urinalysis can indicate colovesicle fistulas. It is important to obtain a CEA level both preoperatively and at approximately 1 month postoperatively. If an elevated preoperative level fails to return to normal, persistent disease is indicated. CEA levels that are elevated well above normal can make one suspicious of liver metastases. A chest radiograph should always be performed to look for lung metastases. Although not uniformly done preoperatively, computed tomography (CT) scans of the abdomen provide very useful information. As many as 30 percent of patients may have occult hepatic metastases that are not palpable at laparotomy and are shown only by CT scanning. Magnetic resonance imaging (MRI) scanning is proving to be even more effective in detecting small metastases in the liver, but it is not equal to CT scanning in detecting extra hepatic metastases. A CT scan also gives useful information relative to retroperitoneal lymph node enlargement, shows the position of both ureters, and indicates any possibility of obstruction as well as the functional status of both kidneys. Also, it can diagnose extramural spread of rectal cancer and may indicate involvement of adjacent organs, especially the urinary bladder. If a CT scan has not been obtained, an intravenous pyelogram (IVP) can give useful information, especially in patients with large right colon cancers or advanced rectosigmoid lesions, in which ureteral or bladder involvement is not uncommon.

Bone scans or lung CT scans do not give sufficient clinical information in asymptomatic patients to warrant their expense.

THERAPY: GENERAL CONSIDERATIONS

Because surgical resection is the only effective treatment for most carcinomas of the colon and for all but early rectal carcinomas, the surgeon's goal in treating localized colon or rectal tumors must be to control the primary tumor and do everything possible to prevent recurrence. Approximately 70 percent of patients present with "totally resectable" primary tumors, but nearly one-half of these patients will eventually die of recurrent or metastatic disease. Obviously, microscopic deposits are left behind or are potentially spread at the

time of the operation. From 30 percent to 50 percent of recurrences are local or regional, and, therefore, potentially avoidable or treatable. A number of predictors of an increased failure rate in colorectal cancer are beyond a surgeon's control. Clinical factors include symptomatic lesions, youth, elevated CEA level, obstruction, perforation, adjacent organ involvement, ulcerated primary tumor, location in rectum, fixed tumor in rectum, and circumferential bowel involvement. Pathologic predictors of failure include poorly differentiated histology; deep penetration of the bowel wall; infiltrating deep margins; mucinous, signet ring, or scirrhous adenocarcinomas; lymphatic and lymph node involvement; and venous perineural invasion. Although all of the preceding factors are beyond the surgeon's control, there is some evidence that surgeons can alter the recurrence and metastatic rate. Modes of spread, whether by direct continuity to surrounding organs, through the peritoneal cavity, through the lymphatic or hematogenous channels, or by direct implantation, are theoretically influenced by surgical techniques. Commonly accepted techniques that can possibly lower the iatrogenic spread of colorectal cancers are minimal manipulation of tumor, wide resection of bowel and mesentery, and en bloc resection of adjacent organs. Techniques of possible importance include isolation of the involved bowel segment with tapes, early high ligation of colonic vessels, mechanical measures such as covering the tumor with gauze or irrigating the bowel lumen with cytotoxic agents, and pelvic lymphadenectomy for advanced rectal cancer. The issue of high or low ligation of the inferior mesenteric artery for patients with rectal or sigmoid carcinoma remains controversial, but most recent reports suggest no significant difference in the recurrence rate or survival between patients having ligation of the inferior mesenteric artery flush with the aorta versus having the ligation and resection go up just to the left colic branch. Certainly, the more extended operations lead to increased morbidity and cannot be recommended until studies show a more clear survival benefit. I isolate the involved bowel and perform an early ligation of colonic vessels whenever possible, but I do not perform colonic irrigations or radical pelvic lymphadenectomy on a routine basis.

Surgical treatment is designed to remove the primary tumor with generous lateral margins as well as all regional lymph nodes and lymphatic channels that can be safely extirpated. Because of the segmental nature of spread from colorectal cancers, the margin of normal bowel distal to the tumor need not be extensive. This is especially true in rectal cancer. Several recent studies show that even 2 cm is sufficient for rectal cancers, but 3 to 5 cm should be obtained whenever possible. Longitudinal spread, more than 1 cm beyond the tumor mass, occurs only in patients with retrograde lymphatic obstruction. Prognosis is poor in those patients no matter what procedure is performed. It is important to maximize the lateral margins of resection in potentially curable patients. If a colon or rectal tumor is adherent to other organs, an en bloc resection is critically important. Peeling tumors away from organs leads to a high rate of local recurrence. En bloc resection adds very little morbidity in the usual situation, and leads to salvage rates nearly comparable to those cases without extension to other organs. Rectal tumors most frequently adhere to the vagina, bladder, prostate, and uterus. Total pelvic exenteration may be indicated when the base of the bladder is involved. Sigmoid tumors adhere to ovaries, pelvic sidewalls, and bladder. Cecal tumors tend to adhere to the abdominal wall or to small bowel.

PREPARATION FOR RESECTION

In recent years, we have abandoned the clear-liquid diet and 3-day bowel preparation in deference to 4 L of Golytely on the evening before operation. Oral neomycin and erythromycin base, 1 g each, are given in three doses the afternoon and evening before resection. This provides an excellent bowel preparation without the economic and nutritional consequences of the 3-day bowel preparation. Ancef, 500 mg IM, is given on call to the operating room, with two additional doses being given postoperatively.

Because recent data consistently show an increased rate of infectious complications and a diminished survival rate in patients who are transfused at any time during their management for colorectal cancer, we avoid transfusions in these patients whenever possible. This often means even elderly patients are treated and discharged with hematocrits as low as the mid-20s.

SPECIFIC TREATMENT RECOMMENDATIONS

Anastomoses in any of the resections for lesions above the peritoneal reflexion can be performed with either a one- or two-layer hand-sewn technique or by use of the staplers. Obstructing lesions in the right colon are commonly treated with a one-stage resection, whereas lesions in the distal transverse colon or beyond are more commonly treated with a preliminary diverting colostomy followed in several days by a primary resection. A subtotal colectomy and ileorectal anastomosis is a reasonable additional option in the latter group of patients.

The surgical management of mid-rectal and low-rectal cancers has changed dramatically in the past 10 to 15 years, with a clear trend toward sphincter-saving procedures. Although several small retrospective studies have suggested a higher recurrence rate and a lower survival rate in patients with sphincter-sparing procedures, a large National Surgical Adjuvant Breast Protocol (NSABP) study has recently shown no difference in survival of comparably staged patients treated with abdominoperineal resection or sphincter-sparing procedures, using either a hand-sewn anastomosis or the EEA stapler. With the use of the EEA stapler or a coloanal anastomosis, sphincter-sparing procedures can be performed for selected carcinomas even in the low rectum if at least a 3-cm distal margin can be obtained. However, most patients with tumors palpable within 5 cm of the anal verge are best treated with abdominoperineal resection unless the tumors are small enough for a local resection. Some of these small tumors can also be treated effectively with primary radiation therapy by the Papillion technique. Fulguration is another treatment option, but local excision or radiation would generally be preferred. Several recent studies have shown that local excision of small rectal tumors can yield excellent long-term cure rates. Local excision has the advantage of histopathologic examination of the resected specimen, which is not the case with fulguration or irradiation. If the locally excised tumor proves to be more deeply invasive than suspected, the patient should undergo a more radical resection if medical contraindications do not exist. In all but the most favorable lesions, irradiation should be strongly considered. Special care must be given to avoiding manipulation of tumors being locally resected to minimize the likelihood of iatrogenic spread. Traction sutures placed 1.5 cm outside the tumor's margin at close intervals around the tumor can avoid excess manipulation. The full-thickness rectal resection should be beyond the traction sutures, with a running one-layer closure being done as the resection proceeds. I reserve local resection for low rectal lesions that are less than 3 cm, polypoid, mobile, well-differentiated histologically, and do not penetrate through the full thickness of the rectal wall. Age or general state of health need not influence one's decision when such restrictive criteria are used. Obviously, in patients who are not considered candidates for general anesthesia, more advanced lesions can be managed by local resection and radiation therapy. Recent advances in transrectal ultrasonography allow more accurate preoperative assessment of the depth of penetration of rectal cancers.

Approximately 20 percent of patients with colorectal cancer present with clinically obvious metastatic disease, most commonly to the liver or lungs. Unless the metastatic disease is extensive and the expected survival is short, a palliative resection of the primary tumor is usually indicated to prevent or treat obstruction, bleeding, perforation, and other complications.

MANAGEMENT OF RECURRENT COLORECTAL CANCER

Follow-up Schedule to Detect Recurrent or Metastatic Colorectal Cancer

Some of the more difficult decisions in the management of patients with colorectal cancer concern those with recurrent or metastatic disease. Because several modern series report encouraging results in the management of these patients, detection of such disease becomes increasingly important. Because approximately 80 percent of these recurrences appear within the first 2 years, we recommend follow-up examinations every 3 months for 2 years, every 4 months the third year, and at 6-month intervals until 5 years, at which time a yearly follow-up is adequate. At each follow-up examination, a careful history and physical examination, including a stool guaiac, should be performed. Determinations of CEA levels are also important at each visit. Colonoscopic exams should be repeated at 6 to 12 months, yearly for 2 or 3 years, followed by examinations every 2 to 3 years if no polyps or recurrences are found. A chest radiograph should be obtained at 6-month intervals for the first 2 years and yearly thereafter.

Surgical Options for Recurrence

Recurrence in colorectal cancer is not always the dismal situation that many surgeons envision. Several biologic and anatomic characteristics related to colorectal cancer favor the prospect of surgical control of recurrent disease. For example, recurrent colorectal cancers are usually slow-growing, the lymphatic extension is usually palpable, and the soft tissues surrounding the recurrence can usually be removed.

Factors in recurrent colorectal cancer that tend to be more favorable are anastomotic recurrences; B2 or B3 (through bowel wall or invading an adjacent organ but with negative nodes) original primary tumors; or implantation recurrences in the colostomy site, perineal scar, abdominal wound, or a drain site. Recurrences in the pericolic fat, pelvic recurrences after abdominoperineal resection, or recurrences less than 6 months from the primary resection all tend to be unfavorable for surgical salvage.

Surgeons should adopt an aggressive approach toward patients with recurrent colorectal cancer unless an unfavorable outcome is certain. We should gear our efforts toward a cure by a radical procedure in selected patients or should look to palliate symptoms whenever possible. Re-exploration in patients with a previously resected colon or rectal cancer is indicated in any patient with a rising CEA level and a negative work-up, including a chest radiograph, an abdominal and pelvic CT scan, a bone scan, and a colonoscopy; isolated pulmonary or hepatic metastases or local recurrences; or unresectable patients in whom obstruction or bleeding can be palliated. One can expect approximately 25 percent of recurrent colorectal cancers to be resectable with curative intent. Several studies have documented that resection of recurrent colorectal cancers with negative margins significantly increases the survival in both length of time and quality of life. However, tumor resections with gross disease left behind (debulking procedures) are rarely, if ever, indicated. Anastomotic recurrences account for 25 percent of all recurrences in colorectal cancer. Most of these present with bleeding or pain, and 50 to 60 percent can be totally resected, with the expectation of nearly a 50 percent 5-year survival if all margins are microscopically clear. This is one area in which close follow-up with stool guaiacs can pay big dividends in salvage. There is increasing enthusiasm for the role of total pelvic exenteration for either advanced primary tumors of the rectum with the base of the bladder involved or for patients with recurrent rectal cancer involving the bladder. The operative mortality is reasonable, and cure rates in the 20 to 30 percent range are being reported.

Metastases from colon or rectal cancers most commonly involve the liver or lungs. Pulmonary metastases from colon cancer are rare in the absence of liver metastases but are more likely from rectal cancers. One should usually consider a preliminary laparoscopy or laparotomy to evaluate the liver before embarking upon a pulmonary resection for metastases from a colorectal cancer, but 5-year cure rates from 10 to 15 percent can be expected from aggressive approaches if the liver is free of metastases. The role of hepatic resection in isolated liver metastases is evolving. It is evident that total resection of single or even multiple metastases can provide a long-term cure. With single metastases, a cure rate on the order of 30 percent is expected. This drops off quickly as the number of lesions increases. There is no evidence that extended resections provide any more success than wedge resections if the tumor can be totally removed with microscopically negative margins. Recent studies support the use of intra-arterial chemotherapy in patients with unresectable hepatic metastases who have no apparent disease outside of the liver. Our enthusiasm is growing for that technique since regimens have evolved that appear to have a high response rate but with much less hepatotoxicity than the former high-dose 5-fluoxyridine program.

COMPLICATIONS IN COLORECTAL CANCER RESECTIONS

Major complications should be relatively unusual in patients having elective resections of primary colon or rectal cancers. Wound infections occur in spite of meticulous bowel preparations and systemic antibiotics, but the incidence should be low. Intra-abdominal abscesses are usually secondary to anastomotic leaks. Delayed hemorrhage secondary to inadequately ligated major vessels should be a rare occurrence. Strictures of EEA-stapled anastomoses are not uncommon, especially when postoperative irradiation is given. These usually occur close to the anus, making dilatation under intravenous sedation relatively straightforward. Rectal resections are frequently associated with some degree of urinary and sexual problems. The voiding difficulty is usually transient, but an adequate lymphatic resection for rectal cancer in men usually produces a permanent loss of potency. This possibility should be discussed in advance with all male patients. In patients with colostomies, devascularization with stenosis, retraction, and peristomal hernias are occasionally seen.

Complications are seen more commonly following resections or palliative procedures for patients with recurrent or metastatic colorectal cancer. Many of these patients have been heavily irradiated or have received chemotherapy, both of which can adversely affect anastomotic and wound healing, hemostasis, and resistance to infection.

RESULTS IN COLORECTAL CANCER

Survival from colorectal cancer relates closely to the stage of disease at the time of diagnosis. Approximately 20 percent of patients have lesions that have not extended through the bowel wall or spread to lymph nodes. Most of these patients are cured with resection alone. Another 30 percent present with clinically obvious metastatic disease. Few of these patients are cured. This leaves 50 percent of patients presenting with localized tumors that have grown through the entire thickness of the bowel wall or have spread to regional lymph nodes. From 30 to 60 percent of these patients can be cured with surgical resection alone. Adjuvant chemotherapy plus levamisole has shown some marginal benefits in two recent studies. Pelvic irradiation diminishes the pelvic recurrence rate in rectal cancers and probably improves overall survival. Survival benefits from the resection of recurrent or metastatic colorectal cancer are often difficult to evaluate, but the improved quality of life is often a definite benefit.

HOPES FOR THE FUTURE

Intraoperative radiation therapy is showing encouraging results in advanced carcinoma of the rectum but is still a research procedure that is not widely available. Our own studies using an autologous tumor cell–bacille Calmette Guérin vaccine (active specific immunotherapy) show some promise for this approach to immune induction in the adjuvant setting. Results of an ongoing national cooperative trial should clarify its potential. Human monoclonal antibodies have the potential for earlier diagnosis of metastases and can possibly deliver radionuclides, chemotherapy, or cell toxins to tumors in doses that could be therapeutic but produce less damage to normal tissue than is the case with conventional delivery.

Remarkable advances in the understanding of the molecular biology of all types of cancer give us renewed hope for radically different and improved forms of therapy in the future.

SUGGESTED READING

Herfarth C, Schlag P, Hohenberger P. Surgical strategies in locoregional recurrences of gastrointestinal cancer. World J Surg 1987; 11:504–510.

Hoover HC, Surdyke MG, Dangel RB, et al. Prospectively randomized trial of adjuvant active-specific immunotherapy for human colorectal cancer. Cancer 1985; 55:236–243.

Lopez MJ, Kraybill WG, Downey RS, et al. Exenterative surgery for locally advanced rectosigmoid cancer. Is it worthwhile? Surgery 1987; 102:644–651.

Pezim ME, Nicholls RJ, Chir M. Survival after high or low ligation of inferior mesenteric artery during curative surgery for rectal cancer. Ann Surg 1984; 200:729–733.

Vassilopoulos PP, Yoon JM, Ledesma EJ, et al. Treatment of recurrence of adenocarcinoma of the colon and rectum at the anastomotic site. Surg Gynecol Obstet 1984; 152:777–780.

COLORECTAL CANCER: RADIATION THERAPY

LEONARD L. GUNDERSON, M.D., M.S.
JAMES A. MARTENSON, M.D.

Irradiation is being used in combination with resection and chemotherapy with increasing frequency in the treatment of colorectal malignancies. At the April 1990 National Institutes of Health Consensus Conference on adjuvant therapy for patients with colon and rectal cancer, the combination of postoperative irradiation and chemotherapy was shown to improve both local control and survival of resected but high-risk rectal cancers and, therefore, was recommended as standard treatment. For patients with totally resected colon cancers who have significant rates of local failure, it was noted that radiation containing combined modality therapies should be tested in clinical trials. Therapeutic gains achieved with combination treatment programs (decrease in local recurrence or metastases, or improvement in survival) might be offset by an unnecessary increase in complications unless physicians select patient group(s) that have definite indications for adjuvant treatment and work closely to optimize delivery of the combined modalities.

The intent of this manuscript is to define indications for adjuvant treatment of large bowel cancer by reviewing patterns of failure after surgical resection and then to discuss results of such treatment. Brief sections on diagnostic evaluation, staging systems, and general management are not intended to be complete, but they present information that is pertinent to safe delivery of combined-modality therapy that includes irradiation.

DIAGNOSTIC EVALUATION

The radiation oncologist is often consulted after the lesion is resected and must then use information obtained from preoperative studies as well as the operative and pathologic findings to design appropriate irradiation fields. Studies that evaluate the local extent of disease should be performed on every patient prior to exploration. These studies should include a digital exam, proctoscopy or colonoscopy, and a barium enema study that includes cross-table lateral views. When lesions are palpable, one should note the inferior extent relative to the anal verge, lesion location (anterior, posterior, and so on), degree of circumference involved, and whether the lesion is clinically mobile or fixed. If low and midrectal lesions are immobile or fixed, computed tomography (CT) of the pelvis can confirm lack of free space between the malignancy and a structure that may be surgically unresectable (i.e., presacrum, pelvic side wall). In such cases, the radiation oncologist should be consulted to help determine if it may be preferable to give 4,500 to 5,000 cGy (rad) prior to resection in an attempt to reduce lesion size and alter implantability of cells that may be spread at the time of resection. Although endoscopy procedures are sufficient for diagnosis, they are of limited value to the radiation oncologist in reconstructing tumor volume in three-dimensional fashion for the purpose of sparing normal structures, and endoscopy should not be done as a substitute for a barium enema study. When endoscopy is performed for either colon or rectal lesions, it would be helpful to describe the lesion's position on the bowel wall, the degree of circumference involved, and whether the lesion is exophytic or ulcerative. If hematuria is present or findings on CT or excretory urogram suggest possible bladder involvement, preoperative cystoscopy should be performed.

PATHOLOGIC INFORMATION AND STAGING SYSTEMS

Although the Dukes' staging system is useful in predicting the outcome of survival after surgery, it is less functional in distinguishing subpopulations of patients at greatest risk for local failure who may benefit from adjuvant radiation. A modification of the Astler-Coller rectal system by Gunderson and Sosin subdivides Astler-Coller stages B_2 and C_2 on the basis of degree of extrarectal or extracolonic involvement: microscopic (m), gross or macroscopic extension (g), or operative adherence to or invasion of surrounding organs or structures (B_3 or C_3). This system has been used to analyze survival and patterns of recurrence after potentially curative surgery and indicates that, within Dukes' stage B and C, there are subgroups of patients with significantly different risks for both survival and local failure.

For lesions that extend beyond the rectal wall, the amount of uninvolved tissue (circumferential or radial margins) may be as important or more important than the degree of extrarectal extension. This type of pathologic information may also be of importance in determining indications for adjuvant irradiation of colonic cancers in anatomically immobile sites. For large bowel cancer at all sites, pathologists should routinely define the extra-luminal extent of tumors, measure the narrowest radial margin, and indicate both in the pathology report.

SURGICAL MANAGEMENT

The objective of surgery is to remove the tumor and primary nodal drainage with as wide a margin around both as is technically feasible and safe. If adjacent organs are involved, they should be removed en bloc with the specimen if associated morbidity would be minimal. If the tumor is adherent to prostate or base of bladder, this principle may be contraindicated because the side effects of pelvic exenteration are excessive. In such instances, it may be preferable to use preoperative external irradiation followed by gross total resection (sparing the organ involved by adherence) and supplemental irradiation with intraoperative electrons to the site of adherence (see later discussion). Small clips should be placed around areas of adherence or residual disease for the purpose of boost-field irradiation. With rectal lesions, the pelvic floor should be reconstructed after resection to minimize the amount of small bowel within the true pelvis, and primary or partial closure of the perineum should be performed after abdominoperineal resection to hasten healing (2 to 6 weeks versus 2 to 3 months) and decrease the interval to postoperative irradiation or chemotherapy.

When deciding which operative procedure is possible and adequate for rectal lesions, the surgeon and pathologist commonly refer to the distal bowel margin (amount of resected normal bowel below the primary lesion), but, as indicated previously, more information needs to be obtained regarding nodal and circumferential (radial) margins. When lesions extend beyond the entire rectal wall, the narrowest transected or dissected surgical margin is often the lateral or anteroposterior margin owing to anatomic limitations (in some colonic sites, gross posterior or lateral tumor extension may also result in narrow or compromised operative margins). When perirectal nodes are involved, there is an increased risk of nodal involvement near the surgeon's mesenteric ligature, or in internal iliac or presacral nodes. However, the surgeon rarely removes or biopsies the latter two node groups, and the pathologist rarely examines the former.

Following moderate doses of preoperative irradiation (4,500 to 5,000 cGy), only abdominoperineal resections were recommended owing to the possibility of an increase in anastomotic leaks. Published data confirm, however, that such doses do not preclude anterior resection and primary anastomosis. An unirradiated loop of large bowel should be utilized for the proximal limb of the anastomosis, with temporary diverting colostomies done only on the basis of operative indications.

PATTERNS OF FAILURE AFTER "CURATIVE RESECTION"

Rectal Cancer

The risk of local recurrence after "curative resection" is related to both disease extension beyond the rectal wall as well as to nodal involvement. The incidence of local recurrence for patients with nodal involvement but tumor confined to the wall (C_1) varies from 20 to 40 percent, which is approximately the same incidence as for those patients with negative nodes but extension beyond the wall (i.e., B_2 and B_3), in whom the risk is 20 to 35 percent. When both bad prognostic factors, nodal involvement and extension beyond the wall (i.e., C_2 and C_3) are present, there is nearly an additive risk of local recurrence varying from 40 to 65 percent in the clinical series and 70 percent in a reoperative series. In a series at Massachusetts General Hospital (MGH), the incidence of both total and local failure in the node-negative patients increased with each degree of extension beyond the wall. In that series and a separate one from M.D. Anderson, the degree of extrarectal extension appeared to be an independent factor influencing the risk of local recurrence even in node-positive patients.

Colon Cancer

Clinical series may underestimate the incidence of local failures with colon cancers, because systemic failures are easier to diagnose on the basis of routine laboratory and radiographic studies, and tumor bed recurrences are less apt to result in symptoms than are recurrent rectal cancers. Over the past decade, there has been inappropriate emphasis on liver-only failures in the design of clinical trials. Although data from clinical series suggest that one-third of patients who develop tumor relapse after curative resection have failures solely in the liver, autopsy and reoperative series suggest this may be less than 10 percent.

Data are being accumulated in autopsy, clinical, and reoperative series to indicate that local recurrence can be a significant problem after resection of colonic as well as rectal lesions. In the MGH series by Willett and co-workers, local recurrence was high at most colon sites with modified Astler-Coller B_3, C_2, and C_3 lesions and at some sites with B_2, but the risk was minimal or nonexistent with many B_2 and most C_1 lesions. In a colorectal reoperative series from the University of Minnesota, failures in the tumor bed with or without nodes were most common with rectal lesions but were not uncommon with primaries at other bowel sites. Peritoneal seeding was least common with rectal primaries (lesions are less accessible to the peritoneal cavity). The incidence of hematogenous failures was similar for all sites, although the distribution differed. With rectal primaries, hematogenous failures were fairly evenly divided between liver and lung due to venous drainage via both the mesenteric and internal iliac routes, but with colon primaries, initial hematogenous failures were usually in the liver (venous drainage via the portal system).

ADJUVANT IRRADIATION: RECTAL CANCER

When both surgery and radiation are indicated in an adjuvant setting, differences of opinion exist regarding the preferred sequence. A theoretical advantage of preoperative irradiation is the potential damaging effect on cells that may be spread locally or distantly at the time of resection. The major advantage of postoperative irradiation is the ability to avoid treatment of patients who have metastatic disease that could not be diagnosed prior to exploration or those at low risk for local recurrence. Only those patients at high risk for local recurrence on the basis of operative and pathologic findings are irradiated. A well-designed combination of preoperative and postoperative irradiation could combine the theoretical advantages of each. For clinically mobile rectal lesions, we do not recommend routine full-dose preoperative irradiation because an excessive number of patients would receive unwarranted irradiation with no or only minimal benefit.

Postoperative Irradiation with and without Chemotherapy: Single-Institution Analyses

In prospective but nonrandomized postoperative series using dose levels of 4,500 to 5,500 cGy in 5 to 6 weeks for high-risk patients (B_{2-3}; C_{1-3}), local recurrence has decreased from an expected 35 to 50 percent with operation alone to 10 to 20 percent in the irradiation series. Distant failures continue to be a problem in 25 to 30 percent of patients in spite of the improvement in local control, and improved systemic therapy is needed.

In a published MGH analysis by Hoskins and co-workers (Table 1), local failure was compared at the 3-year interval from resection in nonrandomized but sequential series for operation alone (103 patients) versus operation and postoperative irradiation (95 patients). A significant reduction in local failure was found for most patients who received irradiation (stages $B_{2[g]}$,

Table 1 United States Adjuvant Postoperative Rectal Trials: Irradiation
and Chemotherapy (MAC B_2, B_3, C_1, C_2, C_3)

Group or Institution	Treatment Regimen	Irradiation Dose (Gy) Schedule	Chemotherapy	No. of Patients	Results or Comments			
Nonrandomized								
MGH	Operation alone	None	None	103	↓ LF at 3 yr XRT vs operation alone (B_2, B_3, C_1, C_2)			
	Operation + XRT	50–60/1.8 FX	5-FU, 500 mg/m², 3 days for week 1 (~15 patients)	165	↑ 5–yr NED SR (B_2, 76% vs 47%) (B_3, 69% vs 27%; C_1, 69% vs 25%)			
					Tumor Local	**Control Distant**	**Survival DFS**	**Advantage Overall**
Randomized (published)								
GTSG 7175	Operation alone	None	None	58	—	—	—	—
	XRT	40 or 48/1.8 Gy Fx	None	50	Yes*	No	Inc	Inc
	CT	None	5-FU + MeCCNU	48	No	Yes†	Inc	Inc
	XRT + CT	40 or 44	5-FU, 500 mg/mg², 3 days for week 1 ± 5 XRT; 5-FU + MeCCNU	46	Yes* $P = 0.04$	Yes†	Yes $P = 0.009$	Yes $P = 0.005$
Mayo/NCCTG 79-47-51	XRT	50.4/28 Fx	None	101	—	—	—	—
	XRT + CT	Same	5-Fu + MeCCNU; 5-FU, 500 mg/m², 3 days for week 1 ± 5 XRT; 5-FU + MeCCNU	103	Yes $P = 0.03$	Yes $P = 0.05$	Yes $P = 0.004$	Yes $P = 0.06$
NSABP RO1	Operation alone	None	None	173	—	—	—	—
	XRT	47/26 Fx	None	177	Yes ($P = 0.06$)	Dec	Equal	Equal
	CT	None	5-FU, MeCCNU, VCR	178	Inc	Equal	Yes $P = 0.006$ Inc	Yes $P = 0.05$ Inc
GTSG 7180	XRT + CT (5-FU)	43.2/24 Fx	5-FU, 500 mg/m², 3 days for week 1 ± 5 XRT; 5-FU	210	No comment in abstract			
	XRT + CT (5-FU MeCCNU)	Same	5-FU + XRT; 5-FU + MeCCNU				—	—

*Local control advantage to XRT versus no XRT; $P = 0.04$.
†Distant control advantage to CT versus no CT.
  Abbreviations: MAC = modified Astler-Coller stage, XRT = external irradiation, Fx = fractions, CT = chemotherapy, LF = local failure, SR = survival, DFS = disease-free SR, Inc = increased survival or tumor control but not statistically significant, Dec = decreased, Yes = marginal or statistically significant improvement, 5-FU = 5-fluorouracil.

B_3, C_1, C_2). In an update of that series by Tepper and colleagues, the irradiated patients continued to have a significantly lower incidence of local failure by stage (only 15 of 165 received 5-fluorouracil during irradiation). Improved 5-year survival with no evidence of disease was found in patients with only a single high-risk factor (i.e., either extension beyond the wall or involved nodes—B_2, B_3, and C_1 lesions). The incidence of local failure in irradiated patients in stage B_2 or B_3 was quite low—8 percent (5 of 60). In node-positive patients, however, the incidence was 20 percent or greater: C_1, 20 percent (2 of 10); C_2, 21 percent (16 of 77); C_3, 53 percent (8 of 15) (if eight C_2 and C_3 patients with diffuse peritoneal seeding are excluded, the incidence of local failure is 18 percent for C_2 [13 of 74] and 30 percent for C_3 [3 of 10]).

With regard to distant failures, the risk appears to be significantly higher in patients with both high-risk pathologic findings (C_2, C_3) as opposed to those with only a single risk factor (B_2, B_3, C_1). In published data

from patients irradiated at MGH or Mayo, the incidence of distant failure was approximately 20 percent with B_2, B_3, and C_1 lesions versus 40 to 60 percent with C_2 or C_3 lesions (MGH: C_2, 38 percent, and C_3, 60 percent; Mayo: C_2, 58 percent). The differences in distant failure rates appeared to translate into a difference in survival, because a 5-year survival range of 70 percent to 90 percent was achieved at both institutions in patients with B_2, B_3, and C_1 disease versus 40 percent of patients with C_2 (MGH and Mayo) and 17 percent with C_3 lesions (MGH).

Postoperative Irradiation with and without Chemotherapy: Randomized Trials in United States

A summary of treatment schema and results is seen in Table 1 for four randomized trials that have been reported in either abstract form or as complete manuscripts. Results are reported as a function of treatment impact on patterns of failure (local, distant) and survival (disease-free, overall). Positive survival results were reported in three of the trials.

A three-arm trial from the National Surgical Adjuvant Breast and Bowel Program (NSABP) compared surgery alone with postoperative irradiation (4,600 to 4,700 cGy in 25 to 27 fractions) and postoperative chemotherapy (5-fluorouracil, MeCCNU, vincristine). An advantage in disease-free survival existed when comparing surgery plus chemotherapy with surgery alone ($P = 0.006$), but neither local failure nor distant metastasis was significantly altered with the addition of chemotherapy. A marginal improvement in overall survival was noted ($P = 0.05$). In patients randomized to receive irradiation, there was a significant decrease in local recurrence from 25 to 16 percent ($P = 0.06$), but this did not translate into an improvement in survival (14 percent of patients randomized to irradiation did not receive such).

Data now exist from two randomized postoperative trials (Gastrointestinal Tumor Study Group [GTSG], Mayo/North Central Cancer Treatment Group [NCCTG]) that document a decrease in local recurrence and improvement in both disease-free and overall survival with combined postoperative irradiation and chemotherapy for patients with disease extension beyond the rectal wall, lymph nodes negative (B_2, B_3); positive lymph nodes, confined to wall (C_1); or both (C_2, C_3). In both trials, bolus 5-fluorouracil was given for 3 days on weeks 1 and 5 of irradiation, and patients received 5-fluorouracil and MeCCNU after (GTSG) or before and after irradiation plus 5-fluorouracil (Mayo/NCCTG).

In the GTSG trial, patients with Dukes' B or C lesions were randomized to a surgery-alone control arm and adjuvant treatment arms of postoperative irradiation (4,000 or 4,800 cGy), postoperative chemotherapy (5-fluorouracil and MeCCNU), or a combination thereof (4,000 or 4,400 cGy). The disease-free survival of all three adjuvant arms was higher than surgery alone. The statistically significant advantages with the combined irradiation/chemotherapy arm were achieved in a comparison with the surgery-alone control arm, with highly significant differences in both disease-free and overall survival ($P = 0.009$ and 0.005), but there was also a nearly significant difference in disease-free survival with irradiation and CT versus irradiation alone ($P = 0.06$). The incidence of local failure as an initial failure pattern was significantly decreased with irradiation versus no irradiation ($P = 0.05$), but the best result was achieved with irradiation and CT (local failure rate of 11 percent versus 20 percent with irradiation alone). No impact on local control was seen with chemotherapy versus no chemotherapy, but an apparent impact on distant failures was noted.

Because GTSG radiation doses were lower than in the major prospective single-institution studies and local recurrence rates were high in the radiation-only arm, there was still uncertainty regarding radiation plus chemotherapy versus radiation alone as the preferred postoperative adjuvant treatment. The randomized trial by the Mayo Clinic and the NCCTG (79-47-51) appears to clarify this uncertainty, because the minimum irradiation dose within the boost field in both the irradiation and irradiation-plus-CT arms was 5,040 cGy in 28 fractions over 5.5 weeks. In this trial, the combined arm achieved statistically significant results when compared with those of the irradiation-only arm. In a 1990 update presented at the National Cancer Institute Large Bowel Consensus Conference, these differences exist with regard to failure patterns (local failure rate of 23.5 percent versus 13 percent; $P = 0.03$; distant failure rate of 39 percent versus 29 percent; $P = 0.05$) as well as disease-free survival and overall survival (disease-free survival rate of 60 percent versus 40 percent at 5 years, $P = 0.004$; overall survival of 58 percent versus 48 percent at 5 years, $P = 0.06$). This is the only randomized trial in which a course of chemotherapy was given before irradiation in an attempt to decrease the incidence of distant failures.

Preliminary results from a second GTSG trial were reported at the 1990 American Society of Clinical Oncology meeting. All patients received irradiation and were randomized to receive further chemotherapy with escalating doses, as tolerated, of either 5-fluorouracil alone or 5-fluorouracil plus MeCCNU. No significant advantages were found in those chosen to receive MeCCNU since both disease free and overall survival at 3 years were better on the escalating 5-fluorouracil arm (54 percent versus 69 percent disease free and 66 percent versus 76 percent overall survival).

Preoperative Adjuvant Irradiation for Rectal Cancer

Preoperative series using a variety of dose and portal arrangements have demonstrated evidence of tumor response by virtue of partial or total regression of the primary lesion. Treatment schema and results of both low- and moderate-dose randomized trials in preoperative irradiation are seen in Table 2. As with postoperative trials, results are evaluated as a function of impact on tumor control (local or distant) and survival (disease-free, overall).

Although survival was improved in selected subgroups of patients in two prospective randomized low-dose series (Princess Margaret Hospital, 500 cGy × 1; or VA hospital, 2,000 to 2,500 cGy in 2 to 2.5 weeks), these results were not duplicated in a recently published Medical Research Council trial that compared these two treatment arms with a surgery-alone control arm. Results from a second VA trial using slightly higher doses of preoperative irradiation (3,150 cGy/13 × 175) did not reveal an advantage to the irradiated group.

Results of three moderate-dose trials are seen in Table 2. Doses delivered were equivalent to 3,960 to 4,400 cGy in standard fractionation. All three demonstrated an improvement in local control in irradiated patients for either the total group (European Organization for Research and Treatment of Cancer [EORTC] — 80 percent versus 65 percent, $P = 0.02$;

Catholic University—85 percent versus 53 percent) or subset analyses (Rotterdam—T_3, T_4 lesions, $P=0.08$; EORTC curative resection—85 percent versus 70 percent, $P=0.003$). Improvements in 5-year survival in irradiated patients were demonstrated for the total group only in the smaller Catholic University trial (73 percent versus 30 percent). Subset analyses revealed suggestive survival advantages in irradiated T_3 and T_4 patients in the Rotterdam series ($P=0.001$) and for patients with curative resection in the EORTC trial (70 percent versus 60 percent, $P=0.08$).

Preoperative Irradiation with and without Postoperative Irradiation

Low-dose preoperative irradiation (500 cGy $\times$ 1 or 5×200 cGy) has been combined with selective postoperative irradiation (4,500 to 5,000 cGy in 25 to 28 fractions) in view of some theoretical advantages over either high-dose preoperative or postoperative irradiation. Recent analyses of series from MGH and Thomas Jefferson University suggest that one can safely delete patients who do not require the postoperative component of irradiation (stages A and B_1 with or without select early $B_{2[m]}$ and C_1 lesions) and yet achieve excellent local control and good survival. In the Thomas Jefferson University series, the addition of the postoperative component significantly reduced both total and local failures in patients with Dukes' B and C lesions when compared with low-dose preoperative irradiation alone (total failure, 52 percent versus 19 percent; local failure, 34 percent versus 6 percent). Although such an approach may be preferable to either high-dose preop-

erative or postoperative irradiation for mobile lesions, it would be difficult to develop a meaningful comparison with high-dose preoperative irradiation because clinical staging is inaccurate at present. A randomized comparison with postoperative irradiation has been completed in a combined Radiation Therapy Oncology Group-Eastern Cooperative Oncology Group (RTOG-ECOG) trial.

ADJUVANT IRRADIATION: COLON CANCER

The use of adjuvant radiation for colon cancer has not been extensive. Several publications from Albert Einstein Hospital discuss the use of a whole-abdomen moving-strip technique for colon cancer with doses paralleling those used for ovarian cancer. This technique was used as an adjuvant for patients with "curative resection" but who were at high risk for local recurrence as well as for patients with proven residual disease. Although results were not compared with those achieved with surgery alone from that institution, the technique did not produce excessive morbidity.

Duttenhaver and co-workers reviewed a series of 80 patients with colon cancer with extension beyond the wall, alone or in combination with nodal involvement, who received adjuvant irradiation at MGH starting in April, 1976. When compared with the surgery-alone group from MGH, local recurrence was decreased in irradiated patients with B_3, C_2, and high-risk B_2 lesions. Actuarial 5-year survival was improved in irradiated patients with modified Astler-Coller stage B_3, C_2, and C_3 lesions.

Table 2 Clinically Resectable Rectal Cancer: Randomized Preoperative Irradiation Trials

Group or Institution	Irradiation Dose/Schedule (cGy)	Delay to Surgery	No. of Patients	Results: Failure Patterns and Survival
Randomized: low-dose (surgery-alone control)				
PMH (two arm)	5.0 × 1	Within 8 hr	111	Increased SR with XRT, Dukes' C
VAH (two arm)	20–25/2 wk	0–10 days	700	Resection in 613, in 414 with CAPR 5-yr SR advantage to XRT (41% vs 28%, $P < 0.02$) Autopsy in 180: disease-free—50% XRT, 30% operation ($P<0.05$)
MRC (three arm)	5.0 × 1 vs 20/10 vs operation alone	0–7 days	824	No difference in failure patterns or SR
VAH (two arm)	31.5/18 × 1.75	0–10 days	361	No difference in LF, DF, or SR
Randomized: moderate-dose (surgery-alone control)				
Rotterdam	34.5/15 × 2.3/19 days	Within 2 wk	100	XRT has advantage over operation with T_3, T_4 lesions Increased SR ($P = 0.001$); decreased LF ($P = 0.08$)
EORTC 40761	34.5/15 × 2.3/19 days	4–15 days	466 (341 curative resection)	Advantage to XRT: 5-yr LC—total, 80% vs 65% ($P = 0.02$); curative, 85% vs 70% ($P = 0.003$); 5-yr SR—curative, 70% vs 60% ($P = 0.08$)
Catholic University Campenas	40/20 × 2.0/4 wk	1 wk	68	Advantage to XRT: LC, 85% vs 53%; DF, 15% vs 32%; 5-yr SR, 73% vs 30%

Abbreviations: LC = local control, LF = local failure, DF = distant failure, CAPR = combined abdominoperineal resection, SR = survival, XRT = irradiation, PMH = Princess Margaret Hospital, VAH = Veterans Administration Hospital, MRC = Medical Research Council.

Results in the MGH series were updated by Willett and co-workers. Of the 133 irradiated patients, only 22 received chemotherapy either during or immediately following irradiation. Local control continued to be better in irradiated patients (Table 3). As was found in the MGH rectal series, the incidence of local recurrence in irradiated B_3 and high-risk B_2 patients was low at 10 percent or less. With C_2 and C_3 patients, although local recurrence was less than with surgery alone, it was still excessive—21 percent and 31 percent, respectively. Improved 5-year survival was suggested with B_3 and C_3 lesions (Table 4).

COMPLICATIONS AND THERAPEUTIC RATIO

A suitable therapeutic ratio between local control and complications is achieved only with close interaction between the surgeon and the radiation oncologist and the use of sophisticated radiation techniques. In the postoperative MGH rectal series with shaped multiple-field irradiation techniques, use of bladder distention, and so on, the incidence of small bowel obstruction requiring operative intervention was essentially equal in the group receiving irradiation and the group who had only the operation: 6 percent versus 5 percent, respectively. In the GTSG rectal trial, severe or worse nonhematologic toxicity occurred in 35 percent of patients on the combined-adjuvant arm versus 16 percent who received radiation alone; two patients in the combined-treatment arm died of complications of enteritis but were free of disease. In the Mayo/MCCTG rectal trial using multiple-field irradiation techniques, the incidence of small bowel problems has been 5 percent or less with either irradiation alone or in combination with chemotherapy.

In the colon adjuvant trial from MGH, doses of 4,500 to 5,500 in 180-cGy fractions were delivered with parallel-opposed techniques. With extrapelvic lesions, decubitus position was used whenever this revealed an advantageous shift in small bowel. Subsequent operative exploration was required for small bowel problems in only 2 of 80 patients (2.5 percent) reported by Duttenhaver and colleagues.

Table 3 Stage versus Total and 5-Year Actuarial Local Control for Colon Cancer: Surgery ± Irradiation (MGH Trial)

	Surgery alone*			Surgery plus radiation†		
		Total local failure			Total local failure	
Stage	No. of Patients	No. (%)	5-yr actuarial	No. of Patients	No. (%)	5-yr actuarial
B_2 (total)	163	18 (11)	10	—	—	—
B_2 (high-risk)	61	13 (21)	—	21‡	2 (10)	10
B_3	83	25 (30)	31	37	2 (5)	8
C_2 (total)	100	32 (32)	36	—	—	—
C_2 (high-risk)	—	—	—	47§	6 (13)	21
C_3	49	24 (49)	53	28	8 (29)	31

*Modified from Willett C, et al. Ann Surg 1984; 200:685.
†Modified from Willett CG, Tepper JE, Skates SJ, et al. Adjuvant postoperative radiation therapy for colonic carcinomas. Ann Surg 1987; 206:694.
‡Only B_2 patients with narrow radial margin were irradiated.
§C_2 mid-sigmoid and mid-transverse were not irradiated.

Table 4 Stage versus 5-Year Actuarial Survival for Colon Cancer: Surgery ± Irradiation (MGH Trial)

	Surgery			Surgery plus Irradiation		
Stage	No. of Patients	Disease-free Survival	Overall Survival	No. of Patients	Disease-free Survival	Overall Survival
B_2 (total vs high-risk)*	163	78	70	21	74	77
B_3	83	64	63	37	77	81
C_2	100	48	44	47	48	47
C_3	49	38	37	28	50	51

Adapted from Willett CG, Tepper JE, Skates SJ, et al. Adjuvant postoperative radiation therapy for colonic carcinoma. Ann Surg 1987; 206:694; with permission.
*Only B_2 patients with narrow radial margins were irradiated.

RADIATION FOR LOCALLY ADVANCED COLORECTAL CANCERS (RESIDUAL, UNRESECTABLE, OR RECURRENT)

Philosophy and Dose of Radiation

Although temporary palliation of unresectable primary or recurrent lesions can be achieved with radiation dose levels as low as 2,000 cGy in 2 weeks, prolongation of palliation requires dose levels of 4,000 to 5,000 cGy in 4 to 5 weeks or higher. Data from other tumor systems suggest that the incidence of permanent local control and possible cure might improve if external-beam doses of 6,000 to 7,000 cGy could be safely delivered in 7 to 8 weeks. At such levels, however, the incidence of radiation-induced small bowel damage will be prohibitive unless information is available regarding the relative position of tumor and small bowel and is used to modify irradiation doses and portals.

Small bowel films can be used to define radiation dose limits, and both the surgeon and radiation oncologist have to be somewhat innovative if small bowel radiation enteritis is to be avoided or minimized. Any operative or irradiation maneuver that can decrease the volume of small bowel and other normal tissues within an anticipated irradiation field is indicated. Doses above 4,500 to 5,000 cGy should not be used unless there is good small bowel mobility or minimal volumes of small bowel in the irradiation field. Doses above 5,500 cGy should be used only if small bowel is completely outside the irradiation portal. Operative techniques, including clip placement and reconstruction procedures, can help the radiation oncologist to use appropriate field reduction after an initial 4,500 to 5,000 cGy (i.e., make the field smaller for an additional 1,500 to 2,000 cGy, yet include tumor and miss small bowel with the aid of lateral fields and bladder distention). A unique combination of the two utilizes an intraoperative electron-beam boost to areas of high risk while dose-limiting tissues are retracted out of the field.

Results

External-beam irradiation has been combined with surgical resection, chemotherapy, or immunotherapy for locally advanced disease (Table 5). When radiation is given after subtotal resection of locally advanced lesions

Table 5 Locally Advanced Adenocarcinoma of Colon and Rectum: External Irradiation ± Chemotherapy or Resection

Group or Institution	Treatment	Irradiation Dose/Schedule	Chemotherapy or Immunotherapy	No. of Patients	Results: Failure Patterns and Survival	
Nonrandomized (Primary Irradiation)						
PMH	XRT alone	4,000–5,000cGy/250 cGy Fx	None	67	LF (91%) and 5-yr actuarial SR (2%)	
Randomized						
Mayo	XRT ± 5-FU	4,000cGy/20 × 200	5-FU, 15 mg/kg, on days 1-3 of XRT	65	Median SR (10.5 vs 16 mo) Advantage to XRT + 5-FU (*P* > 0.05)	
Mayo	XRT ± MER	5,000 cGy/7 wk (2-wk split)	MER	44	LF in 28/31 evaluable (90%); no advantage with MER	
RTOG 76-16	XRT ± CT	XRT only: 4,500–7,000 cGy; 170–180 cGy	None	147	No significant differences; trend to XRT + CT in patients with subtotal resection	
		XRT + CT: 4,500–6,000 cGy	5-FU, 500 mg/m^2, for 3 days on weeks 1 ± 5; 5-FU + MeCCNU			
Nonrandomized (Postoperative Irradiation)					**Percentage LF versus Amount Residual**	
					Microscopic	*Gross*
Albert Einstein	Resection + XRT	4,500–6,000 cGy	None	31	2/13 (15%)	9/18 (50%)
MGH	Same	4,500–7,000 cGy/180-cGy Fx	None or 5-FU, 500 mg/m$_2$, for 3 days on week 1	55	9/30 (30%)	12/23 (52%)
Mayo	Same	4,500–6,000 cGy/180-cGy Fx	None or 5-FU, 500 mg/m^2, for 3 days on weeks 1 ± 5	17	7/10 (70%)	6/7 (86%)
Nonrandomized (Preoperative Irradiation)					*Resectability*	**LF after Resection**
Oregon	XRT ± resection	5,000–6,000 cGy/200-cGy Fx	None	40	50%	45%
Tufts	Same	4,500–6,000 cGy/175 to 200-cGy Fx	None	44	75%	36%
MGH	Same	4,500–5,000 cGy/5–6 wk	None	25	72%	43%

Abbreviations: XRT = irradiation; CT = chemotherapy, Fx = fraction, LF = local failure, MER = Method Extracted Residue of BCG, 5-FU = 5-Fluorouracil.

(5,000 to 7,000 cGy in 180 cGy fractions) or before an attempt at resection for initially unresectable disease (4,500 to 5,000 cGy in 5 to 5.5 weeks preoperatively followed by resection in 3 to 5 weeks), although local control and survival can be obtained in some patients, the risk of local recurrence is too high at 30 to 50 percent. In separate series from Princess Margaret Hospital and the Mayo Clinic using radiation alone or with immunotherapy, local recurrence was 90 percent or greater in evaluable patients.

In an attempt to decrease local recurrence and improve survival, both MGH and Mayo have initiated pilot studies that add an intraoperative electron boost to fractionated external-beam irradiation (4,500 to 5,500 cGy in 5 to 6 weeks) with or without resection. In the initial published MGH report of 32 patients, local control appeared to be improved in both the patients with residual disease and those who were initially unresectable, and survival was better in the latter group when compared with historical controls treated only with preoperative irradiation and resection. In ongoing trials, 4-year actuarial survival was 52 percent in patients who present with locally advanced primary lesions and 25 percent in those with recurrence; these data were in contrast to an expected long-term survival of approximately 5 percent when localized recurrences are treated with standard techniques. In patients with both primary and recurrent disease, both local control and survival are improved if the surgeon has been able to perform a gross total resection prior to intraoperative irradiation (IORT) (Table 6). The incidence of moderate or severe soft-tissue complications has not appeared to increase as a result of the aggressive combinations.

In a published series of 51 patients with locally advanced colorectal cancer treated at Mayo, results parallel those achieved at MGH, with 4-year actuarial survival in 55 percent of patients with primary lesions and 25 percent of patients with recurrent lesions. All local failures have occurred in patients who present with recurrence or have gross residual disease after partial resection. In patients at risk for more than 1 year, the addition of 5-fluorouracil during external irradiation may decrease the risk of local recurrence (1 of 11, or 9 percent, versus 6 of 31, or 19 percent), as has been seen in adjuvant series. Results from an updated Mayo analysis of primary patients at risk for 2 years or more are seen in Table 7. Data suggest that improvements in local control with the addition of IORT may translate into improved survival; this needs to be validated in phase 3 trials.

FUTURE DIRECTIONS

Adjuvant Treatment: Rectal Cancer

The NIH Consensus Conference identified three independent primary scientific end–points by which efficacy of adjuvant treatment of rectal cancer should be evaluated: (1) disease-free survival (time to relapse); (2) overall survival; and (3) incidence of pelvic (local) recurrence. Neither irradiation nor chemotherapy as single adjuvants achieve all suggested criterion of

Table 6 Results of Intraoperative and External Irradiation ± Resection in Primary and Recurrent Adenocarcinoma of Rectum (MGH Trial)

| | | 5-year Actuarial Results | |
Extent of Resection	No. of Patients	Local Control (%)	Survival (%)
Primary tumor	39	81	40
Complete resection	23	88	51
Partial resection	16	68	24
Locally recurrent tumor	28	32	17
Complete resection	12	47	34
Partial resection	16	23	6

From Willett CG, et al. RSNA 1988 categorial course, with permission.

Table 7 Locally Advanced Primary Colorectal Cancer: Results with External Irradiation ± Intraoperative Irradiation (Mayo Clinic)

Treatment	No. of Patients at risk	3-year survival (%)	Local failures No. (%)	Distant failures No. (%)
External*	17	24	13 (76)	10 (59)
External + IORT†	20	50	4 (20)	9 (45)

*All deaths occurred within 30 months (local failure range of 3 to 15 months; distant failure range of 3 to 17 months). (From Schild SE, Martenson JA, Gunderson IL, et al. Long-term survival and patterns of failure after postoperative therapy for subtotally resected rectal adenocarcinoma. Int J Radiat Oncol Biol Phys 1989; 16:459.)
†All at risk for 2 years or longer.

efficacy. Irradiation diminishes the rate of local recurrence in both prospective nonrandomized as well as randomized preoperative and postoperative trials, but this has not translated into an improvement in overall survival. Chemotherapy has produced a significant improvement in disease–free survival and marginal improvement in overall survival in the NSABP trial, but no significant improvement in local control has been seen with adjuvant chemotherapy in any randomized study. Only combined modality postoperative adjuvant treatment has consistently demonstrated efficacy in all parameters as noted in two prospectively randomized trials (GTSG and Mayo/NCCTG). In both studies, 5-FU was given during irradiation, and patients received additional chemotherapy either after irradiation plus 5-FU (GTSG) or both before and after (Mayo/NCCTG).

Despite the advantages found with combined-modality treatment, there is a need to improve both local control and systemic control of disease. In both the GTSG and Mayo/NCCTG trials, although local failure was decreased by half with the combined-modality treatment, the incidence of local failure as initial failure was still 11 to 13 percent. The true incidence of local failure as a component of failure at any time in follow-up is probably 15 percent or greater, even with combinations of irradiation and chemotherapy. The desire would be to reduce this figure to 5 percent or less with acceptable morbidity. In patients with disease extension beyond the rectal wall, it may be more difficult to achieve local control when the surgeon's radial margin is narrow. In both trials, systemic failures as an initial pattern of failure existed in 26 to 29 percent of patients in spite of combined CT and irradiation. There is certainly a need to evaluate the delivery of the most effective systemic therapy during the irradiation component of treatment as well as before and after in order to avoid delays of 2.5 to 3 months between sequences of effective systemic therapy (Table 8). As we attempt to optimize systemic control of disease, we may need more aggressive drug combinations with C_2 and C_3 lesions as opposed to B_2, B_3, and C_1 lesions (all C_1 versus those with < 4 positive nodes).

Future trials need to define optimal combinations of irradiation and chemotherapy (what drugs, route and timing of delivery, sequencing of radiation and chemotherapy, and so forth) and to determine whether some patients can be spared the most aggressive treatment combinations (i.e., limited B_2 and C_1 lesions). There is a need to evaluate which drug(s) and methods should be used during irradiation to enhance its effect and which drugs are necessary to alter systemic patterns of failure. It would be helpful to improve clinical staging so that full-dose preoperative and postoperative radiation could be randomly compared for equivalent disease extent and to define the dose of radiation needed on the basis of the narrowest transected surgical margin (distal or radial). It will be important to determine the role of flow cytometry, peritoneal cytology, and other parameters in predicting patterns of failure and prognosis and to increase the use of autopsies in clinical trials to determine exact patterns of failure as an aid in the design of future studies.

Adjuvant Treatment of Colon Cancer

Selected subsets of patients with colon cancer have local recurrence risks equivalent to those seen with rectal cancer if surgery alone is utilized. In view of the positive results seen with combined irradiation and chemotherapy adjuvant treatment of rectal cancer, encouraging pilot study results with postoperative irradiation of high-risk colon cancer at MGH and the positive results of 5-fluorouracil with levamisole in high-risk adjuvant colon cancer, it would be appropriate to consider an intergroup randomized trial comparing 5-fluorouracil and levamisole with 5-fluorouracil, levamisole, and irradiation in patients at high risk for local recurrence following surgical resection (modified Astler-

Table 8 Treatment Recommendations for Large Bowel Cancers

Clinical Situation	Standard Therapy	Investigative Therapy
Adjuvant		
1. *Rectal Cancer:* Completely resected, but at high risk for local failure (modified Astler-Coller stage B_{2-3}, C_{1-3})	Adjuvant postoperative irradiation plus 5-fluorouracil	Clinical trials with principal goal of determining optimal conbination of irradiation and systemic agents
2. *Colon Cancer:* Completely resected, but at high risk for local failure (modified Astler-Coller stage B_3, C_{2-3}, and selected B_2)	Adjuvant postoperative 5-fluorouracil plus levamisole in node-positive patients	Clinical trials to determine the value of 5-FU and levamisole ± adjuvant irradiation for B_3, C_3, and C_2 lesions
Locally Advanced		
3. *Rectal Cancer:* Locally unresectable for cure owing to tumor fixation	Preoperative external-beam irradiation ± 5-fluorouracil followed by surgical resection if feasible	External-beam irradiation ± chemotherapy or radiation sensitizers followed by maximal surgical removal of residual tumor and intraoperative irradiation with electrons or brachytherapy (Nos. 3 and 4)
4. *Colon and Rectal Cancer:* Incomplete resected or locally recurrent	External-beam irradiation ± 5-fluorouracil	

Coller stages B$_3$, C$_3$, and C$_2$, except mid-sigmoid and mid-transverse).

Locally Advanced Disease

When unresectable or residual disease is treated with a combination of conventional irradiation and resection, local control and long-term survival can be achieved in 30 to 50 percent of patients. The presence of dose-limiting normal tissues, however, prevents delivery of adequate levels of external-beam irradiation in a majority of patients. In early colorectal pilot studies from MGH and Mayo, the addition of an intraoperative electron boost appears to improve both local control and survival. A trial has been initiated in RTOG that randomizes to standard treatment with or without an IORT electron boost.

For locally advanced or recurrent colorectal lesions in which operative resection is not feasible, a combination of external-beam irradiation and chemotherapy can achieve useful palliation in 75 to 80 percent of patients as well as an occasional cure. If lesion size and location are such that intraoperative boosts with electrons or implantation techniques can be safely used to supplement external-beam doses, further gains may be possible (Table 8).

The incidence of distant metastases ranges from 30 to 50 percent in patients who present with locally advanced lesions. The highest rates are seen in patients in whom local control is not achieved or those who present for treatment with locally recurrent as opposed to primary lesions. Effective systemic therapy is needed before long-term survival of 50 percent or more will be achieved in patients with localized recurrence. It is hoped that chemotherapy advances with 5-fluorouracil combined with leucovorin and levamisole will translate into a decrease in distant metastases and improvements in survival when combined with irradiation for patients with locally advanced disease.

Acknowlegement. The author appreciates the efforts of Julie Chambers and the Mayo Typing Service for assistance in the preparation of the manuscript.

SUGGESTED READING

Chan KW, Boey J, Wong SKC. A method of reporting radial invasion and surgical clearance of rectal carcinoma. Histopathology 1983; 9:1,319–1,327.
Duttenhaver JR, Hoskins RB, Gunderson LL, et al. Adjuvant postoperative radiation therapy in the management of adenocarcinoma of the colon. Cancer 1986; 57:955–963.
Fisher B, Wolmark N. Rockette H, et al. Postoperative adjuvant chemotherapy or radiation therapy for rectal cancer: Results from NSABP R-01. J Natl Cancer Inst 1988; 80:21–29.
Gastrointestinal Tumor Study Group. Prolongation of the disease-free interval in surgically resected rectal cancer. N Engl J Med 1985; 312:1,465–1,472.
Gastrointestinal Tumor Study Group. Survival after postoperative combination treatment of rectal cancer. N Engl J Med 1986; 315:1,294–1,295.
Gerard A, Buyse M, Nordlinger B, et al. Preoperative radiotherapy as adjuvant treatment in rectal cancer: Final results of a randomized study (EORTC). Ann Surg 1988; 208:606–614.
Gunderson LL, Martin JK, Beart RW, et al. Intraoperative and external-beam irradiation (IORT) for locally advanced colorectal cancer. Ann Surg 1988; 27:52–60.
Wassif SB, Langenhorst BL, Hop CJ. The contribution of preoperative radiotherapy in the management of borderline operability rectal cancer. In: Salmon SE, Jones SE, eds. Adjuvant therapy of cancer II. New York: Grune & Stratton, 1974; 612–626.

COLORECTAL CANCER: CHEMOTHERAPY

JOHN D. HINES, M.D.
YOUCEF M. RUSTUM, Ph.D.

Colorectal cancer will afflict approximately 155,000 individuals in 1990, and it is the second most prevalent cancer in the United States. Following primary surgical resection of colorectal carcinoma, over one-half of patients will relapse if untreated. Because the 5-year adjusted survival rate is nearly 75 percent for those patients with early localized disease in contrast to 20 percent for those with advanced disease, efforts at early detection are of prime importance. It is anticipated that more widespread application of occult blood screening programs will impact on earlier detection of colorectal cancer.

Because there are, as yet, no identifiable etiologic factors responsible for colorectal cancer, a variety of dietary interventions have been under consideration. Dietary fiber supplementation has received a great deal of attention since the original observations by Burkitt and Painter, who observed a lower incidence of colon cancer in African groups ingesting high-fiber diets. Some case control and population studies in Scandinavia, Israel, and the United States have tended to support the notion that increased dietary fiber may have value in lessening the incidence of the disease.

An alternate way of reducing the risk of developing colorectal carcinoma is to intervene early in high-risk patients. This would include more aggressive application of colonoscopy and polyp removal in patients who have a family history of intestinal polyps, because many of these will eventually become neoplastic. More widespread use of the flexible sigmoidoscope will potentially detect approximately those 40 percent of malignant or premalignant lesions occurring within this anatomic site.

SURGICAL TREATMENT

The following are generally accepted guidelines for pretreatment evaluation of potentially curative colorectal cancer:

1. History and Physical Examination. Particular attention should focus on family history of polyps and cancers. Check for hepatomegaly, adenopathy, and, if a rectal mass is identified, ascertain distance from anal verge and from levators. In women, check carefully for abnormalities of the adnexae and uterus.
2. Laboratory. Obtain a complete blood count, carcinoembryonic antigen (CEA) levels, lactic dehydrogenase (LDH) levels, and urinalysis, and assess electrolytes and liver function.
3. Gastrointestinal-Radiology. Perform colonoscopy and air-contrast barium enema when feasible. Obtain a chest radiograph and, for suspected cancer in low sigmoid or rectal area, a full abdominal and pelvic computed tomography (CT) scan.

Surgery should be considered for all patients with colorectal carcinoma unless morbid medical complications are contradictive. The primary aim of surgery is curative, recognizing that in over half of the patients this will not be feasible. Any suspicious additional lesions must be biopsied to confirm or deny their metastatic nature.

Cancers arising in the cecum, ascending colon, and hepatic flexure require a right hemicolectomy, which includes 10 to 15 cm of the terminal ileum, the right colon, and the right half of the transverse colon. Cancers arising in the transverse colon require both a right hemicolectomy and complete resection of the entire transverse colon and splenic flexure. Cancers arising in the splenic flexure and proximal descending colon require a left hemicolectomy, including resection of left inferior mesenteric artery and vein along with its mesentery and omentum. Cancers in the sigmoid colon may be resected by wide sigmoid resection or with left hemicolectomy. Cancers arising in the low sigmoid or intraperitoneal rectum are treated by a low anterior resection. The very low lying rectal carcinomas, less than 7 cm from the anal verge, are treated by an abdominoperineal resection and a permanent end-sigmoid colostomy. The potential cure rate for node-negative patients ranges from 60 to 80 percent. The potential cure rate for node-positive patients translates to a 5-year survival of 30 percent.

ADJUVANT TREATMENT

Following primary surgical management of colorectal carcinoma, more than one-half of patients can expect a relapse of disease. Adjuvant chemotherapy with 5-fluorouracil, singly or in combination with other agents, has been investigated extensively. A recent meta-analysis concluded that regimens containing 5-fluorouracil employed in adjuvant treatment of colorectal carcinoma were associated with a marginal therapeutic benefit in terms of overall survival. The addition of adjuvant immunotherapy to 5-fluorouracil has attracted interest in an effort to improve the therapeutic outcome of patients with node-positive colon carcinoma.

The antihelminthic drug levamisole, a synthetic phenylimidothiazole, has been recognized for over a decade to possess a number of immunomodulatory properties. A number of clinical trials employing 5-fluorouracil and levamisole have been conducted in colorectal cancer patients with metastatic disease. The results of the randomized controlled studies, comparing 5-fluorouracil as a single agent, failed to demonstrate any advantage of adding levamisole to 5-fluorouracil in metastatic colorectal cancer. Interest in levamisole continues, however, in the adjuvant-disease setting for colon carcinoma. Laurie and colleagues recently published the results of a North Central Cancer Treatment Group (NCCTG) trial comparing 5-fluorouracil and levamisole, levamisole alone, and no further treatment in 398 patients with resected B_2 or C lesions. Patients treated with levamisole and levamisole with 5-fluorouracil had a significant increase in disease-free survival largely due to the benefit conferred on the patients with stage C disease. These results provoked the confirmatory Intergroup trial, which entered 1,296 patients between 1985 and 1987. The most recent interim analysis allowed the data-monitor subcommittee to confirm the salutory impact of 5-fluorouracil and levamisole on survival in patients with node-positive (stage C) disease. The publication of these results has altered the Cooperative Group trials, so that 5-fluorouracil and levamisole became the control arms of the studies. This so called "new standard treatment" arm will be tested against a number of schedules of 5-fluorouracil and leucovorin, with or without levamisole, continuous prolonged infusional 5-fluorouracil, and autologous tumor vaccine. Additionally, the National Cancer Institute has now received FDA approval to make levamisole available to registered physicians for adjuvant 5-fluorouracil and levamisole treatment in patients following resection of stage C colon carcinoma under the Group C Treatment IND mechanism.

Less than 1 percent of all patients with colorectal cancer are entered into randomized trials. In order to better define optimal adjuvant therapy, patient participation is strongly advocated not only in large teaching hospitals but in the community hospital setting. Although the results of the levamisole plus 5-fluorouracil trials are encouraging, it is anticipated that even greater survival benefits await the completion of the current ongoing Intergroup adjuvant trial in colon cancer.

In contrast to the negative impact on colon carcinoma, the adjuvant use of radiation therapy has shown some promising results in rectal cancer. Several uncontrolled trials have suggested that postoperative radiation therapy may be effective in decreasing local tumor recurrence after resection of rectal carcinoma with poor prognoses. The Gastrointestinal Tumor Study Group (GITSG) conducted a randomized, controlled trial of postoperative chemoradiation therapy in surgically treated rectal carcinoma and demonstrated a significant reduction in tumor recurrences among patients receiving radiation (4,000 or 4,400 cGy) combined with 5-fluorouracil and methyl-CCNU chemotherapy compared to control patients treated with surgery alone ($P < 0.009$). Equally important was the demonstration of a survival superiority by the one-sided log rank test ($P < 0.05$). Those patients randomized to receive radiation alone or chemotherapy alone had a survival and recurrence rate that did not statistically differ from control patients. Somewhat similar confirmatory results have been recently reported by the NCCTG. These studies, when combined with others that employed prolonged, continuous infusions of 5-fluorouracil with high-dose radiation, led to the current Intergroup Cooperative Study, which compares four randomized controlled arms: arm 1 employs radiation plus sequential 5-fluorouracil and methyl-CCNU chemotherapy, arm 2 employs sequential 5-fluorouracil and methyl-CCNU chemotherapy plus radiation-protracted 5-fluorouracil, arm 3 consists of sequential 5-fluorouracil chemotherapy plus radiation-bolus 5-fluorouracil, and arm 4 employs sequential 5-fluorouracil infusion. The results of this well-conceived trial should permit more precise delineation of what constitutes optimal adjuvant therapy for node-positive rectal carcinoma.

TREATMENT OF METASTATIC COLORECTAL CANCER

For years, the treatment of cancer patients with anticancer drugs has been largely empirical. The rationale for this approach has partly been due to the lack of sensitive and selective markers and appropriate methodologies for conducting studies that would permit understanding of the mechanisms of action of each drug in individual patients with various malignancies. In most cases, tissue specimens from patients with solid tumors are only available during surgery. 5-fluorouracil has been widely employed as a single agent in varying doses and schedules for the treatment of metastatic colorectal cancers, with singularly unimpressive outcomes. Response rates seldom exceed 20 percent. The empiric addition of other chemotherapy agents such as methotrexate and methyl-CCNU to 5-fluorouracil regimens has not significantly improved upon these results. Because of the wide spectrum of marginal antitumor activity exhibited by 5-fluorouracil, and because of its potential for cytotoxicity through both RNA and DNA pathways, numerous investigators have continued to strive for methods of enhancing the therapeutic selectivity and activity of 5-fluorouracil by combining the drug with other agents. Despite promising preclinical evidence of synergistic cytotoxicity, agents such as methotrexate and thymidine yielded unimpressive clinical trial results when combined with 5-fluorouracil.

During the past 10 years, an increasing body of experimental data has accumulated that demonstrates that the cytotoxic effects of 5-fluorouracil for murine and human leukemias and carcinomas can be amplified in cell culture by increasing the intracellular pools of reduced folate. Subsequent studies performed in human colon carcinoma xenografts in athymic mice conclusively showed an enhanced tumor cytotoxicity when 5-fluorouracil was combined with high micromolar amounts (10 μM) of leucovorin (folinic acid, 5-formyl-tetrahydrofolate). This modulation of 5-fluorouracil by leucovorin appears to result from the stabilization of the ternary complex between fluorodeoxyuridylate (FdUMP), which is the active metabolite of 5-fluorouracil, thymidylate synthetase, and 5-10 methylenetetrahydrofolate (Fig. 1). In murine xenograft models of human colorectal carcinoma, prolonged high-dose infusions of leucovorin are necessary to provide the cellular levels of leucovorin needed to yield maximum enhancement of the ternary complex formation. Thus, by providing colorectal cancer cells with supraphysiologic quantities of reduced folates in the presence of the active metabolite of 5-fluorouracil (FdUMP), drug resistance is reversed, resulting in tumor cell kill. A number of phase 1 and 2 clinical trials quickly evolved that employed varying doses of leucovorin with 5-fluorouracil in metastatic colorectal cancer. The majority of these clinical trials yielded significantly higher response rates than had been previously reported with 5-fluorouracil alone. Subsequently, six phase 3 multi-institutional trials were performed that compared high-dose intravenous leucovorin and 5-fluorouracil in varying doses and schedules to 5-fluorouracil alone. The results of five of these six clinical trials demonstrated the significant therapeutic superiority of the combination regimens. Despite these promising responses, overall survival was prolonged but not to a statistically significant degree. The efficacy of so-called low-dose leucovorin (25 mg per square meter) regimens with 5-fluorouracil remains unclear because of divergent results in two large multicenter clinical trials. The GITSG study compared a low-dose leucovorin/5-fluorouracil arm with a high-dose leucovorin/5-fluorouracil arm developed at Roswell Park Institute (RPCI). This arm used leucovorin at 500 mg per square meter with 5-fluorouracil at 600 mg per square meter weekly for 6 weeks. The high-dose leucovorin/5-fluorouracil arm of the study was clearly superior to the low-dose arm. In contrast, the NCCTG reported that a low-dose leucovorin/5-fluorouracil schedule appeared to yield better results than a high-dose leucovorin/5-fluorouracil arm. Based on the results of these phase 3 trials, a large Intergroup study has been activated that employs two dose schedules of leucovorin/5-fluorouracil, with or without levamisole, as adjuvant

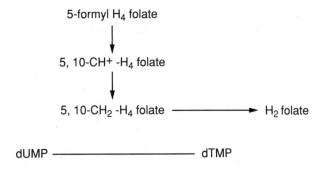

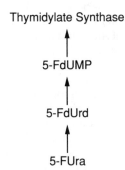

Figure 1 Metabolism of 5 fluorouracil (5-FUra) and modulation of thymidylate synthase inhibition by 5, 10-methylenetetrahydrofolate.

therapy in node-positive colon cancer. One large phase 2 trial has recently been completed that utilized the pharmacokinetic advantages of orally administered high-dose leucovorin with 5-fluorouracil for previously untreated metastatic colorectal cancer. This trial achieved a 48 percent overall response rate with a significant number of complete responders. The median overall survival of these patients exceeded 15 months. The dose and schedule of oral leucovorin and intravenous 5-fluorouracil employed in this trial will be tested in a phase 3 Eastern Cooperative Oncology Group (ECOG) study for metastatic colorectal cancer (vida infra).

Recent preclinical and clinical studies have renewed investigator interest in PALA (*N*-[phosphonacetyl]-L-aspartic acid) as a biochemical modulator for 5-fluorouracil in colorectal cancer. Despite its broad spectrum of clinical antitumor activity against murine solid tumors, PALA as a single agent exhibits no activity in human tumors. Pharmacologic and biochemical studies have demonstrated that PALA can inhibit ACTase (aspartate carbamyl transferase) in normal *and* tumor tissue. Many of the early clinical trials combining PALA and 5-fluorouracil employed an inverse dose relationship with much higher doses of PALA than were needed to modulate 5-fluorouracil. Recently, however, several phase 1 and 2 clinical trials in metastatic colorectal cancer have combined a lower weekly dosage schedule of PALA (250 mg per square meter) with a higher dose of 5-fluorouracil (2.6 to 3.4 g per square meter). The overall objective response rates varied from 40 percent to 50 percent. These clinical response rates in metastatic

colorectal cancer were impressive and are comparable to those reported with high-dose leucovorin and 5-fluorouracil. Currently, the ECOG is mounting a phase 3 clinical trial that compares the following regimens: (1) high-dose intravenous leucovorin/5-fluorouracil (RPCI); (2) high-dose oral leucovorin/5-fluorouracil; (3) PALA/-5-fluorouracil; and (4) a high-dose 5-fluorouracil control arm. The results of this study should provide data that will allow a more rational treatment strategy for the adjuvant setting.

A third class of biomodulating agents that have been under investigation are the interferons. These cytokines have been shown to possess modulation activity for a number of chemotherapeutic agents by increasing their cytotoxic and antiproliferative capabilities. Alpha-interferon, when combined with 5-fluorouracil in tumor cell cultures, will amplify the cytotoxicity of the metabolite FdUMP. Further studies in human colon cancer cell lines demonstrated that the addition of recombinant alpha-interferon (rIFNα) to 5-fluorouracil caused an enhancement of the cytotoxic effects observed with 5-fluorouracil alone. Based on these preclinical observations, a phase 1 pilot study employing rIFNα and 5-fluorouracil for metastatic colorectal cancer was completed by Wadler and associates. There were no responses documented in those patients who had received prior chemotherapy; however, a response rate of 76 percent was documented in 17 previously untreated patients. This response rate dropped to 60 percent when additional patients were enrolled into the study. The estimated 1-year survival rate was estimated to be approximately 60 percent. Because of these promising preliminary results, the ECOG is currently conducting a confirmatory phase 2 clinical trial for previously untreated patients with metastatic colorectal cancer. If this trial does confirm the efficacy of rIFNα and 5-fluorouracil in metastatic disease, the next logical step would be to compare all three biomodulation compounds (leucovorin, PALA, rIFNα) with 5-fluorouracil in a large randomized, controlled clinical trial in metastatic colorectal carcinoma. One or all of these combinations will ultimately be moved into the postsurgical adjuvant setting.

SUGGESTED READING

Ardalan B. A randomized Phase I and II study of short-term infusion of high dose fluorouracil with or without *N*-(phosphonacetyl)-L-aspartic acid in patients with advanced pancreatic and colorectal cancers. J Clin Oncol 1988; 6:1053–1058.

Petrelli N, Douglass HO, Herrera L, et al. The modulation of fluorouracil with leucovorin in metastatic colorectal carcinoma: A prospective randomized Phase III trial. J Clin Oncol 1989; 17:1419–1426.

Rustum YM, McGuire J, eds. Advances in experimental medicine and biology, vol 244. Proceedings of an international symposium on the expanding role of folates and fluoropyrimidines in cancer chemotherapy, Rosewell Park Memorial Institute, Buffalo, NY, April, 1988.

Wadler S, Schwartz EI, Goldman M, et al. Fluorouracil and recombinant alpha-2a-interferon: An active regimen against advanced colorectal carcinoma. J Clin Oncol 1989; 7:1769–1775.

PRIMARY LIVER CANCERS

STANLEY E. ORDER, M.D., Sc.D., F.A.C.R.
GARY B. STILLWAGON, Ph.D., M.D.
DAVID S. ETTINGER, M.D.

Hepatocellular cancer often presents in an insidious manner because the liver can expand and become quite massive without symptoms. Patients fortunate enough to present early with symptoms may be resectable, but the bulk of patients remain nonresectable at presentation.

RESECTABLE HEPATOMA

Following diagnosis by biopsy, resectable patients require careful evaluation with computed tomography (CT), including arteriographic studies, to demonstrate the potential for resection prior to laparotomy. It is our opinion that patients for whom diagnostic studies would indicate resectability are not properly managed if full diagnostic studies are not completed prior to laparotomy. The diagnostic battery should include chest films, a gallium scan for metastatic disease, as well as full tomography and other appropriate studies for metastatic disease. Often, alpha-fetoprotein (AFP) titers are associated with hepatocellular cancer in the differential diagnosis of metastatic versus primary liver tumors; however, one should realize that from 20 to 30 percent of hepatocellular cancers may not have an associated AFT titer elevation, more so in western societies than in the eastern world. Usually cholangiocarcinomas of the liver, another primary liver tumor, are inadvertently discovered when patients are evaluated for hepatocellular cancer. Pathologists, in evaluating liver biopsy specimens, almost always place the proviso of "cannot with certainty distinguish from metastatic disease," thus requiring clinical acumen as part of the evaluation.

Of those patients deemed resectable, a relapse will occur in as high as 90 percent of those resected. Therefore, an arduous, careful CT evaluation on a monthly basis for at least 2 years, as well as serial AFP titers in those patients who are known to be AFP-positive for 3 years, is recommended and followed at our institution. Tumor volumetrics are available from our CT evaluation; we carry out secondary evaluations by taking tape recordings of serial CT slices every 8 mm and by analyzing, pixel by pixel, the entire liver for each return visit for that 2-year duration. As a potential therapeutic prophylaxis, we have carried out hepatitis B vaccination in those patients who are not positive for hepatitis B antigen or antibody, in the hope that prevention of induction factors would occur on the basis of such immunization; however, there is no scientific proof that these assumptions are valid. There may be several causes for relapse following surgical resection, including the following:

1. Relapse at the surgical margins due to technical difficulties with invasive tumors
2. Stimulation by factors that cause regrowth of the normal liver in surgically resected liver, causing regrowth of the tumor
3. Reinduction of tumor in the template of a previously tumor bearing liver

If the patient had an AFP-positive tumor, it has generally been our policy to continue follow up after 2 years on a trimonthly basis with CT scans, utilizing the AFP titer on a monthly basis for at least an additional year. The advantage of such arduous, careful follow-up in the first 3 years following surgery lies in the fact that early relapse, which may be resectable, can be surgically removed prior to presentation with massive or multifocal nonresectable lesions.

NONRESECTABLE HEPATOMA

Various morphologic and biochemical modifiers in nonresectable hepatocellular cancers can indicate the type of clinical approach that should be utilized in the management of the malignancy. For example, high-titer AFP-positive tumors will have a growth rate between 30 and 42 days, and as such will need immediate clinical intervention and cytoreduction if they are to be controlled. This contrasts with hepatocellular tumors that do not have an elevated AFP titer, tumors we have termed *AFP-negative*. These tumors tend to have a slower doubling time, allowing the physician greater opportunity for determining the most effective therapeutic intervention. More classic interpretations, such as well-differentiated or poorly differentiated hepatocellular cancer, also refer to growth rate; the poorly differentiated tumor is associated with elevated AFP titers, and the more well-differentiated tumor is associated with lower titers and less tumor-supportive vasculature. Cirrhosis of the liver may be an important factor in the etiology as well as the treatment of hepatocellular tumors. The diffuse fine cirrhosis of the more classic alcoholic exposure contrasts with the macronodular cirrhosis associated with hepatitis B and seen primarily in the eastern world. The latter has more recently been demonstrated to be associated with hepatitis C as well. The ability to resect, even utilizing wedge resection, may be limited not by the massive size of the tumor but by the density of cirrhosis that may be associated with the primary malignancy in these cases. In our own experience of 100 patients evaluated for hepatitis as a background etiologic factor, 13 percent had hepatitis C and 7 percent had hepatitis B. The remaining patients did not have hepatitis virus as a known etiologic factor.

Active "relapsing" hepatitis must be distinguished, in our opinion, from the presence of hepatitis B antigen or hepatitis B antibody owing to the fact that any cytotoxic measures, whether chemotherapy, radiotherapy, or radiolabeled antibody therapy, may induce relapse of active viral hepatitis in patients with a history of previous viral hepatitis relapse. In such circumstances, liver enzyme levels and poor liver chemistries may lead to a fatal outcome from hepatitis. The literature well documents the extreme danger of attempts to treat patients with hepatocellular cancer who have known active relapses of hepatitis virus infections.

Other etiologic factors, such as hemochromatosis, which is an iron-storage disorder, play a role in considering radiolabeled antibody therapy and potential toxicity as well. For example, the risk of thorotrast toxicity from previous scans or the effects of prolonged irradiation prior to hepatocellular cancer expression, make absolute clinical approaches difficult to formulate. We recommend that use of radiolabeled antiferritin be preceded by a scanning dose to ensure appropriate tumor targeting. We do not recommend the use of radioactive sources and radiation in the treatment of thorotrast-induced hepatoma if other approaches are possible, because tolerance to chronic radiation exposure will be unknown.

Several factors in patients that affect prognosis and therapeutic approaches include the presence or absence of ascites and the presence or absence of jaundice. Ascites clearly demonstrates marked damage to the liver and makes all cytotoxic approaches difficult and less successful. In contrast, although jaundice is certainly a poor prognostic indicator, we have found remission possible in jaundiced patients. *We do not consider adriamycin and 5-fluorouracil administered intravenously to be the drugs of choice in the treatment of nonresectable hepatocellular cancer.* Therefore, we do not consider the inability to treat with adriamycin a significant loss in the management of patients if their bilirubin levels are elevated. Not only is adriamycin ineffective in the treatment of this malignancy but full-dose treatment may reduce the patient's quality of life; moreover, median survival is no greater than 5 to 6 months. For jaundiced patients, we recommend intra-arterial cisplatin as the first-line chemotherapeutic approach in hepatocellular cancer.

The first observations of the value of cisplatin in the primary management of nonresectable hepatocellular cancer were made simultaneously in Finland and Japan. In the United States, randomized prospective studies using intravenous cisplatin clearly indicated the inefficacy of the drug. We carried out studies with external-beam irradiation and intravenous cisplatin followed by intra-arterial cisplatin, and demonstrated that AFP-positive patients who formerly had a 5-month median survival with adriamycin and 5-fluorouracil could achieve a 16-month median survival when using 50 mg per square meter of cisplatin intra-arterially on a monthly basis (Fig. 1). Not only was hematologic toxicity

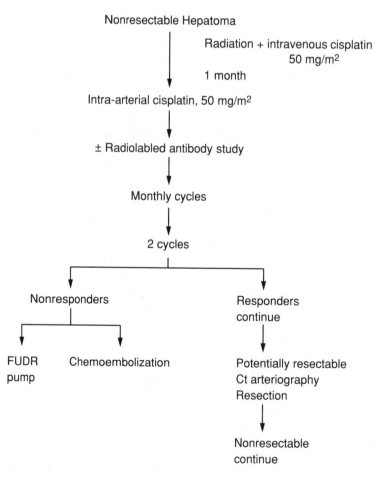

Figure 1 Schema for management of nonresectable hepatocellular cancer.

reduced and the ability to deliver therapy on a monthly basis enhanced but therapeutic reduction of the tumor and improvement in quality of life were obvious. Significantly, some of these patients were frankly jaundiced.

We are presently evaluating the efficacy of integrating intra-arterial cisplatin with iodine-131 antiferritin. We have demonstrated in our laboratory that the low-dose radiation from anti-iodine-131 ferritin combined with cisplatin is more lethal to hepatocellular cancer. This is likely due to shifts in G2 and M phases of the cancer cells as well as to a loss of sublethal repair. It will ultimately be necessary to confirm such findings in a randomized prospective study in order to determine whether the combined treatment further enhances the cytotoxic response in nonresectable hepatoma compared to intra-arterial cisplatin treatment alone.

REMISSION ANALYSIS

We reject the concept that the physical examination of the number of centimeters below the costal margin represents an adequate and scientific review of remission of hepatocellular cancer. A system of tumor volumetric analysis by serial CT scan, requiring complete pixel by pixel evaluation every 8 mm throughout the liver, remains the most objective method of evaluating progression and remission when considered in conjunction with AFP titers, liver chemistries, and physical examination. Clearly, physical examination in the case of cirrhosis with a reduced liver is of no value. It is clear that, in the instance of multifocal or diffuse disease, measurement of 1 diameter of a lesion does not reflect the entire pathophysiologic alteration within the liver. It is also clear that, in patients without an AFP titer, tumor volumetrics is the single objective analysis of tumor remission. Tumor volumetrics becomes a problem sometimes in dense cirrhosis with a diffuse tumor, and magnetic resonance imaging (MRI) may be superior to CT-type analysis. We have made this tumor volumetric analysis available to general hospitals upon request. A grant to aid in training individuals and to obtain the necessary software is available, if the institution pays for the individual physicist to come for the training program.

NEW FRONTIERS IN THE TREATMENT OF NONRESECTABLE HEPATOCELLULAR CANCER

Multiple opportunities with new protocols exist for managing hepatocellular cancer in the future. Bifunctional antibodies, for example, provide new directions in therapy. Bifunctional antibodies have one Fab end that recognizes the tumor and the other end that recognizes the chelate. Administration of the bifunctional antibody can be followed the next day by infusion of the chelate-carrying isotope, creating a higher dose to the tumor-bearing region. Another potentially effective approach is the use of human monoclonal antiferritin, which is presently being investigated in preclinical trials.

Recent laboratory studies of low-dose-rate radiation produced by radiolabeled antibodies indicate increased sensitivity both to chemotherapy and radiation therapy as a result of shifting cells to G2 and M, the more sensitive phases of the cell cycle, as well as a loss of sublethal cellular repair as the radiation is prolonged in time. Exploiting this observation may hold promise for broadening approaches to treatment of nonresectable hepatocellular cancer as well. The precise means by which multimodal applications should be carried out still remain to be determined in a series of studies. It is clear, however, that the further remission is possible. The goal of such multimodal therapy is the conversion of nonresectable hepatoma to resectability. In our present circumstance, long-term survivors beyond 2, 3, and 4 years have been converted to surgical resectability only when radiolabeled antibody is one of the multimodality agents.

INTRAHEPATIC CHOLANGIOCARCINOMA

Most often the diagnosis of a cholangiocarcinoma originating at a primary site in the liver is made following biopsy for presumed hepatocellular cancer. However, the tumor tissue usually stains with anti-CEA, less often with AFP, and rarely with ferritin. Pathologists often add the proviso, "although the tumor represents cholangiocarcinoma, a metastatic adenocarcinoma could not be ruled out." Thus, the physician must have a thorough evaluation of possible primary sites of malignancy prior to acceptance of the final diagnosis.

All of the patients we have seen are nonresectable, with or without metastasis. The work-up, including tumor volumetrics, is similar to that for hepatoma. We treat metastatic lesions conventionally but with full control doses by external radiation and drugs concomitant with liver irradiation to the tumor-bearing region using adriamycin, 15 mg, and 5-fluorouracil, 500 mg, every other treatment day. Total treatment consists of 2,100 rad at 300-rad fractions 4 days a week, followed 1 month later in our initial protocol with 15 mg of adriamycin, 500 mg of 5-fluorouracil, and 20 mCi of iodine-131 anti-CEA on day 1 and 10 mCi on day 5. More recently, we have added 20 mg per square meter of cisplatin. Median survival in the literature for patients with nonresectable cholangiocarcinoma was 4 months; our first trial achieved 6.5 months, and now 10 1/2 months has been realized. The longest survivor lived 4.4 years from the start of treatment.

METASTATIC HEPATOCELLULAR CANCER

Two classes of patients have presented themselves over the last several years with metastatic hepatocellular cancer. They include patients with liver transplants and patients with primary liver tumors that are metastatic. In the former instance, the marked hematopoietic depression, despite good peripheral counts, has always been reflected by the severe hematopoietic toxicity resulting from the use of any chemotherapy or radiolabeled antibody therapy. We have not as yet found a series of agents that can be safely utilized in these patients without significant and unexpected hematologic depression. We presume that the agents necessary to achieve immunosuppression for the liver transplant in part significantly damage the hematopoietic system, therefore limiting the subsequent therapy in these patients. However, external radiation has proved of value when administered in conventional doses to patients with metastatic lesions and liver transplants.

In contrast, those patients presenting with a primary tumor and metastatic disease have responded in more conventional ways to the therapies utilized in the management of their primary and metastatic tumors. Management of metastatic disease in such patients by radiation with chemotherapy or radiolabeled antibody concomitantly to full dose, in addition, in our most recent protocols, to appropriate management of the primary with cisplatin and radiolabeled antibodies, has proved satisfactory. Obviously, with new developing protocols and better agents, further insight will be gained as progress occurs.

Some patients presenting with lung metastasis may achieve several years of remission if their primary tumor is controlled. It has been exceedingly rare for pulmonary metastasis to be the fatal event in advanced hepatocellular cancer. *The focus of treatment should be on the primary tumor and its control.* Most often, conventional radiation or other techniques can control the metastatic lesions.

Intraperitoneal dissemination, similar to ovarian cancer, has occasionally occurred when good local control has been achieved. In such cases, we have found that intraperitoneal radiolabeled antibody (iodine-131 antiferritin) has reduced the AFP titers and led to remission. To date, up to three remission cycles are given monthly. Based on new information, cisplatin will be integrated into future studies.

THE ROLE OF CHEMOEMBOLIZATION

In our opinion, chemoembolization often leads to remission in a significant number of hepatocellular cancers. The difficulty with the procedure is that, after chemoembolization, there is significant limitation for further therapeutic applications. Thus, we have favored intra-arterial cisplatin as the primary approach, with intra-arterial FUDR as a secondary approach, and chemoembolization as a last effort in the management of nonresectable hepatocellular cancer. Our interest in radiolabeled antibody therapy and the fact that the only patients who have been converted from nonresectable to resectable have been those patients treated with radiolabeled antibody have led us to attempt to integrate radiolabeled antibody with the appropriate chemotherapy. As we continue these trials, patients entering our programs first receive cisplatin and radiolabeled antibody treatment; should these fail, they are offered other agents. Chemoembolization is given as the last attempt at remission should all other agents fail. Therapy initiated with chemoembolization cannot include intra-arterial cisplatin and radiolabeled antibody treatment within a reasonable time frame. It is our firm conviction that multimodal therapy will continue to improve results in the management of this hepatocellular cancer. The sequence and best agents remain under evaluation.

It is our belief that best patient management for nonresectable hepatocellular cancer requires patient management in clinical trials rather than by the physician on an individual basis. This is the only way that clinical progress and better therapy can be developed. The preceding therapeutic methods have clearly demonstrated progress in this field from our earlier experience with AFP-positive hepatocellular cancer, in which we had a 5-month median survival regardless of the method of treatment, to a present-day 16-month median survival, and significant improvement in conversion of nonresectable hepatocellular cancer to resectable cancer. At the time of the writing of this report, our first series of successfully treated patients will have remained disease-free for 5 years.

HOW DO WE MANAGE ASCITES?

We do not accept ascites and peripheral edema as status quo if they can possibly be medically managed. Thus, Lasix and Aldactone are used concomitantly to control ascites and edema because it is our impression that both intra-arterial cisplatin and radiolabeled antibody treatment are enhanced by the reduction of a third compartment loss as well as by more complete infusion into the liver. In addition, we advise patients who have either enlarged livers or pressure secondary to ascites to have at least five small meals a day, which will allow them to maintain their nutrition throughout the course of therapy.

HOW IS THE INTRA-ARTERIAL PHASE OF CISPLATIN MANAGEMENT CARRIED OUT?

We initiate intra-arterial cisplatin therapy by threading a catheter in the femoral artery to the hepatic artery, where infusion takes place. This is done monthly times two, before the tumor is evaluated. If there is evidence of tumor remission, an Infusaid pump is considered; should cisplatin prove over the long term to be no longer effective, FUDR could be utilized. The side port could be utilized for cisplatin, and the pump itself could be used for the FUDR, if necessary. Because radiolabeled antibody has no advantage by the direct arterial route, intravenous administration is utilized. The goal of this management remains the conversion of nonresectable hepatocellular cancer to resectable cancer.

SUGGESTED READING

Ettinger DS, Leichner PK, Siegelman SS, et al. Computed tomography assisted volumetric analysis of primary liver tumor as a measure of response to therapy. Am J Clin Oncol 1985; 8:413–418.

Epstein B, Ettinger D, Leichner P, et al. Multimodality cisplatin treatment in nonresectable AFP positive hepatoma: Preliminary results. Int J Radiat Oncol Biol Phys 1989; 17:185.

Order SE, Stillwagon GB, Klein JL, et al. I-131 antiferritin: A new treatment modality in hepatoma: An RTOG study. J Clin Oncol 1985; 3:1573–1582.

Sitzmann JV, Order SE, Klein JL, et al. Conversion by new treatment modalities of nonresectable to resectable hepatocellular cancer. J Clin Oncol 1987; 5:1566–1573.

Stillwagon GB, Order SE, Guse C, et al. 194 Hepatocellular cancers treated by radiation and chemotherapy combinations: Toxicity and response: A Radiation Therapy Oncology Group study. Int J Radiat Oncol Biol Phys 1989; 17:1223–1229.

Tang ZY, Liu MD, Bao YM, et al. Radioimmunotherapy in the multimodality treatment of hepatocellular carcinoma with reference to second look resection. Cancer 1990; 65:211–215.

LUNG CANCER: RADIATION THERAPY

WILLIAM T. SAUSE, M.D.

Lung cancer will cause 142,000 deaths in 1990. Lung cancer deaths represent one-quarter of the cancer deaths in the United States and represent not only a health hazard in the United States but worldwide. Unfortunately, cure rates for lung cancer have ranged between 11 percent and 13 percent over the past 10 years. Although the overall picture is discouraging, the magnitude of this health problem is such that small improvements in treatment can affect large numbers of patients.

Surgical therapy remains the mainstay of curative treatment in this disease. Unfortunately, a minority of patients are candidates for surgery. Cytotoxic chemotherapy has improved, but overall its impact on survival has been small, and toxicity prohibits its general application. Irradiation, although rarely curative, represents a useful tool in the many patients with this disease. The purpose of this chapter is to discuss the application of irradiation in the management of patients with bronchogenic carcinoma.

NON–SMALL-CELL LUNG CANCER

Epithelial tumors of the lung tend to respond to ionizing irradiation in a fashion similar to epithelial neoplasms of other organ sites. Unfortunately, patients with bronchogenic tumors usually present with advanced local regional disease and have a high likelihood of systemic disease. Both factors, the amount of local regional disease and the propensity for distant spread, have a substantial negative impact on the effectiveness of irradiation.

Occasionally, a patient is referred for irradiation who would otherwise be a candidate for surgery. These patients normally exhibit a medical contraindication to operative management. Table 1 depicts results of several

Table 1 Patients Treated with Irradiation

Group	5-Year Survival (%)	
Leiden	16	(38% tumor < 2 cm)
Virginia	17	
Fox Chase	22	(34% tumor < 3 cm)

Table 2 Patients Referred for Irradiation Who Have Locally Advanced Tumor

Author	5-Year Survival (%)
Aristozabel	8
Emami	11
Deeley	6
Guttman	10

Table 3 Patients Treated with Preoperative Irradiation and Subsequent Resection

Author	No Evidence of Tumor in Resected Specimen (%)
Bloedorn	54
Bromley	50
Hellman	70
Shields	25
Total	41

series. Although these results tend to be inferior to surgical resection, they confirm the ability of irradiation to sterilize tumor and provide long-term survival in a group of patients with lung cancer. Many of these patients are elderly or in poor health.

Unfortunately, most patients referred for irradiation have locally advanced tumor. In this setting, the long-term survival with irradiation is poor. Table 2 depicts the results of several series. Most investigators report long-term survival of between 5 percent and 12 percent in this group of patients. Although these results are discouraging, useful information has been gained from these reports that will hopefully direct future studies.

Table 4 Radiation Therapy Oncology Group Trials Using
Irradiation in Lung Cancer

Trial Number	Design	Results
73–01	4,000 cGy split-course 4,000–6,000 cGy continuous	High-toxicity split-course therapy improved local control and short-term survival with higher dose
78–11	6,000 cGy ± levamisole for unresectable cancer	No benefit to levamisole
79–27	Postresection radiation + levamisole	No benefit to levamisole
79–17	6,000 cGy + misonidasole	No benefit to misonidasole
78–14	Large Fx radiation ± misonidasole	No benefit to misonidasole
83–21	6,000 cGy ± thymosin	No benefit to thymosin
83–11	120 cGy bid and 6,000 cGy–7,920 cGy	Improved survival to 6,960 cGy, and no higher toxicity
88–04	Vinblastine/platinum + 6,000 cGy	Good tolerance to vinblastine/platinum + radiation

Table 5 Results of Five Trials Using Chemotherapy and
Radiation Therapy Protocols

Group	Agents	Results
Finnish Lung Cancer Group	Radiation ± CAP	No benefit
Milan	Radiation ± cisplatin/DDP	No benefit
SWOG	Radiation ± Fomi/CAP	No benefit
NCCTG	Radiation ± MACC	No benefit
CALGB	Radiation ± vinblastine/platinum	Benefit to VP

SWOG = Southwest Oncology Group, NCCTG = North Central Cancer Treatment Group, CALGB = Cancer and Leukemia Group B, CAP = Cyclophosphamide Adriamycin Cisplatin, DDP = Cisplatin, FOMI = 5-FU, Oncovin, Mitomycin-C, MACC = Methotrexate, Doxirubicin-Cyclophosphamide–CCNCl.

In the 1960s and 1970s, preoperative external-beam irradiation was applied in many institutions. Table 3 summarizes the results of several surgical series in which preoperative irradiation was utilized. As noted in Table 3, irradiation was able to eradicate the tumor pathologically in approximately one-third to one-half of the patients undergoing surgical resection.

In 1973, the Radiation Therapy Oncology Group (RTOG) initiated a trial randomizing unresectable patients with locoregional tumor to 4,000 cGy split course irradiation versus 4,000 cGy to 6,000 cGy of continuous irradiation. This trial confirmed a dose-response relationship of lung cancer to external-beam irradiation. Not only was local control enhanced but short-term survival improved with escalation of the dose to 6,000 cGy. Unfortunately, overall survival greater than 5 years was not improved by escalating dose in these patients.

Despite improvements in local control with escalating doses, local failure continues to remain a substantial problem in patients undergoing irradiation. Unpublished data from the RTOG suggest that as many as 70 percent of patients receiving 6,000 cGy will ultimately fail in the thorax. Cox has analyzed the sites of failure and causes of death in over 300 patients and found a high incidence of death caused by locally advanced lung cancer.

Data from the preoperative use of irradiation and trials conducted in unresectable patients suggest a dose response of lung cancer to external-beam irradiation. Investigational efforts involving irradiation for lung cancer have attempted to capitalize on the dose-response relationship and increase the biologic effectiveness of irradiation. Whether biologically more effective irradiation will translate into improved local control and survival remains to be answered.

It is impossible to summarize all clinical trials utilizing irradiation in lung cancer. The RTOG has provided leadership and direction for many clinical trials for patients with locally advanced unresectable lung cancer. In general, the design of these trials has paralleled investigational efforts in the use of irradiation in other tumor sites. Table 4 contains the results of some of the RTOG trials conducted in the past 15 years. As previously noted, RTOG 73-01 represented a dose-escalating trial from 4,000 cGy to 6,000 cGy and one arm with 4,000 cGy split-course irradiation. This trial reported a high toxicity to split-course irradiation and improved local control with escalating doses. Detailed analyses of this trial also identified several important prognostic features. Those features most likely associated with improved survival were good Karnofsky performance status and minimal weight loss. These findings were not unique to the RTOG studies, and other groups have noted similar prognostic features.

The RTOG conducted three trials with nonspecific immunologic stimulants using levamisole and thymosin. In these trials, no benefit was noted to the use of these agents. Several trials were also conducted with the use of a hypoxic cell sensitizer, misonidasole. These trials failed to reveal any benefit to the use of this agent.

In 1980, the RTOG embarked on several trials incorporating the use of altered fractionation. These trials were based on the biologic observation suggesting an improvement in the therapeutic ratio with altered fractionation. Preliminary reports from other disease

Figure 1   RTOG 83–11

S	Cell Type	R	Arm 1: Conventional radiation therapy—60 Gy/6 wk
T	Squamous versus other	A	
R		N	Arm 2: Vinblastine weekly × 5 + cisplatin on days 1 and 29 Radiation (as in arm 1) begins day 50
A	Performance Status	D	
T	70–80 versus 90–100	O	
I		M	
F	Stage II, IIIA, IIIB	I	
Y		Z	Arm 3: Hyperfractionated radiation—total dose is 69.6 Gy.
		E	

Table 6   Results of Series in Which Irradiation Has Been Used as an Adjuvant to Surgical Resection

Author	Treatment	Survival (%)	
Green	Surgery	3	
	Radiation therapy	35	
Kirsch	Surgery	0	
	Radiation therapy	23	
Choi	Surgery	8 adenomatous	33 squamous
	Radiation therapy	43 adenomatous	34 squamous
Israel	Surgery	45	
	Radiation therapy	67	

Table 7   Results of Randomized Studies Analyzing Effectiveness of Irradiation Following Surgical Resection

Group	Treatment	Survival (%)
Van Houtte	Surgery	43
	Surgery + radiation therapy	24
Lung Cancer Study Group	Surgery	40
	Surgery + radiation therapy	40

sites also suggested benefit to this approach. RTOG 83-11 was the largest trial conducted incorporating altered fractionation (Figure 1). In this trial, patients were randomized to 120 cGy twice a day in a dose-escalating fashion from 6,000 cGy to 79.2 cGy. The RTOG was able to demonstrate tolerance to these aggressive treatment regimens as well as what appeared to be an improvement in survival at doses of approximately 7,000 cGy.

In the past 10 years, encouraging reports with the use of cytotoxic chemotherapy in lung cancer have stimulated interest in chemotherapy and radiation therapy protocols. Table 5 reflects the results of five such trials. Of the trials depicted, only one trial has shown a benefit in survival as a result of the use of cytotoxic chemotherapy with external-beam irradiation. The Cancer and Leukemia Group B (CALGB) trial randomized patients to 2 months of cisplatin and vinblastine prior to external-beam irradiation versus irradiation alone consisting of 60 Gy. This trial did attribute a statistical benefit in survival to the experimental arm. The RTOG has also conducted a pilot study utilizing vinblastine and platinum with concurrent platinum during the irradiation. This phase 2 trial also suggests a benefit to chemotherapy and irradiation when compared to historic controls. Based on the preliminary results of RTOG 83-11 and the encouraging results of the CALGB trial, the National Cancer Institute has encouraged a high-priority trial for unresectable non–small-cell lung cancer randomizing the experimental arms of hyperfractionated irradiation and chemotherapy with irradiation against standard irradiation consisting of 60 Gy in 6 weeks (Fig. 1).

External-beam irradiation represents a potentially curative modality in patients with non–small-cell lung cancer. Unfortunately, the curative potential is relatively small and related to the amount of tumor in the thorax at presentation and the clinical condition of the patient. A dose-response relationship can be demonstrated to irradiation, and it is hoped that biologic improvement in delivery will improve results.

Irradiation as an adjuvant to surgical resection in non–small-cell lung cancer is an area of controversy. Several retrospective series are reflected in Table 6. Most historical series suggest a benefit to mediastinal irradiation. In these series, irradiation was applied in selective cases with ominous prognostic features. In most instances, these ominous prognostic features include the presence of hilar and mediastinal nodes.

Two randomized studies have also been conducted analyzing the effectiveness of irradiation following surgical resection. These are reflected in Table 7. In the series conducted by Van Houtte, patients with N0 disease were randomized to receive postoperative irra-

Table 8 Results of Prospective Trials Following Irradiation

	No Radiation		Radiation	
Group	Local Control (%)	Survival of 2–3 years (%)	Local Control (%)	Survival of 2–3 years (%)
SEG	45	14	65	20
CALGB	25	8	60	22
National Cancer Institute	55	10	80	25

CALGB = Cancer and Leukemia Group B, SEG = Southeast Oncology Group.

Table 9 Results of Single-Arm Trials Using Irradiation and Chemotherapy Concurrently

Group	Median Survival
Southwest Oncology Group	19 mo
National Cancer Institute	15 mo
University of Pennsylvania	> 24 mo

diation. There was a survival disadvantage to those receiving irradiation following surgical resection. In the Lung Cancer Study Group (LCSG) study, patients with stage II or III disease of squamous histology were randomized to receive irradiation or no irradiation. Unfortunately, only 20 percent of the patients in the LCSG had positive mediastinal nodes. Approximately 100 patients were randomized to each arm. Irradiation did improve local control, but no improvement in overall survival was noted in the study. Irradiation, when utilized following surgical resection, improves local control; however, the impact on survival remains questionable because the two prospectively conducted trials failed to address the issue in patients with N2 disease.

Radiation therapy, if not potentially curative, does have substantial palliative benefit in those patients undergoing treatment. Standard irradiation can induce at least a 50 percent reduction in the visible tumor approximately 60 percent of the time. Twenty percent of patients in RTOG 73-01 exhibited a complete radiographic response to treatment. Although not translating into permanent control, this does translate into good tumor shrinkage and, in many cases, alleviation of discomforting symptoms. A multitude of irradiation schedules have been proposed for patients with locally advanced disease. Many devised treatment schedules can be applied successfully when the goal of treatment is primarily palliative. Schedules that deliver biologically effective treatment and do not socially inconvenience the patient are of great utility. One need not place undue emphasis on the prevention of late complications in this group of patients. Treatment schedules can be more rapid and less socially inconvenient. Irradiation can also offer palliative benefit to those patients with central nervous system and skeletal metastases who are suffering debilitating symptoms.

The use of endobronchial irradiation has paralleled the development of fiberoptic bronchoscopy. Often exophytic tumor masses from bronchogenic carcinoma can cause debilitating symptoms consisting of hemoptysis, cough, and obstruction. Bronchoscopically applied laser therapy can reduce the symptomatic lesion, and irradiation applied endobronchially can further reduce the tumor mass for enhanced palliation. Irradiation delivered in this fashion can be done in two ways. Low-dose-rate endobronchial irradiation requires hospitalization for several days following placement of a radioactive source under endoscopic guidance. Because the radiation is delivered in a low-dose-rate fashion, the patient requires the appliance for several hours, necessitating hospital admission. High-dose-rate endobronchial therapy can be delivered in a matter of minutes on an outpatient basis following bronchoscopic placement. Unfortunately, high-dose-rate equipment is expensive, and the biologic effectiveness is not different from low-dose-rate applications. Investigators from the Mayo Clinic report response rates of 50 percent to 75 percent depending on the presenting symptoms.

SMALL-CELL LUNG CANCER

Small-cell carcinoma of the lung obviously represents a systemic disease. Most modern clinical trials have emphasized questions relative to the systemic management of this illness. Unfortunately, most patients continue to die of this illness, and long-term survival is less than 10 percent.

In the 1960s, the Medical Research Council of the United Kingdom randomized patients with small-cell lung cancer to irradiation versus surgery. At 5 years, 5 percent of the patients were alive, all in the radiotherapeutic arm. Radiation therapy became the standard treatment for small-cell lung cancer. In the 1970s, single-agent chemotherapy and, subsequently, combination chemotherapy steadily improved the median survival of patients with small-cell lung cancer. Unfortunately, aggressive attempts to optimize chemotherapy have failed to improve overall survival. These attempts have included maintenance chemotherapy, reinduction chemotherapy, or late intensification with bone marrow transplant. A plateau in median survival

Figure 2   RTOG 88–15

| Limited-stage small-cell lung cancer | R A N D O M I Z E | Arm 1: DDP/vinblastine/cisplatin × 4 cycles + concurrent standard radiation, 180 cGy qd 4,500 cGy Schedule radiation

Arm 2: DDP/vinblastine/cisplatin × 4 cycles + concurrent MDF TRT-3 150 cGy bid 4,500 cGy Schedule radiation |

DDP = cisplatin, MDF = Multiple Daily Fractions, TRT-3 = Treatment, 3 weeks

Table 10   Results of Studies Using Prophylactic Cranial Irradiation

Author	CNS Relapse	Survival
Cox	No	No
Beiler	Yes	No
Hirsch	No	No
Seydel	Yes	No
Aisner	Yes	No

and overall survival has resulted in renewed interest in local therapy.

Table 8 reflects the results of several prospective trials involving irradiation. Approximately 11 trials have been conducted evaluating the role of irradiation. Taken together, they suggest a small but statistically insignificant benefit to irradiation in limited disease. The three recent trials listed are all prospectively randomized, and all suggest a significant survival as well as local control benefit to irradiation.

Recently, single-arm trials conducted by the Southwest Oncology Group, the University of Pennsylvania, and National Cancer Institute report a substantial improvement in median survival with concurrent chemotherapy and irradiation (Table 9). The University of Pennsylvania and National Cancer Institute trials utilized twice-daily irradiation in an aggressive fashion delivered with concurrent chemotherapy. Because of the enthusiasm with these trials, the Eastern Cooperative Oncology Group (ECOG) and RTOG have embarked on a phase 3 trial analyzing the effectiveness of altered fractionation versus standard irradiation in limited-stage small-cell lung cancer (Fig. 2). It appears as if aggressive irradiation can reproducibly improve the disease-free survival of patients with limited disease. The dose of irradiation, timing of treatment, and selection of chemotherapeutic agents used with irradiation are areas of investigation.

Prophylactic cranial irradiation (PCI) is an area of controversy when analyzing results of small-cell lung cancer. In general, cranial irradiation reduces the incidence of central nervous system failure, but it has had a marginal impact on survival. Table 10 reflects results of several series. Unfortunately, the use of irradiation has contributed to central nervous system toxicity in many patients. Because of the toxicity reported with cranial irradiation and the marginal improvement in survival, PCI should be applied judiciously. Current recommendations would suggest that PCI be reserved for those patients who have completed chemotherapy and are in complete remission. Prophylactic cranial irradiation should be delivered in a conservative fashion, with fraction sizes of 200 to 250 cGy and total doses no greater than 3,000 cGy.

Irradiation is a frequently utilized modality in the treatment of lung cancer. In those good-performance patients with small locoregional tumor burdens, it may be potentially curative. In those patients with a high likelihood of systemic disease or established metastases, irradiation is a potent palliative tool, and symptomatic relief can be achieved in many patients with irradiation. In spite of aggressive modern irradiation, locoregional tumor failure remains a problem in both small-cell and non–small-cell histologies. Our current and future research efforts will attempt to enhance the biologically effective dose of irradiation.

SUGGESTED READING

Cox JD, Azarnia N, Byhardt RW, et al. Altered fractionation: Rationale for the prospective trials of the Radiation Therapy Oncology Group. Lung Cancer 1988; 4:P53–P55.

Dillman RD, Seagren SL, Propert K, et al. Protochemotherapy improves survival in regional non-small cell lung cancer. Proc Am Soc Clin Oncol 1988; 7:195.

Noordijk EMV, Poest Clement E, Hermans J, et al. Radiotherapy as an alternative to surgery in elderly patients with resectable lung cancer. Radiother Oncol 1988; 13:83–89.

Payne DG, Arriagade R, Dombernowsky P, et al. The role of thoracic radiation therapy in small cell carcinoma of the lung: A consensus report. Lung Cancer 1989; 5:135–138.

Perez CA, Stanley K, Rubin P, et al. A prospective randomized study of various irradiation doses and fractionation schedules in the treatment of inoperable non-oat cell carcinoma of the lung. Cancer 1980; 45:2,744–2,753.

LUNG CANCER: CHEMOTHERAPY

RUSSELL F. DEVORE, M.D.
DAVID H. JOHNSON, M.D.

Despite efforts to improve early detection and public health campaigns designed to induce individuals to stop smoking, lung cancer remains the leading cause of cancer-related deaths in the United States. This year alone, approximately 160,000 Americans will be found to have a lung neoplasm and 140,000 will die as a direct result of lung cancer. Even more alarming, the incidence of lung cancer continues to increase, especially among women, and will probably continue to do so through the remainder of this century.

Lung cancer can be divided into two broad categories, small-cell lung cancer (SCLC) and non–small-cell lung cancer (NSCLC). Small-cell lung cancer accounts for 20 to 25 percent of all lung malignancies and is unique in its propensity for early, widespread dissemination. Consequently, SCLC is rarely amenable to surgical treatment. However, because SCLC is highly responsive to a multitude of antineoplastic drugs, it can occasionally be eradicated. Non–small-cell lung cancer, on the other hand, is curable only with surgical resection and is only marginally responsive to chemotherapy. Non–small-cell lung cancer includes squamous (or epidermoid), large-cell, and adenocarcinoma cell types. Unfortunately, most patients with NSCLC present with disease beyond the scope of surgical cure. Thus, both SCLC and NSCLC can be viewed as systemic disease processes that require effective systemic therapies if meaningful progress is to be made in the management of these common malignancies.

Because SCLC and NSCLC differ in clinical presentation, prognosis, therapeutic options, and responsiveness to chemotherapy, they are discussed separately.

SMALL-CELL LUNG CANCER

Small-cell lung cancer is unique among the bronchogenic neoplasms because of its rapid growth rate and proclivity for early, widespread dissemination, and because it is very responsive to chemotherapy and radiation therapy. Prior to 1970, however, SCLC was commonly treated with surgery or radiotherapy. Regardless of which modality was used, most patients quickly developed widespread metastatic disease and few survived longer than 1 year. In the late 1960s, cyclophosphamide was found to improve modestly the median survival of patients with SCLC. Subsequently, numerous antineoplastic agents were found to have activity against this neoplasm, and clinical trials using combination regimens conclusively demonstrated improved long-term survival with intensive combination chemotherapy. As a result, combination chemotherapy has become the cornerstone of SCLC management.

Pre-treatment Evaluation

Pre-treatment evaluation should include confirmation of pathologic diagnosis, complete staging, estimation of prognosis, and an evaluation of the patient's ability to tolerate chemotherapy. Although experienced pathologists have little difficulty distinguishing SCLC from other histologic types of lung cancer, errors in diagnosis can be made as a result of inadequate biopsy material. Intermediate subtype SCLC can be mistaken for NSCLC, particularly when only cytologic material is available for study. Because the distinction has important therapeutic implications, it is imperative that an accurate diagnosis be made. If there is any doubt about the histologic diagnosis, a repeat biopsy with special stains and possibly electron microscopy should be done.

The TNM staging system has not proved useful for SCLC because most patients present with distant metastases (i.e., stage IV using current TNM staging criteria). A simple two-stage classification system dividing patients into limited and extensive-stage categories is more commonly used to determine prognosis and whether local treatment modalities should be incorporated into treatment. Limited-stage patients include those with disease confined to one hemithorax and regional lymph nodes. More importantly, the tumor should be encompassable within a single radiation port. Extensive disease includes patients with tumor beyond these boundaries. A staging evaluation should be done primarily to distinguish between limited-stage and extensive-stage patients. Common sites for metastatic involvement include the central nervous system (10 percent), liver (30 percent), skeleton (25 percent), and bone marrow (25 percent). Recommended staging procedures include a chest roentgenogram, bone marrow biopsy, computed tomography (CT) scans of the head and abdomen, and a radionuclide bone scan. Recently, some investigators have questioned the value of routine assessment of the bone marrow, because the marrow is rarely the sole site of metastatic disease. However, a bone marrow biopsy complements the bone scan and, when positive, is unequivocal proof of metastasis, which cannot be said of any radiographic finding.

In SCLC, performance status and stage are the major pretreatment prognostic factors. Limited-stage patients frequently have a better initial performance status. Nevertheless, nonambulatory patients invariably do less well than ambulatory patients, irrespective of stage. In general, limited-stage patients experience a greater response rate and improved survival when compared to extensive-stage patients. In extensive-stage disease, patients with liver metastases tend to have a poorer prognosis than patients with disease involving other metastatic sites. Also patients with multiple metastatic sites do less well than patients with single sites of metastases. On the other hand, patients with solitary central nervous system involvement at diagnosis apparently do no worse than patients without initial brain involvement. Finally, non–malignancy-related major organ dysfunction can seriously impair a patient's ability to tolerate intense therapy, resulting in increased morbidity and occasionally treatment-related mortality.

Chemotherapy

A number of combination chemotherapy regimens are available for the treatment of SCLC (Table 1). Most of these regimens contain at least three active agents. To achieve optimal response and survival, the active agents must be administered simultaneously and at relatively intensive dosages. The most effective treatment programs require frequent administration of chemotherapy (every 3 to 4 weeks). Ideally, dose should not be compromised during the first two cycles of therapy, especially in those patients being treated with curative intent. The intensity of therapy necessary to effect

maximal results inevitably produces a certain degree of serious toxicity. Some toxicities are related to specific drugs, such as cardiac toxicity with doxorubicin, neurotoxicity with vincristine, and renal toxicity with cisplatin. However, by far the most frequent serious toxicity is neutropenia and infection. Febrile episodes occur in approximately 30 percent of treated patients, and treatment-related mortality, largely due to infection, ranges from 2 to 5 percent.

Using any chemotherapy regimen listed in Table 1, tumor response is observed in 70 to 90 percent of patients. Complete responses occur in approximately one-half of patients with limited disease and up to 30 percent of patients with extensive disease (Table 2). Objective responses are usually noted within 6 to 12 weeks of the start of therapy but may occur after this time. Median survival ranges from 9 to 14 months, depending on the initial disease stage, and approximately 10 to 15 percent of all patients survive disease-free for 2 or more years.

Duration of Therapy

The optimum duration of chemotherapy administration is poorly defined. Investigators have used several different durations of therapy, ranging from 4 to 24 months. Short durations of treatment may be advantageous in terms of reducing acute and chronic treatment-related complications, such as infections and secondary leukemias, but this remains unproved. An Australian study used an induction regimen of cisplatin plus etoposide for 4 cycles followed by either no further chemotherapy or 10 cycles of cyclophosphamide, doxorubicin, and vincristine (CAV). The survival times were no different, but patients given CAV experienced greater toxicity. More recently, a Southeastern Cancer Study Group trial in extensive-stage patients compared four cycles of etoposide with six cycles of CAV and six cycles of CAV alternating with etoposide. Median survivals were virtually identical. These and other data suggest that long durations of treatment are not necessary to optimize treatment outcome.

Alternating Non–Cross-Resistant Chemotherapy

There has been some enthusiasm for using "alternating non–cross-resistant chemotherapy" in the management of SCLC. Although many studies have been

Table 1 Commonly Utilized Combination Chemotherapy Regimens for Small-Cell Lung Cancer

CAV
Cyclophosphamide — 1,000 mg/m² IV on day 1
Doxorubicin (adriamycin) — 45 mg/m² IV on day 1
Vincristine — 2 mg IV on day 1
Repeat cycle every 3 wk

CAE
Cyclophosphamide — 1,000 mg/m² IV on day 1
Doxorubicin (adriamycin) — 45 mg/m² on day 1
Etoposide — 50 mg/m² IV on days 1–5
Repeat cycle every 3 wk

CAVE
Cyclophosphamide — 1,000 mg/m² IV on day 1
Doxorubicin (adriamycin) — 50 mg/m² IV on day 1
Vincristine — 1.5 mg/m² IV on day 1*
Etoposide — 60 mg/m² IV on days 1–5
Repeat cycle every 3–4 wk

EP
Etoposide — 100 mg/m² IV on days 1–3
Cisplatin — 25 mg/m² IV on days 1–3
Repeat cycle every 3 wk
or
Etoposide — 120 mg/m² IV on days 1–3⁺
Cisplatin — 60 mg/m² IV on day 1
Repeat cycle every 3 wk

CAV/EP
CAV as above, alternating every 3 wk with EP (both agents given over 3 days)

EcP
Etoposide — 120 mg/m² IV on days 1–3
Carboplatin — 100 mg/m² IV on days 1–3
Repeat cycle every 4 wk

⁺Etoposide can be given 240 mg/m² PO on days 2 and 3.
*Maximum dose of 2 mg.

Table 2 State-of-the-Art Results of Chemotherapy in Small-Cell Lung Cancer

	Limited Disease	Extensive Disease	All Patients
Complete response	50%	25%	35%
Partial response	30%	50%	40%
Overall response	80%	75%	75%
Median survival	14 mos	7–9 mos	12 mos
2-year survival	15–20%	<2%	5–10%

done, none has yielded a major benefit in median survival. However, in some instances a statistically significant improvement was observed. In analyzing these trials, it would appear that the observed improvement in survival is possibly related to the addition of etoposide and cisplatin rather than a superior strategy of chemotherapy administration. Even in the absence of a survival advantage, however, alternating CAV with etoposide may result in fewer nonhematologic toxicities (such as cardiomyopathy and neurotoxicity), making this an attractive option for this patient population, who often has many coexisting medical illnesses. The cisplatin and etoposide regimen is associated with only modest nonhematologic toxicities.

Combined Modality Treatment

Although combination chemotherapy is unquestionably the cornerstone of SCLC management, thoracic radiotherapy can potentially benefit patients with limited-stage disease. Several randomized studies have yielded a modest improvement in the 2-year survival of patients treated with both thoracic irradiation and chemotherapy compared with chemotherapy alone. The optimum method for combining chemotherapy and thoracic radiotherapy, however, has not been satisfactorily established. Programs employing a concurrent or alternating regimen of chest irradiation appear to yield the best results. It is important that radiotherapy does not delay the administration nor compromise the dose of chemotherapy. Cisplatin plus etoposide appears particularly well suited to concurrent use with radiotherapy because both agents can be given in standard dosages with radiotherapy without excessive, untoward complications. Recent studies indicate this regimen (i.e., cisplatin and etoposide with concurrent chest radiotherapy) can yield 2-year survival rates of 40 percent to 50 percent in SCLC patients with limited disease.

Surgery

Only a small fraction of SCLC patients present with disease that is clinically resectable. In those rare circumstances in which the tumor can be completely resected, however, survival appears to be enhanced. Whether this is a consequence of the surgery or merely a manifestation of the inherent biology of SCLC presenting in this manner is unknown. Such patients should receive adjuvant chemotherapy postoperatively. The role of radiotherapy in this setting is undefined.

Salvage Therapy

Following relapse after initial induction chemotherapy, further treatment is typically less successful. Most salvage regimens effect overall response rates less than 50 percent, and complete responses are rare. Median survival after recurrence is only 2 to 4 months.

Occasionally, however, good responses and prolonged survival can be achieved. Relapsing patients who maintain a relatively good performance status and who have not received any therapy for at least 6 months are more likely to respond to salvage treatment. The highest response rates are seen in CAV failures subsequently treated with etoposide. Unfortunately, the reverse is not true. A trial of therapy with the original induction regimen is warranted in patients who have been progression-free for 12 months or longer. Because patients with recurrent disease cannot be cured with currently available therapy, they can be included in trials of phase 2 agents. Whether this is an optimal arena for testing new agents is a contentious issue.

NON–SMALL-CELL LUNG CANCER

Individuals with NSCLC can be cured only by means of a surgical resection. Unfortunately, even the 30 percent of patients presenting with clinically resectable disease frequently recur with metastases outside the thorax. Consequently, effective systemic treatment is clearly necessary to improve the overall management of NSCLC. Unlike SCLC, however, there are few antineoplastic agents demonstrating a high degree of activity against NSCLC. Although more than 50 single agents have been evaluated during the past two decades, few have yielded a consistent antitumor effect in at least 15 percent of patients (Table 3). Cisplatin, ifosfamide, and mitomycin C are the most active single agents. Vindesine, vinblastine, and etoposide also appear to have modest activity. However, tumor regressions induced with these agents are typically brief and rarely complete. Accordingly, there is no impact on overall survival with single-agent chemotherapy.

Newer agents with possible activity include carboplatin, 10-EDAM (10-ethyl-deaza-amniopterin), trimetrexate (a nonclassical folate), and navelbine (a vinca alkaloid). Each of these agents is undergoing further evaluation.

As is true with other malignancies, response rates improve when multiple-agent regimens are used to treat

Table 3 Single-Agent Activity in Metastatic Non–Small-Cell Lung Cancer

Response Rates > 15%
Cisplatin
Mitomycin C
Ifosfamide

Less Well-Documented Response Rates > 15%
Vinblastine
Vindesine
Etoposide

Response Rates < 15%
Cyclophosphamide
Doxorubicin
Lomustine
Methotrexate
5-Fluorouracil

Table 4 Randomized Trials of Chemotherapy Versus Best Supportive Care or Minimal Therapy in Metastatic Non–Small-Cell Lung Cancer

Group	Therapy	Patients	Response Rate (%)	Median Survival (wk)
Canadian NCI	PV	44	25	32.6+
	CAP	43	15	24.7
	BSC	50	–	17.0*
Australian and United Kingdom	PV	93	28	23.0
	BSC	95	–	16.0
Southeastern Cancer Study Group	PV	125	19	24.7
	MV	122	27	20.4
	mT	128	1	14.8
UCLA	PV1b	22	18	20.4
	BSC	26	12	13.6

Abbreviations: P = cisplatin, V = vindesine, M = mitomycin C, V1b = vinblastine, C = cyclophosphamide, A = doxorubicin, BSC = best supportive care, mT = minimal therapy (i.e., vindesine every 2 weeks).
*P = 0.01.

NSCLC. However, currently available regimens rarely effect an overall response of more than 40 percent, and complete responses typically occur in fewer than 10 percent of patients. Furthermore, in randomized trials comparing combination chemotherapy with "minimal therapy" or "best supportive care" (i.e., palliative radiotherapy and optimal medical management of other malignancy-related problems), survival has *not* been substantially increased (Table 4). Therefore, a strong argument could be made for *not* using chemotherapy in the management of metastatic NSCLC.

On the other hand, despite the lack of major survival benefit, all of the randomized trials listed in Table 4 yielded a modest improvement in survival in the patients treated with chemotherapy (albeit usually without statistical significance). These data suggest that some patients with metastatic disease *may* benefit from a trial of chemotherapy. Such patients must be selected carefully and properly apprised of the potential side effects and goals of treatment.

Patient Selection

The principal factors predicting response to chemotherapy and survival in metastatic non–small-cell lung cancer are performance status, tumor bulk, site of metastases, sex, and age. In most studies, the histologic subtype appears to play very little role in prognosis. Two large series, one from the Eastern Cooperative Oncology Group (ECOG) and the other from Memorial Sloan Kettering Cancer Center, have evaluated prognostic factors with respect to response and survival in patients with chemotherapy-treated metastatic NSCLC. In the ECOG study, several pretreatment factors were associated with survival of 1 year or more, including good performance status; no bone, liver, or subcutaneous metastases; female sex; a histology other than large-cell carcinoma; no weight loss; and no symptoms of shoulder or arm pain. These investigators also observed that patients whose tumor took more than 90 days to exhibit the best response to treatment were more likely to

become long-term survivors than those whose tumor responded quickly (i.e., in less than 30 days).

The Memorial Sloan Kettering group found an improved response duration and survival in patients with a good performance status, no bone metastases, a normal serum lactic dehydrogenase (LDH) level, and female sex. Patients with brain metastases have a median survival time of 3 to 4 months and generally are not considered good candidates for chemotherapy.

Based on these observations, it is reasonable to offer treatment to patients with a good performance status and other favorable prognostic features. Obviously, the limitations of chemotherapy should be discussed frankly. Usually, after two to three cycles of therapy, response and tolerance to treatment can be well assessed. Responding patients with good tolerance of therapy occasionally benefit with an apparent improved quality of life and should continue chemotherapy to maximal tumor response. On the other hand, treatment should be discontinued in the presence of unacceptable toxicity and in those patients who fail to respond after a brief treatment trial. With this approach, one can determine the usefulness of chemotherapy early and eliminate prolonged use of toxic and ineffective treatment.

Chemotherapy Regimens

Owing to the poor results with currently available antineoplastic agents, no one regimen can be considered "standard." Ideally, NSCLC patients with metastatic disease should be treated within the context of a clinical trial. Outside of a clinical trial, it is reasonable to consider any of the regimens outlined in Table 5, keeping in mind all the previously discussed caveats. Cisplatin-based regimens are used most frequently largely as a result of the perception that platinum is the most effective of the available antineoplastic agents.

Toxicity from typical cisplatin-based treatments usually is manageable and less severe in patients with good performance status. Lethal toxicity occurs in less than 5 percent of patients. Nausea, vomiting, and

Table 5 Cisplatin-Containing Regimens Used in Patients with Metastatic Non–Small-Cell Lung Cancer

PE:	Cisplatin, 60–120 mg/m^2 IV, day 1 q3–4wk
	Etoposide, 80–120 mg/m^2 IV, days 1–3 or days 1,3,5 q3–4wks
PV:	Cisplatin, 60–120 mg/m^2 IV, day 1 q4wk
	Vinblastine, 5 mg/m^2 IV, qw × 5, then q2wk
MVP:	Cisplatin, 120 mg/m^2 IV, day 15 and 29, then q6wk
	Vinblastine, 4.5 mg/m^2 IV, days 1, 15, 22, and 29
	Vinblastine, 2.0 mg/m^2 IV, day 8
	Mitomycin C, 8 mg/m^2 IV, days 1, 29, and 71 only
CAP:	Cisplatin, 40–50 mg/m^2 IV, day 1 q4wk
	Adriamycin, 40 mg/m^2 IV, day 1 q4wk
	Cyclophosphamide, 400–600 mg/m^2 IV, day 1 q4wk

Table 6 Tumor Bulk and Chemotherapy Response in Non–Small-Cell Lung Cancer

Regimen	Stage IIIA/B (%)	Stage IV
MVP	53	28
CAP	47	23
EP	56	31

Abbreviations: M = mitomycin C, V = vinca alkaloid, P = cisplatin, C = cyclophosphamide, A = doxorubicin, E = etoposide.

myelosuppression are common, but manageable, in most patients. Significant cisplatin-induced renal toxicity can usually be prevented with careful attention to hydration status.

Combined-Modality Treatment

In preclinical tumor models, chemotherapy is typically most effective in the setting of minimal tumor bulk (i.e., adjuvant therapy postresection or shortly after implantation of a tumor); thus, there is a theoretical attraction for using chemotherapy in NSCLC patients without clinically documented extrathoracic metastases. Recent reports indicate response rates to cisplatin-based chemotherapy in NSCLC patients with locally advanced disease are approximately double those observed in patients with widely metastatic disease (Table 6). This observation has prompted many investigators to explore the utility of combining local modalities of treatment (i.e., surgery and radiotherapy) with chemotherapy.

Approximately one-third of NSCLC patients present with locally advanced and inoperable disease. Traditionally, radiotherapy has been the treatment of choice in this setting. However, a recently completed randomized trial compared radiotherapy alone to treatment with chemotherapy followed by radiotherapy. Chemotherapy included two cycles of cisplatin (100 mg per square meter) on a 4-week basis plus weekly vinblastine (5 mg per square meter) for 5 weeks. Radiotherapy consisted of 60 Gy given over 6 weeks in both treatment arms. Overall response (57 percent versus 40 percent) and median survival (16.5 months versus 8.5 months; $P=0.0028$) were superior in the combined-modality group. These data suggest that cisplatin-based chemotherapy can potentially improve the median survival of patients with locally advanced unresectable NSCLC. However, one should note that similar programs have failed to demonstrate a meaningful survival benefit in pilot studies. Nevertheless, patients with locally advanced, unresectable NSCLC should be considered for multimodality therapy. When possible, this should be done within the context of a clinical trial.

Several investigators have employed chemotherapy in a "neoadjuvant" manner, i.e., prior to surgery, in an attempt to "downstage" patients who clinically appear to be unresectable. Again, such an approach has theoretical attraction and has been proved technically feasible in several single-institution pilot studies. Whether such an approach will improve survival remains to be seen.

SUGGESTED READING

Minna JD, Pass H, Glatstein E, et al. Cancer of the lung. In: DeVita V, Hellman S, Rosenberg SA, eds. Cancer principles and practice of oncology. Philadelphia: JB Lippincott, 1989:591–705.

Mulshine JL, Glatstein E, Ruckdeschel JC. Treatment of non–small cell lung cancer. J Clin Oncol 1986; 4:1704–1715.

Seifter EJ, Ihde DC. Therapy of small cell lung cancer: A perspective on two decades of clinical research. Semin Oncol 1988; 15:278–299.

GENITOURINARY CANCER

EDWARD M. MESSING, M.D., F.A.C.S.

Cancers of the prostate, bladder, and kidney, when taken together, represent the most common cancers in American men and the second most common cause of cancer death. Each is uncommon below the age of 50, and each has a rising incidence with increasing age. As our population lives longer, these malignancies will pose even greater medical challenges. This chapter reviews important issues in the detection, evaluation, and treatment of localized and regional disease for each of these sites. Additionally, the roles of early detection efforts, prevention, and controversial areas in management are discussed.

CANCER OF THE PROSTATE

Epidemiology

There will be over 105,000 new cases of cancer of the prostate diagnosed in American men this year, and 30,000 individuals will die from this disease. Incidence and mortality are significantly higher in blacks than whites and somewhat lower in orientals than whites. Based on autopsy data, however, it is likely that 30 to 50 percent of American men above age 50 have at least a focus of adenocarcinoma within their prostate glands. The vast majority of these individuals, of course, will never have clinically important cancer of the prostate and certainly will not die of this disease. Thus, despite this disease's extreme clinical importance, its relative ubiquity throughout the population poses great challenges not only for clinicians concerned with the needs of their individual patients but for institutional and societal health care planners and students of cancer biology as well.

Presentation and Detection

Despite recent technologic developments (particularly the use of transrectal prostatic ultrasound [TRUS] and prostate-specific antigen [PSA]), the vast majority of men with cancer of the prostate still present with abnormal findings on digital rectal exam (DRE) or obstructive voiding symptoms. The latter, of course, are quite common in middle-aged and elderly men because of benign prostatic hyperplasia (BPH) as well as cancer of the prostate. Roughly 15 to 20 percent of men will already have symptoms of metastatic disease at the time of presentation (e.g., skeletal pain, azotemia due to ureteral obstruction), but these individuals also will often have obstructive voiding symptoms or abnormal DREs.

Once the disease is suspected, biopsy is performed, usually under local anesthesia via a transperineal or transrectal route. Although biopsy is often successful when the needle is guided by the biopsier's finger, recently TRUS-guided biopsies have become increasingly popular because they permit confirmation of needle placement, thereby improving the likelihood of sampling suspicious tissue. Aspiration cytology, when performed and interpreted by an experienced team, will provide as accurate a diagnosis as removing a core of tissue for histologic inspection. Mostly because of sampling and preparation artifacts, needle biopsies, and, to some degree, aspirations, cannot reliably be depended upon to provide information other than whether adenocarcinoma is present. Recently, ultrasonographically guided multiple sampling involving all sectors of the prostate has been advanced as a way of obtaining additional grading and staging information as well as providing an accurate assessment of tumor volume. Initial reports of this technique are promising.

Roughly 10 percent of men who undergo prostatectomy (either by "open" surgery or transurethral resection [TURP]) for bladder outlet obstructive symptoms that were thought preoperatively to be due to BPH will be found to have some adenocarcinoma in the resected gland. Its clinical significance is based on both the volume of cancer found and its histologic grade. Somewhat arbitrarily, these incidentally found tumors have been divided into Stage AI (well-differentiated or moderately differentiated tumors that comprise ≤ 5 percent of resected tissue) and stage AII (any high-grade tumors or those involving over 5 percent of resected tissue). The clinical significance of this distinction will be discussed.

Clinical Staging

Laboratory Tests

Once a diagnosis of cancer of the prostate has been made, a variety of noninvasive staging studies are performed. These include blood tests of hematologic, hepatic, and renal status, and serum markers of cancer of the prostate—prostatic acid phosphatase (PAP), which is assayed by enzymatic techniques, and PSA. Prostate-specific antigen and PAP should be drawn no sooner than at least 48 hours following any prostatic examination and over 10 to 14 days following biopsy or TURP. Currently, enzymatic PAP probably provides the greatest initial staging information because its elevation above 1.5 times the normal maximum value virtually always indicates the presence of extraprostatic malignancy. Although the PSA values probably more accurately reflect tumor volume and stage, they usually are considerably elevated in men with sizable BPH. Thus, except for massive elevations, PSA cannot currently be used for satisfactory staging of individual patients.

Other Studies

Imaging modalities include chest radiograph, technetium-99 scintillation bone scan, and sonographic or radiographic evaluation of the upper urinary tract (to rule out unilateral or bilateral ureteral obstruction). An abdominal/pelvic computed tomography (CT) scan has the additional advantage of evaluating pelvic and retroperineal adenopathy and hepatic architecture as well as inspecting the upper urinary tract. Computed tomography is probably not needed in men with normal PAP, PSA less than 10, and well-differentiated or moderately differentiated lesions that are felt, on DRE or TRUS, to occupy less than half the gland and to be confined to the prostate. If cystoscopy has not previously been performed at the time of biopsy, this examination is mandatory (in the absence of obvious metastases) to assess prostatic growth onto the trigone.

Evaluation of the local tumor is critical in staging and subsequent management decisions. This is performed primarily by DRE and cystoscopy because TRUS and CT have been disappointing for this purpose. The most important examination is that obtained prior to biopsy because trauma artifacts may be indistinguishable on exam from local tumor extension.

Clinical Stages

Cancer of the prostate is divided into four major stages, each with substages: stages AI (T1a) and AII (T1b) have already been defined. These both arise primarily in the transitional rather than the peripheral zones of the prostate. Stage B (T2) tumors are believed to be confined exclusively to the prostate and are subcategorized into BI (0.5 to 1.5 cm in greatest diameter and confined to a single prostatic lobe), BII (a larger nodule involving only one lobe or any tumor crossing the midline), and BIII (any larger tumors). Stage C (T3, T4) tumors extend outside the palpable (or histologic) confines of the prostate, leading into periprostatic fat, trigone, or the seminal vesicles. These again have been subcategorized into CI (minimal extraprostatic extension), which is thought to be surgically removable by radical prostatectomy, or CII (larger than CI). Prostatic tumors can metastasize to pelvic nodes below the bifurcation of the great vessels (DI) or to nodes above this point or hematogenous sites (DII).

Because management decisions are in large part determined by prognosis, which in turn is dictated by stage, accurate clinical staging is critical not only in making individual treatment recommendations but also in interpreting reports of various therapies. However, one should recognize that when pathologic staging is performed (e.g., lymph node dissection or radical prostatectomy), clinical understaging will often be seen (e.g., from approximately 15 percent for clinical B1 lesions to over 50 percent for clinical C). Even more so than for other malignancies, both grade and tumor volume are accurate reflectors of tumor stage; thus, it is particularly likely that a high-grade BII or BIII lesion will be clinically understaged. Although these issues do not always directly influence individual treatment recommendations, they must be considered in the appraisal of treatment options and the realistic expectation of results.

Prognosis

With the exceptions of stages AI and D, little is known about the natural (i.e., untreated) history of cancer of the prostate; hence, prognostic inferences have been made primarily from pathologic staging data.

Stage A

Stage AI tumors have roughly a 10 to 20 percent chance of progressing within 5 to 15 years after TURP when managed expectantly. Alternatively, 25 to 33 percent of clinical stage AII patients already have microscopic pelvic nodal metastases at the time of presentation. Thus, stage AII is a more aggressive disease and should be managed as such.

Stage B

The untreated histories of stage B cancers are much more poorly understood. It is generally believed that because nodal involvement ranges from less than 15 percent (stage BI) to 35 percent (BII/III), there is significant likelihood of eventual demise from a stage B tumor if it is left untreated.

Stage C

Over 50 percent of patients with newly diagnosed clinical stage C tumors will actually have concurrent nodal metastases, indicating their eventual ominous prognosis.

Stage D

Patients with stage DI tumors (confirmed by lymphadenectomy) who undergo no further "curative" treatment to the prostate gland ultimately do poorly, with approximately 60 percent developing hematogenous metastases within 4 years. However, there is no evidence that local treatments to the prostate (either by surgery or radiotherapy) favorably influence survival or even benefit patients by preventing untreatable local symptoms from developing.

Management

There are several difficulties in evaluating the efficacy of available therapies for localized or regional cancer of the prostate. The tumor itself has a long natural history, and most published series have not actually followed patients for more than 10 years. Additionally, because of the length of follow-up needed, many patients have been lost to follow-up. These two problems have led authors to use various statistical methods to project survival. Considering the age of most patients with prostatic cancer and the numerous other causes of demise that they face, data other than actual disease-free survival at 12 to 15 years become suspect. Moreover, with the exception of two studies that will be discussed later, randomized prospective trials comparing competing treatments have not been performed. Thus, we are left to evaluate treatments, and infer information about natural history, from single-armed retrospective studies that often span decades or even generations! Additionally, it is not always clear from most publications when or if hormonal therapy of various sorts has been administered. This issue will be discussed in greater detail in the next chapter, but undoubtedly such treatment will retard disease progression. Finally, most studies were performed prior to PSA being available, and it is likely that they are reporting somewhat optimistic outlooks. With these limitations in mind, we will evaluate available information concerning modalities of management for localized or regional cancer of the prostate.

Stage A-I

Ten to twenty percent of the patients found to have only a focus of adenocarcinoma at the time that they undergo prostatectomy for presumably benign disease will eventually have their cancers progress if left untreated. Therapeutic recommendations range from instituting immediate aggressive local treatment (as for stages AII/B) to observation alone, to performing some restaging procedure(s) and only treating those who have cancer confirmed on rebiopsy. We prefer the last approach because, in several studies, when this is done and patients without cancer found on rebiopsy are observed, fewer than 5 percent ever develop clinically apparent cancer of the prostate. Alternatively, 40 percent to 50 percent of those in whom *any* cancer is documented on rebiopsy (20 to 25 percent of men believed to have stage AI tumors after the initial TURP) will experience progression if left untreated within 5 to 7 years. Rebiopsy can be performed via repeat TURP, although we usually prefer systematic ultrasonically guided transrectal biopsies because, based upon radical prostatectomy studies of Neerhut and colleagues, residual cancer will often reside primarily in the peripheral zones. If more cancer is found (even only a tiny focus), then patients are considered to have stage AII disease.

Stage A-II

Although there are some fundamental anatomic differences between stage AII and stage B cancer of the prostate (primarily that stage A tumors usually arise in the transitional prostatic zone, whereas stage B tumors generally arise more peripherally), because the incidence of nodal metastases is quite similar, it is likely that

each have similar metastatic potentials. Therefore, they are usually both treated identically.

Stage B

The natural history of stage B cancer of the prostate is uncertain. It is likely that there are some patients who can be followed for many years with palpably evident nodules that do not substantially enlarge or metastasize during the period of observation. Unfortunately, currently we have no way of predicting who these fortunate individuals will be, and because from 15 percent to 35 percent of patients with clinical stage B cancers will actually have nodal metastases at diagnosis, a course of "watchful waiting" would seem to run the great risk of allowing other potentially curable lesions to metastasize while under observation. Thus, if the patient's general medical condition would predict 4 to 5 years of reasonably good health, an attempt at definitive cure seems appropriate. Primary curative modalities for organ-confined cancer of the prostate include three forms of radiation therapy or radical prostatectomy. A conference recently held by the National Cancer Institute reached no consensus as to which treatment was preferable, although it is widely held by all that radiotherapy probably offers no better chance of cure than radical surgery.

Radiotherapy

65 Gy of external-beam radiotherapy is normally delivered to the prostatic bed over a 6½ week period through multiple ports. Series from single institutions indicate that roughly 60 percent of evaluable patients will be alive at 10 years. Data for longer periods of time are available from only one institution, in which many patients have been lost to follow-up and cannot be included. The chief complications of this modality include impotence in 30 to 40 percent of men who claim to be potent at the start of treatment and urgency incontinence in 2 percent. Most patients experience some urinary urgency and diarrhea during and shortly after the termination of treatment, but this abates in all but a small percentage. Serious complications, including radiation proctitis, cystitis, myelitis, or dermatitis, can occur but are notably uncommon. In men who have moderate to severe symptoms of bladder outlet obstruction or markedly enlarged and obstructing prostates on endoscopic inspection, a preradiotherapy "channeling" TURP is probably indicated because many of these individuals will develop complete urinary retention early in their course of treatment. If a TURP is *not* performed in these individuals, suprapubic or (continuous or intermittent) urethral catheter bladder drainage will be necessary, thus causing further vesical irritation and, at times, symptoms so incapacitating that radiotherapy has to be terminated. Although some authors have claimed that a preradiotherapy TURP may promote tumor dissemination, there are numerous contrary publications

on the same topic and no prospective information is available to support this contention. Alternatively, because even a benignly enlarged gland will normally regress after completion of radiotherapy, only individuals who are believed to be likely to go into retention during radiotherapy should undergo pretherapy TURP.

Recently, a mixed form of external-beam radiation using neutron therapy combined with the more standard photon beam has been employed in a phase 3 study for more advanced (clinical stage C) cancer of the prostate. The advantages of the neutron beam include greater tissue penetration and less surrounding tissue damage. Theoretically, by mixing the beams, one can achieve sterilization of the field outside the prostate as well as within it. Preliminary reports from the phase 3 study indicate a moderately favorable therapeutic response for the mixed-beam approach, although long-term follow-up and its impact on disease progression and survival are not yet known. Whether such treatments are beneficial for less extensive tumors (stage AII or B) has also not been addressed. Perhaps a further disadvantage is that only a limited number of institutions are presently capable of offering such therapy, thus making it unavailable to most American men.

Interstitial placement of either ^{125}I or ^{198}Au "seeds" has been used for many years. Initially, these isotopes were placed through open surgical approaches (either retropubically or transperineally), but recently methods have become available to deliver them through CT-generated templates, so that only needle incisions are necessary. Normally, individuals are placed in a dorsal lithotomy position after being fully anesthetized. Biplanar fluoroscopy is needed for adequate placement of the seeds. One of the major problems with this technique is that the lithotomy position achieved in the Radiotherapy Department for template simulation is rarely precisely duplicatable in the operating room for actual isotope insertion. Some institutions are attempting to use ultrasonically guided seed placement, and this may permit more precise introduction. Patients remain in the hospital for 72 hours after interstitial irradiation in a lead-lined room. A urethral catheter remains in place during this period and is then removed. Placement in someone who has undergone a recent TURP (e.g., stage AII) is notoriously incomplete because the remaining shell-like prostate gland will not always be able to hold the entire seed, thus allowing it to enter the prostatic urethral lumen and be urinated out. Long-term follow-up from percutaneously placed interstitial radiotherapy is not available. However, series that have used surgically placed ^{125}I do not have as satisfactory 10-year progression-free and disease-free survivals as those using external-beam radiotherapy or radical prostatectomy.

Radical Prostatectomy

There is no argument that if the tumor is truly confined to the prostate gland itself, radical prostatectomy offers at least as good chance of cure as any other therapy. Although single-armed studies with careful follow-up tend to indicate a somewhat better disease-free survival for men treated by radical surgery than by radiotherapy, because some individuals have received adjuvant hormonal therapy and because patients with extraprostatic extension determined pathologically are often not included in outcome, results of many series (other than the two mentioned previously) are at times difficult to interpret. In the only randomized prospective study comparing external-beam radiotherapy with radical prostatectomy, surgery offered substantially better 5- and 7-year disease-free survival rates (87 percent versus 58 percent for 5 years and 78 percent versus 51 percent for 7 years) in patients with pathologically negative pelvic lymph nodes. However, this study has been criticized because of its randomization scheme and potential selection bias in allocation of patients for each treatment group. Furthermore, the group who received radiotherapy appeared to fare worse than most single-institution, single-armed radiotherapy groups from the same era (Table 1).

Radical prostatectomy can be performed through a perineal or retropubic approach. The latter has gained recent favor in large part because it permits simultaneous lymphadenectomy. Both procedures are associated with a 30 to 40 percent impotence rate and a 2 to 5 percent incontinence rate, with both complications being slightly more frequent in individuals who have undergone previous TURP. Additional complications are those normally anticipated for the location and magnitude of surgery (e.g., atelectasis, hemorrhage, wound infection), including lymphadenectomy (e.g., lymphocele, deep venous thrombosis, transient edema of penis or lower extremities). Patients remain hospitalized for 7 days postoperatively and usually have their catheters removed 2 to 3 weeks after surgery. Thereafter, there is a variable period of time in which urinary continence must be regained. Additional long-term complications include urethral stenoses and bladder neck contractures, most of which are easily managed by dilations. Local control rates after radical prostatectomy for histologically confirmed stage B tumors are excellent, with fewer than 10 percent of patients experiencing local recurrence within 10 years.

Pathologic Stage C

In individuals who have undergone radical prostatectomy in which there is extracapsular extension, involvement of the seminal vesicles, or positive surgical margins, the incidence of local recurrence is somewhat higher. This is primarily the case for the latter two, and there are now several series to indicate that, at least over 5 to 7 years, the likelihood of local recurrence in men with surgical margin–negative, seminal vesicle–negative tumors with extracapsular extension is little more than 5 to 7 percent, whereas it is 20 to 25 percent for those individuals with seminal vesicle or surgical margin involvement. Retrospective studies with small numbers of subjects indicate that external-beam radiotherapy to

Table 1 Survival in Clinical Stages A2 and B Prostatic Cancer

Reference	Number of Patients	Treatment	NED Survival (%)**		
			5 years	10 years	15 years
Bagshaw et al (1988)	491	External-beam radiotherapy	81*	60*	34*
Carlton and Scardino (1988)	353	[198]Au + external beam	58	35	
Grossman et al (1982)	155	[125]I interstitial	89‡		
Paulson et al (1989)	56†	External beam	58		
Paulson et al (1989)	41†	Radical prostatectomy	87		
Paulson et al (1990)	368	Radical prostatectomy	80	70	

*Actuarial survival, not NED.
†Randomized prospective study; all patients N0.
‡Actual survival, not NED.
**NED survival = alive without evidence of cancer based on physical examination, radiographic imaging (bone scan, chest x-ray, CT, IVP), and PAP. This does not include the results of PSA determinations, post treatment biopsy of the normal feeling prostate, or postsurgical prostatic bed.

Table 2 Survival in Clinical Stage C Prostatic Cancer

Reference	Number of Patients	Treatment	Survival (%)		
			5 years	10 years	15 years
Bagshaw (1988)	385	External-beam radiotherapy	60*	36*	22*
Scardino (in press)	117	[198]Au + external beam radiotherapy	41 (NED)	19 (NED)	7.5 (NED)
Paulson et al (1984)	40	External-beam radiotherapy†	58		
Paulson et al (1984)	33	Observation and delayed hormones†	60		

*Actuarial survival; may have disease persistence or progression.
†Randomized prospective study. "Nonprogressive" means patients are alive without obvious metastases or symptomatic local growth; however, they may have local residual disease.

the prostatic bed may reduce this incidence. Presently, a controlled prospective intergroup study is underway to evaluate this. Postoperative radiotherapy seems to be well tolerated as long as individuals have already gained continence before it is instituted and the total dose is limited to 60 Gy. However, whether this type of additional local treatment retards or prevents systemic progression is not known. The effect of radiotherapy on potency is also uncertain.

The role of hormonal therapy in the post–radical prostatectomy patient with pathologic stage C disease also has not been adequately evaluated. There are certainly several indirect lines of evidence to indicate that progression will be retarded by the institution of hormonal therapy, but whether this effects prolonged survival is far less certain. It appears now that characteristics other than stage alone, particularly DNA ploidy, may have significant prognostic value in determining who might benefit from early hormonal manipulation. Unfortunately, such information is difficult to ascertain without large amounts of tissue to perform analyses (i.e., specimens obtained by needle biopsies or even TURP usually require sophisticated and time-consuming image analysis techniques that are available only in investigational settings). Presently, several retrospective analyses of archival radical pros-

tatectomy specimens are underway to determine if primarily diploid tumors have a more favorable response to hormonal manipulation than nondiploid-aneuploid ones. When interpreting such information, however, it must be remembered that it is likely that diploid tumors generally have a far better outlook with or without hormonal therapy.

Clinical Stage C

In those individuals with palpable (or ultrasonographically) diagnosed disease outside the prostatic capsule, optimal treatment is not known. Over 50 percent of such individuals will have nodal metastases, thus complicating interpretation of reports of efficacy from any series that lacks pathologic staging of the lymph nodes. With this limitation in mind, series from single institutions report 20 to 35 percent 10-year clinical disease-free survival (without posttreatment biopsy or PSA determinations) for patients with clinical stage C tumors treated by radiotherapy (Table 2). It does appear that good *symptomatic* local control can be achieved by external photon-beam radiotherapy in 80 percent of patients, but a minimum of 60 to 65 Gy needs to be delivered to accomplish this. Lower doses have much higher failure rates.

Further complicating the choice of management in clinical stage C disease are the findings by Paulson and colleagues in a prospective randomized study, that radiotherapy offered no advantage in retarding disease progression or prolonging actual survival over management by observation and hormonal therapy upon progression. Additionally, approximately 25 percent of patients with clinical stage C1 lesions will actually have disease confined to the prostate gland. The use of ultrasonically guided biopsy in suspicious areas outside the gland to confirm extracapsular extension should permit a better pretreatment assessment of this problem. Undoubtedly, some of these patients could undergo technically successful radical prostatectomy, but in view of the high incidence of nodal involvement, the increased incidence of local complications (particularly if anastomatic sites are involved) after radical prostatectomy, and the good symptomatic local control reported for radiotherapy, it is unclear that radical surgery should be the preferred modality for even small-volume clinical stage C disease. Adjuvant therapies such as radiotherapy (if radical surgery *is* performed) or hormonal manipulation have various advocates, but these modalities have not been tested prospectively.

An alternate approach that has been used for many years would be "shrinking" of the palpable tumor by several months of hormonal therapy followed by radical prostatectomy. This undoubtedly allows the surgery to be performed more easily, and although some tumors are pathologically down-staged, it is unclear whether this simply reflects clinical overstaging or pathologic artifact because the majority of cells are killed. More importantly, whether this treatment results in improved local or distant disease control is not known.

Stage D1

For those individuals with nodal metastases that are histologically documented by percutaneous biopsy or lymphadenectomy (or, as recently described, by laparoscopy), there is no evidence that further treatment to the prostate (either by radiotherapy or surgery) offers any particular benefit. Although most of these men progress within 4 or 5 years, it is primarily with systemic disease; local symptoms can be managed by a variety of endoscopic means. Whether these individuals should undergo early hormonal treatment or just be followed carefully until progression occurs is not known.

Post-treatment Assessment

For all stages of cancer of the prostate, regular follow-up throughout a patient's life is needed not only because progression may take many years to become manifest but also because there is a truly effective, albeit not curative, treatment available for progressing disease—endocrine manipulation. Standard evaluations on a semiannual basis include physical exam and lab studies (particularly serum creatinine, PSA, and PAP). Bone scans should probably be performed much less

frequently, and evaluation of the upper urinary tract need only be done as clinically indicated or upon progression (once the initial pretreatment study was negative).

The roles of PSA, TRUS, and repeat prostatic biopsy in determining future management are currently being studied. Prostate-specific antigen probably has its greatest value in the follow-up of patients after definitive therapy to the prostate gland. After radical prostatectomy PSA *invariably* goes down to undetectable levels unless there is persistent or recurrent disease. From the limited data available for postradiotherapy PSA levels, its subsequent elevation from a posttreatment plateau also indicates recurrence and progression. This test is such a sensitive reflector of persistent cancer that some authors have advocated that serial PSA monitoring and physical examinations are the only routine follow-up studies necessary. We have had two patients whose PSA levels remained undetectable after radical prostatectomy while they developed diagnosable and *clinically significant* local recurrence or metastases, which leads us to be skeptical of this recommendation. Furthermore, in those individuals taking hormonal therapy, PSA levels may be markedly depressed while the disease progresses. Despite this, PSA remains a truly valuable tool in assessing therapeutic efficacy.

Prostate-specific antigen is such a sensitive test that it will often become elevated in the absence of any other objective or subjective evidence of disease. This leads to the therapeutic dilemma of whether additional local treatment is appropriate or whether systemic progression has occurred. Moreover, the time interval between initial elevation of PSA and other objective evidence of recurrence or progression is not yet known. Despite this, additional treatments (particularly radiotherapy) have been offered to men after radical prostatectomy whose PSA was initially depressed postoperatively but then rose into the detectable range. Usually, PSA levels will descend again upon treatment, but the duration and permanence of the descent are not known. Undoubtedly, this would imply that at least some of the cancer was within the field of radiotherapy; however, it does not indicate whether there might not be additional tumor outside (or even within) this field that will eventually grow to the size to produce detectable amounts of PSA and indeed cause symptoms. The role of additional local treatment after primary radiotherapy is far less certain. Salvage radical prostatectomy or interstitial radiation can be attempted, but each carries questionable efficacy and certainly greater morbidity than would occur if given prior to radiotherapy.

The role of TRUS on a routine follow-up basis or repeat prostatic biopsy (in the absence of a palpable mass or recurrent local symptoms) is even more ambiguous. Certainly, for the purpose of studies, these monitoring devices are indicated. In routine clinical practice, however, because the efficacy of salvage treatment after initial therapy with "curative" intent is unclear, to make a concerted effort to look for recurrence with such means is highly questionable. The sole exception to this would be in the management of (particularly younger) men with newly diagnosed stage AI prostate cancer who would normally just be observed (vide supra).

BLADDER CANCER

There will be 49,000 new cases of bladder cancer diagnosed in the United States this year and 10,000 deaths due to this disease. The vast majority of these tumors are transitional cell carcinomas (TCCs), and for purposes of this chapter, our emphasis will be on pure TCCs and those TCCs that have squamous or adenomatous elements. As with cancer of the prostate, the incidence of TCC rises with advanced age. It is also far more common in men than women and almost twice as common in American whites as American blacks. However, mortality between races is approximately equal (for respective sexes), an observation that has been presumed to be due to differences in access to health care but may also reflect different exposures or susceptibilities to carcinogenic agents or different biologies of TCC in the two races. Aside from age, sex, and race, exposure to cigarette smoking has long been recognized as an important risk factor, with TCC being approximately four times as common in individuals who are current smokers than in those who have never smoked, and approximately twice as common in former cigarette smokers as in individuals who never smoked. It has also long been recognized that bladder cancer has been associated with exposure to environmental or industrial carcinogens. However, fewer than 20 percent of Americans who will die of bladder cancer this year have known exposures to carcinogens (other than to cigarette smoke).

Pathology

The transitional epithelium lines the urinary tract from the renal calyces to beyond the prostatic urethra; thus, TCC can, and does, arise anywhere in this location. Histologically, and indeed in terms of tumor behavior, transitional cell tumors arising throughout the urinary tract have similar behaviors and prognoses. However, such tumors are 20 times more common in the bladder than in the extravesical urinary tract. For the vast majority of patients, the development of TCC represents a field-change phenomenon, with multiple tumors and numerous recurrences after local treatment being the rule. Awareness of this behavior has strongly influenced management.

Approximately 70 percent of patients with newly diagnosed TCC have tumors that are confined to the epithelium (stage Ta) or that invade only into the underlying lamina propria (stage T1). It is extremely unusual for these superficial tumors to be associated with concomitant metastases; thus, all are theoretically curable by local means. However, once the tumor invades into the muscularis (stage T2, T3a) or through it

(stage T3b), or to neighboring structures (stage T4), the likelihood of recognized (e.g., N+) or unrecognized micrometastases is much higher. Indeed, almost all deaths from bladder cancer occur in individuals who have concomitant or previous muscle-invading bladder tumors. This has been recognized for many decades and has critical prognostic and therapeutic implications.

Diagnosis and Staging

The vast majority of TCCs, in both the bladder and upper urinary tract, are detected because they cause grossly visible or microscopic hematuria. Less frequently, upper tract obstruction or irritable voiding symptoms may also occur, although generally only in more advanced disease. Two features of bladder cancer–induced hematuria have now been documented and must be remembered by clinicians: (1) The degree of hematuria is unrelated to the seriousness of its underlying cause, so that once above some threshold (usually two to three red blood cells per high-power field), the possibility of harboring serious disease is significant. (2) Bladder cancer–induced hematuria is often quite intermittent; thus, once hematuria is recognized, it is unclear whether one can wait for a second specimen to be found to contain hematuria before full urologic evaluation (including intravenous urography, cystoscopy, and bladder wash or urinary cytology) is recommended. In contrast to cancer of the prostate, bladder cancer is almost never found incidentally at autopsy, indicating that it is likely to cause symptoms or more significant problems at some time during a patient's life. Hence, the early detection of TCC and early institution of therapy can never be considered as subjecting patients to unnecessary concern or treatment (as can be strongly argued for incidently detected cancer of the prostate).

Once a cystoscopic examination has revealed that a bladder tumor is present, it should be endoscopically resected in its entirety (transurethral resection of bladder tumor, TURBT). This is not only therapeutic but provides valuable histologic grading and staging information. Additionally, biopsies should be taken from any abnormal or suspicious-looking areas within the bladder as well as from several sites of endoscopically normal appearing mucosa. Because invasion of the prostatic substance or prostatic urethra has a significant impact upon the success of certain therapies, transurethral biopsies of the prostatic urethra are also needed. Any radiologically abnormal appearing areas in the upper urinary tract must also be investigated by obtaining upper tract cytology or direct histologic sampling (through brushing or biopsy) and, if possible, visual inspection through ureteroscopy. Even in the presence of an obvious bladder tumor, bladder lavage cytology is of great value not only to provide a baseline for future management but also because the finding of high-class cytology in the face of a low-grade papillary TCC would indicate the presence of more aggressive tumor elsewhere.

After the initial tumor is resected in its entirety, and the aforementioned histologic, cytologic, and radiographic studies are obtained, a metastatic evaluation, including at least a chest radiograph and, in the presence of high-grade or deeply invasive disease, a CT scan of the abdomen and pelvis and possibly a bone scan, should be undertaken. Such extensive studies may not be needed in the face of low-grade superficial papillary tumors.

Management of Transitional Cell Carcinoma

Superficial Low-Grade Transitional Cell Carcinoma

After initial TURBT and bladder biopsy, findings on histologic inspection will dictate further management. Superficial low-grade tumors, even in the absence of severe epithelial dysplasia or carcinoma in situ (CIS) elsewhere in the bladder and without high-class bladder cytology, will still recur (usually in new locations) after complete endoscopic resection approximately half the time. Recurrences usually happen within the first 2 years after TURBT.

Management generally consists of frequent cystoscopic and cytologic inspections that are performed on an outpatient basis under local anesthesia. Suspicious lesions or obvious tumors require repeat biopsy or resection, and suspicious cytology on follow-up similarly requires numerous biopsies of the bladder and prostatic urethra. Although several forms of intravesical chemo- or immunotherapeutic agents have been found to reduce the frequency of recurrences, these treatments are usually withheld from individuals with newly diagnosed low-grade superficial papillary tumors because, despite a high chance of recurrence, such malignancies rarely progress on subsequent recurrence (no more than 10 percent of patients with grade 1, stage Ta TCC ever develop stage T2 disease). However, if recurrences are frequent (e.g., more than two to three within a 12-month period of time), intravesical installations of any of several agents appear to be efficacious (Table 3). These include thiotepa (30 mg in 30 ml weekly for six to eight treatments and monthly thereafter), mitomycin C (20 to 40 mg in 20 to 40 ml), bacillus Calmette Guérin (BCG) (1 ampule in 50 ml), and perhaps adriamycin (50 mg in 50 ml) — all through similar schedules. Because it is the least expensive and is well tolerated, thiotepa is usually the first drug used. The most common toxicities of these agents are temporary irritable voiding symptoms, bone

marrow suppression (particularly for thiotepa), or fever and a flulike syndrome (for BCG). Occasionally, severe and permanent local symptoms (particularly for mitomycin or for BCG), or sepsis (for BCG) can occur that necessitate cessation of treatment or introduction of antituberculosis medications (for BCG).

High-Risk Superficial Tumors

In individuals with high-grade, large (5 cm or greater in diameter), multiple (three or more), or lamina propria–invading (stage T1) tumors, or in those with high-class cytology, severe epithelial dysplasia, or CIS, the risk of recurrence is slightly higher than with low-grade superficial bladder tumors; more importantly, however, the likelihood of progression to a higher stage upon recurrence is considerably greater. Progression rates range from approximately 20 percent in individuals with moderately or well-differentiated solitary T1 lesions without CIS or high-class cytology to roughly 70 percent in patients with CIS with or without concomitant or prior superficial tumors. Even for individuals at highest risk (e.g., CIS) the use of intravesical instillations of 1 ampule of BCG weekly for 6 to 8 weeks and then monthly has been shown to reduce the likelihood of progression to muscle invasion from approximately 70 percent to 25 percent over a 5-year period. At the present time, prospective randomized studies are underway to evaluate whether BCG is truly more effective than mitomycin C, whether reduction in the dose of BCG or the number of instillations can be done without compromising efficacy, or whether maintenance instillations are beneficial.

Failures of Standard Management

Individuals with low-grade superficial tumors who fail initial treatment (either TURBT or TURBT plus intravesical installations of thiotepa) usually should receive another intravesical agent and can be predicted to have a 30 percent to 50 percent response rate. If failure is with a high-grade superficial lesion or positive cytology, then after extravesical sources of disease are ruled out, intravesical instillations of BCG or mitomycin should be instituted. Individuals with high-risk superficial disease who fail BCG with high-grade recurrences

Table 3 Intravesical Therapy for Superficial Transitional Cell Carcinoma of Bladder

Agent	Prophylaxis of Superficial TCC (ref)	Eradication of Existing Tumors	Ablation of CIS (ref)
Thiotepa	56% (Koontz et al, 1981)	47% (Koontz et al, 1981)	22% (Koontz et al, 1983)
Mitomycin C		45% (De Furia, 1980)	50% (Soloway and Ford, 1983)
Adriamycin	67% (Jacobs et al, 1979)	31% (Duchek, 1980)	67% (Edsmyr et al, 1980)
BCG	60% (Jacobs et al, 1979) −100% (Brosman, 1980)	67% (Martinez-Pineiro, 1980)	75% (Herr et al, 1986)

occasionally respond to a repeat induction course of BCG or other intravesical agents but have a high likelihood of progression to muscle-invading disease with subsequent recurrences. Rules governing when to abandon endoscopic or intravesical modalities are being evaluated. However, patients with high-risk tumors that are not totally eradicated (or recur) by 6 months after the institution of BCG therapy almost invariably develop muscle-invading TCC or succumb to TCC. Thus, at least by that time — and possibly sooner — it would be justified to abandon conservative therapy.

Summary

Superficial bladder tumors, whether high- or low-grade, are initially treated by total endoscopic resection and histologic and cytologic samplings of the remainder of the urinary tract. Because tumor recurrence is extremely common, whether or not intravesical therapies are used patients are cytoscoped initially every 3 months and less frequently if a tumor-free interval of several years is achieved. Because recurrences may happen at any time, surveillance inspections every 12 months are needed throughout a patient's life. In the absence of high-grade or other high-risk lesions, modifications of this treatment plan are dictated by the frequency and "nuisance" of recurrences. Alternatively, if high-risk lesions are present initially or develop subsequently, aggressive treatment is required because the likelihood of progression to muscle-invading disease with lesser modalities is very high.

Rationale for Early Detection Screening

Although 70 percent of patients with newly diagnosed bladder cancers will only have superficial tumors, those with stage T2 disease have little better than a 50 percent chance of being cured even by the most extensive therapies. Unfortunately, only 10 to 15 percent of patients who ever have muscle-invading TCCs have a prior history of superficial tumors. Thus, the extensive surveillance and treatment strategies for superficial disease just discussed, although of great importance to individual patients, are unlikely to reduce bladder cancer mortality significantly — at least until many more tumors destined to become invasive are detected while still confined to a superficial location. For individuals with a very high likelihood of developing a new bladder tumor — such as those with a prior history of superficial tumors — surveillance by regular cystoscopic and cytologic examinations is mandatory. This type of "screening" obviously could not be performed in the asymptomatic individual with no prior history of bladder cancer, but various screening modalities have either been proposed or have actually been carried out with very promising results. At this time, however, there are no prospective studies to indicate that screening, or even early detection, will result in reduced morbidity or mortality from TCC.

Muscle-Invading and Regional Disease

Even when receiving the most extensive local treatment, such as radical cystoprostatectomy and urinary diversion, no more than 65 percent of individuals with stage T2 disease and 40 percent of individuals with stage T3b disease survive 5 years (Table 4). The vast majority of deaths occur because of metastatic TCC; local recurrences develop in no more than 10 percent to 15 percent of all patients (almost all of whom also have concomitant metastases). Thus, it is not a surprise that radiotherapy (20 to 45 Gy) offers no demonstrable efficacy when administered immediately before radical surgery. Although radical external-beam radiotherapy (65 Gy) is capable of curing some patients with invasive TCC, fewer than 50 percent of patients with stage T2 tumors and no more than 25 percent of those with T3 disease are cured by combining radical radiotherapy

Table 4 Five-Year Survival for Invasive Transitional Cell Carcinoma of Bladder*

Reference	Therapy	T2	T2–T3a**	T3a	T3a–T3b**	T3b	Local Recurrence
Goffenet, 1975	Radiotherapy	—	35%	—		20%	50%
Wallace and Bloom, 1976	Radiotherapy	—		—	21%	—	NR
Hope-Stone et al, 1981	Radiotherapy	—		—	38%	—	40%
Freiha, 1990	Radiotherapy	—	30%‡	—		—	62%
Montie et al, 1984	Radical cystectomy	87%		61%		61%	NR
Freiha, 1990	Radical cystectomy	—	65% (NED)	—		—	NR
Freiha, 1990	20–40 Gy preoperative radiotherapy and radical cystectomy	—	59% (NED)	—		—	NR

*Summarized from Droller (1985) and Freiha (1990).
†Eleven percent of survivors required cystectomy.
‡Approximately 25 percent of patients had T3b disease, 70 percent T2–T3a, and 5 percent unknown. Data only reported for all stages.
Abbreviations: NR = not reported.
**Data reported only for combined stages. "T2-T3a" means patients had either T2 or T3a disease; "T3a-T3b" means patients had either T3a or T3b disease. Further breakdown in stage distribution or outcome is not provided in reference.

with "salvage" (upon proven recurrence of TCC) cystectomy. In those relatively rare individuals who have a solitary muscle-invading bladder tumor that is 2 cm or more from the bladder neck without CIS elsewhere, a segmental cystectomy can be performed with as favorable treatment results as total cystectomy.

Systemic Adjuvant Therapy for Invasive Bladder Cancer. Because only 50 percent of patients with stage T2 to stage T3b TCC will be cured by extensive local treatment, and because most patients die of metastases without local recurrence, the possibility that these individuals already have micrometastases at the time of treatment has stimulated attempts at administering systemic therapy in the perioperative period. The advent of cisplatin- and methotrexate-based chemotherapy regimens for metastatic disease has provided the basis for using these in the adjuvant or neoadjuvant setting. At the present time, with the exception of a series with a limited number of patients recently reported by Skinner and colleagues in which a cisplatin-cyclophosphamide-doxorubicin (CisCA) regimen was used after cystectomy, there is no evidence to support the use of adjuvant systemic treatments. A large study comparing a different regimen, methotrexate-vinblastine-doxorubicin-cisplatin (MVAC) plus cystectomy versus cystectomy plus observation (with MVAC upon recurrence), is currently underway in an intergroup setting and should answer this issue.

Because patients with extensive local disease (T4) or regional metastases have a 30 percent or smaller chance of being cured by local modalities alone, these patients constitute a group in whom precystectomy or adjuvant systemic therapy is probably justified. Again, no data from controlled prospective trials are available to support this contention, but the truly ominous prognosis these individuals have and the demonstrated efficacy that current regimens offer for metastatic disease make it reasonable that they be used for extensive regional disease.

Can the Bladder Be Saved in Invasive TCC? In addition to trying to improve the outlook from micrometastases, attempts at bladder salvage in patients with muscle-invading cancer have been undertaken combining cisplatin or cisplatin-methotrexate-vinblastine (CMV) plus radical radiotherapy. Although initial reports from phase 2 studies were encouraging, showing higher local control rates over historical data for radiotherapy (65 to 70 Gy) alone, when these studies were expanded to larger groups, cure rates were not as good as those in contemporary cystectomy series, and many patients could only be cured by having their bladders removed anyway. Thus, although cystectomy has considerable morbidity (a major surgical undertaking, impotence, and the need for a urinary stoma), it currently affords patients the best chance of cure from muscle-invading TCC (see Table 4). Until the intergroup or similar studies are completed, it will not be certain whether additional treatments hold any added benefit.

Reducing the Morbidity of Cystectomy. Three recent surgical developments considerably reduce the morbidity associated with cystoprostatectomy. Walsh and associates described the nerves responsible for potency, which travel posterior to the prostate gland. Adherence to their surgical guidelines to avoid these nerves has allowed potency to be maintained in roughly 70 percent of men who were potent preoperatively and who undergo either radical prostatectomy or cystoprostatectomy. Additionally, the development of various forms of continent urinary diversions (e.g., Kock pouch, Indiana pouch, and so forth) does not necessarily obviate the need for a urinary stoma but does prevent continued loss of urine. Finally, the formation out of bowel of urinary pouches that can be anastomosed to the urethra has permitted the creation of the "neobladder," with which almost all patients achieve daytime urinary continence although enuresis or nocturia often occurs. These surgical developments reduce cystectomy's morbidity but still do not improve its chance of effecting cure. This can only be accomplished by earlier detection or better treatment of micro- and macrometastases.

KIDNEY CANCER

Epidemiology

Renal cell carcinoma (RCC) will be diagnosed in 24,000 Americans this year, and over 10,000 will die from the disease. As with TCC and cancer of the prostate, the incidence of RCC rises with increasing age. Renal cell carcinoma is almost twice as common in men as in women. However, as opposed to cancer of the prostate and TCC, significant differences in the incidence of this disease in various racial, ethnic, or environmentally exposed groups have not been documented. As with most malignancies, there is a slightly higher incidence in current smokers but not nearly to the same degree as is seen for TCC. Recently, exciting studies using genetic probes have demonstrated deletions on the short arm of chromosome 3, perhaps demonstrating loss of suppressor a gene locus and offering possible clues not only to the etiology of RCC but also to identification of individuals at risk. Currently, however, with the exception of an extremely unusual familial form of this entity, only patients with von Hippel-Lindau's syndrome or those who develop renal cystic disease while on hemodialysis are at demonstrated increased risk for contracting RCC.

Renal cell carcinoma is actually a far more common and lethal disease than would be assumed from data based on clinical diagnoses such as those mentioned previously. For example, the elegant autopsy studies of Helsten and colleagues show that nearly 70 percent of RCCs remain undiagnosed during life. However, 25 to 30 percent of those RCCs *incidentally* found at autopsy actually cause death. If one extrapolates these findings to reported mortality data, it is likely that close to 18,000 Americans will actually die of RCC in 1990.

Clinical Presentation, Pathology, and Staging

As with TCC, most RCCs are detected because of hematuria. However, an increasing number of cases are found on imaging studies performed for unrelated reasons (e.g., abdominal ultrasound and CT examinations). This probably explains the relatively recent shift to earlier stage at presentation, with nearly 40 percent of newly diagnosed RCCs now being confined to the kidney (stage I), 20 percent extending extrarenally but confined to Gerota's fascia (stage II), 20 percent extending into the main renal vein, perinephric fat, or regional nodes (stage III), and 20 percent with massive local extension or hematogenous spread (stage IV).

As opposed to both cancer of the prostate and TCC, with the exception of a "sarcomatoid" pattern, which appear in fewer than 10 percent of RCCs, histology offers relatively little prognostic information. Some retrospective reports now indicate that aneuploidy or hyperploidy, as seen on cytometric analysis, carries prognostic information but these observations have yet to be confirmed prospectively.

A peculiarity of pathologic inspection is that a neoplasm histologically identical to RCC, the renal "adenoma," is often found incidentally. Although the autopsy study mentioned before only considered renal tumors to be RCC if they were 3 cm or more in diameter, various authors have reported that those tumors 2 cm or less carry a benign outlook. As has been pointed out by Beckwith and colleagues, however, roughly 7 percent of metastatic RCCs are associated with a primary lesion of less than 2 cm, so that from a histopathologic point of view as well as a logical one, it is uncertain why size alone can be a criterion of benignity. Despite this, there is little doubt that this tumor's pattern of growth remains quite unpredictable. Renal cell carcinomas often reach considerable size and, as documented by reviewing sequential imaging studies, can be present for many years but fail to cause symptoms or to metastasize. Unfortunately, although such cases stand out, they remain decidedly uncommon, for the vast majority of patients with RCC who are not treated succumb to this disease within 2 to 5 years.

Evaluation of a Renal Mass

Whatever imaging modality is originally used, once a renal space-occupying lesion is identified, it is mandatory to determine whether this is a simple cyst, a complex or mixed cyst, or a solid mass. Fewer than 1 percent of sonographically confirmed simple cysts harbor malignancy and, thus, rarely require further workup. Alternatively, 15 to 45 percent of complex cysts and about 90 percent of solid renal masses are malignant. Unfortunately, sampling artifacts make biopsying a complex renal cyst an unproductive exercise in trying to distinguish a benign one from one associated with malignancy. Because most RCCs associated with cysts are hypovascular, renal angiography is also not usually of value. Alternatively, over 80 percent of solid RCCs will contain angiographic abnormalities ("neovascularity") that are highly diagnostic. The two nonmalignant solid renal lesions that can be mistaken for typical RCC from radiographic studies — angiomyolipoma (an hamartomatous lesion) or oncocytoma (a benign neoplasm) — cannot always be distinguished from RCC on preoperative evaluations. Indeed, although angiomyolipomas may have a characteristic appearance on CT scan because of their lipid component, oncocytomas are even histologically very similar to the granular variety of RCC and cannot be diagnosed without examining the entire tumor.

Other renal mass lesions include inflammatory conditions (e.g., abscess, carbuncle, and xangranulomatous pyelonephritis) that are almost always associated with signs and symptoms of infection or a strong infection history. Similarly, although the kidney is often a common site for metastases, these usually occur in multiple locations extremely late in the course of other malignancies; thus, the solitary renal mass is only rarely a metastatic lesion. Lymphomas can involve the kidney, as can TCCs. The latter normally can be distinguished from RCC by retrograde pyelography because all TCCs arise on the urothelial surface. At times, lymphomas are more difficult to distinguish, and, in the presence of massive adenopathy or other signs, biopsy might be justified. However, with this exception or in other very unusual cases, biopsy of a solitary renal mass almost invariably confirms the radiographic diagnosis and is not commonly performed prior to surgery. For this reason, RCC is one of the few neoplasms for which an extensive metastatic evaluation is undertaken prior to obtaining a histologic diagnosis. Because RCCs commonly metastasize to the lungs, retroperitoneal nodes, the liver, and bones, imaging studies such as chest radiograph or CT, abdominal CT, and bone scan are usually performed. Furthermore, because spread through the renal venous tree into the inferior vena cava occurs in about 15 percent of RCCs, radiographic visualization of the vena cava and ipsilateral renal vein (by CT, ultrasound, vena cavography, or nuclear magnetic resonance imaging) preoperatively is mandatory.

Management of Renal Cell Carcinoma

Stage I, II, and III RCCs are all managed by radical nephrectomy. No data are available confirming a salutory effect for radiotherapy on either palliation or cure of RCC either alone or in a pre- or postoperative setting. Furthermore, there is no systemic therapy of enormous efficacy. Thus, treatment for RCC that is resectable is surgical removal. Radical nephrectomy is normally performed through a transperitoneal route in which the renal vessels are ligated prior to manipulation of the tumor and the kidney and all the contents within

Gerota's fascia (including the ipsilateral adrenal gland) are removed en bloc. Regional lymphadenectomy should always be performed because the status of local nodes cannot be determined preoperatively or by gross palpation. Furthermore, unless there is a concerted effort to remove nodes from around the ipsilateral great vessel, almost no nodes will ever be available for histologic review. Although the efficacy of node dissection in terms of cure has yet to be demonstrated, it appears to offer benefit in preventing local recurrence. Indeed, perhaps the greatest advantage of radical nephrectomy as opposed to a lesser procedure is exactly that—achieving local control. Local recurrence of RCC, although seen in only 15 percent of patients undergoing nephrectomy, is very difficult to treat and is usually extremely symptomatic. Node dissection can be performed safely, usually adding 20 minutes to surgery, and does not prolong hospitalization. Accurate knowledge of node status is also critical in determining prognosis and evaluating studies of outcome and adjuvant treatments. Because local recurrence is unmanageable and because subsequent development of RCC in the contralateral kidney is decidedly uncommon (<3 percent to 5 percent), except in situations in which total nephrectomy would lead to severely impaired renal function, procedures that spare renal parenchyma on the involved side should be avoided.

One of the more intriguing aspects in the management of RCC is the recognition that this tumor often spreads as thrombous through the renal vein into the inferior vena cava. Roughly 15 percent of patients with RCC will have vena cava involvement, and extension to the level of the diaphragm and even into the right atrium is not uncommon. Although many patients with vena cava involvement at or above the hepatic veins have concomitant metastases, roughly 50 percent will not at the time of diagnosis. Rather formidable surgical procedures to extract these tumor thrombi have been formulated that often include circulatory arrest or cardiac bypass. Such undertakings are only justified in the absence of hematogenous metastases because, in their presence, death will almost invariably come within 6 to 18 months. Alternately, in patients who lack metastases but have renal vein or vena cava involvement, cure rates of 30 percent to 60 percent have been achieved and, hence, extensive surgical procedures are clearly indicated. Careful preoperative evaluation and consultation with other services (cardiovascular or peripheral vascular surgery and anesthesiology) are needed in performing such surgeries.

Another issue for which there is at least tantalizing information involves the resection of a solitary metastasis and the primary RCC lesion simultaneously. Roughly 15 percent of patients with metastatic RCC will only have a solitary hematogenous metastasis, and complete resection of the primary and metastatic lesion has repeatedly yielded 30 percent 5-year survivals. Systemic therapy has not yet been able to achieve these results. Whether this principle should be extended to the more common situation of multiple metastases is far less certain.

SUGGESTED READING

Bagshaw MA. External beam irradiation of prostatic cancer. In: Coffey DS, Resnick MI, Dorr FA, et al, eds. A multidisciplinary analysis of controversies in the management of prostate cancer. New York: Plenum Press, 1988:85.

Carlton CE Jr., Scardino PT. Long-term results after radioactive gold seed implantation and external beam radiotherapy for localized prostatic cancer. In: Coffey DS, Resnick MI, Dorr FA, et al, eds. A multidisciplinary analysis of controversies in the management of prostate cancer. New York: Plenum Press, 1988:109.

Droller MJ: Transitional cell cancer: Upper tracts and bladder. In: Walsh P, Gittes R, Perlmutter A, Stamey T, eds. Campbell's urology. 5th ed. Philadelphia: WB Saunders, 1985:1343.

Freiha FS. Treatment options for patients with invasive bladder cancer with special reference to bladder substitution with the Stanford pouch. Monogr Urol 1990, 11:34–47.

Grossman HB, Batata M, Hilaris BS, et al. ^{125}I implantation for carcinoma of the prostate. Urology 1982; 20:591.

Hellsten S, Berg T, Wehlin L. Unrecognized renal cell carcinoma: Clinical and diagnostic aspects. Scand J Urol Nephrol 1981; 15:269–272.

Herr HW, Pinsky CM, Whitmore WF, et al. Long-term effects of intravesical bacillus Calmette-Guerin on flat carcinoma in-situ of bladder. J Urol 1986; 135:265–267.

Lieskovsky G, Pritchett R, Skinner DG. Surgical management of renal cell carcinoma. Monogr Urol 1984; 5:98–125.

Messing EM. Early stage bladder cancer. Wisc Med J 1987; 86:14–17.

Paulson DF. Randomized series of treatment with surgery vs. radiation for prostate adenocarcinoma. In: NCI Consensus development conference on the management of clinically localized prostate cancer, 1989:127.

Paulson DF, Hodges GB Jr, Hinshaw W, et al. Radiation therapy versus delayed androgen deprivation for Stage C carcinoma of the prostate. J Urol 1984; 131:901.

Paulson DF, Moul JW, Walther PJ. Radical prostatectomy for clinical T_{1-2} No Mo prostatic adenocarcinoma. Presented at Prostate Cancer: An update. Bloomingdale, IL, June 1990.

Scardino PT. Is radiotherapy effective for locally advanced (Stage C or T3) prostate cancer? In: Murphy GP, Khoury S, eds. Therapeutic progress in urological cancer. New York: Alan R. Liss, (in press).

Walsh PC, Mostwin JL. Radical prostatectomy and cystoprostatectomy with preservation of potency: Results using a new nerve sparing technique. Br J Urol 1984; 56:694–697.

GENITOURINARY CANCER: CHEMOTHERAPY

GEORGE WILDING, M.D.

Cumulatively, cancers of the prostate, bladder, and kidney account for more than 50,000 deaths in the United States each year. These patients die of uncontrolled, metastatic cancer. The role of systemic therapy with cytotoxic agents or hormones in these diseases ranges from minimally useful in renal cell carcinoma to frequently palliative in prostate cancer to very promising in bladder cancer. This chapter reviews the use of systemic therapy in patients with disseminated cancers of the prostate, bladder, and kidney. Many of the drugs noted in the previous chapter as agents used for localized disease are further characterized as to their use and toxicities as applied to patients with metastatic disease. Biologic therapies are covered in the following chapter.

In cases of renal cell carcinoma, the patient and his or her physician must carefully consider the risk-benefit ratio of systemic chemotherapy. There will be many cases in which chemotherapy will be deemed inappropriate. In patients with metastatic prostate cancer, hormone therapy is a well-tolerated front-line therapy that benefits approximately 75 percent of patients in a palliative, not curative, manner. Unfortunately, chemotherapy provides a poor second-line choice but still can account for significant palliation in a portion of patients failing hormone therapy. Advanced cancers of the urothelium, on the other hand, are chemoresponsive tumors, with approximately 50 percent of the patients achieving an objective response to combination chemotherapy. Responders to combination chemotherapy show a prolonged survival over nonresponders. For each disease, we discuss the most effective and widely used treatment(s). In each case, strong consideration should be given to entering the patient on a therapeutic trial when one is available.

BLADDER CANCER

The use of chemotherapy in patients with metastatic cancer of the bladder, specifically transitional cell carcinoma, has been bolstered in recent years by the introduction and development of cisplatin-containing regimens. These regimens have resulted in objective response rates of approximately 50 percent and convey a survival advantage to the responders. In this section, the active single agents are reviewed, and this review is followed by a discussion of the three most commonly used combination regimens.

A considerable number of agents have been tested against transitional cell carcinomas of the bladder and have shown modest activity. This fulfills a basic requirement for the development of successful combination regimens. Namely, active combination therapies usually contain drugs that show activity as single agents in the disease in question. Secondly, the agents constituting a combination should have different mechanisms of action and, whenever possible, not have overlapping toxicity profiles.

As shown in Table 1, cisplatin, methotrexate, vinblastine, and doxorubicin (Adriamycin) all have notable activity against transitional cell carcinomas when used as single agents. Other agents of interest include cyclophosphamide and 5-fluorouracil. Most important, each of these agents has different mechanisms of action and, to some extent, nonoverlapping toxicity profiles, with the exception of myelosuppression, which is common to many cytotoxic drugs. For example, cisplatin acts by covalently binding DNA, thus creating inter- and intrastrand cross-links. Vinblastine is a plant alkaloid that binds to tubulin and inhibits microtubule formation. Adriamycin, on the other hand, intercalates into DNA and acts via free-radical formation or topoisomerase II–dependent damage. Finally, methotrexate, an antifolate, inhibits dihydrofolate reductase and thereby disrupts the synthesis of DNA precursors.

The most active combination of drugs examined for advanced urothelial cancer is the MVAC regimen developed at the Memorial Sloan-Kettering Cancer Center (MSKCC) (Table 2). As noted in Table 2, MVAC employs methotrexate, vinblastine, Adriamycin, and cisplatin. Each of these agents, when administered singly, induce complete or partial response rates of 29, 18, 17 and 30 percent, respectively. The MVAC regimen, although designed to be repeated every 28 days, commonly has a cycle length of 5 weeks or more because of myelosuppression.

In one series of 83 evaluable patients with bidimensionally measurable, advanced transitional cell carcinoma, an overall complete remission (CR) rate of 37 percent was observed (31 patients). Of these patients, 11 achieved a clinically proven CR, and 10 patients were converted to a CR via surgical removal of all residual

Table 1 Single-Agent Trials in Previously Treated and Untreated Patients with Advanced Urothelial Tract Tumors

Drugs	No. of Patients	Complete and Partial Remissions (%)
Cisplatin	320	30 (25–35)*
Cyclophosphamide	26	7 (0–17)
Doxorubicin	248	17(12–23)
5-Fluorouracil	105	15(18–22)
Methotrexate	236	29(23–25)
Vinblastine	38	16 (4–28)

*Numbers in parentheses indicate range of 95 percent confidence intervals.

Table modified from Yagoda A. Chemotherapy of urothelial tract tumors. Cancer 1987; 60:574–585; with permission.

Table 2 Methotrexate, Vinblastine, Adriamycin, and Cisplatin (MVAC) for Metastatic Transitional Cell Carcinoma

Drug	Schedule (day)*			
	1	2	15†	22†
Methotrexate (30 mg/m²)	X		X	X
Vinblastine (3 mg/m²)		X	X	X
Adriamycin (30 mg/m²)		X		
Cisplatin (70 mg/m²)		X		

*The cycle repeats in 28 days. See Steinberg CN, Yagoda A, Scher HI, et al. MVAC (methotrexate, vinblastine, doxorubicin [Adriamycin], and cisplatin) for advanced transitional cell carcinoma of the urothelium. J Urol 1988; 139:461–469 for dose modifications.
†No drugs were administered when mucositis was present, while blood cell count was less than 2,500 per microliter, or platelet count was less than 100,000 per microliter.

disease. The median duration of response of patients achieving a CR was 37 months, with 55 percent of the patients achieving CR alive at 40 months' follow-up. The estimated probability of surviving 2 and 3 years was 71 percent and 54 percent, respectively.

Thirty-one percent of patients achieved a partial remission (PR), with a median duration of response of 8 months and 11 months for survival. Of interest, half of the patients with PRs failed at sites other than those involved at presentation, although all of the patients with PRs initially had extensive disease. Nonresponders had a median survival of 7 months. Responding patients received five to six cycles of therapy. The MVAC regimen does not appear to be active in non–transitional cell urothelial tumors.

After a median follow-up of 40 months, 78 percent of the 57 CR/PR patients had developed brain metastases. This was the only site of relapse in 5 of the 10 patients. Median survival was only 2 months after the diagnosis of a brain metastasis.

The MVAC regimen induces a wide variety of toxicities. White blood cell nadirs less than 200 per microliter were observed in as many as 32 percent of the cycles, whereas 41 percent of the patients suffered some degree of mucositis. Nausea and vomiting were universal despite antiemetics, and hemoglobin dropped more than 2 g per 100 ml in 76 percent of the patients. High-grade thrombocytopenia (< 50,000 per microliter) occurred in only 5 percent of the patients, whereas grade 1 neurotoxicity occurred in 3 percent and higher than grade 1 renal toxicity occurred in 6 percent of patients. Because no drugs were administered when mucositis was present, the white blood cell count was less than 2,500 per microliter or the platelet count was less than 100,000 per microliter, the median cycle length was 5 weeks or more, and as little as one-third of the patients received both the day 15 and day 22 treatments. The drug-related death rate was 4 percent.

In general, the overall 68 percent response rate reported by the MSKCC group suggests that MVAC is the most active combination regimen studied thus far. Interim analysis of an Eastern Cooperative Oncology Group (ECOG study) comparing MVAC to cisplatin alone has confirmed the superiority of MVAC over cisplatin. However, the overall response rate of the MVAC arm was only 33 percent, whereas the response rate for cisplatin alone was 9 percent. Because myelosuppression and mucositis are the dose-limiting toxicities of the MVAC regimen, attempts are being made to ameliorate these side effects via the use of G-CSF or GM-CSF (colony-stimulating factor). In addition, if successful, these factors may permit administration of full doses per schedule.

Starting in 1981, Torti and his colleagues in the Northern California Oncology Group (NCOG) initiated therapy of patients with advanced urothelial cancers with the combination of cisplatin, methotrexate, and vinblastine (CMV) (Table 3). All patients had measurable disease, had not received any prior systemic therapy, and had a creatinine clearance greater than 50 ml per minute. Cycles were scheduled for every 21 days.

Sixty-two evaluable patients were treated. Twenty-six percent achieved a complete response, and, when surgically consolidated CRs were taken into account, the overall CR ratio was 34 percent. Complete responders received a median of six cycles of therapy. The median survival of patients who relapsed was 14 months.

Toxicity of the CMV regimen consisted primarily of myelosuppression and renal toxicity. Approximately 25 percent of the patients had creatinine levels rise above 2 mg per deciliter, and half of the patients required dose modifications owing to a decreased creatinine clearance. Although 14 patients developed severe leukopenia (white blood cell count < 1,000 per microliter) and 2 died with bacteremia, some of these patients, including the 2 that died, received methotrexate (40 mg per square meter) at doses higher than those used in the current regimen. Gastrointestinal toxicities were minor. As with MVAC, central nervous system (CNS) relapses have been noted in CNS to the CMV regimen, again raising the issue of whether the CNS is a sanctuary.

The CMV regimen appears to achieve a CR rate similar to MVAC and offers several advantages. First, it does not contain Adriamycin and therefore may be more appropriate for use in patients with cardiac dysfunction. Second, it involves a 3-week versus 4-week cycling period

Table 3 Cisplatin, Methotrexate, and Vinblastine (CMV) for Metastatic Transitional Cell Carcinoma

	Schedule*		
Drug	Day 1	Day 2	Day 8
Cisplatin (100 mg/m^2)		X	
Methotrexate (30 mg/m^2)	X		X
Vinblastine (4 mg/m^2)	X		X

*The cycle repeats in 21 days. See Harker WG, Meyers FJ, Freiha FS, et al. Cisplatin, methotrexate, and vinblastine (CMV): An effective chemotherapy regimen for metastatic transitional cell carcinoma of the urinary tract. A Northern California Oncology Group Study. J Clin Oncol 1985; 3:1463–1470 for dose modifications.

Table 4 Cisplatin, Cyclophosphamide and Adriamycin for Metastatic Transitional Cell Carcinoma

	Schedule*	
Drug	Day 1	Day 2
Cisplatin† (70–100 mg/m^2)		X
Cyclophosphamide (650 mg/m^2)	X	
Adriamycin (50 mg/m^2)	X	

*The cycle repeats in 21 to 48 days. See Khandekar JD, Elson RJ, DeWys WD, et al. Comparative activity and toxicity of *cis*-disammine dichloroplatinum (DDP) and a combination of doxorubicin, cyclophosphamide and DDP in disseminated transitional cell carcinoma of the urinary tract. J Clin Oncol 1985; 3:539–545 for dose modifications.
†Accompanied by mannitol-forced diuresis.

with a single (day 8) interval drug administration schedule versus the day 15 and day 22 dosing schedule used in MVAC. Randomized comparison of CMV versus MVAC is not available. Given the shorter cycle period for CMV, the difficulty in administering both the day 15 and day 22 MVAC doses, and the frequent delay of subsequent cycles, which effectively lengthens MVAC to a 5-week regimen, it would appear that CMV is the more dose-intense regimen for cisplatin, methotrexate, and vinblastine. It is not known if Adriamycin sufficiently compensates for the lower dose intensity of the other three agents in the MVAC regimen.

Logothetis and his colleagues at the M.D. Anderson Cancer Center have established an extensive experience with a cisplatin, cyclophosphamide, and Adriamycin (CISCA) regimen (Table 4). In a series of 97 patients with unresectable urothelial cancers, 28 percent achieved a CR, whereas an additional 28 percent had PR for a PR/CR rate of 56 percent overall. Responses were seen in 11 of 20 cases (55 percent) with mixed histologies containing transitional cell carcinoma as well as spindle cell, adenocarcinoma, or squamous cell histologies. One of the advantages of this regimen is that it does not require interval administration of drugs during the middle weeks of each cycle as seen with the MVAC and CMV regimens. One disadvantage of CISCA is that it contains Adriamycin, which may be problematic in some patients with cardiac dysfunction. More importantly, it replaces vinblastine and methotrexate, two of the more active single agents, with cyclophosphamide, which appears to be less active than either of these agents when used as a single agent. A recent study by Logothetis and colleagues comparing CISCA to MVAC has confirmed that MVAC is the more active of the two regimens.

Transitional cell carcinoma of the upper urinary tract (ureter and renal pelvis) is rare, accounting for less than 5 percent of all urothelial tumors. However, metastatic transitional cell carcinoma of the upper urinary tract is aggressive and uniformly fatal. Few series of uniformly treated patients are available. Logothetis has reported on the treatment of 24 patients with upper urinary tract transitional cell tumors treated with CISCA or other regimens such as MVAC. The overall response rate was 38 percent (five PR and four CR). No significant

differences in response were noted between the 10 patients treated with CISCA and 8 treated with MVAC.

PROSTATE CANCER

Prostate cancer is diagnosed in more than 100,000 men in the United States each year and accounts for 30,000 cancer deaths yearly. It is the most prevalent solid tumor in American men. Approximately 50 percent of the new cases will present with metastatic prostate cancer (stages D1 and D2), whereas another 10 percent will have disease extending through the capsule of the prostate gland (stage C). In addition, approximately 20 percent of men with clinical stage A2 disease and 30 percent or more of men with clinical B2 disease have positive lymph nodes on lymphadenectomy, making them pathologically stage D1. At the present time, metastatic prostate cancer is not curable. Fortunately, metastatic prostate cancer can be effectively palliated via a number of available hormonal therapies. However, all patients with disseminated prostate cancer ultimately suffer and die from hormone-independent cancer. The purpose of this section is to (1) outline the currently available hormone therapies used as front-line treatment for metastatic prostate cancer; (2) review second-line hormone manipulations, and (3) summarize the status of cytotoxic chemotherapy in this disease (Table 5).

The mainstay of hormone therapy for metastatic prostate cancer is bilateral orchiectomy. Proven by Higgins in the 1940s to be an effective palliative therapy, this treatment remains the "gold standard" by which other hormone therapies are measured. Orchiectomy removes the primary source of testosterone in men, the testicles. Its advantages are that it is a one-time treatment that removes concerns of compliance, drug delivery and metabolism, and drug toxicity. In addition, compared to the newer therapies, it remains relatively inexpensive (e.g., the cost of bilateral orchiectomy performed on an outpatient basis in the Midwest is approximately $1,200 to $1,500). Although it is certainly irreversible, there exists a viewpoint that even after hormone failure a patient should be maintained in an orchiectomized state. The rationale for this approach

Table 5 Endocrine Therapies for Metastatic Prostate Cancer (Stage D2)

Therapy	Dose	Common Side Effects*	Patient Cost†
LHRH agonist			
Leuprolide (Lupron Depot)	7.5 mg IM q28d	Hot flashes, impotence, bone pain (early)	$300/mo
Goserelin (Zoladex)	3.75 mg SC q28d		
Flutamide‡	250 mg PO q8hr	Gynecomastia, diarrhea	$200–250/mo
DES	1 mg PO qd	Impotence, gynecomastia, cardiovascular,§ thromboembolic§	<$10/mo
Bilateral orchiectomy		Impotence, psychologic effects	$1,000–1,500 once
Secondary therapies:			
Ketoconazole	200–400 mg PO tid	Gastrointestinal intolerance, adrenal insufficiency**	$300–350/mo
Megesterol acetate	40 mg PO qid	Impotence, thromboembolic, gynecomastia	$50–100/mo
Hydrocortisone	20 mg PO bid	Fluid retention	$10–20/mo

*The most common side effects are listed and should not be considered comprehensive.
†Patient costs are estimates from practice in Wisconsin and can vary considerably.
‡Flutamide has been approved for use with an LHRH agonist to ameliorate the first response.
§Cardiovascular includes edema, congestive heart failure, myocardial infarction, and arrest. Thromboembolic includes vein thrombosis, pulmonary embolism, and cerebrovascular accident.
**Hydrocortisone replacement is commonly given with ketoconaide therapy because of the high incidence of adrenal insufficiency.

maintains that although a patient's tumor may no longer be dependent for growth on testosterone, it still may be responsive to testosterone stimulation. The most common side effect of orchiectomy is impotence and loss of libido. The Veterans Administration Cooperative Urologic Research Group (VACRRG) studies from the initiation of hormone therapy for stage D2 prostate cancer patients is commonly delayed until absence of symptoms. Some patients and physicians may find it more suitable to initiate hormone treatment earlier in the course of a patient's disease.

The psychological effects of orchiectomy are always raised when discussing side effects. When Cassileth and colleagues obtained baseline questionnaires on 147 patients with stage D2 prostate cancer, 78 percent chose a medical form of therapy, the luteinizing hormone–releasing hormone (LHRH) agonist Zoladex, over orchiectomy. Thirty-six percent of the patients choosing Zoladex chose it "to avoid surgery," whereas 32 percent of those choosing orchiectomy did so because of "convenience."

Diethylstilbestrol (DES) was studied extensively in the VACURG studies of the 1960s. One of the primary conclusions from this series of studies was that DES, 5 mg per day, was equivalent in its antitumor palliative effects to orchiectomy, although it also accounted for a high incidence of thrombotic events and cardiovascular deaths, and 1 mg per day was equivalent to 5 mg per day of DES and resulted in fewer thrombotic events. However, there was a trend towards more cardiac and thrombotic events in the group taking 1 mg of DES per day (36/155) versus the placebo arm (26/143). Diethylstilbestrol, 3 mg per day, came into use because it resulted in testosterone levels equivalent to those following orchiectomy, although it is *not* more efficacious than 1 mg of DES per day as an antitumor agent; 3 mg per day of DES is clearly associated with an increased number of thrombotic events. The com-

bination of DES and orchiectomy provides no antitumor advantage over either alone. This is understandable if DES has no direct effect on prostate cancer cells but acts solely by shutting off LH release from the pituitary, and thereby testosterone production by the testes, thus achieving a medical orchiectomy. Other side effects of DES that are troublesome to patients are breast tenderness and enlargement as well as loss of libido. Financially, DES is inexpensive, at less than $10 per month. With the cardiovascular and thrombotic risks of DES, 3 mg per day, the suggestion of increased risks with even 1 mg per day of DES, and the availability of alternative and equivalent medical therapies, one needs to seriously consider discarding DES as the medical therapeutic option of choice in favor of the therapies outlined below.

With the discovery of the decapeptide LHRH, a large number of analogues were synthesized and analyzed in comparison to the native peptide. Native LHRH has a half-life in the blood stream of only several minutes and is released from the hypothalamus in pulses approximately every hour. By substituting D-amino acids at the 6 position and by adding groups such as an ethylamide group to the carboxy terminus, the half-life of many analogues was increased to hours, and, in some instances, the binding affinity of the analogue for the LHRH receptor was also increased. After release from the hypothalamus, LHRH binds to cell-surface receptors in the pituitary. The receptor-hormone complex stimulates the production and release of LH into the circulation. The binding of LH to its receptors on Leydig cells in the testes induces the production of testosterone. Because the pituitary cells normally function under pulsatile stimulation by native LHRH, the prolonged activity of the LHRH agonists results in constitutive rather than pulsatile exposure to the LHRH analogues and leads to a desensitization of the pituitary cells to LHRH stimulation. Consequently, LH levels fall, and testosterone production by the Leydig cells decreases dramatically.

Initial clinical trials compared daily subcutaneous injections of an LHRH agonist, leuprolide, 1 mg per day, to DES, 1 mg three times a day, in men with stage D2 prostate cancer. At 12 weeks, there was no difference in the number of responders or the number of men who progressed. At the end of 1 year, there was no significant difference in survival between the two treatments.

With the development of depot formulations of leuprolide (Depot Lupron) and goserelin (Zoladex), treatment with monthly injections of LHRH agonists became more attractive to patients and compliance improved. In trials of Zoladex versus orchiectomy for the treatment of patients with advanced prostate cancer, there was no significant difference between treatment groups with regard to subjective and objective responses, endocrine responses, clinical effects, side effects, time to treatment failures and death, or survival after similar median follow-up periods. In a comparison of Zoladex versus DES, 1 mg PO three times a day, response duration and survival were similar; however, there was a more rapid response to treatment in the Zoladex group. Because these compounds are agonists, during the first 2 weeks of treatment, LH and testosterone levels rise before they fall; this has been called the flare response. Therefore, patients with impending spinal cord compression or urinary obstruction should not be started on LHRH agonists alone. Concomitant treatment with an effective antiandrogen, such as flutamide, can attenuate the flare response in most patients. In the Zoladex studies, although 11 of 300 Zoladex patients had increased bone pain, no patient required discontinuation of treatment during the initial stages of treatment. On the other hand, 15 percent of the patients receiving DES had their treatment discontinued during the first 3 months of treatment because of toxicity. Sixteen of 126 DES patients suffered vascular symptoms or complications.

Although the testes produce greater than 90 percent of the circulating androgens in men, the adrenal glands make and secrete weak androgens that can be converted in one or two enzymatic steps to testosterone. Therefore, the concept of combining an LHRH agonist or orchiectomy with an antiandrogen was developed in an attempt to achieve maximal androgen blockade. One of the larger randomized studies examining complete androgen blockage was the National Cancer Institute–sponsored intergroup trial comparing the use of leuprolide, an LHRH agonist, administered subcutaneously daily with either a placebo or the nonsteroidal antiandrogen flutamide. More than 600 patients were admitted to the study. The 300 patients receiving leuprolide and flutamide had a longer progression-free survival (16.5 versus 13.9 months; $P = 0.039$) and an increase in the median length of survival (35.6 versus 28.3 months; $P = 0.035$) compared to the 300 patients receiving leuprolide alone. Most striking was the improved survival of the 41 patients with minimal metastatic disease who were treated with the combination regimen versus leuprolide and placebo. If confirmed, this would support earlier intervention with hormone therapy in patients with metastatic prostate cancer. Of interest, the patients receiving the combination therapy showed the greatest improvement in symptoms during the first 12 weeks of therapy, suggesting that amelioration of possible LHRH agonist induced flare effects during this period. Thirteen percent of the patients taking flutamide complained of diarrhea compared to 4% in the control group.

Primary hormone therapy ultimately fails in all patients as hormone-independent disease emerges. Secondary attempts at hormone manipulation yield palliative results, generally subjective in nature, in approximately 20 percent of patients and are of short duration. Second-line therapies are usually aimed at reducing adrenal androgen production. The agents most often used include hydrocortisone, 20 to 40 mg per day; ketoconazole, 200 to 400 mg PO three times a day (steroidogenesis inhibitor); and flutamide.

Cytotoxic chemotherapy has shown a low level of activity in patients who have failed primary hormone therapy. There is no proven benefit of chemotherapy as a front-line therapy. Likewise, combination chemotherapy has not proved superior to single agents, which is reflective of the lack of active agents. Although the survival of patients failing their first hormone therapy is approximately 12 months, patients receiving chemotherapy have a median survival of 6 months.

Although a large number of agents have been tested, few have shown activity. Cyclophosphamide, 5-fluorouracil, cisplatin, and others have shown objective response rates of 10 percent or less. Adriamycin given as a weekly injection of 20 mg per square meter is generally well tolerated and has proven to be of palliative benefit in terms of stabilization of disease, diminished pain, or improved performance status in approximately half the patients treated. However, responses are short-lived (approximately 3 months), and objective responses are infrequent (10). Survival is not improved.

A variety of problems complicate the task of finding active cytotoxic agents for prostate cancer. First, because prostate cancer occurs in an elderly population with a median age of 70, patients commonly have concomitant medical problems, particularly pulmonary, cardiovascular, and renal problems, that predispose them to the side effects of chemotherapy and commonly prevent the administration of optimal chemotherapy doses. Secondly, most patients with metastatic prostate cancer have an impaired bone marrow reserve because of bone metastases or prior radiation therapy. This factor, again, leads to poor tolerance of cytotoxic therapy, particularly with agents with hematologic toxicities. Finally, only 5 percent to 15 percent of patients with metastatic prostate cancer have bidimensionally measurable disease; most have diffuse bone disease that may be evaluable but not measurable. Some have advocated entry of only patients with bidimensionally measurable disease into phase 2 drug studies to avoid this problem.

Failure of primary hormone therapy heralds the end of our ability to control systemic disease effectively. Our inability to overcome hormone independence and drug resistance highlights the need to place patients on investigative trials whenever possible.

RENAL CANCER

In general, the treatment of renal cell carcinoma with chemotherapy has not been shown to increase survival. The most active agent in this disease appears to be vinblastine, 0.2 to 0.3 mg per kilogram per week, with an objective response rate of approximately 15 percent. Responders to vinblastine do have an improved survival. The resistance of renal cell cancers to chemotherapy may be related to the expression of the multiple drug resistance gene *mdr*, which codes for a transport glycoprotein called p170. This protein is located in the cell membrane and serves as an efflux pump capable of ejecting many types of xenobiotics and toxins from cells expressing p170. Normal renal tubular epithelial cells constitutively express the *mdr* gene. Likewise, renal cell carcinomas that are derived from renal tubular epithelial cells commonly express the *mdr* gene. Ongoing clinical trials are assessing the ability of agents such as verapamil, amiodarone, antihistamines, steroid agents, and tamoxifen to inhibit p170 function and thereby reverse the multiple drug resistance phenotype. In view of the dismal performance of cytotoxics in the disease, all patients with metastatic renal cell carcinoma should be considered for entry into trials examining the efficacy of new agents, modulation of existing agents such as vinblastine, or development of biologic therapies (see next chapter). Because of their proven, though limited, efficacies, regimens containing vinblastine, alpha-interferon or interleukin-2 frequently are administered to eligible patients sometime during the course of their disease.

Hormonal therapy in the form of progestational agents such as Megace have anecdotally been reported to be of benefit in renal cell carcinoma. Clinical trials, however, have failed to confirm activity for steroid hormones in this disease. No eligible patient should be denied access to investigational cytotoxic or biologic therapy to be treated with hormonal agents.

Supported by NIH grant R29-CA50590 and by the Veterans Administration.

SUGGESTED READING

Bladder Cancer

Harker WG, Meyers FJ, Freiha FS, et al. Cisplatin, methotrexate, and vinblastine (CMV): An effective chemotherapy regimen for metastatic transitional cell carcinoma of the urinary tract. A Northern California Oncology Group Study. J Clin Oncol 1985; 3:1463–1470.

Khandekar JD, Elson RJ, DeWys WD, et al. Comparative activity and toxicity of *cis*diammine dichloroplatinum (DDP) and a combination of doxorubicin, cyclophosphamide and DDP in disseminated transitional cell carcinoma of the urinary tract. J Clin Oncol 1985; 3:539–545.

Sternberg CN, Yagoda A, Scher HI, et al. MVAC (methotrexate, vinblastine, doxorubicin and cisplatin) for advanced transitional cell carcinoma of the urothelium. J Urol 1988; 139:461–469.

Yagoda A. Chemotherapy of urothelial tract tumors. Cancer 1987; 60:574–575.

Prostate Cancer

Byar DP. Proceedings: The Veterans Administration Cooperative Urological Research Group's studies of cancer of the prostate. Cancer 1973; 32:1,126–1,130.

Cassileth BR, Soloway MS, Vogelzang NJ, et al. Patients' choice of treatment in stage D1 prostate cancer. Urology (S) 1989; XXXIII: 57–62.

Crawford ED, Eisenberger MA, McLeod DG, et al. A controlled trial of leuprolide with and without flutamide in prostatic carcinoma. N Engl J Med 1989; 321:419–424.

Eisenberger MA, Simon R, O'Dwyer PJ, et al. A reevaluation of nonhormonal cytotoxic chemotherapy in the treatment of prostatic carcinoma. J Clin Oncol 1985; 3:827–841.

Henrikkson P, Linde B, Edhag O. Deleterious effects of low-dose estrogen therapy on coronary status in patients with prostatic cancer. Eur Heart J 1987; 8:779–784.

Labrie F, DuPont A, Belanger A. Complete androgen blockade for the treatment of prostate cancer. In: DeVita VT Jr, Hollman S, Rosenberg SA, eds. Important advances in oncology. Philadelphia: JB Lippincott, 1985:193–217.

Peeling WB. Phase III studies to compare goserelin (Zoladex) with orchiectomy and with diethylstilbestrol in treatment of prostatic carcinoma. Urology (S) 1989: XXXIII:45–51.

Raghaven D. Non-hormone chemotherapy for prostate cancer: Principles of treatment and application to the testing of new drugs. Semin Oncol 1988; 15:371–389.

Kidney Cancer

Fojo AT, Shen DW, Mickley LA, et al. Intrinsic drug resistance in human kidney cancer is associated with expression of a human multidrug-resistance gene. J Clin Oncol 1987; 5:1,922–1,927.

Harris DT. Hormonal therapy and chemotherapy of renal cell carcinoma. Semin Oncol 1983; 10:422–430.

Hrushesky WJ, Murphy GP. Current status of the therapy of advanced renal carcinoma. J Surg Oncol 1977; 9:277–288.

BIOLOGIC RESPONSE MODIFIERS IN THE TREATMENT OF GENITOURINARY CANCER

PETER C. KOHLER, M.D., Ph.D.
PAUL M. SONDEL, M.D., Ph.D.

Biologic response modifiers (BRMs) represent what may become a fourth modality in the treatment of cancer. Biologic response modifiers encompass an ever-expanding number of treatment approaches whose mechanisms of action involve augmentation or amplification of a normal host response (either immunologic or hematopoietic) or alteration in the tumor susceptibility to various mechanisms of killing. Evidence to suggest a role of BRM in the treatment of genitourinary malignancies includes the prognostic implications of the ABO blood group surface antigens and the Thomsen-Friedenreich (T) antigen in bladder cancer; the detection of circulating levels of several cytokines following intravesical bacillus Calmette Guefin (BCG); and the intriguing but rare reports of spontaneous regressions of metastatic renal cancer, believed to be a result of host immune response. A more thorough description of BRMs is provided in the chapter by Drs. Albertini and Schiller.

BLADDER CANCER

With an estimated 40,000 new cases per year, bladder cancer is the second most common carcinoma of the GU tract. The majority of patients (75 percent) with bladder cancer have disease that is of low stage or superficial at diagnosis (stages Tis, Ta, and T_1) and can be effectively treated by transurethral resections. Long-term survival with this approach occurs in 80 percent of patients, but only half are cured. Following the initial transurethral resection, the chance of subsequent superficial tumors or the development of muscle-invading disease will be dependent on the number of tumors, grade, and initial stage. Intravesical therapy has been shown to be an effective means of treating known residual disease. It is also an effective prophylactic agent, having been shown to decrease the recurrence of superficial bladder cancers.

Bacillus Calmette Guefin acts as a nonspecific stimulator of the immune system. The use of intravesical BCG has been shown to be an effective therapy for residual disease and for tumor prophylaxis. The mechanism of action for intravesical BCG is unknown, but it may be through a local inflammatory reaction that denudes the mucosa or secondary to a systemic immunologic response to BCG antigens. Following administration of BCG, circulating levels of interferon, interleukins-1 and 2, and tumor necrosis factor (TNF) have been detected.

For patients with gross disease, intravesical BCG can achieve a complete response in 70 percent of newly diagnosed patients and 50 percent of patients who have failed therapy with thiotepa or mitomycin. Intravesical BCG has also been shown to reduce the rate of relapse, improve relapse-free survival, and prevent the development of invasive carcinoma following a transurethral resection. In a meta-analysis performed by Laudone and Herr involving 1,600 patients enrolled in 10 controlled clinical trials, the recurrence rate at 1 year following transurethral resection ranged from 36 to 67 percent. Compared to transurethral resection, a less than 10 percent reduction in the rate of recurrence was seen with thiotepa, a 10 to 20 percent reduction with mitomycin and doxorubicin, and a greater than 40 percent reduction with BCG. Recently, BCG has been approved by the FDA for use in patients with carcinoma in situ, in whom it is felt to be the intravesical agent of choice.

Toxicity secondary to intravesical BCG is usually local and due to an intense inflammatory reaction; it includes hematuria, urinary frequency, and dysuria. Systemic side effects are much less common and include temperature higher than 103°F (3.9 percent), pneumonitis (1 percent), hepatitis (1 percent), arthralgias or arthritis (0.5 percent), and skin rash (0.4 percent). Its use is contraindicated in patients who are immunosuppressed or who have an active tuberculosis infection. Antituberculosis agents have been used for patients with severe local reactions and those suspected of developing systemic infection ("BCGosis").

Alpha-interferon has also undergone initial testing in the treatment of superficial bladder cancer. The Northern California Oncology Group has conducted a phase 1 study testing interferon in high-risk patients. Escalation of the interferon was stopped at 10^9 U owing to formulation problems; no dose-limiting toxicities were seen. Of 19 patients with carcinoma in situ, 6 (32 percent) had a complete response documented by cytology and biopsy and 5 (26 percent) had a partial response. Three of the patients remained disease-free in excess of 1 year with no maintenance treatment. Responses were seen over the complete dose range tested, including the initial dose of 50×10^6 U.

Other BRMs studied in the treatment of superficial bladder cancer include Poly I:C, an interferon inducer. Although no difference in recurrence rates was documented between patients treated with transurethral resection alone and those given Poly I:C following transurethral resection, there was an improved survival in the experimental group. In those patients treated with Poly I:C who remained disease-free, a two- to eight-fold elevation in serum interferon level was detected. Interleukin-2 (IL-2) has also undergone preliminary testing in superficial bladder cancer. The number of patients treated at this point is too small to draw any conclusions.

RENAL CANCER

Disappointing results with chemotherapy and in vitro and in vivo evidence linking regression of metastatic renal cancers to activity of the immune system have led to a large number of trials using BRMs in renal cancer. Nonspecific immune stimulators, including BCG, xenogeneic immune RNA, transfer factor, and thymosin fraction 5 have undergone limited testing. Despite small numbers of patients and impure materials, these studies showed some evidence of clinical activity in patients with advanced disease, including a few patients who achieved a complete response.

Research into the use of specific antitumor immunotherapy has included autologous tumor vaccines and monoclonal antibodies (MoAb). Although tumor-specific antigens on renal cancer cells have not yet been found, a number of surface antigens that are more selectively expressed on these tumor cells and that most likely represent differentiation antigens have been identified. Studies utilizing autologous tumor cells combined with nonspecific immune augmenting agents, which include: tuberculin, phytohemagglutinin (PHA), BCG, *Corynebacterium parvum*, cimetidine, and cyclophosphamide, have shown occasional responses in limited testing.

The use of MoAb for staging and therapy is under active investigation. Problems that will need to be solved include the heterogeneity of the surface antigens expressed by tumor cells, the development of the human anti-mouse antibody (HAMA) response due to sensitization from murine immunoglobulins, and whether the most effective means of achieving antitumor activity will be by linking the MoAb with a radionuclide, toxin, or drug. Each of these issues is undergoing active investigation.

Interferons have undergone extensive clinical testing in patients with metastatic renal cancer. Quesada and colleagues reported the first evidence of antitumor activity in 1983 using a partially purified alpha-interferon. Five partial responses were seen in 19 patients treated with 3 million units (MU) of daily intramuscular injections. Studies conducted with recombinant alpha-interferon have since been done that investigate a wide dose range (1 to 50 MU) and varying schedules and routes of administration. Response rates ranged from 5 percent to 27 percent, with a duration of response of 3 to 16 months. In the majority of studies, a complete response rate of less than 10 percent was reported. Response rates for the subtypes of alpha-interferon do not appear to be significantly different (19 percent human leukocyte interferon, 17 percent partially purified lymphoblastoid interferon, and 14 percent recombinant interferon).

Despite the number of trials, the optimal dose, schedule, and route for administering interferon have not been determined; however, some conclusions can be drawn from the data derived from the testing of recombinant human alpha-interferon. Intermediate- and high-dose regimens (10 to 20 MU) generally have a higher response rate than low-dose regimens (1 to 2 MU). The duration of therapy may be an important variable because, in many cases, responses are first seen only after several months of treatment. Tumor burden and sites of metastases may be important factors in predicting response. Although responses have been reported to occur more frequently in patients who have their primary tumor resected, it has not been conclusively shown in randomized studies that a nephrectomy is necessary to achieve a response. The majority of responses occur in patients with disease confined to the lung and mediastinum. Responses in the liver, bone, brain, or renal primary are rare. Neutralizing antibodies develop in a significant number of patients treated with recombinant interferon. The effect of these antibodies on antitumor activity is unclear.

Fewer clinical trials in renal cancer have been conducted with beta-interferon or gamma-interferon. It does not appear that either has clinical activity any greater than alpha-interferon and results with gamma-interferon suggest inferior response rates. Combinations of alpha-interferon with other BRMs (gamma-interferon, diflouromethylornithine [DFMO], and double-stranded RNA) and cytotoxic agents (primarily vinblastine) were similarly shown to be no more effective than single-agent alpha-interferon alone, and were associated with increased toxicity.

INTERLEUKIN-2

In 1976, Morgan, Ruscetti, and Gallo first described an immunologic hormone initially called T-cell growth factor (TCGF). The development of recombinant techniques has allowed production of the active component in TCGF, interleukin-2 (IL-2). Produced by helper T cells in response to mitogenic or antigenic stimulation, IL-2 serves as a stimulus for key components of both the cellular and humoral arms of the immune response. Incubation of peripheral blood lymphocytes in IL-2 results in the generation of activated cells (LAK cells) that are capable of lysing tumor cells with relative sparing of normal tissues.

Interleukin-2 alone or combined with ex vivo–generated autologous LAK cells has undergone clinical testing in patients with metastatic renal cancer (Table 1). The largest of the studies has been conducted at the Surgery Branch of the National Cancer Institute under the direction of Dr. Steven Rosenberg. Confirmatory studies have also been done through participating institutions in the Extramural LAK Working Group. Patients in both studies were treated with 100,000 U per kilogram of IL-2 by intravenous bolus every 8 hours for five consecutive days to stimulate LAK precursors. Harvesting was then done by leukopheresis. The collected peripheral blood lymphocytes were then incubated in IL-2 for 3 to 4 days to increase LAK activity. Treatment was begun at day 12 with infusion of the collected LAK cells combined with additional IL-2 to maintain viability of the LAK cells.

Table 1 Maximum Tolerated Doses of Selected
Interleukin-2 Treatment Regimens*

Group or Institution	Dose and Schedule
National Cancer Institute	10^5 U/kg IV bolus q8h on days 1–5 and 13–17
Seattle	30×10^6 U/m^2/day IV; 2- and 24-hr infusion weekly
Tufts	10^6 U/m^2 IV bolus weekly
Illinois Cancer Council	3×10^7 U/m^2 24-hr continuous infusion twice weekly
University of Chicago	4.5×10^6 U/m^2 24-hr continuous infusion weekly $\times$ 6
Wisconsin	3×10^6 U/m^2/day/IV continuous infusion 4 days/wk $\times$ 4 consecutive weeks

*Treatment regimens using IL-2 alone at a variety of cancer centers.

An overall response rate of 35 percent was seen in the initial 72 patients with metastatic renal cancer treated with LAK and IL-2 at the National Cancer Institute. Eight (11 percent) of these patients achieved a complete response. Fifty-four patients with metastatic renal cancer were treated with a similar IL-2 regimen without the administration of ex vivo–generated LAK cells. The overall response rate was 22 percent, with four (8 percent) complete responses. In the Extramural LAK Working Group, 32 patients with renal cancer were treated using the National Cancer Institute's IL-2 and LAK regimen. A 16 percent response rate was reported, with two (6 percent) patients achieving a complete response. Of note is the durability of the complete responses in both studies, which have, in some instances, exceeded a year. As seen with interferon, factors that appear to favor response include low tumor burden and metastatic disease confined to the lungs.

In both of these trials, the toxicity associated with therapy was substantial, and intensive care unit support was necessary for many patients. Major side effects included hypotension, fever, renal failure, fluid retention, and pulmonary edema. Many of the severe clinical problems associated with treatment are due to a capillary-leak syndrome felt to be caused by endothelial damage by LAK cells and by the release of other cytokines such as TNF and gamma-interferon. Although nonsteroidal anti-inflammatory agents such as indomethacin are commonly used to ameliorate the fever associated with treatment, there is some evidence to suggest that this may exacerbate the renal insufficiency induced by treatment with IL-2. Immunosuppressive agents such as dexamethasone can significantly decrease the toxicity associated with IL-2, but at a cost of decreased efficacy.

In an attempt to reduce toxicity and improve therapeutic effects, alternative approaches to those carried out by the National Cancer Institute have been undertaken. The administration of IL-2 by continuous infusion was thought to offer several advantages. Interleukin-2 has a short half-life (5 to 7 minutes), and once activated, LAK cells are dependent on its continued presence to maintain activity. Therefore, by providing a constant exposure to IL-2, an enhancement in in vivo LAK activity might be seen. Toxicity might also be lessened with continuous infusion by avoiding the high peak levels of IL-2 occurring with bolus infusion. In addition, the immunologic effects associated with IL-2 therapy, like the toxicity, dissipate quickly once IL-2 is stopped. This suggests that longer periods of treatment, with breaks for recovery, might provide a more tolerable, yet efficacious, therapy.

These factors led to the approach taken at the University of Wisconsin, where patients are treated with repeated cycles of IL-2 either alone or in combination with ex vivo autologous LAK cells. A striking enhancement in LAK activity is seen following 4 weeks of treatment (each week consists of 4 days of continuous infusion of IL-2 followed by 3 days of rest). The toxicity associated with this approach has been acceptable. In the initial report, 3 of the 14 patients (21 percent) with metastatic renal cancer who were treated with 3×10^6 U per square meter achieved a partial response. Studies combining LAK cells with this schedule of IL-2 are now in progress.

Although dramatic individual responses have been reported with IL-2 alone or in combination with LAK cells, it is becoming increasingly clear that the complete response rate with this approach is low. This has led to studies investigating alternative ways of utilizing IL-2. Tumor-infiltrating lymphocytes that have been obtained from a resected tumor and have greater specificity are being tested with IL-2. Other combinations currently under study include the addition of chemotherapy, other BRMs, including interferon (alpha, beta, and gamma), TNF, and MoAbs to IL-2 regimens. Regional therapy is being tested on patients with nodal metastases from head and neck carcinomas. It is also being tested as intravesical therapy for superficial bladder carcinomas.

SUGGESTED READING

Buzaid AC, Todd MB. Therapeutic options in renal carcinoma. Semin Oncol (Suppl 1) 1989; 16(1):12–19.

Hawkins MJ. IL-2/LAK: Current status and possible future directions. PPO Updates 1989; 3(8).

Herr HW, Laudone VP, Whitmore WF. An overview of intravesical therapy for superficial bladder cancer. J Urol 1987; 38:1,363–1,368.

Quesada JR. Biologic response modifiers in the therapy of metastatic renal cell carcinoma. Semin Oncol 1988; 15(4):396–407.

Rosenberg SA. Adoptive immunotherapy for cancer. Sci Am 1990; May:62–69.

Sosman JA, Hank JA, Sondel PM. In vivo activation of lymphokine-activated killer activity with interleukin-2: Prospects for combination therapies. Semin Oncol (Suppl 1) 1990; 17(1):22–30.

Torti FM, Lum BL. Superficial carcinoma of the bladder: Natural history and the role of interferons. Semin Oncol (Suppl 2) 1986; 13(3):57–60.

TESTICULAR CANCER

PATRICK J. LOEHRER, Sr., M.D.

Over the past two decades, the therapeutic approach and prognosis of patients with germ cell neoplasms have vastly improved. Improvement in staging of patients, reliable serum markers (beta-subunit human chorionic gonadotropin, and alpha-fetoprotein), and, most importantly, the development of effective cisplatin-based combination chemotherapy have been the major factors behind the progress in the outcome of patients with this disease. Over 95 percent of those diagnosed with testicular cancer should be curable with proper treatment, including 80 percent of those patients who present with disseminated germ cell neoplasms. This chapter focuses upon the recent advances and current controversies in the treatment of early and advanced-stage germ cell neoplasms.

NON-SEMINOMATOUS GERM CELL TUMORS

Histologically, germ cell neoplasms can be divided into two categories: seminoma and nonseminomatous germ cell tumors (embryonal carcinoma, yolk sac carcinoma, teratoma, choriocarcinoma, or any combination). The distinction between seminoma and nonseminomatous germ cell tumor (NSGCT) is most important for those patients with early stage disease. For early stage disease, radiotherapy remains the treatment of choice for seminoma while NSGCT is primarily managed by surgery.

The clinical staging of patients with testicular cancer is as follows: stage A (or I), which is limited to the testis alone; stage B (or II), which includes spread to the retroperitoneal lymph node structures; and, finally, stage C (or III), which includes supradiaphragmatic extension, and pulmonary or other visceral organ involvement. Approximately 20 percent of patients with NSGCT will present with stage C; the remaining 80 percent of patients will be evenly distributed between stages A and B.

The emphasis on staging work-up should be directed towards detecting whether a patient has advanced stage B or stage C disease (in which initial treatment is primarily chemotherapy) or whether a patient has an early stage NSGCT, which is generally treated with primary retroperitoneal lymph node dissection (RPLND) or, in some settings, surveillance. Evaluation should include a careful history and physical examination, with particular attention paid to the supraclavicular lymph nodes, roentgenographic examinations, including a chest radiograph (computed tomography [CT] scan of the chest, if chest radiograph is normal), and abdominal CT scan. Serum alpha-fetoprotein (AFP) and beta-subunit human chorionic gonadotropin (BHCG) should also be obtained. Whereas 90 percent of those patients with recurrent NSGCT testicular cancer will demonstrate an elevation in one or both of these serum markers, approximately 30 percent of patients with clinical stage A disease will have retroperitoneal lymph node involvement despite normal serum markers.

CLINICAL STAGE A DISEASE

The time-honored approach for a patient presenting with clinical stage A testicular cancer is a RPLND. Properly performed, this modality cures approximately 50 to 60 percent of patients with carcinoma involving the lymph nodes, with a less than 1 percent chance of local recurrence. Approximately 10 percent of pathologic stage A patients and 40 to 50 percent of resected stage B patients will develop recurrent disease. When followed closely with a monthly chest radiograph and serum markers during the first year and every 2 months during the second year, virtually all those patients who develop recurrent disease will have minimal metastatic disease, for which the cure rate with cisplatin combination chemotherapy is 99 percent or greater.

One of the major drawbacks of a traditional bilateral RPLND as initial treatment of clinical stage A patients is that 70 percent of patients will undergo this operation "needlessly" (i.e., without documentation of retroperitoneal metastases). In addition, bilateral RPLND will uniformly produce retrograde ejaculation and sterility. Modifications of the RPLND have improved the ability to maintain antegrade ejaculation in over 80 percent of patients. Dr. Donohue and his associates at Indiana University have recently developed a nerve-sparing RPLND in which the sympathetic nerves are carefully dissected, which enables one to maintain normal ejaculatory function and, thus, significantly minimizes the morbidity from treatment.

The concept of initial observation in lieu of surgery for clinical stage A testicular cancer stems from the aforementioned concerns of surgically induced ejaculatory dysfunction as well as the tremendous success seen with chemotherapy for patients with advanced disease. Dr. Peckham and his colleagues in England initially introduced the concept of surveillance only for patients with clinical stage A disease. Similar trials have been instigated here in the United States in which such patients carefully followed with radiographs and markers every month and CT scans of the abdomen every 2 months had the anticipated 30 percent recurrence rate. In some series, patients also were followed by lymphangiograms. Multivariant analysis has suggested several prognostic factors that predict relapse for clinical stage A patients, including invasion of the venous and lymphatic vessels, absence of yolk sac elements, and presence of undifferentiated (embryonal carcinoma) tumor. However, the time to relapse differs from that for patients undergoing RPLND as primary therapy because there is a continuous (4 percent per year) relapse rate beyond 2 years.

One of the major concerns regarding surveillance for patients with stage A testicular cancer is the reliability of patient and supportive service. Computed tomography scans must be of excellent quality and interpreted by skilled radiologists. For those patients who recur with bulky abdominal disease and pulmonary metastases, a less favorable outcome with subsequent chemotherapy is achieved. Surveillance for patients with stage A disease remains an option *only* for the most highly motivated group of patients and physicians who maintain a rigorous follow-up schedule that includes frequent CT scans of the abdomen. A modified RPLND, performed by a skilled urologist, remains the standard for the majority of patients. Efforts to delineate those patients clearly destined to benefit from RPLND are underway.

STAGE B DISEASE

As mentioned previously, stage B testicular cancer is defined as disease that has spread to the retroperitoneal lymph nodes. Stage B disease can be subdivided into B1 (microscopic only), B2 (macroscopic but less than 10 cm), or B3 (palpable, or ≥ 10 cm). Indications for surgical intervention for those patients with stage B disease have been modified in the postcisplatin chemotherapy era. Nonetheless, RPLND alone in such patients is associated with a 50-70 percent relapse-free survival. Stage B disease represents one of the few malignancies with such a cure rate in the face of lymphatic involvement.

ADJUVANT THERAPY

In light of the effectiveness of the chemotherapy in metastatic disease, the issue of adjuvant therapy in patients with resected stage B disease was addressed by the Testicular Cancer Intergroup Study. Following RPLND, 195 patients with completely resected stage B disease were randomized to observation only or to receive two postoperative courses consisting of cisplatin, vinblastine, and bleomycin (PVB) or a variation (VAB-6). This study confirmed that patients treated with surgery alone had a relapse rate of approximately 48 percent. All but three patients were subsequently cured with four cycles of systemic chemotherapy upon disease recurrence. In the patients who received two cycles of adjuvant therapy, there have been two recurrences and one cancer death. Thus, the overall survival of 98 to 99 percent was not significantly different between the two arms. This study demonstrated that two cycles of adjuvant chemotherapy would virtually eliminate the chance for disease recurrence; however, similar long-term results were attainable with those patients who were carefully followed with monthly chest radiographs and serum markers alone. It is important to recognize, however, that two cycles of adjuvant therapy do not supplant an "inadequate" RPLND. Patients who may

undergo a "debulking" procedure should be treated with more aggressive combination chemotherapy (three or four cycles of therapy) as if they had metastatic disease.

Patients with early stage B disease as manifested by elevated markers followed by orchiectomy or minimal abnormalities on CT scans, present a mild therapeutic dilemma. Some investigators are exploring the option of giving systemic chemotherapy to such patients while reserving surgery for those patients who have persistent residual disease. In general, those patients who present with lymph nodes measuring 3 cm or less in greatest diameter should generally be referred to a competent urologist for a RPLND.

STAGE C DISEASE

In patients who present with advanced testicular cancer, combination chemotherapy is the mainstay of treatment. The dramatic change in therapeutic outcome during the past 15 to 20 years has been outlined in several reviews. The single, most important breakthrough came with the discovery of cisplatin and its activity in patients with refractory testicular cancer. Prior to the utilization of cisplatin, various regimens demonstrated objective remissions, but only rare patients attained durable, complete remissions. In 1974, Dr. Einhorn at Indiana University combined cisplatin with the active drug combination of vinblastine and bleomycin (PVB) (Table 1). The rationale for PVB included single-agent activity, different mechanisms of action, and differing dose-limiting toxicities for each of the three drugs. In the first 47 patients treated, 70 percent attained a complete remission, and an additional 11 percent were rendered free of disease with surgical extirpation of residual disease, which revealed teratoma of persistent carcinoma. The additional cycles of chemotherapy were administered in those patients with resected carcinomas. Fifty-seven percent of these patients remain continually free of disease.

Numerous trials have been done under the auspices of Indiana University and the Southeastern Cancer Study Group over subsequent years (Table 2). Random prospective trials demonstrated that lowering the dose of vinblastine was associated with less myelosuppression without adverse impact on overall survival. Further trials failed to demonstrate an improvement in response rate or survival with the addition of doxorubicin (a mildly active drug) to induction therapy or maintenance

Table 1 Original PVB Regimen

Agent	Dosage
Cisplatin	20 mg/m^2/days 1–5 every 3 wk × 4
Vinblastine	0.2 mg/kg day 1 and 2 every 3 wk × 4
Bleomycin	30 U IV push weekly × 12

Maintenance vinblastine, 0.3 mg/kg monthly × 21 mo

Table 2 Results of Sequential PVB Studies at Indiana University

Study No. (Yr)	No. of Patients	No. with CR (%)	NED with Surgery (%)	Now NED (%)
1 (1974–1976)	47	33 (70)	5 (11)	25 (57)
2 (1976–1978)	78	51 (65)	13 (17)	57 (73)
3 (1978–1981)	147	92 (63)	31 (21)	117 (80)

Table 3 Treatment Arms of Southeastern Cancer Study Group Trial Comparing PVB and PVP-16B

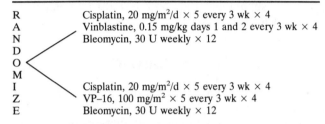

R
A
N
D
O
M
I
Z
E

Cisplatin, 20 mg/m²/d × 5 every 3 wk × 4
Vinblastine, 0.15 mg/kg days 1 and 2 every 3 wk × 4
Bleomycin, 30 U weekly × 12

Cisplatin, 20 mg/m²/d × 5 every 3 wk × 4
VP–16, 100 mg/m² × 5 every 3 wk × 4
Bleomycin, 30 U weekly × 12

Table 4 Indiana University Staging System for Disseminated Testicular Cancer

Minimal Extent
1. Elevated markers only
2. Cervical nodes (± nonpalpable retroperitoneal nodes)
3. Unresectable nonpalpable retroperitoneal disease
4. Fewer than five pulmonary metastases per lung field and largest < 2 cm (± nonpalpable retroperitoneal nodes)

Moderate Extent
1. Palpable abdominal mass only (no supradiaphragmatic disease)
2. Moderate pulmonary metastases: 5–10 metastases per lung field and largest <3 cm *or* solitary pulmonary metastases of any size >2 cm (± nonpalpable retroperitoneal disease)

Advanced Extent
1. Advanced pulmonary metastases: primary mediastinal nonseminomatous germ cell tumor *or* >10 pulmonary metastases per lung field, *or* multiple pulmonary metastases with largest >3 cm (± nonpalpable retroperitoneal disease)
2. Palpable abdominal mass plus supradiaphragmatic disease
3. Liver, bone, or central nervous system metastases

vinblastine therapy. As such, the initial 2-year regimen was shortened to a brief 12 weeks of therapy.

THE ETOPOSIDE ERA

Although 70 percent of patients would be cured of their disease with PVB, a cohort of patients would be candidates for salvage chemotherapy. For patients progressing on cisplatin, no drug, with the exception of etoposide, demonstrated single-agent activity. Based on preclinical data demonstrating synergy of cisplatin/VP-16, this combination was used as initial salvage therapy in patients failing to be cured with initial PVB therapy. Approximately 25 to 30 percent of such patients were subsequently cured. This formed the basis of a prospective randomized trial that compared PVB to cisplatin plus etoposide plus bleomycin (PVP-16B) (Table 3). Eighty-nine of 121 (73.5 percent) patients who were treated with PVB obtained a complete remission or were rendered disease-free following resection of teratoma or carcinoma. This compared to 102 of 123 (83 percent) patients who were treated with PVP-16B. Although hematologic toxicity was comparable in both groups of patients, neuromuscular side effects, including paresthesias, myalgias, and abdominal cramps, were significantly less in those patients receiving etoposide. Furthermore, for those patients with advanced disease, the PVB-16B regimen was associated with a significantly improved survival. As such, PVB-16B has become the preferred induction chemotherapy for metastatic disease.

Evaluation of patients with disseminated germ cell tumors treated with PVB-16B has led to various staging systems that have estimated prognosis. The Indiana University Staging System (Table 4) separated those patients with good-risk (minimal and moderate) disease (over 90 percent cure rate) from those patients with advanced disease (a 50 to 60 percent cure rate) (Table 5).

Table 5 Disease-Free Status in Advanced Testicular Cancer According to Indiana Staging System, 1978–1983

Minimal	Moderate	Advanced
102/103 (99%)	50/55 (91%)	43/81 (53%)

Subsequent research strategies have turned to minimizing toxicity for those patients with good-risk disease while looking at more innovative and intense therapy for patients with poor prognosis.

GOOD-RISK TESTICULAR CANCER

The Southeast Cancer Study Group recently completed a trial to evaluate the optimal duration of therapy with good-risk disease. In 184 patients with minimal or moderate disease, therapy was either the standard *four* cycles of PVB-16B over 12 weeks or *three* cycles of the same regimen over 9 weeks. Ninety-three of 96 (97 percent) patients randomized to receive four cycles of therapy achieved a disease-free status compared to 86 of 88 (98 percent) patients receiving three cycles. Overall, 91 percent and 92 percent of the patients, respectively, remain continuously free of disease with three and four cycles, respectively. Thus, therapy could be shortened to three cycles of therapy, or just 9 weeks, in patients with good-risk disease.

Alternative treatment strategies in good-risk disease have looked at the omission of bleomycin. In a trial reported by the Australian Germ Cell Neoplasm Trial Group, 104 patients received either PVB alone or without weekly doses of bleomycin. In another trial performed by investigators at Memorial Sloan-Kettering Cancer Center, 140 good-risk patients were randomized to receive VAB-6 or four cycles of cisplatin plus etoposide alone. The largest trial in good-risk disease has been performed by the European Organization for Research on Treatment of Cancer in which patients were randomized to receive cisplatin plus etoposide (120 mg per square meter on days 1, 3, and 5) alone or with weekly bleomycin. Although the initial two trials have reportedly shown no advantage with the addition of bleomycin, the latter trial is still ongoing, with the suggestion of an increased recurrence rate for those patients who did not receive bleomycin. Preliminary results from the Eastern Cooperative Oncology Group trial also suggest a higher recurrence rate for patients who did not receive bleomycin. Until further results emerge from these trials, one cannot advocate the omission of bleomycin, particularly when administered with only three cycles of VP-16 for patients with good-risk disease.

POOR-RISK PATIENTS

Dose intensity is a concept that has permeated the thinking of many researchers in medical oncology. Indeed, when one retrospectively reviews data in germ cell neoplasms, an improved survival is observed in those patients who receive more intense cisplatin (33 mg per square meter per week versus ≤ 25 mg per square meter per week) dosage. In one prospective randomized trial performed by the Southwest Oncology Group, patients who received 120 mg per square meter of cisplatin had a significant improvement in response rate and overall survival compared to patients treated with 75 mg per square meter (both receiving vinblastine and bleomycin). Whether further escalation of cisplatin dosage might improve the therapeutic outcome is uncertain. Dr. Ozols and his colleagues at the National Cancer Institute reported the feasibilies of ultra-high dosages of cisplatin (40 mg per square meter daily for 5 days) in combination with etoposide, bleomycin, and vinblastine. In a prospective randomized trial comparing this regimen with PVB, an improvement in response rate and survival was noted in patients treated with the high-dose regimen. However, it was unclear whether the improvement in survival in this latter study was associated with the intense dosage of cisplatin or the addition of etoposide.

As a consequence, a prospective randomized trial was performed by the Southeastern Cancer Study Group, Indiana University, and the Southwest Oncology Group in which patients were randomly assigned to receive cisplatin at two dosages (20 mg per square meter versus 40 mg per square meter daily for five days) with the identical dosages of etoposide (100 mg per square meter daily for 5 days) and bleomycin (30 U per

week × 12). From October, 1984, through August, 1989, 150 patients with advanced germ cell tumors were entered on this protocol. Forty-four of 68 patients treated with the high-dose cisplatin (65 percent) achieved a disease status with chemotherapy or resection of teratoma and carcinoma compared to 51 of 73 (70 percent) treated with standard-dose therapy. Significantly greater neurologic and hematologic toxicity was associated with the more intense regimen. Thus, doubling the dose of cisplatin, the most effective single agent in germ cell malignancies, did not improve the therapeutic outcome of such patients. An ongoing intergroup trial is currently evaluating the role of ifosfamide in patients with advanced disease.

SALVAGE THERAPY

Despite the success of cisplatin combination chemotherapy over the past 15 years, approximately 20 to 30 percent of patients will be candidates for salvage chemotherapy. Testicular cancer has served as a gateway of testing new active compounds, including cisplatin and etoposide. The majority of patients who currently enter phase II trials for refractory germ cell tumors have been heavily pretreated. In our experience, only two drugs, etoposide and ifosfamide, have demonstrated activity in cisplatin-refractory patients.

Although virtually all patients respond to initial induction chemotherapy, early recognition of resistance is important. Observation of the decline of serum markers provides some early clues. For instance, a log reduction of BHCG should occur with each successive course of this therapy (e.g., 10,000, 1,000, 100, 10 ...). Salvage regimens can be successfully implemented before the overt development of resistance to cisplatin, as manifested by rising markers on therapy.

Occasionally, patients may be misdirected for initiation of salvage therapy based on false impressions of tumor progression either with growing benign teratoma on therapy, false elevations of serum markers with BHCG (marijuana, cross-reactivity with luteinizing hormone, antibodies), or alpha-fetoprotein (hepatitis). Occasionally, pseudonodules may occur with bleomycin and may mimic metastatic disease. Furthermore, persistent elevation of markers may occur with cancer within the brain or testis, which may serve as a sanctuary site.

Ifosfamide is an oxazaphosphorine analogue of cyclophosphamide and was found to be active in cisplatin-refractory patients by investigators in Europe and in Indiana. Like etoposide used in the salvage setting, however, single-agent ifosfamide failed to produce durable complete remissions. In a trial initiated in 1983, 56 patients who were previously treated with cisplatin, vinblastine, and VP-16 were treated with a regimen of cisplatin, ifosfamide, and either vinblastine (VeIP) or etoposide (VIP). Overall, 20 (36 percent) patients achieved disease-free status. Nineteen of these patients remained disease-free for 16 to 63 months, and 9 patients remained continuously free of disease. The curative potential of ifosfamide as part of third-line therapy is unprecedented in the postcisplatin era, and it led to the current evaluation of ifosfamide in first-line therapy for patients with advanced disease.

Extending the preclinical observations of synergy of cisplatin plus VP-16, a further dose-intensification model of high-dosage carboplatin (900 to 2,000 mg per square meter) plus etoposide (1.2 g per square meter) followed by autologous bone marrow transplant was initiated at Indiana University. In 20 highly refractory patients receiving this therapy, durable complete remission was attained in 5 patients. Current trials evaluating this approach as part of initial salvage therapy are ongoing.

TOXICITY OF CHEMOTHERAPY

The acute toxicity associated with chemotherapy is well recognized. Although nephrotoxicity was a serious problem in early phase II trials with cisplatin, with adequate pretreatment and posttreatment hydration, it is relatively uncommon that clinically significant nephrotoxicity occurs. Nonetheless, one should be cautious with concurrent use of other nephrotoxic agents, including contrast dyes and aminoglycosides.

Nausea and emesis have remained relative problems for patients treated with cisplatin combination chemotherapy. However, this has largely been abrogated with the use of combination antiemetic therapies as well as newer serotonin agonists that minimize and can frequently eliminate nausea and vomiting associated with cisplatin. Raynaud's phenomena has been reported with vinblastine and bleomycin therapy and appears to be enhanced with cisplatin. Persistent paresthesia is dose-related with therapy. Although there is some controversy as to potential cardiovascular complications of cisplatin combination chemotherapy, a recent analysis of patients who were treated on the Testicular Intergroup trial revealed no significant difference between those patients observed versus those who receive adjuvant therapy or who develop recurrent disease.

The majority of patients who present with disseminated germ cell tumors will be severely oligospermic or azospermic. Following four cycles of PVB, 96 percent of patients are azospermic. With time, however, approximately half of patients will have normal sperm counts and motilities. Thus far, no congenital abnormalities have been known in the wives of patients who have successfully had children.

In a recent review of 207 patients with a minimal follow-up of 5 years, we noted relatively few long-term severe side effects other than sterility and Raynaud's function. Late recurrences of cancer and leukemia are generally not observed in the absence of the use of more classic alkylating agents other than cisplatin. Late recurrences beyond 2 years are unusual in testicular cancer and have generally been associated with those patients who have had resection of benign teratoma or persistent abdominal disease, which would imply residual teratoma. There is, however, a close association between mediastinal germ cell malignancies and acute megakaryocytic leukemia that is not treatment-related.

SEMINOMAS

As mentioned previously, early stage seminoma can be treated with radiation therapy in lieu of a RPLND with a 95 percent cure rate. Some patients with pure seminoma may have low levels of BHCG; in general, such patients would be treated as if they had seminoma without elevation of markers. Any patient, however, who has nonseminomatous elements or an elevated AFP should be treated as a similarly staged patient with NSGCT.

Some controversy exists regarding the role of observation for clinical stage A patients. Dr. Thomas and her associates in Canada have recently demonstrated that a recurrence rate of clinical stage I seminoma patients is much less frequent than previously appreciated (less than 10 percent). Yet, other investigators are concerned with the surveillance policy for patients with seminoma who may recur with more advanced disease because they differ from NSGCT in that they rarely have elevated serum markers on recurrence.

In patients with bulky stage B disease, controversy exists regarding the most appropriate treatment approach. Approximately 60 percent of patients will be cured with infradiaphragmatic radiotherapy alone. For those who recur following radiotherapy, cisplatin-based chemotherapy should be successful for the vast majority. Prophylactic mediastinal radiotherapy does not appear to improve the cure rate for stage B disease, but it will significantly impair the ability to give full-dosage chemotherapy in those patients failing to be cured. In previously untreated patients with bulky stage B seminoma, chemotherapy without radiotherapy would expect to cure over 90 percent of cases. As such, infradiaphragmatic or cisplatin combination chemotherapy is a viable alternative for patients with bulky stage B disease.

Cisplatin-based combination chemotherapy is the treatment of choice for patients with advanced seminoma who have a similar prognosis as those patients with similarly staged NSGCT. Extensive prior radiotherapy (mediastinal and infradiaphragmatic) and extent of disease appear to impact prognosis adversely. Management of seminoma patients with residual bulky disease following chemotherapy is unclear. Some data suggest that patients with residual masses that are 3 cm or larger have a greater chance of having persistent carcinoma. In such cases, resection may be difficult; thus, careful observation by serial CT scans is a viable option. Accepted and investigative approaches for treatment of Seminoma and NSGCT are demonstrated in Table 6.

EXTRAGONADAL GERM CELL TUMORS

Although commonly arising in the testis, germ cell tumors may arise at various midline structures, such as

Table 6 Treatment Recommendations

Clinical Setting	Standard Therapy	Investigative Therapy
Nonseminomatous Germ Cell Tumor (NSGCT)		
Stage A	Retroperitoneal lymphad-enopathy (modified or nerve-sparing)	Surveillance (including first year): CT scan of abdomen every 2 mo, chest radiogram and markers (AFP, BHCG, LDH) qmo × 1 yr. Second year: Abdominal CT q4mo with chest radiograph and serum markers every 2 mo
Stage B1 or B2 (S/P RPLND)	Observation with PVP-16B on relapse or two cycles of PVP-16B as adjuvant	None
Stage B3 or C		
Minimal or moderate	PVP-16B × three cycles or cisplatin plus etoposide × four cycles plus resection of residual disease	Ongoing trials to minimize toxicity
Advanced	PVP-16B × four cycles plus resection of residual disease	Clinical trials ongoing, such as VIP (etoposide, ifosfamide plus cisplatin) versus PVP-16B Early integration of high-dose chemotherapy with autologous bone marrow transplant
Seminoma		
Stage A	Infradiaphragmatic radio-therapy (2,500 cGy)	Surveillance (including first year): CT scan of abdomen every 2 mo, chest radiograph and markers (AFP, BHCG, LDH) qmo × 1 yr. Second year: Abdominal CT q4mo with chest radiograph and serum markers every 2 mo.
Stage B1 or B2	Infradiaphragmatic radio-therapy (2,500 cGy)	
Stage B3 (palpable or > 10 cm)	Infradiaphragmatic radio-therapy or cisplatin-based combination chemotherapy	Management of residual mass of ≥ cm is contro-versial (observe, resect, radiotherapy)
Stage C	PVP-16B × 4 cycles or other cisplatin-based combination therapy	Same as NSGCT clinical trials; based on tumor extent ("good risk" vs. "poor risk")

the mediastinum, retroperitoneum, pineal gland, prostate, or thymus. Although historically patients with extragonadal germ cell tumors present with more advanced disease, they have a similar chemosensitive response as their counterparts with testicular cancer.

Primary mediastinal germ cell tumors appear unique in their propensity to present with more advanced disease as well as their association with chromosomal abnormalities and atypical syndromes. A close association with Klinefelter's syndrome and primary mediastinal tumors has been recently elucidated. Furthermore, non–germ cell malignancies (e.g., sarcomatous elements, adenocarcinoma), acute megakaryocytic leukemia, and other myelodysplastic disorders occur much more frequently in patients with mediastinal germ cell tumors than in patients with germ cell neoplasms of testicular origin.

Extragonadal germ cell tumors must be considered in the differential diagnosis of a patient with a carcinoma of unknown primary. Therefore, serum HCG and AFP should be performed, particularly in those patients who are young presenting with mediastinal or retroperitoneal tumors. An empiric trial of PVP-16B for such patients should be strongly considered. Approximately 50 to 60 percent of patients with extragonadal germ cell tumors should be cured with cisplatin combination chemotherapy with complete excision of residual disease being extremely important.

Supported in part by PHS MO1 RR00-750-06.

SUGGESTED READING

Einhorn LH. Testicular cancer as a model for curable neoplasm: The Richard and Hinda Rosenthal Foundation Award Lecture. Cancer Res 1981; 41:3,275–3,280.

Loehrer PJ, Sledge GW, Einhorn L. Heterogeneity among germ cell tumors of the testis. Semin Oncol 1985:304–316.

Loehrer PJ, Williams SD, Einhorn LH. Testicular cancer: The quest continues. J Natl Cancer Inst 1988; 80(17):1373–1382.

Williams SD, Birch R, Einhorn LH, et al. Disseminated germ cell tumors: Chemotherapy with cisplatin plus bleomycin plus either vinblastine or etoposide. A trial of the Southeastern Cancer Study Group. N Engl J Med 1987; 316:1,435–1,440.

Williams SD, Stablein DM, Einhorn LH, et al. Immediate adjuvant chemotherapy versus observation with treatment at relapse in pathological stage II testicular cancer. N Engl J Med 1987; 317: 1,433–1,438.

UTERINE AND ENDOMETRIAL CANCER

GEORGE D. MALKASIAN Jr., M.D.

Over the years, the American Cancer Society has predicted the number of new cases of endometrial cancer expected in any single year and the number of anticipated deaths from that cancer in that particular year. In 1977, the number of anticipated new cases was 27,000, with new cases rising to 39,000 in 1983 and 1984 but declining to 37,000 in 1985; 35,000 in 1987; 34,000 in 1989; and 33,000 in 1991. The number of anticipated deaths from the disease in 1983 was 3,400, declining to 2,900 in 1987, only to rise to 5,500 in 1991. This is an 89.7 percent rise in anticipated deaths in 4 years, a finding that to date has gone unexplained. In 1991, it is anticipated that endometrial cancer will account for 46.0 percent of all new primary genital cancers and about 23.4 percent of all deaths from cancers arising in these organs. Compared to the 1989 figures of 47 percent and 12 percent, respectively, the increase in deaths is striking, making this a disease not to be taken lightly. In 1985, data showed that the probability of a woman's developing endometrial cancer was 3.3 percent if she was born in 1975 and 2.4 percent if she was born in 1985.

RISK FACTORS

Hormones

An analysis of women who had used combination oral contraceptives at some time in their lives showed a relative risk of occurrence of endometrial carcinoma of 0.5 percent when compared with women who had never used oral contraceptives. This protective effect took place when combination oral contraceptives had been used for a minimum of 12 months, and it persisted for at least 10 years after the cessation of their use. The relative risk decreased most significantly in nulliparous users (to 0.4 percent when compared with nulliparous never users). On this basis alone, the authors of the study predicted a drop of about 2,000 cases per year in the population at risk.

A case control study of the relationship between exogenous estrogens and endometrial carcinoma identified a 2.3 percent risk when any estrogen had been used for longer than 6 months. In this study, the risk of conjugated estrogens used for any duration was 2.0 percent; when estrogens were used for 6 or more months, this rose to 4.9 percent; when used for 1 year or more, it was 5.3 percent; when used for 2 years or more, it was 8.3 percent; and when used for more than 3 years, it was 7.9 percent. This study also demonstrated that, whereas doses of 0.625 mg per day for 6

months or more were associated with a risk of 1.4 percent, doses of 1.25 mg per day for 6 months or more promoted an increase to 7.2 percent. The risk for 6 or more months of uninterrupted estrogen use is 7.9 percent.

Studies relating the use of sequential contraceptives to endometrial carcinoma are consistent. These all suggest that the 16 days of unopposed estrogen followed by 5 days of a weak progestin do not allow the estrogen effect to be counteracted by the progestin.

Studies of higher dose progestin for longer periods show the incidence of endometrial cancer to be 390:100,000 in estrogen users alone and 49:100,000 among estrogen-progestin users. These figures are compared with 245:100,000 in nonhormone users in the population at large. This same study reports the occurrence of carcinoma among estrogen-progestin users when the progestin had been used for 6 to 10 days, but no cases of carcinoma had been identified in women who had used a progestin for 14 days per cycle. The associations between endometrial carcinoma and feminizing ovarian tumors and between endometrial carcinoma and polycystic ovarian syndrome are both statistically much greater than chance. This increased risk emphasizes the need to sample the endometrium whenever either of these ovarian situations is encountered.

Other Risk Factors

Endometrial cancer occurs significantly more often in patients who are obese or nulliparous. When obesity is defined as 30 percent or more above the upper limit of ideal weight for height and frame, the relative risk of endometrial cancer is 3.5 percent. The relative risk for nulliparous patients is 1.8 percent. The attributable risk or etiologic fraction (the percentage of the total cases that would not have occurred if the factors under consideration had been absent) is calculated at 9.0 percent for long-term use of estrogens but 25.0 percent for obesity and 19.0 percent for nulliparity. This study shows the risk factors of obesity, nulliparity, and unopposed exogenous estrogen exposure to be additive.

Gallbladder disease, hypertension, and diabetes are frequently listed among the risk factors associated with endometrial carcinoma. Mayo Clinic studies demonstrate these conditions to reflect the referral base group under study more commonly. The incidence of these factors in local county patients reflects the occurrence of these diseases in the county population at large. For example, when diabetes was evaluated, the expected and/or observed numbers were 4.3 and 3, respectively, for the local county, 4.0 and 7 for Southeastern Minnesota, 5.3 and 14 for a 100-mile radius referral, 15.7 and 28 for a 500-mile referral, and 22.8 and 45 when referred from beyond that distance.

Pelvic radiation is a risk factor in patients with mesodermal mixed sarcomas of the uterus. Approximately 20 percent of the patients with this histologic subtype have received such treatment.

PATHOLOGY

Reviews of pathology material from uterine cancer registries have identified three subtypes of endometrial carcinoma with very favorable prognoses. These are adenoacanthoma, adenocarcinoma with no defined specific features, and secretory carcinoma. All of these have 5-year survival rates for stage I of 87.5 percent, 79.8 percent, and 86.6 percent, respectively. Patients with secretory carcinoma have a 13.6 percent fatal recurrence rate after 5 years. The three subtypes with a significantly less favorable prognosis are papillary carcinoma, mixed adenosquamous carcinoma, and clear cell type. These latter three subtypes together constitute approximately 17 percent of all endometrial carcinomas. The 5-year survival rates in stage I patients with these subtypes are 69.7 percent, 53.1 percent, and 44.2 percent, respectively.

A number of authors subdivide the papillary adenocarcinomas into two clinicopathologic types—well differentiated and papillary serous adenocarcinoma. The reported 5-year survival rates for these two subtypes are strikingly different (100 percent and 24 percent, respectively).

Mesodermal mixed tumors of the uterus constitute a group of mesodermal mixed sarcomas and carcinosarcomas. When evaluated as separate entities, the 5-year survival rates are similar at approximately 50 percent. If the lesions are grade 1 or 2 and confined to the myometrium, 5-year survival is reported at 60 percent. Higher grade lesions or those with increased depth of penetration have a decreased 5-year survival of 25 percent.

RECEPTORS

A study of cytosol steroid receptor levels in 213 postmenopausal patients with endometrial cancer showed (1) a negative correlation of estrogen receptors (ER) and progesterone receptors (PR) with grade, (2) ER and PR levels positively correlated with each other, and (3) neither ER nor PR levels correlated with age. Survival in early endometrial cancers showed significant relation to ER positive status and PR positive status. Another study found the same correlation of ER positive and PR positive status with survival to exist within patients with metastatic and recurrent endometrial cancer. An inverse relationship has been shown between ER and PR status and epidermal growth factor receptors in endometrial carcinomas.

TUMOR MARKERS

Lipid associated sialic acid (LASA), CA125, and NB/70K were studied. In patients with papillary serous endometrial carcinoma, 61.5 percent have elevated serum CA125 preoperatively, 66.6 percent have elevated LASA, and 63.6 percent have elevated NB/70K. The majority of those with elevated titers had extra uterine spread. One study has shown a significant correlation of CA125 levels with depth of penetration of tumor with the uterine wall. TAG 72 has been shown to be elevated in 30 percent of patients with metastatic endometrial carcinoma as were 65 percent of CA15-3 levels in these patients.

STAGING

In 1971, the Cancer Committee of the International Federation of Gynecology and Obstetrics (FIGO) published a staging categorization for endometrial carcinoma based on clinical evaluation and description (Table 1). Although this FIGO scheme has some clinical usefulness, by today's standards it has some definite deficiencies. For example, in this FIGO classification, the depth of invasion of the myometrium is not defined, and the amount of tumor is not quantitated. Peritoneal cytologic and nodal evaluation (both important staging characteristics) are not properly integrated in this classification. The definitive staging procedures should include (1) sampling of the peritoneal fluid present on entering the peritoneal cavity; (2) assessment of the extent of neoplastic spread; (3) sampling of the pelvic and/or para-aortic nodes; (4) evaluation of the myometrial penetration, i.e., inner, middle, or outer one-third; and (5) description of the cellular subtype and grade. This type of staging is addressed when employing surgery as the first-line treatment approach and then with information from steps 1 through 5 in planning the adjuvant therapy. A common error in clinical versus surgical staging became apparent when 52 patients with surgical stage II disease were evaluated. Of this group, only 24 had been clinically staged correctly. The remainder had been designated as having stage I disease. Further, 23 patients clinically diagnosed with stage II disease were found, in fact, to have stage I disease when the specimen was pathologically evaluated. Table 2 demonstrates the influence of grade of tumor and its

Table 1 Staging of Carcinoma of the Corpus Uteri—Federation of Gynecology and Obstetrics Cancer Committee, January 1971

Stage 0   Carcinoma in situ
Stage 1   Carcinoma confined to the corpus
   Stage IA—length of uterine cavity is 8 cm or less
   Stage IB—length of uterine cavity is greater than 8 cm
   All stage I cases to be graded as follows:
      G1—highly differentiated adenomatous carcinomas
      G2—differentiated adenomatous carcinomas with partly solid
         areas
      G3—predominantly solid or entirely undifferentiated carcinoma
Stage II   Carcinoma involves corpus and cervix
Stage III   Carcinoma extends outside the uterus but not outside
   the true pelvis
Stage IV   Carcinoma extends outside the true pelvis or obviously
   involves mucosa of the bladder or rectum. (Bulbous edema as
   such does not itself constitute stage IV disease)

Table 2 Myometrial Invasion

Stage and Grade	Depth of Invasion (%)		
	Inner Third	Middle Third	Outer Third
IA			
G1	89.5	5.8	4.7
G2	69.1	20.4	10.5
G3	60.0	17.1	22.9
IB			
G1	87.1	8.2	4.7
G2	61.1	16.7	22.2
G3	52.0	16.0	32.0
Total	76.8	12.7	10.5

correlation with penetration of the myometrium in the most recent Mayo Clinic series of stage I patients. It is evident that the separation of patients into stages IA and IB is an artificial one. A staging categorization for endometrial carcinoma addressing these problems is currently being developed.

A study of the relationship of pathologic grade and myometrial penetration with the frequency of involvement of pelvic and aortic nodes was done by the Gynecological Oncology Group. This study provided the data derived from the FIGO clinical staging and the use of surgical staging. Overall, there was a 23 to 25 percent occurrence of pelvic nodal metastasis with grade 3 tumors and superficial myometrial invasion. Further, about 45 percent of these had aortic nodal involvement. Patients with grade 1 disease and deep invasion had positive pelvic nodes 25 percent of the time, although no aortic nodal involvement was reported. Grade 3 tumors with deep myometrial invasion showed 42 to 43 percent pelvic node involvement and 30 to 35 percent aortic nodal involvement. When the tumor was confined to the endometrium, there was minimal nodal involvement (0 to 1.7 percent) for all practical purposes. When adenocarcinomas, adenoacanthomas, and adenosquamous carcinomas were compared for grade and depth of penetration, they behaved in a similar fashion. Finally the data show that if the sampled pelvic nodes are negative, the number of positive aortic nodes is very small. A little over half of the positive nodes reported were palpable.

An estimated 15 percent of stage I carcinomas have positive peritoneal cytologic findings. The recurrence rate in patients with positive cytology is nearly fourfold greater than in that of patients with negative results. The presence of positive cytology in this group of patients, therefore, is of major concern and justifies more aggressive adjuvant therapy considerations.

Table 3 shows the relationship of survival to stage in the two Mayo Clinic series in which the primary approach was extended extrafacial abdominal hysterectomy staying medial to the ureters. In connection with this, bilateral salpingo-oophorectomy was done and palpable nodes were sampled. Two things were evident in this table: (1) the FIGO categories of IA and IB are not of practical use, and (2) the survival did not improve over the two 10-year intervals.

Table 3 Survival Rates According to Stage and Grade — Mayo Clinic Study

Stage	Series 1 1953–1962		Series 2 1963–1972	
	No. Patients	5-Year Survival	No. Patients	5-Year Survival
IA	324	83.0	400	92.0
G1	209	88	197	92.7
G2	92	76.1	168	86.5
G3	23	65.2	35	68.2
IB	85	78.9	177	81.3
G1	40	97.5	90	89.6
G2	29	75.9	60	76.4
G3	16	37.5	27	62.9
II	24	75.0	23	69.2
III	44	59.1	—	—
IV	46	13.0	—	—
Total	523	73.8	600	—

Table 4 Myometrial Invasion and 5-Year Survival

Stage and Grade	Depth of Invasion (%)		
	Inner Third	Middle Third	Outer Third
IA			
G1	93.7	83.3	92.3
G2	89.0	71.9	82.4
G3	76.3	60.0	56.3
IB			
G1	93.7	83.3	92.3
G2	87.9	67.0	57.0
G3	76.3	60.0	56.3

Table 4 correlates the grade and depth of penetration with 5-year survival in stage I patients in the later Mayo series. It is again evident that both the grade and depth of cellular penetration are the important prognostic factors rather than the subcategories of stage I and other disease characteristics.

Evaluation of patients with surgical stage II disease shows two factors to be of importance in survival: (1) grade of disease, and (2) the extent of involvement of the endometrial cavity. The 5-year survival rate is 100 percent for those with grade I lesions, 75 percent for those with grade 2 lesions, and 50 percent for those with grade 3 lesions. When less than 50 percent of the endometrial cavity is involved, the 5-year survival is 100 percent and falls to 54 percent if a larger amount of the cavity is involved.

THERAPEUTIC APPROACH

The primary approach to all stage I lesions is wide extrafacial hysterectomy with surgical development and removal of a generous vaginal cuff, bilateral salpingo-oophorectomy, pelvic node sampling, and peritoneal cytologic examination done on fluid removed when the abdomen is first opened. Estrogen and progesterone receptor studies should be performed. Depending on the pathologic grade of the tumor, depth of cellular invasion, the presence of positive cytology and/or positive pelvic and/or aortic nodes, additional treatment considerations should be provided as follows: patients who have stages IA and IB grade 1 lesions, regardless of the depth of penetration, should have no further treatment unless (1) the cytologic findings are positive, in which case, chromic phosphate (^{32}P) is used when possible; or (2) the nodes are positive, in which case, appropriate pelvic and aortic areas are irradiated.

Patients with stages IA and IB grade 2 lesions with penetration beyond the inner one-third of the myometrium and/or positive nodes should receive pelvic irradiation approximating 5,000 cGy with appropriate nodal boosts. These patients who are node-negative but whose cytologic findings are positive should be considered for intraperitoneal radioactive phosphate (^{32}P) treatment.

Patients with stages IA and IB grade 3 lesions of any depth of invasion or whose lesions are of papillary, adenosquamous, or clear cell type with or without positive nodes should be considered for whole abdominopelvic irradiation, as described by Martinez.

Patients with stage II lesions should be treated by Wertheim hysterectomy with bilateral salpingo–oophorectomy and bilateral pelvic node resection. Surgical sampling and pathologic review of para-aortic nodes should be done if pelvic nodes are metastatically involved. No further treatment is recommended if the lymph nodes are negative on pathologic review. If metastatic nodal disease is present, pelvic radiation with appropriate nodal radiation should be provided. If there are positive cytologic findings and positive nodes are present, whole abdominopelvic radiation is administered in accordance with the Martinez technique.

The question of estrogen replacement is frequently discussed following surgery for carcinoma of the endometrium, particularly in the premenopausal and perimenopausal patient. Today, replacement therapy is generally contraindicated. A restrospective evaluation was done of 47 patients receiving estrogen. Thirty-seven used it vaginally, 7 received it orally, and 6 used estrogen both orally and vaginally for at least 3 months, starting at a median of 15 months after surgery. They reported no increased incidence of recurrence. Another retrospective review of 44 patients with clinical stage I endometrial carcinoma treated with oral estrogen replacement for a median duration of 64 months showed no recurrent endometrial cancer and no intercurrent deaths. These patients had low-grade tumors, less than one-half myometrial penetration, and no metastases to lymph nodes or other organs. Despite the absence of a prospective randomized trial to demonstrate the safety of estrogen replacement therapy, a recent survey of gynecologic oncologists showed them to be using such therapy in these patients. This led to the following statement's being issued by the American College of Obstetricians and Gynecologists:

There are no definitive data to support specific recommendations regarding the use of estrogen in women previously treated for endometrial carcinoma. However, responses from a survey of members of the Society of Gynecologic Oncologists indicate that 83% of the respondents approved using estrogen replacement therapy in patients with stage I, grade 1 endometrial cancer; 56% favored using estrogen in cases of stage I, grade II cancer; and 39% would use estrogen in cases of stage I, grade III cancer. The Committee on Gynecologic Practice has concluded that in women with a history of endometrial carcinoma, estrogens could be used for the same indications as for any other women, except that the selection of appropriate candidates should be based on prognostic indicators and the risk the patient is willing to assume. If the patient is free of tumor, estrogen replacement therapy cannot result in recurrence. If an estrogen-dependent neoplasm is harbored somewhere in her body, it will eventually recur; however, estrogen replacement may result in an earlier recurrence. Prognostic predictors (depth of invasion, degree of differentiation, and cell type) will assist the physician in describing the risks of persistent tumor to the patient.

In the absence of estrogen replacement therapy:
1. A well-differentiated neoplasm of endometrioid cell type with superficial invasion would render a risk of persistent disease of approximately 5%.
2. A moderately differentiated neoplasm of endometrioid cell type with up to one-half myometrial invasion would render a 10–15% risk of persistent disease. The risk would increase to 20–30% for adenosquamous cell type and to approximately 50% for serous papillary tumors.
3. A poorly differentiated neoplasm, regardless of cell type, with invasion of over one-half of the myometrium, would render a 40–50% risk of persistent disease.

Because the metabolic changes of estrogen deficiency are significant, the woman should be given complete information, including counseling about alternative therapies, to enable her to make an informed decision. For some women the sense of well-being afforded by amelioration of menopausal symptoms or the need to treat atrophic vaginitis or osteoporosis may outweigh the risk of stimulating tumor growth.

The need for progestational agents in addition to estrogen is unknown at present.

If only control of vasomotor symptoms is sought, this can be done quite nicely with a progestogen.

Radioactive chromic phosphate (^{32}P) has been shown to be effective in patients with microscopic metastatic residual endometrial carcinoma of the peritoneal cavity. Of patients so treated, 10 of the 15 survived for more than 5 years tumor-free. A joint study addressing this aspect of treatment reports that 10 of 26 patients with positive peritoneal cytologic findings and no other abdominal disease had recurrent disease when no treatment was used beyond the primary surgery. When a similar group of 23 patients with positive peritoneal cytology was studied with intra-abdominal ^{32}P, only three recurrences were observed. A study of 567 surgically treated stage I patients showed that 7 percent of the patients with negative peritoneal cytology and 32 percent of those with positive peritoneal cytology developed recurrences. This is highly significant.

In stage I disease, an evaluation of adjuvant progesterone in the form of 6 methyl-17 hydroxyprogesterone, 1,000 mg, was given within 24 hours of surgery and followed by 500 mg per week for 14 weeks. A randomized, control, placebo-treated group of patients with stage I disease was followed for the same period. Over 5 years, the recurrence rate was identical in the two groups. These patients did not have estrogen and/or progesterone receptor studies done, and such information in a subsequent study would be important. CA125 levels were studied in 15 patients with recurrent carcinoma of the endometrium. Of these, six had levels over 35 U per milliliter. In those patients with positive levels at the time of recurrence, the test appears to be a means of following response to treatment.

In recent flow cytometric DNA analyses of stage I endometrial carcinoma, the overall 5-year progression-free survival for patients with grade 1 and 2 lesions was 90 percent. Stratification by DNA diploid and DNA nondiploid patterns revealed progression-free survivals of 94 and 64 percent, respectively. Patients with positive peritoneal cytologic findings and a diploid pattern had no relapses, whereas patients with positive peritoneal cytologic findings and a nondiploid pattern had recurrences of their tumors. When DNA content and receptor content of tumors are known, it has been shown that the aneuploid tumors with high ER levels and without myometrial invasion beyond the inner one-third have a relapse rate of 18 percent and aneuploid tumors, poorly differentiated without elevated ER levels or myometrial invasion, have a relapse rate of 44 percent.

When the site of recurrent disease was evaluated in patients with stage I lesions, 2 of 8 with grade 1 lesions, 19 of 27 with grade 2 lesions, and 6 of 17 with grade 3 lesions had recurrences in the abdomen and/or pelvis, where irradiation could have been a useful adjuvant treatment. The remaining lesions recurred outside the abdomen or pelvis, either singly or as multiple sites of recurrence. These findings point out the need for adjuvant therapy in high risk cases, i.e., patients with grade 3 lesions of any pathologic type or adenosquamous, papillary, or clear cell histologic lesions.

When recurrent disease is isolated and amenable to surgery, this is our primary salvage procedure. If surgery is not feasible, radiation therapy is the next choice. Our experience has also demonstrated that radiation therapy has been particularly useful in controlling pain from metastatic disease to bone.

Progesterone treatment for recurrence or advanced primary disease attained popularity in the early 1960s. The most recent evaluation of this form of therapy in our institution shows that these agents have induced an 11.2 percent response in 155 patients so treated. The response rates were 40 percent for Broder's grade 1 tumors, 17.5 percent for Broder's grade 2 tumors, and 2.4 percent for Broder's grade 3 lesions.

No Broder's grade 4 tumors responded to progesterone. The survivals from the onset of hormone treatment were 40 percent at 1 year, 19 percent at 2 years, and 8 percent at 5 years. The data show that survival was dependent on the differentiation of the tumor, the tumor volume, and the interval from the time of initial treatment to the onset of progesterone therapy. The progestogens used were 17 hydroxyprogesterone caproate, 6,17 dimethyl-6-dehydroprogesterone, and 6-methyl, 6-dehydroprogesterone acetate. None of these produced results better or worse than the others.

In a number of patients who failed to respond to progesterones, an alternative hormonal treatment has been evaluated. Of 46 patients who received tamoxifen, 20 mg per day, 22 failed to respond to progestogens. None of these patients responded to the tamoxifen. There were five responses to tamoxifen among the 24 patients who had not previously been treated with a progestogen.

The soft agar colony formation assay for in vitro testing of sensitivity to gynecologic malignancies was evaluated in 47 patients with carcinoma of the endometrium. Of these, 13 showed positive assay, and 149 drugs were evaluated, with 20 sampled drugs showing sensitivity. The drugs indicating sensitivity in vitro did not behave in a similar fashion in vivo.

Cytotoxic agents used to date have had minimal antitumor activity and have not been particularly useful. The combined programs such as cyclophosphamide, doxorubicin, and cisplatin have reported 10 to 30 percent objective response rates for 1 to 3 months with no significant improvement in survival. One study reported a 40 percent objective response rate to high-dose carboplatin for 1 month. Partial disease regressions have been seen in 28 percent of patients treated with moderate doses of carboplatin for a median of 128 days. A combination of methotrexate, vinblastine, doxorubicin, and cisplatin has shown only minimal response in patients with recurrent and/or metastatic disease independent of whether these tumors had not encountered, encountered, responded to, or not responded to progesterones. Further active antitumor agents are needed for these malignancies, and new trials of any promising agents should be encouraged.

FOLLOW-UP

Follow-up evaluations are scheduled every 3 to 4 months during the first year after primary therapy, every 6 months for the next 2 years, and yearly thereafter. During these follow-up examinations, in addition to screening for recurrent endometrial carcinoma, it is necessary to keep in mind the fact that the relative risk of subsequent breast cancer is 1.3 percent in this population. The increase was noted in patients who had the risk factors common to breast cancer, that is, nulliparity and obesity. Alternatively, the nonobese parous patient with endometrial carcinoma did not seem to be at risk for breast cancer. A temporal relationship exists for those at risk in that the increased incidence occurred 5 or more years after their treatment for endometrial cancer. A borderline increased risk for colon cancer also seems to be present for these patients. However, this is greatest in the first 5 years after therapy. On this basis, periodic mammograms and hemoquant screening of these patients is appropriate. An unusual occurrence of primary carcinoma of the lung was found 10 or more years after treatment for endometrial carcinoma, thereby pointing out the necessity of biopsying all lung lesions occurring late after primary therapy of endometrial cancer before treating them as recurrences.

Current Studies

The areas of interest under prospective study at present are (1) the prospective evaluation of treatment modalities for patients with other poor histologic and anatomic prognostic factors, (2) the evaluation of treatment modalities for patients with stage I, grade 3 disease, (3) the chemotherapeutic manipulation of advanced primary or recurrent disease, (4) the prospective evaluation of estrogen replacement therapy in patients at low risk of recurrence, (5) the value of receptor studies, (6) further flow cytometric studies incorporating the information with postsurgery treatment protocols, and (7) the incorporation and use of tumor markers for monitoring of treatment responses.

SUGGESTED READING

Borazjani G, Twiggs LB, Leung BS, et al. Prognostic significance of steroid receptors measured in primary metastatic and recurrent endometrial carcinoma. Am J Obstet Gynecol 1989; 161:1253–1257.

Britton LC, Wilson TO, Gaffey TA, et al. Flow cytometric DNA analysis of stage I endometrial carcinoma. Gynecol Oncol 1989; 34:317–322.

Chambers JT, MacLusky N, Eisenfield A, et al. Estrogen and progestin receptor levels as prognosticators for survival in endometrial cancer. Gynecol Oncol 1988; 31:65–77.

Christopherson WM, Alberhasky RC, Connelly PJ. Carcinoma of the endometrium. II. Papillary adenocarcinoma: a clinical pathological study of 46 cases. Am J Clin Pathol 1982; 77:534–540.

Christopherson WM, Connelly PJ, Alberhasky RC. Carcinoma of the endometrium. V. An analysis of prognosticators in patients with favorable subtypes and stage I disease. Cancer 1983; 51:1705–1709.

Creasman WT, Disaia PJ, Blessing J, et al. Prognostic significance of peritoneal cytology in patients with endometrial cancer and preliminary data concerning therapy with intraperitoneal radiopharmaceuticals. Am J Obstet Gynecol 1981; 141:921–927.

Fountain KS, Malkasian GD Jr. Radioactive colloidal gold in the treatment of endometrial cancer: Mayo Clinic experience 1951–1976. Cancer 1981; 47:2430–2432.

Gambrell RD Jr. Prevention of endometrial cancer with progestogens. Maturitas 1986; 8:159–168.

Kukura V, Zaninovic I, Hrdina B. Concentrations of CA-125 tumor marker in endometrial carcinoma. Gynecol Oncol 1990; 37:388–389.

Lee RB, Burke TW, Park RC. Estrogen replacement therapy following treatment for stage I endometrial carcinoma. Gynecol Oncol 1990; 36:189–191.

Lindahl B, Alm P, Ferno M, et al. Prognostic value of steroid receptor concentration and flow cytometrical DNA measurements in stage I-II endometrial carcinoma. Acta Oncol 1989; 28:595–599.

Llorens MA, Bermejo MJ, Salcedo MC, et al. Epidermal growth factor receptors in human breast and endometrial carcinomas. J Steroid Biochem 1989; 34:505–509.

Malkasian GD Jr, Decker DG. Adjuvant progesterone therapy for stage I endometrial carcinoma. Int J Gynaecol Obstet 1978; 16:48–49.

Malkasian GD Jr, Annegers JF, Fountain KS. Carcinoma of the endometrium: stage I. Am J Obstet Gynecol 1980; 136:872–888.

Malkasian GD Jr. Management of uterine and other gynecologic sarcomas. In: Williams CJ, Whitehouse JMA, eds. Cancer of the female reproductive system. Chichester, England: John Wiley & Sons, 1985:273.

Malkasian GD Jr, Podratz KC, Stanhope CR, et al. CA 125 in gynecologic practice. Am J Obstet Gynecol 1986; 155:515–518.

McDonald TW, Annegers JF, O'Fallon WM, et al. Exogenous estrogen and endometrial carcinoma: case-control and incidence study. Am J Obstet Gynecol 1977; 127:572–580.

Martinez A, Schray MF, Howes AE, Bagshaw MA. Postoperative radiation therapy in epithelial ovarian cancer: the curative role based on 24 year experience. J Clin Oncol 1985; 3:901–911.

Podratz KC, O'Brien PC, Malkasian GD Jr, et al. Effects of progestational agents in treatment of endometrial carcinoma. Obstet Gynecol 1985; 66:106–110.

Soper JT, Berchuck AB, Olt GJ, et al. Preoperative evaluation of serum CA 125, TAG 72, and CA 15-3 in patients with endometrial carcinoma. Am J Obstet Gynecol 1990; 163:1204–1209.

Tseng PC, Sprance HE, Carcangiu ML, et al. CA 125, NB/70K, and lipid-associated sialic acid in monitoring uterine papillary serous carcinoma. Obstet Gynecol 1989; 74:384–387.

Turner DA, Gershencon DM, Atkinson N, et al. The prognostic significance of peritoneal cytology for stage I endometrial cancer. Obstet Gynecol 1989; 74: 775–780.

Wallin TE, Malkasian GD Jr, Gaffey TA, et al. Stage II cancer of the endometrium: a pathologic and clinical study. Gynecol Oncol 1984; 18:1–17.

OVARIAN CANCER: SURGERY

GEORGE C. LEWIS Jr., M.D.

Surgery continues to play a vital role in the management of ovarian cancer, but as with other modalities, the role of surgery continues to change. For many years, the uterine corpus, the uterine cervix, and the ovaries have been the most common primary sites for pelvic genital malignancies. During the same years, there has been a steady evolution in the management of these malignancies, but this same evolution has led to a therapeutic dichotomy of surgical approach between ovarian cancer and the others. This is especially true for cervical and uterine neoplasia because surgery has been recognized as playing more of a primary therapeutic role with an achievable objective of cure, whereas surgery for ovarian cancer still plays an adjuvant or subservient role.

Surgery for ovarian cancer comes in many guises and is used for many purposes. In cervical and uterine malignancies, for the vast majority of patients today, surgery diagnoses and cures. The surgical management of the majority of patients in the United States with cervical and uterine cancer could be considered practically standardized; not so for ovarian cancer. This sharp contrast of surgical approaches depends more on the pathophysiology of the malignancies than it does upon any technical aspect of surgery. A lymph node dissection for cervical, endometrial, or ovarian cancer may be technically performed in almost the same manner for all three types of malignancy, differing only in degree of node removal for invasive cervical cancer. The same procedure is much less likely to be used for ovarian cancer than it is for endometrial and cervical cancer because the usual extensive spread of ovarian tumor physically can preclude node sampling, or the massive disease can make the contribution of node dissection quite trivial.

Much more extensive intraperitoneal surgery should be anticipated for primary ovarian cancer than for cervical or endometrial cancer. In fact, the majority of patients with ovarian cancer should have a preoperative bowel preparation as employed for any colon surgery.

A number of parameters have a major influence on the pathogenesis of ovarian cancer and its treatment. The relatively dense barriers of the normal cervical and uterine tissues and the greater clinical accessibility of their tumors mean that disease may be more curable by surgery. Ovarian cancer starting deep within the pelvis and migrating over the constantly shifting, lubricated peritoneal surfaces will involve a lot more of the anatomic territory of the abdomen and pelvis than could be postulated for a comparable growth of endometrial or cervical cancer. Indeed, for over 90 percent of patients with ovarian cancer, because of actual or presumed spread, surgery alone will offer no cure; in reality, surgery's challenge is how to increase the effectiveness of other modalities.

Before turning to surgery's role for ovarian cancer, consideration must be given to patterns of spread and a few other factors, such as cell type and grade, as related to prognosis, surgical decisions, and selections of other modalities. For brevity, consideration will be limited to epithelial tumors, because most ovarian tumors are epithelial, and usually behavior of other cell types resembles that of epithelial cancer.

Malignant epithelial growths may arise as de novo intra- or extra-ovarian, within a benign tumor, or in conjunction with tumors of low malignant potential. Regardless of how they may originate, the surgical staging will be the same, whereas the extent of therapeutic effort may vary. The site of origin is not necessarily solitary; it may be multifocal, especially for extra-ovarian tumors. The surgeon's observations and biopsy or removal of ovarian tissues are relevant to determining the possible site of origin, the grade, and the true stage of the disease; all relate to prognosis and subsequent therapeutic decisions.

Well-differentiated tumors and tumors of low malignant potential are relatively nonaggressive and are less likely to disseminate early in their development. In contrast, poorly differentiated tumors tend to disseminate early. Any grade of ovarian tumor, once growing on the surface of the ovary, penetrating it, or rupturing it, can then spread promptly over surfaces or traverse lymphatic channels to pelvic and para-aortic nodes. Gravity and peritoneal fluid flow paths to the diaphragm influence tumor cell migration to specific sites that are considered high risk. For apparently "early" malignancy, the tumor in high-risk sites will frequently be occult, and the surgeon is obligated to perform random tissue biopsies or cytologic sampling from grossly normal tissues at high risk. These sources for cells or tissues include peritoneal fluid or washings, the walls of the posterior pelvic cul de sac, the peritoneum over the bladder, the paracolic gutters, the undersurface of the diaphragm, particularly the right, and the omentum. In patients with minimal or no residual disease at the end of surgery, pelvic and para-aortic nodes must be sampled. When first-glance impressions suggest that no extra-ovarian disease exists, the surgeon must not assume that there is no tumor spread. The surgeon must search the abdominal and pelvic contents visually and by palpation. The ovarian site must not be automatically assumed to be the primary site, and other locations must be checked, such as stomach, colon, pancreas, and appendix, with its adjacent lymph nodes. Checking the appendix is especially important if the tumor is mucinous or a carcinoid, in which case an incidental appendectomy would be justified. Thorough sampling includes ascitic fluid or, in its absence, washings of the pelvis, each paracolic gutter, and the under-surface of the diaphragm. Sampling should be done in all cases, even with obvious effusions, because not all ascitic fluid contains cancer cells, especially from patients with no apparent extra-ovarian cancer. Note that normal saline should not be used for irrigation; instead, irrigation should be done with Ringer's lactate solution for optimal cell presentation. The collective process of exploration, peritoneal biopsies, node sampling, omentectomy, and peritoneal washings is called surgical staging or a staging laparotomy, and it is normally associated with removal of reproductive tract structures.

Just as it is necessary to biopsy apparently normal tissues, it is just as important not to assume that everything that looks like cancer is. This is most likely to happen in patients who have had previous operations who present with scattered small lesions that resemble metastases but that might possibly be granuloma. At the very least, simple biopsy with frozen section is required.

Peritoneal defects caused by node and peritoneal sampling need not be closed, because there seems to be no increase in adhesions as a result and the practice helps reduce the incidence of later lymphocele and hematoma formation. The resulting temporary increase in peritoneal fluid should be handled by intra-abdominal Jackson-Pratt drains, which can also help warn of intra-abdominal hemorrhage or infection and may assist in controlling ascites until the first course of chemotherapy. The drain can be pulled by the third or fourth day in the absence of ascites.

The surgeon dealing with more than apparent stage I disease should anticipate the possibility for bowel resection to prevent or avoid obstruction by ordering appropriate preoperative bowel preparation. Although it is true that ovarian cancer metastases, being superficial, often can be peeled off vital structures, too often it may be necessary to tackle large volumes whose removal is made possible by bowel resection. This tumor mass reduction of varying extent is generically labeled *debulking*.

Recurrent tumor poses some different challenges. Scarring from prior node dissection may preclude subsequent sampling, except for needle aspiration. Adhesions can limit re-exploration. Adhesions at the site of prior tumor resection should be lysed, and suspicious areas biopsied; if there are no suspicious areas, random sampling of adhesions is needed. Obviously, this lysis process has to be tempered by concerns about bowel laceration and fistulae. Residual omentum should be sampled, especially if there are no gross lesions. Thorough exploration and random sampling are required to establish the malignancy of gross disease and to uncover occult disease. For primary and subsequent surgeries, the dictated notes should describe size and location of lesions on opening and closing the abdomen. Finally, if not done previously, thought should be given at subsequent surgery to intraperitoneal catheter placement as an access route for sampling and therapy.

PRIMARY SURGERY

Minimal Disease

Minimal disease, for practical purposes, is malignancy confined to one or both ovaries as established by surgical staging. Because minimal ovarian cancer is encountered infrequently, its preoperative diagnosis can be easily overlooked until the open abdomen or the

pathology report provides the correct diagnosis. Minimal disease has the potential for traps for patient and surgeon; as a result, surgery for early primary malignancy has to be highly individualized. Of course, the simplest management is to think of cancer early in the preoperative work-up. With this foresight, it is possible to make the correct vertical incision and to perform the appropriate staging. For the surgeon who is not accustomed to staging laparotomies and especially node dissections and omentectomy, it is essential to work with an experienced surgeon or to refer the patient to a surgeon with such expertise.

For frozen sections of an ovary, pathologists may be understandably reluctant to diagnose cancer immediately, especially if the tumor is well differentiated or borderline. When, on frozen section, a benign or noncommittal diagnosis is obtained for a patient of any age, the staging surgery may have to be delayed; for young individuals, removal of the uterus and adnexa may also be delayed until the final diagnosis is determined. If the pathologist later diagnoses malignancy, the patient must complete the required surgery (1) for staging and prognosis, (2) for adjuvant treatment selection, and (3) to improve response and potential for cure. With proper staging to establish a true stage IA or stage IB malignancy, patients should expect greater than 85 percent 5-year survival often from surgery alone. Correct staging identifies disease risk categories and permits optimal matching of risk and therapy.

The standard surgical therapy for minimal ovarian cancer is a total hysterectomy and bilateral salpingo-oophorectomy plus a staging laparotomy as previously described. However, there can be some exceptions, such as the young patient, including premenarchal women with stage IA grade 1 epithelial cancer or a similar stage of germ cell tumor. There must be no capsule rupture, no capsule penetration by tumor, and no surface malignancy. For these patients, a unilateral oophorectomy with preservation of the remaining uterus and adnexa is acceptable, providing the staging laparotomy is negative. One additional step that is not universally accepted is a wedge biopsy of the opposite, seemingly benign, ovary to search for any malignancy. With such surgery, better than 90 percent survival may be anticipated for epithelial cancer without adjuvant chemotherapy; close to 100 percent survival may be expected for germ cell tumors with adjuvant chemotherapy.

The current trend in surgery for benign adnexal disease is to use operative laser laparoscopy, which has been claimed to be cost-effective and probably has decreased overall morbidity and mortality. Laparoscopic surgery can result in the removal (intact, morcellated, or vaporized) of all sorts of adnexal masses. With the potential for cancer cell dissemination during removal, however, there may be iatrogenic tumor spread, and certainly laparoscopy is not a staging laparotomy. A negative laparoscopic examination will not account for many sites, including the extraperitoneal ones. For the patient with microscopic disease, optimal potential for cure means optimal surgical evaluation. "Diagnostic" needling of ovarian cystic masses guided by palpation, laparoscopy, or ultrasonography, although readily accomplished, cannot substitute for an incision through which intact tumor can be removed and the abdominopelvic contents appraised completely. Occasionally, a massive cyst obstructs all attempts at removal and has to be decompressed. This is best done within a purse-string tie around a small trochar or a 16- to 18-gauge needle that is inserted through a thick-walled section of the tumor. Obviously, the area should be isolated before needling and irrigated afterward.

Intermediate Disease

Patients with positive ascites (stages IC and IIC) and individuals with disease beyond the ovary but "confined" to the pelvis (stage IIA and B) constitute an intermediate category between stages IA and B and stages III and IV. Patients identified as being in this category can anticipate reasonable probability of tumor control—a luxury not afforded patients with the advanced stages of disease. This probability for better prognosis can vanish when the random sampling of staging laparotomy uncovers occult extrapelvic lesions. At surgery, 15 percent to 20 percent of the patients who have disease initially resembling stage I or stage II will be found to have extrapelvic spread.

With the possible exception of a unilateral germ cell tumor, surgery for this category of disease must be total hysterectomy, bilateral salpingo-oophorectomy, and staging laparotomy. For some patients who are quite young, cure may be achieved while conserving uterus and one adnexa, providing staging laparotomy and complete gross debulking are accomplished and later followed by adjuvant chemotherapy.

After debulking a stage II bulky cancer, every effort should be made to end up with gross residual disease not over 0.5 cm in its largest diameter. Experience to date suggests that this is the ideal minimal residual to strive for with any required debulking. Extraperitoneal resection may be needed to accomplish debulking, sometimes by peeling tumor off pelvic structures and sometimes by partial bowel or bladder resections. Surgical stapling techniques and bowel preparation can reduce the need for ostomies. If needed, the distal ureter can be resected and the new distal end implanted in the bladder. Usually, preoperative findings suggest that major resection and bowel preparation should be considered. If all gross disease is resected, the surgeon should consider the placement of an intraperitoneal catheter with a reservoir or a Tenkoff catheter for later intraperitoneal therapy. Of course, extensive adhesions may preclude such an option. Frozen section or grossly positive nodes also preclude this route for therapy. When there is residual gross disease regardless of surgical stage, the operative notes need to provide size and location of lesions.

Extensive Disease

This category of ovarian neoplasia, for surgical purposes, includes all patients with disease outside the pelvis except patients with malignant ascites as their only extra-ovarian disease. This is a broad category ranging from a single microscopic peritoneal focus of cancer to metastases in liver or extra-abdominal sites. Most patients will present with large, widespread tumor masses that should be debulked as much as possible. Successful debulking appears to identify individuals with responsive disease or to alter conditions that render the disease more susceptible to chemotherapy, a sort of unsolved riddle as to why debulking provides apparent benefit. Optimum results depend on the optimal tumor reduction described previously. Debulking is not without its hazards, and for patients with large-volume disease, transfusion and bowel resection, along with their potential hazards, should be expected.

Because of the potential value of debulking, one should consider surgical management of advanced ovarian cancer as involving a number of options. The best category is stage III cancer by virtue of microscopic peritoneal implants only. The second-best category is gross stage III disease that is initially less than 0.5 cm in diameter or larger masses that can be debulked to an ideal residual. The third category is incompletely resectable intra-abdominal and pelvic lesions with no liver or extra-abdominal metastases, but in this situation, there is no hope of ideal debulking. The fourth category includes various degrees of resectable disease and extra-abdominal or liver metastases. Debulking for these patients probably increases the palliative value of chemotherapy, but the outcome will be determined by the distant metastases. The least favorable category is technically inoperable disease. The surgeon will be fortunate to get a tissue sample, and therapy by any other modality will mostly be palliative.

The patient classed as stage IIIA only because of microscopic findings needs no more than the staging laparotomy, hysterectomy, and bilateral salpingo-oophorectomy used for diagnosis and treatment of early stage disease, but unlike some of the stage IA patients cured by surgery alone, this patient will require chemotherapy. One should consider placing a catheter for intraperitoneal therapy for later access.

For patients who have bulky disease that is resectable, the major objective should be to achieve the ideal residual tumor. When the surgeon realizes the ideal reduction is attainable, there should be no hesitation in performing bowel resections and anastomoses. Portions of pancreas, a wedge of liver, the spleen, and other sites may be included. Metastatic nodal lesions should be included in the debulking. If there is no gross nodal involvement, patients having successful intra-abdominal debulking should have node sampling. This may not be practical at the end of an extensive debulking operation, especially with large blood losses. For these same patients, other aspects of standard staging, such as peritoneal biopsies, add nothing further and may be omitted.

When gross lesions are not reducible to an ideal minimum residual, the surgeon should perform maximum debulking and complete standard pelvic surgery, including total hysterectomy and bilateral salpingo-oophorectomy. For these patients, supracervical hysterectomy is justified to avoid bowel and bladder injury, which may occur as a result of digging the cervix out of a tumor-bound pelvis. Serious consideration should be given to bowel bypass and resection, but only to avoid forthcoming obstruction. This extent of surgery appears worthwhile even for stage IV disease; if nothing else, the surgery may prolong palliation by chemotherapy and avoid or delay appearance of intestinal obstruction, the usual terminal event for such malignancies.

Risk-benefit judgments must come into play for patients who are technically inoperable because of massive disease in order to avoid replacing death from cancer with death as a result of therapy. A limited incision can permit biopsy of what looks like ovarian tissue or masses arising from ovaries. Patients with extensive abdominal disease, ascites or pleural effusion, and a poor functional status may have only thoracentesis, paracentesis, or both for palliation and to confirm malignancy. These technically inoperable patients all have poor prognosis and minimal expected response to any therapy.

Bulky disease is not always nonresectable, and surgeons should at least keep in mind the surface nature of many tumor implants and think of resecting colon or small intestine to achieve a major degree of debulking. A patient with extensive tumor involvement of the colon can be handled by colectomy and any required additional debulking to decrease her chance of intra-abdominal recurrence following adjuvant chemotherapy.

NONPRIMARY SURGERY

Several categories of surgery may come into play after a patient has initiated or completed her primary therapy.

COMPLETION OF PRIMARY SURGERY

The patient may come to require completion of the primary surgical attempt in two ways. In the first case, the surgeon is surprised by the final positive pathology report, which is received several days after surgery, because he or she presumed benign disease or the frozen section was benign and staging was not done, or because the surgeon, presuming cancer metastases, failed to perform surgical staging, even though later biopsies are reported negative. In each of these situations, a return to the operating room is a must.

The second indication for completion of indicated surgery occurs when the nononcologic surgeons realize that the primary operative situation is not one they are prepared to carry out because no one is available to consult or the patient was not prepared for or did not consent to the required surgery. The operation is stopped at this point. The patient is then referred to another surgeon for a second procedure.

DEBULKING AFTER NONSURGICAL THERAPY

Two situations might lead to "primary"-type surgery being performed after another modality has been employed. The first is to plan to take those patients who have been found to be nonresectable by gynecologic oncologists and give them two or three cycles of intensive chemotherapy; for those patients who at least do not show progression, reoperate and attempt to carry out the previously impossible surgery. If the surgery is successful, the patient goes on to further chemotherapy; if surgery is not possible, then the patient is referred to another research program. Such surgery after limited chemotherapy is still investigational.

In the second situation, a patient who was considered inoperable surprisingly proves extremely responsive to chemotherapy; she appears operable and makes the unanticipated return to the operating room. The aggressiveness of this secondary surgery should be identical to a primary operation, with the anticipation of returning to chemotherapy after successful surgery.

SURGERY FOR COMPLICATIONS OF DISEASE OR THERAPY

The normal progression of ovarian cancer has the potential for intestinal obstruction at any time. Post-surgical adhesions can also be the source for obstruction. The real cause of ileus, nausea, vomiting, distention, and other sequelae of obstruction from cancer or therapy may not be known until the patient is re-explored and corrective measures instituted. During the primary surgery, the surgeon may perform the necessary preventive bypass surgery to avoid anticipated obstruction. Disease and adhesion formation are not that predictable, however, and the patient may need bowel resection, bypass operations, ostomies, ileostomies, and lysis of adhesions at any time during her illness.

In relatively late disease, when the patient has little to gain from any therapy, the potential operations come down to those that will provide temporary improvement in the quality of life, such as a gastrostomy instead of a nasogastric tube or a Baker tube in small bowel to provide temporary drainage or nutritional support. Needless to say, every operation raises the potential for another return to the operating room for similar surgery. Decisions as to aggressive management have to be based on the patient's functional status and prior treatment. When a patient has had total abdominal radiation, the surgeon should be most cautious about opening the abdomen again for any reason.

The disease or surgery can be the source of another dreaded complication, fistula formation. Management of fistulae will take into consideration a host of factors, and it will depend mostly on what can be done about the disease and the wishes of the informed patient. One can do bypass procedures with fairly consistent success when the etiology is not primarily the cancer, but even then success will depend on prior surgery, prior radiation, tumor burden, and the patient's nutritional status. In general, in optimistic situations in which there is potential for at least a few months of reasonable quality of life, a patient may do well on tubal drainage and hyperalimentation. With stable malignancy and chronic fistula formation(s), bypass surgery may be considered after prolonged trials of nonsurgical support that fail. There is no simple formula for resolving these most vexing problems.

The conscientious surgeon has to think very hard about where to draw the line on repetitious surgery. Sometimes the patient helps by refusing to go further; sometimes the family makes it worse by pushing for "everything to be done." Sometimes neither the patient nor the family has faced reality, or the surgeon is equally nonrealistic and feels that everything has to be done. The decision has to be based on the informed patient's wishes, the potential for any meaningful therapy after the operation, and the status of the supporting team of family and friends. A think session of supporting services, physician, family, and, most important, the patient can often work out solutions that exclude surgery and would be hard to accept otherwise.

PLANNED RE-EXPLORATION

The most common planned re-exploration is the "second-look" operation. This procedure is one that is performed after the apparently successful completion of all the planned primary therapy. The patient should have reasonable risk of persistent disease and potential for secondary therapy if required. A patient with high primary cure potential stage IA, grade 1 or one with low malignant potential stage I, is not a candidate. Generally, a second look is a diagnostic laparotomy, and its objectives include direct surgical and pathologic evaluation of a patient's abdomen and pelvis to define tumor status, location and debulking of tumor, facilitation of secondary therapeutic approaches through provision of access routes to or markers of persistent tumor, and provision of corrective surgery if needed (close colostomies, lyse adhesions, and so forth). Some surgeons who stress surgical evaluation while minimizing other objectives have touted laparoscopy rather than laparotomy. Unless the laparoscopy is positive, it must be associated with a laparotomy to evaluate everything thoroughly, including nodes. Laparoscopy would offer only minimal opportunity for debulking, would have limited value in marker or access-route placement, and would not be a means for most corrective surgery.

The selection of such planned re-exploration should be guided by the first objective noted. The patient should show no persistent disease clinically. For the tumor marker CA-125, this means a value less than 100 U. There must be some planned potential gain for the patient through alternative therapy for cure or prolongation of useful life based on the outcome of the surgery. The other indications for the second look simply increase the value of the first objective. For minimal or no gross residual tumor, catheter placement can provide access for radioisotopes or chemotherapy. Ostomy revision or closure can be conveniently tied to second-look surgery.

ADJUNCTIVE SURGERY

A host of procedures may come up for consideration under a variety of circumstances. Commonly employed is subclavian catheter placement for vascular access with multiple planned operations, repeated intravenous toxic drugs, and long-term nutritional support. The procedure can be done simply under local anesthesia, the implant can continue for months, and risks are limited to thrombophlebitis, infection, pneumothorax, and cardiac injury or arrythmia. Intraperitoneal drains may be for intraperitoneal radioisotopes and chemotherapy and for peritoneal cell sampling. These access routes and therapies may be associated with ileus, organ injury, infection, and other hazards of abdominal surgery, but they allow much higher concentrations of therapeutic agents at peritoneal tumor sites.

Fluid collections frequently must be drained by paracentesis or thoracentesis. For paracentesis, a simple plastic tube from a 14- to 18-gauge intravenous needle (Longdwell and Intracath, e.g.) can be slipped into the peritoneal cavity under a local anesthesia. The plastic tube is then connected to intravenous tubing and drained by gravity into discarded empty intravenous solution bags. For thoracentesis, a standard disposable set with vacuum bottles is very effective, but pneumothorax is a hazard. With repeated pleural effusion, a chest tube placement and tetracycline for formation of adhesions may be needed to slow or stop the process. The same situation in the abdomen is not dealt with so easily. In the past, there were attempts to drain the abdomen by way of jugular veins, but there have been problems with defibrination, shock, and ultimately mechanical failure before there was any benefit.

For every surgical step in ovarian cancer surgery, one must decide how far to go. The patient wants everything to prolong life, the relatives want something done, and the surgeon likes to perform miracles. However, a few people with prolonged, tortuous lives can bring grave doubt to the conscientious surgeon. Possibly the toughest and most debatable issue is how far to go with adjunctive surgery in terms of resection of obstructed bowel, ostomies, and bypass. There comes a time in doing these procedures for the inevitable bowel problems when one has to stop and think about what the patient gains if relief is very temporary, the patient declines anyway, and the hospital environment gets more depressing.

With primary surgery, the patient's chances are best if both surgeon and patient include ovarian cancer in treatment plans, if the surgeon is qualified to make decisions and to do what's required, and if the surgery is thoughtfully associated with subsequent management. The greatest opportunity for a successful outcome depends almost entirely on the overall conduct of the primary therapy, whether it is single or multiple modality. Secondary therapy, because it is unlikely to offer cure or prolonged tumor control, has to be guided by considerations of quality of life and the balance of risk versus benefit. Ultimately, the most important guideline for selecting surgical or therapeutic options is this: Will the patient benefit? Surgery can play a major role, and surgeons can offer the best outcome to each patient if the question is asked and the answer is properly applied to subsequent therapeutic decisions.

SUGGESTED READING

Buchsbaum HJ, Brady MF, Delgado G, et al. Surgical staging of ovarian carcinoma: A Gynecologic Oncology Group study. Surg Gynecol Obstet 1989; 169:226–232.

Creasman WT, Gall S, Bundy B, et al. Second-look laparotomy in the patient with minimal residual stage III ovarian cancer (Gynecologic Oncology Group study). Obstet Gynecol 1989; 35:375–382.

Delgado G, Oram DH, Petrilli ES. Stage III epithelial ovarian cancer: The role of maximal surgical reduction. Gynecol Oncol 1984; 18:293–298.

Tazelaar HD, Bostwick DG, Ballon SC, et al. Conservative treatment of borderline ovarian tumors. Obstet Gynecol 1985; 66:417–422.

Young RC, Walton LA, Ellenberg SS, et al. Adjuvant therapy in stage I and II epithelial ovarian cancer: Results of two prospective randomized trials. N Engl J Med 1990; 322:1,021–1,027.

OVARIAN CANCER: CHEMOTHERAPY

ROBERT F. OZOLS, M.D., Ph.D.

Ovarian cancer is the most fatal gynecologic malignancy in women in the United States. Approximately 20,000 new cases will be diagnosed yearly, and there will be nearly 12,000 deaths. The vast majority of ovarian tumors are derived from the coelomic epithelium, and the most common histologic type is serous cystadenocarcinoma. Other epithelial tumor histologic types include mucinous cystadenocarcinoma, endometrioid carcinoma, undifferentiated carcinoma, and clear cell carcinoma. Approximately 10 percent of epithelial tumors are classified as germ cell or sex-cord stromal tumors (primarily granulosa cell and Sertoli-Leydig cell tumors).

The incidence of epithelial ovarian carcinoma increases with age, with 80 percent of the women being diagnosed after menopause. There are no specific signs or symptoms of ovarian cancer. Among the common symptoms are pelvic pressure, vague abdominal pain, alterations in bowel function, and abdominal distention. Ovarian cancer tends to remain confined to the peritoneal cavity during its entire clinical course, although pleural involvement and liver involvement occur in 5 percent to 10 percent of cases.

Screening for ovarian cancer has been hampered by a lack of an identifiable high-risk group of patients and by the absence of sufficiently sensitive and specific diagnostic tests. Although there are kindreds in whom ovarian cancer is transmitted as a dominant gene, these ovarian cancer families are rare, and only several hundred families have thus far been identified. The pathogenesis of ovarian cancer also is unclear. It has been postulated that "incessant ovulation" leads to an aberrant repair process in the ovarian surface epithelium that leads to the development of the tumor. In support of this hypothesis is the observation that factors that decrease the number of ovulatory cycles, such as pregnancy, lactation, and some oral contraceptives, have a protective effect against ovarian cancer. Although serum levels of CA-125, ultrasound examinations, including transvaginal sonography, and routine pelvic exams may be useful in monitoring women at high risk for ovarian cancer, it has not been established that these techniques are capable of diagnosing women at an earlier stage of disease. It seems prudent that all women over the age of 40 should have yearly pelvic exams and that women in high-risk categories should additionally be evaluated using ultrasonography and serum CA-125 levels.

DIAGNOSIS AND INITIAL EVALUATION

When the diagnosis of epithelial ovarian cancer is suspected, the initial staging work-up should include chest radiograph, computed tomography (CT) scan and ultrasound of the abdomen, serum CA-125 levels, and radiographic studies of the gastrointestinal system in symptomatic women. Surgery plays a critical role in the initial staging and therapeutic approach to women with ovarian cancer. The staging laparotomy should be exhaustive and include a midline incision that extends above the umbilicus. This enables the surgeon to visualize and examine the peritoneal contents in a systematic fashion. The primary tumor must be carefully examined for presence of capsular integrity, tumor excrescences, and dense adhesions. A bilateral salpingo-oophorectomy hysterectomy and partial omentectomy should be performed. All peritoneal surfaces should be closely inspected, and biopsies should be obtained from suspicious areas. Blind biopsies from the abdominal wall and the right diaphragm may also be useful. The retroperitoneal lymph nodes should be carefully evaluated and biopsies performed. Peritoneal washings should be obtained if there is no ascites present. The currently used International Federation of Gynecology and Obstetrics (FIGO) staging system for epithelial ovarian

Table 1 Staging of Ovarian Cancer

Stage I	Growth limited to the ovaries.	
	Stage IA	Growth limited to one ovary; no ascites; no tumor on the external surface; capsule intact
	Stage IB	Growth limited to both ovaries; no ascites; no tumor on the external surfaces, capsules intact
	Stage IC*	Tumor either stage IA or IB but with tumor on the surface of one or both ovaries; or with capsule ruptured; or with ascites present containing malignant cells or with positive peritoneal washings
Stage II	Growth involving one or both ovaries with pelvic extension.	
	Stage IIA	Extension or metastases to the uterus or tubes
	Stage IIB	Extension to other pelvic tissues
	Stage IIC*	Tumor either stage IIA or IIB but with tumor on the surface of one or both ovaries; or with capsule(s) ruptured; or with ascites present containing malignant cells or with positive peritoneal washings
Stage III	Tumor involving one or both ovaries with peritoneal implants outside the pelvis or positive retroperitoneal or inguinal nodes. Superficial liver metastasis equals Stage III. Tumor is limited to the true pelvis but with histologically verified malignant extension to small bowel or omentum.	
	Stage IIIA	Tumor grossly limited to the true pelvis with negative nodes but with histologically confirmed microscopic seeding of abdominal peritoneal surfaces
	Stage IIIB	Tumor of one or both ovaries with histologically confirmed implants of abdominal peritoneal surfaces, none exceeding 2 cm in diameter; nodes negative
	Stage IIIC	Abdominal implants >2 cm in diameter or positive retroperitoneal or inguinal nodes
Stage IV	Growth involving one or both ovaries with distant metastasis. If pleural effusion is present, there must be positive cytologic test results to allot a case to stage IV. Parenchymal liver metastasis equals stage IV.	

*In order to evaluate the impact on prognosis of the different criteria for allotting cases to stage IC or IIC, it would be of value to know if rupture of the capsule was (1) spontaneous or (2) caused by the surgeon and if the source of malignant cells detected was (1) peritoneal washings or (2) ascites.

carcinoma is detailed in Table 1. In addition to accurately staging the patient, the goal of surgery is to remove as much disease as possible, because the volume of residual disease at the time chemotherapy is initiated is a major prognostic factor for achievement of a complete remission. Consequently, cytoreductive surgery should be attempted in all patients with epithelial ovarian cancer.

Within limited-stage ovarian cancer (stage I and stage II), survival is correlated with the presence of well-defined clinicopathologic factors. Among the factors associated with a favorable prognosis are well-differentiated (or moderately well differentiated) histology, disease confined to the ovaries, absence of malignant ascites or cytologically positive peritoneal washings, no excrescences on the tumor capsule, and the absence of dense adhesions. Factors associated with a less favorable outcome in limited-stage ovarian cancer include a poorly differentiated tumor, malignant ascites or cytologically positive cells in peritoneal washings, the presence of dense adhesions, and a ruptured capsule or extracystic excrescences. Limited-stage disease repre-

sents a clinically important minority of patients with ovarian carcinoma. The vast majority (80 to 85 percent) of women will have widespread intra-abdominal disease (FIGO stage III) at the time of diagnosis; however, between 2,000 and 3,000 (10–15%) women will have limited-stage disease. Stage IV disease has a distinctly worse prognosis as does the presence of bulky residual disease (any tumor mass greater than 2 cm in diameter). In addition, it has recently been demonstrated that amplification of the Her-2/neu oncogene also confers an unfavorable prognosis in patients with advanced disease.

With more accurate staging and improved treatments, there has been a modest overall improvement in survival for patients with epithelial ovarian cancer. For patients with limited-stage favorable disease, 5-year survivals are approaching 95 percent. In contrast, for women with limited-stage disease and unfavorable clinicopathologic features, 5-year survival is approximately 80 percent. In patients with advanced ovarian cancer, the overall 5-year survival has increased to 15 to 20 percent. Consequently, although progress has been made with more aggressive surgery and new chemotherapy regimens, the majority of patients with advanced ovarian cancer still die of their disease.

TREATMENT OF LIMITED-STAGE DISEASE

The treatment approach for patients with limited-stage ovarian cancer is based upon clinicopathologic parameters determined after the initial careful staging laparotomy. In those patients with favorable prognostic characteristics, it has recently been demonstrated that adjuvant therapy with intermittent melphalan is not necessary, because 5-year survival is approximately 95 percent with surgery alone. It has also been demonstrated in a prospective randomized trial that the 5-year survival was identical in patients with unfavorable parameters treated with either intermittent melphalan or intraperitoneal $_{32}$P. The toxicity of melphalan (myelosuppression, and gastrointestinal toxicity) was significantly greater than the toxicities observed with intraperitoneal $_{32}$P; consequently, the latter treatment has been adopted by the Gynecologic Oncology Group as the standard form of treatment against which an intensive combination chemotherapy regimen is currently being evaluated. Patients with unfavorable-prognosis limited-stage disease are randomized to receive either intraperitoneal $_{32}$P or three cycles of cisplatin (100 mg per square meter) plus cyclophosphamide (1,000 mg per square meter). For those patients not entering this clinical trial, it seems prudent to use the same approach as for patients with advanced epithelial ovarian cancer.

TREATMENT OF ADVANCED DISEASE

Ovarian cancer is a highly drug-sensitive tumor. The most active agents in this disease are platinum complexes, and their use with bifunctional alkylating agents such as cyclophosphamide remains the treatment of choice. Although single-agent melphalan is well tolerated and has produced objective responses in patients with advanced disease in the past, there is currently little, if any, justification for its continued use due to the availability of more active combinations.

A series of clinical trials have been performed evaluating the contribution of cisplatin and adriamycin to the combination chemotherapy of patients with advanced ovarian cancer. The two-drug regimen of cisplatin plus cyclophosphamide has been prospectively compared to the three-drug regimen of cyclophosphamide, adriamycin, and cisplatin or to the CHAP-5 regimen (cyclophosphamide, hexamethylmelamine, adriamycin, and cisplatin). Although in some trials adriamycin-containing combinations have produced higher response rates, there is no significant improvement in survival, and the two-drug combination of cisplatin and cyclophosphamide has been considered the treatment of choice.

Retrospective studies have suggested that the dose-intensity (milligrams per square meter of drug per week) of cisplatin is an important factor in achieving optimal results in patients with advanced disease. However, prospective evaluation of high-dose cisplatin regimens has been limited by the toxicity of cisplatin. Cisplatin, particularly at high doses, is associated with nephrotoxicity, severe nausea and vomiting, myelosuppression, and a dose-limiting peripheral neuropathy. Patients receiving cisplatin and cyclophosphamide should be routinely monitored with weekly white blood cell counts and careful neurologic examinations. Unfortunately, the peripheral neuropathy can be delayed in onset and can progress even after the cessation of cisplatin therapy. The nephrotoxicity can usually be well managed using aggressive hydration techniques and is no longer considered dose-limiting.

The second-generation cisplatin analogue carboplatin has essentially replaced cisplatin in the treatment of patients with advanced ovarian cancer. Carboplatin is nonnephrotoxic, has less nausea and vomiting, and is essentially devoid of neurotoxicity. However, it does have more myelosuppression, particularly thrombocytopenia, than the parent compound. Both carboplatin and cisplatin share the same active intermediate; consequently, there is almost complete cross-resistance between these two agents. Patients who are resistant to cisplatin therapy have less than a 10 percent chance of responding to carboplatin treatment.

Carboplatin is excreted extensively in the urine within the first 24 hours of administration. Although it is nonnephrotoxic, patients with a decreased clearance of carboplatin on the basis of altered renal function will have substantially more hematologic toxicity. Consequently, dose adjustments for carboplatin should be made in patients who have severe renal dysfunction or a prior history of chemotherapy, or who are elderly.

Formulas have been derived that can be used to help calculate a dose that will produce a desired degree of thrombocytopenia based upon patient's history of prior chemotherapy and the creatinine clearance or glomerular filtration rate. However, in clinical trials comparing carboplatin combinations versus cisplatin combinations in previously untreated patients with advanced ovarian cancer, formulas were not used routinely to select dosage. The initial dose of carboplatin was 300 to 350 mg per square meter in these trials, and doses were adjusted on the basis of thrombocytopenia after the first course. On the basis of prospective randomized trials that have demonstrated equal efficacy of carboplatin regimens compared to cisplatin regimens as well as markedly less toxicity, the combination of carboplatin plus cyclophosphamide can be considered the treatment of choice for patients with advanced ovarian cancer (Table 2). The carboplatin dose should be 300 to 350 mg per square meter, and the cyclophosphamide dose, 600 mg per square meter. If a formula is not used to calculate the dosage, the dosage of carboplatin can be adjusted after the first course. If the platelet count does not decrease to below 100,000, the dose of carboplatin on the second cycle can be increased by 25 percent to 33 percent. If, on the other hand, the platelet toxicity is severe, the dose of carboplatin can be decreased.

Table 2 Cisplatin and Carboplatin in Advanced Ovarian Cancer

Drug Combination	Schedule	Duration of Treatment
Cisplatin (100 mg/m²) plus cyclophosphamide (600 mg/m²)	Cycles every 28 days. Cisplatin, either 20 mg/m² qd × 5 or 100 mg/m² on day 1. Cyclophosphamide on day 1.	Six cycles for either combination
Carboplatin (300–350 mg/m²) plus cyclophosphamide (600 mg/m²)	Both drugs on day 1 of 28 day cycles.	

Induction therapy with carboplatin plus cyclophosphamide should be administered on a monthly basis for six cycles. There is no evidence that additional therapy will increase the complete remission rate or prolong survival.

SECONDARY CYTOREDUCTION

After their initial surgery, approximately 25 to 40 percent of patients will have bulky residual ovarian cancer. Patients who cannot be effectively cytoreduced at the time of diagnosis have approximately a 10 percent chance of achieving a complete remission with chemotherapy. The feasibility and efficacy of secondary or delayed cytoreduction surgery after two to three cycles of induction chemotherapy have been studied. Unfortunately, although a short course of chemotherapy increases the number of patients who can be surgically cytoreduced, survival is not improved and remains substantially worse compared to that of patients who undergo successful cytoreductive surgery at the time of diagnosis. Furthermore, there also appears to be no significant role for cytoreductive surgery in patients after completion of a full six cycles of induction chemotherapy. Surgery after initial chemotherapy is primarily indicated for palliation of intestinal obstructions.

COMBINED-MODALITY APPROACHES WITH RADIATION THERAPY

In previous untreated patients with small-volume residual disease, it has been demonstrated that pelvic plus abdominal radiation therapy can produce similar survival to what has been observed with combination chemotherapy. Abdominal radiation therapy is not effective in previously untreated patients with bulky residual ovarian cancer. There has not been a prospective randomized trial comparing radiation versus chemotherapy in patients with advanced ovarian cancer who have been optimally surgically cytoreduced. Although abdominal radiation is effective in previously untreated patients with small-volume disease, it appears to have little role in the treatment of patients after induction chemotherapy. Numerous uncontrolled trials have uti-

lized radiotherapy in patients who have documented residual disease after induction chemotherapy. In these trials, only patients with microscopic disease had prolonged survival. Furthermore, abdominal radiation therapy in this situation is usually associated with a considerable toxicity that is primarily related to effects on the gastrointestinal tract.

It has been suggested that whole abdominal radiation therapy may have a role in patients with microscopic disease at second-look surgery or in patients who have a negative second look but who are at a high risk for relapse. The overall relapse rate in patients who achieve a complete remission is approximately 30 percent to 50 percent. Risk factors for relapse from a negative second-look laparotomy include a high-grade tumor or the presence of bulky disease prior to the initiation of chemotherapy. It has been speculated that whole abdominal radiation therapy may decrease the relapse rate in this group of patients, although no prospective trial has demonstrated the efficacy of any form of treatment in decreasing the relapse rate.

INTRAPERITONEAL CHEMOTHERAPY

Ovarian cancer remains confined to the abdominal cavity virtually throughout its entire clinical course. In an effort to increase the delivery of chemotherapeutic agents directly to the tumor, phase 1 and pharmacologic studies have evaluated the role of intraperitoneal chemotherapy in patients with ovarian cancer. It has been demonstrated that the intraperitoneal administration of most drugs active in ovarian cancer is associated with a pharmacologic advantage. Administration of drugs directly into the peritoneal cavity leads to higher levels in the fluid bathing of tumor cells than can be achieved in the systemic circulation. Furthermore, with drugs such as cisplatin, it has been demonstrated that cytotoxic concentrations of the drug can also be achieved in the systemic circulation. Consequently, in theory, after intraperitoneal administration, a peritoneal tumor is exposed to high levels of drug that can directly diffuse into the outer layers of the tumor mass, and the inner core of the tumor can be effectively treated by cytotoxic drug concentrations via the microcirculation. Although clinical studies have demonstrated that intraperitoneal therapy is technically feasible, the role of intraperitoneal therapy in the management of patients with ovarian cancer remains to be established.

In initial trials, a Tenckhoff catheter was used for peritoneal access. More recently, however, totally implantable Port-a-cath systems have been used that are associated with a lower complication rate and increased patient acceptance. However, intraperitoneal catheters are still associated with significant toxicities, including bowel perforation, sepsis, and outflow obstruction.

Cisplatin has been the most single active agent when used intraperitoneally in patients with residual ovarian cancer. Approximately 30 percent of patients who have small-volume residual disease at second-look laparotomy can be converted into a complete remission by the intraperitoneal administration of cisplatin or cisplatin-based combinations. In uncontrolled trials a 74 percent 5-year survival has been reported in patients with small-volume residual disease who have received intraperitoneal platinum or platinum-containing combinations. The combination of platinum plus VP-16 appears to be the most active regimen currently reported for patients with residual ovarian cancer.

Prospective randomized trials are currently in progress in previously untreated patients with small-volume residual disease comparing intraperitoneal platinum and intravenous cisplatin. Patients are randomized to receive either intraperitoneal cisplatin or intravenous cisplatin at a dose of 100 mg per square meter, and all patients receive intravenous cyclophosphamide at 1,000 mg per square meter. Furthermore, pilot clinical trials are also in progress evaluating alternating cycles of intravenous chemotherapy and intraperitoneal chemotherapy. Until the completion of such trials, intraperitoneal chemotherapy should be considered an investigational procedure.

SECOND-LOOK SURGERY

The role of second-look surgery following completion of induction chemotherapy is itself controversial. It is clear that second-look surgery has no therapeutic role. The only reason for a second-look procedure is if subsequent therapy will depend on findings at the exploratory laparotomy. Patients who have evidence of residual disease after induction chemotherapy, including a persistently elevated CA-125 or radiographic or clinical evidence of residual masses, should not routinely undergo a second-look laparotomy but instead should be treated with salvage regimens. Approximately 25 percent to 35 percent of patients who are clinically disease-free at the completion of induction therapy will be found to have residual disease at a second-look laparotomy.

A currently acceptable approach is to use intraperitoneal chemotherapy for that group of patients who have small-volume residual disease after induction chemotherapy. Clinical trials are currently in progress to determine whether intraperitoneal therapy can prevent relapses in patients who achieve a negative second-look laparotomy. Although intraperitoneal ^{32}P, whole abdominal radiation, intraperitoneal chemotherapy, or systemic chemotherapy have been advocated by some investigators to prevent or decrease the relapse rate in patients who achieve a negative second look, currently there are no prospective data that document that the relapse rate can be decreased by any type of therapy.

SALVAGE CHEMOTHERAPY

Salvage chemotherapy has generally been ineffective in patients with recurrent ovarian cancer. In most trials, single-agent therapy or combination chemotherapy has produced clinical complete remissions in less than 10 percent of patients, and overall survival has been in the range of 4 to 6 months. However, several agents (Table 3) have recently been reported to have significant activity in previously treated patients. Carboplatin's activity depends on the patient's prior response to cisplatin-based chemotherapy. In patients with a prior response to cisplatin-based chemotherapy, carboplatin produces an objective response rate of 28 percent. In contrast, in patients with tumors resistant to cisplatin, carboplatin produces only a 5 percent objective response rate. Ifosfamide is an alkylating agent whose clinical development was initially limited by severe hemorrhagic cystitis. However, the availability of mesna, which protects the uroepithelium from the toxic metabolites of ifosfamide, has permitted a more in-depth evaluation of ifosfamide in ovarian cancer and in other tumors. Ifosfamide as a single agent produces objective responses in approximately 20 percent of previously treated patients. Taxol is a diterpene plant alkaloid that has a novel mechanism of action—inhibition of cell division by preventing depolymerization of microtubules. In a recent phase 2 trial, Taxol was demonstrated to have significant activity in previously treated patients with ovarian cancer. Hexamethylmelamine has been available for many years but recently has been shown to have activity in patients who received prior treatment with cisplatin.

Patients most likely to respond to salvage chemotherapy are those patients who had an excellent initial response to prior induction therapy and a long disease-free interval. These patients should be treated at relapse with a platinum drug. Upon a second relapse, they can be treated with non–platinum-containing salvage chemotherapy. Patients who do not respond to initial induction chemotherapy are unlikely to respond to other salvage therapies and should be treated with new investigational approaches.

INVESTIGATIONAL TREATMENTS

High-dose Chemotherapy

The availability of carboplatin should permit a more careful evaluation of the importance of dose intensity of

Table 3 Second-line Therapy of Cisplatin-Treated Ovarian
Cancer Patients

Drug	Dose	Response Rate (%)
Taxol	110–250 mg/m^2 24-hr continuous infusion qmo	30
Ifosfamide	1.2 g/m^2 IV qd 1–5	20
Hexamethylmelamine	400 mg PO qd × 14 every month	15 CR
Carboplatin	300–1,000 mg/m^2	(28, 16, 5)*

*Response to second-line carboplatin is dependent upon prior response to cisplatin: 28 percent for responders, 16 percent for patients who did not respond, and 5 percent for patients with disease progression while on cisplatin.
Abbreviation: CR = complete response.

platinum complexes in patients with advanced disease. Clinical trials of high-dose carboplatin with granulocyte-macrophage colony-stimulating factor (GMCSF) or granulocyte colony-stimulating factor (GCSF) or with autologous bone marrow support are in progress. Additional studies are evaluating the role of carboplatin combined with cisplatin. Dose escalations in these latter platinum complex trials may be facilitated by agents that decrease their toxicity (e.g., WR2721, to potentially protect against neurotoxicity and myelosuppression, and the ACTH analogue ORG2766, to protect against neurotoxicity). Until the clinical trials are completed, the current recommendation is to administer cisplatin at 100 mg per square meter per cycle, and if carboplatin is used in its place, at a starting dose of 300 to 350 mg per square meter per cycle.

New Drug Combinations

Clinical pilot studies of new combination regimens will soon be initiated. Among the new combinations to be tested are carboplatin plus ifosfamide, cisplatin plus taxol, and carboplatin plus cyclophosphamide plus hexamethylmelamine.

Biologic Agents

Ovarian cancer is well suited for the study of biologic agents and biologic response modifiers. Ovarian cancer cells express antigens, and access to the peritoneal cavity permits assessment of the immune response following biologic treatments. Clinical trials are in progress evaluating the toxicity and efficacy of monoclonal antibody-immunotoxin conjugates in patients with refractory ovarian cancer. These studies are based on prior demonstration in preclinical models of human ovarian cancer that immunotoxins have marked antitumor effects. Monoclonal antibodies have been directed against either tumor-associated antigens or the transferrin receptor. The transferrin receptor is primarily expressed in dividing cells, and in the abdominal cavity, only malignant cells should be expressing this receptor. Toxins used in these studies have included recombinant ricin A chain as well as *Pseudomonas* exotoxin. Addi-

tional studies linking radioisotopes to monoclonal antibodies are also in progress.

It has also been demonstrated that a combination of interleukin-2 and lymphokine-activated killer cells (LAK) is effective in a murine model of human ovarian cancer. Based upon these observations, clinical trials have evaluated interleukin-2 plus LAK in patients with residual ovarian cancer. Although activity has been reported, enthusiasm for this approach has been dampened by the severe intraperitoneal toxicity. The intraperitoneal administration of interferon also has been shown to produce responses in patients with small-volume disease. Although biologic approaches have activity, improved efficacy and decreased toxicity remain the goals of experimental protocols.

Reversal of Drug Resistance

The biochemical basis for drug resistance in ovarian cancer remains to be completely established. However, it has been demonstrated in preclinical models of ovarian cancer that resistance to cisplatin and alkylating agents is associated with increased glutathione levels and in an increased DNA repair capacity. In preclinical systems, it has been demonstrated that inhibition of glutathione synthesis with buthionine sulfoximine, an irreversible inhibitor of the key enzyme in the biosynthesis of glutathione, leads to the potentiation of cytotoxicity of alkylating agents and platinum compounds. Furthermore, inhibition of DNA repair with drugs such as aphidicolin, an inhibitor of DNA polymerase alpha, also potentiates the cytotoxicity of cisplatin in drug-resistant tumor cells. Based upon these preclinical observations, clinical trials of agents that can reverse drug resistance, such as buthionine sulfoximine, have recently been initiated.

NONEPITHELIAL OVARIAN TUMORS

Ovarian Germ Cell Tumors

Cisplatin-based regimens have led to a dramatic improvement in the prognosis of women with germ cell tumors of the ovary. These tumors occur more frequently in younger patients than epithelial ovarian carcinomas. Patients usually present with symptoms resulting from a pelvic mass, such as urinary frequency and lower abdominal pain or pressure. Serum alpha-fetoprotein (AFP) and human chorionic gonadotropin (HCG) can be detected frequently in patients with germ cell tumors and are useful in the diagnosis and monitoring of patients after surgery.

The most common malignant germ cell tumor of the ovary is a dysgerminoma. Approximately 75 percent of patients are diagnosed with stage I disease, and 10 percent of patients have bilateral tumors. A unilateral salpingo-oophorectomy can be performed if the patient desires fertility. The dysgerminoma tumor has long been known to be highly sensitive to radiation therapy, which frequently has been administered when the tumor has metastasized. More recently, it has been demonstrated that the combination of cisplatin, velban, and bleomycin (PVB) is also effective therapy for patients with metastatic germ cell tumors of the ovary. Furthermore, it has been demonstrated that replacement of vinblastine by etoposide in this regimen leads to less toxicity and possibly more efficacy; consequently, the BEP regimen (cisplatin, etoposide, and bleomycin) can be considered the regimen of choice for women with metastatic germ cell tumors of the ovary.

Immature teratomas are the second most common germ cell malignancy. Bilateral ovarian involvement is rare, and a unilateral salpingo-oophorectomy can be performed to preserve fertility. Adjuvant chemotherapy has been shown to be successful, and patients with stage IA, grades 2 to 3 lesions, should be treated with the BEP regimen with three to four cycles. Patients with stage IA, grade 1 lesions have an excellent prognosis, and adjuvant therapy is not indicated. Similarly, patients with endodermal sinus tumors are initially treated with unilateral salpingo-oophorectomy. All patients with an endodermal sinus tumor of the ovary are treated postoperatively with BEP chemotherapy.

Sex-Cord Stromal Tumors

This group of tumors include granulosa cell tumors and Sertoli-Leydig cell tumors. The granulosa cell tumors are often estrogen-secreting and are associated with endometrial carcinoma. Most granulosa cell tumors are diagnosed at an early stage, although tumors may recur years after the initial diagnosis. There is no evidence that either radiation or chemotherapy after surgical removal of the tumor prevents recurrences. Similarly, Sertoli-Leydig cell tumors, which frequently present with virilization owing to the production of androgens, are also treated with surgery alone in most instances. Chemotherapy has been reserved for patients with persistent or recurrent disease.

Borderline Tumors of the Ovary

Borderline tumors represent a clearly identifiable subset of epithelial tumors of the ovary that have a markedly superior prognosis compared to invasive carcinomas of the ovary. These tumors have also been termed tumors of low malignant potential and are histologically characterized by the absence of invasion into stromal tissues. In contrast to invasive carcinomas of the ovary, the majority of patients with borderline tumors present with stage I disease. The primary modality of treatment for borderline tumors is surgery. Surgery usually consists of a bilateral salpingo-oophorectomy and hysterectomy. In stage I disease, there is no demonstrated efficacy for adjuvant therapy. A unilateral salpingo-oophorectomy may be adequate therapy for patients in whom fertility is of concern. It has not been established that postoperative chemotherapy is beneficial for those patients who present with advanced-stage disease. The primary approach is to remove as much disease as possible. The disease has a long natural history, and even in patients with advanced disease, deaths from borderline tumors are uncommon in the first 5 years. Consequently, patients with advanced disease have frequently been managed with surgery as needed to deal with symptoms. The Gynecologic Oncology Group is conducting a protocol to determine the role of chemotherapy in patients with recurrent advanced borderline tumors. The current recommendation would be to reserve chemotherapy for those patients with recurrent disease who cannot undergo successful surgical cytoreduction.

SUGGESTED READING

Chambers JT. Borderline ovarian tumors: A review of treatment. Yale J Biol Med 1989; 62:351–365.

Hamilton TC, Ozols RF, Longo DL. Biologic therapy for the treatment of malignant common epithelial tumors of the ovary. Cancer 1987; 8:2,054.

Howell SB, Zimm S, Markman M, et al. Long-term survival of advanced refractory ovarian carcinoma patients with small-volume disease treated with intraperitoneal chemotherapy. J Clin Oncol 1987; 5:1,607–1,612.

Neijt JP, ten Bokkel Huinink WW, van der Burg MEL, et al. Randomized trial comparing two combination chemotherapy regimens (CHAP-5 v CP) in advanced ovarian carcinoma. J Clin Oncol 1987; 5:1,157–1,168.

Omura GA, Bundy BN, Berek JS, et al. Randomized trial of cyclophosphamide plus cisplatin with or without doxorubicin in ovarian carcinoma: A Gynecologic Oncology Group Study. J Clin Oncol 1989; 7:457–465.

Ozols RF, Young RC. Ovarian cancer. In: Haskell CM, ed. Current problems in cancer. Chicago: Year Book Medical Publishers, 1987:59–122.

Rozencweig M, Martin A, Beltangady M, et al. Randomized trial of carboplatin versus cisplatin in advanced ovarian cancer. In: Bunn PA Jr, Canetta R, Ozols RF, et al, eds. Carboplatin: Current perspectives and future directions. Philadelphia: WB Saunders, 1990: 175–186.

Williams SD, Blessing JA, Moore DH, et al. Cisplatin, vinblastine, and bleomycin in advanced and recurrent ovarian germ-cell tumors. Ann Intern Med 1989; 111:22–27.

Young RC, Walton LA, Ellenberg SS, et al. Adjuvant therapy in stage I and stage II epithelial ovarian cancer. N Engl J Med 1990; 322:1021–1027.

HODGKIN'S DISEASE: RADIATION THERAPY

JOHN D. EARLE, M.D.

This chapter reviews the current status of radiation therapy in the treatment of Hodgkin's disease. Space limitations require omission of a great deal of detail. Included is only that which is necessary for the subject described in the title with an emphasis on areas of controversy. It should be remembered that 10-year overall survival for stage I and II Hodgkin's disease is 91 percent and that 10-year disease-free survival is 81 percent. Thus, the process to be described in evaluating and treating patients with Hodgkin's disease is well established and provides an extremely favorable outlook in most cases. From the largest single institution's experience with Hodgkin's disease, it is estimated that 75 percent of patients presenting with previously untreated Hodgkin's disease present with stages I, II, and IIIA. These are usually best managed with radiation therapy and, therefore, are the subject of this discussion.

EVALUATION

Patients usually present with lymphadenopathy. An occasional patient will present with symptoms such as pruritus, night sweats, or fever, but usually a palpable lymph node brings the patient to the attention of the physician. Biopsy of an accessible lymph node is the procedure of choice and an experienced hematopathologist will classify patients included in this chapter as having nodular sclerosing, lymphocyte predominance, mixed cellularity, or lymphocyte depletion Hodgkin's disease. It appears that, carefully staged, these do not differ in prognosis, stage for stage. Generally speaking, lymphocyte predominance, nodular sclerosing, mixed cellularity, and lymphocyte depleted Hodgkin's disease will present with more advanced stages in that order and to that extent have increasingly worse prognoses.

The evaluation of the patient with Hodgkin's disease begins with a careful history, examining the circumstances of presentation. But, in addition, systemic symptoms of fatigue, night sweats, weight loss, fever, or pruritus are important. The extent, nature, periodicity, and timing are all important in staging as will be noted later. Any symptom of compromised respiratory function should be noted. Physical examination should include careful mapping of the lymph nodes, specifying size and location by lymph node regions. Figure 1 details the lymph node regions used in the staging of Hodgkin's disease. Note that the spleen, thymus, and Waldeyer's ring are treated as lymph nodes. Evaluation of the skin may reveal excoriations seen in occasional patients with intense pruritus. Palpation of the abdomen for abdom-

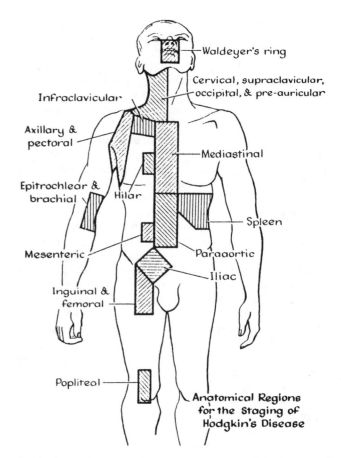

Figure 1 Lymph node regions used in the staging of Hodgkin's disease.

inal masses, hepatomegaly, splenomegaly, in addition to iliac, inguinal, and femoral lymph nodes, and percussion over the spine or pelvis to detect bone percussion tenderness should be performed. Laboratory evaluation should include complete blood count with attention to anemia, leukopenia, and inadequacy of platelets. In addition, a sedimentation rate may provide a useful marker in follow-up evaluation. Liver function tests complete the essential laboratory evaluation. Bilateral iliac crest bone marrow needle biopsies should be obtained at this point. The occasional positive biopsy will allow elimination of many of the following studies where appropriate. Imaging studies that should be accomplished include a PA and lateral chest x-ray. In most instances, the anterior mediastinal mass present in many patients with Hodgkin's disease can be detected on this study. However, it has become increasingly apparent that mediastinal adenopathy may not be detected with these routine tests. A computed tomography (CT) scan of the chest is indispensable when evaluating the mediastinum for smaller volume adenopathy in patients with Hodgkin's disease. The location and character of such masses are critical to the radiation oncologist. It is possible to have an anterior mediastinal mass which, lying anteriorly, protrudes laterally beyond the medial edge of the usual pulmonary block and which may not be detected by routine chest x-rays. This may well have led to some of the mediastinal failures occasionally seen in the past.

The lymphangiogram (LAG) is absolutely mandatory in the adequate evaluation of the patient with Hodgkin's disease. Internal architecture of abdominal lymph nodes may be diagnostically abnormal in the absence of enlargement of these lymph nodes. Thus, the CT scan may reveal normal lymph nodes that can be clearly detected as abnormal on lymphangiogram. However, abdominal-pelvic CT can supplement the lymphangiogram and may reveal hepatic, splenic, or upper abdominal lymphadenopathy otherwise undetectable. The LAG allows the radiation oncologist to tightly tailor the radiation portals about the periaortic, iliac, inguinal, and femoral nodes more closely than any other imaging procedure. Further, contrast will usually be diagnostic for many months allowing excellent accuracy for an extended period following for the minimal cost of a lumbar spine x-ray series. Immunization against pneumococci should be performed before a patient is subjected to laparotomy and splenectomy. Staging laparotomy is still the usual procedure in patients who have proceeded this far in staging and are still considered candidates for curative radiotherapy. The staging laparotomy should not be considered routine and must be performed by a surgeon experienced in *this* procedure. The necessity of careful liver biopsy, splenectomy, palpation, and biopsy of representative lymph nodes are all part of this procedure. The radiation oncologist and/or diagnostic radiologist should have discussed questionable lymph nodes with the surgeon. A young woman, unless a discussion and a decision otherwise was made prior to surgery, should have oophoropexy.

STAGING

Formal assignment of stage may be accomplished at this point. Table 1 defines stages I through IV. In addition, absence of fever, night sweats, or weight loss is denoted by an A. The presence of any one of these symptoms is denoted by a B. Other symptoms have been associated with Hodgkin's disease, but the triad of unexplained fever, night sweats, and unexplained loss of 10 percent or more of body weight are those recognized by the generally accepted Ann Arbor staging classification. If extension to non-lymph node tissues is present, these may be designated by E. This E designation is for extralymphatic extension or involvement so limited that it can be adequately treated with definitive radiotherapy. Finally, clinical staging is denoted by CS preceding the stage number and pathologic staging by PS.

RADIATION THERAPY

As noted above, radiation therapy is the treatment of choice for most patients with stage I, II, and IIIA Hodgkin's disease. Modern radiation therapy utilizing 4

Table 1 Staging Hodgkin's Disease

Stage	Definition
I	Involvement of a single lymph node region (I) or of a single extrahepatic organ or site (I_E)
II	Involvement of two or more lymph node regions on the same side of the diaphragm (II), or localized involvement of an extralymphatic organ or site and of one or more lymph node regions on the same side of the diaphragm (II_E)
III	Involvement of lymph node regions on both sides of the diaphragm (III), which may also be accompanied by involvement of the spleen (III_S) or by localized involvement of an extralymphatic organ or site (III_E) or both (III_{SE})
IV	Diffuse or disseminated involvement of one or more extralymphatic organs or tissues, with or without associated lymph node involvement

The absence or presence of fever, night sweats, and/or the unexplained loss of 10 percent or more of body weight in the 6 months preceding admission are to be denoted in all cases by the suffix letters A or B, respectively.

Adapted from Carbone PP, Kaplan HS, Musshoff K, et al. Report of the Committee on Hodgkin's Disease. Workshop on the Staging of Hodgkin's Disease. Ann Arbor, Michigan, April 1971.

to 10 MV x-rays at extended distances of 80 to 100 cm with individually tailored blocking are utilized to treat anterior and posterior opposed fields each day. Most patients are managed with a mantle or inverted Y field for stage I or stage II presentations with few lymph node regions involved. More extensive involvement above the diaphragm is frequently treated with a mantle and periaortic, splenic pedicle and upper iliac "spade" field. Care is taken in determining the distance between abutting fields. Daily doses approach 200 cGy per day at midplane, frequently beginning with lower doses. Frequent port films are taken during the course of treatment, at least weekly. Adjustments may be made on the basis of these. Further adjustments may be appropriate as bulky disease shrinks. Weekly blood counts are obtained as white count and platelet count will fall during the course of treatment. Interruptions are not usually necessary, particularly in patients who have had splenectomies. Hematologic reserves are usually higher than in unsplenectomized patients.

Total doses of 4,000 cGy are usual for sites of involvement, whereas 3,600 cGy is adequate for prophylactic treatment. It may be that even the latter dose is more than necessary. Additionally, a small boost may be given to sites of bulky disease. Careful monitoring by the radiation oncologist is required during the administration of this course of treatment. Considerable expertise, technical excellence, and formal quality control are required. Specific circumstances may require particular attention during the course of administration of radiation therapy.

Patients presenting with large mediastinal masses are approached in a variety of ways. In many institutions, even the bulkiest of mediastinal masses is treated with radiation. Larger fields, smaller daily doses and interruption of treatment at 1,500 cGy to allow for resolution are the usual procedures. Should shrinkage allow large enough blocks that adequate protection of the lungs can be accomplished, radiation is continued as the primary treatment modality.

Another difficult problem is the patient in whom mediastinal disease has been demonstrated to involve the pericardium. Adequate treatment involves high dose to the entire heart in this circumstance. Because this may lead to unacceptable complication rates, such patients are frequently managed primarily with chemotherapy. As noted, should the very large mediastinal mass fail to resolve after 1500 cGy, these patients also are managed primarily with chemotherapy. We recognize the high likelihood that these patients fail when the mediastinal mass is greater than one-third the diameter of the thoracic cage. However, this has not resulted in a diminution in survival and thus this criterion, by itself, is insufficient to warrant management primarily with chemotherapy. Kaplan has called attention to the fact that the small frequency of failure in each individual lymph node region is multiplied such that at approximately 6 to 7 regions involved, the likelihood of failure is so high that consideration of chemotherapy should be given.

Splenic involvement with more than five nodules is another circumstance in which primary management with chemotherapy rather than radiation therapy is appropriate. Some have treated the liver with radiation in this setting, but because this leads to increased risk of toxicity in the liver and does not address the increased likelihood of failure in other sites, many choose to administer chemotherapy to these patients.

There are several groups of patients in whom laparotomy is not required. Liebenhaut has pointed out that women with clinical stage IA disease, men with clinical stage IA disease in whom only lymphocyte-predominance Hodgkin's disease is present, and patients with clinical stage IA disease presenting in the mediastinum only are all extremely favorable prognostic groups that have less than 5 percent likelihood of disease below the diaphragm or of requiring chemotherapy and may be treated with a mantle only without a laparotomy. The patients who are pregnant when Hodgkin's disease is discovered should be treated in a major medical center with experience dealing with these patients. The usual evaluation and management may be appropriate following therapeutic abortion. However, modern radiotherapy equipment, careful shielding, careful evaluation of predicted doses from phantom measurements and confirmation of these expected doses with diodes during treatment, all supervised by experienced physicists, have allowed mantle treatment. Fetal doses during the mid-trimester in the range of 1 to 5 cGy have been our experience. Normal delivery or cesarean section when a viable infant is detected by the obstetrician has resulted in normal offspring, completion of staging, and resumption of appropriate, uncomplicated management of the mother.

Acute effects of radiation therapy that a patient will first encounter may include nausea. Problematic nausea is less likely in treatment of the chest than in treatment of the upper abdomen. The likelihood of symptomatic nausea seems to be reduced if the initial treatments are 50 percent of the intended daily dose. Adequate explanations and support seem to help avoid this side effect. In some instances, however, nausea is persistent and of sufficient magnitude to warrant antiemetics. As treatment proceeds, patients note a sense of malaise or loss of the feeling of wellbeing. Frank fatigue, the need to nap or retire earlier in the evening is common. The fatigue persists for up to 6 weeks following completion of radiation therapy.

In treatment of the mantle, particularly if full dose is used from the outset, acute parotitis may be noted after the first or second treatment. This symptom is self-limited and rapidly disappears, but it can be very frightening to a patient. Another effect on the salivary glands is to diminish the flow of saliva and thicken secretions. This effect increases during the first several weeks of treatment. All patients should have careful dental prophylaxis at the inception of therapy in order to avoid the caries that can decimate dentition if adequate prophylaxis is not obtained.

Hair loss within the irradiated fields begins by the second week and will be fairly complete at the conclusion of treatment to the affected area. Fine hair begins to return by approximately 6 weeks after therapy. A very rare patient will have persistent or recurrent hair loss within the treated area. In some instances the regrowing hair will be lighter or darker or of a different texture.

Irritation of the skin within fields intersecting the skin, especially in a skin fold or in tangential fashion, can manifest erythema or moist desquamation. Irritation and erythema respond quickly to 1 percent hydrocortisone ointment. Wet reactions are best treated with Domeboro's solution.

Few patients will sustain hematologic depressions requiring interruption of therapy for white counts below 2,000 or platelet counts below 50,000. Should this occur, it is most apt to occur about 2,000 cGy into the last lymph node regions to be treated. In the usual case this would coincide with the last portion of treatment to the inverted Y or periaortic nodal region, after mantle therapy initially. Recovery is usually rapid requiring a week or 10 days of interruption in therapy.

Radiation effects on the small bowel are minimal. Occasional patients will suffer some diarrhea during the latter portion of abdominal irradiation. Crampy abdominal pain may be a signal of irritation to the small bowel or an early warning of small bowel obstruction secondary to adhesions caused by the laparotomy perhaps augmented by the subsequent radiation therapy. This is relatively uncommon, however.

FOLLOW-UP

Continuing follow-up of patients after therapy should involve the radiation oncologist. A number of sequelae of treatment peculiar to these patients are familiar to most radiation oncologists. Radiation exposure to many of the salivary glands alters the salivary flow as well as the chemical environment in the mouth. Dental caries can result unless careful dental prophylaxis has taken place prior to treatment. Pulmonary toxicity given the careful shielding of the lungs mentioned above is an infrequent occurrence. Risk of such side effects of treatment as clinically significant pulmonary symptoms should occur in 3 percent or less of the patients. These symptoms can occur between 6 weeks and 6 months after therapy, but are more frequent in the shorter time interval. Administration and sudden cessation of steroids may trigger pulmonary symptoms in an otherwise asymptomatic patient at anytime after radiation therapy. Treatment of severe symptoms requires systemic steroids and should be embarked upon with caution and the knowledge that steroid administration will require careful monitoring and extremely careful, slow tapering. Cardiac complications should be rare in patients managed with the equally weighted deeply penetrating beams at lower daily and total doses recommended above.

Nearly 50 percent of patients who are treated with a mantle following a lymphangiogram will have chemical signs of hypothyroidism. Approximately half of these will demonstrate clinically significant hypothyroidism. As noted above, affects of radiation on the bone marrow treated during the course of extended field or total nodal irradiation are associated with significant depression of bone marrow reserves. These recover over time, but care in following patients with more than the usual attention to the possibility of infections, such as meningitis or pneumonia, are required. Episodes of herpes zoster infection are much more frequent in these patients than in the general population. Conservative treatment is usually indicated, but patients should be alerted to the possibility of dissemination, which will require greater care and, perhaps, more active treatment.

With careful shielding of the testicles, including primary collimation, outboard collimation, and testicular shields, the dose to the testes should be restricted to a few cGy. Adequate marking of the ovaries and care in positioning the central pelvic blocks should restrict the dose to the female gonads to a level that will preserve fertility, although more than an order of magnitude higher dose will be received by the ovaries in women than by the testes in men. Our usual advice to young people who wish to have children is to take birth control measures for 2 years after this course of treatment. There is no evidence that irradiation of a parent prior to conception leads to abnormalities in the offspring in the human being. However, the theoretical possibility and the fragmentary evidence in animals suggest the above conservative approach is reasonable.

Table 2 Hodgkin's Disease Survival at 5 and 10 Years: Stanford

Stage	Survival		Relapse-free Survival	
	5 year	10 year	5 year	10 year
I	90.3	79.1	78.5	73.8
II	87.6	74.0	69.1	66.2
IIIA	84.7	65.9	71.3	62.8
IIIB	66.0	47.2	47.2	42.6

Data from Kaplan HS. Hodgkin's disease. 2nd ed. Cambridge, MA: Harvard University Press, 1980.

There is no question about the increase in second malignancies seen in patients successfully managed with radiation therapy for Hodgkin's disease. Coleman and others have reviewed the Stanford data and documented such increases in a number of the more common malignancies. The actuarial risk appears to be about 10 percent over the first decade but may be considerably higher for patients treated with chemotherapy. Leukemias and non-Hodgkin's lymphomas, as well as solid tumors such as lung, skin, gynecologic, bladder, colon, prostate, and skin neoplasms have been reported. Caution ascribing causation is required, but investigation of potentially less toxic treatment is clearly indicated.

Table 2 summarizes the percent 5- and 10-year overall survival and relapse-free survival observed in the 1225 patients treated at Stanford. Results are somewhat better for the 923 patients that were laparotomy staged.

SUGGESTED READING

Carbone PP, Kaplan HS, Musshoff K, et al. Report of the Committee on Hodgkin's Disease. Cancer Res 1971; 31:1860–1861.

Coleman CN. Secondary neoplasms in patients treated for cancer: Etiology and perspective. Radiat Res 1982; 92:188–200.

Horning SJ, Hoppe RT, Kaplan HS, Rosenberg SA. Female reproductive potential after treatment for Hodgkin's disease. N Engl J Med 1981; 304:1377–1382.

Kaplan HS. Hodgkin's disease. 2nd ed. Cambridge, MA: Harvard University Press, 1980.

Leibenhaut MH, Hoppe RT, Efron B, et al. Prognostic indicators of laparotomy findings in clinical stage I-II supradiaphragmatic Hodgkin's disease. J Clin Oncol 1989; 7:81–91.

Pedrick TJ, Hoppe RT. Recovery of spermatogenesis following pelvic irradiation for Hodgkin's disease. Int J Radiat Oncol Biol Phys 1986; 12:117–121.

Tarbell NJ, Thompson L, Mauch P. Thoracic irradiation in Hodgkin's disease: Disease control and long-term complications. Int J Radiat Oncol Biol Phys 1990; 18:275–281.

Watchie J, Coleman CN, Raffin TA, et al. Minimal long-term cardiopulmonary dysfunction following treatment for Hodgkin's disease. Int J Radiat Oncol Biol Phys 1987; 13:517–524.

HODGKIN'S DISEASE: CHEMOTHERAPY

GIANNI BONADONNA, M.D.

Over the past two decades, treatment of Hodgkin's disease has evolved considerably through innovations in the management of various stages. The impact of various treatments on the 5-, 10-, and 15-year results is now being balanced against delayed morbidity, such as organ damage and second malignancies, produced by the intensity of therapy or the prolonged delivery of given drugs.

Clinicians should be aware that certain procedures or indications that were routine in the past decade (e.g., staging laparotomy, primary radiotherapy for all subsets of patients with nodal disease) should now find more flexible applications in the light of new prognostic factors. Past and present experience confirms that the complexity of clinical evaluation and the modern, sophisticated treatment modalities demand considerable technical resources and qualified personnel. Practicing physicians should therefore carefully and honestly evaluate whether their own experience and the facilities available to them are adequate. If not, patient referral to specialized centers remains a wise professional response.

PROPER STAGING

Proper staging is still important for selecting patients suitable for curative radiotherapy and those who are candidates for a systemic treatment program with or without irradiation.

The Ann Arbor staging classification was reviewed in 1989 at Cotswolds and modified in light of experience gained in its use and new techniques for evaluating Hodgkin's disease. It was particularly recommended that (1) computed tomography (CT) be included as a technique for evaluating intrathoracic and infradiaphragmatic lymph nodes; (2) the criteria for clinical involvement of the spleen and liver be modified to include evidence of focal defects with two imaging techniques, and that abnormalities of liver functions be ignored; (3) the suffix "X" to designate bulky disease (greater than 10 cm maximum dimension) be introduced; and (4) a new category of response to therapy, unconfirmed/uncertain complete remission (CR [u]), be introduced to accommodate the difficulty of persistent radiologic abnormalities of uncertain significance.

Table 1 outlines the procedures necessary to carry out correct clinical (CS) and pathologic (PS) staging. In particular, staging laparotomy should be performed only if management decisions depend on the histologic identification of occult abdominal disease and in particular a positive spleen. Thus, laparotomy remains, at present, a necessary procedure in CS IA and IIA without bulky mediastinal adenopathy as the 10-year relapse-free survival of PS IA and IIA treated with subtotal nodal radiotherapy alone is 70 to 85 percent. To histologically document hepatic involvement by Hodgkin's disease today, we can recommend either laparoscopy with multiple biopsies or needle biopsy of suspicious lesion(s) on liver CT scanning. Splenectomy is contraindicated in a child younger than 5 years because of increased risk of fulminant septicemia. Most of the above mentioned studies should be repeated once the initial treatment is completed to assess the status of complete remission properly or restaging in the presence of a single recurrence.

PROGNOSTIC FACTORS

The results of clinical trials performed during the last decade have allowed us to reconsider the various prognostic variables. The major unfavorable prognostic factor is tumor mass (e.g., bulky mediastinal lymphoma, multiple extranodal involvement, five or more splenic nodules). The biologic implications of large tumor volume have been extensively studied: the greater the tumor cell population, the more likely it is to contain significant numbers of various classes of drug resistant cells. Modern clinical research should improve the correct assessment and even quantitation of tumor volume. Disease progression while on chemotherapy or short-term complete remission despite intensive multiple drug regimens indicates poor prognosis because of primary cell resistance. In general, prognosis is inversely related to age, because children and young adults fare better than older people. In particular, patients older than 60 years of age often present with advanced disease and other medical problems that cause difficulties in the proper staging and treatment of their disease. Recent observations have confirmed that lymphocyte depleted Hodgkin's disease is a rare but very aggressive form of lymphoma whose prognosis is still unfavorable because of widespread nodal and extranodal involvement. The presence of B symptoms carries, in general, unfavorable prognostic significance, especially in patients with more advanced disease. Patients with stage IIB disease appear to have an adverse prognosis when they manifest all three systemic symptoms; this finding is often associated with bulky mediastinal disease. Males almost always have a less favorable prognosis compared with that of females.

PRINCIPLES OF TREATMENT

In patients with limited disease after adequate staging (PS I-IIA), the aim of current therapy is to provide a high cure rate within a short period of time and with limited morbidity. In patients with advanced Hodgkin's disease (stage IIIB-IV), the aim of therapy is

Table 1   Essential Procedures for Proper Staging in Addition to History
and Physical Examination

Radiologic examinations.   (1) Chest roentgenogram with mass/thoracic ratio (measurement of the largest transverse diameter of mediastinal mass and the transverse diameter of the thorax at the level T5-T6 on a standing posteroanterior film). (2) Computed tomography (CT) of the thorax, abdomen, and pelvis with intravenous contrast if necessary, with images at 1 cm intervals. (3) Bipedal lymphography. It may not be essential to have both CT and lymphography. For retroperitoneal nodes below L2 and smaller than 1.5 cm, lymphography may clearly be helpful.

Special imaging studies.   (1) Isotope scanning (e.g. gallium for extent of nodal involvement or technetium for involvement of bone). (2) Ultrasonography. (3) Magnetic resonance imaging (MRI). (4) Other imaging studies necessary to resolve the significance of symptoms or physical signs.

Laboratory tests.   Complete blood count, erythrosedimentation rate, renal and liver function tests, including LDH, serum uric acid (including absolute lymphocyte count), and copper.

Core needle biopsy from posterior iliac crest.   Biopsy should be bilateral, especially in the presence of CS III and in patients with systemic symptoms.

Staging laparotomy with splenectomy and multiple biopsies of hepatic and abdominal lymph nodes in CS I-II if therapeutic decision depends on the identification of occult abdominal involvement.

Needle or surgical biopsy of any suspicious extranodal (e.g., osseous, pulmonary, cutaneous) lesion(s).

Cytologic examination of any effusion.

to achieve durable complete remission, in most cases through effective full dose polydrug regimens at the expense of acceptable morbidity. Because a fraction of patients with advanced lymphoma are not cured by drugs, most probably due to primary tumor cell resistance, more attention should be given to the potential of alternating treatments, that is, alternating non-cross resistant drug regimens in stage IV and alternating chemotherapy with radiotherapy to the site(s) of initial bulky disease. For the management of the intermediate stages (IIB-III), more than one treatment option is available, and in the selection of optimal therapy, physicians should take into consideration some of the known prognostic variables such as disease extent (bulky adenopathy, stage IIIA versus III$_2$A) and systemic symptoms.

Patients resistant to primary drug therapy pose problems because current salvage treatments (second and third line chemotherapy as well as high dose chemotherapy with autologous bone marrow transplantation) appear to induce durable complete response in only a limited number of selected patients.

GUIDELINES TO PRIMARY TREATMENT

Stage IA-IIA With No Bulky Adenopathy

Following staging laparotomy, patients with supradiaphragmatic disease and no bulky mediastinum are treated with subtotal nodal irradiation delivered with high energy equipment at conventional tumoricidal doses (involved areas—40 to 44 Gy, uninvolved areas—35 Gy). In rare cases (4 to 5 percent) with subdiaphragmatic nonbulky Hodgkin's disease, radio-

therapy is administered through an inverted Y field including the splenic pedicle in stage I, and through total nodal irradiation (including the mediastinum) in stage II, respectively. With this strategy, the 10-year relapse-free survival (RFS) ranges from 70 to 85 percent; total survival following salvage chemotherapy in relapsing patients ranges from 80 to 95 percent. Late relapses (i.e., 3 years or more after completion of radiotherapy) are 10 to 13 percent, and they occur more often in patients with stage I disease and a nodular sclerosis histology. In patients not subjected to staging laparotomy, subtotal or total nodal irradiation including a splenic port, RFS may be inferior, but total survival remains similar because, in both situations, the ability to salvage patients with combination chemotherapy after they relapse from radiotherapy is excellent.

Stage IB-IIB with No Bulky Adenopathy

In patients treated as those with the same stage and no systemic symptoms, the 10-year freedom relapse is comparatively lower, but most cases can be salvaged with optimal chemotherapy. However, in a small subset of stage IIB patients presenting with all three systemic symptoms, prognosis is extremely poor since the 5-year freedom from relapse rate is only about 40 percent. In this subset, staging laparotomy is superfluous, and combined modality therapy is recommended. In all other patients with nonbulky, true (i.e., after laparotomy) stage IB-IIB disease with a solitary systemic symptom, subtotal or total nodal radiotherapy appears the treatment of choice and can yield a 10-year RFS of 80 percent or over.

Stage II (A and B) With Bulky Adenopathy ("X") and Limited Extranodal Extension

With few exceptions, the majority of oncologists agree that this stage group should now be managed with combined modality therapy. In general, patients present with multiple supradiaphragmatic nodal groups involved and may have extension of tumor into the lung, pericardium, or chest wall. Staging includes only lymphography or CT and two needle bone marrow biopsies. Because effective combination chemotherapy is able to induce prompt tumor shrinkage of compressive symptoms from mediastinal-hilar adenopathy, medical treatment should precede irradiation; radiotherapy can be delivered at conventional tumoricidal doses as mantle or subtotal nodal irradiation including spleen once three to four cycles of the selected combination are completed (i.e., MOPP or one of its variants, ABVD, MOPP alternated with ABVD; see Table 2). Utilizing this strategy, most patients begin the radiation program in complete or almost complete clinical remission, thus avoiding the pulmonary sequelae following primary irradiation of huge mediastinal-hilar adenopathy. With a combined modality approach, both 5- and 10-year RFS and survival rates are about 75 percent.

Stage IIIA

There is still debate as how to treat this patient subset properly, which includes various prognostic groups depending on the extent and the bulkiness of disease. If, through careful surgical staging, patients with CS I or CS II show histologic involvement limited to the lymphatic structures in the upper abdomen that accompany the celiac-axis group of arteries (substage III_1), subtotal or total nodal irradiation can represent the treatment of choice for patients with no bulky adenopathy and minimal splenic involvement (less than five positive nodules). In fact, the overall survival results, inclusive of salvage chemotherapy for relapsing patients are comparable with those reported with PS IIA.

The controversy arises when there is involvement of low para-aortic nodes and iliac nodes (substage III_2). Based on the results of numerous trials utilizing systemic drug therapy, when the lymphographic patterns appear typical for retroperitoneal node involvement, most clinicians avoid staging laparotomy and utilize combination chemotherapy with or without radiotherapy. In the past, a common approach involved total nodal irradiation followed by chemotherapy (usually six cycles of MOPP), but this form of treatment carried a high risk of acute leukemia even if irradiation was limited to involved fields. A more recent approach consists first in the delivery of three to four cycles of combination chemotherapy to be followed by total nodal or involved-field irradiation with 30 to 35 Gy if the patient achieves complete or almost complete remission after drug therapy. This approach is particularly useful in patients with extensive Hodgkin's disease and in the presence of bulky mediastinum or para-aortic nodes. In the experience of the Milan Cancer Institute, ABVD plus radiotherapy yielded superior 7-year results (94 percent) when randomly compared to MOPP plus radiotherapy (67 percent) and was associated with minimal (0.7%) leukemogenesis, irreversible gonadal dysfunction, and cardiac toxicity. In light of modern concepts about drug resistant tumor cells, it appears highly questionable whether further chemotherapy, utilizing the same drug regimen, after completion of the irradiation program is strategically important to influence the duration of complete remission. On the contrary, chemotherapy after extensive irradiation must often be delivered through low dose regimens because of prolonged myelosuppression and may increase the incidence of treatment related sequelae. To make combined treatment even more tolerable as far as myelosuppression is concerned, one may utilize the so-called ping-pong strategy devised at Stanford University, that is the delivery of two cycles of combination chemotherapy alternating with the irradiation of two lymph node regions, starting with central nodal areas. Regardless of the treatment sequence utilized, the frequence of durable complete remission appears invariably superior following combined modality therapy (over 80 percent) compared to total nodal irradiation alone (less than 50 percent). Thus, combined modality appears to be the most effective means to maximize, through the first treatment approach, the chances of cure of stage IIIA disease when low retroperitoneal nodes are positive as well as when extensive splenic involvement (5 or more positive nodules) and/or bulky adenopathy are present.

Over the past 15 years, there have been several attempts to treat stage IIIA disease with combination chemotherapy alone, usually MOPP. With the exception of the results achieved at the National Cancer Institute, both incidence and duration of complete remission following MOPP alone are, in general, inferior compared with combined modality therapy, and the majority of relapses occur in the original sites of disease. In the light of more recent findings on the efficacy of Adriamycin-containing regimens, it remains to be demonstrated whether current 5-year results could be further improved by relatively short-term treatment (e.g., four cycles) with ABVD or MOPP-ABVD followed by involved field radiotherapy.

Stage IIIB

It remains unresolved at present whether the optimal management of this stage group is combined modality therapy, as above described for stage III_2A, or intensive combination chemotherapy with or without irradiation to the lymphoid regions presenting with bulky disease. The results from the Milan Cancer Institute utilizing ABVD for three cycles followed by subtotal or total nodal irradiation appear excellent: complete remission in 92 percent of cases and 85 percent RFS at 7 years (no bulky lymphoma 96 percent, bulky lymphoma 81 percent). These findings appear superior to those reported after a single drug combination (e.g., MOPP) alone and comparable, though devoid of acute leukemia and sterility, to the results achieved with combined modality therapy utilizing MOPP or similar regimens.

Stage IV (A and B)

This stage group is best managed with intensive, full dose combination chemotherapy. However, it may be possible that irradiation limited to the site(s) of initial bulky disease can further optimize the long-term RFS.

MOPP has been the most widely used drug combination in clinical practice. However, in recent years, the administration of MOPP has been alternated monthly with ABVD (MOPP-ABVD) in the attempt to overcome the problem of primary drug resistance. The largest experience has been achieved so far by investigators of the Milan Cancer Institute. In their first study, they have shown that there was a superiority of alternating chemotherapy compared to MOPP alone in terms of complete remission (89 percent versus 74 percent), freedom from progression (65 percent versus 36 percent), 8-year relapse-free (73 percent versus 45 percent), and total survival (84 percent versus 64 percent). In particular, the superiority of alternating chemotherapy was evident in the subsets known to be prognostically unfavorable or less affected by MOPP chemotherapy (i.e., age over 40 years, systemic symptoms, nodular sclerosis, and bulky lymphoma). Almost identical results were obtained in a subsequent trial carried out by the Milan Cancer Institute. The superiority of MOPP-ABVD over MOPP alone in stage IV has been confirmed by investigators of Cancer and Acute Leukemia Group B.

The alternating treatment is simple to administer (Table 2). MOPP is administered at the classic dose schedule, both when used alone or when alternated with ABVD. Prednisone is administered on cycles 1, 4, 7, and 10. The ABVD regimen is started on day 29 from the initiation of the previous MOPP cycle. All four drugs are given simultaneously as rapid intravenous injections on day 1 and 15 of each cycle. After each ABVD treatment, patients are given no other therapy for an additional 14 days. On day 29 from the initiation of ABVD, the next cycle of MOPP is started. Thus each treatment cycle of both drug regimens takes approximately 1 month. MOPP-ABVD should be administered until complete clinical remission is achieved (median five cycles) followed, after bone marrow and liver biopsies if these organs were known to be involved prior to therapy, by two consolidation cycles (MOPP and ABVD). It is important to administer full dose chemotherapy of both regimens unless peripheral leukocytes are below 3,500 per cubic millimeter and/or platelets below 100,000 per cubic millimeter, respectively, on the planned day of drug administration. In this case, physicians can decide whether to delay therapy for a few days or give chemotherapy, thereby reducing temporarily by 50 percent the dose of mechlorethamine, procarbazine, Adriamycin, and vinblastine. About 40 percent of patients manifest a leukocyte fall to less than 2,500 per

Table 2 MOPP and ABVD Regimens

Combination	Dose (mg/m²)	Days of Treatment	Frequency
MOPP			
Mechlorethamine	6 IV	1 and 8	
Vincristine	1.4 IV	1 and 8	q 28 days
Procarbazine	100 PO	1 to 14	
Prednisone*	40 PO	1 to 14	
ABVD			
Adriamycin	25 IV	1 and 15	
Bleomycin	10 IV	1 and 15	q 28 days
Vinblastine	6 IV	1 and 15	
Dacarbazine	375 IV	1 and 15	

*On cycle 1, 4, 7.

cubic millimeter; a platelet fall to under 75,000 per cubic millimeter can be observed only in 15 percent of cases. Complete or almost complete alopecia occurs in only 17 to 20 percent of patients, and severe peripheral neuropathy in 7 percent, respectively. Vomiting is more frequent and severe after ABVD compared to MOPP.

SALVAGE THERAPY

Relapse from Primary Radiotherapy

After proper restaging, further irradiation can be delivered, if technically feasible, to patients with isolated marginal or true recurrence followed by combination chemotherapy. Recent results from the Milan Cancer Institute suggest that Adriamycin containing regimens (ABVD, MOPP-ABVD) can yield superior results compared to MOPP (complete remission 90 percent versus 75 percent, 7-year RFS 80 percent versus 55 percent, survival 80 percent versus 45 percent). Whenever possible, as in stage IV disease, chemotherapy should be administered for a minimum of six cycles or to complete tumor remission plus two consolidation cycles.

Relapse from MOPP

If the duration of first complete remissions is longer than 12 months, retreatment with MOPP remains the standard approach; it can yield a second complete remission in about 80 percent of patients, and in 75 to 85 percent of cases remission is durable. The same strategy is recommended in patients relapsing from other polydrug regimens. Patients relapsing from MOPP but in whom duration of first complete remission is less than 12 months as well as patients who do not achieve complete remission or show progressive disease during primary chemotherapy require treatment with non-cross resistant regimens. The most widely used salvage chemotherapy in MOPP resistant patients is ABVD. Treatment should be given at full dose to complete remission plus two consolidation cycles. The complete response rate is about 50 percent, and the likelihood of attaining complete remission is higher or lower in relation to A or B symptoms as well as to the anatomic extent of disease. Approximately 20 percent of all MOPP resistant patients remain disease-free at 5 years or more. Comparable results are being obtained with other Adriamycin containing regimens if treatment is promptly instituted at the time of recurrent or progressive lymphoma.

Relapse from MOPP-ABVD

Patients should be retreated with the same alternating sequence if duration of first complete remission is longer than 12 months. Physicians should avoid risk of cumulative doses of Adriamycin (over 550 mg per square meter) and of bleomycin (over 200 mg per square meter). In patients with shorter duration of complete remission, CEP is recommended for a minimum of six cycles. The dose schedule is as follows: CCNU—80 mg per square meter orally, on day 1, etoposide 100 mg per square meter orally or intravenously from day 1 through 5, prednimustine 60 mg per square meter orally from day 1 through 5. All drugs are recycled on day 28. Prednimustine can be replaced by an equivalent dose of chlorambucil and prednisone. Complete remission can be achieved in about 40 percent and the 5-year survival is 20 percent.

Salvage with ABMT

In recent years, high dose chemotherapy with autologous bone marrow transplantation (ABMT) has been applied to patients with advanced Hodgkin's disease in relapse or refractory to first or second line chemotherapy. One of the different drug regimens tested so far consists of cyclophosphamide 5 g per square meter, BCNU 600 mg per square meter, and etoposide 400 mg per square meter with total body irradiation. If patients are properly selected (i.e., with age less than 50 years, with no prior radiotherapy, and in first relapse from primary chemotherapy), complete remission can be achieved in more than two-thirds of cases. In this type of patient, the actual RFS rate remains to be determined, but is expected to be in excess of 50 percent at 3 years. Because of severe myelosuppression for about 2 weeks and the persisting uncertainty about patients who may benefit from high dose chemotherapy with ABMT, this form of intensive treatment should be administered at present in specialized centers.

CHEMOTHERAPY IN EARLY STAGES

There is no standard role of chemotherapy in the management of stage I-II of Hodgkin's disease. However, chemotherapy may be indicated under certain circumstances, as summarized in Table 3. Full dose or wide field irradiation in children and adolescents would result in unacceptable bone and muscle growth abnormalities. Pediatric patients are now being treated with combination chemotherapy combined with involved

Table 3 Indications for Primary Chemotherapy in the Management of Early Stage Hodgkin's Disease

If irradiation cannot or should not be given in full tumoricidal doses, or to appropriate (usually subtotal nodal) fields.
If diagnostic or staging information is inadequate by plan or circumstances.
If appropriate staging and irradiation would result in less than half of the patients enjoying prolonged recurrence-free survival.
If the acute toxicity and long-term complications of chemotherapy can be reduced significantly.

field, low dose radiotherapy, and regardless of stage, 90 percent or more are alive at 10 years. As previously mentioned, another group of patients is those with bulky mediastinal adenopathy extending to the surrounding organs or all three B symptoms. If staging laparotomy is unavailable or considered unacceptable because of the patient's age, medical condition, or the therapeutic philosophy, chemotherapy should be given. If well-tolerated chemotherapy regimens were available, which after adequate long-term experience were associated with low or no leukemia or other neoplasm risk and low or no sterility risk, then chemotherapy would be the preferred treatment. The ABVD combination may represent an effective drug regimen devoid of chronic organ damage. The major disadvantages remain severe nausea and vomiting in at least half of patients. However, at present, it remains to be demonstrated whether a milder chemotherapy will be safer, more tolerable, and as effective as ABVD.

TREATMENT RELATED MORBIDITY

The most serious consequence of curative therapy for Hodgkin's disease is the emergence of second malignancies. Most common among these are acute, nonlymphocytic leukemia, myelodysplastic syndromes including preleukemia, and diffuse aggressive lymphomas. In patients treated with MOPP or one of its variants, i.e., treatment including alkylating agents, procarbazine, or nitrosourea derivatives (BCNU, CCNU), the risk of leukemia within 10 years is 3 to 4 percent. This risk seems to be increased when patients are older than 40 years at the time of systemic treatment and when combined treatment modality is utilized, especially if salvage MOPP is given after radiation failure (over 15 percent). The overall risk of non-Hodgkin's lymphoma is about 2 percent. The risk of developing a secondary solid tumor is continuing to increase beyond 10 years (a finding not seen with leukemia), and the risk is highest in older patients; approximately two-thirds of the tumors have occurred so far in the radiation therapy field. Since the selection of agents may be important (ABVD does not appear to be as toxic as MOPP in terms of the development of secondary leukemias), the accrual of more data from patients who receive alternate drug regimens is essential in assessing the relative carcinogenicity of the treatment modalities.

Gonadal dysfunction represents another important iatrogenic toxicity that considerably affects the quality of life in patients with Hodgkin's disease. A few cycles of MOPP or MOPP-like combinations induce azoospermia in 90 to 100 percent of patients, and this finding is associated with germinal hyperplasia and increased FSH levels, with normal levels of LH and testosterone. In addition, only 10 to 20 percent of patients eventually show recovery of spermatogenesis after long periods of time, even up to 10 years. About half of women become amenorrheic, and premature ovarian failure appears dependent upon age (over 30 years: 75 to 85 percent; under 30 years: about 20 percent). This is most probably related to the total dose of drugs, and is a progressive rather than an all-or-none phenomenon. The Milan Cancer Institute has reported that the administration of ABVD chemotherapy produces only a limited and transient germ cell toxicity in males and no drug induced amenorrhea. Thus, to circumvent chemotherapy induced sterility, the use of drug regimens not containing alkylating agents, procarbazine, or nitrosourea derivatives is highly recommended. An alternative for males undergoing MOPP or MOPP-ABVD combinations is represented by sperm storage prior to chemotherapy; however, both physicians and patients should be aware that about one-third of male patients with Hodgkin's disease have low sperm count or sperm motility before starting cytotoxic treatment. The usefulness of the administration of analogues of gonadotropin releasing hormone in males or oral contraceptives in premenopausal women remains to be fully confirmed. Libido tends to decrease after both the diagnosis of Hodgkin's disease and treatment with combination chemotherapy. There is no evidence of teratogenicity in patients treated for Hodgkin's disease.

Pericarditis, both acute and chronic, is the most common symptomatic cardiovascular complication of mediastinal irradiation. The incidence of pericarditis is related to the dose, dose rate, and volume irradiated. Clinically evident pericarditis occurs in about 15 percent following anteroposterior fields from a linear accelerator to a mean mediastinal dose of 44 Gy. Pericardial effusions develop in 25 percent to 30 percent of patients within 2 years of radiation. Surgical stripping of the pericardium remains the only definitive therapy for chronic constrictive pericarditis. Radiation induced myocardial fibrosis at the subclinical level occurs in over 50 percent of irradiated patients. Chronic cardiomyopathy may occur after anthracycline administration only if the cumulative dose of Adriamycin exceeds 400 to 450 mg per square meter. At the Milan Cancer Institute, cardiac evaluation of patients treated with ABVD plus irradiation failed to detect any clinical and laboratory abnormalities up to 8 years from starting ABVD chemotherapy (maximum cumulative dose of Adriamycin: 300 mg per square meter).

Acute radiation pneumonitis and chronic restrictive fibrosis are the most important pulmonary complications of mantle irradiation. Both are related to the total dose, dose rate, and volume of lung tissue irradiated. The overall incidence is about 20 percent. Patients with relapsed Hodgkin's disease who receive total body irradiation in preparation for bone marrow transplantation are also at risk for developing pneumonitis. The drugs with greatest potential for pulmonary toxicity are bleomycin and BCNU. In patients treated with ABVD plus radiotherapy, overt bleomycin related lung toxicity is uncommon, and no pulmonary damage was seen in patients given MOPP-ABVD.

SUGGESTED READING

Bonadonna G, Santoro A, Gianni MA, et al. Primary and salvage chemotherapy in advanced Hodgkin's disease: the Milan Cancer Institute experience. Ann Oncol 1991; 2 (Suppl. 1):9–16.

Bookman MA, Longo DL. Concomitant illness in patients treated for Hodgkin's disease. Cancer Treat Rev 1986; 13:77–11.

Coltman CA Jr (Guest Editor). Hodgkin's Disease. Semin Oncol 1990; 17:641–771.

Lister TA, Crowther D, Sutcliffe SD, et al. Report of a Committee convened to discuss the evaluation and staging of patients with Hodgkin's disease: Cotswolds Meeting. J Clin Oncol 1989; 7:1630–1636.

Rosenberg SA. The continuing challenge of Hodgkin's disease. Ann Oncol 1991; (Suppl. 2):29–31.

NON-HODGKIN'S LYMPHOMA: RADIATION THERAPY

SHIAO Y. WOO, M.D.
LILLIAN M. FULLER, M.D.

The role of the radiation oncologist in managing patients with non-Hodgkin's lymphomas has changed dramatically in the past two decades. Until combination chemotherapy regimens were developed, radiotherapy was the only effective treatment for patients with this type of cancer. Before 1950, when treatment was administered with orthovoltage equipment, it was generally only palliative in intent. In 1950, however, a report by Lenz showed that lymphosarcoma of the tonsil could be cured with radiotherapy. Then, following Peters' report, also in 1950, that early stage Hodgkin's disease could be cured with radiotherapy, radiotherapists became interested in treating patients for non-Hodgkin's lymphomas definitively and in exploring the value of prophylactic treatment, including total lymphoid irradiation. A significant number of patients with early stage non-Hodgkin's lymphomas were cured, but radiotherapy was seldom effective for patients with advanced-stage disease. Today, with effective combination chemotherapy regimens and combined-modality programs, the prognosis for patients with all stages of diffuse non-Hodgkin's lymphomas has changed dramatically.

Treatment results for patients with non-Hodgkin's lymphomas may also be attributed to new pathologic classifications, which correlate morphologic findings with prognosis, and to the development of better diagnostic imaging procedures. Retrospective and prospective studies designed to identify prognostic factors have also served to improve results. At The University of Texas M.D. Anderson Cancer Center, a weekly lymphoma planning clinic and response conference organized by the Lymphoma Service and attended by hematopathologists, radiologists, medical oncologists, and radiation oncologists has proved to be an excellent forum for exchange of information and treatment decisions for all patients admitted to the service. In addition to a disease-oriented examination prior to any treatment, information obtained from diagnostic imaging procedures is crucial for planning a radiotherapy field.

Before effective chemotherapy became available, large-volume radiotherapy techniques were used to encompass involved regions and potential areas of spread. Today, prophylactic treatment is seldom indicated and may be detrimental to patients participating in combined-modality programs. Unnecessary inclusion of bone marrow in the radiotherapy fields, for example, may lower a patient's tolerance for chemotherapy. Certain chemotherapeutic agents, moreover, tend to alter the tolerance for irradiation in normal tissues such as the mucous membranes. Computed tomography (CT) and various field-shaping devices have made it possible to execute very precise therapy. This is particularly important for patients on programs that contain chemotherapy.

Current treatment programs for non-Hodgkin's lymphomas are based on both the histopathologic classification and on the stage or extent of the disease. Except for treatment of patients with stage I and II presentations, management of patients with low-grade lymphomas, and particularly follicular small cleaved cell and mixed subtypes, remains controversial. This is so because advanced disease is considered incurable by current treatment modalities. Management of the diffuse lymphomas, which are curable regardless of stage, is less controversial. Issues center on the relative merits of the various chemotherapeutic combinations and on the role of radiotherapy.

THE DIFFUSE LYMPHOMAS

Diffuse Large-Cell Lymphomas

Most patients with diffuse large-cell lymphomas (DLCL) are adults; about half present with apparently localized disease, and of these almost half have extranodal manifestations. When treated with radiotherapy alone, most patients with stage I or II disease will develop disseminated disease within 6 months to 1 year. Because of patient selection, survival rates reported by major institutions have varied significantly. During the 1960s, the policy of the Lymphoma Section in our institution was to treat all patients presenting with stage I or II disease (including those with large abdominal masses who accounted for about one-third of our patient population) with involved-field radiotherapy. Our overall 5-year survival rate for 91 consecutively treated patients was 26 percent. Corresponding results of 38 percent for stage I or IE disease were slightly better. Because we believe that certain categories of patients, notably those with extranodal disease, could have a more favorable prognosis, we decided to evaluate our results for disease presenting in the major extranodal sites, namely Waldeyer's ring, the paranasal sinuses, the thyroid gland, and the stomach. To define the extent of disease more precisely, lymphomas in the head and neck were staged according to the TNM System of the American Joint Committee. While we were conducting these retrospective studies, we added staging laparotomy to the diagnostic armamentarium for patients with localized disease to determine the effect of more precise staging on results.

In these retrospective studies, tumor volume was found to have the most important influence on outcome in patients with localized extranodal head and neck disease. Our 10-year survival rate for patients with T1 or T2 lesions in Waldeyer's ring, without involvement of the cervical nodes, was 70 percent; for those patients with T3 or T4 disease, the survival rate was 55 percent. If the disease had spread to the cervical nodes, the patients'

10-year survival rates dropped to between 20 percent and 40 percent. For those with T1 or T2 lesions originating in the paranasal sinuses, the survival rates were 80 percent, compared with 20 percent for those with more extensive disease. Results for patients with lymphomas originating in the thyroid gland were generally better than for those with disease in Waldeyer's ring or the paranasal sinuses. Twelve patients whose disease did not extend beyond the cervical nodes were surviving free of disease, but only one of three patients with mediastinal involvement survived.

Staging laparotomy is no longer used routinely as an investigative procedure for patients with clinically staged I or II disease. Our experience with a selected patient population with laparotomy-staged I or II disease that was treated with involved-field radiotherapy was that results for patients with stage I or IE disease were excellent, but less satisfactory for those with stages II or IIE disease. Other investigators reported similar results for patients treated with subtotal nodal or total nodal irradiation.

Combination Chemotherapy and Radiotherapy: Stages I and II

In the late 1970s and early 1980s, interest turned to treating patients who had stage I or II DLCL with combination chemotherapy only. From small patient series, Miller and Cabanillas reported improved results for combination chemotherapy over those achieved with radiation alone. However, the incidence of recurrence in initial sites of disease was significant, particularly in patients with bulky involvement.

Currently, the trend in treating stage I and II DLCL is to add radiotherapy to combination chemotherapy regimens that contain doxorubicin. Analyzed by stage, the best results of treatment for stage I disease were reported by investigators at the National Cancer Insti-

tute, who used a combination chemotherapy program popularly known as proMACE-MOPP. This consists of prednisone, methotrexate, doxorubicin, cyclophosphamide, etoposide (proMACE) for induction, and nitrogen mustard, vincristine, procarbazine, and prednisone (MOPP) followed by involved-field radiotherapy for consolidation. Ninety-six patients treated according to this regimen achieved complete remissions, and none has had a relapse during a median follow-up of 42 months. Investigators from Arizona and from Vancouver who pooled their data for patients with stage I or II disease treated with CHOP (cyclophosphamide, doxorubicin, vincristine, prednisone) chemotherapy and involved-field radiotherapy reported a 5-year relapse-free survival rate of 83 percent. Our 10-year survival rate using CHOP-Bleo (CHOP low dose bleomycin) and regional radiotherapy in a "sandwich" technique for patients with stage I or II disease was 78 percent. When we analyzed our results for patients with stage I disease according to tumor burden (Table 1) and lactic dehydrogenase (LDH) level, we found that for patients at low risk of relapse (Table 2), the 10-year survival rate was 90 percent. It was 65 percent for those at high risk. The corresponding result for patients at intermediate risk was 75 percent. Corresponding results for stage II patients were 75 percent, 60 percent, and 37 percent. Our 10-year survival rates of 90 percent for patients with favorable stage I presentations support the policy of investigators in Vancouver of treating such patients with only three cycles of CHOP followed by involved-field radiotherapy.

Gastric Lymphomas: Stages IE and IIE

Our approach to treating patients with stage IE and IIE lymphomas of the stomach is the same as our overall treatment programs for stage I and II disease using CHOP-Bleo and radiotherapy. However, because treat-

Table 1 Criteria for Estimating Total Tumor Burden from Combinations of Extent of Involvement in Nodal and Extranodal Disease Sites

| | Nodal Regions | Extranodal Sites | |
Total Tumor Burden	Number of Regions with Extensive Disease	Number of Sites with Extensive Disease	Number of Sites with Focal Disease
Low	0	0	± 1 or 2
Intermediate	1	0	± 1
	0	1	±1
High*	1	1	—
	2	—	—
	—	2	—
	1	—	2
	—	1	2
	—	—	3

*Criteria for high tumor burden inlcude five possible combinations as shown.
From Velasquez WS, Jagannath S, Tucker SL, et al. Risk classification as the basis for clinical staging of diffuse large-cell lymphoma derived from 10-year survival data. Blood 1989; 74(2): 551; with permission.

Table 2 Prognostic Model for Diffuse Large-Cell Lymphoma Based on Extent of Tumor Burden and Lactic Dehydrogenase Levels*

Tumor Burden	Score	LDH	Score	Total Score	Risk Group
Low	0	Normal	0	0	A
Low	0	High	1	1	B
Intermediate	1	Normal	0	1	B
Intermediate	1	High	1	2	C
High	2	Normal	0	2	C
High	2	High	1	3	D

*Risk groups were determined by adding the assigned scores for tumor burden and LDH.
From Velasquez WS, Jagannath S, Tucker SL, et al. Risk classification as the basis for clinical staging of diffuse large-cell lymphoma derived from 10-year survival data. Blood 1989; 74(2): 555; with permission.

ment of this site is so controversial, we believe it merits separate discussion. Except for lymphomas of the stomach, surgical intervention has had only a minor role in the treatment of the lymphomatous diseases. As a result of persuasive reports, subtotal gastrectomy has been widely accepted as the appropriate treatment for stomach lymphoma preceding administration of chemotherapy, radiotherapy, or both. Avoiding the alleged risk of perforation secondary to chemotherapy or radiotherapy has been cited as an advantage of primary surgical intervention. The disadvantages of subtotal gastrectomy, including malabsorption syndrome and a 10 to 20 percent risk of perioperative mortality, have not been emphasized. Moreover, at diagnosis, a significant number of patients, 20 percent of those with stage IE disease and 40 percent of those with stage IIE disease, have nonresectable lesions.

In our experience, subtotal gastrectomy is seldom necessary for either diagnosis or treatment of gastric lymphomas. Improvements in endoscopic technology and in interpretation of small biopsy specimens have virtually eliminated the need for diagnostic laparotomy with gastrectomy. In our last report, among 35 patients treated with CHOP-Bleo and radiotherapy without gastrectomy, the 5-year survival rate was 70 percent, and the corresponding disease-free survival rate was 60 percent (Fig. 1). From our experience, we believe that the appropriate initial treatment for gastric lymphomas is chemotherapy followed with radiotherapy, rather than gastrectomy, which should be reserved for salvage.

Primary Central Nervous System Lymphomas

Most primary central nervous system lymphomas are diffuse large-cell lymphomas that present in the brain as either solitary or multiple lesions. Small non–cleaved cell lymphomas have been reported, however, usually in patients with acquired immunodeficiency syndrome (AIDS) or other immunodeficiency diseases. Most brain lymphomas respond to definitive radiation. However, the duration of response is generally short. A recent Radiation Therapy Oncology Group (RTOG) study showed a 2-year survival of 30 percent for patients treated with 40 Gy to the entire brain, followed by a

boost of 10 to 20 Gy directed to specific lesions. Other investigators reporting on combined-modality therapy have suggested that the addition of chemotherapy, particularly regimens containing methotrexate, may produce better results than those achieved with radiotherapy alone. We are currently investigating whether hyperfractionated radiotherapy will further improve results in patients treated with alternating chemotherapeutic regimens.

Stages III and IV

The mainstay of treatment for patients with stage III and IV disease is chemotherapy, the role of radiation not being well defined. However, because it is well known that radiation alone can eradicate localized areas of disease, it is only logical to integrate radiation into chemotherapy programs, using it for sites of initial bulky disease or areas of residual disease after aggressive chemotherapy. For all stage III patients treated with the "sandwich" technique of CHOP-Bleo chemotherapy and involved-field radiotherapy, our 10-year survival rate was 50 percent. The corresponding result for patients with stage IV disease who generally had less bulky disease was 50 percent after treatment with chemotherapy. Currently, we are using more intensive chemotherapy for all patients with high tumor burdens or high LDH levels, regardless of stage, who are at significant risk of relapse when treated with CHOP-Bleo chemotherapy and radiotherapy (Fig. 2). Such patients receive radiotherapy to initial areas of bulky disease or residual disease following chemotherapy. Whether this approach will improve our results for high-risk patients with stage III and stage IV disease remains to be seen.

HIGH-GRADE LYMPHOMAS

Lymphoblastic Lymphomas

Most patients with lymphoblastic lymphomas are children. Although many present with mediastinal masses, the disease usually disseminates rapidly, so that initial aggressive chemotherapy is mandatory for survival. Although the addition of radiotherapy may de-

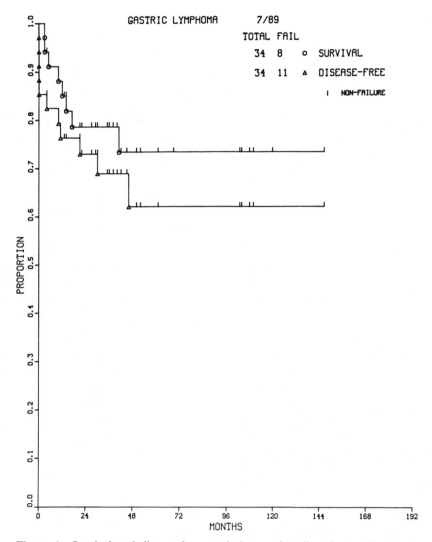

Figure 1 Survival and disease-free survival rates for all patients with gastric lymphoma (Kaplan-Meier method of analysis). (From Maor MH, Velasquez WS, Fuller LM, et al. Stomach conservation in stages IE and IIE gastric non-Hodgkin's lymphoma. J Clin Oncol 1990; 8(2):268; with permission.)

crease the possibility of mediastinal recurrence, it has not influenced the cure rate and therefore should only be given in emergency situations.

Prophylactic cranial irradiation has been useful in preventing central nervous system relapse. In the Stanford experience, 31 percent of patients developed central nervous system relapse when prophylactic treatment of the central nervous system was limited to methotrexate given systemically and intrathecally. Since cranial irradiation was added, no patient developed a relapse in the central nervous system. Today, cranial irradiation (24 Gy) is recognized as a necessary component of standard treatment for lymphoblastic lymphoma. However, radiation limited to the cranium is not sufficient for patients who have meningeal involvement at diagnosis or at relapse. The entire craniospinal axis must be treated in such patients.

Small Non–Cleaved Cell Lymphomas (Burkitt's and Non-Burkitt's)

Chemotherapy is the mainstay of all treatment programs for small non–cleaved cell lymphomas. In the treatment of patients with endemic African Burkitt's lymphoma, hyperfractionated radiotherapy has been shown to improve survival rates over those achieved with conventional radiotherapy. However, in nonendemic Burkitt's and non-Burkitt's lymphoma, the role of radiotherapy is unclear, except for emergency situations in which radiotherapy is mandatory for relieving symptoms caused by superior vena caval syndrome, compression of the airway, orbital proptosis, or cranial nerve palsies. Because intrathecal chemotherapy is as effective as combined-modality therapy in preventing relapse in the central nervous system, prophylactic craniospinal irradiation is no longer used.

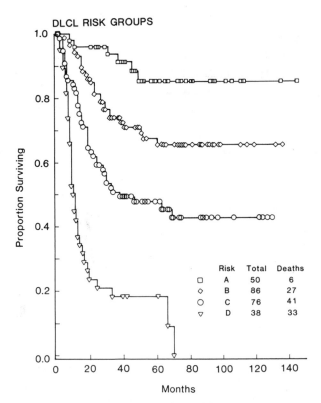

Figure 2 Survival according to risk groups A, B, C, and D for patients with diffuse large-cell lymphoma (DLCL). Differences in survivals between risk groups were statistically significant ($P < 0.01$). (From Velasquez WS, Jagannath S, Tucker SL, et al. Risk classification as the basis for clinical staging of diffuse large-cell lymphoma derived from 10-year survival data. Blood 1989; 74(2):555; with permission.)

However, total-body irradiation is used in some preparatory regimens for patients selected for bone marrow transplantation.

LOW-GRADE LYMPHOMAS

Most low-grade lymphomas are follicular small cleaved cell or mixed types. In the majority of patients, these diseases are generalized at the time of diagnosis. No more than 25 percent of patients present with stage I or II disease. The corresponding incidence for laparotomy-staged patients is approximately 6 percent.

Stages I and II

Investigators from the Princess Margaret Hospital, Stanford University, the M.D. Anderson Cancer Center, and the National Cancer Institute in Milan have reported 10-year relapse-free survivals of 37 to 55 percent, with survivals of approximately 65 percent for large series of patients with stage I or II disease treated with involved-field, extended-field, or total lymphoid irradiation to doses on the order of 30 to 45 Gy. In the Stanford series, patients who received total lym-

phoid irradiation had a better freedom-from-relapse rate than those who received involved-field or extended-field irradiation, suggesting that subdiaphragmatic irradiation is indicated for clinically staged patients treated with irradiation only. For patients who were laparotomy-staged, however, involved-field radiotherapy produced results similar to those achieved with total lymphoid irradiation in clinically staged patients.

The impact of adjuvant chemotherapy is uncertain in treatment of patients with clinically staged I or II disease. A retrospective review of patients treated at the M.D. Anderson Cancer Center showed that patients who received CVP (cyclophosphamide, vincristine, prednisone) or CHOP chemotherapy and involved-field radiotherapy had a better 5-year relapse-free survival rate (64 percent) than those who received radiotherapy alone (37 percent). Although several prospective studies have not shown any significant difference in freedom from relapse between patients treated with CVP (cyclophosphamide, vincristine, prednisone) chemotherapy and extended-field irradiation and those treated with irradiation alone, the Milan study demonstrated improved survival for patients treated on a combined-modality program. It appears that treatment with either total lymphoid irradiation or with chemotherapy and involved-field radiotherapy for patients with clinically staged I or II disease can produce results that are equal to those achieved with regional radiotherapy for laparotomy-staged patients.

Stage III

Treatment philosophies have varied from "watch and wait" to aggressive combined-modality therapy for patients with stage III and stage IV disease. Total lymphoid irradiation or combined-modality treatment has been reported to produce prolonged disease-free survivals in a subset of patients with stage III disease. These are patients who have low tumor burdens, normal LDH levels, and no "B" symptoms. Cox, who was then at Wisconsin, and Paryani, from Stanford, both reported 5-year relapse-free survival rates of 61 percent and 41 percent, respectively, after total lymphoid irradiation. At the M.D. Anderson Cancer Center, patients with favorable features treated with CHOP-Bleo chemotherapy and radiotherapy had a relapse-free survival rate of 73 percent at 5 years and 68 percent at 7 years. Those with unfavorable features, however, including bulky abdominal disease, had a relapse-free survival rate of only 33 percent at 7 years.

Current studies purport to test the value of such biologic compounds as interferon when added to combined-modality treatment programs. However, no highly effective therapy has been established for patients with extensive disease. It would seem appropriate, therefore, to enter such patients in clinical trials in which aggressive combined-modality treatment or bone marrow transplantation is used.

Stage IV

Although aggressive treatment seems to improve relapse-free survival for patients with stage IV disease, whether such treatment can alter survival has not been proved. Nevertheless, new trials of very aggressive therapy, including bone marrow transplantation, seem warranted. Radiation, as an effective single agent, probably should be integrated into such programs.

SUGGESTED READING

Coleman CN, Picozzi VJ Jr, Cox RS, et al. Treatment of lymphoblastic lymphoma in adults. J Clin Oncol 1986; 4(11):1,628–1,637.

Cox JD, Komaki R, Kun LE, et al. Stage III nodular lymphoreticular tumors (non-Hodgkin's lymphoma): Results of central lymphatic irradiation. Cancer 1981; 47:2,247–2,252.

Fuller LM, Hagemeister FB, Sullivan MP, et al. Hodgkin's disease and non-Hodgkin's lymphomas in adults and children. New York: Raven Press, 1988.

Jones SE, Miller TP, Connors JM. Long-term follow-up and analysis of prognostic factors for patients with limited stage diffuse large-cell lymphoma treated with initial chemotherapy with or without adjuvant radiotherapy. J Clin Oncol 1989; 7(9):1,186–1,191.

Kantarjian HM, McLaughlin P, Fuller LM, et al. Follicular large cell lymphoma: Analysis and prognostic factors in 62 patients. J Clin Oncol 1984; 2(7):811–819.

Longo DL, Glatstein E, Duffey PL, et al. Treatment of localized aggressive lymphomas with combination chemotherapy followed by involved-field Radiation Therapy. J Clin Oncol 1989; 7(9):1,295–1,302.

Maor MH, Velasquez WS, Fuller LM, et al. Stomach conservation in stages IE and IIE gastric non-Hodgkin's lymphoma. J Clin Oncol 1990; 8(2):266–271.

Paranyi SB, Hoppe RT, Cox RS, et al. The role of radiation therapy in the management of stage III follicular lymphomas. J Clin Oncol 1984; 2(7):841–848.

Velasquez WS, Jagannath S, Tucker SL, et al. Risk classification as the basis for clinical staging of diffuse large-cell lymphoma derived from 10-year survival data. Blood 1989; 74(2):551–557.

Young RC, Longo DL, Glatstein E, et al. The treatment of indolent lymphomas: Watchful waiting v. aggressive combined modality treatment. Semin Hematol 1988; 25(suppl 2):11–16.

NON-HODGKIN'S LYMPHOMA—UNFAVORABLE DISEASE: CHEMOTHERAPY

MICHAEL V. SEIDEN, M.D., Ph.D.
GEORGE P. CANELLOS, M.D.

The biologic heterogeneity of the malignant lymphocyte in non-Hodgkin's lymphoma is enormous. Survival of patients with non-Hodgkin's lymphoma may span decades, with little or no treatment, or may be limited to months, despite very aggressive therapy. Appropriate management of the disease requires an appreciation of the biologic diversity seen in non-Hodgkin's lymphoma as well as the ability to subclassify lymphomas accurately into prognostic groups. Of the approximately 30,000 new cases of non-Hodgkin's lymphoma this year, about 50 percent will fall into an unfavorable prognostic group, requiring the prompt initiation of therapy.

Since the 1950s, there has been considerable interest in clinicopathologic correlation in lymphoma, and several different classification schemes have been developed to help separate the aggressive lymphomas from the low-grade or indolent lymphomas. Presently, the International Working Formulation has been accepted as a useful histopathologic classification system of non-Hodgkin's lymphoma, although review of the literature requires knowledge of the modified Rappaport classification system and, to a lesser extent, the Lukes-Collins scheme as well. Table 1 lists the high-grade lymphomas by their Rappaport and Working Formulation classifications. In the latter, diffuse large-cell lymphoma (DLCL) is considered an intermediate-grade lymphoma, whereas it is classified as a high-grade lymphoma under the term of *diffuse histiocytic lymphoma* in the modified Rappaport classification. A review of 1,153 consecutive cases of non-Hodgkin's lymphoma demonstrated DLCL in 20 percent, immunoblastic lymphoma in 9 percent, and lymphoblastic and small non–cleaved cell each representing about 5 percent of the total group.

Staging studies should be aimed at defining extent of disease as well as clinical assessable sites of disease. Data are accumulating to indicate that high-dose radionucleotide gallium scanning is a useful diagnostic tool for identifying active disease in nodal and extranodal sites, including areas not easily assessed by conventional radiographs or computed tomography (CT). Bone marrow biopsy, although not usually positive, should be performed as part of initial staging. Cerebrospinal fluid examination is indicated in the setting of abnormal neurologic complaints or in diffuse undifferentiated or lymphoblastic lymphoma. Lymphomatous involvement of Waldeyer's ring, thyroid, or lacrimal glands should be accompanied by evaluation of the upper gastrointestinal tract because of known association between these two areas. Bipedal lymphangiogram and exploratory laparotomy are almost never required except in unusual circumstances. Finally, because misdiagnosis and misclassification of lymphoid malignancies remain common problems, all pathologic material should be reviewed by an experienced hematopathologist. Repeat biopsy is justified in equivocal situations in which immunoperox-

Table 1 Rappaport and Working Formulation Classifications
of High-Grade Lymphomas

Rappaport Classification	Working Formulation Equivalent
Unfavorable-Prognosis Lymphoma	Intermediate-Grade Lymphoma
Diffuse histiocytic	Diffuse large-cell, Cleaved/non–cleaved cell
	High-Grade Lymphoma
Diffuse undifferentiated	Diffuse large-cell, Immunoblastic, Small non–cleaved cell
Lymphoblastic	Lymphoblastic

idase or flow cytometric studies will serve to clarify the immunophenotypes. The use of molecular biologic studies for immunoglobulin and T-cell receptor B-chain gene rearrangement may occasionally be useful in circumstances in which clonality is uncertain.

CHEMOTHERAPY FOR DIFFUSE LARGE-CELL LYMPHOMA

In DLCL, pathologically confirmed, nonbulky stage I disease may be cured with radiation therapy as a sole modality. Other high-grade lymphomas as well as bulky stage I and higher stage DLCL will require multiagent chemotherapy with or without radiotherapy. Prior to the initiation of therapy, it is important that the patient undergo a complete staging evaluation. High-grade lymphoma tends to disseminate early in its natural history and may present with multiple noncontiguous sites of disease. Trials evaluating most of the effective chemotherapy regimens are reported under the diagnostic heading of diffuse histiocytic lymphoma. Nevertheless, many of the conclusions can be applied to DLCL, immunoblastic lymphoma, and most intermediate-grade lymphomas. The unique biology of lymphoblastic lymphoma usually sets it apart from DLCL. Immunoblastic lymphomas are a new classification and were previously included within the diffuse histiocytic lymphoma category in the Rappaport classification. The treatment of diffuse undifferentiated (small non–cleaved cell) lymphomas is discussed in a later chapter.

In the 1960s, initial studies with the regimens MOPP* and C-MOPP demonstrated that a significant fraction of patients could achieve indefinite long-term disease-free survival. These studies reported long-term survivors in only 30 percent of the total group, with the remaining patients having short-lived complete responses, partial responses, or no response. These studies emphasize that only complete responders achieved significant survival benefit, with incomplete responders generally surviving less than 1 year, which was similar to the nonresponders. The substitution of adriamycin (hydroxy-daunorubicin) for procarbazine in

the C-MOPP regimen generated the CHOP regimen, in which all chemotherapy was given on the first day of a 21- to 28-day cycle and tended to be very well tolerated (Table 2). Complete remission rates with CHOP are approximately 50 percent, with about 80 percent of complete responders achieving long-term remission. An attempt to improve initial complete response and cure of high-grade non-Hodgkin's lymphoma has led to many modifications of the CHOP regimen. Three general themes, each with an experimental basis, have been used. The first was to add additional active agents to the CHOP regimen with the hope that these additional agents would further increase cell kill. Ideally, added agents should have different mechanisms of action, resistance, and toxicity. Because CHOP is associated with moderate myelosuppression, additional agents should ideally not add to myelosuppression. Bleomycin and methotrexate with leucovorin rescue fulfilled the preceding criteria and led to M-CHOP, m-BACOD, CHOP-Bleo, and BACOP regimens. Often bleomycin or methotrexate was added at mid-cycle in an attempt to prevent early tumor regrowth and increase tumor kill per cycle. The initial reports of complete response to CHOP-Bleo and BACOP were approximately 75 percent, with about 50 percent or more achieving long-term survival. Although historical comparisons between these CHOP variants with CHOP alone have suggested a superiority of the former, randomized trials comparing the newer variants to CHOP have only recently been undertaken.

A second approach entailed dose intensification. Intensification can be accomplished by either increasing drug dose or by shortening the time interval between doses. Simple escalation of the doses of cyclophosphamide and adriamycin in CHOP-Bleo demonstrated no benefit when compared to standard CHOP-Bleo. Second-generation CHOP-based regimens, such as M-BACOD and MACOP-B, employed both escalation and frequent dosing intervals. In M-BACOD, essentially standard CHOP-Bleo (dexamethasone instead of prednisone), is given on day 1. On day 14, high-dose methotrexate (3 g per square meter) followed with leucovorin rescue is given. Long-term follow-up data following M-BACOD demonstrated a 72 percent complete response rate, with 50 percent of patients alive and free of disease at 8 years. In an attempt to reduce the

---

*For all abbreviations, see Table 2 for definitions.

Table 2 Commonly Used Chemotherapy Regimens
for Diffuse Large-Cell Lymphoma

CHOP

Cyclophosphamide	750 mg/m^2	Day 1
Doxorubicin	50 mg/m^2	Day 1
Vincristine	1.4 mg/m^2	Day 1 (maximum 2 mg)
Prednisone	50 mg/m^2	Days 1–5

Repeat cycles every 21–28 days, usually six cycles, or two cycles past CR.

m-BACOD

Cyclophosphamide	600 mg/m^2	Day 1
Doxorubicin	45 mg/m^2	Day 1
Vincristine	1 mg/m^2	Day 1
Dexamethasone	6 mg/m^2	Days 1–5
Bleomycin	4 units/m^2	Day 1
Methotrexate	200 mg/m^2	Days 8, 15
Leucovorin rescue	10 mg/m^2	Days 9, 10, 16, 17 four doses each day

Repeat cycles every 21 days.

MACOP-B

Cyclophosphamide	350 mg/m^2	Days 1, 15
Doxorubicin	50 mg/m^2	Days 1, 15
Vincristine	1.4 mg/m^2	Days 8, 22
Methotrexate	400 mg/m^2	Day 8
Leucovorin rescue	15 mg	Days 9, 10–six doses
Bleomycin	10 mg/m^2	Day 22
Prednisone	75 mg	Every day throughout the treatment
Cotrimoxazole	2	Daily

Repeat cycles every 28 days for a total of three cycles.

COP-BLAM III

Cyclophosphamide	350 mg/m^2	Day 1 of cycle A and B
Doxorubicin	35 mg/m^2	Day 1 of cycle A and B
Prednisone	40 mg/m^2	Days 1–5 of cycle A and B
Bleomycin	7.5 mg/m^2	Day 1 of cycle A only (bolus)
Bleomycin	7.5 mg/m^2/day	Days 1–5 of cycle A only (continuous drip)
Vincristine	1 mg/m^2/day	Days 1–2 cycle A (continuous infusion) and day 1 (bolus) only cycle B
Procarbazine	100 mg/m^2	Days 1–5 of cycle A and B

Cycles alternate every 21 days between A and B for a total of 12 cycles.

ProMACE-CYTABOM

Cyclophosphamide	650 mg/m^2	Day 1
Doxorubicin	25 mg/m^2	Day 1
Etoposide	120 mg/m^2	Day 1
Cytarabine	300 mg/m^2	Day 8
Bleomycin	5 units/m^2	Day 8
Vincristine	1.4 mg/m^2	Day 8
Methotrexate	120 mg/m^2	Day 8
Prednisone	60 mg/m^2	Days 1–14
Cotrimazole	2 bid	Days 1–21

Cycles repeated every 21 days for a total of six cycles.

Continued.

toxicity of the M-BACOD regimen, standard-dose methotrexate (200 mg per square meter) replaced high-dose methotrexate, giving the m-BACOD regimen. A historical comparison of m-BACOD with M-BACOD has recently demonstrated that both regimens generate similar survival statistics.

MACOP-B uses most of the same drugs as m-BACOD, except that prednisone replaces dexamethasone. In MACOP-B, treatment is condensed so that 6 months of therapy is completed in 3 months. Scheduling includes cyclophosphamide and doxorubicin given every other week, with rescued methotrexate, vincristine, and bleomycin being given on intervening weeks so that patients receive therapy weekly for 12 weeks. Long-term results reveal a 52 percent complete response (CR) rate, and approximately 50 percent of patients are alive at 3

Table 2 Commonly Used Chemotherapy Regimens
for Diffuse Large-Cell Lymphoma — cont'd

Pro-MACE-MOPP

Cyclophosphamide	650 mg/m²	Days 1, 8
Doxorubicin	25 mg/m²	Days 1, 8
Etoposide	120 mg/m²	Days 1, 8
Methotrexate	1.5 mg/m²	Day 15
Leucovorin	50 mg/m²	Day 16 every 6 hours for five doses
Prednisone	60 mg/m²	Days 1–5

Cycle length is 28 days. Use flexible number of cycles until CR or maximal response, then change to:

Nitrogen mustard	6 mg/m²	Days 1, 8
Vincristine	1.5 mg/m²	Days 1, 8
Procarbazine	100 mg/m²	Days 1–14
Prednisone	60 mg/m²	Days 1–14

Cycle length is 28 days with variable cycle number. Normally, the cycles of MOPP are equal to the cycles of ProMACE.

years, similar to that seen with m/M-BACOD. Toxicity of m/M-BACOD and MACOP-B is significant. Mucositis, pulmonary toxicity, congestive heart failure, and septic deaths may occur with these regimens. In m-BACOD, 35 percent had severe myelosuppression, 18 percent had pulmonary toxicity requiring the discontinuation of bleomycin, and 35 percent had severe mucositis. Toxicity was even more severe in MACOP-B, with a 7 percent toxic death rate, a 75 percent incidence of mucositis, a 42 percent incidence of parasthesias secondary to vincristine, and a 20 percent incidence of serious gastrointestinal bleeding, presumably secondary to 12 weeks of continual steroids. Obviously, increased toxicity seen in these regimens is only warranted if these regimens prove to be superior to CHOP alone. Historical comparison of survival seen with CHOP versus m/M-BACOD or MACOP-B suggests a modest advantage favoring the later regimens, although there is a possibility that patient selection could explain these differences.

The addition of procarbazine to a slightly dose-reduced CHOP-Bleo regimen yielded the program COP-BLAM. Subsequent modifications of COP-BLAM have included the use of continuous-infusion bleomycin and vincristine, leading to COP-BLAM III, which has demonstrated an 84 percent CR rate. Like the other dose-intensive CHOP variants, toxicity has been significant. ProMACE-CYTABOM uses the six drugs found in M-BACOP and adds cytosine arabinoside and etoposide. ProMACE is given on day 1 and CYTABOM on day 8 of each 21-day cycle. Initial reports have demonstrated a high CR rate of 84 percent, with a very respectable 63 percent 3-year, disease-free survival. Like COP-BLAM III and ProMACE-MOPP, toxicity has been a very significant concern.

The third approach involves the use of multidrug protocols given in an induction/consolidation schema. This approach attempts to solve the problem of drug resistance by first treating with a four- or five-drug regimen in an induction phase, followed by a second four- or five-drug regimen using a separate set of lymphoma-active drugs in a consolidation cycle. The number of cycles in the induction/consolidation phases

Table 3 Reported Response Rates and Survival for Treatment Regimens in Non-Hodgkin's Lymphoma

Regimen	Complete Response (%)	Disease-free Survival (%)	
		2 yr	5 yr
CHOP	40–65	35–60	30–55
m–BACOD	61–70	52	47
MACOP–B	50–81	30–65	NA
COP–BLAM III	84	67	NA
ProMACE–CYTABOM	84	63	NA
ProMACE–MOPP	75–80	50–55	NA

Abbreviation: NA = not available.

are flexible and hence have been termed *flexi-therapy*. ProMACE-MOPP is a flexi-therapy that combines prednisone, methotrexate, adriamycin, cyclophosphamide, and etoposide as a five-drug induction regimen. After two or three cycles of ProMACE induction, therapy is changed to standard MOPP, which includes three drugs not found in ProMACE. This regimen resulted in a 96 percent response rate, with a 74 percent CR rate at the National Cancer Institute. Doses of cyclophosphamide are high, and myelosuppression is the major dose-limiting toxicity, with a 10 percent septic death rate. A prospective randomized comparison of ProMACE-MOPP with ProMACE-CYTABOM has demonstrated similar response and survival figures but lower toxicity with the ProMACE-CYTABOM regimen.

Table 3 reviews the overall CR rates and disease-free survival rates of some of the common chemotherapy regimens used in DLCL. Although many of the more recent regimens present very impressive response and survival rates, it is premature to assume that they have demonstrated an advantage over standard CHOP. First, follow-up of patients in the later regimens has been short, with many patients used in analysis followed for less than 2 years. Secondly, most reports using the later regimens have been single-arm institutional studies without concurrent CHOP controls. Indeed, the few randomized studies comparing CHOP to CHOP variants have been performed in cooperative groups and revealed no differences. The newer programs show a rather consistent result of approximately half of the patients surviving disease-free over extended periods.

Single-institution studies tend to include patients who are younger, with better performance status than community-based cooperative group trials. Comparisons must be stratified by known prognostic factors such as age, stage, performance status, and extent or bulk of disease. Until that is done, definitive statements cannot be made concerning the impact of the newer variants compared to CHOP, which remains a widely used "standard" regimen. Clinicians resolved to use CHOP as a standard regimen should be encouraged to use full doses of cyclophosphamide and doxorubicin as originally described.

PROGNOSTIC FACTORS

Analysis of long-term results of a number of regimens according to presenting clinical characteristics has served to define those factors that may predict the overall results of a cohort of patients (Table 4). A recent analysis of a large group of patients treated at the Dana-Farber with m/M-BACOD revealed that performance status, extranodal sites of disease, and largest mass dimensions could accurately define prognostic groups. Patients with excellent performance status, one or less extranodal site of disease, and no mass larger than 10 cm in diameter had a good result, with a CR rate of 88 percent and a 5-year survival of 75 percent. Patients with a poor performance status, numerous extranodal sites, or masses larger than 10 cm in diameter did poorly, with only a 36 percent CR rate and a 17 percent 5-year survival. In addition, serum LDH may contribute further prognostic information. A universally accepted prognos-

tic scheme is needed by which to compare the results of various treatment programs. Patients within the favorable prognostic group have a high cure rate with standard CHOP or CHOP variant. The poor-prognosis group will certainly require newer and more intensive approaches, including perhaps bone marrow or hematopoietic growth factor support to overcome myelosuppression, which is associated with newer dose-intensive regimens.

EVALUATION OF RESPONSE

Restaging studies at 3 months will usually reveal the majority of patients destined to be in complete remission. Patients who respond slowly tend to have less durable remissions despite having subsequent cycles of chemotherapy. Repeat staging studies after three cycles of therapy may provide a useful guideline for the progress of therapy. Residual masses that become gallium-negative may reflect a CR that is occurring prior to complete resolution of necrotic or fibrotic masses.

SECOND-LINE OR SALVAGE THERAPY FOR RELAPSED AND REFRACTORY LARGE-CELL LYMPHOMA

Approximately half of all patients with DLCL will either fail to achieve initial complete remission (primary

Table 4 Prognostic Factors

	Good Prognosis	Poor Prognosis
Clinical Factors		
Clinical stage	1–2	3–4
Performance status	0–1	2–4
B symptoms	No	Yes
Size of largest mass	< 10 cm	> 10 cm
Extranodal disease	0–1 site	> 1 site
CNS lymphoma	No	Yes
Bone marrow lymphoma	No	Yes
Age	< 65	> 65
Serologic Factors		
Lactate dehydrogenase	Normal	Elevated
Beta-2 microglobulin	Normal	Elevated
HIV	Negative	Positive
Pathologic Markers		
Ki-67	< 60% +	> 60% +
Cell phenotype	B cell	T cell
Cytogenetics	3p duplication	2p +, BCL-2
Proliferative index	< 10% S phase	> 20% S phase
Aneuploidy	Absent	Present

Table 5 Salvage Chemotherapy in Non–Hodgkin's Lymphoma

MIME		
Methyl–GAG	500 mg/m^2	Days 1, 14
Ifosfamide	1 g/m^2/d	Days 1–5
Methotrexate	30 mg/m^2	Day 3
Etoposide	100 mg/m^2/d	Days 1–3
DHAP		
Dexamethasone	40 mg/m^2/d	Days 1–4
Cytarabine	2 g/m^2	Day 2 × 2 doses
Cisplatin	100 mg/m^2	Day 1 continuously
Cycles repeated every 21–28 days.		
ESAP		
Etoposide	40 mg/m^2/d	Days 1–4
Solumedrol	500 mg/m^2	Days 1–4
Cytarabine	2 gm/m^2	Day 5
Cisplatin	25 mg/m^2/d	Days 1–4
Cycles repeated every 21 days.		continuously
NOAC		
Mitoxantrone	10 mg/m^2/d	Days 2,3
Cytarabine	3 g/m^2	Day 1 × 2 doses
Cycles repeated every 21–35 days.		
Hydroxyurea–Cytarabine		
Hydroxyurea	500 mg	Day 1 every 6 hr × four doses
Cytarabine	100 mg/m^2/d	Days 1–4 continuously
Hydroxyurea	500 mg	Days 5–28 every 4 hr

refractory) or relapse from complete remission within 36 months of diagnosis. The efficacy of second-line therapy is dependent on several clinical factors, i.e., age, performance status, extent of disease, disease-free interval, and nature of initial therapy. Most salvage regimens that employ newer agents achieve a CR in 20 to 30 percent of patients but are usually followed by a high relapse rate. Less than 20 percent of patients remain continuously free of disease in their second CR. Table 5 lists some of the more commonly used second-line multidrug regimens. The MIME regimen (see Table 5) has demonstrated a 24 percent CR rate with an additional 36 percent of patients achieving a partial response. The median duration of freedom from relapse was 15 months for the complete responders. Initial response and duration of response to front-line therapy were useful prognostic markers in determining the probability of response to MIME. Relapse off therapy was more likely to predict a response to MIME as compared to primary refractory patients. At 2 years of follow-up, a low proportion of patients are alive and free of disease. Further follow-up for MIME and the other salvage regimens is needed. Patients who either fail to achieve a CR with initial therapy or who are in early relapse may benefit from high-dose therapy and bone marrow or peripheral stem cell support.

AGGRESSIVE LYMPHOMA AND THE ACQUIRED IMMUNODEFICIENCY SYNDROME

Non-Hodgkin's lymphoma is increased in many of the congenital immunodeficiency states and, more recently, in the patients with the acquired immunodeficiency syndrome (AIDS). High-grade lymphomas, primary central nervous system lymphoma, and systemic lymphoma with central nervous system involvement are all over-represented in persons seropositive for human immunodeficiency virus (HIV).

Treatment of lymphoma in the HIV patients is still evolving. A large number of CHOP-based regimens have been used therapeutically, and essentially all of these have demonstrated a 30 to 50 percent CR rate, with some patients remaining free of lymphoma for more than 2 years. Almost without exception, the long-term survivors have come from a subgroup of HIV-positive patients with good performance status and no history of opportunistic infection prior to their non-Hodgkin's lymphoma. Treatment does not seem to accelerate their immunologic deterioration. Complete responses can be durable, and indeed, patients achieving a CR are at higher risk of dying from AIDS-related opportunistic infections than recurrent lymphoma. A high fraction of AIDS-related lymphoma presents as central nervous system disease, leading to intensification of CHOP regimens with high-dose methotrexate and cytarabine. The myelosuppressive effect of these dose-intensive regimens is particularly severe in this immunocompromised population. In particular, patients with previous opportunistic infection and low peripheral helper lymphocyte (CD 4+) counts do very poorly, with median survival of only a few months.

LYMPHOBLASTIC LYMPHOMA

Lymphoblastic lymphoma is a high-grade diffuse lymphoma, usually of thymic phenotype. It usually presents in young men as a mediastinal mass and superior vena cava obstruction syndrome. There is a relatively high frequency of bone marrow and central nervous system involvement at diagnosis. A large fraction of patients have the CALLA (common acute lymphocytic leukemia antigen) and TDT (terminal deoxytransferase) molecules on the tumor cell surface. Acute lymphocytic leukemia may present with anterior mediastinal adenopathy and identical immunophenotypes, suggesting that lymphoblastic lymphoma represents a malignancy whose biology is intermediate between non-Hodgkin's lymphoma and acute lymphocytic leukemia. The microscopic appearance of biopsied tissues is indistinguishable from acute lymphocytic leukemia.

The treatment of lymphoblastic lymphoma requires intensive multiagent chemotherapy, including intrathecal methotrexate and central nervous system irradiation as well as consolidation therapy and maintenance therapy, similar to high-risk acute lymphocytic leukemia treatment protocols (Table 6). Patients presenting with localized disease, a normal LDH, and without extranodal or central nervous system disease represent a favorable prognostic group, with the large majority achieving long-term disease-free survival. Those presenting with high LDH central nervous system involvement, or extensive bone marrow or extralymphatic involvement are rarely cured with currently used regimens. Treatment for these poor-prognosis patients is uncertain. Early experience with dose intensive cyclophosphamide combined with high-risk acute lymphocytic leukemia protocols has been promising. The use of bone marrow transplant to consolidate first complete remission in high-risk patients has some optimistic support from Europe.

IMMUNOBLASTIC LYMPHOMA

Immunoblastic lymphoma (or immunoblastic sarcoma) was previously a subset of DLCL in the modified Rappaport classification. It is defined as an independent subgroup of high-grade lymphomas in the Working Formulation. It is relatively uncommon, representing 10 percent or less of the cases of non-Hodgkin's lymphoma. B-cell and thymic cell immunophenotypes have been described. Pathology is complex, with plasmacytoid, clear cell, pleomorphic, epitheloid (Lennert's lymphoma), and Ki1+variants having been described. Despite their histologic complexity, all possess an aggressive clinical behavior.

Patients tend to be older, with a mean age of 60.

Table 6 Treatment Protocols for Lymphoblastic Lymphoma

Stanford Protocol for Lymphoblastic Lymphoma (Low Risk)

Cyclophosphamide	400 mg/m² × 3 d	Weeks 1,4,9,12,15,18
Doxorubicin	50 mg/m²	Weeks 1,4,9,12,15,18
Vincristine	2 mg	Weeks 1–6,9,12,15,18
Prednisone	40 mg/m²	Weeks 1–4, then taper
L–Asparaginase	6,000 U/m² × 5	Week 4
Methotrexate	12 mg IT	Week 3, then × 5 during RT
Whole–brain radiation therapy	2,400 rad (12 fractions)	Weeks 5–7
6–Mercaptopurine	75 mg/m² daily	Weeks 21–52
Methotrexate	30 mg/m² weekly	Weeks 21–52

Stanford Protocol for Lymphoblastic Lymphoma (High Risk)

Cyclophosphamide	400 mg/m² × 3 days	Weeks 1,4,12,18,24
Adriamycin	50 mg/m²	Weeks 1,4,12,18,24
Vincristine	2 mg	Weeks 1–6, 12,13,18,19, 24,25
Prednisone	50 mg/m²	Weeks 1–2, 12–13, 18–19, 24–25
C–Asparaginase	6,000 U/m² MWF	Weeks 1–5, then 12–13, 18–19, 24–25
Methotrexate	12 mg IT	Weeks 1, 4–8
Whole–brain radiation therapy	2,400 rad (× 12 fractions)	Weeks 6–8
Cytarabine	300 mg/m² M W F	Weeks 9,15,21
VM–26	165 mg/m² M W F	Weeks 9,15,21
Methotrexate	200 mg/m²	Weeks 10,16,22
Leucovorin rescue	10 mg/m²	Weeks 10,16,22 × 6 doses
6–Mercaptopurine	75 mg/m² daily	Weeks 27–104
Methotrexate	30 mg/m²	Weeks 27–104
Trimethoprim/ sulfamethoxazole	2 BID daily	Weeks 1–26
Ketoconazole	200 mg daily	Weeks 1–26

M W F = Monday, Wednesday, Friday; IT = Intrathecal

Interestingly, about one-third of patients will have an underlying pre-existing immunologic disorder. Patients with immunoblastic lymphoma may have histories of allergic (chronic urticaria), autoimmune (Sjögren's syndrome, Hashimoto's thyroiditis, celiac sprue), or lymphoproliferative diseases (chronic lymphocytic leukemia, myeloma, angioimmunoblastic lymphadenopathy). Although leukopenia is common at presentation with both the T-cell and B-cell immunoblastic lymphoma, polyclonal hypergammaglobulinemia is commonly seen in only the T-cell variant. Most patients present with advanced-stage disease and unusual sites of presentation (bone, liver, central nervous system) have been reported.

Because of the advanced age of most patients, its relative rarity, and coexisting lymphoproliferative malignancies, the prognosis is poor. There are no large series of patients treated in a similar fashion. In general, this group has responded poorly to multiagent chemo-therapy. Generally, fewer than 50 percent of patients can be expected to achieve CR, with a minority of patients surviving 2 years. In most series, patients with the thymic immunoblastic lymphoma, such as Lennert's lymphoma, will have a poorer outcome than those with the B-cell types.

SUGGESTED READING

DeVita VT, Jaffe E, Mauch P, et al. Lymphocytic lymphomas. In: DeVita VT, Hellman S, Rosenberg SA, eds. Cancer: Principles and practice of oncology. Philadelphia: JB Lippincott, 1989.

Levine AM. Lymphoma in acquired immunodeficiency syndrome. Semin Oncol 1990; 17:104–112.

Levine AM, Taylor CR, Schneider DR, et al. Immunoblastic sarcoma of T-cell versus B-cell origin. I. Clinical features. Blood 1981; 58:52–60.

Picozzi VJ, Coleman CN. Lymphoblastic lymphoma. Semin Oncol 1990; 17:996.

INDOLENT LYMPHOMAS: CHEMOTHERAPY

MICHAEL SPIRITOS, M.D.
PETER A. CASSILETH, M.D.

The non-Hodgkin's lymphomas are an extremely heterogeneous group of neoplasms whose clinical course varies based on the histologic type. Over the past several decades, several pathologic classifications have been proposed that categorize these entities by their morphologic appearance, lymph node architecture, cell of origin, or immunophenotype. Pathologists and clinicians have had difficulty translating the different subtypes from one classification to another. A Working Formulation was therefore developed that allowed such translation and generated three major categories that grouped 10 histologic subtypes by differences in survival. The three groupings are labelled low, intermediate, and high grade, which correlates with their respective favorable, intermediate, or unfavorable prognoses for survival. The low-grade lymphomas comprise three histologic subtypes: small lymphocytic (SL), follicular small cleaved (FSCL), and follicular mixed small and large cell (FML). These correlate with the older Rappaport classification of diffuse lymphocytic well-differentiated (DLWD), nodular lymphocytic poorly differentiated (NLPD), and nodular mixed lymphoma (NML), respectively. This chapter focuses on the chemotherapeutic management of these low-grade or indolent lymphomas. However, it should be noted that early studies often included other histologic subtypes under the heading of favorable lymphomas, including follicular large cell (nodular histiocytic lymphoma) and diffuse small cleaved (diffuse lymphocytic poorly differentiated). These latter subtypes are currently included in the intermediate-grade lymphomas and are not discussed here.

The low-grade lymphomas as a group have a median survival of approximately 7 years. This compares favorably with the median survivorships of the intermediate-and high-grade lymphomas of 2.5 and 1 year, respectively. The plot of relapse-free survival after chemotherapy-induced remission shows other differences between these groups. The relapse curve has an early constant slope in the low-grade lymphomas. The more aggressive subtypes display biphasic curves with a pattern of early relapse (associated with short survival) followed by a plateau and only rare relapses after 3 to 4 years. In low-grade lymphomas, remissions inevitably are followed by relapses, the degree of response to chemotherapy (partial versus complete responses) does not correlate with survival, and cures are rare. In contrast, the intensive treatment of the more aggressive lymphomas leads to durable remissions and cures in a substantial proportion of patients.

INCIDENCE AND NATURAL HISTORY

There are approximately 30,000 cases of non-Hodgkin's lymphoma (NHL) seen in the United States annually. Of the low-grade lymphomas, FSCL is the most common, comprising approximately 20 to 25 percent of all NHL. The FML histologic type comprises 10 percent of all NHL and is twice as frequent as SL. The median age of patients at diagnosis is 50 to 60 years. It is rare for the indolent lymphomas to present within the first two decades of life.

Low-grade lymphomas typically present with progressive, nontender lymph node enlargement, usually slowly increasing in size over months to years, at times achieving significant bulk. Some patients exhibit waxing and waning lymph node size. As will be discussed later, more than 75 percent of patients present with disseminated disease, either stage III or IV. Bone marrow and liver are the most commonly involved extralymphatic sites.

An important biologic feature of the indolent lymphomas is their tendency to become clinically more aggressive with time. This can occur without a change in histologic pattern, but in approximately one-third of patients, it is associated with histologic transformation to intermediate- or high-grade subtypes. Clinical and histologic transformation are marked by decreased responsiveness to chemotherapy, and a median survival from the time of transformation less than 1 year.

DIAGNOSIS

Although subtypes of NHL are classified on the basis of morphologic criteria alone, further characterization of the indolent lymphomas by surface marker, molecular, or chromosomal analysis is frequently performed. The malignant cells are almost invariably found to be of B-cell origin. Southern analysis with probes for the immunoglobulin genes demonstrate uniform rearrangements consistent with a monoclonal B-cell population. Chromosomal analysis of the follicular lymphomas reveals the presence of the t(14;18) translocation in more than 75 percent of patients.

Staging of the low-grade lymphomas is usually based on clinical evaluation, without resorting to laparotomy, utilizing the Ann Arbor classification devised for Hodgkin's disease. At presentation, more than 50 percent of patients demonstrate advanced stages of disease (III or IV). Of patients with clinical stage I or II who are subjected to staging laparotomy, 40 to 50 percent are found to have disease below the diaphragm. Among the three histologic subtypes of indolent lymphoma, bone marrow involvement is most common in SL and least common in FML, occurring in 70 percent and 30 percent of patients, respectively. Conversely, apparently localized disease occurs more frequently in FML, less often in FSCL, and rarely in SL. Despite the frequent finding of advanced stage at presentation, the indolent lymphomas are associated with long survival.

The extensive involvement at diagnosis appears to reflect the capacity of the small malignant lymphocytes to circulate and readily populate a wide variety of organs.

EARLY STAGE DISEASE

Although this discussion focuses on the chemotherapeutic management of the low-grade lymphomas, it is important to note that primary radiation therapy may be the treatment of choice for stages I and II. Truly limited stage indolent lymphoma occurs very infrequently. Local radiation therapy in doses of 3,500 to 4,000 cGy causes complete remissions in virtually all such patients. With this approach, 5-year disease-free survivals range from 40 to 83 percent, and overall survival is 69 to 100 percent. In two studies with median follow-up greater than 5 years, late relapses are rare and survival curves flatten, suggesting curability of limited disease after local radiation therapy. Extended-field ports do not provide better survival than generous involved field radiation. Younger patients with stage I disease fare better than older patients or patients with stage II disease. Few studies of the combination of chemotherapy and local radiation in limited-stage indolent lymphoma have been conducted. A few nonrandomized studies claim improved disease-free survival when systemic therapy is added to local radiation therapy but no improvement in overall survival.

ADVANCED-STAGE DISEASE

For patients with stages III and IV, and most of the patients presenting with clinical stage II (representing 85 to 90 percent of the indolent lymphomas), chemotherapy is the treatment of choice. Treatment regimens range from single alkylating agents to aggressive adriamycin-containing combination chemotherapy. An analysis of the literature does not define a clear chemotherapy program of choice for these patients; rather, one selects an optimal individual approach based upon clinical presentation and patient characteristics.

Single-agent alkylator chemotherapy is effective for indolent lymphomas with minimal toxicity; therefore, it should be considered the standard against which newer approaches are evaluated. Table 1 summarizes the results of studies of single-agent therapy. The overall complete remission (CR) rate is 52 percent. Median survival varies from 20 months to more than 5 years and does not correlate with the frequency of CR induction. The variability in long-term outcome in different studies is due to variations in patient population. Patients with FSCL survive longer than patients with FML, and patients with asymptomatic disease live longer than symptomatic patients. Outcome will necessarily vary depending on the distribution of these, and other, characteristics. Because patients with indolent lymphomas have long survival, lengthy follow-up is required to assess outcome accurately. This is especially problematic if one wishes to demonstrate improvement in the tail of the survival curve, when it may be possible to demonstrate a plateau (potential cures).

Most of the studies of single-agent therapy used relatively modest doses, usually as a daily oral dose. The two studies at the bottom of Table 1 employed intermittent high-dose therapy (chlorambucil, 80 mg per square meter over 5 days orally, and cyclophosphamide, 2.5 to 5.0 g per square meter over 5 days intravenously). A number of patients in these two trials had poor prognostic features, contributing to the low CR rates. Nevertheless, single-agent alkylator therapy by intermittent high doses does not appear to have an advantage over modest daily oral doses. At the same time, one has to consider that the risks of alkylating agent-induced secondary acute leukemia may be lower after pulse therapy than after long-term chronic administration.

Detailed analysis of other single-agent alkylator

Table 1 Results of Therapy with Single Agents

Drug	No. of Patients	CR Rate (%)	Survival (years)	Study
CYT or CHL	38	40	50% at 2½‡	Stanford
CYT	13	47	50% at 2½	Minnesota
BCNU ± Pred vs CYT ± Pred*	97	47	83% at 2	Eastern Cooperative Oncology Group
CHL	60	68	—	St. Bart's
CHL	67	65	50% at 3¾	Capetown
CYT or CHL	17	64	60% at 4	Stanford
CYT or CHL	20	55	90% at 2½	Stanford
CHL†	33	33	60% at 5	Yale
CYT + MED†	22	27	50% at 1¼	St. Bart's
Weighted Mean		52		

Abbreviations: CYT = cyclophosphamide; CHL = chlorambucil; MED = methylprednisolone, PRED = prednisone.
*Followed by randomization in CR to maintenance CHL or BCNU, CYT, PRED, and vincristine.
†High-dose pulse therapy.
‡Median survival for patients with FSCL; median survival was 20 months for patients with FML.

therapy studies leads to the following conclusions: CRs are achieved in more than one-half of treated patients; maximal benefit from low-dose therapy may require 9 to 12 months (or more) of treatment; and therapy is well tolerated with a minimum of side effects. After partial remission (PR) or CR is achieved and therapy is discontinued, one observes a pattern of continuous relapse. Finally, the response to therapy does not correlate with survival; patients in PR have the same survival as patients in CR.

In an attempt to improve on these results, combination chemotherapy has been extensively evaluated in the management of the indolent lymphomas. Results from nonrandomized studies, using cyclophosphamide, vincristine, and prednisone (CVP), are listed in Table 2. The addition of vincristine and prednisone to the alkylating agent, cyclophosphamide, in these regimens yields CR rates (in the range of 60 to 80 percent) higher than those obtained with single-agent chemotherapy. Several randomized as well as nonrandomized trials comparing a CVP-type of regimen with single-agent alkylator therapy have been performed (Table 3). These studies fail to demonstrate a survival difference between CVP and single-agent therapy despite a higher CR rate and shorter time to CR with CVP therapy. Given the small number of patients in these studies, a modest but

meaningful difference in survival could have been missed.

Attempts to improve response rates by means of chemotherapy combinations more intensive than CVP have generally been unsuccessful and have added toxicity. Unfortunately, few studies have been randomized. Table 4 lists the response rates to these regimens. The most common combinations employ CVP in conjunction with BCNU (BCVP), adriamycin (CHOP), or procarbazine (COPP). The Eastern Cooperative Oncology Group study, randomizing patients to receive CP, COPP, or BCVP, found equivalent pathologically documented complete response rates of 54 percent, 56 percent, and 53 percent, respectively. Overall survival at 5 years was similar among all three groups, but progression-free survival was significantly better for the COPP regimen. Both BCVP and COPP were more toxic than CP and entailed significantly greater leukopenia and nausea and vomiting. The same study included 52 patients with FML. In these patients, CP, COPP, and BCVP produced similar CR rates and no significant differences in disease-free or overall survival.

Although adriamycin is an important component in the successful treatment of high-grade lymphomas, its value in the low-grade lymphomas is unclear because it has not been adequately evaluated in randomized trials. In a retrospective review of follicular lymphomas, including some patients with follicular large-cell lymphoma who were treated at M.D. Anderson on several combination-chemotherapy protocols over an 11-year period, a logistic regression model suggested that adriamycin-containing regimens were associated with significantly better CR and overall survival. However,

Table 2 Results of CVP Combination Chemotherapy

No. of Patients	CR Rate (%)	Survival (years)
30	40	96% at 2
23	83	65% at 5
41	61	50% at 2½
31	50	73% at 2
37	54	60% at 5
Weighted Mean	57	

Abbreviation: CVP = cyclophosphamide, vincristine, and prednisone.

Table 3 Results of Comparative Chemotherapy Trials

Therapy	N	CR Rate (%)	Survival (years)
CHL		68	
vs	104	(P = <0.01)	50% at 9
CVP		89	
C-V-P		47	50% at 2
vs	29	(NS)	
CVP		82	50% at 3
CHL		13	
vs	66	(NS)	72% at 2½
CVP		37	
CHL		64	
vs	34	(NS)	
CVP		88	
Weighted Mean		73	

Abbreviations: C-V-P = sequential administration of each drug singly after progression; NS = not significant; CHL = chlorambucil; vs = randomized study.

Table 4 Results of Intensive Chemotherapy Programs

Therapy	No. of Patients	CR Rate (%)	Survival (years)
COP*P	34	50	—
COP*P	13	16	—
COP*P		56	70% at 5
vs			
CP	128*	54	63% at 5
vs			
BCVP		53	58% at 5
COP*P		61	
vs			
CP	52†	65	
vs			
BCVP		50	
BCVP	42	42	
CHOP-B*	16	62	72% at 2
B*ACOP	11	82	
COPA		70	54% at 3
vs	41		
CVP		65	69% at 5
BCVP Mlp	35	88	90% at 5

Abbreviations: C = cyclophosphamide, O = vincristine, P = prednisone, P* = procarbazine, B = BCNU, H or A = adriamycin, B* = bleomycin, Mlp = melphalan.
*Patients with FSCL in Eastern Cooperative Oncology Group study.
†Patients with FML in Eastern Cooperative Oncology Group study.

another partially randomized study from Paris comparing patients with FSCL treated with CVP, with or without adriamycin, demonstrated no difference in response rates or survival. Other trials of aggressive regimens adding bleomycin to adriamycin and CVP have, in small numbers of patients with indolent lymphomas, demonstrated that CR rates are in the range of 60 to 80 percent. However, a pattern of continuous relapse is still noted, and toxicity is significantly greater than that seen with either CVP or single-agent therapy.

Increasing the intensity of chemotherapy by use of higher doses of individual agents used in combination does speed the time to response and may even prolong the time to relapse. Peculiarly, however, and unlike most other cancers, these responses to treatment of patients with indolent lymphomas do not translate into increased survival. After CR, relapses still occur, indicating persistence of the malignant clone of lymphocytes. Biologically, survival is determined by the ultimate transformation of these lymphomas into clinically aggressive disease. Except perhaps for the FML subtype, which is discussed later, chemotherapy is, by definition, palliative.

Radiotherapy, either total body or total nodal, is effective in the management of advanced-stage indolent lymphomas. Nonrandomized trials report CR rates of 80 to 100 percent. Most of these studies did not require rebiopsy of involved visceral sites to document CR, as is done in chemotherapy trials. This may contribute to the high CR rate noted in radiation therapy trials. Four randomized trials comparing radiotherapy to chemotherapy are listed in Table 5. Response rates and survival are equivalent with the two modalities in these small trials. It should be noted that upon failure, patients who receive initial total-body radiotherapy are often poorly

tolerant of subsequent chemotherapy because of impaired marrow reserve.

In patients treated initially with chemotherapy, failures tend to occur in sites of previously documented disease, suggesting that it is more effective in controlling microscopic than bulk disease. Relapse after TNI (total nodal irradiation) usually occurs outside the treatment portals, indicating that local treatment fails to control the disease systemically. The value of combined-modality therapy was evaluated at Stanford, randomizing patients to receive either chronic oral single-agent alkylator therapy, CVP for 2 years beyond CR, or CVP before and after TNI in a "sandwich" fashion. Response rates and 30-month survival data were equivalent, with a pattern of continuous late relapse demonstrable for all groups. Combined-modality therapy does not appear to be better than chemotherapy alone.

OBSERVATION

In the 1970s, Rosenberg at Stanford began to follow a number of asymptomatic or minimally symptomatic patients with newly diagnosed advanced indolent lymphoma without any initial therapy. Patients received involved-field radiotherapy as needed for locally progressive disease. The institution of chemotherapy was reserved until the patient developed constitutional symptoms or the disease showed rapid progression, threatened a vital organ, or extended beyond a reasonably encompassing radiation therapy port. Patients who were selected for observation gave a history of slowly progressive lymph node enlargement associated with either advanced patient age or concurrent medical problems that could complicate chemotherapy. In their initial report of 44 patients with stage III or IV indolent lymphoma, most eventually required systemic therapy, although the median time to treatment was 37 months. When survival of this group of treatment-deferred patients was compared to 112 patients treated on protocols during the same years, the overall 4-year survivals (77 percent versus 83 percent, respectively) were similar. The Stanford group later reported on a total of 83 patients whose treatment was deferred. Median follow-up of these patients was 50 months. Spontaneous regressions of disease occurred in 23 percent of patients after a median 8 months observation, and one-third of these were clinical CRs. Therapy was required in 61 percent of the entire group at a median of 3 years of observation. Median time to initiation of treatment was longer for SL (6 years) and FSCL (4 years) than for FML (16 months). The overall actuarial median survival was 11 years, but it was significantly greater for patients with FSCL than for FML. The incidence of histologic transformation in these patients was similar to a group of comparable patients receiving chemotherapy on protocol during the same period.

In an attempt to confirm Stanford's results, the National Cancer Institute conducted a randomized trial of 84 patients comparing initial observation to an

Table 5 Randomized Trials of Chemotherapy Versus Radiation Therapy

Treatment	No. of Patients	CR Rate (%)	Survival (years)
CHL		65	50% at 4½
vs	67		
TBI		53	50% at 4½
CYT or CHL		64	60% at 4
vs			
CVP	51	88	90% at 4
vs			
TBI		71	90% at 4
CVP		67	
vs	44		—
TBI		75	
CVP (FSCL)		62	
or			50% at >5
COPP (FML)	75		
vs			
TNI or TBI		85	50% at >5

Abbreviatons: CHL = chlorambucil; TBI = total-body irradiation; CYT = cyclophosphamide; CVP = cyclophosphamide, vincristine and prednisone; COPP = cyclophosphamide, vincristine, procarbazine, and prednisone; TNI = total nodal irradiation.

aggressive combined-modality approach consisting of Pro-MACE/MOPP (prednisone, methotrexate, doxorubicin, cyclophosphamide, etoposide/nitrogen mustard, vincristine, procarbazine, prednisone) chemotherapy and 2,400 cGy of total nodal radiation. The patients randomized to initial observation were treated palliatively, when feasible, with involved-field radiotherapy to control local disease manifestations. When these patients later experienced symptomatic or rapidly progressive disease, they were then treated with the same combined-modality program. Of the 41 patients observed without therapy, 16 required local radiotherapy and 18 crossed over to systemic treatment at a median of 34 months. Approximately one-half of the patients have received no therapy at a median 2 years of follow-up. The CR rate was 78 percent for patients randomized to initial treatment, and the median duration of CR is more than 45 months. In contrast, the CR rate was only 43 percent for those 18 patients on observation initially who later received therapy. Nevertheless, with short follow-up, overall survival is similar in the two treatment arms — 83 percent at 5 years. An update of this trial with extended survival data is needed to determine whether early, aggressive therapy alters the long-term outcome in the indolent lymphomas. Because of the small number of patients in each arm, survival differences between them will have to be substantial to be significantly different. As expected, the combined-modality regimen was toxic, and, to date, four patients (10 percent) developed other malignancies. The incidence of secondary cancer in the treated patients versus the potential for improved survival is an important consideration in choosing to treat with combined-modality therapy.

The preceding discussion of the low-grade lymphomas has considered the three subtypes SL, FSCL, and FML to be equivalent, based upon their similar natural histories. Because FSCL constitutes 60 to 70 percent of the indolent lymphomas, and few studies evaluate more than 100 patients, it is difficult to document significant biologic differences between subtypes, although they undoubtedly exist.

IS FML CURABLE?

The National Cancer Institute, in a 1977 review of 80 patients with FSCL and FML treated with either CVP or COPP combination chemotherapy, noted better survival rate in patients with FML than in those with FSCL. Of 24 FML patients treated with COPP, the CR rate was 77 percent and only 4 of 18 CRs relapsed at a median follow-up of 3 years. The survival curve had a plateau that suggested possible cures. In contrast, in 49 patients with FSCL, nearly all of whom were treated with CVP, the survival curve demonstrated the typical pattern of continuous late relapse. In a later report of these patients with median follow-up of 7 years, the expected 5-year disease-free survival in NML is 57 percent with a median CR duration of greater than 7 years. Although late relapses were seen, the survival curve still demon-strates a plateau and is significantly better than that for FSCL patients treated with CVP. In two other studies of single-agent chemotherapy, FML was noted to have significantly longer CR duration than FSCL. As noted earlier, a randomized study (see Table 4) by the Eastern Cooperative Oncology Group, failed to show any differences in disease-free or overall survival between combinations of varying intensity in either FML or FSCL. Moreover, in a retrospective review of four Eastern Cooperative Oncology Group trials involving the treatment of 80 patients with FML, the 2-year survival was found to be inferior to patients with FSCL. However, it should be noted that in FSCL, the 2-year survival for patients achieving CR (88 percent), did not differ from patients achieving PR (83 percent). In contrast, in FML, the 2-year survival was 85 percent for patients achieving CR versus 33 percent for patients achieving PR. Whether FML is curable by chemotherapy remains controversial.

EXPERIMENTAL APPROACHES

In addition to the wide range of effective chemotherapeutic drugs in the indolent lymphomas, the activity of a number of biologic response modifiers has been demonstrated. Recombinant alpha-interferon has been given in a variety of doses and schedules, as shown in Table 6. Response rates are approximately 40 percent, but only 10 percent are complete. The median response duration is usually brief — 6 to 12 months. Response to recombinant alpha-interferon does not correlate with histology, stage, symptoms, bulk of disease, or prior therapy. Although the optimal dose and schedule of interferon are unknown, it appears that lower doses are as effective as higher, more toxic, doses. Trials of chemotherapy combined with alpha-interferon are ongoing. At present, the use of interferon remains experimental.

Monoclonal antibodies are another potential treatment for the low-grade lymphomas. Anti-idiotype antibodies have been custom-made for patients and infused in doses ranging from 400 to 15,500 mg. Only a small number of patients have been treated to date; responses approximate 50 percent, but CR is rare. In a murine model, the combination of alpha-interferon and monoclonal antibodies was synergistic because interferon seemed to counter the emergence of idiotype-negative clones that appear when antibodies are used alone. Investigators at Stanford used this combination in 11

Table 6 Results of Alpha-Interferon Trials

Dose	No. of Patients	CR (%)	PR (%)
3–198 × 10⁶ U q3d	5	0	20
9–86 × 10⁶ U biw	6	0	33
3–50 × 10⁶ U daily	17	12	24
50 × 10⁶ U tiw	24	16	38
12 × 10⁶ U tiw	16	6	38
Weighted Mean		10	33

patients and achieved 2 CRs and 7 PRs. The median duration of response was 7 months (range of 2 to >24 months). There was no difference in the emergence of idiotype-negative clones when compared to patients treated with antibodies alone.

High-dose chemoradiotherapy with bone marrow rescue has an established role as curative salvage therapy in the management of the intermediate- and high-grade NHLs. To date, these trials have included very few patients with indolent histologies to allow comment on its role in the relapsed or refractory setting. Because of favorable early data from the National Cancer Institute's aggressive ProMACE-MOPP/TNI regimen, some centers are evaluating bone marrow transplantation in previously untreated patients with indolent lymphomas.

Acknowledgment. The authors thank Ms. Helene Heintzelman for her skilled preparation of this manuscript.

SUGGESTED READING

Gallagher CJ, Gregory WM, Jones AE, et al. Follicular lymphoma: Prognostic factors for response and survival. J Clin Oncol 1986; 4:1,470–1,480.

Glick JH, Barnes JM, Ezdinli EZ, et al. Nodular mixed lymphoma: Results of a randomized trial failing to confirm prolonged disease-free survival with COPP chemotherapy. Blood 1981; 58:920–925.

Horning SJ, Rosenberg SA. The natural history of initially untreated low-grade non-Hodgkin's lymphomas. N Engl J Med 1984; 311: 1,471–1,475.

Portlock CS. Management of the low-grade non-Hodgkin's lymphomas. Semin Oncol 1990; 17:51–59.

Rosenberg SA, et al. The Non-Hodgkin's Lymphoma Pathologic Classification Project: National Cancer Institute sponsored study of classifications of non-Hodgkin's lymphomas: Summary and description of a working formulation for clinical usage. Cancer 1982; 49:2,112–2,135.

Young RC, Longo DL, Glatstein E, et al. The treatment of indolent lymphomas: Watchful waiting versus aggressive combined modality treatment. Semin Oncol 1988; 25:11–16.

Young RC, Johnson RE, Canellos GP, et al. Advanced lymphocytic lymphoma: Randomized comparisons of chemotherapy and radiotherapy, alone or in combination. Cancer Treat Rep 1977; 61: 1,153–1,159.

SMALL, NONCLEAVED CELL LYMPHOMAS

VINAY JAIN, M.B., B.S.
IAN MAGRATH, M.B. B.S., F.R.C.P., F.R.C. Path.

The small, noncleaved cell lymphomas are rapidly growing tumors of the B-cell lineage of the lymphoid system. Histologically, they consist of a uniform population of cells that have a high nuclear-to-cytoplasmic ratio, round or oval noncleaved nuclei containing two to five nucleoli, and very basic cytoplasm. In the Rappaport system, these lymphomas fall under the rubric of "undifferentiated" lymphomas and are divided into Burkitt's and non-Burkitt's subtypes according to rather ill-defined histomorphologic criteria: The Burkitt's subtype is composed of more uniform cells, and contains fewer cells with a single large nucleolus than the non-Burkitt's subtype. The small, noncleaved cell lymphomas are found predominantly in children and constitute 30 to 50 percent of all childhood lymphomas in Europe and the United States. In the course of the last decade, however, the incidence of this variety of high-grade lymphoma has dramatically increased in young, adult men owing to the current acquired immunodeficiency syndrome (AIDS) pandemic.

CLINICAL FEATURES

In Africa, where the tumor was first described, the maxilla and mandible are the most common sites of involvement, jaw tumors being present in almost 70 percent of all patients. In the United States and Europe, the abdomen is the most common site of involvement, abdominal tumors being present in approximately 90 percent of patients at the time of presentation. The presenting features include abdominal swelling, pain, a change in bowel habits, vomiting, or gastrointestinal bleeding. Other sites frequently involved include the bone marrow, central nervous system, breast, testis, ovary, bone, and lymph nodes. Pleural effusion and ascites are not infrequently seen, and tumor deposits have been described, on occasion, in almost all organs and tissues of the body.

INITIAL WORK-UP

Once a patient with a diagnosis of small, noncleaved cell lymphoma has been identified, it is of the utmost importance to complete the staging work-up within the

Table 1 Investigations Required for Staging a Patient with Small, Noncleaved Cell Lymphoma

Essential Studies
  Complete blood count
  Chemistry
    Serum electrolytes
    Blood urea nitrogen and creatinine
    Liver enzymes
    Serum LDH
    Serum uric acid
  Bone marrow biopsy and aspirate
  CSF examination (cytocentrifuge)
  Imaging studies
    Chest radiograph
    Abdominal computed tomography
    Gallium-67 scan

Optional studies
  Bone scan
  Chest computed tomography
  Abdominal ultrasound (liver, spleen, kidneys, pelvis)*

Research studies
  Serum, interleukin-2 receptor
  Magnetic resonance imaging scan (for bone marrow involvement)

*This may be the study of choice in children with little intra-abdominal fat. It can be useful in distinguishing between bowel and tumor, which is not always possible on computed tomography scan.

next 24 to 48 hours. The tumor has a rapid doubling time (the theoretical doubling time is as short as 24 hours), and delay in therapy permits the tumor to grow, thus increasing the immediate risk of complications and diminishing the chances of a successful outcome. The investigations required for staging are listed in Table 1.

STAGING

Staging systems are based on the extent and resectability of the tumor at presentation and take into account the adverse prognosis of patients with bone marrow and central nervous system involvement. The two most commonly used staging systems are given in Table 2. Serum lactic dehydrogenase (LDH) correlates well with tumor bulk, and a serum LDH greater than 350 is taken as a sign of extensive disease.

MANAGEMENT

Combination chemotherapy is the primary treatment modality for all stages of small, noncleaved cell lymphoma. Steady progress has been achieved, over the past 30 years, in increasing the curability of this

Table 2 Staging Systems for Small, Noncleaved Cell Lymphoma

Staging System	Stage	Definition
St. Jude	I	Single tumor (extranodal)
		Single anatomic area (nodal), excluding mediastinum or abdomen
	II	Single tumor (extranodal) with regional lymph node involvement
		Primary gastrointestinal tumor completely resected
		On same side of diaphragm: Two or more nodal areas Two single tumors (extranodal)
	III	On both sides of the diaphragm: Two single tumors (extranodal) Two or more nodal areas
		All primary intrathoracic tumors
		All extensive primary intra-abdominal disease
		All primary epidural or paraspinal tumors
	IV	Any of the above with initial CNS or bone marrow involvement ($<25\%$)
National Cancer Institute*	I	Single extra-abdominal tumor
	IR	Resected ($<90\%$) intra-abdominal tumor
	II	Multiple extra-abdominal sites, excluding bone marrow and CNS
	IIIA	Unresected intra-abdominal tumor
	IIIB	Intra- and extra-abdominal tumor except bone marrow
	IVA	Bone marrow involvement without abdominal or CNS tumor
	IVB	Bone marrow and abdominal tumor or CNS disease

*Adapted from Magrath IT. Small, noncleaved cell lymphomas. In: Magrath IT, ed. The non-Hodgkin's lymphomas. London: Edward Arnold, 1989:256–275.

otherwise rapidly fatal malignancy. Almost all patients with limited-stage disease can expect to be cured, and a majority of patients with advanced disease, including those with involvement of the bone marrow and central nervous system (CNS), are being cured with current regimens. Surgery has a limited, but defined, role, primarily in lymphomas presenting as an abdominal mass. In such patients, surgery is necessary to establish histology and may be used to debulk the tumor and prevent or treat complications (e.g., gastrointestinal bleeding). Radiation therapy is rarely necessary in the small, noncleaved cell lymphomas. Radiation to bulk disease has not been shown to improve curability compared to chemotherapy alone. It may, however, reduce the tolerance of the bone marrow to chemotherapy, thus precluding the delivery of the desired doses of drugs, and introduce additional toxicity. In patients with testicular involvement, in which penetration of drug to all parts of the tumor may be suboptimal, local radiation therapy may be of benefit, in combination with systemic chemotherapy.

Complications from Tumor Masses

In spite of the urgency of initiating therapy, it may be necessary to deal with complications resulting from tumor masses before any therapy is given. Patients with a high tumor burden may have associated metabolic abnormalities that, if uncorrected before chemotherapy, may lead to fatal electrolyte disturbances. Other patients may present with life-threatening complications owing to the location and bulk of the tumor (Table 3), which require urgent intervention.

Mediastinal (uncommon in the small, noncleaved cell lymphomas) or pharyngeal masses can lead to *superior vena caval compression* and *airway obstruction*. Tracheotomy may be needed if symptomatic airway obstruction is present, but emergency radiation therapy, although traditionally used in this situation, should be withheld in most patients because it does not improve

Table 3 Small, Noncleaved Cell Lymphoma Presentations Requiring Emergency Intervention

Intrathoracic masses
  Airway obstruction
  Superior vena caval obstruction
  Cardiac tamponade
  Cardiac arrhythmias

Intra-abdominal masses
  Gastrointestinal bleeding
  Bowel obstruction
  Renal obstruction
  Inferior vena cava obstruction

Intracranial masses
  Increased intracranial tension

Epidural masses
  Paraplegia

the long-term outcome and increases the risk of pulmonary and cardiac toxicity. Its use should be reserved for patients who have not had any symptomatic improvement within a few days of starting chemotherapy. It is worth noting that, in patients in whom minimal response to chemotherapy is observed (a rare situation), radiotherapy can be, at best, palliative. In almost all patients, the immediate initiation of appropriate chemotherapy leads to a rapid diminution of tumor size with corresponding improvement in symptoms.

Surgical intervention should be considered in patients presenting with *gastrointestinal bleeding*, both for control of bleeding as well as for tumor debulking and establishment of histology. *Ureteric obstruction*, on the other hand, can best be managed by hemodialysis (to normalize serum electrolytes, uric acid, urea, and creatinine) followed by appropriate chemotherapy. Placement of ureteral stents and nephrostomy tubes is not normally recommended because it may lead to perforation or leakage, thus increasing the risk of infection and delaying chemotherapy. Such an approach may be appropriate, however, in the absence of facilities for hemodialysis.

Intra-abdominal *venous obstruction* may occur as a result of extrinsic venous compression by the tumor, with or without an associated intraluminal thrombus. Anticoagulation in this situation may be hazardous owing to the increased risk of gastrointestinal bleeding, particularly if thrombocytopenia occurs after chemotherapy. An inferior vena cava filter should be considered in such patients to prevent pulmonary embolization.

Cardiac tamponade from large malignant pericardial effusions may lead to severe hemodynamic compromise. This should be managed by pericardiocentesis and the placement of a pericardial catheter, along with institution of specific chemotherapy. Surgery with construction of a pericardial window is not generally necessary, because of the exquisite chemosensitivity of the tumor.

Correction of Metabolic Abnormalities

The high growth fraction and rapid doubling time of the small, noncleaved cell lymphomas lead to accumulation of cellular breakdown products in the circulation.

Prior to therapy, this is manifested as hyperuricemia, which may be sufficiently severe that there is associated oliguric renal failure. Institution of chemotherapy in this setting can lead to a sudden and potentially lethal increase in serum potassium, because potassium released from tumor cells cannot be excreted efficiently in the absence of an adequate urine flow. The situation is compounded by an increase in the urinary burden of oxypurines and phosphates, consequent upon rapid tumor lysis, with deposition of these compounds in the renal tubules and consequent worsening of renal function and hyperkalemia. Therefore, it is imperative to correct the underlying metabolic abnormalities as rapidly as possible and to ensure that the kidney is capable of excreting high fluid volumes before initiating tumor-specific chemotherapy.

Aggressive alkaline diuresis and high doses of allopurinol (10 mg per kilogram) should be started promptly. Allopurinol inhibits xanthine oxidase and causes part of the uric acid to be excreted as xanthine and hypoxanthine. In this way, a higher total purine load can be excreted by the kidney without exceeding the dissolving capacity of urine for any particular purine metabolite. A high urine outflow (up to 250 cc per square meter per hour) is needed to permit the excretion of the high solute burden caused by lysis of malignant cells, which will occur once chemotherapy is commenced. Some patients may not be able to excrete all the fluids administered to them before and during chemotherapy, particularly in the presence of renal deposits of uric acid that persist from previous hyperuricemia, or of "third spacing," caused by the presence of pleural or peritoneal tumor infiltration with effusions or venous obstruction. In this situation, vigorous hydration should be accompanied by the administration of diuretics and monitoring of either central venous or, preferably, pulmonary capillary wedge pressure. If patients are unable to maintain an adequate urine flow despite fluids and diuretics or have acute renal failure or ureteral obstruction (not uncommon in the presence of large intra-abdominal mass), hemodialysis should be instituted promptly. Because of the need for intensive physiologic and biochemical monitoring, patients with extensive disease are best managed in an intensive care unit during the initial period of chemotherapy.

Bicarbonate is used in fluids administered before chemotherapy because the solubility of most purine metabolites is much higher at an alkaline pH. Once chemotherapy is started, bicarbonate should not be given, as it lowers the solubility of phosphates and may cause their precipitation in renal tubules. Bicarbonate can also increase the likelihood of tetany in the hypocalcemic patient (hypocalcemia accompanies hyperphosphatemia), but use of intravenous calcium infusions should be avoided, except in life-threatening situations, because of the risk of calcium deposition in soft tissues. Symptomatic hypocalcemia in the presence of hyperphosphatemia is best managed by hemodialysis.

Chemotherapy

Combination chemotherapy regimens can cure a majority of patients with small, noncleaved cell lymphoma. Most current regimens consist of intensive doses of alkylating agents (cyclophosphamide, sometimes alternating with ifosfamide) given in combination with other agents active in lymphomas (especially methotrexate, vincristine, anthracyclines, epipodophyllotoxins, and cytarabine). Sequential treatment cycles are given as soon as recovery of granulocyte counts occurs, to maximize dose intensity and minimize the duration of therapy.

Intrathecal prophylaxis with methotrexate, with or without cytarabine, is usually given to all patients, although patients with very limited disease or completely resected intra-abdominal tumor rarely have CNS recurrence. Systemic high-dose methotrexate or cytarabine can also achieve effective drug levels in the cerebrospinal fluid and may decrease the chances of a CNS relapse. Radiation is not recommended for routine CNS prophylaxis.

Individual Regimens

High-dose cyclophosphamide, in combination with intermediate- or high-dose methotrexate, remains the mainstay of most regimens. The COMP protocol, designed by the Children's Cancer Group (Fig. 1), consists of a high dose of cyclophosphamide (1.2 g per square meter at induction, 1 g per square meter for subsequent cycles) in combination with intermediate-dose methotrexate (300 mg per square meter), weekly vincristine (1.4 mg per square meter), and daily prednisone. Intrathecal methotrexate is used for CNS prophylaxis. Radiation is given to sites of bulk disease, although, as discussed previously, there is no evidence that radiation improves the outcome, although it may reduce the delivered dose intensity. The National Cancer Institute (NCI) 77-04 protocol (Fig. 2) differs from COMP primarily in the addition of adriamycin (40 mg per square meter) and use of a higher dose of methotrexate (2,760 mg per square meter, infused intravenously over 42 hours) followed by leucovorin rescue. Both intrathecal cytarabine and methotrexate are given for CNS prophylaxis. Both these protocols require 15 to 18 months to be completed (although only six cycles of protocol 7704 are given for patients with limited disease). A modified version of NCI 77-04 (protocol 85-C-67) includes a total of only six cycles for all patients.

The "total therapy B" protocol from St. Jude's Children's Hospital can be completed in 5 to 6 months (Fig. 3). It consists of a higher dose of cyclophosphamide (1.8 g per square meter given in six divided doses) followed by vincristine (1.5 mg per square meter) and adriamycin (50 mg per square meter) in cycle A. Cycle B consists of high-dose methotrexate (1 g per square meter infused over 24 hours) with leucovorin rescue followed by an intravenous cytarabine infusion (400 mg per square meter over 48 hours, escalated in subsequent cycles to 800, 1,600, and 3,200 mg per square meter). Both intrathecal methotrexate and cytarabine are given for CNS prophylaxis.

If patients are matched for age and tumor burden, all of the above regimens yield similar results. Some 85 to 95 percent of patients with low serum LDH levels (<350) will achieve a durable complete remission, and patients with St. Jude stage III disease will achieve 60 to 80 percent long-term survival. Patients with bone marrow or CNS involvement (stage IV disease) at presentation, however, have a considerably worse prognosis.

Recently, the German BFM86 and the French SFOP regimens have produced remarkably good results in patients with bone marrow or CNS involvement at presentation. The German BFM86 regimen (Fig. 4) consists of a preparative cytoreductive phase of cyclo-

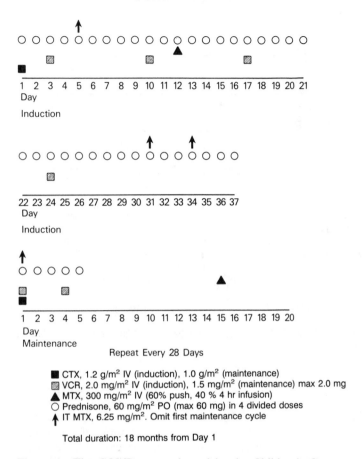

Figure 1 The COMP protocol used by the Children's Cancer Group. This protocol includes radiation to sites of bulk disease.

phosphamide (five daily doses of 200 mg per square meter). This is followed by cycle A, which consists of ifosfamide (800 mg per square meter a day for 5 days), methotrexate (500 mg per square meter infused over 24 hours), cytarabine (600 mg per square meter in four divided doses) and VM26 (200 mg per square meter in two divided doses). Cycle A is followed by cycle B, which contains the same dose of methotrexate, cyclophosphamide (1,000 mg per square meter in five daily doses) in place of ifosfamide, and adriamycin (25 mg per square meter). Intrathecal prophylaxis is conducted with three drugs (methotrexate, cytarabine, and prednisone). Oral glucocorticoids (prednisone or dexamethasone) are given in each cycle. A total of four cycles (two of A and two of B) are given after the preparatory cycle. Patients with bone marrow involvement are given a higher dose of methotrexate (5 g per square meter over 24 hours) and one dose of vincristine (1.5 mg per square meter). The regimen takes 4 months to complete. Early data with this regimen are quite encouraging, with an 81 percent disease-free survival in 45 patients treated with stage IV disease.

The SFOP 86 regimen designed by the French Pediatric Oncology Society consists of a preinduction cycle (with vincristine and cyclophosphamide), two induction cycles (with very high doses of cyclophosphamide and methotrexate), two consolidation cycles (with cytarabine and VP-16), and four maintenance cycles. Cranial radiation (24 cGy) is given during the first maintenance cycle, although whether cranial irradiation actually improves survival remains to be demonstrated. With this regimen, a remarkably good event-free survival of 72 percent has been reported in 23 patients with stage IV small, noncleaved cell lymphoma who had CNS involvement at presentation.

The Pediatric Oncology Group regimen for stage IV disease consists of an initial cycle consisting of cyclophosphamide (1.8 g per square meter in six divided doses) followed by Adriamycin (50 mg per square meter) and vincristine (1.5 mg per square meter) and accompanied by intrathecal methotrexate and cytarabine. This cycle is followed by a regimen that includes high-dose methotrexate (1 g per square meter) and high-dose cytarabine (12 g per square meter in four divided doses). A total of eight cycles are given (four of each). Six to eight months are required to complete the regimen. Again, results are encouraging, because 51 percent of 30 patients with bone marrow involvement who were

PROTOCOL 77-04

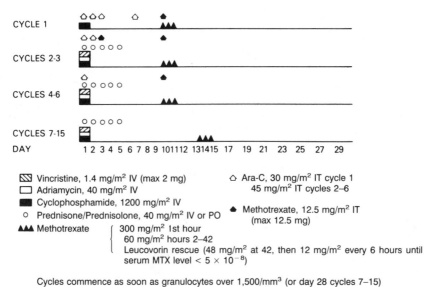

Figure 2 The 7704 protocol of the National Cancer Institute. Radiation is not routinely included.

treated on this regimen achieved durable complete remissions. The preceding three regimens have produced the best results so far reported in stage IV small, noncleaved cell lymphoma.

Patients with localized or completely resected disease have an excellent prognosis, and 90 percent can be cured. In these patients, as few as 6 weeks of therapy, as given in BFM protocol 83/86, for example, is sufficient. At the NCI, such patients are currently treated with three cycles of therapy, which can be completed in 9 weeks.

LYMPHOMA IN THE IMMUNOCOMPROMISED HOST

Lymphomas have been seen with increasing frequency in immunosuppressed individuals, especially patients undergoing organ transplantation or those suffering from AIDS. These lymphomas are predominantly immunoblastic or small, noncleaved cell type by histology. In contrast to patients without an underlying immunodeficiency disease, most patients present with "B" symptoms (fever, night sweats, and weight loss). Tumors frequently occur in atypical, extranodal sites, including the parotid gland, heart, lung, and eye. There is a 20-fold increase in the incidence of CNS involvement, and it is not unusual for patients to present with an isolated intracerebral mass. Other relatively frequent presentations include hepatomegaly, isolated cutaneous involvement, intramuscular infiltration, massive ascites, or involvement of other sites infrequently associated with lymphoma.

The management of these patients poses a dilemma. Conventional, intensive chemotherapy regimens are poorly tolerated in patients who have already manifested other stigmata of AIDS-related complex (ARC) or AIDS, and lead to an increased incidence of life-threatening infectious complications. In fact, AIDS patients treated on more intense regimens (i.e., with higher doses of cyclophosphamide) have had a poorer overall survival than those treated with conventional regimens such as CHOP or mBACOD.* Smaller doses of chemotherapy, on the other hand, are usually ineffective. Efforts are being made to design regimens that address the special problems faced by these patients (e.g., a much higher risk of CNS relapse).

The treatment of lymphoma in an immunocompromised host should be individualized. Patients with no history of opportunistic infections and a reasonably well-preserved immune system (T4 cell count >500 per microliter in adults) may be treated as intensively as nonimmunocompromised patients. Cotrimoxazole or aerosolized pentamidine should be used as prophylaxis against *Pneumocystis carinii* pneumonia. In patients with AIDS, antiretroviral therapy should be continued, if possible, during and after the treatment period. Patients with advanced immunosuppression and a history of multiple opportunistic infections should be treated in a palliative fashion, with the goal of treatment being relief of symptoms and improvement of quality of life. CHOP or a similar regimen provides a reasonable choice, particularly as it is still unknown whether this regimen is inferior to subsequently designed regimens. Other special considerations relating to the chemotherapy of

---

*Abbreviations are defined in Table 2 of the chapter, *Non-Hodgkin's Lymphoma — Unfavorable Disease: Chemotherapy.*

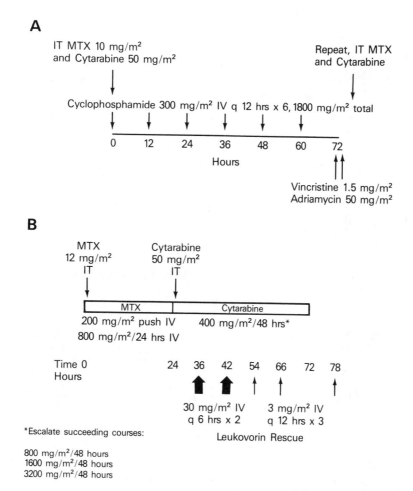

Figure 3 Total therapy B protocol from St. Jude's Children's Hospital.

AIDS-associated lymphomas include the avoidance of bleomycin in patients with pulmonary infections or compromise and the avoidance of prednisone in patients with mycobacterial infections. Radiation therapy should be used for intracerebral lymphomas.

Most patients with AIDS-associated lymphoma, or other iatrogenic forms of immunosuppression, do poorly despite therapy and die within a few months of diagnosis, either from their underlying immunodeficiency or from lymphoma. Occasional patients, particularly those who were asymptomatic prior to lymphoma development, will achieve durable complete remissions, emphasizing the need for individualizing therapy. This is not true for the majority of patients, however, and it is for this reason that there is a powerful incentive, with AIDS patients, to attempt to develop treatment using noncytotoxic agents (e.g., immunotoxins, lymphokines or antilymphokines).

LYMPHOPROLIFERATIVE SYNDROME ASSOCIATED WITH EPSTEIN-BARR VIRUS

Immunosuppressed individuals may be unable to mount an appropriate immune response to Epstein-Barr virus infection. This sometimes results in a lymphopro-

liferative syndrome presenting with generalized lymphadenopathy and organ infiltration. Histologically, these tumors range from polymorphic B-cell hyperplasia to frank immunoblastic lymphoma. Regardless of the type, however, these lymphoproliferations will be fatal if left untreated. In some patients, reversal of immunosuppression may lead to regression of lymphoproliferation. Alpha-interferon (2 million units per square meter every day for a week and then three times a week) and intravenous immunoglobulins (400 to 500 mg per kilogram for 3 days and then every 1 to 3 weeks) have been shown to induce remissions in some patients. Chemotherapy, although not invariably effective, may be necessary in patients who do not respond to the aforementioned measures.

TREATMENT OF RELAPSED PATIENTS

The prognosis for patients who relapse with small, noncleaved cell lymphoma after modern chemotherapy is generally poor. Patients who relapse after achieving a remission with initial chemotherapy do tend to have a better chance of achieving a second remission with salvage chemotherapy. Current approaches for the

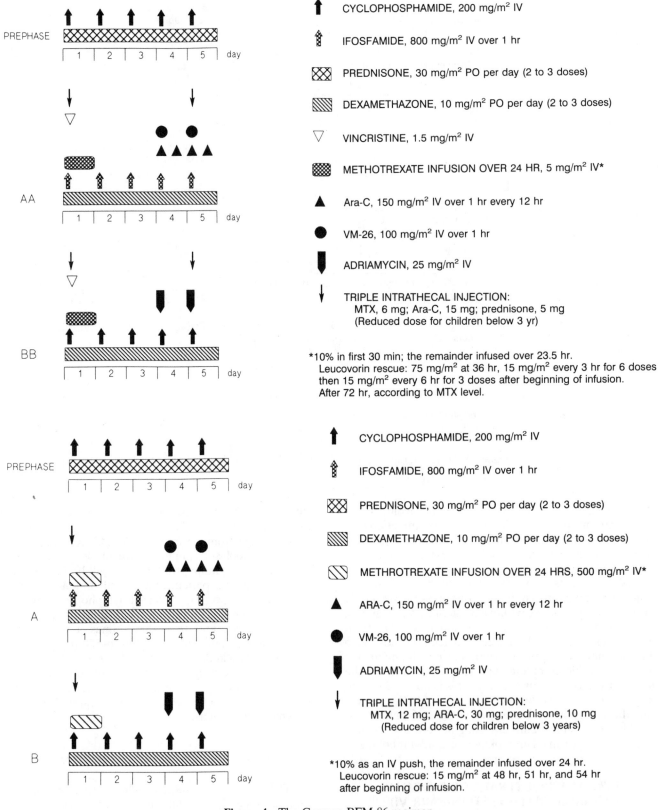

Figure 4 The German BFM 86 regimen.

management of these patients include high-dose chemotherapy with hematopoietic growth factors or autologous bone marrow salvage. Cures have been reported in patients treated with the BACT (BCNU, 200 mg per square meter IV on day 1; cytarabine, 200 mg per square meter IV on days 2 to 5; cyclophosphamide, 45 mg per kilogram on days 2 to 5; and 6-thioguanine, 200 mg per square meter on days 2 to 5) or BEAM (BCNU, 300 mg per square meter on day 1; cytarabine, 200 mg per square meter on days 2 to 5; melphalan, 140 mg per square meter on day 6; and etoposide, 200 mg per square meter on days 2 to 5). Attempts should be made to enroll relapsed patients on experimental, high-dose treatment protocols.

Drug Administration and Toxicity

Ifosfamide and, to a lesser extent, cyclophosphamide can cause hemorrhagic cystitis. Mesna is routinely given to patients during and after ifosfamide for prevention of this complication. Methotrexate metabolism differs significantly from patient to patient. In patients receiving high-dose methotrexate, serum levels should be monitored, and leucovorin rescue should be continued until methotrexate levels are less than 5×10^{-8} M. Patients with massive ascites, pleural effusion, or other large fluid collections need extended monitoring of methotrexate levels and prolonged leucovorin rescue because methotrexate accumulates in these fluids and can cause prolonged neutropenia. In patients with renal impairment, the dose of methotrexate may need to be modified, or methotrexate may be withheld completely.

Early signs of neuropathy should be looked for in all patients, and vincristine should be modified or withheld if significant peripheral neuropathy is evident. High-dose cytarabine can cause confusion and cerebellar dysfunction. Cytarabine is excreted in tears and causes conjunctivitis, which may be prevented by instillation of dexamethasone eyedrops. Intrathecal methotrexate can lead to arachnoiditis.

Almost all patients on current regimens will have absolute neutropenia during each cycle of chemotherapy. This leads to a significant morbidity and occasional mortality from infective complications. Besides bacterial infections, infections with fungi (*Candida* and *Aspergillus*) and viruses (cytomegalovirus) can prove to be a problem. Patients with hepatosplenic candidiasis may present with high spiking fevers and abnormal liver function tests. Candidiasis needs to be diagnosed early and treated intensively with amphotericin B. Cytomegalovirus infection, if it is causing pneumonitis, should be treated with ganciclovir and intravenous immunoglobulin.

Stomatitis and mucositis are frequently seen and are mainly due to methotrexate, although adriamycin often contributes. Good oral hygiene is essential. Frequent mouth washes with bicarbonate or a mixture of Maalox, lidocaine, and diphenhydramine (Benadryl) are helpful.

Adequate nutrition is important for a successful outcome. If patients are unable to eat owing to mucositis or profound anorexia, and there is sufficient weight loss, hyperalimentation may be considered.

Late Effects of Treatment

Impaired reproductive function and risk of second malignancies are the most common long-term complications. Many male children undergoing lymphoma chemotherapy will become infertile, although the risk is lower for prepubertal children. Women younger than 20 years of age have a much lower incidence of infertility, and most will retain normal reproductive function. Second malignancies are not seen frequently, although one British study has reported an 8.6 percent incidence of second malignancies. Cranial irradiation along with high-dose methotrexate has been associated with leukoencephalopathy and impaired intellectual and psychological development. Current protocols, however, do not routinely incorporate cranial irradiation.

ASSESSMENT OF RESPONSE

Small, noncleaved cell lymphomas are exquisitely chemosensitive, and there is a rapid reduction in tumor size within a few days of initiating chemotherapy. Most responding patients (approximately 90 percent) achieve a complete remission by the first or the second cycle of therapy. Patients should be followed after each cycle by repeating all abnormal radiologic studies, gallium scan, and bone marrow biopsies. Serum LDH levels usually correlate with the tumor burden, and a progressive increase in serum LDH after an initial decline is an ominous sign. Such patients should be thoroughly evaluated for evidence of relapse. Relapse in small, noncleaved cell lymphoma occurs, almost invariably, within the first year from the start of treatment. Patients who are disease-free 1 year after commencing chemotherapy can, therefore, be considered to be cured.

SUGGESTED READING

Magrath IT. Small noncleaved cell lymphomas. In: Magrath IT, ed. The non-Hodgkin's lymphomas. London: Edward Arnold, 1989: 256–275.

Magrath IT. Malignant non-Hodgkin's lymphomas. In: Pizzo PA, Poplack DG, eds. The principles and practice of pediatric oncology. Philadelphia: JB Lippincott, 1989:415–457.

PERIPHERAL T-CELL LYMPHOMA AND ADULT T-CELL LYMPHOMA/LEUKEMIA

ANN-LII CHENG, M.D.
IH-JEN SU, M.D., Ph.D.

Neoplasms of postthymic T cells include several relatively new pathologic entities of emerging clinical importance (Table 1). New diagnostic tools such as immunohistochemistry, cytogenetics, and analysis of gene rearrangement have helped ascertain that a wide variety of lymphoproliferative diseases are clonal proliferations of mature T cells and should be reclassified in the expanding family of peripheral T-cell lymphomas (PTCL). It is important for physicians to recognize this entity and understand the evolving concept of management. Knowledge is accumulating about the natural history, tumor biology, and response to treatment of PTCL; however, two basic questions remain unanswered. First, should PTCL be treated in the same way as its B-cell counterpart? Second, are conventional classification systems of non-Hodgkin's lymphoma (NHL) also applicable to PTCL? In this chapter, we discuss our current approaches to both PTCL and the closely related HTLV-1-associated adult T-cell lymphoma/leukemia (ATLL).

PERIPHERAL T-CELL LYMPHOMA

Peripheral T-cell lymphoma was first recognized as a distinct histologic entity in 1975, but the full spectrum of this disorder has not been appreciated until recently. It is estimated that 20 to 30 percent of diffuse aggressive lymphomas in the United States belong to this entity. In some far Eastern countries, including Japan (HTLV-1–nonedemic area) and Taiwan, PTCL constitutes 30 to 40 percent of diffuse aggressive lymphomas and becomes one of the major lymphomas in these areas because follicular lymphomas are rare. Chronic Epstein-Barr virus (EBV) infection and evidence of the EBV genome in neoplastic T cells have been reported in some cases. A causal relationship has not been established.

Classification

A well-accepted clinicopathologic classification of PTCL has yet to be developed. Currently, we find it helpful to describe it in two different ways (Table 1).

In 10 to 30 percent of cases the characteristic distribution of the neoplastic T cells or the exuberant proliferation of the reactive cells dominates the histologic picture to form specific histologic patterns. The homing nature and cytokine secretion of the neoplastic T cells are two of the major mechanisms contributing to

Table 1 Classification of Postthymic T-Cell Malignancies

Peripheral T-cell lymphoma
  Classification by histologic patterns:
  Nonspecific type
  Specific types
    Angiocentric type PTCL
    AILD-like PTCL
    MH-like PTCL
    Lennert's lymphoma
    Others (T-zone, HD-like, etc.)

  Classification by modified working formulation:
  Small- and medium-sized cell
  Mixed-cell
  Large-cell/immunoblastic cell
  Others (multilobated, signet ring, etc.)

Adult T-cell lymphoma/leukemia (HTLV-1 related)

Mycosis fungoides/Sezary syndrome (cutaneous T-cell lymphoma)

T-cell chronic lymphocytic leukemia

T-cell chronic prolymphocytic leukemia

Abbreviations: AILD = angioimmunoblastic lymphadenopathy with dysproteinemia, MH = malignant histiocytosis, HD = Hodgkin's disease.

these histologic characteristics. These entities are usually associated with distinct clinicopathologic manifestations. Their disease course can be better anticipated by these patterns rather than by the histologic gradings of the neoplastic T cells. The remaining 70 to 90 percent of PTCL usually contain a mild to moderate amount of infiltrating epithelioid cells, histiocytes, eosinophils, plasma cells, and vascular endothelial cells and are classified as nonspecific-type PTCL (see Table 1).

The grading concept of PTCL is still a matter of debate. In our experience, the working formulation classification, although not as powerful as it is in B-cell lymphoma, is still useful for survival prognostication of PTCL. In our series, the overall survival of the small- and medium-sized cell group is significantly better than that of the large-cell and immunoblastic cell group.

Clinicopathologic Features and Treatment Guidelines

Many specific subtypes of PTCL, such as AILD (angioimmunoblastic lymphadenopathy with dysproteinemia)-like, angiocentric-type, or MH (malignant histocytosis)-like subtypes, have recently been recognized as distinct categories of PTCL. Their response to NHL-like or other therapeutic protocols has yet to be evaluated by ongoing clinical trials. Therefore, it would be prudent at this moment to consider the treatment of these entities separately, especially in early stages of disease. In general, tumor behavior of specific subtypes of PTCL diverges remarkably in early stages of disease, but as the diseases progress, they usually become indistinguishable from one another. This phenomenon probably reflects dedifferentiation of the neoplastic cells, as evidenced by the observation that specific patterns of PTCL tend to transform into nonspecific ones.

Regardless of the heterogeneous histology, an important clinical feature shared by most PTCL is the characteristic poor response of recurrent tumors to second-line chemotherapy. In contrast to low-grade B-cell lymphomas, in which the protracted disease course is often incurable but associated with repeated response to chemotherapy, a low-grade PTCL is often curable but develops drug resistance rapidly if it fails first-line therapy.

Nonspecific PTCL

This entity represents 70 to 90 percent of the PTCL patients. It is characterized by B symptoms (50 to 60 percent), advanced staging (70 to 80 percent), lymphadenopathy (80 to 90 percent), bone marrow involvement (30 to 40 percent), hepatomegaly (30 to 40 percent), splenomegaly (10 to 20 percent), lung and pleura involvement (10 to 20 percent), and skin involvement (10 to 20 percent). Diagnosis requires immunophenotype or T-cell receptor gene rearrangement analysis to document the clonal origin of the neoplastic T cells.

Although the prognosis varies greatly, most investigators suggest that this group of patients be treated with intensive combination chemotherapy regardless of the morphologic gradings. In our experience, a standard CHOP regimen may result in complete remission in 50 to 60 percent of the patients, and approximately half of these can be expected to have a durable disease-free survival. Evidence to date suggests that patients treated with less intensive chemotherapy have a much less favorable outcome. One important reason for poor survival of undertreated patients is that the disease usually progresses rapidly and becomes refractory to subsequent chemotherapy after failing first-line drugs. The Nebraska Lymphoma Study Group, in a prospective study comparing PTCL with its B-cell counterpart, revealed a particularly poor prognostic group of stage IV PTCL in which no complete remissions or 3-year-survival patients were seen. This observation was consistent with our current view that drug resistance develops rapidly in the residual tumor of PTCL. It is therefore reasonable to consider protocols with increased intensity as the first-line treatment. For example, BACOP/L17M, a chemotherapeutic protocol with intensive consolidation and maintenance program, has been reported by investigators from the University of Hong Kong to improve significantly the complete remission and overall survival rates of PTCL patients. However, a longer period of follow-up is necessary for that study.

The role of radiotherapy in PTCL is limited because most patients present with advanced clinical stage and, in other cases, there is often occult systemic disease. However, long survival induced by single-modality radiotherapy has been reported sporadically. We recommend that definitive radiotherapy be reserved only for patients who have localized disease and cannot tolerate intensive chemotherapy.

Angiocentric-type PTCL

Two major clinical entities, i.e., polymorphic reticulosis of upper respiratory tract and lymphomatoid granulomatosis of lungs and skin, are included in this category. They fall into a pathologic spectrum described by Jaffe as angiocentric immunoproliferative lesion. Many of the previously considered "prelymphomatous" conditions are now thought to represent early stages of angiocentric-type PTCL. Clinically, some of the patients may have a protracted course, but most of them die of relentless progression of disease.

Polymorphic reticulosis of upper respiratory tract tends to affect middle-age men. A mild clustering in the Mongolian ethnic groups has been seen. The clinical picture is characterized by local destructions of the nose, paranasal sinuses, palates, and nasopharynx. This condition was previously included in an ambiguous category of lethal or nonhealing midline granuloma. Systemic symptoms of fever, weight loss, and night sweats are seen in approximately 60 percent of the patients. Because of the location, chance of early detection is high. However, pathologic diagnosis is frequently hampered by extensive necrosis of the tumor. Repeated biopsy and careful review of specimens are critical. Localized disease is highly treatable by radiotherapy. Smalley and colleagues reviewed the results of 34 patients treated at the Mayo Clinic that suggested that a minimum dose of 42 Gy is necessary to achieve long-term local control. A generous treatment volume to include adjacent structures was recommended, as a 20 percent marginal-failure rate was observed in their series. Prophylactic irradiation to clinically uninvolved lymph nodes is considered controversial; chance of recurrence at these sites is about 10 percent. In general, a durable remission can be produced by radiotherapy alone in approximately 70 percent of the patients presenting with localized disease. Distant metastases frequently involve skin, lung, brain, and kidney. In our experience, distant metastases are extremely difficult to salvage by chemotherapy. Clinical trials with new modalities of treatment are needed for these situations. Solitary metastasis in lungs or brain may occasionally be salvaged by local resection or radiation.

Patients with pulmonary lymphomatoid granulomatosis present with nonspecific complaints of fever, weight loss, shortness of breath, cough, and hemoptysis. Radiologic findings include unilateral or bilateral, single or multiple poorly marginated nodules or masses with occasional interstitial infiltrates or pleural effusions. This entity is associated with frequent regional lymph node involvement and extrapulmonary recurrence. Therefore, local treatment with surgical resection or radiotherapy is generally not adequate. As for aggressive NHL, systemic chemotherapy is the favored approach. Patients treated initially with conservative chemotherapy are often compromised in their ability to achieve a complete remission. For example, investigators at the

National Cancer Institute reported the results of a protocol in which cyclophosphamide, 2 mg per kilogram per day, and prednisolone, 1 mg per kilogram per day, were used. In 15 patients with lower-grade lymphomatoid granulomatosis, 7 achieved durable remission. Only one of the eight patients who had failed this protocol was able to achieve complete remission by second-line intensive chemotherapy. Conversely, six of eight patients with high-grade angiocentric PTCL achieved complete remission by intensive protocols, including C-MOPP, ProMACE-MOPP, and ProMACE-CytaBOM.* Distant metastases frequently involve liver, skin, brain and kidney. Tumors refractory to chemotherapy are often still relatively sensitive to radiotherapy. Successful salvage and palliation with aggressive radiotherapy have been reported.

AILD-like PTCL

Angioimmunoblastic lymphadenopathy with dysproteinemia (AILD), originally described by Frizzera in 1974, is characterized clinically as having a predilection for the elderly and an association with generalized lymphadenopathy, hepatosplenomegaly, skin rashes, fever, hypergammaglobulinemia, autoantibodies, hemolytic anemia, and thrombocytopenia. In approximately 80 percent of AILD, clonal perforation of mature T cells can be demonstrated by chromosome abnormalities ($+3$, $+5$) or T-cell receptor gene arrangement analysis. These features strongly favor a diagnosis of AILD-like PTCL. True AILD and AILD-like PTCL may belong to the same disease spectrum. Evidence suggests that the latter represents a selective clonal expansion of the abnormal cells and clones of the former. A small percentage of patients with AILD-like PTCL may have a protracted course or go into remission spontaneously. The majority of the patients, however, die in 2 years or transform into an aggressive-type PTCL.

Treatment is hampered by the generally aggressive nature of the disease, and the relatively advanced age and immunodeficiency state of the patients. Conventional treatment with steroids or simple combination with cyclophosphamide produces a 30 to 50 percent complete remission rate. The median survival is only 10 to 20 months. A trend toward longer survival has been observed by using more intensive chemotherapy. A large prospective study at Kiel University used prednisolone as a single agent to treat patients presenting with stable disease and used an intensive chemotherapy protocol (COP-BLAM/IMVP-16) to treat patients presenting with progressive disease or those who had already failed the steroid therapy. The results showed a 29 percent complete remission for the prednisolone arm and a 37 to 57 percent complete remission for the intensive chemotherapy arm. The duration of remission lasted only a few months in most cases. In our experience, treatment with prednisolone alone is usually insufficient. It is used as a temporary measure to treat patients whose general condition prohibits the use of combination chemotherapy. However, intensive chemotherapy should be given with extreme caution and, if possible, in the early phase of the disease so as to avoid exacerbating the immunodeficiency state that is frequently associated with the late phase of AILD-like PTCL. Infection by microorganisms is one of the leading causes of death in this disease entity. Prophylactic use of antibiotics against *Pneumocystis carinii*, mycobacterium, herpes virus, and fungi is frequently necessary. Further studies are needed to investigate the response of this group of PTCL to either standard chemotherapeutic protocols used for NHL or empiric therapies designed to control the protean cytokine-induced reactions that probably play an important role in the pathogenesis of the disease.

MH-like PTCL

Histiocytic medullary reticulosis (HMR) was first described in 1939 as a clinicopathologic entity characterized by fever, weight loss, hepatosplenomegaly, lymphadenopathy, and profound pancytopenia due to widespread tissue infiltration by phagocytizing histiocytes. This condition was later considered synonymous with malignant histiocytosis (MH), a systemic malignancy derived from cells of the mononuclear phagocytic system. It is now clear that at least 50 percent of the previously diagnosed cases of MH are actually MH-like PTCL. True MH is rare.

Peripheral T-cell lymphoma may be associated with hemophagocytosis in two different ways. First, it may elaborate cytokines capable of activating benign histiocytes, which in turn cause the hemophagocytosis. This represents the most common mechanism. Second, a rare T-gamma lymphoma may have direct phagocytosis of red blood cells by the neoplastic T-gamma cells. Clinically, most cases of MH-like PTCL present with a syndrome indistinguishable from true MH. Rarely, some angiocentric-type PTCL may transform into MH-like PTCL as a terminal event. The latter condition should be carefully differentiated from infection-associated phagocytosis syndrome.

To date, little is known about the difference in treatment response between MH-like PTCL and true MH; however, it is reasonable to treat the former as an advanced aggressive lymphoma. The preliminary results suggest a complete remission rate of approximately 30 percent with CHOP or its equivalent. The prognosis is generally poor in adult patients. Again, as in AILD-like PTCL, efforts to control the secretion or biologic actions of cytokines represents an important direction for future investigations.

Lennert's (Lymphoepithelioid Cell) Lymphoma

Lymphoepithelioid cell lymphoma was first described by Lennert in 1968. It is characterized histologically by a prominent population of epithelioid histiocytes that may be intimately mixed with lymphoid cells or

---

*Abbreviations are defined in Table 2 of the chapter *Non-Hodgkin's Lymphoma — Unfavorable Disease: Chemotherapy.*

form discrete granulomas. This entity represents a subtype of PTCL composed of cells with a differentiated T-helper cell phenotype.

Clinically, patients tend to be older and have disseminated disease at presentation, with involvement of liver, spleen, bone marrow, and retroperitoneal or other lymph nodes. Prognosis is variable, and some patients may have a prolonged clinical course. In the majority of patients, however, its clinical course is indistinguishable from that of nonspecific PTCL, and these patients should be treated as such.

Others

Hodgkin's disease–like PTCL and T-zone lymphoma are frequently considered as specific subtypes of PTCL. In our experience, the clinical picture of these two entities is not different from that of the nonspecific PTCL, and can be handled as such. However, it is of practical importance to make the correct diagnosis of HD-like PTCL because their response to a Hodgkin's disease–oriented protocol is typically poor. A retrospective study from the National Cancer Institute has redesignated 10 of 39 lymphocyte-depletion type Hodgkin's disease as NHL. By using the MOPP protocol, complete remissions were achieved in only three patients, and median survival was 7 months. It is estimated that approximately 10 to 20 percent of cases previously diagnosed as Hodgkin's disease are actually PTCL.

Future Perspectives

Understanding the nature of the biologic behavior of neoplastic T cells remains a key to improving the clinical management of PTCL. One of the clues is to identify the protean humoral factors secreted by these cells and their subsequent biologic effects in complicated cellular interactions. This will be of practical importance in the management of certain specific types of PTCL.

Drug selection and administration schedules in treatment of PTCL may not follow the same principles that currently work well in the B-cell lymphomas. Prospective studies are needed to clarify if there are any basic differences in the response to chemotherapy between PTCL and its B-cell counterpart. Clinical trials to discover protocols that have specificity for PTCL should be pursued.

ADULT T-CELL LYMPHOMA/LEUKEMIA

Adult T-cell lymphoma/leukemia is a unique T-cell malignancy caused by the human T-cell lymphotropic virus type-1 (HTLV-1). Geographic, ethnic, and familial clustering are noted in HTLV-1 infection. Endemic areas include southwestern Japan, central Africa, and the Caribbean basin. Blacks in the southeastern section of the United States represent an ethnic clustering. Infection by both HTLV-1 and human immunodeficiency virus type-1 (HIV-1) has become increasingly prevalent, particularly among intravenous drug users.

Routes of transmission include vertical transmission from mother to child and horizontal transmission by sexual intercourse or blood transfusion. Sporadic cases of HTLV-1 infection and ATLL have been reported from almost everywhere in the world.

Diagnosis of ATLL depends on identification of characteristic multilobated ATLL cells in the peripheral blood. In all cases, the serum is positive for anti-HTLV-1 antibodies, and the ATLL cells contain the proviral DNA of HTLV-1. The pathognomonic ATLL cells have helper/inducer immunophenotype but also have functions of suppressor/cytotoxic T cells. At presentation, about 60 percent of patients have ATLL cells, but eventually almost all patients will have them in their peripheral blood. Histomorphologic and immunophenotypic study of the tumor tissues is not sufficient to differentiate ATLL from HTLV-1(-) PTCL. Because HTLV-1 infection can also induce a mild immunodeficiency state, opportunistic infections with *Pneumocystis carinii*, *Candida* spp, and *Strongyloides stercoralis* are frequently encountered. To date, no effective antiviral agents against HTLV-1 are available. Specific management of ATLL depends on the presenting clinical syndromes of the patients.

Clinical Syndromes

The host responses to infection with HTLV-1 can be classified into several categories.

Carrier State

These patients are asymptomatic. There may be an increase in serum immunoglobulin, and, despite normal leukocyte counts and differentials, the percentage of CD2(+) and Tac (+) cells is elevated. The chance of ATLL developing after seroconversion is 0.01 percent to 0.1 percent per year. The incubation period is usually more than 20 years.

Subclinical ATLL

These patients are almost entirely asymptomatic and are distinguished by a mild proliferation of abnormal-appearing lymphocytes. Minor lymphadenopathy, transient fever, or rash may develop, but the patients generally feel well. In about half of the patients, abnormal lymphocytosis will resolve without residual disease. The remainder will have persistence of this pattern or will show progression to a more acute form of the disease.

Chronic/Smoldering ATLL

About one-third of the clinically apparent ATLL falls into this category. These patients have skin lesions (erythema, papules, and nodules), abnormal lymphocytosis, and mild bone marrow involvement. Hypergammaglobulinemia is common. Hepatosplenomegaly, persistent lymphadenopathy, and hypercalcemia are typically absent. Reported overall survival of this group is 22 to 180 months. About 40 percent of patients will progress to acute ATLL.

Acute/Subacute ATLL

Most clinically apparent cases of ATLL belong to this category. The clinical picture is characterized by skin lesions, generalized lymphadenopathy, hepatosplenonomegaly, hypercalcemia, lymphomatous meningitis, and elevated leukocyte count with multilobated lymphocytes. The patients present with complaints of fever, rash, weakness, cough, abdominal pain, lymphadenopathy, and disturbances of consciousness. Anemia and thrombocytopenia are infrequent and mild.

Treatment

The carrier state and subclinical and chronic forms of ATLL should not be treated unless patients are under clinical trials of empiric therapies. Currently, chemotherapy is the standard mode of treatment for acute/subacute ATLL. Protocols similar to those used in aggressive NHL are frequently adopted. Investigators at the National Cancer Institute treated 10 patients with combination-chemotherapy protocols (e.g., ProMACE-MOPP, CHOP, COMLA) and achieved a prompt complete remission in 7 patients. Unfortunately, the duration of remission was typically short; five of these seven patients had relapsed by a median time of 13 months. Relapse or exacerbation was frequently associated with the emergence of a more immature phenotype. Reports from other investigators suggested that survival might be improved by more intensive chemotherapy, but more experience is necessary before this can be concluded.

Several empiric therapies have reported sporadic success. Among these, interferons, 2-deoxycor-

fomycin, azidothymidine, and toxin or radioactive-element–conjugated anti-Tac antibodies are under active investigation. We recommend that patients who relapse from combination chemotherapy should have a trial of one of these empiric therapies.

Future Perspectives

Development of effective vaccination and antiviral agents against the HTLV family remains the ultimate solution to the problem of HTLV infections.

Unsatisfactory results of the current treatments may be improved by combined-modality approaches. For example, preliminary encouraging results have come from a new treatment in which chemotherapy was administered first to decrease the tumor burden, and this was followed by interferons to produce a remission. Combinations including chemotherapy with biologic response modifiers or other modes of therapy should also be addressed in the future.

SUGGESTED READING

Armitage JO, Greer JP, Levine AM, et al. Peripheral T-cell lymphoma. Cancer 1989; 63:158–163.
Broder S, Bunn PA, Jaffe ES, et al. T-cell lymphoproliferative syndrome associated with human T-cell leukemia/lymphoma virus. Ann Intern Med 1984; 100:543–557.
Jaffe ES. Pathologic and clinical spectrum of post-thymic T-cell malignancies. Cancer Invest 1984; 2:413–425.
Jones JF, Shurin S, Abramowsky C, et al. T-cell lymphomas containing Epstein-Barr viral DNA in patients with chronic Epstein-Barr virus infections. N Engl J Med 1988; 318:733–741.
Kim JH, Durack DT. Manifestations of human T-lymphotropic virus type 1 infection. Am J Med 1988; 84:919–928.

MELANOMA: SURGERY

S. EVA SINGLETARY, M.D.
CHARLES M. BALCH, M.D., F.A.C.S.

Although melanoma currently represents only 1 to 3 percent of all malignancies in the United States, the incidence is doubling every 6 to 10 years. In 1935, only 1 in 1,500 individuals developed melanoma. By 1987, the incidence rate increased to 1 in 135, and by the year 2,000, the estimated rate is expected to be 1 in 90. Despite this dramatic increase in the number of cases, melanoma is a potentially curable cancer if diagnosed and properly treated at an early stage.

Guidelines and treatment options for surgical management are based on knowledge of the natural history of the disease, prognostic factors for metastasis and survival, staging of the disease by clinical and radiologic parameters, and operative risks. In early stage melanoma, tumor thickness is the primary criterion in determining the surgical approach for both the primary site and the regional lymph nodes. In patients with clinical evidence of metastases in regional nodes or at solitary distant sites, surgery is usually still indicated for local disease control and possible prolongation of life.

STAGING SYSTEM

The original melanoma staging system involved three stages: stage I, for localized melanoma; stage II, for regional metastasis; and stage III, for distant metastasis. A major limitation of this system is that currently the majority of patients (85 percent or more) diagnosed as having melanoma have stage I disease. The new staging system (Table 1) adopted by the American Joint Committee on Cancer (AJCC) is based on the microstaging of the primary melanoma and knowledge of patterns of metastasis (Fig. 1).

Table 1 Staging for Melanoma: American Joint Committee on Cancer

Stage	Criteria
IA	Localized melanoma ≤0.75 mm thick or Clark's level 2* (T1, N0, M0)
IB	Localized melanoma 0.76 mm to 1.5 mm thick or Clark's level III* (T2, N0, M0)
IIA	Localized melanoma > 1.5 mm but ≤ 4.0 mm thick or Clark's level IV* (T3, N0, M0)
IIB	Localized melanoma > 4.0 mm thick or Clark's level V* (T4, N0, M0)
III	Limited nodal metastases involving only one regional lymph node basin or fewer than five intransit metastates but no nodal metastases (any T, N1, M0)
IV	Advanced regional metastases (any T, N2, M0) or any distant metastases (any T, any N, M1 or M2)

*When the thickness and level of invasion criteria do not match the same T classification, thickness of lesion should take precedence.

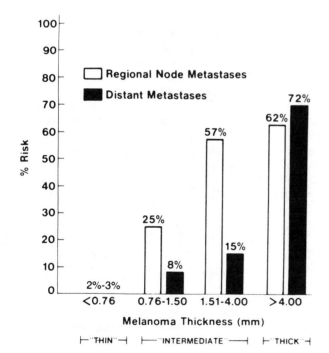

Figure 1 Estimated biologic risk that microscopic metastases will become clinically evident in regional nodes (within 3 years) and at distant sites (within 5 years) for melanomas subgrouped by thickness categories. (From Balch CM. Surgical management of regional lymph nodes in cutaneous melanoma. J Am Acad Dermatol 1980; 3:511–524; with permission.)

Stages I and II consist of clinically localized disease; these stages are subdivided into A and B according to Breslow's tumor thickness and Clark's levels of invasion. Patients with stage III disease have nodal metastases in a single lymph node basin, whereas those with stage IV melanoma have one of the following: (1) distant metastases; (2) nodal metastases involving two or more lymph node basins; (3) five or more intransit metastases; or (4) nodal metastases either larger than 5 cm in diameter or fixed to the surrounding tissues.

METASTATIC EVALUATION

A complete history and physical examination are the most important initial steps in determining appropriate therapy. Although melanoma can metastasize to virtually any organ or tissue, knowledge of the patterns of metastasis will help the physician focus on the site most likely to harbor disease. The regional lymph nodes are the most common site of metastases, followed by skin, subcutaneous tissue, and lung. Other potential sites of metastasis are the liver, brain, bone, and gastrointestinal tract. In the absence of symptoms or signs of metastasis, a minimum number of laboratory and radiologic tests should be ordered because their diagnostic yield is low and not cost-effective.

Clinical follow-up after treatment of the melanoma is based on the same principle. The frequency of clinic visits is dictated by the tumor thickness and stage of the melanoma. For thin melanomas less than 1 mm thick, biannual examinations should be sufficient because the risk of metastasis is low. Patients with melanomas thicker than 1 mm or with regional metastases should be examined more frequently: every 3 months during the first 2 years, every 6 months until 5 years, and then once a year throughout their lifetime.

PRIMARY MELANOMA

Biopsy Technique

Whether excisional or incisional, the biopsy must be full-thickness, including the subcutaneous tissue, to determine accurately the thickness and level of invasion of the melanoma. Any lesion suspected to be a melanoma should never be shaved or curetted for diagnosis.

The preferred procedure is an excisional biopsy with an elliptic incision including a narrow margin (2 mm) of normal-appearing skin. The orientation of the biopsy incision should be in the direction of lymphatic drainage to the nearest regional nodal basin. A properly placed biopsy scar facilitates a subsequent wide excision and primary closure and often avoids the need for a skin graft.

For large lesions or those in critical locations, such as the face, hands, or feet, an incisional biopsy with a scalpel or a 6-mm punch dermatome may be performed. The biopsy specimen should be a full-thickness wedge or core of skin and subcutaneous tissue from the most raised or irregular area of the lesion.

Surgical Margins

The surgical margins of excision are determined by the tumor's thickness, which most accurately predicts the likelihood of recurrence. Although a noninvasive lesion, melanoma in situ (Clark's level 1 or atypical melanocytic hyperplasia) should be excised with at least a 0.5-mm margin to prevent a local recurrence. For invasive melanomas less than 1 mm thick, both randomized and nonrandomized studies indicate that a 1-cm margin should be sufficient and safe.

The optimal margin for melanomas thicker than 1 mm is controversial. Results of the World Health Organization's randomized study of 612 evaluable patients demonstrated no significant differences in local recurrence or survival rates in patients with melanomas less than 2 mm thick who had a 1-cm margin of excision as compared with a 3-cm margin. However, there were four local recurrences in patients with melanomas 1 to 2 mm thick that had been excised with a 1-cm margin.

If one considers a local recurrence to be a retained primary lesion, then local recurrence must be considered a failure of surgical therapy (i.e., too narrow a margin). However, a local recurrence may also reflect the first evidence of occult disseminated metastases, and wider resection may not influence survival outcome. Patients at highest risk for local recurrences are those with melanomas located on the scalp, face, hand, or foot (5 percent to 12 percent local recurrence rate) or melanomas at least 4 mm thick (13 percent) or with ulceration (11 percent). The prognosis after treatment of a local recurrence is poor: 80 percent of these patients eventually die of distant metastases. Therefore, surgical guidelines for excision margins (Table 2) should be adjusted for individual patients based on the collective importance of prognostic factors. When the primary is appropriately excised, the overall risk for a local recurrence is extremely low: 3.2 percent in a collected series involving 3,520 patients and less than 1 percent for melanomas thinner than 1 mm.

Surgical Excision Technique

An elliptic incision should be used to excise the primary melanoma. The long axis or length of the incision should be in the direction of lymphatic drainage and should be approximately three to four times the width of the incision to allow primary closure. The width of the incision is the measured margin from the lateral edge of the previous biopsy scar. Because the lymphatics drain to the regional nodes in the subcutaneous tissue superficial to the deep fascia, excision of the fascia would not affect the incidence of local recurrence or intransit disease. In a retrospective review at The University of Texas M. D. Anderson Cancer Center, no significant differences in the incidence and site of subsequent recurrence or in survival were seen in 107 patients in whom the fascia was excised compared with 95 patients in whom the fascia was left intact. If the primary melanoma is very thick, however, one should consider excising the fascia to obtain a histologically negative deep margin. Pigmented nonabsorbable sutures should not be used in the closure because they could be confused with a possible local recurrence. Skin grafts should be avoided either by primary closure or the rotation of skin flaps. The cosmetic outcome of the scar and its acceptance by the patient have been shown to be inversely correlated with the degree of surgical indentation or depression and not with the length of the scar.

Special Sites

Fingers and Toes

Melanomas on the fingers and toes are usually treated by amputation. Depending on the extensiveness of nail bed or paronychial involvement and on the location of the lesion's proximal border, an amputation should be performed proximal to the distal interphalangeal joint of the fingers or the thumb with at least a 1-cm skin margin. For large lesions outside the confines of the nail bed or with associated satellites, a metacarpophalangeal joint amputation (ray amputation) is necessary. A ray amputation of the entire digit should be performed for a melanoma located on a toe because there is no significant effect on function and better local control may be achieved.

Sole of the Foot

Because melanomas on the plantar surface of the foot often involve a large area, split-thickness skin grafts are often needed to cover the defect. It is important to preserve the deep fascia over the extensor tendons to ensure support of the skin graft. A portion of the heel or ball of the foot should also be retained for weight bearing, if feasible. Amputations of the foot are seldom necessary.

Ear

A wedge excision or partial amputation is performed after confirming the diagnosis with an excisional or punch biopsy. If possible, the upper part of the ear should be preserved for patients who wear glasses. For

Table 2 Recommended Skin Margins for Excising Melanomas of Different Types

Type of Melanoma	Margins (cm)*
In situ	0.5–1
< 1 mm thick	1
≥ 1 mm thick	2–3
Lentigo maligna	1

*For anatomic sites where these margins cannot be used, the widest practical margin of excision is acceptable.

large recurrences or initial widespread disease, a total amputation of the ear may be required. An ear prosthesis may offer both cosmetic and functional rehabilitation.

Face

Lentigo maligna melanomas are typically located on the face or neck in older patients with sun-damaged skin. Because this histologic melanoma type has a low risk for recurrence, a 1-cm excision margin is adequate.

Breast

Margins of excision of a breast melanoma should be based on tumor thickness, as with any other anatomic location. Removal of the entire breast is unnecessary.

REGIONAL NODAL METASTASES

Of melanomas that have the inherent potential to metastasize, 85 percent will disseminate via lymphatic drainage to the regional lymph nodes. Patients can be categorized into three groups based on thickness of the primary melanoma to estimate quantitatively the risk of regional or distant metastatic disease. Thin melanomas (less than 1 mm thick) are associated with localized disease and only a 2 percent to 4 percent risk for metastasis to regional or distant sites. However, men with thin trunk lesions have up to a 10 percent risk of developing metastases. Patients with intermediate-thickness melanomas (1 to 4 mm thick) have a risk of up to 60 percent for regional metastases but a relatively low risk (less than 20 percent) for distant disease. Patients with thick melanomas (4 mm or greater) have not only a high risk for regional node metastases (greater than 60 percent) but also a high risk for occult distant metastatic disease (greater than 70 percent). Other risk factors for each patient must also be taken into account. Patients with ulcerative melanomas have a higher risk for metastases than those with nonulcerative melanomas do, even when matched for other prognostic parameters, such as tumor thickness. Extremity melanomas in women have a lower metastatic potential than lesions of equivalent thickness on the extremities of men. Patients with melanomas located on the trunk or head and neck areas fare worse regardless of sex than patients with tumors at other sites.

Clinically Negative Regional Lymph Nodes

The efficacy of elective lymph node dissection to remove suspected microscopic or clinically occult metastatic melanoma is still controversial. Several prospective but nonrandomized trials of elective node dissections involving over 2,000 stage I melanoma patients treated at the University of Alabama in Birmingham, the University of Sydney in Australia, and Duke Medical Center in North Carolina have demonstrated an improved survival rate in patients with intermediate-

thickness melanomas (1 to 4 mm). The results from the Alabama and Sydney trials show this increased survival rate for all patients with intermediate-thickness melanomas of the trunk, head, and neck. The benefit of elective node dissection in patients with extremity melanomas was greater in men than in women.

However, randomized prospective studies from the World Health Organization and from the Mayo Clinic did not show improved survival of patients with extremity or truncal melanomas who underwent elective node dissection compared with patients treated with wide excision alone. Because these randomized trials have not been completely accepted because of the stratification criteria used, a new randomized prospective study of elective node dissection for intermediate-thickness melanomas at all sites is in progress by cooperative cancer centers in the United States and Canada.

Clinically Positive Regional Lymph Nodes

If clinical examination reveals any adenopathy in the regional nodal basin that is suspected of harboring metastatic disease, surgical excision of the nodal metastases will provide the most effective treatment for achieving local control and possible cure. If the clinical examination is equivocal and close observation is not reliable, then fine-needle biopsy or open biopsy may be performed.

A complete lymph node dissection that removes all nodal and lymphatic tissue within the anatomically defined region is necessary. When a cervical node contains metastasis and the melanoma is located on the face, ear, or anterior scalp, both a superficial parotidectomy and a modified or complete neck dissection should be performed. When an axillary node contains metastatic disease, removal of not only level 1 and 2 axillary nodes (lateral and posterior to the pectoralis minor muscle) but also level 3 nodes (medial to the pectoralis minor muscle) should be undertaken. If the primary melanoma is located on the posterior trunk, the subscapular nodes should also be included in the dissection. When the inguinal lymph nodes are involved, a dissection of the nodes in the femoral triangle and above the inguinal ligament is usually appropriate. Controversy exists whether the additional removal of the iliac and

Table 3 Relationship of Positive Iliac-Obturator Nodes to 5-Year Survival

Series	Total Patients*	5-Year Survivors
Memorial Sloan-Kettering	46	4
Columbia University	4	0
University of California (LA)	24	4†
Roswell Park Memorial Institute	18	1
Royal Marsden Hospital	47	3
Netherlands Cancer Institute	23	3
M.D. Anderson Cancer Center	15	4

*All patients had iliac-obturator nodal metastases.
†One with distant metastasis.

obturator nodes is indicated (Table 3). Some series have reported an occasional long-term survivor in patients with iliac or obturator nodal metastases. Others have demonstrated that iliac-obturator node dissection may benefit only patients who have microscopic metastases in the inguinal region (a 9 percent to 20 percent 5-year survival rate). However, data from both M. D. Anderson Cancer Center and Memorial Sloan-Kettering Cancer Center did not indicate that the extent of inguinal lymphadenectomy influenced survival rates. Removal of the iliac and obturator lymph nodes may be considered in selected patients in whom the risk of surgery is relatively low to maximize local disease control and to avoid impending symptoms of iliac vein obstruction or pressure on the obturator or femoral nerves.

Although no adjuvant therapy thus far has been found effective against AJCC (American Joint Committee on Cancer) stage III melanoma, participation in ongoing and future clinical trials is imperative for these patients because of their dismal prognoses. In the M. D. Anderson Cancer Center series of 1,001 melanoma patients with regional nodal metastases, the goal of cure by node dissection was rarely achieved, as reflected by the low 5- and 10-year survival rates of 33 percent and 28 percent, respectively. Distant metastases after node dissection remained the major problem, confirming that the metastatic involvement of regional lymph nodes implies the presence of subclinical disseminated disease in most patients. This risk of distant metastases depended on the extent of tumor burden (Fig. 2). The occurrence of distant disease was significantly lower in patients with a single involved node (60 percent with distant metastasis) than in patients with multiple positive nodes (80 percent, $P < 0.00001$). The presence of

disease outside the lymph node capsule also increased the risk of distant metastases (81 percent, $P < 0.05$). Data from The University of Alabama and University of Sydney Melanoma Unit's series of 551 patients with nodal metastases also demonstrated a direct correlation between the number of nodal metastases and survival. Only patients with one positive node had a reasonable expectation of cure: 40 percent were alive at 10 years, whereas only 13 percent of patients with two or more nodal metastases were alive at 10 years. Ulceration of the primary melanoma was also found to be an important prognostic factor independent of the number of positive nodes. The 3-year survival rate for patients with nodal metastases who also had ulcerative primary melanomas was only 29 percent, compared with 61 percent for patients with nodal disease but nonulcerative melanomas ($P = 0.0002$). The most favorable prognosis was seen in patients with one positive node and no ulceration of the primary melanoma; this group had a 50 percent 10-year survival rate.

Recurrent Nodal Metastases After Node Dissection

Tumor recurrence within or adjacent to the area of a previous lymph node dissection is usually seen in one of two clinical settings. In the first, a patient who is known to have undergone an initial complete lymph node dissection presents with recurrent nodal disease at the peripheral boundaries of the previously dissected nodal basin. Local excision of the recurrence and surrounding soft tissue with histologically negative margins is the appropriate treatment choice. In the second setting, a patient who had an incomplete prior lymph node dissection or no dissection presents with a

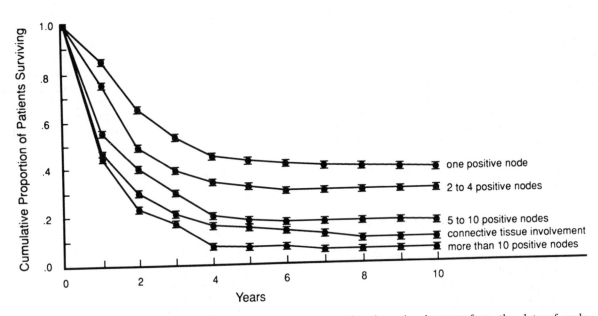

Figure 2 Survival rate by number of positive nodes or connective tissue involvement from the date of node dissection to the date of last follow-up or death. (From Calabro A, Singletary SE, Balch CM. Patterns of relapse in 1001 consecutive patients with melanoma nodal metastases. Arch Surg 1989; 124:1,051–1,055; with permission.)

"skipped" metastasis to an adjacent nodal basin. Usually these recurrences can be excised in continuity with a lymph node dissection of the nearby nodal basin. For example, if a patient presents with a nodal metastasis in the infraclavicular region from a primary melanoma on the shoulder, an axillary node dissection should be performed in addition to excision of the infraclavicular nodal metastasis. If the recurrence represents multiple positive nodes or invasion into adjacent structures, however, surgical resection can be confined to the area of involvement and the use of adjuvant irradiation to yield better local disease control can be considered. The use of radical surgery, e.g., forequarter amputation or hemipelvectomy, should be very limited. The anticipated benefit of relieving symptoms should substantially exceed the risk of the operation itself, and the goal of prolonging life should not severely limit the patient's quality of life.

Of 1,001 patients who underwent regional node dissection for histologically positive melanoma metastases at M. D. Anderson Cancer Center, tumor recurrence within the regional nodal basin (Table 4) occurred in 162 patients: 17 percent of 287 who had cervical node dissections, 15 percent of 438 with axillary dissections, and 17 percent of 276 with inguinal or ilioinguinal dissections. The two factors that had an independent and statistically significant correlation with recurrence were the number of nodal metastases ($P = 0.00001$) and the presence or absence of connective tissue involvement ($P = 0.001$). Recurrence within the previously dissected nodal basin occurred in 9 percent of 360 patients with 1 positive node, 15 percent of 340 patients with 2 to 4 positive nodes, 17 percent of 130 patients with 5 to 10 positive nodes, 33 percent of 100 patients with more than 10 positive nodes, and 29 percent of 71 patients with matted nodes. Of 113 patients who had tumor involvement of the surrounding connective tissue, 28 percent relapsed within the node-

dissection field, compared with 15 percent of patients without involvement of tissues surrounding the nodes. Clinical decision making regarding surgical treatment options requires judgment about whether the potential benefits outweigh the risks for an individual melanoma patient. Of the 162 patients in the M. D. Anderson series who developed recurrence within the nodal basin after node dissection, the 5- and 10-year survival rates were only 11 percent and 5 percent, respectively.

INTRANSIT METASTASES

Metastases from malignant melanoma that arise in the lymphatics or soft tissues between the site of the primary melanoma and the first major regional nodal basin have been termed *intransits*. Arbitrary definitions of the distance from the primary site for a metastasis to be described as an intransit, a satellite, or a local recurrence have created confusion in previous staging systems and in the evaluation of treatment modalities. For example, intransits occurring within 3 cm or 5 cm from a primary melanoma site were defined as "satellites" according to the definitions of individual institutions. A multifactorial analysis of 135 melanoma patients presenting with regional cutaneous metastases at M. D. Anderson Cancer Center demonstrated that the distance from the primary site was not the key prognostic factor in patient outcome. The most important predictor of survival was the histologic location of the intransit (Fig. 3). Patients whose intransit metastases were confined to the subcutaneous tissue had a more virulent disease than patients who had intradermal intransits. Age at diagnosis, site of the primary melanoma, and the number or size of intransits did not affect the patient's prognosis in this study. However, in the Tulane Medical Center series, the number of intransits was significant: patients with four or fewer lesions had a better outcome than those with five or more. The presence of concomitant regional nodal metastases was also associated with a lower survival rate, dependent on the number of positive nodes.

Currently, intransits occur in relatively few melanoma patients, approximately 2 to 3 percent. The previously reported occurrence rates of 10 to 20 percent indicate that most melanomas treated in the 1960s and early 1970s were thicker, more ulcerated, and often associated with nodal metastases — all risk factors for the development of intransits.

Although intransit metastasis is often a signal of potential distant disease, an individual patient may derive palliation and sometimes cure from aggressive local therapy. Treatment options depend on the number, anatomic location, size, and distribution of intransits; the presence of disease at other sites; and the medical condition of the patient.

Isolated limb perfusion with regional chemotherapy and hyperthermia is probably the most effective treatment for extremity intransits. However, patients with large skin-grafted defects that are greater than one-third

Table 4 Incidence of Regional Nodal Basin Recurrence After Node Dissection in 1,001 Melanoma Patients According to Extent of Nodal Involvement

Risk Factor	Patients with Recurrence in Nodal Basin (%)	P Value
No. of positive nodes*		
1 only	9	
2–4	15	<0.05*
5–10	17	<0.05*
>10	33	<0.0005*
Matted	29	<0.001*
Extranodal disease		
Absent	15	
Present	28	<0.001

*Pairwise comparison with one positive node.
From Calabro A, Singletary SE, Balch CM. Patterns of relapse in 1001 consecutive patients with melanoma nodal metastases. Arch Surg 1989; 124: 1,051–1,055; with permission.

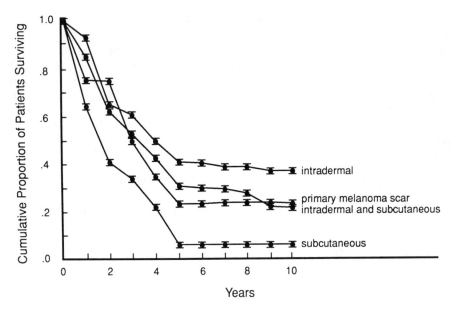

Figure 3 Patient survival from the date of treatment of regional cutaneous metastases to the date of last follow-up visit or death, categorized by the histologic location of metastases: intradermal, primary melanoma scar, intradermal and subcutaneous, and subcutaneous. (From Singletary SE, Tucker SL, Boddie AW. Multivariate analysis of prognostic factors in regional cutaneous metastases of extremity melanoma. Cancer 1988; 61:1,437–1,440; with permission.)

of the extremity circumference are not suitable candidates because the skin graft may function as a tourniquet if postperfusion edema of the extremity develops. Similarly, technical difficulties in cannulating the vessels of patients with severe arteriosclerotic disease may occur with possible disruption of calcified plaques.

Another alternative is the use of intra-arterial chemotherapy infusion via percutaneous angiography. The experience at M. D. Anderson Cancer Center with intra-arterial infusion of cisplatin alone or with dacarbazine as salvage therapy demonstrated an overall response rate of 37 percent. However, most of the responses were partial remissions of short duration, and the rate was comparable to response rates from 9 percent to 42.5 percent reported for the intravenous administration of similar drug regimens. The best long-term results were seen in those patients who responded to infusion chemotherapy and then subsequently underwent surgical excision.

Another regional modality that may provide significant palliative benefit with occasional prolonged regional control is the use of high-dose radiation (greater than 4 Gy per fraction). Hyperthermia of 42°C to 43°C prior to or during radiotherapy may enhance the response rate. Current studies include the use of radiosensitizers such as misonidazole or the specific targeting of melanoma cells to spare normal tissue destruction. For example, thermal neutron therapy utilizes boron-10 to absorb thermal neutrons in melanoma cells by conjugation with compounds, such as chlorpromazine, that have a high affinity for melanin.

Recent progress in the immunobiologic study of melanoma may also provide more innovative approaches such as melanoma-specific tumor cell vaccines, activated tumor-infiltrating lymphocytes, or immunotoxic conjugates against melanoma-associated antigens.

Systemic chemotherapy with dacarbazine or in combination with other drugs has shown little effect in maintaining control of disease. Although amputation of an extremity is seldom indicated, radical surgery may often provide effective palliation for the patient who has severe symptoms such as pain, bleeding, and odor from uncontrollable tumor burden. Aggressive regional treatment of intransits has resulted in median survival rates ranging from 19 months to 42 months, but the majority of patients eventually succumb to systemic metastases.

RESECTABLE DISTANT METASTASES

The goals of surgical excision of distant metastases are relief of symptoms, prolongation of life, and clinical staging to determine subsequent treatment. The anticipated benefit should exceed the operative risk of the surgery itself. The obvious limitation of surgery is that it is a local form of therapy and, therefore, should be confined to lesions that are accessible and limited in number and to selected patients on whom the operation can be safely performed.

Lung Metastases

Surgical excision of solitary pulmonary metastases in asymptomatic patients may be indicated if the tumor has a relatively slow growth rate and whole-lung tomograms or computed tomography (CT) scans demonstrate no other disease. The median survival following this procedure ranges from 16 to 24 months, with 5-year survival rates of 12 to 21 percent. The operation is usually safe, with a 1 percent mortality, but patients should be carefully selected because only a minority will benefit. Another indication for thoracotomy is to confirm that a solitary lesion does not represent a second primary malignancy or a benign process.

The extent of resection is determined by the location and number of metastases and the pulmonary function status. A wedge or segmental resection is usually sufficient, but a lobectomy may be required for larger or more central lesions or if a primary lung carcinoma is found. A pneumonectomy is rarely indicated.

Brain Metastases

For solitary and surgically accessible brain metastases, a craniotomy is a relatively safe procedure (operative mortality of approximately 5 percent) that alleviates symptoms in most patients and prevents further neurologic damage. Caution should be used to prevent tumor spillage because metastases in the scalp incision occur in about 10 percent of patients. Corticosteroids and whole-brain irradiation are generally used postoperatively.

Survival is determined by the neurologic status at the time of surgery and by the presence of metastases at other sites. The average survival after surgery is 6 months, with a range from 2 to 20 months. Rarely, a few patients will live 3 to 5 years or longer after surgery.

Gastrointestinal Metastases

Surgery is usually the only alternative for most patients with the acute complications of obstruction, perforation, or massive bleeding caused by gastrointestinal metastases. The decision to operate depends on the patient's overall clinical condition, but symptoms can be successfully alleviated in most cases, with an average survival of 4 to 8 months. In a few patients, surgical excision of symptomatic isolated gastric or intestinal metastases has achieved survival of up to 2 to 5 years.

Obstruction is usually caused by large polypoid submucosal lesions that mechanically obstruct the bowel or act as the lead point for intussusception. These lesions can usually be excised with a limited bowel resection or, depending on the site and number of lesions, through enterotomies. In patients with extensive disease, only lesions causing immediate symptoms should be removed or bypassed.

Massive or repeated episodes of hemorrhage requiring transfusions are uncommon and most likely are due to gastric metastases. Repeated transfusions for continued hemorrhage burden both patient and physician with the difficult decision of when to suspend treatment. Partial gastrectomy or sometimes a more extended operation may often provide the best and quickest form of palliation.

Skin, Subcutaneous Tissue, or Distant Lymph Node Metastases

Surgical excision is the treatment of choice for isolated distant metastases in the skin, subcutaneous tissues, and lymph nodes. Sequential metastases in these areas may also be effectively treated by surgery unless the lesions become numerous or appear in short succession or in surgically inaccessible sites. In this situation, palliative irradiation for regional control may be considered.

SUGGESTED READING

Balch CM, Houghton A, Peters L. Cutaneous melanoma. In: DeVita VT, ed. Cancer: Principles and practice of oncology. 3rd ed. Philadelphia: JB Lippincott, 1989:1,499–1,542.

Balch CM, Milton GW, eds. Cutaneous melanoma: Clinical management and treatment results worldwide. Philadelphia: JB Lippincott, 1985.

Calabro A, Singletary SE, Balch CM. Patterns of relapse in 1001 consecutive patients with melanoma nodal metastases. Arch Surg 1989; 124:1,051–1,055.

Feun LG, Gutterman J, Burgess MA, et al. The natural history of resectable metastatic melanoma (stage IV A melanoma). Cancer 1982; 50:1,656–1,663.

Singletary SE, Tucker SL, Boddie AW. Multivariate analysis of prognostic factors in regional cutaneous metastases of extremity melanoma. Cancer 1988; 61:1,437–1,440.

Veronesi I, Cascinelli N, Adamus J, et al. Thin stage I primary cutaneous malignant melanoma: Comparison of excision with margins of 1 or 3 cm. N Engl J Med 1988; 318:1,159–1,162.

SARCOMA: SURGERY

F. KRISTIAN STORM, M.D., F.A.C.S.

Soft-tissue sarcomas account for approximately 1 percent of solid cancers, with an incidence of 2 per 100,000, that effect 6,000 individuals in the United States per year. These tumors are characterized by their aggressive local behavior and are among the most difficult malignancies to eradicate at their primary site. Moreover, prognosis is often dependent on whether or not a local recurrence develops. Because the presence of local recurrence more than doubles the likelihood that a person will die of the disease, and because nearly two-thirds of patients who develop distant metastases are found to have concomitant local recurrence, initial treatment of the primary lesion is of paramount importance.

Although the treatment of sarcomas should be multimodal, the role of surgery and appropriate surgical techniques in this tumor cannot be overstated and should be well understood by the practitioner undertaking the care of such patients.

STAGING

The staging of soft-tissue sarcomas is unique. With the exceptions of regional and distant involvements, the histopathologic *grade* of the tumor (based on cytologic criteria, number of mitoses, and the degree of necrosis) determines the *stage* of the patient (Table 1). As a working construct, grade 1 tumors (G1) are considered

low grade and grade 2 (G2) and grade 3 (G3) high grade, and the corresponding patients are considered at low or high risk for local recurrence and metastases. The grade of malignancy has greater bearing on treatment planning and prognosis than the histopathologic variety of sarcoma. In general, tumors of the same grade are managed similarly, irrespective of their apparent cell of origin.

Although staging applies to all patients, the location of the tumor is the determinant of presentation, evaluation, biopsy technique, and operative management.

EXTREMITY SARCOMA

Presentation and Differential Diagnosis

Patients with soft-tissue sarcoma most often present with a painless mass of weeks to many months in duration. There is often a history of trauma or "muscle strain" that has led to a delay in diagnosis. Soft-tissue masses that are firm, fixed to underlying or adjacent tissue, or recently increasing in size should be biopsied immediately. It should be underscored that traumatic intramuscular hematomas should virtually resolve within 6 weeks; failure of resolution should raise suspicion of bleeding or necrosis within a soft-tissue tumor, warranting biopsy.

A rare but important presentation of sarcoma is "spontaneous pneumothorax" in an otherwise apparently healthy individual. Sarcomas most frequently metastasize to the lung, often only to the periphery of the lung, which is not well visualized on plain chest radiograph or chest tomograms and can result in disruption of the visceral pleura and tension pneumothorax. A blood-tinged effusion should raise concern, and once the lung is re-expanded, a computed tomography (CT) scan of the chest should be obtained to look

Table 1 Clinical Staging of Sarcoma*

Patient Stage	Tumor Grade (G)†	Tumor Size (T)†	Lymph Nodes (N)	Distant Metastases (M)
IA	G1	T_1	N_0	M_0
IB	G1	T_2	N_0	M_0
IIA	G2	T_1	N_0	M_0
IIB	G2	T_2	N_0	M_0
IIIA	G3	T_1	N_0	M_0
IIIB	G3	T_2	N_0	M_0
IIIC	Any G	Any T	N_1	M_0
IVA	Any G	Any T	Any N	Bone, nerve, vessel invasion
IVB	Any G	Any T	Any N	M_1

*This table depicts the original American Joint Committee on Cancer Staging clinical staging system (1977), upon which most of the trials to date have been based. Histopathologic tumor grade determined patient stage: G1, G2, and G3 tumors were stage I, II and III patients, respectively. Tumors 5 cm or smaller were substage A; tumors larger than 5 cm were substage B. Patients with lymph node metastases were stage IIIC; those with bone, nerve, and vessel invasion, IVA; and those with distant metastases, IVB.

The second edition of the staging system (1983) used T_3 to denote tumors with bone, nerve, or vessel invasion.

The current third edition (1988) has eliminated the T_3 designation. Stage IIIC has also been eliminated, and N_1 now categorizes a case as stage IVA. Stage IVA has been redefined as any G, any T, N_1, M_0. Stage IVB remains M_1. Tumors that invade local structures are not separately specified.

†Tumor characteristics: G1 = well-differentiated, low-grade; G2 = moderately, well differentiated, intermediate-grade; G3 = poorly differentiated, undifferentiated, high-grade; T_1 = ≤ 5 cm; T_2 = >5 cm.

for small peripheral metastatic nodules. Effusion cytology in this setting is rarely helpful.

Biopsy Technique

Fine-needle aspiration biopsy or core-needle biopsy (Tru-Cut) is rarely useful in the diagnosis of primary soft-tissue masses. An open biopsy is usually required to provide an adequate tissue sample to evaluate these tumors fully, which tend to be histologically heterogeneous within the same specimen.

Open biopsy of a suspected sarcoma should always be performed in the operating room. The principle of open biopsy of such masses involves obtaining a representative sample of the most viable part of the neoplasm with minimal disruption of tissue planes. The biopsy incision should always be placed in the long axis of the extremity and carefully situated such that the biopsy site can be widely excised and incorporated within a subsequent wide excision should it prove necessary. Sarcomas tend to be vascular, and strict attention needs to be given to thorough hemostasis to prevent regional seeding of tumor cells along an expanding hematoma.

A frozen section should be obtained on a portion of the sample to assure that viable and diagnostic tissue has been obtained for paraffin section evaluation. "Touch preps" and a portion of fresh tissue fixed for electron microscopy should be requested.

Preoperative Work-up

Once the diagnosis of soft-tissue sarcoma is made, an orderly evaluation of the patient should be undertaken to evaluate local, regional, and distant sites of potential tumor spread. A CT scan with contrast is required for all deep lesions. A magnetic resonance imaging (MRI) scan usually provides additional useful information in surgical planning, and an arteriogram can be helpful in selected patients. A careful physical examination of regional lymph nodes is mandatory because a few percent of high-grade lesions will manifest clinically positive nodal metastases warranting lymphadenectomy. A bone scan may disclose rare synchronous asymptomatic bone metastases. A CT scan of the chest is mandatory for full evaluation of the lung, the most common site of metastatic disease.

Neoadjuvant Therapy

Neoadjuvant (preoperative) multimodality therapy should be considered in the treatment plan of any intermediate or high-grade soft-tissue sarcoma (G2 and G3 lesions) and in adequately treated recurrent lesions regardless of grade.

Preoperative chemotherapy and radiotherapy have been shown to reduce significantly the incidence of local recurrence (Table 2). Although various protocols exist, there is a substantial body of evidence supporting the use of intra-arterial or intravenous adriamycin (90 mgm total dose) followed by 350 cGy $\times$ 8 (2,800 cGy total dose) immediately before surgery. This frequently results in tumor shrinkage and reduction in tumor viability. It is believed to enhance local resectability as well as improve local disease eradication.

Operative Technique

Surgery, with the aid of neoadjuvant chemotherapy and preoperative or postoperative radiotherapy, can lead to salvage of more than 95 percent of limbs.

Table 2 Results of Surgery for Sarcomas in Extremities

	Year	No. of Patients	Local Recurrence (%)	Limb Salvage (%)	Complications (%)	Complications Requiring Surgery (%)	Wound Slough (%)	Fractures (%)	Follow Up (median)	Irradiation Dose (cGy)
Amputation	1972–1976	21	3/21 (14)	0						
Wide excision	1972–1976	11	4/11 (36)	?	14/63 (22)					
Excision and irradiation	1972–1976	31	7/31 (23)	?						2.6 × 30
Preoperatively, 35 Gy and IA adriamycin	1974–1984	77	4/77 (5)	74/77 (96)	33/77 (43)	18/77 (23)	15/77 (20)	8/77 (10)	96 mo	3.5 × 10
Preoperatively, 17.5 Gy and IA adriamycin	1981–1984	137	17/137 (12)	130/137 (95)	35/137 (26)	8/137 (6)		2/137 (2)	48 mo	3.5 × 5
Preoperatively, 28 Gy and IA adriamcyin	1984–1987	97	5/97 (5)	95/97 (98)	23/97 (24)	10/97 (10)			24 mo	3.5 × 8
Preoperatively, 28 Gy and IA adriamycin	1984–1988	44	3/44 (7)	43/44 (98)	8/44 (18)				36 mo	3.5 × 8
versus										
Preoperatively, 28 Gy and IV adriamycin		52	5/52 (8)	52/52 (100)	5/52 (10)					

Adapted from Eilber, FR. (UCLA Medical School), 1990; with permission.

Successful surgery depends on complete knowledge of the three-dimensional anatomy of the area treated and a thorough understanding of the locoregional biology of the tumor itself. Sarcomas are "pushing" tumors that traverse along fascial planes and muscle bundles, and along nerves and vessels. Although neurovascular structures are themselves rarely invaded, the perineurium or adventitia may be the only excision margin, and it should be removed meticulously en bloc with the specimen.

Enucleation

Enucleation, also known as intralesional debulking, limited-margin excision, or, more commonly, shelling out of tumor, is mentioned only to be condemned. Sarcomas are characterized by a pseudocapsule that unfortunately lends itself to this inappropriate procedure; however, it should be underscored that this capsule is comprised of compressed, alive tumor cells that are, in fact, the most viable and, thus, the most virulent portion of the tumor. Violation of this plane should be considered in only the smallest and most superficial of lesions, and then only for purposes of diagnosis (excisional biopsy) and never as definitive surgical therapy. Enucleation alone results in 100 percent local recurrence.

Wide Excision

Wide excision, also referred to as monobloc excision, tridimensional excision, or radical excision of sarcoma, encompasses the prior biopsy site and the tumor plus a variable and undefined margin of surrounding normal soft tissue. In practice, 10-cm proximal and distal margins, with at least one normal muscle or fascial barrier between the greatest extent of the tumor and the resection plane, are sought-after goals. One should realize that essential neurovascular structures may limit these margins in some areas. Although preoperative neoadjuvant therapy may well have rendered these margins sterile, the surgeon is encouraged to employ frozen sections liberally on close margins or else sacrifice these structures in lieu of function. This form of resection is designed to provide total tumor removal while preserving a useful extremity, and it relies heavily on the contribution of multimodal therapy. However, the surgeon should be prepared to resect significant portions of major muscle groups and have a clear concept of the functional outcome of his or her undertaking.

Compartment Resection

Compartment resection, also known as muscle group resection, is an en bloc removal of all adjacent muscle bundles from origin to insertion. This operation is now used rarely, and then only when several contiguous muscle groups are involved with tumor or tumor has invaded neurovascular structures or bone, or when one is dealing with recurrent tumor after failed multimodality therapy. Functional deficits are often significant.

Amputation

Amputation is reserved for medically debilitated or infirm patients who cannot withstand a lengthy operative procedure and a demanding postoperative rehabilitative program. It is also used for local palliation of symptoms in selected patients with refractory or inoperable metastatic disease.

Results of Therapy

Surgery Alone

Surgical resection as a single treatment modality results in an unacceptably high incidence of local recurrence that usually results in the death of the patient. Experience from patients treated with surgery alone into the late 1960s indicated local recurrence rates from 50 to 90 percent, which provoked surgeons to use amputation more frequently as the standard of care. Even with amputative therapy, however, minimum local recurrence rates in the stump remained at least 15 percent, indicating the need for other treatment options.

Combination Surgery and Radiotherapy

The addition of radiation therapy, in the forms of brachytherapy or external-beam therapy, has reduced significantly the incidence of local recurrence, particularly for smaller lesions distal to the elbow or knee. Preoperative or postoperative adjuvant radiotherapy is indicated in patients with intermediate and high-grade soft-tissue sarcomas and in selected cases of low-grade tumors (see the following chapter, *Sarcoma: Combined-Modality Approaches*).

Combination Surgery and Neoadjuvant Chemoradiotherapy

Over the past decade, limb salvage surgery with an acceptably low incidence of local recurrence has been associated with the use of preoperative intra-arterial adriamycin and radiation. A recent prospective randomized trial indicates that the drug may be given intravenously without compromising treatment. The incidence of local recurrence and the number of wound complications appear to be highly dependent on radiation dose (see Table 2).

TRUNCAL SARCOMA

Sarcomas arising within the body wall, shoulder girdle, and pelvic girdle should be treated similarly to soft-tissue tumors in extremities, with curative intent. The role of neoadjuvant therapy is less well defined for tumors arising within these areas, but this therapy is frequently employed in anticipation of tumor shrinkage and a reduced incidence of local recurrence, as occurs in extremity sarcomas (see Table 2).

Operatively, chest and abdominal wall resection and reconstruction are often required. Tumors involving the shoulder may require some form of interscapulothoracic amputation in which a functional forearm and hand are preserved. Tumors of the pelvis may require segmental or ipsilateral internal hemipelvectomy, and the surgeon should adhere to the principles of soft-tissue sarcoma surgery outlined earlier, with the intent toward limb salvage. In such patients, consent for amputation is also obtained in the event that the location and extent of the tumor found at operation preclude complete resection or necessitate removal of vital neurovascular structures that would render the limb insensate and otherwise functionally useless.

RETROPERITONEAL SARCOMA

Presentation and Differential Diagnosis

In combined series of patients with a retroperitoneal neoplasm (n = 675), 18 percent have proved to be benign and 82 percent malignant, a 4:1 ratio favoring the likelihood of cancer in a patient presenting with an isolated retroperitoneal tumor. Of those with cancer, 55 percent were sarcoma, with the remaining 45 percent representing lymphoma, urogenital malignancy, or some less common cancer.

A palpable mass is present in 80 to 90 percent of patients who frequently present with vague, poorly localized abdominal discomfort and increasing abdominal girth. Neurologic symptoms from nerve root compression occur in 30 percent of patients, benign ascites from portal vein obstruction in 15 percent, and various gastrointestinal symptoms from invasion or, more commonly, displacement in 10 percent.

Evaluation of a Retroperitoneal Mass

Based on the initial clinical diagnosis of a retroperitoneal mass, patients should undergo a gastrointestinal series, barium enema, intravenous pyelogram, and chest radiograph to rule out other nonneoplastic etiologies, information that will also prove quite useful if the diagnosis of sarcoma is established later. If suspicion of sarcoma remains high, the patient should undergo abdominal CT scan with contrast to evaluate the location and extent of the mass as well as the proximity or involvement of adjacent organs, and to evaluate the liver (a common site of metastases from retroperitoneal sarcomas). Magnetic resonance imaging may be useful in selected cases. If a primary retroperitoneal tumor appears likely, an aortogram to delineate vascular invasion, vessel displacement, and location of major tumor-feeding vessels is generally indicated. The results of the aortogram may also dictate the need for an inferior vena cavagram. Once these tests have been

performed and the etiology of the mass remains undetermined, biopsy is indicated.

Biopsy Technique

Unfortunately, fine-needle aspiration biopsy and core-needle biopsy are of limited value in the diagnosis of retroperitoneal neoplasms. Laparotomy with a carefully performed open biopsy is almost always necessary to define the nature of the tumor, whether it be sarcoma, lymphoma, a urogenital malignancy, or some rare neoplasm.

The method of biopsy is of utmost importance to prevent contamination of the peritoneal cavity with tumor cells. A wound-edge plastic barrier should be utilized and the tumor bed isolated with an abundance of laparotomy gauze packs. A controlled incisional biopsy should be obtained, and a portion should be frozen to confirm the presence of viable tissue sufficient for diagnosis. If a definitive diagnosis cannot be made on frozen tissue, the patient's incision should be closed to await permanent sections. In any event, the tumor incisional biopsy site should be meticulously closed with thorough hemostasis. Intra-abdominal sarcomatosis virtually never occurs without an antecedent history of biopsy, suggesting a cause-effect relationship that warrants extreme caution to prevent peritoneal tumor seeding during biopsy.

Operative Technique

All histopathologic varieties of sarcoma are found in the retroperitoneum: liposarcoma, 23 percent; fibrosarcoma, 19 percent; leiomyosarcoma, 16 percent; neurosarcoma, 12 percent; undifferentiated sarcoma, 16 percent; and other rarer sarcomas, 14 percent (data from combined series, n = 449). Retroperitoneal sarcomas are characterized by their aggressive local behavior and involvement with contiguous organs and structures. Unlike soft-tissue sarcomas of the extremities, that generally remain confined within fascial barriers and muscle groups, sarcomas arising within the retroperitoneum are invariably large and uncontained.

Preoperative preparation of the patient should include a complete oral antibiotic bowel prep, systemic antibiotics, correction of attendant anemia to a hematocrit of 40 percent, and adequate blood availability, in anticipation of major organ resections and potentially massive intraoperative blood loss. A preoperative intravenous pyelogram should show bilateral functioning kidneys in the event of ipsilateral nephrectomy, and the location of ureters may need to be defined by preoperative stent placement. A nasogastric tube, bladder catheter, central venous access, and arterial monitoring are mandatory.

Patients undergoing definitive resection of a retroperitoneal sarcoma should be approached either through a long midline incision from xyphoid to pubis or through a diagonal "saber-slash" incision across the midline traversing the flank, either of which may be extended into the chest. A flank approach is contraindicated because the vascular supply to these tumors invariably arises from midline vessels, which should be controlled at the start of the procedure. The first maneuver in determining resectability frequently requires determination of a free dissection plane adjacent to the aorta (left-sided tumors) or vena cava (right-sided tumors) extended dorsally through the ileopsoas muscles adjacent to the spine. This will determine whether the tumor has traversed along lumbar vessels or nerves through the spinal foramen into the dural space, which may mitigate against curative resection. Because tumor compression results in extensive venous collaterals, the lower inferior vena cava can ordinarily be resected with impunity; however, a subadventitial dissection of aorta or cava is usually possible.

The surgeon must be prepared to undertake major organ resections, not infrequently including the hemidiaphragm, stomach, pancreas, colon, liver, kidney, and so forth. Dissection should always be in normal tissue. The tumor should never be compressed, because dehiscence may occur through cystic or necrotic areas. Aspiration of large cystic areas may facilitate resection, but this should be done through a double purse-string suture and an aspirating trocar under high vacuum to prevent tumor spill and seeding of the peritoneum.

Reconstruction of the diaphragm, chest, and abdominal wall often requires interposition of synthetic mesh and creative plastic surgery that exploits the available anatomy.

Results

Surgery Alone

From combined series of patients explored for retroperitoneal sarcoma (n = 360), 30 percent have been found to be unresectable and underwent biopsy only, 20 percent were partially resectable, and only 50 percent had complete resection of all gross tumor. The basis of unresectability has included the extent of the tumor, sarcomatosis or malignant ascites, nerve root or major vascular involvement (e.g., superior mesenteric artery), pelvic sidewall involvement, bone invasion, or hepatic metastases.

In patients who were completely resected (combined series, n = 204), 90 percent had disease recurrence. Life table analysis showed 40 percent recurrence by 2 years, 70 percent by 5 years, and 90 percent by 10 years; 85 percent had local disease recurrence, and 35 percent had distant metastases, generally to liver or lung. Local recurrence almost invariably resulted in the death of the patient.

These data confirm the locally aggressive nature of sarcomas arising within the retroperitoneum and indicate the need for more comprehensive locoregional therapy.

Combination Surgery and Radiotherapy

Radiotherapy for unresected (biopsy only) and partially resected patients has had little impact on outcome. Adjuvant radiotherapy in patients who have had resection of all gross disease has, to date, shown essentially no benefit.

Combination Surgery and Neoadjuvant Chemoradiotherapy

Preoperative intravenous adriamycin (90 mgm total dose over 3 days) and 3,500 to 4,000 cGy (standard fraction) are being studied in an attempt to reduce local recurrence and, thus, enhance survival; however, data are too preliminary for conclusions to be drawn.

PULMONARY METASTASES

Surgery may be of benefit in selected patients with lung metastases from soft-tissue sarcoma. Unfortunately, recurrence of the primary tumor is often heralded by pulmonary metastases; thus, complete re-evaluation of the primary site should be undertaken if distant metastases become evident. Wedge or segmental resection is the operation performed most frequently; 30 to 40 percent 5-year survival is expected. The major determinant of prognosis after resection is the tumor doubling time (TDT) of the pulmonary nodules. With a slow TDT of greater than 40 days, median survival has been as high as 44 months. With a rapid TDT of less than 20 days median survival is only 14 months, not unlike unresected disease. Studies are in progress to evaluate rapidly growing tumors that respond to chemotherapy with prolongation of TDT followed by resection. Unpublished reports indicate that some cases benefit from this approach, but statistics are not yet available. It is clear, however, that even isolated lung metastases with a short TDT that are refractory to chemotherapy do not benefit from pulmonary resection. Pulmonary resection of metastatic disease should also never be undertaken until complete remission of the primary sarcoma has been assured.

SUGGESTED READING

Arlen M, Marcove R, eds. Surgical management of soft-tissue sarcomas. Philadelphia: WB Saunders, 1987.

Eilber F, Morton D, eds. Soft-tissue sarcomas. Orlando: Grune & Stratton, 1987.

Karakousis C, ed. Soft-tissue sarcomas. Semin Surg Oncol, 1988; 4(1).

Shiu M, Brennan M, eds. Surgical management of soft-tissue sarcoma. Philadelphia: Lea & Febiger, 1989.

Sugarbaker P, Nicholson T, eds. Atlas of extremity sarcoma surgery. Philadelphia: JB Lippincott, 1984.

SARCOMA: COMBINED-MODALITY APPROACHES

TIMOTHY J. KINSELLA, M.D.
REY RODRIGUEZ, M.D.

Soft-tissue sarcomas are malignant neoplasms that arise from mesodermally derived tissues. They are relatively uncommon, with an incidence of 5,700 cases (0.5 percent of new cancer cases) estimated for 1990 in the United States. Because of widespread distribution of soft tissues, sarcomas can arise in a variety of anatomic sites. These tumors have a wide spectrum of histologic types classified on the basis of the putative cell of origin, but they are usually considered together because of similar behavioral characteristics. Treatment and prognosis are based on factors other than histologic subtype. Independent prognostic factors include malignancy grade, tumor size, intratumor vascular invasion, and DNA aneuploidy.

In about 90 percent of cases, sarcomas present as an apparently localized soft-tissue mass with no evidence of metastasis. However, these tumors expand locally, creating a pseudocapsule of the compressed adjacent normal tissue. The pseudocapsule is virtually always invaded by tumor cells, with spread along muscle and fascial planes, blood vessels, and nerves. Because of this, a local recurrence can develop at a surprising distance from the original tumor. High-grade tumors have a propensity for early systemic dissemination, particularly to the lung. These factors account for a substantial mortality (3,100 estimated deaths in 1990 in the United States). Clinical advances in the treatment of soft-tissue sarcomas have been hampered by the difficulty of accruing adequate numbers of patients for prospective, randomized therapeutic trials and by the multiple tumor sites, which influence the treatment options. However, evolution of management during the past decades has resulted in substantial improvement in local control and long-term survival. These improved results are related to more thorough staging, precise radiotherapeutic techniques, and the use of aggressive combined-modality therapy.

SOFT-TISSUE SARCOMAS OF THE EXTREMITIES

Approximately 60 percent of soft-tissue sarcomas occur in the extremities, with lower extremity lesions predominating in a ratio of 3:1 compared to upper extremity tumors. Because these tumors have a pseudocapsule, it often appears that minimal surgical procedures would likely be sufficient for achieving local control. Historically, many patients were treated with limited excision. However, various reports demonstrated unacceptable high local failure rates (50 to 93 percent), and these practices were abandoned. Therefore, a trend developed toward more aggressive surgery, with amputation or radical compartmental excision being adopted as the procedures of choice. These surgical procedures resulted in marked improvement in local failure rates (2 to 34 percent). Unfortunately, significant functional and cosmetic impairment were observed.

With the advent of radiotherapy, it was attempted to use this modality to enhance treatment of sarcomas. Initial results were disappointing because tumors often regressed slowly or incompletely after radiation. These tumors gained the reputation of being "radioresistant." Residual masses at times never changed or regressed slowly after treatment. However, under microscopic examination, these masses could be shown to be sterilized of tumor. Interest returned after it was realized that the tumors were not truly radioresistant; most tumors were simply too large and bulky to be treated with radiation alone without exceeding normal tissue tolerance. Since the pioneering work of Cade in the 1950s, radiation therapy plus limited surgical resection has been used to improve local control. Surgery is used to remove the primary tumor mass, and the radiation is used to treat microscopic tumor extension. This combined approach yields better functional and cosmetic results, with local control rates comparable to or better than those achieved by radical surgery (Table 1).

A number of approaches have been proposed for combined-modality therapy. These include preoperative radiation, postoperative radiation, preoperative radiation with regional chemotherapy, and adjuvant chemotherapy. Although these general strategies are now well established, the precise technique by which to obtain optimal tumor control while minimizing normal tissue morbidity is under active investigation.

Preoperative Radiotherapy

There is a good rationale for preoperative irradiation. Even when treating a large tumor mass, preoperative radiation to a dose of 45 to 50 Gy may inactivate greater than 99 percent (up to 2 logs of cell kill) of the tumor cells. This will decrease the likelihood of tumor implantation during surgery. Also, tumor cells that may

Table 1 Local Control of Sarcomas for Various Treatments*

Treatment	5-Year Local Control (%)
Local resection	7–50
Radical excision	66–98
Preoperative irradiation followed by resection	83–95
Preoperative regional chemotherapy and irradiation followed by resection	82–96
Surgical excision followed by irradiation	78–92

*Data were obtained from various series.

have been shed into the circulation would be unlikely to be viable and to establish distant metastases. With preoperative radiation, the oncologist needs to treat only tissues thought to be at risk for tumor involvement, and radiation fields need not encompass areas to be manipulated by the surgeon, as is the case in postoperative therapy. The largest advantage of preoperative radiation may be that some patients who would have needed an amputation if surgery were done initially may be eligible for conservative treatment. Radiation therapy administered preoperatively may allow the surgeon to decrease the extent of the surgical procedure and to perform a limb-preserving operation. Even if the tumor mass does not decrease in size after irradiation, the tumor may consist pathologically of necrotic debris with little viable tumor. A potential difficulty with preoperative radiation is delayed healing of the surgical wound, although if good surgical and radiotherapeutic techniques are used, primary healing should occur. Several series demonstrate that planned preoperative radiation therapy in patients with high-grade sarcoma can yield excellent results, with 5-year disease-free survival of 56 to 74 percent and local control rates of 83 to 95 percent.

Postoperative Radiotherapy

Postoperative radiotherapy has several theoretical advantages. These include immediate surgery, avoidance of radiation-induced delays in wound healing, and availability of a large specimen for histopathologic investigation with definite interpretation of tumor size and extension. With this technique, however, the initial postoperative treatment volume should include the wound, which is usually a larger volume than would have been treated preoperatively. Several retrospective, single-institution series have been reported utilizing this approach. The 5-year results include a disease-free survival of 60 to 68 percent and a local control rate of 78 to 92 percent. The National Cancer Institute conducted a randomized, prospective trial that evaluated limb-sparing surgery with postoperative radiation and compared it with amputation in patients with high-grade extremity sarcomas. The local control rate was somewhat better for the amputation arm; however, this was not reflected in survival rates. Similar rates of disease-free and overall survival were observed beween groups. In the limb-sparing group, 85 percent of patients maintained a functional limb.

Preoperative Radiotherapy with Regional Chemotherapy

The discovery and clinical application of doxorubicin significantly modified the treatment of soft-tissue sarcomas. Since 1974, Eilber and associates at UCLA have used preoperative intra-arterial doxorubicin and radiation for the management of extremity sarcomas. The rationale for this approach was to deliver regionally an active chemotherapeutic agent that had direct cyto-

toxicity and potential radiosensitization. A total of 344 patients with high-grade extremity soft-tissue sarcomas were treated in sequential protocols. The first protocol consisted of intra-arterial doxorubicin, 30 mg per day, for 3 consecutive days, followed by radiation therapy to a dose of 35 Gy at 3.5 Gy per fraction, followed by surgical resection. Of the 77 patients treated, the local recurrence rate was 6 percent with a minimum follow-up of 7 years. However, the complication rate in this protocol was 35 percent. These complications consisted mainly of bone fractures and wound sloughs. In order to reduce the complications, the second protocol was conducted. This protocol involved 137 patients treated with intra-arterial doxorubicin at the same doses, followed by 17.5 Gy of radiation at 3.5 Gy per fraction. Although the complication rate decreased, the local recurrence rate increased to 13 percent. Therefore, in the third protocol, patients were treated with preoperative doxorubicin, followed by radiation to a dose of 28 Gy. The recurrence rate decreased to 7 percent with a similar rate of complications. In addition, this protocol randomized patients to intra-arterial versus intravenous doxorubicin. There was no difference in the local recurrence rate. Therefore, these protocols showed that there was a dose-response relationship to radiation and that intra-arterial infusion was not superior to the intravenous route. A most recent protocol utilized *cis*-platinum, 120 mg per square meter, followed by doxorubicin infusion and radiation to 28 Gy. The preliminary results showed an improved local recurrence rate of 4 percent. Overall, the limb salvage rate of these protocols has been greater than 96 percent, and the local tumor control is 91 percent.

No clinical trial has compared the "UCLA approach" to conventional fractionated irradiation for extremity sarcomas, but our guess is that it would yield comparable local control, at best, but with poorer extremity function. In light of these concerns, we are reluctant to recommend this approach of preoperative chemoradiotherapy for patients with extremity sarcoma outside of a randomized, prospective trial.

Radiation Therapy Technique

To achieve local control and a good functional result, the radiation treatment must be delivered in a precise manner. A planning computed tomography (CT) scan of the extremity is mandatory. A dose of 60 to 65 Gy (routine fractionation) is commonly prescribed using a shrinking-field technique. The initial field should encompass all areas with a significant probability of microscopic tumor included. We usually treat the whole compartment involved, while avoiding treatment of the entire cross-section of the extremity, which can result in problems with edema, pain, and loss of function. Because extremity sarcomas tend to grow in a longitudinal fashion, often 5 to 10 cm are added beyond the proximal and distal margins of the tumors. We routinely use opposed fields (anteroposterior/posterior-anterior or obliques) and radiation with energies ranging from 4 to 6 mv. Extremity immobilization using customized molds is an important component of radiation treatment planning.

Adjuvant Chemotherapy

Despite adequate local control, a significant proportion of patients (40 to 60 percent) with high-grade soft-tissue sarcomas will ultimately have recurrences and die from metastatic disease, usually in the lung. Adjuvant chemotherapy has been proposed in an effort to eradicate micrometastasis. Several trials have been reported evaluating its role. Only randomized, prospective studies will be presented because the survival in the control arms of randomized studies has been superior to those of historical controls.

There is controversy as to whether single-agent (doxorubicin) or multiagent chemotherapy is superior. Gherlinzoni and colleagues, at the Instituto Orthopedica Rizzoli, randomized patients to receive doxorubicin, 75 mg per square meter, every 3 weeks for six cycles in the adjuvant arm versus observation after primary treatment. With a median follow-up of 28 months in 59 patients, the disease-free survival was 79.1 percent in the adjuvant arm and 54.3 percent in the control arm. A subsequent report confirmed the disease-free advantage (68 percent versus 41.5 percent, $P < 0.02$) and noted a survival advantage as well (87.5 percent versus 67.5 percent, $P < 0.02$).

However, other randomized trials of adjuvant, single-agent doxorubicin in patients with high-grade soft-tissue extremity sarcomas have failed to demonstrate either a significant overall survival or disease-free survival benefit. At UCLA, Eilber and co-workers randomized 119 patients with grade 3 extremity sarcoma to observation versus doxorubicin (450 mg per square meter) given over five monthly cycles after preoperative intra-arterial doxorubicin and radiation therapy. No difference was noted in disease-free survival (58 percent versus 54 percent) and overall survival (84 percent versus 80 percent) after a median follow-up of 28 months. There was a slightly higher frequency of local recurrences in the control group, but this was not statistically significant.

The Scandinavian sarcoma group randomized 240 patients with resectable, localized high-grade sarcomas to adjuvant doxorubicin (60 mg per m^2 for nine cycles) and observation after primary therapy. With a median follow-up of 40 months, there was no significant difference in overall or disease-free survival between groups. Trials conducted at Dana Farber Cancer Institute/ Massachusetts General Hospital and the Eastern Cooperative Oncology Group (ECOG) also showed no survival or disease-free survival benefit in the doxorubicin group.

At the M.D. Anderson Tumor Institute, 47 patients with high-grade sarcoma were randomized to observation versus combination chemotherapy with cyclophosphamide, doxorubicin, vincristine, and actinomycin-D for seven cycles. Primary therapy included conservative

surgical excision and postoperative radiotherapy. The disease-free survival in the chemotherapy group was 85 percent at 2 years, 60 percent at 5 years, and 55 percent at 10 years, which was significantly superior to that of the observation group, which experienced disease-free survival of 57 percent, 35 percent, and 35 percent, respectively. However, overall survival was not significantly improved.

At the National Cancer Institute, 67 patients with extremity sarcomas were randomized to observation versus combination chemotherapy with cyclophosphamide, doxorubicin, methotrexate, and leucovorin rescue after treatment of their primary sarcoma. At 7.1 years median follow-up, the 5-year disease-free survival and overall survival were 75 percent and 82 percent, respectively, in the chemotherapy group; these rates were superior to those seen in the observation group (54 percent and 60 percent, respectively). The high dose of doxorubicin utilized in this trial was associated with significant cardiac toxicity. A subsequent trial comparing the same chemotherapy regimen with a reduced doxorubicin dose and no methotrexate regimen showed no difference in disease-free or overall survival between the two arms. Importantly, treatment-related cardiotoxicity was reduced in the low-dose regimen.

Edmonson and co-workers, from the Mayo Clinic, randomized patients to eight cycles of vincristine, cyclophosphamide, and actinomycin D alternating with vincristine, doxorubicin, and DTIC after complete excision. No radiation therapy was utilized. They noted no survival advantage for the chemotherapy group, although those patients experienced some delay in the development of distant metastasis and required fewer salvage surgical procedures for excision of metastasis. Local failure was 30 percent in the two arms of this study, underscoring the need for adjuvant irradiation.

The European Organization for Research on Treatment of Cancer (EORTC) conducted a multi-institutional study randomizing 225 patients to observation versus combination chemotherapy with CYVADIC (cyclophosphamide, vincristine, doxorubicin, and DTIC) for eight cycles. All patients received postoperative irradiation. The 3-year disease-free survival was 67 percent for the chemotherapy group versus 52 percent for the control patients. However, overall survival was not significantly improved.

In summary, the value of adjuvant chemotherapy for patients with high-grade soft-tissue sarcomas of the extremity is unresolved. Although some trials showed a disease-free survival advantage, other trials have not confirmed these findings. Prolonged survival benefit has not been observed with extended follow-up in any randomized study.

NONEXTREMITY SARCOMAS

Approximately 40 percent of soft-tissue sarcomas occur in nonextremity sites. The surgical approach to these tumors is tempered by the inability to perform an ablative (amputation) or, in some cases, a radical procedure (compartmental resection). Adjacent vital structures often constrain the surgeon to local excision with limited margins of resection. Because of the difficulty with obtaining wide, negative margins, adjuvant therapy is often recommended.

Since 1977, the National Cancer Institute has conducted a randomized, prospective study of patients with high-grade sarcoma of the head and neck, breast, and trunk. Thirty-one patients were randomized after surgical resection and postoperative radiotherapy to adjuvant combination chemotherapy (doxorubicin, cyclophosphamide, and methotrexate) versus observation. The results revealed a 3-year actuarial disease-free survival in the chemotherapy arm of 77 percent compared to 49 percent in the control group ($P = 0.075$). There was no significant benefit in overall survival. Subset analysis demonstrated that the group of patients with sarcoma of the trunk demonstrated the greatest benefit from chemotherapy.

Retroperitoneal tumors are more difficult to manage. Most of these tumors are large (greater than 10 cm) and locally advanced at diagnosis. They surround vital structures, which often precludes satisfactory wide excision. In addition, adjacent radiosensitive organs, particularly the bowel and kidneys, limit the delivery of postoperative radiotherapy to significant doses. At the National Cancer Institute, combined-modality studies were performed with resectable soft-tissue sarcomas of the retroperitoneum. After surgical resection and high-dose postoperative radiation, 15 patients were randomized to receive or not receive adjuvant doxorubicin, cytoxan, and methotrexate. The 2-year actuarial survival, disease-free survival, or locoregional control was not improved in the chemotherapy arm. In addition, there was significant morbidity, primarily related to bowel injury.

In an attempt to improve locoregional control and reduce bowel injury associated with external-beam radiation, a randomized, prospective trial was carried out comparing postoperative conventional high-dose external-beam radiation therapy (50 to 55 Gy) versus intraoperative radiation (20 Gy) plus low-dose external-beam radiation (35 to 40 Gy). Intraoperative radiation was used at the time of surgery and permitted a high single dose of electron-beam therapy to be delivered directly to the tumor bed after moving as many incidental structures as possible out of the radiation field. The therapy in the intraoperative arm was better tolerated with less acute toxicity. At 5-year follow-up, there was a trend towards an improved in-field local control in the experimental arm. However, no improvement in disease-free or overall survival was seen.

NONRESECTABLE SARCOMAS

When soft-tissue sarcomas are judged to be technically unresectable, or when the patient is medically inoperable, such patients are treated with palliative intent by many physicians. The rationale behind this strategy is partially based on the traditional belief that soft-tissue sarcomas are radioresistant. In 1951, Sir Stanford Cade was among the first to report encouraging results in the treatment of sarcoma by radiation alone. Subsequently, others have shown that radiation therapy alone can achieve local control in patients with sarcomas. Tepper and Suit treated 36 patients with radiation alone. The 5-year overall survival rate was 28 percent, and local control was 44 percent. There was an inverse relationship between tumor size and the ability to obtain tumor control. It was concluded that local control can be achieved by radiation alone but that it usually requires aggressive treatment with very high doses of radiation, which carry significant risk of adverse sequelae.

At the National Cancer Institute, in an attempt to improve tumor response and minimize late, radiation-induced complications, patients with unresectable sarcomas were treated with hyperfractionated, high-dose external-beam radiation (65 to 75 cGy in twice-daily fractions over 7 to 9 weeks) combined with continuous infusion of iododeoxyuridine, a nonhypoxic radiosensitizer. Of the 28 patients treated, 5 had complete tumor response, 14 had a partial objective response, and in 6 patients, the tumor size remained stable. Local tumor control that lasted for the patients' remaining life was achieved in 17 of 28 patients. It seems that radiotherapy alone for selected patients with unresectable (or inoperable) sarcoma can result in local control. Although preliminary results of hyperfractionated external-beam radiation and radiosensitizers are encouraging, their definite role awaits the results of controlled, randomized trials that are just beginning.

SUGGESTED READING

Chang AE, Kinsella T, Glatstein E, et al. Adjuvant chemotherapy for patients with high-grade soft-tissue sarcomas of the extremity. J Clin Oncol 1988; 6:1,491–1,500.

Eilber FR, Morton DL, Eckhardt T, et al. Limb salvage for skeletal and soft-tissue sarcomas: Multidisciplinary preoperative therapy. Cancer 1984; 53:2,579–2,584.

Glenn J, Kinsella T, Glatstein E, et al. A randomized prospective trial of adjuvant chemotherapy in adults with soft-tissue sarcomas of the head and neck, breast and trunk. Cancer 1985; 55:1,206–1,214.

Glenn J, Sindelar WF, Kinsella T, et al. Results of multimodality therapy of resectable soft-tissue sarcomas of the retroperitoneum. Surgery 1985; 97:316–324.

Kinsella TJ, Glatstein E. Clinical experience with intravenous radiosensitizers in unresectable sarcomas. Cancer 1987; 59:908–915.

Kinsella TJ, Sindelar WF, Lack E, et al. Preliminary results of a randomized study of adjuvant radiation therapy in resectable adult retroperitoneal soft-tissue sarcomas. J Clin Oncol 1988; 6:18–25.

Rosenberg SA, Tepper J, Glatstein E, et al. Prospective randomized evaluations of (1) limb-sparing surgery plus radiation therapy compared with amputation and (2) the role of adjuvant chemotherapy. Ann Surg 1982; 196:305–315.

Suit H, Proppe K, Mankin M, et al. Preoperative radiation therapy for sarcoma of soft tissue. Cancer 1981; 47:2,269–2,274.

SARCOMA: CHEMOTHERAPY

MARK M. ZALUPSKI, M.D.
LAURENCE H. BAKER, D.O.

The treatment of patients with soft-tissue sarcoma presents a significant challenge because of a number of factors associated with this tumor. Soft-tissue sarcoma is uncommon, accounting for only 1 percent of all cancers diagnosed annually in the United States. Yet, within this group of uncommon cancers, there is great heterogeneity in behavior. Soft-tissue sarcoma occurs in patients of all ages, and in all body sites, in a sometimes confusing variety of histologies and histopathologic grades. Physicians in surgery, orthopedics, radiation oncology, pathology, and pediatric and medical oncology are all involved in the treatment of this disease. The intent of therapy in the majority of patients with soft-tissue sarcoma is curative, but the cancer can be fatal, and there is increased morbidity and mortality when soft-tissue sarcoma is managed inappropriately. This variety of histologies and presentations, in association with its rarity, places soft-tissue sarcoma among the least well understood and poorly treated of all cancers.

Progress made in the management of this tumor has primarily resulted from the establishment of centers with a particular interest in this group of diseases that emphasize a multidisciplinary approach to treatment. The creation of sarcoma intergroups to develop and direct clinical trials has led to improvements in the therapy of this disease. Nevertheless, despite progress, the prognosis of patients with these diseases, especially metastatic disease, has not improved markedly.

Efforts to further improve the care of patients with sarcomas focus on continued entry and participation in clinical trials. Clinical trials offer the best treatment strategies for patients with these diseases and should be considered in every instance. Identification and development of new therapies is only possible through the process of clinical trials. Finally, basic research into the biology of these cancers, which will translate into major progress in the fundamental understanding of this disease, is facilitated by referral and entry into clinical trials.

PATHOLOGY AND PROGNOSTIC FACTORS

The histologic classification of soft-tissue sarcomas is based on the benign mesenchymal counterpart of the presumed malignant cell of origin. Inconsistencies in this classification and variation in the reported frequency of sarcoma types are due to interobserver differences in assignment of type and the existence of sarcomas that remain unclassified. Although the histologic type of soft-tissue sarcoma is associated with patient prognosis, it appears that the histologic grade of the tumor is of greater significance.

A number of investigators have shown strong correlations with histopathologic grade and disease-free interval and overall survival for specific histologic types and within mixed series of soft-tissue sarcomas. The importance of histopathologic grade was recognized by a task force on the staging of this disease that recommended the inclusion of grade into the staging system. Histopathologists assign sarcoma grade based on mitotic rate, extent of necrosis, vascularity, tumor matrix, nuclear pleomorphism, and tumor cellularity. The precision of this grading is dependent on the experience of the pathologist; it is hindered by tumor heterogeneity and the subjectivity of the characteristics that determine grade. In an attempt to define the reproducibility of grading and the assignment of tissue type, Coindre and colleagues reported only 75 percent consensus regarding grade and 61 percent agreement regarding type between a study and reference group of pathologists. Nevertheless, even with this inherent imprecision, the designation of grade has been shown to be the most important variable in predicting the subsequent behavior of soft-tissue sarcomas. The grade of soft-tissue sarcoma is reported, depending on the institution, on a two-, three-, or four-grade scale. The three-grade system is used most commonly and will be employed in all subsequent comments regarding grade in this chapter.

Clinical treatment decisions are based primarily on grade, although other factors have also been shown to influence therapy and prognosis. Both site and size of the tumor are important in determining local therapy and also have prognostic value independent of histopathologic grade. Similarly, the depth and compartmentalization of the tumor influence the outcome of therapy in this disease. In most instances, the histopathologic type of sarcoma is not as important in therapy or prognosis as the other factors just discussed. Exceptions to this statement include types that are uniformly high grade (e.g., rhabdomyosarcoma) or types in which standard therapy approaches have been demonstrated to be ineffective (e.g., gastrointestinal leiomyosarcomas).

PRIMARY MANAGEMENT

Although the treatment of soft-tissue sarcomas needs to be individualized, a few principles are generally applicable. Because of the propensity of soft-tissue sarcomas to recur locally and the tendency for treatment to result in loss of function, primary therapy must be carefully considered and executed. To obtain local control, radical surgical margins are necessary when surgery is the sole primary therapy in soft-tissue sarcoma. The demonstration of comparable local control with wide surgical margins and radiation therapy has led to functional as well as anticancer considerations when planning primary therapy. Increasing application of preoperative therapies, including radiation and chemotherapy, appears to be achieving a degree of local control previously seen only with radical operations. Theoretical advantages to preoperative therapies, in addition to functional considerations, include earlier exposure of potential micrometastasis to systemic chemotherapy and in vivo assessment of the effectiveness of therapy through evaluation of histopathologic necrosis and other experimental parameters. The relative value of the different approaches to local therapy can only be assessed in a cooperative clinical trial. The details of local therapies are covered elsewhere in this text.

Sarcomas arising in visceral sites deserve special consideration regarding primary therapy. Owing to their internal location, visceral sarcomas are generally advanced when diagnosed, and the surgical principles regarding compartmental resection of sarcomas are often not applicable because of the lack of natural barriers to sarcoma extension. The effective use of adjunctive radiotherapy is made more difficult in this situation because of the radiosensitive organs in the field at risk for recurrence. The use of adjuvant chemotherapy has not been shown to be of value in this setting. Alternative approaches in delivering radiotherapy, such as brachytherapy and the use of radiosensitizers, as well as innovative sequencing and delivery of chemotherapy need to be explored as additional therapies to surgery.

ADJUVANT THERAPY

The decision to use systemic adjuvant therapy in surgically resected soft-tissue sarcomas primarily depends on histopathologic grade. The randomized and nonrandomized adjuvant studies that have thus far been conducted suggest benefit for adjuvant chemotherapy in soft-tissue sarcoma of the extremity and high-grade lesions. Currently, adjuvant chemotherapy cannot be recommended for low- or intermediate-grade lesions that have received adequate primary treatment. The use of adjuvant chemotherapy in high-grade lesions is considered investigational and, optimally, should be given in a study setting only. If an adjuvant study is not available, treatment of patients with high-grade, extremity, or truncal lesions that are greater than 5 cm in size is probably warranted from the available data.

The current Sarcoma Intergroup adjuvant study is a randomized study for grade 3 soft-tissue sarcomas in which therapy is divided into local treatment, followed by randomization to adjuvant chemotherapy or no further treatment. The local therapy of the patient entered on this study can consist of any of four options determined by the treating physicians. Radical resection, wide excision followed by postoperative radiotherapy, wide excision with pre- and postoperative radiotherapy, or intra-arterial doxorubicin followed by preoperative radiotherapy and wide excision are all acceptable local therapies. Patients are stratified for postoperative care prior to randomization by type of disease (primary versus local recurrence), dominant disease site, tumor size, local therapy, and whether tissue is available for biologic study. Patients receiving adjuvant chemotherapy are treated with six cycles of doxorubicin, dacarbazine (DTIC), and ifosfamide. The primary objective of this trial is to determine whether adjuvant chemotherapy can improve overall survival and disease-free survival of selected patients with soft-tissue sarcomas. Important features of this trial include patient eligibility limited to those with high-grade lesions only; a short, dose-intense period of chemotherapy; and the biologic studies that will be performed on tumor specimens. It is hoped that the potentially significant findings of the trial will overcome possible reluctance of treating physicians and patients to accept random assignment to treatment or no further therapy.

METASTATIC DISEASE

Soft-tissue sarcoma is one of the few metastatic solid tumors that can be cured. Aggressive use of surgery for pulmonary metastasis results in long-term survival in up to 25 percent of patients treated in this manner. Larger chemotherapy series also report that approximately one-third of patients who achieve complete remission with chemotherapy have long-term disease-free survival and may be cured. In an attempt to increase the number of patients cured, the use of more aggressive therapies in metastatic soft-tissue sarcoma, including multimodality therapy, appears warranted.

The majority of patients with metastatic soft-tissue sarcoma develop metastasis to the lungs. A surgical approach to pulmonary metastasis should always be considered. Some series of metastatectomy in this disease report up to a 20 percent 5-year disease free survival after surgical resection. The doubling time of the metastatic nodules, the number of metastases, and the disease-free interval all influence the likelihood of cure with surgery in this setting. Patients, however, should not be denied surgical consideration on the basis of these criteria. Patients with bilateral pulmonary disease, extrapulmonary disease, or synchronous metastatic disease should not be considered categorically unresectable. As improvements are made in the systemic therapy of sarcoma, the role of surgery in metastatic disease will likely increase.

In some of the surgical series discussed previously, it is unclear what role, if any, chemotherapy had in the patient's postoperative treatment. A portion of patients who fail following pulmonary metastatectomy do so because of progression of unrecognized micrometastatic lesions. It has also been reported that patients achieving partial response to chemotherapy who are subsequently rendered disease-free through surgery have an equivalent survival to those patients who achieve a complete response to chemotherapy alone. We have adopted the approach of treating our patients with pulmonary metastasis with two or more cycles of chemotherapy prior to surgical resection. Patients demonstrating a partial or minor response are continued postoperatively with the same combination in an effort to eliminate microscopic foci of disease. Patients without response or those with disease progression need not be treated postoperatively or can be treated with different drugs after surgery in an attempt to consolidate the remission obtained through surgery. The optimal approach to combining surgery and chemotherapy in the metastatic disease setting is insufficiently understood and needs to be studied further.

The value of chemotherapy in soft-tissue sarcoma is contingent on the perspective with which one examines the data. The introduction of doxorubicin led to complete responses in metastatic soft-tissue sarcoma and ushered in a period of increasingly complex and toxic combination programs. Early studies reported response rates of 50 percent or greater, with complete response rates of up to 15 percent with doxorubicin-based combinations. More recent cooperative group trials report response rates that are one-half of those previously observed, and many question the value of administering combination chemotherapy in this disease. The agents deemed useful in the treatment of soft-tissue sarcoma will be reviewed, and our current thoughts on combination therapy will be presented.

The single most active chemotherapeutic agent in the treatment of soft-tissue sarcoma is doxorubicin. The activity of doxorubicin in this disease was identified soon after its clinical introduction. It remains the cornerstone of chemotherapy in this disease. The response rate in soft-tissue sarcoma to single-agent doxorubicin ranges from 15 to 35 percent. Complete responses, some of long duration, have also been observed with doxorubicin alone. A dose-response relationship with this drug in soft-tissue sarcoma has long been recognized, and was again seen in a recent Southwest Oncology Group (SWOG) trial. In this trial, the dose of doxorubicin received as a percentage of dose intended was related to response rate, with data presented in Table 1 for those patients receiving three cycles of therapy. A similar relationship between dose intensity received and improved response rate was noted for patients receiving two courses of therapy. In order to maximize the benefit of doxorubicin in this disease, attention to dose intensity must be observed.

The utility of doxorubicin in this disease is limited by the cumulative cardiotoxicity produced by this drug. It appears that doxorubicin can be given to a greater cumulative dose by 96-hour infusion and with a lower risk of cardiotoxicity than at comparable doses delivered by bolus therapy. A SWOG trial comparing doxorubicin and DTIC by bolus and infusional schedules demonstrated no difference in response rate or survival between arms, but it revealed decreased cardiac toxicity in the infusion arm. We believe doxorubicin delivered by 96-hour continuous intravenous infusion is the preferred schedule for the drug. Used as a single agent, it can be given in doses from 60 to 90 mg per square meter depending on patient tolerance.

Ifosfamide has also been shown to be an important drug in the treatment of soft-tissue sarcoma. Phase 2 studies in soft-tissue sarcoma with ifosfamide have demonstrated response rates of 20 to 40 percent. It is significant that responses have been observed in patients who have progressed on doxorubicin. Additionally, ifosfamide is the only single agent besides doxorubicin

Table 1 Doxorubicin Dose Intensity Related to Response

Dose-Intensity Doxorubicin Received/Intended	Complete and Partial Response Rate (%)
< or ≥ 80%	15 versus 27
< or ≥ 90%	19 versus 28
< or ≥ 100%	20 versus 31

SWOG 8024: Patients receiving at least three cycles of therapy (n = 171).

that reliably produces complete response in this disease.

Ifosfamide has been administered as a single agent in sarcoma in cycles consisting of one to five days. With larger daily doses of 3 g per square meter or greater, serious neurotoxicity has been reported. In order to maximize dose and safety, ifosfamide should be given over three to five days with a total dose of 7.5 to 10.0 g per square meter per cycle. In an attempt to further decrease neurotoxicity, infusional delivery of ifosfamide has been studied, with less neurotoxicity noted as a result. There is some sentiment, however, that infusional delivery of ifosfamide may decrease efficacy. Whether infusional schedules compromise response is currently not clear and is under evaluation. Ifosfamide should always be given with attention to hydration and using the uroprotector Mesna to prevent urothelial toxicity.

Dacarbazine has been identified to have a low level of activity in soft-tissue sarcoma and in patients who have progressed on doxorubicin. Although response rates to single-agent DTIC in soft-tissue sarcoma are less than 20 percent and complete responses are rarely observed, the agent is currently used in combination therapy. It has been suggested that DTIC is active in gastrointestinal leiomyosarcomas, a subtype resistant to doxorubicin, but this has not been well studied.

Other commercially available agents that have been extensively used and studied, primarily in combination therapy, are cyclophosphamide, methotrexate, actinomycin-D, and vincristine. The true response rates of any of these drugs in adult soft-tissue sarcomas is probably less than 15 percent. Cyclophosphamide, compared to ifosfamide in a recent European trial, demonstrated an 8 percent response rate. Reviewing published reports, methotrexate appears to have greater activity in standard doses than in high-dose regimens, a paradoxical finding explained by small, single-institution studies. Actinomycin-D and vincristine as single agents have been studied in very few adult patients, but when used in combination therapy, they appear to add very little, if anything, to doxorubicin.

Cisplatin does not appear to be active in this group of diseases, with the exception of uterine sarcomas. A recent SWOG study, which attempted dose intensification of cisplatin, did not demonstrate improved response. Etoposide, mitomycin-D, and miscellaneous other agents, despite showing minimal single-agent activity in this disease, are being evaluated in various combinations at some centers.

In the majority of patients who develop metastatic

disease, the initial chemotherapeutic approach involves combination chemotherapy. Although a number of studies utilizing combination chemotherapy in this disease are reported in the literature, the greatest experience is with doxorubicin-based combinations. The highest response rates reported with doxorubicin-based combinations also include DTIC, cyclophosphamide, and vincristine.

The SWOG has conducted sequential trials with doxorubicin combinations. The first randomized trial compared doxorubicin, cyclophosphamide, vincristine, and either DTIC or actinomycin-D. The arm containing DTIC demonstrated improved response and survival. The second randomized trial compared doxorubicin and DTIC to doxorubicin, DTIC, and either cyclophosphamide or vincristine. There were no significant differences in response or survival between any of the three arms. As a result of these sequential studies, the two-drug combination of doxorubicin and DTIC became the standard SWOG combination in soft-tissue sarcoma.

The value of DTIC in this disease has been questioned by some. Borden and colleagues reported a trial conducted by the Eastern Cooperative Oncology Group (ECOG) in which single-agent doxorubicin in two schedules was compared to doxorubicin and DTIC. Although the response rate in the combination was significantly higher, survival in the three arms was not different and toxicity, primarily gastrointestinal, was higher in the DTIC-containing regimen. The authors concluded that the addition of DTIC to doxorubicin was not warranted owing to an increase in toxicity with no appreciable change in survival.

The lack of a survival advantage in the preceding trials is not surprising given the low response rates seen in the study. Any benefit from the combination on survival in responders is lost when the effect is diluted by nonresponders. Improved response rate and duration of response should be the primary goals of therapy in a disease in which overall response rates are low, and in which a complete response or a partial response, which can be converted to complete through surgery, may be of long duration. In the first study reported by SWOG using the doxorubicin-DTIC combination, 25 complete remissions were seen, with the majority of complete responders living 3 years or longer. As mentioned previously, several larger chemotherapy series have reported that approximately one-third of complete responders continue to be disease-free and may be cured. Because of preceding analysis, we interpret the role of DTIC as important in this disease. Additionally, the gastrointestinal toxicity of DTIC can be considerably lessened by administering the drug through 96-hour continuous infusion. In the majority of patients given chemotherapy for metastatic soft-tissue sarcoma, doxorubicin should be combined with DTIC.

Our standard treatment approach in patients with metastatic soft-tissue sarcoma has been doxorubicin, 60 mg per square meter, and DTIC, 1 g per square meter, infused together over 96 hours. Outpatient therapy is possible in the majority of patients thus treated, and the decreased cardiac toxicity of the infusional schedule permits continued therapy in those responding. Reports from the Dana Farber Cancer Institute of increased response rates with the three-drug combination of doxorubicin, DTIC, and ifosfamide prompted a randomized trial in metastatic sarcoma comparing the three-drug combination to doxorubicin and DTIC. The addition of ifosfamide, 2.0 g per square meter infused over 72 hours, to the doxorubicin-DTIC treatment program increases the inconvenience and toxicity of therapy, but it will probably also favorably influence response. Continuing analysis of this recently completed Sarcoma Intergroup trial will be helpful in determining future directions for chemotherapy in this disease.*

FUTURE DIRECTIONS

The demonstrated dose-response relationship seen in the soft-tissue sarcomas makes intensification of therapy a reasonable approach to improve the outcome in this disease. Myelosuppression, with its attendant complications, is the predominant toxicity of the doxorubicin, DTIC, and ifosfamide combination. Granulocyte-macrophage colony-stimulating factor (GM-CSF) has been piloted with the three-drug combination and was shown to lessen the severity and shorten the interval of myelosuppression. Whether these effects of GM-CSF are sustainable, and the toxicities of the treatment tolerable during continuing therapy, needs to be determined. The low incidence of clinical bone marrow metastasis in soft-tissue sarcoma and the younger population of patients afflicted with this disease suggest the use of high-dose chemotherapy with autologous bone marrow rescue as a possible therapy. The curative potential of autologous transplant in metastatic sarcoma appears promising for some histologies and is under investigation in a number of centers. Until these and other new approaches become more available, the use of doxorubicin-based combination chemotherapy, with careful attention to dose intensity and availability of medical support for complications of therapy, remains the optimal approach to patients with metastatic disease.

Biologic therapy may also play a role in the treatment of soft-tissue sarcoma in the coming decade. Interferons, interleukins, colony-stimulating factors, and immunotoxins will be evaluated as therapies in this disease. The real value of many of these agents may be as adjuvant therapy or in combination with chemotherapy.

We are entering an era in oncology in which the cellular biology of a patient's tumor will likely influence the choice and effectiveness of treatment. In metastatic disease, for instance, assessment of the likelihood of response to chemotherapy by detection and quantitation of drug resistance may allow modifications of therapy to circumvent or overcome that resistance. The next generation of adjuvant trials will likely target subgroups

---

*The Sarcoma Intergroup adjuvant trial described in the adjuvant therapy section was closed in late 1990 due to lack of accrual.

of patients based on parameters other than, or at least in addition to, histopathologic grade. Characterization of tumor phenotypes that predict for micrometastasis or for tendency to local recurrence will permit adequate treatment for all and avoid overtreatment for some. The near future certainly holds the promise of a greater basic understanding of soft-tissue sarcoma and, consequently, significant improvements in their therapy.

SUGGESTED READING

Antman KH, Ryan L, Elias A, et al. Response to ifosfamide and Mesna: 124 previously treated patients with metastatic or unresectable sarcoma. J Clin Oncol 1989; 7:126–131.

Baker LH, Frank J, Fine G, et al. Combination chemotherapy using adriamycin, DTIC, cyclophosphamide, and actinomycin D for advanced soft-tissue sarcoma: A randomized comparative trial. A Phase III, Southwest Oncology Group study (7613). J Clin Oncol 1987; 5:851–861.

Borden EC, Amato DA, Rosenbaum C, et al. Randomized comparison of three adriamycin regimens for metastatic soft-tissue sarcomas. J Clin Oncol 1987; 5:840–850.

Ryan JR, Baker LH, eds. Proceedings of the international symposium on sarcomas, October, 1987. Recent concepts in sarcoma treatment. Dordrecht, The Netherlands: Kluwer Academic Publishers, 1988.

THYROID AND ADRENAL GLAND CANCER

JOHN HORTON, M.B., Ch.B., F.A.C.P.

Carcinoma of the thyroid gland affects almost 11,000 inhabitants of the United States each year, with an approximate 3:1 ratio between women and men. It accounts for 90 percent of all endocrine malignancies and causes 1,000 deaths annually. Known etiologic factors include radiation, especially in childhood, hereditary, and, possibly, goiter, iodine deficiency, or excess. Medullary thyroid cancer, inherited by an autosomal dominant effect in 20 percent of cases, occurs in familial medullary thyroid carcinoma, multiple endocrine neoplasia MEN-2a, and MEN-2b. The prognosis for the majority of patients with thyroid cancer is related to age and is generally very good. The significant exception to this rule is one of the most rapidly fatal human cancers, anaplastic carcinoma.

Pathology and Spread

The majority of primary malignant tumors of the thyroid are of glandular epithelial origin and are carcinomas. The relative incidence of the four most common histologic varieties is shown in Table 1. Metastases to the thyroid gland most often originate from primary carcinomas of the lung and kidney or from malignant melanomas.

Determination of whether a slowly growing thyroid nodule is a benign adenoma or a malignant tumor is sometimes difficult by histologic examination alone. Evidence of invasion of blood vessels or transgression of tumor excision margins is helpful in establishing the latter entity. Malignant papillary lesions are often multifocal, a factor that, along with direct extension into contiguous structures in the neck and age over 45, is associated with an inferior prognosis. Lymph node metastases in the neck do not affect the prognosis for papillary carcinoma but confer inferior survival statistics for medullary tumors. Follicular carcinomas usually have a relatively uniform microfollicular pattern and infrequent node metastasis. Hurthle cell (or oxyphil cell) tumors are a subtype of follicular neoplasms. Only about 2 percent of benign Hurthle cell adenomas become malignant. Medullary carcinomas, which occur most often in the fifth and sixth decades of life, are tumors of the calcitonin-secreting C cells. They are bilateral in patients with familial medullary carcinoma (MEN-2a and MEN-2b) but usually unilateral with the sporadic disease. The prognosis is worse for older patients with familial or large tumors, or when distant metastasis has occurred. Anaplastic carcinoma can now reliably be differentiated from lymphoma and poorly differentiated medullary carcinoma by histochemical means, and it has a uniformly poor disease prognosis. This tumor often originates from pre-existing thyroid cancer in the elderly.

Table 1 Characteristics of Thyroid Cancer in the United States

Histologic type	Incidence (%)	Approximate Survival	
		5 yr (%)	10 yr (%)
Papillary	60	90–95	75–92
Follicular*	25	75–95	66–90
Medullary	3	60–80	40–60
Anaplastic	12	0	0

*Includes Hurthle cell.

Evaluation of the Thyroid Nodule

Thyroid nodules are present in 4 percent to 7 percent of the adult general population and in about 25 percent of those who were exposed to radiation in childhood. Radiation exposure increases the likelihood of malignant change from about 15 percent in nonexposed subjects to about 40 percent in exposed subjects. The finding of enlarged cervical lymph nodes increases the chance that the nodule is malignant. Laboratory tests are generally unhelpful in diagnosis, although sequential thyroglobulin determinations are used in following patients with radiation exposure. Serum calcitonin measurements, sometimes combined with provocation using calcium or pentagastrin, are invaluable for the diagnosis of medullary tumors.

Exogenous suppression of thyroid-stimulating hormone (TSH) using thyroid hormone is often associated with shrinkage of solitary nodules. This does not rule out malignancy. Radionuclide scanning, using ^{123}I or ^{99m}Tc–pertechnetate, can only be used to predict the likelihood of malignancy based on the functional status of the nodule and does not successfully discriminate between benign and malignant nodules. Ultrasound accurately measures the size and number of nodules and determines whether they are solid or cystic. Fine-needle aspiration is now widely used as a safe, inexpensive, and reasonably sensitive and specific diagnostic tool when performed and evaluated by experts. Large or rapidly growing tumors, in which there is suspicion for lymphoma or anaplastic carcinoma, may be better assessed using a cutting-needle biopsy. A flow diagram that summarizes an approach to evaluation of a thyroid nodule is shown in Figure 1.

Surgery

Surgical resection is performed when a thyroid nodule is suspicious for or diagnosed as carcinoma.

Known benign nodules are not excised. Excision of the ipsilateral thyroid lobe is the procedure of choice for the lobe with the nodule. Isthmus lesions are resected along with the closest thyroid lobe. If frozen section demonstrates a well-differentiated carcinoma, a near-total thyroidectomy is performed, leaving a small portion of thyroid on the contralateral side to preserve parathyroid glands and the recurrent laryngeal nerve. There is greater morbidity from total thyroidectomy, and, at least in patients under 45 who have small tumors, it is not associated with longer survival. Older patients with larger, more aggressive, or metastatic well-differentiated tumors benefit from total or near-total thyroidectomy because this lessens the required ^{131}I dose for subsequent total thyroid ablation.

Hurthle cell tumors and medullary carcinomas are handled surgically in a similar fashion to the well-differentiated papillary and follicular tumors. The majority of anaplastic tumors are unresectable at presentation, but surgical resection is indicated for small tumors (Tables 2 and 3).

Adjuvant Therapy

Prescription of thyroid hormone for patients who have had resection of a well-differentiated thyroid cancer suppresses TSH levels and decreases the recurrence of radiation-induced thyroid carcinoma, although a beneficial effect on survival has not clearly been demonstrated. Similarly, the use of postoperative ^{131}I therapy has decreased recurrence rates but has not increased survival. Therapy with ^{131}I using ablative doses in the range of 30 to 100 mCi, is considered in patients over 45 and in those whose tumors are multiple, locally invasive, and over 2.5 cm in size. It is not of value in patients with medullary carcinoma because the C cells themselves do not concentrate the radionuclide.

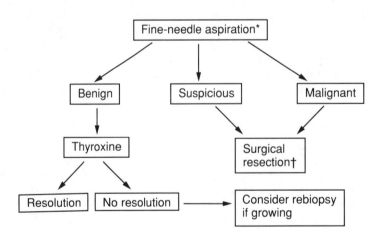

Figure 1 Algorithm for management of a thyroid nodule.

*Consider cutting-needle biopsy for large or rapidly growing tumors.

†Special considerations may apply for thyroid lymphoma or anaplastic carcinoma.

Anaplastic Thyroid Cancer

Surgery is indicated for small tumors. Radiotherapy alone has not been effective, but a combination of hyperfractionated radiation (5,760 cGy given at 160 cGy per treatment twice daily for 3 days each week over 40 days) plus doxorubicin, 10 mg per square meter IV weekly, has been reported to be transiently effective in eight of nine patients so treated.

Metastatic Disease (Well-Differentiated Tumors)

Locally recurrent or persistent disease in the neck is surgically excised if feasible, although formal radical neck dissection is not usually required. External-beam radiation may be helpful for less differentiated recurrent or locally advanced lesions that do not take up [131]I. Metastatic disease to the lung may be silent, and may be diagnosed only by postoperative radionuclide uptake studies. It is often controlled for years or decades by ^{131}I, although patients who have metastases to bone have a less favorable prognosis. Many clinicians use doses of 100 to 200 mCi, and this may be repeated several times. Toxicity includes hematologic suppression, nausea and vomiting, pulmonary fibrosis, and, later, leukemia. Surgical resection is considered for isolated metastases, and external-beam radiation is used for localized symptomatic tumors that do not take up [131]I.

Because papillary and follicular metastases that take up ^{131}I usually respond very well to ablation with ^{131}I, such tumors are treated with ^{131}I and not with chemotherapy. Chemotherapy for metastatic well-differentiated or anaplastic thyroid carcinoma is often ineffective, and conflicting data exist as to whether the combination of doxorubicin (60 mg per square meter IV every 3 weeks) and cisplatin (40 mg per square meter IV every 3 weeks) is more effective than doxorubicin (60 mg per square meter every 3 weeks) alone. A combination of doxorubicin, bleomycin, vincristine, and melphalan has produced four responses in 11 patients treated. A combination of dacarbazine and 5-fluorouracil, given daily for 5 days every four weeks, has produced a complete response in one patient with a sporadic medullary thyroid cancer.

Table 2 Management of Medullary Thyroid Cancer

Rule out pheochromocytoma
Localized tumor: total thyroidectomy plus central node dissection
Localized inaccessible tumors: external-beam radiation
Metastasis with diarrhea: debulking surgery, somatostatin analogue

Table 3 Management of Anaplastic Thyroid Carcinoma

Small tumors (minority): surgical resection
Large tumors (majority): radiation plus doxorubicin
Disseminated disease: chemotherapy trials, supportive care

ADRENAL GLAND CANCER

Diagnosis and management of tumors of the adrenal gland provide challenges to a variety of medical practitioners. Tumors can present with symptoms of corticosteroid excess, masculinization or feminization, or hypertension, or they may be silent. Hyperplasia, benign tumors, or malignant neoplasms may occur, the last causing additional morbidity because of local extension or metastatic spread. Proper management first requires the definition of any endocrine abnormality that is present. Then, the cause is established, followed by treatment of both the tumor and, when required, the hormonal abnormality.

Benign adenomas of the adrenal gland are common, but adrenocortical carcinomas are rare, having an estimated annual incidence of only two per million. Nevertheless, hyperplasia and benign and malignant tumors can cause appreciable morbidity and mortality. Widespread use of computed tomography (CT) and magnetic resonance imaging (MRI) of the upper abdomen as part of the staging process for patients with other carcinomas and for evaluation of benign diseases has brought to light a high incidence of incidental tumors in the adrenal gland that require appropriate diagnosis and management.

Pathology

Metastases from primary carcinomas of other sites are the most common adrenal neoplasms, with lung and breast cancer being the principal offenders in the United States. Histologic documentation of their presence is rarely required, and they rarely produce clinically significant morbidity. Hyperplasia and primary tumors of the adrenal gland may involve either the cortex or the medulla of the adrenal gland.

Adrenal Cortex

The normal adrenal gland weighs between 3 and 6 g. In pituitary-based hypercortisolism (Cushing's disease), the glands become hyperplastic and enlarge to approximately twice their normal size, with a widened inner zone of the zona reticularis and a sharply demarcated outer zone of clear cells. The adrenals are usually larger in patients with the ectopic adrenocorticotropic hormone (ACTH) syndrome. Adrenal adenomas are benign neoplasms of adrenal cortical cells. They rarely exceed 5 cm in largest diameter and only rarely demonstrate cellular pleomorphism and tumor necrosis. They can produce the Cushing's syndrome, hyperaldosteronism, or, rarely, adrenogenital syndromes, but usually are nonfunctional.

Adrenocortical carcinomas have a bimodal age incidence, with peaks below age 5 and in the fourth and fifth decades. The tumors are generally larger than benign adenomas. Indeed, a diameter of over 5 cm is one criterion used to make the sometimes difficult differentiation between a benign and a malignant neoplasm.

Tumor necrosis, hemorrhage, vascular invasion, and mitoses are diagnostic of malignancy, as is the presence of nodal or distant metastatic disease. Cells with large nuclei and nucleoli are consistent with malignancy, and the presence of broad fibrous bands denotes a predilection for metastatic spread. Feminizing or masculinizing syndromes are more often seen with malignant rather than benign tumors, and malignant tumors often produce combinations of hormones, including aldosterone. They enlarge and invade locally and metastasize to lymph nodes (68 percent), the lung (42 percent), and bone (26 percent). Table 4 presents the most current staging system.

Adrenal Medulla

Pheochromocytomas are rare tumors that arise in chromaffin cells in the adrenal medulla and elsewhere. They secrete catecholamines, which induce hypertension. Ninety percent of pheochromocytomas originate in the adrenal medulla. The rest most often arise in the organ of Zucherkandl, which is located adjacent to the aortic bifurcation, in the carotid body, in the hilum of the kidney, or in the bladder. Bilateral adrenal pheochromocytomas occur in the MEN-2a and MEN-2b syndromes, and familial pheochromocytoma has been described. Approximately 25 percent of patients with the von Hippel-Lindau syndrome develop the disease. Malignant change, which occurs in about 10 percent of all tumors, is more often associated with an extra-adrenal primary site, and malignant tumors tend to be larger than their benign counterparts. Differentiation between benign and malignant tumors using histopathologic criteria alone is often difficult. The findings of extensive necrosis and aneuploidy suggest malignancy. Metastatic patterns are similar to those of malignant adrenal cortical tumors.

The Asymptomatic Adrenal Nodule

Adrenal masses are commonly discovered radiographically during the initial staging or follow-up of

Table 4 Staging for Carcinoma of the Adrenal Gland

Criteria
T_1	Tumor ≤ 5 cm, invasion absent
T_2	Tumor > 5 cm, invasion absent
T_3	Tumor outside adrenal in fat
T_4	Tumor invading adjacent organs
N_0	No involved lymph nodes
N_1	Involved lymph nodes
M_0	No distant metastases
M_1	Distant metastases

Stage
I	T_1, N_0, M_0
II	T_2, N_0, M_0
III	T_1 or $T_2 N_1 M_0$, $T_3 N_0 M_0$
IV	Any T, any N M_1, T_3, T_4, N_1

patients with known cancer, particularly lung cancer. Further diagnostic studies in this clinical situation are often not required. An unexpected adrenal mass may be detected on 0.6 percent of abdominal CT scans done for other reasons. In this situation, work-up and management need to be done with the recognition that the majority of these asymptomatic masses are both benign and nonfunctional. A history and physical examination are performed to evaluate for Cushing's syndrome, hypertension, masculinization or feminization, weight loss, or an occult neoplasm. Laboratory evaluation may include a 24-hour urine test for 17-hydroxy and 17-ketosteroids, catecholamines, and a 1 mg dexamethasone suppression test. Sex hormone levels are measured only if there is clinical evidence of masculinization or feminization. Aldosterone levels are performed if hypertension or hypokalemia is present. Magnetic resonance imaging can distinguish between adrenal metastases and nonfunctioning adenomas, and pheochromocytomas appear bright on the T_2-weighted image. The combination of MRI and biochemical assessment usually provides reliable information on the character of an adrenal mass. Fine-needle aspiration of an adrenal nodule may produce severe morbidity, and is generally not required.

Management

The most common cause of symptomatic hypercortisolism is iatrogenic administration of corticosteroids. Dose tapering and cessation are effective management. The symptoms and clinical findings associated with the Cushing's syndrome are well known and will not be discussed here. The diagnosis is established when biochemical evidence of a pituitary-dependent hypercortisolism is made, and management is focused on the pituitary. Studies may include a dexamethasone suppression test, CT of the pituitary sella, ACTH gradients in petrosal sinus blood, adrenal CT or MRI, or iodocholesterol imaging of the adrenals. The details of an appropriate work-up have recently been reviewed and are referenced in the Suggested Reading list. Patients with the ectopic ACTH syndrome respond best to control of the tumor that is secreting the ACTH. The hypertension and hypokalemia of the Conn syndrome associated with adrenal adenomas respond well to spironolactone or amiloride plus hypotension-inducing agents. Unilateral adrenalectomy is performed when an adrenal aldosteronoma is demonstrated.

Adenoma of the Adrenal Cortex

Resection of the adrenal gland containing the adenoma is curative. Small tumors can be resected using a posterior approach, but when tumors exceed 6 cm in size, an anterior or flank approach is preferred because the tumor is more likely to be malignant. Corticosteroid replacement is required during surgery and for several months thereafter.

Carcinoma of the Adrenal Cortex

Preoperative staging work-up includes a chest radiograph or CT of the chest, and imaging of the mass and the remainder of the abdomen and pelvis by CT and MRI. This allows evaluation for distant metastatic disease, vena caval blood flow, and the number of functional kidneys present. Complete surgical resection of the tumor and adrenal, when feasible, is the indicated treatment. Involved contiguous structures are also resected, in part or in toto. If complete resection is not possible, surgical tumor debulking may reduce local complications and those due to hormone secretion. Surgery is also indicated for selected isolated metastases.

Follow-up of treated patients includes monthly monitoring of the appropriate abnormal steroid secretion as well as intermittent repeat of imaging studies. Evidence of recurrence or progression prompts studies to delineate the site and extent of the spread and consideration of additional surgical resection or radiation for localized tumors. Induction of a complete remission in this way is unusual, and o,p-DDD (mitotane) is often prescribed. This drug, by a direct effect on steroid metabolism, reduces plasma cortisol and urine 17-ketosteroids in about two-thirds of patients treated and induces objective tumor shrinkage in about one-third. Complete responses occur rarely, but a few long-term survivors are reported.

Treatment is usually initiated in divided doses of 2 to 6 g daily and increased to maximal tolerance. Doses resulting in serum levels greater than 14 μg per milliliter are preferred to maximize antitumor effects. The drug often induces gastrointestinal (80 percent), neuromuscular (50 percent), and skin rash (15 percent) complications. These sharply limit the clinical effectiveness of this drug. Mitotane greatly enhances the metabolism of dexamethasone, so high doses of this agent, together with the mineralocorticoid Florinef, are required to provide an adequate and necessary corticosteroid-replacement program. Good data do not exist to support use of this agent alone as an adjuvant in patients with completely resected disease. Combining cisplatin (75 to 100 mg per square meter) with mitotane has produced a 25 percent incidence of responses lasting a median of 4 months.

Of the other cytotoxic regimens that have been used to palliate metastatic disease, cisplatin (40 mg per square meter) plus etoposide (100 mg per square meter), both given daily intravenously for 3 days, may be the current optimal approach, with five of six patients having responded to this or a similar regimen. Doxorubicin and alkylating agent-based combinations have been less effective. Suramin plus hydrocortisone, an experimental approach, has also produced responses.

Benign Pheochromocytoma

Once the primary site of tumor has been established, preoperative preparation for tumor resection includes alpha-adrenergic blockade, usually with phenoxybenzamine in doses sufficient to control the hypertension. Careful hemodynamic monitoring is required during surgical resection. Hypertensive episodes are controlled by short-acting drugs such as nitroprusside. Exploration of the entire abdomen is required because multiple tumors may be present.

Malignant Pheochromocytomas

Preoperative work-up includes an appropriate delineation of local tumor extent and a search for distant metastases in the lung, lymph nodes, and liver. Complete surgical resection, whenever possible, is the preferred initial treatment, and isolated metastases can be managed by surgical resection or radiation therapy. Hypertensive symptoms may be controlled by catecholamine blockade. Follow-up imaging using ^{131}I-M1BG has a high specificity for metastases, and trials of this agent used for treatment have started. Standard chemotherapeutic approaches are largely ineffective, but a combination of cyclophosphamide (750 mg per square meter IV on day 1), vincristine (1.4 mg per square meter IV on day 2), and dacarbazine (600 mg per square meter IV on days 1 and 2) has produced both objective responses and decreased urinary catecholamine excretion. This treatment program was developed for neuroblastoma, a tumor having several similarities to pheochromocytoma. One could speculate whether there might be a role for high-dose chemotherapy with autologous bone marrow rescue for some "good-risk" patients with malignant pheochromocytoma, analogous to the demonstrated role for this aggressive approach in some patients with neuroblastoma.

SUGGESTED READING

Ahuja S, Ernst H. Chemotherapy of thyroid carcinoma. J Endocrin Invest 1987; 10:303–310.

Barkan AL, ed. Medical therapy of endocrine tumors. Endocrinol Metab Clin North Am 1989; 18(2).

Copeland PM. The incidentally discovered adrenal mass. Ann Intern Med 1983; 98:940–945.

Goolden AW. The use of radioactive iodine in thyroid carcinoma. Eur J Cancer Clin Oncol 1988; 24:339–343.

Kaye TB, Crapo L. The Cushing syndrome: An update on diagnostic tests. Ann Intern Med 1990; 112:434–444.

Kim JH, Leeper RD. Treatment of locally advanced thyroid carcinoma with combination doxorubicin and radiation therapy. Cancer 1987; 60:2,372–2,375.

Luton JP, Cerdas S, Billaud L, et al. Clinical features of adrenocortical carcinoma, prognostic factors, and the effect of mitotane therapy. N Engl J Med 1990; 322:1,195–1,201.

NEUROENDOCRINE CANCER

SCOT C. REMICK, M.D.

Neuroendocrine carcinoma comprises an eclectic group of tumors with variable biology and natural history. At one end of the spectrum of this disease entity is the incidental finding of a carcinoid tumor less than 1 cm in the resected appendix from which long-term survival or cure is certain. It is common to see patients with extensive hepatic metastases from carcinoid tumor who are nutritionally replete, enjoy good functional status, and survive without therapy for many years. The clinical course of patients with extrapulmonary small-cell carcinoma is reminiscent of small-cell lung cancer, which is characterized by early and widespread metastases and survival frequently recorded in months.

Carcinoid tumor, islet cell carcinoma, medullary thyroid carcinoma, pheochromocytoma, melanoma, and small-cell carcinoma in pulmonary and extrapulmonary sites are to be considered neuroendocrine tumors. These tumors are rare (Table 1) and are characterized by their affinity for silver histochemical stains, the production of biogenic amines and polypeptide hormones, and the presence of neurosecretory granules upon ultrastructural examination. These tumors are found in all parts of the body. It remains useful to consider these tumors as part of the amine precursor and decarboxylation (APUD) system of Pearse, the tumors of which originate from the neural crest. Emerging data suggest that some tumors may be of endodermal origin. The attractiveness of the APUD concept is that it most readily explains the diversity of sites in which these tumors are found.

The protean manifestations of neuroendocrine carcinoma present a unique challenge to the diagnostician. The therapeutic approach to patients with these tumors is equally challenging and variable. The remainder of this discussion focuses on the treatment of gastrointestinal carcinoid tumor and the malignant carcinoid syndrome, islet cell carcinoma, and extrapulmonary small-cell carcinoma.

GASTROINTESTINAL CARCINOID TUMOR

Carcinoid tumors are most frequently found in the appendix. Isolated appendiceal carcinoids of less than 1 cm in diameter are essentially cured by simple appendectomy. Similarly, rectal carcinoid tumors of less than 1 cm in diameter are treated by fulguration or local excision. No periodic clinical follow-up or biologic determination of urine 5-hydroxyindoleacetic acid (5HIAA) is required, and the patient is informed that he or she is cured.

Primary carcinoid tumors of greater than 2 cm in diameter of the appendix or rectum are treated with more aggressive surgical procedures. Right hemicolectomy for appendiceal lesions and low anterior or abdominoperineal resection for rectal lesions is recommended, as there is a greater than 80% chance of subsequent dissemination.

For primary tumors of between 1 and 2 cm, definitive surgical recommendations cannot be made. It is known that the larger the tumor, the greater the likelihood that there are regional or distant metastases. Therefore, for lesions approaching 2 cm, the degree of local invasion, presence of regional lymph node metastases, age of the patient, and operative risk will determine the necessity for more aggressive surgical procedures. It is reported in the literature that appendiceal lesions of between 1 and 1.4 cm in diameter can probably be safely treated by simple appendectomy. If appendectomy is performed for lesions between 1.5 and 2 cm or wide local excision is employed for rectal lesions between 1 and 2 cm, these patients should be carefully followed.

It is less common to identify small lesions of less than 1 cm in diameter within the small intestine because they usually originate deep within the mucosa where they are not likely to cause symptoms. It is known that when such small lesions are identified, they have a much greater tendency toward dissemination than their appendiceal counterpart. Up to 15 percent of lesions between 0.5 to 0.9 cm and 60 percent of lesions 1 to 1.4 cm metastasize. Therefore, wide excision with en bloc resection of adjacent lymph node mesentery is recommended.

Small gastric and duodenal carcinoids can be excised locally. Subtotal gastrectomy with omentectomy or pancreatoduodenectomy may be advisable for larger and invasive tumors. An unusual feature of gastric (7 percent) and small intestinal carcinoids (29 percent) is their tendency for multicentricity. The operator must be alert to this, and the occurrence of multicentric lesions may further dictate the type of surgical procedure.

The occasional patient with more remote nodal involvement, extensive regional invasion, or peritoneal implants may benefit with good survival (71 percent 5-year survival) from complete surgical excision of all tumor. There is no role for debulking surgery or partial resection of tumor. An exception is made for the patient with known metastatic disease who presents with a clinical history of chronic and intermittent small bowel obstruction. Given the often protracted natural history of this disease, select patients may derive significant relief of abdominal pain by exploratory laparotomy. Resection of isolated hepatic metastases may also be of significant symptomatic benefit or even curative in

Table 1 Approximate Annual Incidence of Neuroendocrine Carcinoma

	No. of cases
Islet cell carcinoma (gastrinoma and insulinoma)	400
Carcinoid tumors of small intestine	600
Extrapulmonary small-cell carcinoma	1,000

selected patients. There is no role for adjuvant chemotherapy in all patients who have undergone complete and possibly curative resection of gastrointestinal carcinoid tumor.

MALIGNANT CARCINOID SYNDROME

There is no agreement on when treatment should be started in patients with the malignant carcinoid syndrome. Diarrhea and flushing are the most common and troublesome symptoms encountered. Asthma as an initial manifestation of the syndrome is very rare, and carcinoid heart disease, which affects approximately 20 percent of patients, is a late complication. Poor prognostic features of this disease include impairment of liver function, very high levels of urinary 5HIAA (150 mg or more per 24 hours), and clinical evidence of carcinoid heart disease, for which more aggressive intervention is warranted. It is known that the urinary 5HIAA level correlates very well with tumor burden and is a useful marker to follow in patients on therapy.

Simple Measures

There is a hierarchal therapeutic approach in this disease, as outlined in Figure 1. At the outset, no therapy is warranted for mild symptoms, and patients intuitively avoid precipitants of flush such as various foods, alcohol, stress, or exercise. A variety of pharmacologic agents

have been tried to no avail for the control of flushing. Mild diarrhea is frequently responsive to codeine, tincture of opium, diphenoxylate, or loperamide. Cyproheptadine, a serotonin and histamine antagonist, may also relieve diarrhea in the occasional patient. This medication is usually begun at a dose of 4 mg three times daily and adjusted accordingly up to a maximum dose of 0.5 mg per kilogram per day. Major side effects of all antidiarrheals and cyproheptadine are drowsiness and fatigue. Appropriate bronchodilator and diuretic therapy is warranted for the management of bronchospasm and right-sided heart failure, respectively. Select patients with severe carcinoid heart disease may benefit from valve replacement. A careful assessment of the status of the patient's malignant disease and operative risk is imperative in these instances.

Somatostatin Analogue

With the availability of octreotide acetate (SMS 201-995), a long-acting somastostatin analogue, patients with the malignant carcinoid syndrome are more successfully palliated. It is appropriate to initiate such therapy in patients who have failed simpler measures. Both flushing and diarrhea are promptly relieved in the majority of patients (88 percent). Seventy-two percent of patients demonstrated a 50 percent or greater reduction in urinary 5HIAA, and objective tumor regression is occasionally seen. The median duration of biochemical response is 12 months, and the majority of patients

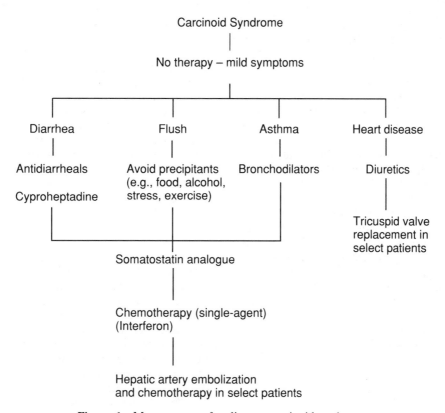

Figure 1 Management of malignant carcinoid syndrome.

experienced relief of flushing or diarrhea over a period of 4 to 18 months.

The drug is administered subcutaneously, usually in a test dose of 50 μg once or twice daily that is escalated to 150 μg three times daily. An occasional patient may derive benefit from lower dosages or require higher dosages up to 1,500 μg total daily dose. The drug is usually well tolerated, and side effects in the initial clinical trial were limited to transient hyperglycemia and steatorrhea. Other side effects may include pain at the injection site, nausea, and vomiting.

Chemotherapy

Chemotherapy is reserved for patients who have failed treatment with the long-acting somatostatin analogue or have a very high tumor burden from which they are symptomatic. No standard therapy can be recommended in this setting because responses, when seen, are usually partial and not durable, and toxicity is frequent. Single-agent objective response rates for 5-fluorouracil, doxorubicin, and dacarbazine are in the 20 percent range. When chemotherapy is initiated, it is usually with 5-fluorouracil or doxorubicin. Combination chemotherapy, usually with streptozotocin and 5-fluorouracil, does not yield superior objective response rates. Streptozotocin has the advantage of not being myelosuppressive, but it is very emetogenic, and renal insufficiency and proteinuria are common side effects. The streptozotocin and 5-fluorouracil regimen may be of use in the patient who, despite failing single-agent chemotherapy, maintains a good performance status and may not have received one or two of the drugs in the combination.

In patients failing chemotherapy, a variety of approaches have been evaluated to a limited extent. Hepatic artery ligation results in prompt relief of symptoms and cytoreduction but a median duration of response of less than 5 months. Hepatic artery infusion of 5-fluorouracil is not efficacious. Currently, hepatic artery embolization followed by chemotherapy is under investigation. Interferon is an alternative therapeutic approach that has been reported to relieve symptoms of carcinoid syndrome, but it is associated with a 10 percent objective response rate. There is no role for the use of tamoxifen in the treatment of carcinoid.

There is no reported chemotherapy regimen that prolongs survival in patients with malignant carcinoid syndrome. Because the natural history of this disease is often protracted—median survival from time of first flush (38 months) and first elevated 5HIAA (23 months)—the initiation of chemotherapy must be carefully reviewed in terms of potential benefit and risk to the individual patient. If a clinical trial is available for treating a patient this is to be encouraged. The more common therapeutic regimens and their side effects are outlined in Table 2.

Carcinoid Crisis

Carcinoid crisis is a rare but potentially life-threatening complication of the malignant carcinoid syndrome. Manifestations of carcinoid crisis may include prolonged cutaneous flushing, hypertension, severe hypotension, tachycardia, arrhythmia, light-headedness, and coma. These events may occur spontaneously but are usually precipitated by severe stress, such as the induction of anesthesia, surgery, or initiation of chemotherapy.

The somatostatin analogue is a useful antidote in the management of carcinoid crisis. It is advisable in patients with florid carcinoid syndrome or elevated urinary 5HIAA greater than 150 μg per 24 hours to have initial chemotherapy dosages reduced by 50 percent. The administration of the somatostatin analogue prior to starting chemotherapy may be an acceptable alternative and permit 100 percent dosing. Similarly, the prophylactic administration of somatostatin analogue in dosages of 150 to 200 μg every 6 to 8 hours for a day or two prior to surgery and 250 to 500 μg 1 to 2 hours before more urgent surgery has been reported to be successful. The intravenous administration of somatostatin analogue has also been reported to reverse profound hypotension associated with the induction of anesthesia. This medication should be readily available in the operating room at all times for patients with the carcinoid syndrome.

ISLET CELL CARCINOMA

Several points regarding the biology of islet cell and carcinoid tumors are worthy of mention. The clinical diagnosis of islet cell carcinoma, of which gastrinoma and insulinoma are most common, is established by the presence of a pancreatic nodule or mass and the associated endocrine syndrome. Islet cell carcinoma is pathologically indistinguishable from carcinoid tumor. It is reasonable to assume that, in the absence of elevated urinary 5HIAA and in the presence of histopathologic confirmation of neuroendocrine hepatic metastases, the clinical diagnosis is islet cell carcinoma. This notion has therapeutic implications. Islet cell tumors are more likely than carcinoid tumors to produce clinical endocrine syndromes from very small primary tumor masses and in the absence of hepatic metastases. Islet cell tumors like carcinoid tumors may also be mutlicentric. The clinician should be alert to the fact that islet cell tumors sometimes occur as part of the multiple endocrine neoplasia syndrome type 1.

The therapeutic principles employed in the management of islet cell carcinoma are similar to those in carcinoid tumor. Surgery is indicated for locoregional disease, which may be curative. Significant palliation and perhaps prolonged survival may result in select patients who have undergone complete resection of extensive intra-abdominal tumor. Regionally directed hepatic artery embolization may also be of palliative benefit. Further elaboration of the supportive and primary therapy for the various hormonal syndromes and islet cell tumors is beyond the scope of this discussion.

The medical oncologist is usually consulted for the management of progressive symptomatic and metastatic disease. In this circumstance, the use of the somatostatin

Table 2 Treatment Regimens in Neuroendocrine Carcinoma

Regimen	Dose	Major Side Effects	Comment
Carcinoid Syndrome and Symptomatic Islet Cell Carcinoma			
Somatostatin analogue (SMS 201–995)	150 µg SQ tid	Transient hyperglycemia, steatorrhea, pain at injection site, nausea, and vomiting	This is very well tolerated with prompt relief of symptoms. Some patients may require lower or higher dosages
Carcinoid Tumor			
5-Fluorouracil	500 mg/m² IV on days 1–5; repeat cycle q5wk	Myelosuppression, stomatitis	
Doxorubicin	60 mg/m² IV on day 1; repeat cycle q3wk	Myelosuppression, stomatitis, cardiotoxicity	This is not advisable in patients with carcinoid heart disease
Dacarbazine	250 mg/m² IV on days 1–5; repeat cycle q4–5wk	Myelosuppression, nausea, and vomiting	
Streptozotocin and 5-Fluorouracil			
Streptozotocin	500 mg/m²/day IV on days 1–5	Nausea and vomiting, renal insufficiency, proteinuria, myelosuppression, stomatitis	Combination chemotherapy does not yield superior objective response rates
5-Fluorouracil	400 mg/m²/day IV on days 1–5; 36–40; repeat cycle q10wk		
Islet Cell Carcinoma			
Streptozotocin and 5-Fluorouracil			
Streptozotocin	500 mg/m²/day IV on days 1–5	Nausea and vomiting, renal insufficiency, proteinuria, myelosuppression, stomatitis	Streptozotocin and 5-fluorouracil yield superior objective response rate and suggestive survival advantage versus streptozotocin alone
5-Fluorouracil	400 mg/m²/day IV on days 1–5; repeat cycle q6wk		
Extrapulmonary Small-Cell Carcinoma			
CAV			
Cyclophosphamide	1,000 mg/m² IV on day 1	Myelosuppression, cardiotoxicity, neuropathy	This is easy to administer as outpatient
Doxorubicin	50 mg/m² IV on day 1		
Vincristine	1.4 mg/m² IV on day 1; repeat cycle q3wk		
VP-16 and DDP			
Etoposide	100 mg/m² IV on days 1–3	Myelosuppression, renal and neurotoxicity	Closely monitor renal function. It is usually given to inpatients. Alternative regimen: VP-16, 100 mg/m² IV on day 1, with VP-16, 200 mg/m² PO divided dose on days 2 and 3, and cisplatin, 60–75 mg/m² IV on day 1.
Cisplatin	25 mg/m² IV on days 1–3; repeat cycle q3wk		

analogue may be of value, and the dosages employed are as previously described (see Table 2). Interferon may also have a therapeutic role in the management of this disease. Islet cell carcinoma appears to be more responsive to cytotoxic chemotherapy than carcinoid tumor. Objective response rates to streptozotocin range from 30 to 50 percent in this disease. Combination chemotherapy with streptozotocin and 5-fluorouracil (see Table 2) has been reported to produce a significantly better objective response rate (63 percent) when compared to streptozotocin alone (33 percent) and a suggestive survival advantage. Encouraging results with a combination of streptozotocin and doxorubicin have also been reported

in the literature. Given the apparent sensitivity of islet cell carcinoma to streptozotocin and streptozotocin-based combination regimens, it is important to consider this diagnosis in a patient with a hepatic neuroendocrine carcinoma, particularly in the absence of an elevated urinary 5HIAA.

EXTRAPULMONARY SMALL-CELL CARCINOMA

By definition, patients with extrapulmonary small-cell cancer have a histologic diagnosis of small-cell carcinoma, a normal plain radiograph and computed tomography (CT) scan of the chest, and a normal sputum cytology or negative bronchoscopy. An exception is made for the patient who may have abnormal roentgenographic studies of the chest, histologically documented small-cell cancer of the esophagus, and a normal tracheobronchial tree upon bronchoscopic examination.

Patients with extrapulmonary small-cell cancer are clinically staged in a similar fashion to those with small-cell carcinoma of the lung. In limited disease, tumor is confined to a localized anatomic region with or without regional lymphatic involvement. Spread of disease beyond locoregional boundaries is considered extensive disease. Table 3 outlines the required studies to be performed in the clinical staging of patients with extrapulmonary small-cell cancer.

Extrapulmonary small-cell neoplasms have been reported throughout the body. The natural history of these tumors in some sites appears to differ from that of small-cell lung carcinoma. Prolonged survival has been reported when tumors have been primarily managed with local modalities of surgery and radiation in contrast to small-cell lung cancer. Prolonged survival, when reported, is usually in patients with primary head and neck tumors. From review of the literature, patients with extrapulmonary small-cell cancer are not uniformly treated. It is also difficult to evaluate therapeutic strategies, because patients are not comparably staged. Only a minority of patients are treated with systemic combination chemotherapy.

The chemotherapeutic regimens used in treating extrapulmonary small-cell cancer are the same as those employed in small-cell lung carcinoma, which are outlined in Table 2. In general, patients with extensive disease in any site are best managed initially with combination chemotherapy. Radiotherapy may also provide effective palliation in many sites. The greatest challenge to the medical oncologist is to define the optimal therapy, usually combined-modality therapy, in patients with limited disease. The remainder of this discussion will outline therapeutic recommendations for

limited-disease extra-pulmonary small-cell cancer for a variety of primary sites.

Head and Neck, Esophagus, and Cervix

Primary small-cell cancers of the head and neck are not uncommon. The majority of patients with small-cell cancer of the head and neck have been treated with local modalities of surgery, radiation, or both. Some patients have enjoyed prolonged survival in the absence of systemic chemotherapy. In a small series of patients with small-cell tumors of the minor salivary glands, 30 percent survived 5 years. Impressive 5- and 10-year survival rates have been reported in patients with paranasal neuroendocrine tumors. Median survival of patients with small-cell cancer of the hypopharynx, larynx, and trachea is between 7 and 11 months.

Considering the preceding survival data, patients with primary small-cell tumors of the hypopharynx, larynx, and trachea should be initially treated with systemic combination chemotherapy. The natural history of disease in these sites closely mimics that in the lung. For limited-disease primary tumors of the minor and major salivary glands, parotid gland, paranasal sinus, and nasopharynx, attempts at complete surgical resection are undertaken and followed by adjuvant radiotherapy. For unresectable disease, primary radiotherapy is administered and followed by surgical exploration, if possible, as this may result in local eradication of disease.

A special consideration is the patient who presents with cervical lymph node metastasis with an unknown primary tumor. After an appropriate negative evaluation, as outlined in Table 3, that includes triple endoscopy, definitive radiotherapy should be administered. Irradiation of 45 to 50 cGy should be given in parallel opposed lateral fields to cover all of the neck nodal regions and an anterior field to cover the lower cervical nodes. The field is subsequently narrowed to include a boost approaching 60 to 70 cGy to the nasopharynx, oropharynx, base of the tongue, and hypopharynx.

The role of chemotherapy in extrapulmonary small-cell cancer of the head and neck, as in other sites of the body, needs to be defined. A rational consideration might be to administer adjuvant chemotherapy to patients who are a good medical risk and to all patients who have residual disease after local modalities of therapy. Whether chemotherapy will appreciably improve survival in patients with limited disease who were treated with local modalities of therapy remains to be answered.

Median survival of small-cell cancer of the esophagus is regarded as 3 months. The esophagus is the most common site of this disease within the gastrointestinal tract. Historically, surgery has been the primary mode of therapy. Radiation therapy is effective for palliation and local control. Increasing reports of the use of primary chemotherapy in the management of this disease are appearing. Given the aggressive clinical course and poor survival, patients with this disease should be treated with systemic combination chemotherapy initially, regardless of stage. In patients thought to have anaplastic or

Table 3 Staging Evaluation for Extrapulmonary Small-Cell Carcinoma

Recommended
  Chest radiograph
  Chest and abdominal/pelvic computer tomography scan
  Bone marrow aspiration and biopsy (to confirm limited disease)
  Sputum cytology or bronchoscopy

Optional
  Bone scan
  Head computed tomography scan

Special Considerations by Primary Site
  Head and neck: direct laryngoscopy, bronchoscopy, and
    esophagoscopy
  Esophagus: upper endoscopy and bronchoscopy
  Cervix: pelvic examination and intravenous pyelogram
  Urinary bladder: cytoscopy
  Colon and rectum: lower endoscopy

undifferentiated carcinomas of the esophagus, it is important to consider that this may represent a nonpulmonary small-cell cancer. Perhaps with earlier recognition of this entity and the use of chemotherapy, the otherwise grim prognosis in these patients may be improved.

Histologic subtypes of cervical carcinoma are of prognostic significance. Small-cell carcinoma has the poorest prognosis. This latter group is divided into neuroendocrine and squamous or epithelial small-cell variants. True neuroendocrine small-cell carcinoma of the cervix may be the most common nonpulmonary site of this disease and appears to pursue a more aggressive clinical course than other histologic types of cervical cancer.

Therapy for cervical small-cell cancer has included surgery, radiation, or both. More recent reports of true neuroendocrine cervical small-cell carcinoma report 5-year survival rates between 10 and 20 percent. It is known that radiotherapy is superior to radical surgery in preventing local recurrence and that the former modality is not effective in salvaging patients who relapse postoperatively. The use of systemic chemotherapy in advanced disease, although not widely reported, has been discouraging. Small-cell tumors of the cervix do not appear to be as chemosensitive as their pulmonary counterpart. It is advisable to manage patients who are diagnosed with small-cell cervical carcinoma aggressively. Given the relatively young age and good medical condition of the majority of women with this disease, initial therapy should include radical surgery, radiation, or both, and this should be followed by adjuvant chemotherapy.

Colon, Rectum, and Pancreas

Early studies of small-cell carcinoma of the large intestine have observed 10-year survival rates in approximately 40 percent of patients who underwent curative resection. More recent reports have not observed such favorable outcome, because the majority of patients presented with metastatic disease and median survival was 5 months. Surgery has been the primary mode of therapy. There is little information about adjuvant radiation in patients having undergone surgical resection of primary rectal small-cell carcinoma. The role of chemotherapy in both colon and rectal cancer is not well defined, but its use is increasingly reported in patients with advanced disease, with activity comparable to that for lung cancer. Therefore, all patients with colorectal small-cell cancer should be explored with the intention of primary resection. In patients with primary colon cancers, adjuvant combination chemotherapy is appropriate. In those with primary rectal lesions, adjuvant radiotherapy should be considered and possibly followed by a course of consolidation chemotherapy.

Small-cell carcinomas of the pancreas are rare and are characterized by a very rapid clinical course. This problem is not unlike adenocarcinoma in this site, where early detection rarely occurs. Surgery is not recommended, and patients are best approached with systemic therapy.

Uterus, Kidney, Prostate, and Urinary Bladder

For the limited number of patients with small-cell carcinoma of the uterus and kidney, surgery has been the mainstay of therapy. Mean survival is approximately 1 year and only a few patients have received chemotherapy. For a young patient with small primary tumors, aggressive surgery followed by adjuvant combination chemotherapy may be appropriate.

Small-cell carcinoma of the prostate and urinary bladder is increasingly recognized. Small-cell cancer in these sites is frequently admixed with adenocarcinoma and transitional cell carcinoma. The small-cell component generally portends a poor prognosis.

Surgery has been most commonly employed in patients with small-cell carcinoma of the prostate. Whether small-cell cancer in this gland is responsive to hormonal manipulation remains to be defined, although one would not expect it to be. Similarly, the chemoresponsiveness of small-cell prostate cancer is largely unknown. For patients with disease confined to the prostate, local modalities of treatment are initially recommended, and the role of adjuvant therapies, both hormonal and cytotoxic, needs to be explored.

For patients with small-cell carcinoma of the urinary bladder, local modalities of therapy alone, cystectomy, radiation, or both are probably inadequate as primary therapy. This disease tends to pursue an aggressive clinical course, with widespread metastases and survival recorded in months. A combined-modality approach employing combination chemotherapy in patients with disease confined to the urinary bladder appears warranted.

Extrapulmonary small-cell cancer is a distinct clinicopathologic entity from small-cell anaplastic carcinoma of the lung. Experience with chemotherapy as primary, adjuvant, or consolidative treatment for extrapulmonary small-cell cancer is limited. Presentations limited to a single extrapulmonary site represent a challenge to the clinician. Optimal integration of all modalities of treatment (surgery, radiation, and chemotherapy) is appropriate, although the specific sequence remains to be defined. Patients with extensive metastatic disease are best approached with primary systemic combination chemotherapy.

SUGGESTED READING

Kvols LK, Moertel CG, O'Connell MJ, et al. Treatment of the malignant carcinoid syndrome: Evaluation of a long-acting somatostatin analogue. N Engl J Med 1986; 315:663–666.

Levenson RM, Ihde DC, Matthews MJ, et al. Small-cell carcinoma presenting as an extrapulmonary neoplasm: Sites of origin and response to chemotherapy. J Natl Cancer Inst 1981; 67:607–612.

Marsh HM, Martin JK Jr, Kvols LK, et al. Carcinoid crisis during anesthesia: Successful treatment with a somatostatin analogue. Anesthesiology 1987; 66:89–91.

Moertel CG. An odyssey in the land of small tumors. J Clin Oncol 1987; 5:1,503–1,522.

Moertel CG, Hanley JA, Johnson LA. Streptozocin alone compared with streptozocin plus fluorouracil in the treatment of advanced islet-cell carcinoma. N Engl J Med 1980; 303:1,189–1,194.

Remick SC, Hafez GR, Carbone PP. Extrapulmonary small-cell carcinoma: A review of the literature with emphasis on therapy and outcome. Medicine 1987; 66:457–471.

CANCER OF UNKNOWN PRIMARY SITE

F. ANTHONY GRECO, M.D.
JOHN D. HAINSWORTH, M.D.

Patients with metastatic cancer and no obvious primary site are relatively common, accounting for about 5 to 10 percent of all cancer patients. Until recently, this group of patients attracted little attention, because their prognosis was uniformly poor, regardless of treatment. However, effective therapy is now available for many types of advanced cancer, so it is not surprising that some carcinomas of unknown primary site are very sensitive to chemotherapeutic agents. The clinician must approach each patient with carcinoma of unknown primary site with the objectives to identify patients with treatable malignancies, using both clinical and pathologic criteria, and to avoid superfluous diagnostic procedures and inappropriate treatment in patients with unresponsive neoplasms.

The typical patient with cancer of unknown primary site develops symptoms at a metastatic site; routine history, physical examination, chest radiograph, and laboratory studies fail to identify the primary site. In this clinical setting, light microscopic examination of the biopsy specimen usually identifies one of four major categories: (1) poorly differentiated neoplasm; (2) adenocarcinoma; (3) squamous carcinoma; or (4) poorly differentiated carcinoma. These four groups identified by light microscopic examination vary with respect to clinical characteristics, recommended diagnostic evaluation, treatment, and prognosis.

POORLY DIFFERENTIATED NEOPLASMS OF UNKNOWN PRIMARY SITE

The diagnosis of poorly differentiated "neoplasm" can describe a large number of neoplasms, many of which are highly responsive to systemic therapy. The diagnosis implies the inability of the pathologist to distinguish between carcinoma and other cancers, such as lymphoma, sarcoma, and melanoma. Further evalu-

ation is always necessary in these patients and frequently results in a more precise diagnosis, often with specific therapeutic implications. The most common cause of a nonspecific pathologic diagnosis is an inadequate biopsy. Fine-needle aspiration biopsy usually provides inadequate amounts of tissue for the initial diagnosis of metastatic cancer, because histology is poorly preserved and adequate material is not available for special studies. Often, a specific and more definitive diagnosis can be made by obtaining a larger biopsy. Some pathologic studies require special processing of the biopsy specimen; therefore, close communication with the surgeon and pathologist is important if repeat biopsy is performed.

Occasionally, light microscopic examination alone fails to provide a diagnosis more specific than poorly differentiated neoplasm or poorly differentiated carcinoma, even when a large, adequately preserved biospy specimen is available. Immunoperoxidase staining and electron microscopy are indicated for further examination of the neoplasm. Immunoperoxidase staining is now widely available, and a number of useful stains have been developed (common leukocyte antigen, epithelial membrane antigen, keratins, vimentin, S-100, prostate specific antigen, neuron-specific enolase, and others). Because these stains are not usually specific, they should not be used alone to make a diagnosis; however, they are frequently useful in conjunction with the light microscopic examination and clinical features. These stains can suggest the diagnosis of lymphoma, melanoma, neuroendocrine carcinoma, sarcoma, or germ cell tumor. However, some neoplasms can only be classified as carcinomas, whereas in up to 30 percent of patients, immunoperoxidase staining gives inconclusive results.

The examination of cellular ultrastructure by electron microscopy can also provide important information in the differential diagnosis of poorly differentiated neoplasms. The important distinction between lymphoma and carcinoma can be made in most instances. Other important ultrastructural findings include neurosecretory granules (neuroendocrine tumors such as small-cell lung cancer, carcinoid tumors, neuroblastoma), premelanosomes (melanoma), and intracellular lumina/surface microvilli (adenocarcinoma).

Two specific chromosomal rearrangements associated with solid tumors have recently been identified. A large percentage of germ cell tumors (both testicular and extragonadal) have an isochromosome of the short arm of chromosome 12 (il2p). Peripheral neuroepithelioma and Ewing's tumor share a specific chromosomal translocation (11;22). In the future, the recognition of additional specific chromosomal abnormalities may facilitate the identification of tumor lineage or origin in other patients.

ADENOCARCINOMA OF UNKNOWN PRIMARY SITE

Clinical Features and Natural History

About 70 percent of all carcinomas of unknown primary site are adenocarcinomas. The typical patient with this diagnosis is elderly and has metastatic tumor at multiple sites. The most common sites of involvement are the liver, lungs, and bones, but many other sites are also involved.

In most patients, the clinical course is dominated by symptoms related to the sites of metastases. The primary site becomes obvious during the clinical course in only 15 to 20 percent of patients. At autopsy, however, a primary site can be detected in 60 to 80 percent of patients. The most common primary sites are pancreas and lung, accounting for approximately 40 percent of all cases; other gastrointestinal sites (stomach, colon, liver) are also frequent. Adenocarcinomas of the breast and prostate, which occur commonly in the general population, are infrequently identified in this group of patients.

Pathology

The diagnosis of adenocarcinoma is based on the formation of glandular structures by neoplastic cells and is usually made without difficulty using light microscopy. All adenocarcinomas share these histologic features; therefore, the site of origin usually cannot be ascertained. Specialized pathologic evaluation infrequently provides useful additional information; one exception is the immunoperoxidase stain for prostate-specific antigen, which is quite specific for prostate cancer and should be used in men with suggestive clinical findings. Immunoperoxidase stains for estrogen receptors are also available and should be considered in women with metastatic adenocarcinoma in whom estrogen and progesterone receptors were not obtained.

The histopathologic diagnosis of poorly differentiated adenocarcinoma should be viewed differently because these patients may vary both with respect to tumor biology and responsiveness to systemic therapy. This diagnosis is made when only minimal glandular formation is seen by light microscopy. Sometimes, the diagnosis is based on a positive mucin stain alone in a tumor that would otherwise be called poorly differentiated carcinoma. Additional pathologic study with electron microscopy and immunoperoxidase stains should be performed on these tumors. Evaluation and treatment of these patients are similar to that of patients with poorly differentiated carcinoma.

Diagnostic Evaluation

A summary of the recommended methods of evaluation for this group of patients is outlined in Table 1. All patients with adenocarcinoma of unknown primary site should undergo a thorough history and physical examination (including pelvic examination in women), standard laboratory screening tests (complete blood count, SMA18, and urinalysis), and chest radiograph. Serum acid phosphatase level should be measured in men, and all women should have mammography, because palliative therapy is available for patients with advanced prostate or breast cancer. Computed tomography of the abdomen can identify the primary site in 20 to 35 percent of patients and should probably be included in the routine evaluation. Additional radiologic

Table 1 Evaluation of Patients with Adenocarcinoma of Unknown Primary Site

Histopathology	Clinical Evaluation*	Special Pathologic Studies	Subgroups with Treatable Tumors	Prognosis
Well-differentiated adenocarcinoma	CT scan of abdomen; acid phosphatase (men); mammograms (women); additional radiologic studies to evaluate abnormal symptoms, signs, laboratory values	Men: prostate-specific antigen (immunoperoxidase) Women: estrogen receptor, progesterone receptor	Women with axillary node metastasis Women with peritoneal carcinomatosis Men with blastic bone metastasis	Poor for entire group, (median survival = 4 mo); better for treatable subgroups
Poorly differentiated carcinoma and poorly differentiated adenocarcinoma	CT scan of abdomen, chest; serum HCG, AFP; additional radiologic studies to evaluate abnormal symptoms, signs, laboratory values	Immunoperoxidase staining; electron microscopy	Neuroendocrine tumors Predominant tumor location in mediastinum, retroperitoneum, lymph nodes	Variable—about 15% curable with cisplatin-based chemotherapy; many others receive useful palliation
Squamous carcinoma (cervical lymph nodes)	Direct laryngoscopy with visualization of nasopharynx; fiberoptic bronchoscopy	—	Nodes located in high or mid-cervical region	30 to 50% long-term survival with radical surgery or radiotherapy

*In addition to history, physical examination, blood counts, serum chemistries and chest radiography.

evaluation should evaluate clues and abnormalities identified by history, physical examination, or routine laboratory studies; radiologic evaluation of asymptomatic areas is rarely useful.

Treatment and Prognosis

Therapy for patients with adenocarcinoma of unknown primary site depends on the recognition, based on clinical features, of certain treatable patient subgroups. Women who have adenocarcinoma involving axillary lymph nodes should be suspected of having breast cancer. Documentation of estrogen receptors in the tumor tissue is strong supportive evidence for this diagnosis. Women who have no evidence of other metastatic sites may have stage II breast cancer and are therefore potentially curable with appropriate therapy. Even when physical examination is negative, 50 to 60 percent of women have a small, primary breast tumor found following mastectomy. Therapy includes a simple mastectomy and axillary node dissection; radiation therapy to the breast and axilla may be an equally effective alternative. Women with other metastatic sites in addition to axillary lymph nodes may have metastatic breast cancer; treatment with either hormonal therapy or combination chemotherapy is often of major palliative benefit.

Women with peritoneal carcinomatosis have tumors that can at times be treated effectively using the guidelines established for ovarian cancer. Some of these women may have unrecognized ovarian cancer; however, excellent treatment results can also be achieved in women who have had previous oophorectomy or normal ovaries. Therapy should include laparotomy with attempted surgical cytoreduction, followed by combination chemotherapy, which is known to be useful for ovarian carcinoma. With optimal treatment, median survival in this group is about 2 years; 15 percent of patients achieve long-term, disease-free survival.

Men with blastic bone metastases, elevated serum acid phosphatase level, or tumor staining with prostate-specific antigen should be suspected of having prostate adenocarcinoma. Hormonal therapy may provide effective palliation.

For the remainder of patients with metastatic adenocarcinoma of unknown primary site, treatment is relatively ineffective. This is not surprising, because the majority of these patients have primary sites in either the lung or the gastrointestinal tract, that are relatively unresponsive to systemic therapy. Treatment with a variety of chemotherapeutic agents, used either singly or in combination, produces low response rates (5 to 30 percent) and has little impact on the short median survival of 3 to 6 months. Regimens with partial response rates of 20 to 30 percent include 5-fluorouracil, doxorubicin, and mitomycin-C, and cisplatin and etoposide. Responses with these regimens are usually partial and persist for only a few months. Although a brief trial of such treatment is reasonable, it is also appropriate to treat these patients with symptomatic care alone, particularly if they are elderly or debilitated.

SQUAMOUS CARCINOMA OF UNKNOWN PRIMARY SITE

Squamous carcinoma at a metastatic site is unusual in the absence of an obvious primary site. Effective treatment is available for some of these patients, and appropriate evaluation is important.

Cervical lymph nodes are the most common metastatic site for squamous carcinoma of unknown primary site. Patients are usually middle-aged or elderly and have a history of substantial tobacco use. Patients with squamous carcinoma in upper or mid-cervical lymph nodes should be suspected of having a primary tumor in the head and neck region. They should have thorough examination of the oropharynx, nasopharynx, hypopharynx, larynx, and upper esophagus by direct laryngoscopy, and any suspicious areas should be biopsied. Patients with squamous carcinoma involving the lower cervical or supraclavicular lymph nodes are more likely to have lung cancer, and fiberoptic bronchoscopy is indicated if the head and neck examination and chest radiograph are unrevealing.

For patients with no identified primary site, treatment should be given to the involved neck. Similar treatment results have been obtained with radical neck dissection, high-dose radiation therapy, or a combination of these modalities. In patients with high or mid-cervical adenopathy, 3-year survival after such treatment ranges from 35 to 60 percent. These patients probably have clinically undetectable primaries in the head and neck, which are effectively treated with the local metastatic disease. Long-term survival is poor for patients with lower cervical or supraclavicular adenopathy, probably because most of these patients have lung cancer. However, a small group (10 to 15 percent) achieve long-term survival after local treatment to the cervical area.

Squamous carcinoma appearing in inguinal lymph nodes usually arises from primaries in the genital or anorectal areas. Women should undergo careful examination of the vulva, vagina, and cervix, with biopsy of any suspicious areas. Men should have careful inspection of the penis. The anorectal area should be examined by digital examination and anoscopy in both sexes, with biopsy of suspicious areas. Finding a primary site in these patients is important, because therapy of carcinomas of the vulva, vagina, cervix, and anus may be curative even after spread to regional lymph nodes.

Metastatic squamous carcinoma in other visceral sites almost always represents metastatic lung cancer. The clinician should be suspicious of the diagnosis of poorly differentiated squamous carcinoma, particularly if other clinical features are unusual for lung cancer (i.e., young patient, nonsmoker, unusual metastatic site). One should consider additional pathologic evaluation with immunoperoxidase studies or electron microscopy as well as a trial of therapy as described later for patients with poorly differentiated carcinoma. If clinical features suggest the possibility of a lung cancer, computed tomography of the chest and fiberoptic bronchoscopy are appropriate.

POORLY DIFFERENTIATED CARCINOMA OF UNKNOWN PRIMARY SITE

Approximately 25 percent of carcinomas of unknown primary site have a poorly differentiated histology. In the past, patients with this diagnosis were not considered separately from the larger group with adenocarcinoma of unknown primary site and were assumed to have similar poor response to treatment and short survival. Increasing evidence indicates that these patients form a distinct group with respect to clinical features, tumor biology, and responsiveness to systemic therapy. All patients in this group should be evaluated carefully. Some have extremely responsive neoplasms, and some are curable with appropriate systemic therapy.

Clinical Characteristics

These patients are frequently younger than patients with well-differentiated adenocarcinoma of unknown primary site and often give a history of rapid progression of symptoms and have objective evidence of rapid tumor growth. Tumor in lymph nodes, mediastinum, and retroperitoneum is more common in this group, although many sites can be involved with metastases.

Pathology

Patients with a light microscopic diagnosis of poorly differentiated carcinoma should undergo additional pathologic study with immunoperoxidase staining and electron microscopy as described for patients with poorly differentiated neoplasms. These studies can suggest unsuspected diagnoses in up to 25 percent of this patient group, including some for which a specific therapy is available (e.g., lymphoma, neuroendocrine tumors, Ewing's tumor).

Diagnostic Evaluation

The initial diagnostic evaluation of these patients should be similar to that described for patients with adenocarcinoma of unknown primary site (see Table 1). Computed tomography of the chest and abdomen should be performed owing to the frequency with which these tumors involve the mediastinum and retroperitoneum. Measurement of the serum tumor markers human chorionic gonadotropin (HCG) and alpha-fetoprotein is essential in all patients, because elevated levels of these substances suggest the diagnosis of a germ cell tumor.

Treatment

When a specific diagnosis of a treatable neoplasm is made on the basis of specialized pathologic study, patients should be treated appropriately. In addition, patients with elevated levels of HCG or alpha-fetoprotein should be treated with combination chemotherapy effective against germ cell tumors, even if this histologic diagnosis cannot be made definitively.

The majority of patients in this group will have no diagnosis more specific than poorly differentiated carcinoma or poorly differentiated adenocarcinoma and will have normal serum tumor markers. Some of these patients have highly responsive neoplasms, and up to 30 percent will have complete response to combination chemotherapy with intensive cisplatin-based regimens such as those used in the treatment of germ cell tumors. Approximately 50 percent of the complete responders (15 percent of the entire group) have prolonged disease-free survival. Clinical features associated with chemotherapy responsiveness include location of tumor in the mediastinum, retroperitoneum, or lymph nodes (as opposed to other visceral sites), and younger age. Chemotherapy-responsive tumors cannot always be reliably predicted using clinical and pathologic criteria; therefore, it is reasonable to give all patients in this group a trial of cisplatin-based chemotherapy. A trial of one or two courses should be administered, followed by re-evaluation for response; responders should receive a total of four courses, whereas nonresponders should be removed from treatment.

A subset of patients have neuroendocrine features identified only by electron microscopy or immunoperoxidase staining. The nature of these tumors is unclear; some patients may have unrecognized small-cell lung cancer, but approximately 50 percent of patients in this group are nonsmokers, making the diagnosis of small-cell lung cancer unlikely. Although optimal therapy for these patients is undefined, a high response rate can be achieved using cisplatin-based combination chemotherapy. Some achieve complete response to therapy, and a small percentage are long-term survivors.

SUGGESTED READING

Greco FA, Vaughn WK, Hainsworth JD. Advanced poorly differentiated carcinoma of unknown primary site: Recognition of a treatable syndrome. Ann Intern Med 1986; 104:547.

Hainsworth JD, Dial TW, Greco FA. Curative combination chemotherapy for patients with advanced poorly differentiated carcinoma of unknown primary site. Am J Clin Oncol 1988; 11:138.

Hainsworth JD, Johnson DH, Greco FA. Poorly differentiated neuroendocrine carcinoma of unknown primary site: A newly recognized clinicopathologic entity. Ann Intern Med 1988; 109:364.

Patel J, Nemoto T, Rosner D, et al. Axillary lymph node metastasis from an occult breast cancer. Cancer 1981; 47:2923.

Strnad CM, Grosh WW, Baxter J, et al. Peritoneal carcinomatosis of unknown primary site in women: A distinctive subset of adenocarcinoma. Ann Intern Med 1989; 111:213.

PEDIATRIC SOLID TUMORS

PAUL S. GAYNON, M.D.

Cancer in infants, children, and adolescents is rare compared to cancer in adults. It has an annual incidence of 12.7 cases per year among 100,000 children younger than 15 years of age. However, cancer is still the second leading cause of death among young people, after accidents and excluding neonatal complications. Modern multimodality therapy results in cure for over 60 percent of those afflicted. In 1950, the cancer mortality rate among children was 8.0 per 100,000 and in 1982, 4.3 per 100,000. The participation of a majority of newly diagnosed children in the United States in formal clinical trials has contributed to the progress seen thus far and has lent credence to a claim that gains in the treatment of childhood malignancy are reflected sooner in national mortality statistics than in the medical literature. By the year 2000, 1 in 1,000 young adults will be a survivor of childhood cancer.

Children are best treated in a major center under the care of a multidisciplinary team of experienced pediatric health care professionals, including oncologists, surgeons, pathologists, radiotherapists, diagnostic radiologists, oncology nurses, psychologists, and social workers, in order to arrive most rapidly at the correct diagnosis, establish the extent of disease, determine the plan of treatment with the best chance for cure and the least potential for late sequelae, and provide thorough explanation and age-appropriate education and ongoing psychosocial support to the child and his or her family. Such a setting provides access to facilities for pediatric intensive care, pediatric anesthesia, and the variety of pediatric subspecialists. In major centers, inpatient pediatric nurses are most likely to be familiar with chemotherapy and its complications, with central venous line care, and with the psychosocial needs of children with cancer and their families. In a university center, families have the best opportunity to participate in the formal clinical trials that assure state-of-the-art treatment and have led to past improvement in outcome.

Irradiation dosage must be modified with regard to patient age. Chemotherapy dosage is generally based on surface area. However, such an approach tends to produce excess toxicity in infants and toddlers, for whom dosage per unit body weight needs to be considered. Intrathecal dosage may best be based on age rather than weight or surface area.

BRAIN TUMORS

Brain tumors are the single largest category of childhood solid tumors, accounting for 19 percent of new cancer cases and 25 percent of cancer deaths and for 27 percent of new solid tumor cases and 42 percent of solid tumor deaths. In adults, supratentorial tumors predominate. In children, 57 percent are infratentorial; 48 percent involve the cerebellum and fourth ventricle, and 9 percent involve the brain stem. Forty-three percent are supratentorial, 27 percent involve the cerebral hemispheres, and 16 percent involve midline structures. Symptoms correlate with the site of the tumor.

Medulloblastoma

Medulloblastoma is the most common tumor involving the cerebellum and fourth ventricle and comprises 23 percent of pediatric brain tumors. Patients frequently present with hydrocephalus. Increased ventricular pressure should be reduced by ventriculostomy prior to craniotomy in order to prevent herniation, whether or not a permanent ventriculoperitoneal shunt is planned. At presentation, myelography demonstrates subarachnoid dissemination in more than 30 percent of patients.

Conventional therapy has included surgery and irradiation. With surgery and irradiation limited to the cranium, cure was rare. With surgery and craniospinal irradiation, 50 percent to 60 percent of patients will survive 5 years. Over the course of their illness, 5 percent of children may have metastases outside of the central nervous system.

Between 1976 and 1981, the Children's Cancer Study Group (CCSG) and the International Society of Pediatric Oncology (SIOP) evaluated adjuvant chemotherapy following completion of craniospinal irradiation therapy. The CCSG excluded children less than 2 years of age and employed vincristine, CCNU, and prednisone. The SIOP included children less than 2 years of age and studied vincristine and CCNU. On the CCSG trial, the 54-month progression-free survival (PFS) was 59 percent for patients assigned to adjuvant therapy and 49 percent for those assigned to no adjuvant therapy; on the SIOP trial, the PFS was 55 percent and 43 percent, respectively. Statistical significance was marginal. In both trials, however, patients with more extensive disease (Chang stages T_{3-4}, M_{1-4}) appeared to obtain greater benefit from adjuvant therapy than those patients with more limited disease (Chang stage T_1 to T_2, M_0).

The present CCSG trial for children with extensive local disease or any evidence of metastatic spread compares pre- and postirradiation "8-in-1" chemotherapy (Table 1) to postirradiation chemotherapy with vincristine, CCNU, and prednisone, as employed in the previous trial. In similar patients, SIOP is employing high-dose methotrexate, procarbazine, and vincristine preirradiation and vincristine and CCNU postirradiation. The Pediatric Oncology Group (POG) is testing the value of postirradiation adjuvant therapy with MOPP chemotherapy as employed in Hodgkin's disease.

In a joint CCSG-POG study, children with more limited local disease and no evidence of metastatic spread will receive surgery and craniospinal irradiation either at a dose of 25 cGy or 35 cGy. All patients will receive 50 cGy to the posterior fossa.

Table 1 Eight-in-One Chemotherapy (14 to 28-Day Cycle)

Hour 0

Vincristine	1.5 mg/m² (max 2.0 mg)
Methylprednisolone	300 mg/m² repeat hour 6 and 12
CCNU	75 mg/m²

Hour 1

Procarbazine	75 mg/m²

Hour 2

Hydroxyurea	3,000 mg/m² for malignant astrocytoma
	1,500 mg/m² for medulloblastoma

Hour 3–9

Cisplatin	90 mg/m² for malignant astrocytoma
	60 mg/m² for medulloblastoma

Hour 9

Cytosine arabinoside	300 mg/m²

Hour 12

DTIC	150 mg/m² for malignant astrocytoma
Cyclophosphamide	300 mg/m² for medulloblastoma

Infants and children younger than 4 years of age are more likely to have more advanced disease at presentation than older children. Even after adjustment for "T" and "M" stage, however, younger children have had a worse outcome in several trials. In addition, the neuropsychological and endocrinologic sequelae of brain irradiation are more severe in younger children. A number of investigators have recommended primary treatment with surgery and chemotherapy for infants, omitting or modifying radiation therapy. The radiation dose may be reduced and administration limited to the posterior fossa or delayed until completion of planned chemotherapy.

Low-Grade Astrocytoma

Surgery is the mainstay of therapy for low-grade astrocytoma. Supratentorial astrocytomas constitute 36 percent of pediatric brain tumors. Two-thirds are histologically low grade—grade 1 or 2. The National Cancer Institute's Surveillance, Epidemiology, and End Results Program (SEER) reports an overall 71 percent 5-year survival. Survival is better for patients with optic gliomas and hypothalamic gliomas and worse for patients with cerebral hemisphere gliomas. Cerebellar astrocytomas constitute 12 percent of pediatric brain tumors. Most are histologically grade 1, with a few being grade 2. Seventy-five percent are classified as juvenile (synonyms: pilocytic, microcystic); 25 percent are classified as diffuse and appear indistinguishable from adult cerebellar astrocytoma. The SEER reports a 91 percent 5-year survival for children with cerebellar astrocytoma. Outcome is significantly worse for patients with diffuse cerebellar astrocytoma. Surgery alone may be adequate when a complete resection has been obtained. After less complete resections, local irradiation is commonly administered, although clear evidence of efficacy is lacking. The CCSG is mounting a study in which children older

than 5 years of age with low-grade astrocytoma and incomplete resection will be randomly assigned to receive or not to receive adjuvant radiation therapy.

Children with neurofibromatosis are at increased risk for development of a variety of malignancies, including central nervous system malignancies, especially optic glioma. The natural history of these patients is poorly documented. Some have reported that children with neurofibromatosis and optic glioma have a more benign course than others with histologically identical lesions but without neurofibromatosis. Others have found otherwise. Routine magnetic resonance imaging (MRI) scanning has frequently demonstrated abnormalities in asymptomatic children with neurofibromatosis. At present, surgery, irradiation therapy, and chemotherapy are best deferred until clinical or radiographic progression occurs in children with neurofibromatosis who are asymptomatic.

High-Grade or Malignant Supratentorial Astrocytoma

The SEER reports a 35 percent 5-year survival for children with high-grade or malignant supratentorial astrocytoma diagnosed between 1973 and 1980. These tumors constitute about 11 percent of pediatric brain tumors. Local recurrence is common despite surgery and radiation therapy. Between 1976 and 1981, CCSG investigators randomly assigned 58 children with malignant astrocytoma (18 grade 3 and 40 grade 4) to receive or not to receive adjuvant vincristine, CCNU, and prednisone after surgery and radiation therapy. The 5-year PFS was 46 percent for the adjuvant chemotherapy group and 18 percent for the no-adjuvant-therapy group. This difference was statistically significant and persisted after correction for various known prognostic factors. Survival was better for patients who had total, subtotal, or partial resection than for patients who had only biopsy. The current CCSG trial is testing pre- and postirradiation "8-in-1" chemotherapy. In "8-in-1" for malignant astrocytoma, DTIC replaces cyclophosphamide (see Table 1). Current recommendations for therapy include aggressive surgery, local radiation therapy, and chemotherapy. Again, radiation therapy may be omitted, modified, or delayed for infants.

Brain-Stem Gliomas

Brain-stem gliomas constitute 9 percent of pediatric malignancies. The SEER reports an 18 percent 5-year survival. Biopsy and determination of histologic malignancy may be useful for patients with findings suggestive of a better prognosis, namely, patients with no cranial nerve palsies at presentation and isodense rather than hypodense lesions on unenhanced computed tomography (CT) scan. Even with CT and MRI, diagnosis is not infallible. Biopsy, either via craniotomy or CT-guided stereotactic techniques, should be performed if imaging studies suggest a benign process, e.g., arteriovenous malformation, paracytic cyst, encephalitis, or tuberculoma, or a less usual malignant process, e.g., ependymoma or medulloblastoma. Subtotal resection may be of therapeutic value if the lesion is exophytic, has a significant cystic component, or lies at the medullocervical junction. The role of surgery in a patient with a typical intrinsic pontine lesion is unclear at present.

With conventional aggressive radiation therapy, the consistent problem has been local recurrence. No benefit has been demonstrated for adjuvant chemotherapy with vincristine, prednisone, and CCNU. Current attention is focused on the use of hyperfractionated irradiation. Rapidly proliferating neoplastic cells are more sensitive to irradiation than are the more slowly proliferating glial and vascular tissues. Normal cells are better able to repair sublethal irradiation damage than are neoplastic cells. Therefore, more frequent and smaller irradiation doses exploit this difference by allowing nonneoplastic tissues to repair sublethal damage. At this writing, a dose of 78 cGy is under study.

LYMPHOMA

Lymphomas account for 17 percent of childhood solid tumors and 12 percent of tumor deaths. Forty-three percent of children with lymphoma have Hodgkin's disease, and 57 percent of children have non-Hodgkin's lymphoma. The SEER found 5-year survivals of 84 percent and 51 percent for children with Hodgkin's disease and non-Hodgkin's lymphoma who were diagnosed between 1976 and 1981. Recent experience is likely better. Lymphomas are uncommon in early childhood.

In pediatric lymphoma, surgery and proper handling of an adequate volume of biopsy material is critical primarily for diagnosis, not treatment. Diagnosis requires removal of an entire node so that nodal architecture as well as cell morphology might be examined. Children frequently have reactive inguinal nodes, whether they have lymphoma or not, and despite concerns about cosmesis, enlarged cervical, supraclavicular, or axillary nodes may yield a diagnosis more reliably. However, children with resectable abdominal non-Hodgkin's lymphoma do benefit from gross total excision. Such lymphomas are generally nonlymphoblastic.

Hodgkin's Disease

Pediatric Hodgkin's disease is similar to Hodgkin's disease in adults, except that lymphocyte depletion histology is rarely seen. Children are more tolerant of myelosuppressive chemotherapy than are adults, but they are more vulnerable to the growth-limiting effects of radiation therapy. Because long-term survival is expected with a variety of therapeutic strategies, late sequelae of therapy such as infertility, coronary artery disease, pulmonary fibrosis, hypothyroidism, anthracycline cardiotoxicity, and secondary malignancies become primary concerns. Splenectomy places patients at lifelong risk for overwhelming sepsis and may increase the incidence of secondary leukemias.

Non-Hodgkin's Lymphomas

Pediatric non-Hodgkin's lymphomas are generally divided into two groups by histology for purposes of treatment: diffuse lymphoblastic lymphoma and diffuse nonlymphoblastic lymphoma. Some prefer to divide nonlymphoblastic lymphomas into large-cell lymphoma and "undifferentiated" lymphoma, which includes both Burkitt's lymphoma and non-Burkitt's types. Nodular histology is extraordinarily rare. Formal surgical staging is rarely indicated.

Lymphoblastic lymphomas constitute about 38 percent of the cases of pediatric non-Hodgkin's lymphoma. They usually arise from lymphatic sites above the diaphragm. A mediastinal presentation is most frequent. Such patients are at risk for sudden tracheal compression and respiratory embarrassment. Rapid diagnosis, prompt staging, and early initiation of specific therapy is useful. Emergency mediastinal irradiation may be lifesaving. Patients with more than 25 percent marrow blasts and FAB L1 or L2 morphology are generally thought to have acute lymphoblastic leukemia, despite the presence of a "lymphomatous mass." Patients with lymphoblastic lymphoma are treated aggressively whether they have localized disease (Murphy stage I or II) or the more common disseminated disease (Murphy stage III or IV). A recently completed trial compared the conventional 10-drug LSA2L2 regimen with a simplified, less toxic, experimental regimen called ADCOMP (Table 2) and found a 70 percent 4-year event-free survival with either. Both regimens employed central nervous system prophylaxis with intrathecal chemotherapy and no prophylactic cranial irradiation. Although this study employed irradiation therapy to sites of original extra-abdominal bulky disease, the role of irradiation therapy is controversial.

"Undifferentiated" lymphoma (Burkitt's and non-Burkitt's) usually arises in the abdomen or in the head and neck region. Children with massive abdominal disease and elevated lactic dehydrogenase (LDH) levels are at highest risk for tumor lysis syndrome, i.e., hyperuricemia, hyperphosphatemia, hypocalcemia, and renal failure. Large-cell lymphoma usually arises in the mediastinum or in the head and neck region. In a seminal randomized trial, the 10-drug LSA2L2 regimen was shown to be superior to the simpler, less toxic COMP regimen (Table 3) for children with lymphoblastic lymphoma. However, for children with nonlymphoblastic lymphoma, i.e., "undifferentiated" or large-cell lymphoma, COMP was shown to be superior to LSA2L2. Children with localized disease (Murphy stage I or II) or grossly resected abdominal disease have achieved a 4-year event-free survival of greater than 90 percent with six 1-month cycles of COMP and no radiation therapy. In the past, surgery and radiation therapy were curative for fewer than half of such patients. Patients with more advanced disease receive 18 1-month cycles of COMP. Outcome is less satisfactory, as only 57 percent of patients survive disease-free at 2 years. Marrow or central nervous system disease at diagnosis is a grave finding in children with nonlymphoblastic lymphoma but

Table 2 ADCOMP for Lymphoblastic Lymphoma

	Dose	Schedule
Induction (35-day course)		
Cyclophosphamide	1,200 mg/m^2 IV	Day 0
Vincristine	2.0 mg/m^2 IV	Days 2, 9, 16, 23
Prednisone	60 mg/m^2/day PO	Days 2–29
Daunomycin	60 mg/m^2 IV	Day 16
L-Asparaginase	6,000 U/m^2 × 9 MWF IM	Days 16–34
Cytosine arabinoside	Dose by age; IT	Day 0
Methotrexate	Dose by age; IT	Days 16, 30
Radiation therapy to extra-abdominal sites of bulky disease		
Maintenance (10 courses; 42 days/course)		
Cyclophosphamide	1,000 mg/m^2 IV	Day 0
Vincristine	1.5 mg/m^2 IV	Days 0, 14
Prednisone	60 mg/m^2/day PO	Days 0–4
Methotrexate	300 mg/m^2 IV; 60% IV push + 40% over 4 hrs	Day 14
Daunomycin	30 mg/m^2 IV	Day 28
Methotrexate	Dose by age; IT	Day 0

IT = Intrathecal.

Table 3 (D)COMP for Nonlymphoblastic Non-Hodgkin's Lymphoma

	Dose	Schedule
Induction (28 day course)		
Cyclophosphamide	1,200 mg/m^2 IV	Day 0
Vincristine	2.0 mg/m^2 IV	Days 2, 9, 16, 23
Prednisone	60 mg/m^2 PO	Days 2–29
Methotrexate	300 mg/m^2 IV; 60% IV push + 40% over 4 hrs	Day 16
Daunomycin	50 mg/m^2 IV	Day 16
Cytosine arabinoside	Dose by age; IT	Day 0
Methotrexate	Dose by age; IT	Day 16
Maintenance (15 courses; 28 days/course)		
Cyclophosphamide	1,000 mg/m^2 IV	Day 0
Vincristine	1.5 mg/m^2 IV	Days 0, 14
Prednisone	60 mg/m^2/day PO	Days 0–4
Methotrexate	300 mg/m^2 IV; 60% IV push + 40% over 4 hrs	Day 14
Daunomycin	50 mg/m^2 IV; maximum cumulative dose, 350 mg/m^2	Day 14
Methotrexate	Dose by age; IT	Day 0

IT = Intrathecal.

not in those with lymphoblastic lymphoma. Recently, daunomycin was added to COMP for patients with advanced disease in order to produce the DCOMP regimen (see Table 3).

NEUROBLASTOMA

Neuroblastoma, ganglioneuroblastoma, and ganglioneuroma account for 12 percent of pediatric solid tumors and 19 percent of tumor deaths. The SEER found that 50 percent of children diagnosed between 1976 and 1981 survived 5 years.

Two-thirds of patients are younger than 4 years old at diagnosis, and two-thirds of tumors arise in the abdomen or pelvis from the medulla of the adrenal glands or from paraspinal sympathetic ganglia. Two-thirds of patients with neuroblastoma have disseminated disease—generally bone or bone marrow metastases—at diagnosis. Iodine-123 metaiodobenzylguanidine scanning may identify skeletal metastases not demonstrated on technetium-99m-methylene disphosphonate bone scan or skeletal radiographs and, unfortunately, vice versa. Bone marrow immunocytochemistry may identify marrow metastases not demonstrated by conventional microscopic examination of a bone marrow biopsy. Tumors frequently excrete catecholamine metabolites such as vanillylmandelic acid (VMA) and homovanillic acid (HVA). Patients with marrow disease and elevated urinary catecholamines do not require open biopsy for diagnosis. Poor outcome is associated with age older than 1 year, disseminated disease, elevated serum ferritin level, deletions or re-arrangements of the distal part of the short arm of chromosome 1, near-diploid or hypotetraploid modal chromosome number, or *N-myc* gene amplification. Better outcome is associated with age younger than 1 year and thoracic primaries. These factors are highly interrelated, and the independent significance of each is unknown.

Surgical resection is highly curative for children of any age with localized disease, Evans stage I or II. The 5-year survival is on the order of 90 percent. In general, no role has remained for irradiation therapy, even following incomplete resection. A minority of children with Evans stage II disease have been shown to have tumors with gene amplification of *N-myc;* their outcome is more similar to that of children with disseminated disease than it is to that of others with localized disease.

A minority of patients have dumbbell lesions at presentation and actual or potential spinal cord compression. The clinician must be alert and differentiate refusal to walk because of bone pain from inability to walk secondary to spinal cord compression. Radiographs of the vertebrae may demonstrate erosion. A MRI scan of the spine with gadolinium contrast may demonstrate an intraspinous mass in addition to the more obvious abdominal mass. The intraspinous mass may swell and precipitate or exacerbate cord compression when the intra-abdominal mass is manipulated at surgery. These tumors should be approached by a combined surgical and neurosurgical team. Some have employed laminectomy and postoperative irradiation. Others have employed a chemotherapy regimen including cyclophosphamide, 150 mg per square meter per day on days 0 to 6, and adriamycin, 35 mg per square meter on day 7, in order to avoid the sequelae of laminectomy and spinal irradiation in young children.

Infants who are younger than 1 year of age and have localized disease have a similarly excellent outcome. In addition, infants with Evans stage I or II primaries and liver, skin, or bone marrow metastases but with no bony lesions on skeletal survey are likely to experience spontaneous remission without specific therapy. When therapy is required, e.g., for respiratory embarrassment secondary to massive hepatomegaly, the least treatment necessary to alleviate symptoms is chosen. Among this group, an elevated serum ferritin or gene amplification of *N-myc* identifies a subgroup of infants with poorer outcome. Among infants with large primary tumors (Evans stage III) or disseminated disease with bony lesions, perhaps 50 percent will be long-term survivors with aggressive multimodality therapy.

Although neuroblastoma is highly responsive to chemotherapy and irradiation therapy, responses may be transient and outcome is less satisfactory for older children with advanced disease. Patients with regional disease benefit from intensive chemotherapy, aggressive surgical resection, often following initial chemotherapy, and irradiation therapy. Neuroblastoma is a highly infiltrative tumor, and initial resection is often impossible. Table 4 depicts a chemotherapy regimen currently em-

Table 4 CCG-321P2 for Advanced Neuroblastoma (28-Day Cycles)

Agent	Dose	Schedule
Cisplatin	60 mg/m² IV	Day 0
Etoposide	100 mg/m² IV	Days 2, 5
Adriamycin	30 mg/m² IV	Day 2
Cyclophosphamide	900 mg/m² IV	Days 3,4

ployed by the CCSG for children aged greater than 1 year. With intensive chemotherapy such as MADDOC, which is used at the Dana Farber Cancer Institute, "6-in-1," or "P2," which is depicted in Table 4, aggressive surgery, and consolidative irradiation therapy, perhaps half of Evans stage III patients will be long-term survivors.

In the past, children older than 1 year of age with disseminated neuroblastoma had a 2-year progression-free survival of less than 10 percent. Ablative chemoradiotherapy with purged autologous marrow rescue (bone marrow transplant) has been employed following initial conventional chemotherapy, aggressive surgical debulking, and careful application of irradiation therapy to sites of initial disease prior to any recurrence in the first progression-free interval. Two-year progression-free survivals on the order of 50 percent have been reported. With more recent intensive, although nonablative regimens, results may be similar. With previous chemotherapy, immunocytochemistry usually demonstrated persistent marrow neuroblastoma. With more recent regimens, immunocytochemistry frequently finds no marrow neuroblastoma. Both POG and CCSG are conducting trials to compare the results of ablative therapy with purged autologous marrow rescue and intensive chemotherapy. Cytokines and chemoprotectants may allow further intensification of therapy in the future.

When neuroblastoma is diagnosed in infants younger than 1 year of age, it is usually localized and lacks the laboratory markers for rapid progression, e.g., elevated serum ferritin level, gene amplification of *N-myc,* and so on. With quantitative assays of urinary VMA and HVA, one can identify infants with neuroblastoma with a sensitivity greater than 90 percent. Such a program was initiated in Kyoto City in Japan. Over 400,000 infants were screened, and 25 cases of neuroblastoma were identified. Survival from neuroblastoma increased from 17 to 75 percent without any significant change in treatment strategies. Researchers at the University of Minnesota and in Ontario, Canada, are working jointly to corroborate these exciting findings.

WILMS' TUMOR

Kidney tumors constitute 9 percent of pediatric solid tumors and contribute to 6 percent of tumor deaths. The SEER reports that the 5-year survival for children diagnosed between the years 1976 and 1981 was 76 percent. The vast majority are classified under the rubric of Wilms' tumor. Wilms' tumor is rare at birth and the modal age is 3 years. Where neuroblastoma is usually disseminated at presentation, Wilms' tumor is localized in about 80 percent of cases and resectable. Wilms' tumor metastasizes to regional and distant lymph nodes, lung, and liver. Certain histologic variants, namely clear-cell tumor of the kidney, metastasizes to bone.

Children with Wilms' tumor are frequently hypertensive at presentation, unlike children with neuroblastoma. Radiographically, Wilms' tumor results in distortion of the affected kidney, whereas neuroblastoma classically results in displacement of the affected kidney. Both kidneys may be involved simultaneously in about 5 percent of cases. Wilms' tumor may appear in the other kidney at a later time or metachronously in another 5 percent of cases. Abdominal CT provides an excellent means for examination of the contralateral kidney and the liver. Abdominal ultrasound is invaluable for examination for the renal vein and vena cava for tumor invasion. A CT scan of the chest may be better obtained before surgery because atelectases may appear after anesthesia and complicate interpretation.

Treatment begins with surgical excision of the tumor. An abdominothoracic approach may be required. Assistance from cardiovascular surgery may be required to remove tumor from the vena cava and right atrium. The integrity of Gerota's fascia is maintained. Suspicious abdominal lymph nodes are resected. Careful pathologic examination yields the histologic subtype and extent of regional tumor involvement. Histologies are divided into favorable (80 percent) and unfavorable (20 percent). Unfavorable histologies include anaplastic, clear-cell, and rhabdoid tumors. Children with the rare rhabdoid tumor frequently have simultaneous or metachronous brain tumors and a dismal prognosis.

Table 5 details current recommendations by histology and stage, largely derived from the National Wilms' Tumor Study III. Tumor bed irradiation is reserved for patients with local extension, local tumor spill, or unfavorable histology. Whole-abdominal irradiation is employed only with gross abdominal involvement or extensive contamination of peritoneal surfaces. Bilateral lung irradiation is employed for children with lung metastases. Children with liver metastases receive whole-liver irradiation.

Children with favorable histology and stage I or II disease receive vincristine and actinomycin D. National Wilms' Tumor Study II showed that patients with stage II and III disease had a better outcome when they received adriamycin in addition to vincristine and actinomycin D. However, the comparison was not "isotoxic." Patients who received adriamycin received twice as many courses of therapy as did patients who received only vincristine and actinomycin D. In National Wilms' Tumor Study IV, the comparison was isotoxic, and no benefit was shown for adriamycin among children with stage II disease. National Wilms' Tumor Study IV showed no added benefit for cyclophosphamide.

Chemotherapy should begin promptly, but intraoperative administration is no longer in vogue. Chemotherapy should be initiated within 1 week of surgery after

Table 5 Wilms' Tumor

Stage I; favorable histology (or anaplastic)
    AMD weeks 0, 5, 13, 24
    VCR weekly × 10 then days 0, 4 of each AMD course
No irradiation
Stage II; favorable histology
    AMD weeks 0, 5, 13, 22, 31, 40, 49, 58
    VCR weekly × 10 then weekly × 6 wk on weeks 15, 23, 33, 42, 51, 60
No irradiation
Stages I, II; unfavorable histology
Stage III
Stage IV*
    AMD weeks 0, 13, 26, 39, 52, 65
    VCR weekly × 10 then days 0, 4 of each AMD course
    ADR weeks 6, 19, 32, 45, 58
Local irradiation
*Abdominal irradiation as per local stage:
    VCR, 1.5 mg/m^2 IV (max 2.0 mg);
    AMD, 15 μg/kg/d IV × 5 days (max 500 μg);
    ADR, 20 mg/m^2 IV × 3 days

Abbreviations: VCR = vincristine, AMD = actinomycin D, ADR = adriamycin.

recovery from postoperative illeus and reinstitution of oral alimentation.

Patients with favorable histology and stages I, II, III, and IV disease have projected 3-year disease-free survival rates of 93 percent, 82 percent, 79 percent, and 67 percent, respectively. The outcome of stage IV patients may depend on the bulk of metastatic disease. Some argue that lung metastases identified on CT scan but not found on chest radiograph require no specific therapy. Patients with unfavorable histology have projected disease-free survival rates of 53 percent, 61 percent, 25 percent, and 7 percent, respectively. Children with stage I anaplastic tumors may not, in reality, be at any greater risk of relapse than patients with stage I favorable histology.

In the future, phase 2 activity reported for carboplatin and for the combination of ifosfamide and etoposide may be translated into better therapy for stage IV patients with favorable histology and patients with unfavorable histology.

RHABDOMYOSARCOMA AND RELATED TUMORS

Soft-tissue sarcomas constitute 9 percent of pediatric solid tumors and account for 8 percent of tumor deaths. For purposes of the Intergroup Rhabdomyosarcoma Study (IRS) and for purposes of therapy in general, histologically similar small, round, blue cell tumors such as "undifferentiated sarcoma" and extraosseus Ewing's sarcoma are grouped with the histologic variants of rhabdomyosarcoma. Spindle cell tumors, such as fibrosarcoma and malignant fibrous histiocytoma, are usually considered separately. The SEER found a 58 percent 5-year survival for children with soft-tissue sarcoma who were diagnosed between 1976 and 1981.

Rhabdomyosarcoma arises most frequently in the head and neck region or genitourinary tract of younger children and the extremities or trunk of adolescents. Three variants are described: embryonal (including sarcoma botryoides), alveolar, and pleomorphic. Embryonal histology is considered favorable. Alveolar and undifferentiated histology is considered unfavorable. Pleomorphic histology is unusual in children. Therapy and its chance for success depend on the site, extent of resection, stage, and histopathology of the tumor.

Group 1 tumors are confined to the muscle or organ of origin and are completely resected. Contiguous involvement of adjacent structures by infiltration outside of the muscle or structure of origin is allowed, except for lymph nodes, providing that all tumor has been completely excised. Microscopic confirmation is required. Patients with favorable histology receive postoperative "cyclic sequential" vincristine and actinomycin D for 1 year and no radiation therapy (Table 6). The 3-year disease-free survival was 83 percent on IRS III.

Group 2 tumors have evidence of regional spread but remain amenable to gross total excision. Patients with paratesticular primaries, e.g., spermatic cord, epididymus, testis, or testicular tunic, have an excellent outcome. Patients with parameningeal primaries, e.g., nasopharynx, paranasal sinus, middle ear, mastoid, or pterygopalatine-infratemporal fossa, require special attention to the possibility of meningeal spread. Patients with favorable histology receive postoperative radiation therapy (41.4 cGy) starting on day 14 following initiation of "cyclic sequential" vincristine and actinomycin D. The 3-year disease-free survival was 77 percent on IRS II. The IRS III demonstrated no additional benefit for adriamycin.

Patients with unfavorable-histology group 1 and 2 tumors receive postoperative "pulse VAC" chemotherapy with vincristine, actinomycin D, and cyclophosphamide (Table 7). Postoperative radiation therapy begins on day 42. The 4-year progression-free survival was about 65 percent. No clear benefit has yet been shown from the addition of adriamycin and cisplatin on IRS III.

Group 3 tumors have evidence of regional spread without distant metastases and gross residual disease after definitive surgery. Patients with favorable-histology rhabdomyosarcoma of nonparameningeal head and neck sites, e.g., orbit, eyelid, scalp, parotid gland, oral cavity, larynx, oropharynx, or cheek, have an excellent prognosis when treated with vincristine, actinomycin D, and radiation therapy as above. Patients with parameningeal primaries and overt intracranial involvement benefit from "prophylactic" whole-brain radiation and intrathecal chemotherapy. Irradiation of the tumor and a margin of adjacent meninges appears adequate for patients with parameningeal primaries but without overt intracranial extension. Intrathecal therapy is not necessary without erosion of the base of the skull or cranial nerve abnormalities.

In patients with group 3 tumors of the dome of bladder, vagina, or uterus, the bladder may often be preserved. Interval excision after 20 weeks of chemotherapy is usually adequate and replaces immediate exenteration. Pelvic irradiation is generally unnecessary. If complete response has not been obtained with initial chemotherapy and limited surgery, then irradiation is recommended. Children with group 3 tumors of the prostate, bladder neck, or bladder trigone ("central" lesions) have rarely achieved an adequate response to chemotherapy alone. In these patients, early application of local irradiation is recommended in order to preserve the bladder.

The IRS III found no added benefit for the addition of cisplatin and adriamycin or cisplatin and etoposide to "pulse VAC" chemotherapy (see Table 7) and radiation therapy for group 3 or group 4 (metastatic). In addition, the experimental regimens appeared more toxic than the control "pulse VAC" regimen. The 3-year disease-free survival rate was 62 percent for group 3 and 11 percent for group 4. The IRS limits cyclophosphamide to 10 mg per kilogram per day to 3 days in each pulse because of concerns about toxicity. Other versions have prescribed 5 to 7 days of cyclophosphamide in each pulse and repeated pulses monthly. The IRS IV will investigate ifosfamide (with mesna uroprotection) and etoposide.

OSTEOGENIC SARCOMA

Osteogenic sarcoma constitutes about 4 percent of pediatric solid tumors. Patients tend to be adolescents and young adults. Men predominate in a ratio of 1.6 to 1. The SEER found 5-year survivals of 26 percent for children diagnosed between 1967 and 1973 and 43 percent for children diagnosed between 1973 and 1981. Classical osteogenic sarcoma must be differentiated from parosteal osteogenic sarcoma and periosteal osteogenic sarcoma. About one-half of tumors arise in the femurs. The humerus and the tibia are two of the more frequent sites. Jaw lesions tend to have a good outcome.

With amputation alone, 85 percent of patients with apparently localized osteogenic sarcoma will have metastases within 1 year after amputation. Two recently completed randomized trials have confirmed the value of postoperative chemotherapy in preventing or delaying the appearance of metastases.

Disarticulation was once the therapy of choice for femoral lesions. Now transosseus amputation with care-

Table 6 Rhabdomyosarcoma and Related Tumors

Cyclic sequential vincristine (VCR) and actinomycin D (AMD)
AMD	Weeks 0, 9, 18, 27, 36, 45
VCR	Weekly × 6 wks, weeks 3, 12, 21, 30, 39, 48

Pulse VAC
VCR	Weekly × 10 then day 0 + 4 of each AMD course
AMD	Weeks 0, 12, then q4wk to 2 yr
CYCLO	10 mg/kg/day IV × 3 days on weeks 0, 12, and q4wk
VCR	Vincristine, 2.0 mg/m² (max 2.0 mg)
AMD	Actinomycin D, 15 μg/kg/day × 5 days (max 500 μg/day)
CYCLO	Cyclophosphamide

Table 7 Osteogenic Sarcoma

	Dose	Schedule
Induction Therapy (135 days)		
Preoperative chemotherapy		
Methotrexate and citrovorum rescue* IV		Days 0, 7, 35, 42
Vincristine	1.5 mg/m² (max 2 mg)	Days 1, 8, 36, 43
Bleomycin	1.5 U/m² IV	
Cyclophosphamide	600 mg/m² IV	BCD on days 14, 15
Actinomycin D	600 mg/m² IV (max 1.25 mg)	
Surgery		
Postoperative chemotherapy		
BCD (see above)		Day 63
Methotrexate and citrovorum rescue		Days 84, 91, 121, 128
Vincristine	1.5 mg/m² IV (max 2.0 mg)	Days 85, 92, 122, 129
Adriamycin		Days 98, 99, 100
Maintenance Therapy		
Regimen A (grade 1 or 2 histologic response), 3 cycles 63 days each		
Adriamycin	30 mg/m² IV	Days 0, 1, 21, 22
Cisplatin	120 mg/m² IV	Days 0, 21
BCD (see above)		Days 42, 43
Regimen B (grade 3 or 4 histologic response), 3 cycles 77, 42, and 42 days each		
BCD (see above)		Days 0, 1
Methotrexate and citrovorum rescue		Days 21, 28, 56, 63 (first cycle only)
Vincristine	1.5 mg/m² (max 2.0 mg)	Days 22, 29, 37, 64 (first cycle only)
Adriamycin	30 mg/m² IV	Days 35, 36, 37 (cycle 1) Days 21, 22, 23 (cycles 2, 3)

*High-dose methotrexate, 8 g/m² for age > 12 years or 12 g/m² for age ≤ 12 years (min 12 g and max 18 g).

ful delineation of the extent of involvement and good margins is now fully adequate for most cases and functionally superior. Much current effort is focused on achieving limb salvage.

Chemotherapy prior to definitive surgery (neoadjuvant chemotherapy) was originally introduced in order to allow time for the construction of a prosthesis in order to facilitate limb salvage. One hears the argument that local recurrence is no more common after limb salvage than after amputation. Despite the obvious cosmetic appeal of limb salvage, three considerations should be kept in mind. First, limb-salvage patients are selected from among other patients. They generally are older and have smaller and more distal tumors and thus perhaps should have a better outcome than those for whom limb salvage is not offered. In one trial, patients who underwent preoperative chemotherapy, limb salvage, and postoperative chemotherapy had an outcome inferior to that of patients who underwent immediate amputation and postoperative chemotherapy. Secondly, in some cases, amputation may afford better function than limb salvage, e.g., below-knee amputation versus limb salvage for a tibial lesion. Thirdly, the complications of limb salvage surgery, e.g., infection and slow healing in a poorly perfused limb, may delay or interrupt the chemotherapy necessary to prevent metastases. Some clinicians are certainly more sanguine. In cases in which surgical extirpation is not feasible, radiation therapy may be employed.

About 25 percent of patients have metastatic disease at diagnosis; 85 percent have only lung metastases. Aggressive surgical management appears warranted, with meticulous resection of metastases either before or after the initiation of chemotherapy. Repeated thoracotomies may be necessary. Cure is possible for a minority of patients.

A variety of chemotherapeutic regimens have been employed with similar results. All effective regimens employ adriamycin. High-dose methotrexate (2.5 to 12 g per square meter) with leucovorin rescue, cisplatin, and vincristine are commonly employed. Children less than 12 years of age require higher doses of methotrexate in order to achieve levels similar to those obtained in older patients. No randomized study has yet shown that high-dose methotrexate is superior to lower-dose methotrexate.

The response to preoperative chemotherapy can be assessed at definitive surgery and used to select subsequent chemotherapy. Although patients with a "good" histologic response may have a consistently better outcome than patients with a "poor" histologic response, the effectiveness of this approach for "poor" responders or on the overall outcome has not been demonstrated. The value of the combination of bleomycin, actinomycin D, and cyclophosphamide (BCD) is controversial. The phase 2 activity of the combination of ifosfamide and etoposide has generated much interest. Table 6 depicts

Table 8 Ewing's Sarcoma

	Dose		Schedule
Induction Phase			
Vincristine	2.0 mg/m^2	IV (max 2.0 mg)	Weeks 0, 3, 6
Adriamycin	75 mg/m^2	IV	Weeks 0, 3, 6
Cyclophosphamide	1,200 mg/m^2	IV	Weeks 0, 3, 6
Local Therapy Phase			
Surgery or radiation therapy			
Vincristine	2.0 mg/m^2	IV (max 2.0 mg)	Weeks 9, 12, 13, 14, 15
Adriamycin	75 mg/m^2	IV	Weeks 9
Cyclophosphamide	1,200 mg/m^2	IV	Weeks 9, 12, 15
Maintenance			
Vincristine	2.0 mg/m^2	IV (max 2.0 mg)	Week 18 and q3wk × 11
Adriamycin	75 mg/m^2	IV	Week 18 only
Actinomycin D	1.25 mg/m^2	IV	Week 21 and q3wk × 10
Cyclophosphamide	1,200 mg/m^2	IV	Week 18 and q3wk × 10

the chemotherapy schema used in a recently completed CCSG study. This trial assigned therapy based on response to preoperative chemotherapy and obtained a 61 percent 2-year PFS for children with localized osteogenic sarcoma of an extremity.

A minority of patients may achieve cure after metastasis with aggressive surgery, including multiple thoracotomies as necessary and chemotherapy. Bony metastases are ominous. Patients with unilateral pulmonary metastases more than 1 year after diagnosis have the best outcome, although substantial palliation and prolongation of life can be obtained for others.

EWING'S SARCOMA OF BONE

Ewing's sarcoma constitutes about 3 percent of pediatric solid tumors. As with osteogenic sarcoma, patients tend to be adolescents and young adults. Ewing's sarcoma is rare among blacks. The most common sites of involvement are the pelvic bones, femur, humerus, and ribs. Ewing's sarcoma is a small, round, blue cell tumor and can be difficult to distinguish histologically from neuroblastoma, rhabdomyosarcoma, and lymphoma. Cytogenetics shows a consistent 11:22 translocation, which is also found in primitive neuroectodermal tumor. The SEER found a 23 percent 5-year survival for children diagnosed between 1967 and 1973 and a 48 percent 5-year survival for children diagnosed between 1973 and 1981. Thirty percent of patients may have metastases at diagnosis.

As with osteogenic sarcoma, 90 percent of patients with apparently localized disease will metastasize within 1 year despite effective local therapy. With the use of adjuvant chemotherapy, the incidence of metastases is markedly decreased. Unlike rhabdomyosarcoma, adriamycin is a critical component of therapy. Cyclophosphamide, actinomycin D, and vincristine are usually employed. Phase 2 activity has been demonstrated for 5-fluorouracil and for the combination of ifosfamide and etoposide.

In the past, surgery was limited to the initial diagnostic biopsy. Radiation therapy was employed for local control. The treatment port included the entire bone affected, and treatment was delayed in order to allow chemotherapy to reduce the bulk of tumor to be treated and to reduce tumor anoxia. However, despite doses as high as 70 cGy and with effective chemotherapy that prevented distant metastases for many patients, perhaps 15 percent of patients had local recurrence. Amputation was reserved for lesions involving the lower extremity of a child younger than 10 years of age, hands or feet, expendable bones such as the rib, clavicle, wing of scapula, or fibula, or following chronic osteomyelitis in an irradiated limb.

Data have accumulated that surgical excision contributes to local control and PFS. In the guidelines of the Third Intergroup Ewing's Sarcoma Study (IESS), patients with extremity lesions and actual or impending pathologic fractures are candidates for immediate amputation. Surgical excision is recommended after initial chemotherapy and before radiation therapy if such can be accomplished without functional impairment. Surgery may have fewer sequelae than radiation therapy in young children because of the effect of radiation on bone growth.

Radiation therapy is delayed a minimum of 9 weeks from diagnosis. Radiation therapy *is not* administered to patients who have undergone complete resections with adequate margins. Patients with no resection or gross residual disease receive 5,580 cGy. Patients with microscopic residual disease receive 5,040 cGy. A tailored port with 1-cm margins is employed rather than whole-bone irradiation. The impact of this approach to local control is yet to be demonstrated.

Patients with pulmonary metastases receive bilateral pulmonary irradiation. All metastatic sites are irradiated, except bone marrow.

In summary, patients undergo an initial surgical biopsy or amputation and then receive combination chemotherapy for 9 weeks. Tumor status is then reassessed, and patients then undergo surgery or radiation therapy and complete an additional 8 months of chemotherapy. The IESS III control chemotherapy regimen is depicted in Table 8. The IESS III is studying the added value of ifosfamide and etoposide.

The distal extremity, jaw, skull, face, clavicle, vertebra, and scapula are believed to be favorable sites, the rib is intermediate, and the proximal extremities, pelvis, and sacrum are unfavorable sites. On IESS II, however, patients with localized disease and pelvic or sacral primaries, which conventionally are unfavorable sites, had a 5-year survival of 75 percent. Patients with localized disease and primaries other than pelvic or sacral bones had a 5-year survival of about 60 percent. Perhaps 30 percent of patients with metastatic disease at diagnosis survived for 5 years; these were almost exclusively patients with metastases solely to the lung.

SUGGESTED READING

National Cancer Institute, Physicians Data Query System, Bethesda, MD.

Nesbit ME. Advances and management of solid tumors in children. Cancer 1990; 65:696–702.

University of Southern California, Children's Cancer Study Group Protocols, Pasadena, CA.

Young JL, Gloeckler Ries L, Silverberg E, et al. Cancer incidence, survival, and mortality for children younger than 15 years. Cancer 1986; 58:598–602.

AIDS AND CANCER

JUDITH A. LUCE, M.D.
JOHN L. ZIEGLER, M.D.

The recognition of an association between infection with the human immunodeficiency virus (HIV) and the occurrence of specific malignancies began with the first descriptions of Kaposi's sarcoma in homosexual men in 1981. Since that time, although a broad understanding of the pathogenesis of acquired immunodeficiency syndrome (AIDS) has been achieved, little more has been learned about the mechanisms of oncogenesis in HIV-infected individuals.

Both Kaposi's sarcoma and non-Hodgkin's lymphomas are now established as AIDS-related cancers, and their importance in AIDS is reflected in their impact on cancer statistics in endemic urban areas. In the San Francisco Bay area, e.g., Kaposi's sarcoma had become the fourth most common cancer in men by 1986, and the same statistical source registers a clear increase in the incidence of non-Hodgkin's lymphoma.

There are four important clinical aspects in the management of AIDS patients with cancer: (1) alterations in the natural history of the tumor due to the underlying immunodeficiency; (2) consideration of an AIDS diagnosis in patients with cancer who are at risk for AIDS; (3) treatment strategy with respect to iatrogenic immune suppression; and (4) the use of prophylactic measures to avert opportunistic infections in AIDS patients undergoing cancer therapy.

KAPOSI'S SARCOMA

From its original description in elderly men from eastern Europe and the Mediterranean basin, to the reports of endemic occurrence in Africa, Kaposi's sarcoma has usually been described as an indolent malignancy. Skin involvement was usually confined to the lower extremities, and even when tumors became bulky and ulcerated, responses to simple forms of chemotherapy were described as rapid and often complete. However, childhood cases in Africa were more aggressive, more likely to involve lymph nodes and viscera, and more lethal. In the immunocompromised HIV-infected host, this disease often pursues a multicentric, more aggressive course that is characterized by visceral spread and more rapid demise. The pathogenesis of Kaposi's sarcoma is unknown. The current theories about its origin suggest that it is a lymphoendothelial tumor and that it is a proliferative disease arising under the influence of some trophic substance produced in response to HIV infection. Whether the multicentric lesions represent metastases from some clonal growth or nonclonal multicentric primaries has never been proven.

A formal staging system has only recently been devised for this malignancy, perhaps because of its lack of predictable, organized spread. Investigators have identified prognostic factors that predict for more indolent or more aggressive disease behavior. Krown and colleagues have divided patients into two risk groups, which are outlined in Table 1. High-risk patients have an expected median survival of less than 6 months, and low-risk patients in excess of 1 year. Kaposi's sarcoma may present as a first manifestation of AIDS in individuals whose CD4 ("helper" T cell) counts are still relatively high; these patients often have superior performance status and other features that permit longer survival. Procedures for staging are usually confined to careful physical examination, documentation of all areas of skin or lymph node involvement, chest radiographs, complete blood count, chemistries, and staging of HIV infection with CD4 cell count or serum beta$_2$-microglobulin. Further clinical examinations are dictated only by symptoms; Kaposi's sarcoma may be present in other viscera in an asymptomatic state. There is no benefit to extensive evaluation in the absence of symptoms. Careful evaluation for concomitant opportunistic infections is also important.

Treatment of Kaposi's sarcoma has never been shown to affect the survival of HIV-infected patients. Nevertheless, there are important clinical reasons for initiating therapy. Palliation of symptoms, especially pain, ulceration, and lymphedema, is useful. Cosmetic considerations are often important because of the social problems encountered by AIDS patients. Disseminated or visceral disease may require treatment because of regional symptoms such as diarrhea or dyspnea, organ obstruction, or systemic symptoms such as fever.

Local forms of treatment include intracutaneous or intralesional therapies such as vinblastine and tumor necrosis factor. Topical treatments such as laser photo-therapy or radiation therapy are also available. Radiation therapy produces tumor regression and excellent palliation of local symptoms such as edema, pain, and ulceration; this may be achieved with very low doses. Single doses of 800 to 1,200 cGy of superficial therapy with electron beam palliate skin lesions well. Areas such as lymph nodes may require greater dose depth and higher doses. The University of California San Francisco (UCSF) experience suggests that small fractions are better tolerated than more conventional dose fractionation, and that doses in excess of 3,000 cGy are rarely required. Pulmonary Kaposi's sarcoma may be palliated transiently with ten 150-cGy fractions.

Individuals with HIV infection are particularly sensitive to local tissue toxicity from radiotherapy. Areas such as the oral and rectal mucosa and foot are particularly sensitive, and indeed local toxicity is dose-limiting. Toxicity to these tissues is unusual when single fractions are used, but becomes universal with conventional fractions and doses over approximately 1,500 cGy.

Systemic therapies that are effective in Kaposi's sarcoma are oulined in Table 2. Most of the response rates reported in this table were obtained in single-arm trials. Weekly alternating vinca alkaloid therapy, a regimen based on the African treatment experience, is well tolerated systemically, although it may be accom-

Table 1 Staging of Kaposi's Sarcoma

Good Risk (All of the Following)	Poor Risk (Any of the Following)
Cutaneous focus, and/or lymph nodes and/or minimal oral disease	Tumor edema or ulceration, gastro-intestinal nodes, or other visceral Kaposi's sarcoma, extensive oral Kaposi's sarcoma
CD4 cell count ≥ 200uL	CD4 cell count < 200 uL
No "B" symptoms	"B" symptoms (fever, sweats, weight loss)
No prior opportunistic infection or thrush	History of opportunistic infection or thrush
Performance status ≥ 70	Performance status < 70
No other HIV-related illness	Other HIV-related illness (e.g., neurologic, lymphoma)

From Krown SE, Metroka C, Wernz JC, for the AIDS Clinical Trials Group Oncology Subcommittee. Kaposi's sarcoma in the acquired immune deficiency syndrome: A proposal for uniform evaluation, response, and staging criteria. J Clin Oncol 1989; 7:1201; with permission.

panied by significant marrow suppression and neuropathy. This regimen may even be managed in conjunction with zidovudine antiretroviral treatment, provided the latter drug is given at levels of 500 to 600 mg per day in divided doses. The three-drug ABV regimen has been reported as particularly effective in pulmonary Kaposi's sarcoma; however, complete responses are not common, and radiographic regression unusual. Bleomycin and vinblastine have been used in combination to avoid anthracycline toxicity; doxorubicin has been an effective single agent in patients unable to tolerate further vinca alkaloids or bleomycin. Etoposide has single-agent activity; it has not yet been reported in combination regimens. Alpha-interferon has activity comparable to chemotherapy, although it has the disadvantage of parenteral administration and marked systemic toxicity at the doses that have proven effective for Kaposi's sarcoma.

Toxicity of chemotherapy for Kaposi's sarcoma is due mostly to marrow suppression. Approximately one-third of patients on the low-dose regimens, such as alternating vincristine-vinblastine, may be expected to have transient neutropenia requiring dose modification. Approximately one-third became severely anemic, requiring transfusion on this combination plus higher doses of zidovudine (1,200 mg per day). Dose adjustments for marrow suppression should be made if the neutrophil count falls below 1,000 per microliter. Fever and neutropenia are rare when blood counts are watched carefully and doses modified. Systemic symptoms of fever, fatigue, myalgias, and weight loss are common problems with the use of alpha-interferon, and are usually dose-limiting.

Results of treatment for Kaposi's sarcoma are not often dramatic. Local treatment may result in transient complete regressions of local lesions, but systemic therapy rarely produces complete responses. Response rates are higher in patients with lower tumor burdens.

Table 2 Regimens for Kaposi's Sarcoma

Agent	Dose/Schedule	Response (Overall) (%)
Etoposide	150 mg/m^2 IV daily × 3 q28d	76
Vinblastine	6 mg/m^2 IV weekly, or 0.1 mg/kg IV weekly	75
Vincristine	1.2 mg/m^2 IV weekly, or 2.0 mg IV weekly	65
Alternating vincas (every other week)	0.1 mg/kg IV vinblastine, alternating with 2.0 mg vincristine IV	40–50
Alpha-interferon	10–40 million units SQ or IM, qd × 5d weekly, qd tiw	40
Adriamycin	10–20 mg/m^2 IV q1–2wk	> 70
Bleomycin	10 mg/m^2 IV qwk	> 70
ABV	Adriamycin, 10–20 mg/m^2 IV q2k Bleomycin, 10 mg/m^2 IV q2wk Vincristine, 1.4 mg/m^2 IV q2wk	79
BV	Same as above, minus adriamycin	> 70

Palliation of symptoms and stabilization of disease may be satisfactory outcomes for patients who tolerate the treatment well. Definitive therapy awaits the discovery of the trophic agent that produces this proliferative disease.

NON-HODGKIN'S LYMPHOMA

The epidemic of non-Hodgkin's lymphoma (NHL) occurring in HIV-infected individuals has certain unique characteristics. All of the AIDS-related NHL cases described to date have been diffuse intermediate- and high-grade lymphomas of three types: large-cell lymphoma, immunoblastic lymphoma, and small, non-cleaved (either Burkitt's type or non-Burkitt's type) lymphoma. They are characterized by rapid onset and high frequency of extranodal involvement, especially in the marrow, liver, central nervous system (CNS), gastrointestinal tract, and lungs. Primary CNS lymphomas are a frequent subset of this population.

The causative agent of AIDS-associated NHL has not been found, although the search for infectious agents or trophic substances has been intense. Clearly, AIDS-associated NHL is due to neither HIV itself, which is not present in the malignant cells, nor to Epstein-Barr virus, although the latter has been found in some NHLs (especially in the CNS).

Staging of AIDS-associated NHL should be thorough, both because the disease is most often extensive and in order to rule out concomitant opportunistic infection. Staging at UCSF includes CT scans of the brain, chest, and abdomen, full laboratory evaluation, bilateral bone marrow biopsies, and lumbar puncture for cerebrospinal fluid cytology. Although fine-needle aspiration is sufficient to make the diagnosis of lymphoma in the vast majority of AIDS-associated cases, formal tissue biopsies may be useful for other reasons, including diagnosis of opportunistic infection.

Treatment of AIDS-associated NHL has been frustrated by the poor tolerance of HIV-infected pa-tients of marrow-suppressing and immunosuppressing regimens. Some general principles are clear: regional therapy with radiation alone is not adequate; the CNS must be treated prophylactically in all patients (and is involved in a significant minority); and the nontreatment option should be considered for persons who already have very advanced AIDS, for whom treatment is of no proven benefit.

Two basic strategies have been pursued in the treatment of AIDS-related NHL. Clearly, the disease responds, often rapidly and completely, to conventional cytotoxic chemotherapy. The first strategy attempts to find multiagent regimens using marrow-sparing drugs and lowered doses to reduce toxicity to tolerable levels. The low-dose m-BACOD regimen of Levine and colleagues is one such attempt, and is outlined in Table 3. Overall response rates are lower than reported in standard dose regimens in nonimmunosuppressed patients, with 52 percent of patients achieving complete remission, and disease-free survival is less than 8 months. Neutropenia less than 1,000 per microliter occurred in 25 percent of patients.

Table 3 Regimens for AIDS-Associated Non-Hodgkin's Lymphoma

CHOP/GMCSF: Kaplan, San Francisco General Hospital
Cyclophosphamide	1,000 mg/m^2 on day 1
Doxorubicin	40 mg/m^2 on day 1
Vincristine	2 mg on day 1 q21d
Prednisone	100 mg/m^2 on days 1–5
GM–CSF	10–20 µg/kg/day on days 4–13

Low-dose m-BACOD: Levine, USC, and AIDS Clinical Trials Group
Bleomycin	4 mg/m^2 on day 1
Doxorubicin	25 mg/m^2 on day 1
Cyclophosphamide	300 mg/m^2 on day 1 q21d
Vincristine	1.4 mg/m^2 on day 1
Dexamethasone	6 mg/m^2 on days 1–5
Methotrexate	200 mg/m^2 on day 15
Leucovorin	10 mg/m^2 q6hr × 6; start 24 hr after methotrexate

A second strategy reported by Kaplan and associates employs more standard doses of CHOP chemotherapy with granulocyte- macrophage colony-stimulating factor (GM-CSF) to avoid severe neutropenia. This regimen has proved to be safe and effective in reducing the severity of neutropenia and the incidence of fever and hospitalization. To date, more than 60 percent of patients have complete responses, and median survival is not yet clear. Fewer than 25 percent of patients developed fever and neutropenia during each cycle. Side effects of GM-CSF include fever, myalgia, rash, and headache. A prospective comparison of these two differing strategies will be undertaken. Salvage therapy with a variety of agents has been attempted, but significant prolongation of survival has been elusive.

Patients who have stage II, III, or IV disease are treated to complete remission plus two cycles, or to six cycles altogether, or to failure of therapy due to either intolerable toxicity or relapse. More detailed information about the precise duration of therapy is lacking. Patients who have meningeal involvement at diagnosis have been treated with either methotrexate or combinations of methotrexate and cytosine arabinoside, given intrathecally in conventional doses. Prophylactic intrathecal therapy is recommended for all patients with advanced-stage disease; this therapy may be given concurrently with systemic chemotherapy, and methotrexate has been the preferred drug. The precise number of treatments and precise frequency of therapy have varied in reports, but for prophylaxis, six weekly doses are used at UCSF; patients with meningeal involvement receive biweekly therapy.

Localized AIDS-associated NHL has been treated with sequential systemic chemotherapy and involved-field radiotherapy with tolerable side effects and a high fraction of complete responses. Recurrence is usually at sites distant from the primary disease. Primary CNS lymphoma has been treated with radiotherapy in conventional doses and fractionation. Systemic adjuvant chemotherapy for this disease is experimental, and no useful data are available.

AIDS-associated NHL has a very poor prognosis overall; however, great variation among different groups of patients has been observed. Persons who had a prior AIDS diagnosis have the worst prognosis; they usually have a median survival of approximately 3 to 4 months, but this is reduced to only weeks if the patients have poor performance status at diagnosis. If NHL is the first manifestation of AIDS, and patients have a good performance status, survival appears to be roughly the same as survival for any other first AIDS diagnosis, which, in most centers, is from 12 to 18 months. Survival of AIDS-related primary CNS lymphoma is poor, however, averaging less than 6 months.

OTHER CANCERS

No other malignancies have been clearly associated with HIV infection, but two are seen commonly enough in HIV-infected individuals to merit further discussion.

Anal carcinoma has been slowly increasing in incidence in the United States for nearly 20 years, and, in some reports, particularly in homosexual men. This disease may be caused by human papilloma virus infection and appears in association with anal condylomata, but the role of immunosuppression (by any mechanism) in its pathogenesis is unproven. Anal carcinoma has been reported in a significant number of HIV-infected individuals; both cloacogenic carcinoma and squamous carcinoma are seen. Management is complicated by the poor tolerance of HIV-infected individuals for radiotherapy and chemotherapy, which is the preferred treatment regimen in most institutions. Schecter and colleagues at San Francisco General Hospital have therefore sought to treat HIV-infected patients with anal carcinoma predominantly with surgery, with acceptable outcome and morbidity (equal to chemotherapy and radiotherapy-treated patients at that institution). Radiotherapy as postsurgical consolidation has occasionally been undertaken, with tolerable results when small fractions and a protracted schedule are used.

Hodgkin's disease, which has a peak in incidence in the same age group as the majority of HIV-infected persons, has also been reported in the setting of HIV infection. The outcome is poor, with a median survival of approximately 1 year. Patients with Hodgkin's disease and HIV infection tend to have advanced disease and are more likely to have unfavorable histology (e.g., lymphocyte-depleted) than non–HIV-infected persons. In Kaplan's experience at San Francisco General Hospital, patients also tolerated conventional chemotherapy extremely poorly, attaining an average of only 40 percent of the prescribed doses of MOPP and ABVD chemotherapy. Based on this experience, Kaplan and colleagues are exploring a regimen with less hematopoietic toxicity; others are pursuing the use of GM-CSF and conventional dose regimens.

Other malignancies that may coincide with HIV infection have been reported, including chronic lymphocytic leukemia, multiple myeloma, testicular carcinoma, and squamous carcinomas of the oropharynx and esophagus. Lung cancer and gastrointestinal malignancies have been observed at San Francisco General Hospital in HIV-infected patients. Guidelines for the treatment of these diseases can be extrapolated from the experience with other AIDS malignancies.

Nontreatment is a reasonable option in patients with far-advanced AIDS. Palliation with radiotherapy, which is used in small fractions and with attention paid to mucosal toxicity, is indicated for symptomatic disease. When surgical cure can be effected, this approach is rational for patients who have no specific contraindications. There are no data to date that suggest that surgical intervention worsens the prognosis of HIV-infected persons. Chemotherapy may be used with great caution, given the frequency of significant marrow suppression. However, the chemotherapy experience in HIV-infected patients with other malignancies has been poor, suggesting that a conservative approach to management is justified.

SUPPORTIVE CARE

Additional supportive care of patients with AIDS malignancies is important to prevent complications of therapy and, it is hoped, to improve survival. Antiretroviral therapy, of proven benefit in prolonging survival in AIDS, is recommended for patients with both Kaposi's sarcoma and lymphoma. Zidovudine treatment, 500 to 600 mg per day PO in divided doses, has been tolerated by patients on low-dose chemotherapy for Kaposi's sarcoma. Patients with lymphoma are placed on the same dose orally after completion of the chemotherapy. In general, the tumors do not respond to zidovudine alone, although patients may improve symptomatically.

Prophylaxis for *Pneumocystis carinii* pneumonia is an additional supportive therapy that has been shown to reduce morbidity in AIDS, and it may be undertaken concurrently with therapy for AIDS malignancies. A number of regimens have been used for prophylaxis, including aerosol Pentamidine, parenteral Pentamidine, dapsone, and trimethoprim-sulfamethoxazole. The latter drug has a high rate of side effects, including allergic and marrow-suppressing effects, and is the least well tolerated of the regimens.

Indwelling central venous catheters have been used for administration of therapy in AIDS patients. Although complicated by a high rate of local infections in patients using them daily for parenteral nutrition or gancyclovir, they have been generally well tolerated by patients with AIDS and cancer.

Neutropenia and fever due to chemotherapy are common complications in AIDS malignancies, especially lymphoma. Although it is likely, based on early results from San Francisco, that this frequent complication may be ameliorated by the use of GM-CSF, the San Francisco experience also suggests that this complication is not a particularly severe one. There have been no deaths in more than 160 hospitalizations for fever and neutropenia, and the rate of development of bacteremia does not appear to be greater than that reported for non–HIV-infected persons. Also, the duration of neutropenia is not particularly prolonged when lymphoma therapy is used as described previously. Broad-spectrum antibiotics and routine supportive care are appropriate. AIDS-related opportunistic infections must be considered in all febrile neutropenic patients, but initial empiric antifungal or anti-*Pneumocystis carinii* therapy is not justified initially unless symptoms, signs, or laboratory data suggest such infections are likely.

Methods to avoid or prevent mucositis and mucosal *Candida* infection in HIV-infected patients undergoing radiation therapy and chemotherapy may prove useful, but they have not been studied in formal trials.

Appropriate nutritional, emotional, and social support are important in all HIV-infected individuals.

RISK OF AIDS IN CANCER PATIENTS

Exposure to AIDS by way of transfusion is a concern of many cancer patients. The current Centers for Disease Control estimate of the risk of HIV infection in screened blood is approximately 1 in 100,000. The screening test widely used is an ELISA assay, which may be negative during the first few weeks after infection of a potential blood donor. Other methods of screening out high-risk individuals are routinely employed by most blood banks, and the combined effectiveness of this practice and ELISA screening has been estimated by Cumming and colleagues to result in a risk of 1 in 150,000. Testing for viral RNA or DNA, based on polymerase chain reaction, is not in widespread use, because of technical reasons. Avoidance of unnecessary transfusion and use of single donor rather than pooled blood products remain sound clinical practices. All newly diagnosed hemophiliacs or HIV-negative hemophiliacs should be treated with monoclonal or heat-treated factor VIII preparations.

SUGGESTED READING

Chak LY, Gill PS, Levin AM, et al. Radiation therapy for acquired immunodeficiency syndrome-related Kaposi's sarcoma. J Clin Oncol 1988; 6:863.

Crombleholme T, Schecter W, Wilson W. Anal carcinoma: Changes in incidence, natural history and treatment: A 26-year review of the UCSF-SFGH experience. Proc ASCO 1989; 8:13.

Cumming PD, Wallace EL, Schorr JB, et al. Exposure of patients to human immunodeficiency virus through the transfusion of blood components that test antibody-negative. N Engl J Med 1989; 321:941.

Gill PS, Akil B, Colletti P, et al. Pulmonary Kaposi's sarcoma: Clinical findings and results of therapy. Am J Med 1989; 87:57.

Gill P, Levine A, Krailo M, et al. AIDS-related malignant lymphoma: Results of prospective clinical trials. J Clin Oncol 1987; 5:1,322.

Kaplan LD, Abrams DI, Feigal E, et al. AIDS-associated non-Hodgkin's lymphoma in San Francisco. JAMA 1989; 261:719.

Kaplan L, Kahn J, Grossberg D, et al. Importance of schedule in the administration of recombinant human granulocyte-monocyte colony stimulating factor (rGM-CSF) to patients with HIV-associated B-cell lymphoma. Proc ASCO 1990; 9:996.

Knowles DM, Chamulak GA, Subar M, et al. Lymphoid neoplasia associated with the acquired immunodeficiency syndrome (AIDS): The New York University Medical Center experience with 105 patients (1981-1986). Ann Intern Med 1988; 108:744.

Krown SE, Metroka C, Wernz JC, for the AIDS Clinical Trials Group Oncology Subcommittee. Kaposi's sarcoma in the acquired immune deficiency syndrome: A proposal for uniform evaluation, response, and staging criteria. J Clin Oncol 1989; 7:1201.

Levine A, Wernz J, Kaplan L, et al. Low-dose chemotherapy with CNS prophylaxis and AZT maintenance for AIDS related lymphoma: Preliminary results of a multi-institution study. Proc ASCO 1989; 8:18a.

Rosenblum ML, Levy RM, Bredesen DE, et al. Primary central nervous system lymphomas in patients with AIDS. Ann Neurol (Suppl) 1988; 23:S13.

Ziegler JL, Beckstead JH, Volbering P, et al. High-grade non-Hodgkin's lymphoma in 90 homosexual men: Relationship to generalized lymphadenopathy and acquired immunodeficiency syndrome. N Engl J Med 1984; 311:565.

BRAIN TUMORS

JACK M. ROZENTAL, M.D., PH.D.

In 1990, approximately 17,000 primary central nervous system (CNS) neoplasms will be diagnosed in the United States (Table 1). The annual incidence for primary brain tumors in the United States is approximately 8.2 per 100,000 population. Age-specific incidence rates for intracranial neoplasms exhibit two peaks, one in childhood and another in adults between the ages of 45 and 75 years. In children, CNS tumors comprise the most frequent solid tumors and are the second most common malignancy. Approximately two-thirds of CNS tumors in children are in the posterior fossa; 25 percent are medulloblastomas, 21 percent are astrocytomas, and 20 percent are glioblastomas. About two-thirds of CNS tumors in adults are hemispheric; about 20 percent are meningiomas, usually a tumor of relatively benign histology. Gliomas account for approximately 60 percent of the primary brain tumors in adults; malignant gliomas (anaplastic astrocytoma and glioblastoma multiforme) account for more than 90 percent of those and will be the focus of this chapter.

The prognosis for patients with malignant gliomas remains poor; approximately 75 percent of such patients die within 1 year of diagnosis. Present day multimodal treatments have failed to increase the median survival time of such patients much beyond 1 year. By the time it is diagnosed, the tumor has already undergone at least 30 doublings and probably more if one considers that extensive cell death occurs within growing tumors. Only between three and six further doublings are required for the intracranial tumor burden to become lethal. Thus, when a malignant brain tumor is diagnosed, it is already "mature," heterogeneous, and has progressed through roughly 85 percent of its life cycle. Clearly, the odds for therapeutic success are small to begin with, and they are worse when tumors are already large and widely infiltrative when discovered.

Aggressive treatment of malignant brain tumors is best initiated as soon as possible after the diagnosis has been established. The standard treatment modalities available for use against malignant brain neoplasms are surgery, ionizing radiation, and chemotherapy. Immunotherapy, photodynamic therapy (PDT), and hyperthermia are currently experimental but have potential for future applications. In attempts to effect a cure, most glioma treatment protocols include several complementary approaches.

PROGNOSTIC FACTORS

Several well-established prognostic factors affect the outcome of patients with malignant gliomas. These are important to assess the likelihood that an individual patient will benefit from treatment and minimize iatrogenic complications if the probability of a favorable outcome is small. A substantial body of evidence suggests that younger patients with malignant gliomas survive longer than older patients regardless of treatment. Patients younger than 45 years have the best prognosis, whereas there is no good evidence that chemotherapy, for example, is of any benefit to patients over 65 years of age. Patients whose presurgical Karnofsky performance scores are higher than 70 also have a better prognosis. Some consider performance status more important than the extent of surgical resection as a determinant of outcome. In addition, performance status frequently influences patient selection for treatment and therefore may bias the results of clinical trials. Both the postoperative tumor area and the tumor area 9 weeks after irradiation are of prognostic significance; patients with smaller residual tumors live longer. Improved histopathologic classification of tumors (see Table 1) has enhanced our ability to stratify patients entered in clinical trials and thus better assess the effect of treatment. For example, the accurate diagnosis of anaplastic astrocytoma and glioblastoma multiforme has identified the former as a subgroup of patients with a better response to treatment and with a longer median survival than patients with glioblastoma. The labeling index of the tumor (determined with bromodeoxyuridine or with the Ki-67 antibody) is an independent variable that may also be of prognostic importance. A labeling index of less than 3 percent appears to correlate with longer survival.

SURGERY

The indications for surgery, and some potential complications, are listed in Table 2. Surgical interven-

---

Table 1 Neuroepithelial Brain Tumors

Astrocytic tumors: astrocytoma (fibrillary, protoplasmic, gemistocytic), anaplastic astrocytoma, glioblastoma (giant-cell glioblastoma, gliosarcoma), pilocytic astrocytoma, pleomorphic xanthoastrocytoma, subependymal giant-cell astrocytoma

Oligodendroglial tumors: oligodendroglioma, anaplastic oligodendroglioma

Ependymal tumors: ependymoma (cellular, papillary, epithelial, clear cell), anaplastic ependymoma, myxopapillary ependymoma, subependymoma

Mixed gliomas

Choroid plexus tumors: choroid plexus papilloma, choroid plexus carcinoma

Neuroepithelial tumors of uncertain origin: astroblastoma, polar spongioblastoma, gliomatosis cerebri

Neuronal and mixed neuronal-glial tumors: gangliocytoma, dysplastic gangliocytoma of cerebellum (Lhermitte-Duclos), desmoplastic infantile ganglioglioma, dysembryoplastic neuroepithelial tumor, ganglioglioma, anaplastic ganglioglioma, central neurocytoma, olfactory neuroblastoma

Pineal tumors: pineocytoma, pineoblastoma

Embryonal tumors: medulloepithelioma, neuroblastoma, ependymoblastoma, retinoblastoma, primitive neuroectodermal tumors (PNETs) with multipotent differentiation: (a) medulloblastoma, (b) cerebral or spinal PNETs

(Condensed from the WHO–1990 Classification)

tion is carried out at the earliest possible time on patients who are candidates for surgery. In good hands, the surgical mortality rate from a craniotomy should be less than 1 percent and the morbidity rate no more than 10 percent. Stereotactic techniques, in which biopsy specimens are obtained through burr holes, which are drilled with the patient under local anesthesia, have been made possible by the development of computers and have revolutionized brain tumor surgery. With stereotaxy it is no longer necessary to subject all patients to craniotomy, a major source of morbidity, for diagnosis. Deep-seated and brainstem tumors, which were previously considered inaccessible, are now amenable to stereotactic biopsy and occasional partial debulking. The postoperative course of patients after a stereotactic biopsy is short and relatively free from complications, so the time and cost of hospitalization are decreased. Furthermore, aggressive treatment can be started early, when the patient is in good condition; for example, a patient undergoing brain irradiation is less likely to develop wound healing problems after a burr hole is drilled than after a craniotomy.

A persistent and not easily resolved argument relates to the effect of the extent of surgical resection of supratentorial malignant gliomas on patient survival and quality of life. Some clinicians argue that patient survival is significantly longer and better following extensive (gross "total") removal of tumor than in patients who undergo a limited (subtotal) resection or biopsy. Others argue that total tumor removal is unlikely regardless of the extent of resection; therefore, they opt for a biopsy to establish a tissue diagnosis and minimize operative morbidity, and proceed with adjuvant treatments (radiation and chemotherapy). Among patients entered in adjuvant therapy trials, survival of those who undergo biopsy does not appear to be shorter than survival of patients who have had a gross total resection of tumor. Clinical treatment trials, however, have not been controlled for tumor location and extent of resection.

Although 80 to 90 percent of malignant gliomas recur within 2 cm of the original tumor margin, it has been demonstrated that in at least 40 percent of patients isolated tumor cells infiltrate the brain beyond the perimeter of abnormal signal on the T_2-weighted image

of a magnetic resonance (MR) scan taken at the time of diagnosis. Because surgical resections rarely, if ever, extend to the perimeter of abnormal signal on the T_2-weighted image of the MR scan, it is evident that surgery alone will not cure these tumors. Furthermore, there is no proof that gross total resections of tumor achieve a 1-log to 2-log (90 to 99 percent) cell kill, as frequently assumed. The effects of surgical cytoreduction on the cell-cycle kinetics of residual tumor are not known.

There are some clear-cut indications for proceeding with craniotomy and gross total tumor excision. An excision with generous margins (i.e., lobectomy) of a polar tumor located in a noneloquent area of brain is indicated; this is a situation in which long-term survival can potentially be achieved with adjuvant therapy. Gross ("total" or "subtotal") excision should be considered for the relief of increased intracranial pressure (Table 3) in patients who are at risk for cerebral herniation. Additionally, patients with large intracranial masses may not respond to steroid quickly enough or to a significant degree. In these circumstances, relief of the intracranial pressure may improve patient performance status enough to allow consideration of further adjuvant treatments.

Several contemporary surgical techniques are available to enhance tumor removal, but their impact on patient survival is unknown. The carbon dioxide laser light can be used for cutting, coagulation, and tumor evaporation. Intraoperative ultrasound can be used to help localize lesions. The ultrasonic aspirator can aid in atraumatic tumor resections. Intraoperative brain mapping can be used to extend the margins of tumor resection while avoiding eloquent regions of the brain. Electrocorticography may be used to identify a refractory seizure focus adjacent to the tumor, which may be included in the resection.

Tumor recurrence is almost inevitable in patients with malignant gliomas regardless of the initial treatment. Functional deterioration and death are rapid after tumor progression or recurrence unless further treatment is given and is effective. Several recent clinical studies indicate that reoperation should be considered for patients with recurrent malignant glioma. If patients are properly selected, operative morbidity and mortality are no greater than those for a first surgery. The median duration of high-quality survival can double from about 12 weeks to 24 weeks after reoperation. In the setting of

Table 2 Surgery for Brain Tumors

Indications	Precise histopathologic diagnosis
	Cytoreduction
	Relieve intracranial pressure
	From tumor mass effect
	From obstructive hydrocephalus, which
	requires a shunt
Complications	Swelling of the brain
	Hemorrhage into the tumor bed
	Communicating hydrocephalus
	Cerebral abscess
	Wound infection
	Seizures
	Syndrome of inappropriate antidiuretic
	hormone (SIADH)

Table 3 Symptoms and Signs of Increased Intracranial Pressure

Headaches (initially they awaken the patient)
Vomiting (occasionally "projectile," i.e., without nausea)
Dizziness or giddiness
Changes in mental function (psychomotor asthenia)
Papilledema
Increased blood pressure and slowed pulse (Cushing's reflex)
Cranial nerve palsies (Nerve VI palsy is the most frequent)
Stupor and coma

recurrent disease, tumor cytoreduction and relief of increased intracranial pressure can provide an added interval during which additional adjuvant treatment can be contemplated and initiated. Performance status will not improve following a second surgery; therefore, patients whose condition has deteriorated significantly should not be made to endure pointless procedures.

CORTICOSTEROID

Corticosteroids are not cytotoxic against gliomas, but they rapidly decrease the tumor mass effect and the intracranial pressure; for these reasons they are universally useful in the management of patients with brain tumors. The most commonly employed corticosteroid in neuro-oncology is dexamethasone (Decadron). Dexamethasone decreases cerebral blood flow and blood volume and probably causes vasoconstriction of cerebral vessels in patients with malignant gliomas. It also decreases the permeability of tumor capillaries to small hydrophilic molecules, resulting in a reduction of cerebral edema. In this fashion, dexamethasone not only decreases the volume of the intracranial contents and the mass effect generated by the tumor but also protects the brain from the acute effects of ionizing radiation.

The conventional dosage of dexamethasone is described in Table 4. Dramatic symptomatic and functional improvement can begin within a few hours of the first intravenous injection of dexamethasone. Maximum symptomatic improvement is achieved between 3 and 14 days after treatment is started. Dexamethasone is a toxic drug (Table 5); therefore, it is tapered as tolerated, but slowly, once the patient's neurologic condition has stabilized and definitive treatment has been initiated. It is usually safe to start tapering dexamethasone after surgical debulking or about 1 week after brain irradiation has begun. The objective of tapering the steroid is to discontinue the drug altogether or to maintain the lowest dose that prevents further functional deterioration. Many patients become steroid dependent, so if deterioration occurs while dexamethasone is being tapered, the dose must be readjusted. There is no absolute limit to the upper dose of dexamethasone that can be prescribed (see Table 4), rather practical considerations and the toxic effects of steroids (see Table 5) dictate individual dose ceilings.

The pharmacologic half-life of dexamethasone is between 2 and 3 hours after either oral or intravenous administration; the beneficial effects of a dose, however, may last 24 hours or more. Although it is customary to switch from intravenous to oral dexamethasone at the same dose, the oral bioavailability of the drug varies from 10 percent to 98 percent, so dosage adjustments may be required. The concurrent administration of dexamethasone with diphenylhydantoin (Dilantin) may lower plasma dexamethasone levels by up to 70 percent; the clinical relevance of this interaction is unknown. Toxic effects from dexamethasone are common (see Table 5) and may be severe; their incidence is higher if the plasma albumin levels are depressed, so the importance of an adequate diet cannot be overemphasized.

CHEMOTHERAPY

Clinical trials have demonstrated that chemotherapy, when it is used as an adjuvant to surgery and radiation therapy, increases the proportion of patients with malignant gliomas who are long-term survivors (longer than 18 months). Unfortunately, because the best regimens (single drugs or multidrug combinations) are active in only about 35 percent of patients, the impact of chemotherapy on the median survival time (MST) is minimal. The chemotherapy regimens commonly used at present consist of carmustine (BCNU) or procarbazine (Table 6). Recently, the combination of procarbazine,

Table 4 Use of Dexamethasone

Condition	Dose
For mild to moderate neurologic dysfunction	4 mg orally or IV every 6 hours
For acute neurologic deterioration	10 mg IV bolus followed by 4 mg IV every 6 hours until the neurologic condition has stabilized; administration is then oral
Tapering dexamethasone	Initially may decrease the dose to 4 mg tid for 5 to 10 days. If the patient remains stable, decrease the total daily dose by 2 mg increments every 5 to 10 days until the total daily dose is 6 mg/d, then decrease the total daily dose in 1 mg increments as tolerated

Table 5 Toxic Effects of Dexamethasone and Their Treatment

Toxic Effect	Treatment
Hyperglycemia	Control diet or use insulin as necessary
Gastrointestinal bleeding and/or perforation	Prophylaxis with H_2-receptor blockers (ranitidine or cimetidine)
Steroid mania or psychosis	May respond to haloperidol and/or benzodiazepines
Immunosuppression and opportunistic infections	Vigilance and treatment as appropriate
Fluid and electrolyte imbalance	Frequent laboratory studies and patient weights; may require diuretic
Adrenal suppression	Of most concern in patients under stress and while tapering, so taper slowly
Hiccups	Haloperidol
Thromboembolism	Anticoagulation
Myopathic weakness	These and the toxic effects listed above respond to decreasing doses of dexamethasone
Cushing's syndrome	
Impaired wound healing	
Negative nitrogen balance	
Petechiae and ecchymoses	

Table 6 Conventional Chemotherapy Regimens

Carmustine*	200 mg/m² IV repeated every 6 weeks for 1 year
Procarbazine	150 mg/m²/day orally in 3 or 4 divided doses for 28 days repeated every 8 weeks for 1 year
PCV†	
Lomustine	110 mg/m² orally on day 1
Procarbazine	60 mg/m²/day orally on days 8 to 21
Vincristine	1.4 mg/m² IV on days 8 and 29
	This protocol is repeated every 6 to 8 weeks for 1 year

*Carmustine, procarbazine, and PCV are usually administered after brain irradiation, but the first dose of carmustine may optionally be administered prior to brain irradiation.

†Hydroxyurea (400 mg/M²), given orally every 6 hours every other day during radiation therapy, may be added to this regimen.

Table 7 Antiemetic Regimens for Chemotherapy

Condition	Regimen
For mild to moderate symptoms	Diphenhydramine, 50 mg orally or 25 mg IV once 30 minutes before chemotherapy
	Prochlorperazine, 20 mg orally or 10 mg IV 30 minutes before chemotherapy and every 6 hours as needed
For severe symptoms	Diphenhydramine, 50 mg orally or 25 mg IV once 30 minutes before chemotherapy
	Lorazepam, 1 mg orally or IV
	Haloperidol, 1 mg orally or IV Lorazepam and haloperidol are given together 30 minutes before chemotherapy and then orally as needed every 3 to 4 hours during the first day and every 6 hours thereafter if needed

lomustine (CCNU), and vincristine (PCV) administered after radiotherapy (see Table 6) has proved to be of benefit, especially for patients with anaplastic astrocytomas. A suitable antiemetic regimen (Table 7) should always be incorporated into the chemotherapy protocol.

Complicated, unconventional chemotherapy regimens, such as the eight-drugs-in-one-day regimen or NCOG 6G91 (Table 8) offer no clear therapeutic advantage over simpler, conventional chemotherapy protocols and may carry an added risk of toxic side-effects. The major drawback of multidrug regimens may relate to the need for an initial reduction in the dosage of the individual drugs (relative to their conventional dose when used as single agents) to administer combinations of such toxic drugs. Toxicity often dictates further dosage reductions in significant numbers of patients, which further compromises the intensity and effectiveness of multidrug combinations (Table 9).

Carmustine

The Brain Tumor Cooperative Group (BTCG) established the combination of carmustine (BCNU) and

Table 8 Two Unconventional Chemotherapy Regimens (drug doses in mg/m²)

Eight-Drugs-In-One-Day Regimen

Methylprednisolone, 300
Vincristine (max 2.0 mg), 1.5
Lomustine, 75
Procarbazine, 75
Hydroxyurea, 3,000
Cisplatin, 90
Cytosine arabinoside, 300
Dacarbazine, 150

Northern California Oncology Group (NCOG) 6G91†

Before Radiation
  5-Fluorouracil (1g/m²/day) IV on Days 1-3
  Lomustine (110 mg/m² orally) on Day 7
During Radiation
  Radiation: 45 Gy to whole-brain plus a 15 Gy boost (begin 3-7 days after lomustine)
  Hydroxyurea (300 mg/m² every 4 hours × 4 doses) on Monday and Wednesday
  Misonidazole (0.5 g/m²) before each radiation therapy fraction
After Radiation
  Procarbazine (130 mg/m²/day orally × 28 days)
  Vincristine (1.5 mg/m² IV × 1 day/wk × 4) starting 1 week after completion of procarbazine
  Carmustine (200 mg/m² IV × 1 day) 10 to 14 days after completion of the procarbazine and vincristine cycle
  5-Fluorouracil (1 g/m²/day × 3) IV starting 10 to 14 days after completion of BCNU

*2 cycles of preirradiation chemotherapy are administered at 2 to 3 week intervals; brain irradiation starts 2 weeks after the second cycle of chemotherapy; up to 8 cycles of postirradiation chemotherapy are administered at monthly intervals starting 2 weeks after brain irradiation.

†3 cycles of postirradiation chemotherapy are administered at 4 to 5 week intervals

Table 9 Toxic Effects of Some Chemotherapeutic Agents

Toxic Effects	Chemotherapeutic Agents
Myelosuppression	Carmustine, Lomustine, Procarbazine
Peripheral neuropathy	Vincristine, Cisplatin, Procarbazine
Encephalopathy	Carmustine, Lomustine, Methotrexate, Cytarabine, 5-Fluorouracil, Procarbazine
Myelopathy	Methotrexate, Cytarabine, Thiotepa
Gastrointestinal	Carmustine, Lomustine, Procarbazine
Lung, kidney, liver, etc may be affected by all drugs	

radiotherapy as the standard against which treatments for malignant glioma are measured (see Table 6). The BTCG reported that the MST of patients with malignant gliomas was 14 weeks if the tumor was only surgically debulked. MST increased to between 36 and 50 weeks if whole-brain irradiation was used as an adjuvant to surgery. BCNU did not appreciably influence the MST because only a minority of patients responded to the drug. However, BCNU increased the percentage of patients who survived 18 months or longer from less than 5 percent to about 20 percent. The BTCG further demonstrated that procarbazine plus radiotherapy (see Table 6) was an effective treatment of malignant gliomas although it offered no survival advantage over BCNU plus radiotherapy. Lomustine (CCNU), a nitrosourea which may be taken orally, also has shown activity against malignant gliomas in some trials.

Several investigators have attempted to enhance the therapeutic potential of BCNU with innovative protocols. Unfortunately, no protocol to date has significantly improved the survival rates obtained with intravenous BCNU plus radiotherapy.

Intracarotid BCNU

Intracarotid (usually into the supraophthalmic portion of the carotid artery) BCNU achieves intratumoral drug levels 4 to 380 times greater than those obtained with the same doses administered intravenously, because of the high clearance rate of intravenous BCNU. Intracarotid BCNU also may limit the incidence of systemic toxic effects from the drug. However, leukoencephalopathy and catheter-related complications among patients treated with intracarotid BCNU occur in approximately 50 percent of patients. Nonuniform drug delivery (streaming) occurs at low infusion rates and may result in a regional drug concentration at least five times greater than expected, provoking sporadic focal brain and retinal toxicity. Despite the high intratumoral levels achieved, a number of clinical trials have failed to establish a clear therapeutic advantage for intraarterial BCNU; its use as routine therapy for malignant gliomas is not warranted at present.

High-Dose Chemotherapy with Bone Marrow Rescue

The numerous toxic effects of BCNU, myelosuppression in particular, preclude taking advantage of the steep dose–response effect exhibited by this alkylating agent because maximally effective drug doses are also the most toxic. Autologous bone marrow transplantation shortens the period of marrow aplasia induced by intensive, high-dose therapy and represents an example of high dose-intensity treatment. This treatment approach has been applied chiefly to patients whose tumors recur after more conventional treatment. Response rates to marrow-ablative doses of chemotherapy (BCNU at 600 to 1400 mg per m^2) may be higher than when drugs are used at more standard doses. Nonetheless, a very high incidence of fatal systemic toxic effects limits the practicality of this approach for brain tumor treatment. Since BCNU cannot sterilize malignant gliomas even though high intratumoral levels are reached following intracarotid administration, it appears unlikely that marrow-ablative high-dose therapy with BCNU alone will achieve a cure. A pilot study of marrow-ablative doses of BCNU in combination with etoposide (VP-16) and thiotepa is in progress at the Memorial Sloan-Kettering Cancer Center (Table 10).

Table 10 Marrow-Ablative Chemotherapy Regimen*

For newly diagnosed tumors
  BCNU—600 mg/m^2 (100 mg/M^2 every 12 hours × 6 doses)
  VP-16—250 mg/m^2/d × 3 days
  Thiotepa—300 mg/m^2/d × 3 days
For recurrent tumors, depending on histology
  Carboplatin—500 mg/m^2/d × 3 days may be substituted
    for BCNU

*Jonathan Finlay, M.D., Personal communication, 1990.

For reviews of other drugs and drug combinations used to treat malignant gliomas the reader is directed to the suggested reading list at the end of this chapter.

Intracarotid Chemotherapy Following Blood–Brain Barrier Disruption

Major controversy in neuro-oncology surrounds the treatment of brain tumors with intracarotid chemotherapy following blood–brain barrier disruption (BBBD) with hyperosmotic agents. Proponents of this treatment approach report both high response rates and relatively low morbidity rates among heterogeneous groups of patients with intracranial neoplasms of diverse types. Either hyperosmotic mannitol or Renografin-76 can be used to produce BBBD. The incidence of seizures may be less after BBBD with Renografin-76.

A series of experiments in animal models contests the ability of BBBD to increase the amount of chemotherapy delivered to brain tumors. In animal model systems, BBBD has resulted in up to 105-fold increases in the cortical permeability to small hydrophilic molecules and to cytotoxic drugs but only a 1.7- to 13-fold increase in the permeability of the tumor to those agents. Therefore, the net effect of this treatment is to reverse the tumor-to-cortex permeability relationship for both small hydrophilic molecules and for cytotoxic drugs. Thus, a sink effect increases the delivery of water-soluble chemotherapeutic agents to the brain parenchyma; drug delivery to the tumor itself, whose capillaries present little or no barrier to the passage of serum proteins, remains essentially unchanged. As many as 90 percent of treated gliomas recur within 2 cm of the initial tumor margin; therefore, it appears that BBBD merely increases the exposure of brain to toxic chemicals without providing a clear therapeutic benefit. In this context, BBBD is probably detrimental. In the case of lipophilic drugs, whose access to tumors is mainly dependent on blood flow and not capillary permeability, a cogent argument for drug administration with concomitant BBBD does not exist. Additionally, as many as 50 percent of tumor microvessels in an animal model may not be perfused with blood. The significance of this finding to the intravenous, intracarotid, or intracarotid after BBBD routes of drug administration remains undetermined.

There is no good evidence that a blood–tumor barrier significantly restricts the uptake of chemotherapy by tumors. Among others, the concentrations of

3-deazauridine, N-phosphoacetyl L-aspartic acid (PALA), IMPY, mitoguazone, diaziquone (AZQ), vinblastine, AMSA, epipodophyllotoxin (VP-16), VM-26, cisplatin, pentamethylmelamine, tiazofurin, and mitoxantrone attainable in human brain tumors following systemic administration have been studied. All drugs attained potentially cytotoxic concentrations within the tumors. Moderately high concentrations of drugs were found within the first centimeter of the brain adjacent to tumor, but beyond that concentrations decreased rapidly with increasing distance into normal brain. Thus, even drugs that do not normally enter the CNS could be active against malignant brain tumors and should not be excluded from therapeutic drug trials. The concentrations of thio-tepa in the brain parenchyma of dogs after administration by intravenous bolus, intravenous infusion, intracarotid bolus, and intracarotid bolus following BBBD with hyperosmolar mannitol have been monitored. Following intravenous infusion, the thiotepa concentration in brain parenchyma was consistently higher than in simultaneously sampled cerebrospinal fluid and plasma. This was true both at the end of the infusion (peak level) and 180 minutes after the infusion (wash-out level). Peak concentrations after the infusion were 7 to 16 times higher than after an intravenous bolus and of the same magnitude as achieved after intracarotid administration with barrier disruption. This suggests that after prolonged intravenous infusions cytotoxic drugs might reach the same tumor concentrations as achieved after intracarotid administration with or without BBBD.

Controlled trials using blood–brain barrier disruption versus systemic or intracarotid infusions of the same drug without barrier disruption have not yet been reported. Until a controlled trial is performed in an adequate number of patients, this treatment approach will remain controversial and the issue of its usefulness unresolved. Preliminary studies indicate that the vascular permeability pattern of a tumor, determined quantitatively on rapid, sequential contrast-enhanced computed tomography (CT) scans, may partially determine its response to chemotherapy. This concept is being tested clinically at the Evanston Hospital (Evanston, IL).

Polyanhydride Wafers Impregnated with BCNU

Recently, a nonrandomized phase I trial using direct intratumoral implants of BCNU-containing wafers was completed. The implants were well tolerated, there was no increase in surgical morbidity or mortality, and survival was longer than for historical re-operated control patients. The BCNU-containing wafers are a biodegradable polyanhydride polymer with varying amounts of sialic acid. The amount of sialic acid in the polymer determines the rate at which BCNU is released, which typically extends over a period of weeks. Local concentrations of BCNU are high and fall off quickly with increasing distance from the site of implantation. A multi-institution, randomized, double-blinded, phase III trial of intracavitary BCNU-containing wafers implanted

at the time of surgical debulking is presently underway (Nicholas Vick, MD, personal communication, 1990).

RADIATION THERAPY

Brain irradiation is the most clearly effective modality for the treatment of malignant gliomas. The ability of radiation to prolong patient survival has been demonstrated in numerous excellent, controlled, prospective and retrospective clinical studies. Nonetheless, several important questions surround the use of brain irradiation, namely: What volume of brain should be irradiated? Do radiation doses greater than 60 Gy further increase local tumor control? Are radiation sensitizers capable of potentiating the effect of radiation?

Patient survival and tumor response to radiotherapy are dose related up to about 60 Gy (administered in 180 to 200 cGy fractions). Using conventional fractionation schemas, doses greater than 60 Gy significantly increase the incidence of late radiotherapy-related complications (Table 11). Chemotherapy, especially when administered by the intracarotid route, intrathecally, or simultaneously with radiation, may further lower the brain's tolerance to ionizing radiation.

If the volume of irradiated brain includes only the contrast-enhancing margin of the tumor (determined by CT) plus a 1-cm margin, a significant volume of tumor is missed in almost 100 percent of patients. If the volume of irradiated brain includes the tumor plus the margin of edematous brain plus a 1-cm margin, a significant volume of tumor is still missed in 45 percent of patients. If the volume of irradiated brain is increased to include the tumor plus the margin of edematous brain plus a 3-cm margin, the full tumor volume usually is covered. Several retrospective clinical studies have failed to demonstrate a survival advantage for patients treated

Table 11 Nervous System Complications of Ionizing Radiation

Acute reactions (occur during radiation and are probably due to edema)
  Increased intracranial pressure
  Exacerbation of symptoms or signs
  These usually respond to steroids
Early Delayed Reactions (occur a few weeks to months after radiation)
  Somnolence and lethargy
  Cerebellar signs
  Neurologic deterioration
  These are usually transient and do not require treatment
Late Reactions (occur months to years after radiation)
  Mild impairment of function
  Cerebral atrophy
  Mineralizing microangiopathy
  Focal brain necrosis
  Dementia
  Endocrine dysfunction
  Cranial nerve palsies
  Spinal cord injury
  Death

with whole-brain irradiation compared with those treated to the involved field (determined on a contrast-enhanced CT scan) plus a "generous" margin. Regardless of the irradiated volume, 80 to 90 percent of patients still fail within 2-cm of the originally determined tumor margin. Although isolated tumor cells that extend beyond the margin of either CT- or MR-determined abnormalities are demonstrable in a large proportion of patients, it does not seem that marginal tumor miss by radiation is clinically important. A more important factor determining radioresistance may relate to the proportion of hypoxic cells within the tumor. Hypoxic cells are relatively more radioresistant to the cytotoxic effects of ionizing radiation than well-oxygenated cells. Tumors may contain between 1 and 30 percent of hypoxic cells. The unfortunate reality is that conventionally delivered brain irradiation fails to control the bulk of local neoplasm.

Several strategies have emerged from attempts to overcome radioresistance and improve local tumor control; these include hyperfractionation, use of hypoxic and nonhypoxic cell radiosensitizers, stereotactic irradiation, and brachytherapy. Hyperfractionation is a technique wherein smaller fractions of radiation (about 120 cGy per fraction) are delivered two or more times per day. This allows a higher total dose to be delivered in a shorter time and attempts to approximate the continuous low dose of irradiation achieved by brachytherapy techniques. Delivering lower radiation doses per fraction also decreases the oxygen-enhancement ratio, thus decreasing the relative radioresistance conferred to the tumor by hypoxic cells. Additionally, rapidly cycling tumor cells are slower to repair sublethal damage than are normal cells, which are therefore relatively spared. Hyperfractionation trials conducted by the Radiation Therapy Oncology Group (RTOG) have achieved total doses up to 81.6 Gy but failed to produce any appreciable survival gain. At a dose of 81.6 Gy, some patients died from radiation related complications (see Table 11). Therefore, despite the theoretic advantages of hyperfractionating radiation, a plateau of radiation dose versus response appears to have been reached.

Attempts at modification of the biologic response of tissues to radiation by radiosensitizing drugs is under investigation. These compounds have affinity for electrons and, in a low oxygen-tension environment, fix the DNA damage produced by radiation. The use of radiosensitizing drugs is aimed at achieving a substantial differential effect (therapeutic gain) resulting in sensitization of hypoxic tumor cells to ionizing radiation. Initial results from the laboratory suggested that therapeutic gains of 1.5- to 2.0-fold could be expected with this strategy. It now appears that actual clinical therapeutic gains may be more on the order of 1.1 to 1.2. It is doubtful that a 10 to 20 percent increase in radiosensitivity of the up to 30 percent of the tumor which is hypoxic is sufficient to produce a substantial impact on patient survival. Two classes of chemical radiosensitizers have been tested clinically: the nitroimidazoles (metronidazole and misonidazole) and the halogenated pyrim-

idine analogs (bromodeoxyuridine [BrUrd] and iododeoxyuridine [IdUrd]). The halogenated pyrimidine compounds are analogs of the nucleoside thymidine. Although the exact mechanism by which halogenated pyrimidines cause radiosensitization is not known, it most likely results from their direct incorporation into DNA in place of thymidine.

Incorporation of radiosensitizing agents into clinical trials has not yet resulted in unequivocally improved survival. However, preliminary results of a clinical trial testing a continuous intracarotid infusion of BrUrd appear promising. In addition, an RTOG-sponsored trial of conventional brain irradiation plus a continuous intravenous infusion of IdUrd is currently underway. Dose-limiting systemic toxicity from radiosensitizing drugs affects chiefly the bone marrow and gastrointestinal tract, but significant local toxicity (within the radiation field) does not generally occur. Hydroxyurea, cisplatin, and carboplatin also bind to DNA and may be potentially useful radiosensitizing agents. A new class of oxygen-carrying compounds, perfluorochemicals, is also undergoing clinical testing.

Exposure of the brain to a large single fraction of radiation can potentially sterilize a tumor. However, use of large fractions also reduces the therapeutic ratio of the treatment and results in serious short- and long-term complications (see Table 11). One solution to this problem is the use of precisely collimated beams of radiation that intersect at the center of the tumor after entering from several points distributed over the skull—this is the basis of stereotactic radiotherapy.

During stereotactic radiotherapy a single high dose of radiation is targeted to a small target volume of tumor and adjacent brain while minimal amounts are delivered to the normal brain. A stereotactic system is applied to immobilize the head and to obtain the precise stereotactic coordinates for treatment. Tumor measurements in three dimensions (anteroposterior, lateral, and rostrocaudal) are determined after a contrast-enhanced CT scan. A point representing the center of the tumor is selected on the central slice (the central tumor target point) and the stereotactic coordinates of the point are obtained to generate a three-dimensional reconstruction of the patient's head. This three-dimensional model is used to calculate the number and diameter of the treatment arcs, start and stop angles for the linear accelerator gantry, and couch angles appropriate for the selected treatment cone size. A cone 0.5 cm larger than the maximum tumor diameter is generally used. The isodose line covering the periphery of the tumor, represented by the 80 percent isodose line in the patients, is used for prescription. The total dose prescribed to this line is extrapolated so as to stay below the 1 percentile necrosis level for each cone size. Deep single lesions whose maximum diameters range between 0.5 cm and 3.5 cm are ideal for stereotactic treatment. The volume of normal brain that ultimately receives therapeutic doses of radiation when the diameter of the treated lesion is larger than 3.5 cm makes the likelihood of subsequent complications unacceptably high. Radiation doses on the order of 15 to 27.5 Gy are routinely delivered to the central tumor target point using a modified linear accelerator. Precise data regarding the efficacy of this technique are not yet available, although it is reported to be useful in the treatment of metastatic brain lesions. We have found stereotactic treatment of malignant gliomas useful as a boost either before or after conventionally fractionated brain irradiation.

Brachytherapy is an alternative means of delivering a high dose of radiation while relatively sparing the surrounding normal tissue. Interstitial brachytherapy consists of the implantation into the tumor bed of radioactive isotopes, the most common of which are high-activity iodine 125 (^{125}I) and iridium 192 (^{192}Ir). Upon decay, ^{125}I emits low-energy beta and gamma rays, which are quickly attenuated in tissue, thus limiting the exposure of normal brain to radiation. Iridium 192 emits gamma rays upon decay. Tumors may be considered for implantation if they are small (less than 5 cm in diameter), well circumscribed, and relatively superficial, and if the patient has a Karnofsky performance score of at least 70. Relative contraindications for treatment with brachytherapy include large (maximum diameter greater than 5 cm) or diffuse, multifocal or "butterfly" tumors, tumors that have spread to the subarachnoid space, and tumors located in the diencephalon or posterior fossa.

Tumor targets are selected from an enhanced CT scan. Iodine 125 implants with an activity of 30 to 50 mCi are afterloaded with the patient under local anesthesia into prepositioned catheters whose location is determined from a CT stereotaxy system. The number of catheters and the number and strengths of the individual sources are chosen so the implants deliver 30 to 60 cGy per hour to the periphery of the contrast-enhancing lesion plus a 0.5-cm margin. A "minimum tumor dose" is calculated for this rim of tumor; the volume contained within the rim receives a radiation dose higher than the calculated minimum. After the desired dose has been delivered, the catheters are removed with the patient under local anesthesia.

Iridium 192 implants allow for similar pre-planning, afterloading, and removal at the patient's bedside. Because of the ready availability of a large spectrum of source intensities, ^{192}Ir implants can be tailored very specifically to contour the tumor surface with a substantially smaller dose gradient. Generally, radiation boosts of up to 60 Gy are delivered with brachytherapy.

Another innovative procedure by which tumors might be more effectively irradiated consists of the systemic injection of tumor-specific monoclonal antibodies conjugated to radioactive compounds (for example, yttrium 90 [^{90}Y], a beta emitter). Theoretically, radiation can be delivered directly to the tumor bed in continuous low dose-rates. Two major problems hamper the clinical application of this procedure: (1) monoclonal antibodies specific enough to localize only to the tumor are not yet available; and (2) the dose-rate achievable with currently available technology is on the order of 10 cGy per hour, which is too low to stop cell proliferation. An approximately 30- to 35-fold increase in the total radiation dose delivered to the tumor with radioactive monoclonal antibodies is still required to sterilize neoplasms.

At present, a conventional approach to brain irradiation is both effective and easily accomplished. Radiation is individualized after a planning CT and radiation is delivered in multiple field arrangements, usually isocentric, with beams of megavoltage energy. Thus, using parallel opposed fields, 45 to 50 Gy in 180 to 200 cGy fractions are delivered to the tumor plus a 2- to 3-cm margin beyond the edema followed by a boost of 10 to 15 Gy depending on tumor size.

IMMUNOTHERAPY

Patients with malignant gliomas have a relative state of immunodeficiency at the time their tumor is diagnosed. This immune status is characterized by a decreased number of circulating T cells, cutaneous anergy to common skin-test antigens, depression of lymphocyte blastogenic responsiveness to mitogens and alloantigens, and the presence of circulating humoral immune suppressor factors. In addition, cultured human glioblastoma secretes an interleukin-1–like factor that inhibits interleukin-2 (IL-2)–dependent proliferation of T cells as well as the induction of alloreactive cytotoxic T cells. A humoral immune inhibitory factor from the transforming growth factor beta (TGFβ) family, TGFβ-2, has been purified from patients with malignant gliomas. TGFβ-2 inhibits the proliferative response to IL-2 of tumor infiltrating lymphocytes (TILs) derived from glioblastomas by up to 85 percent. This inhibition can be overcome by increasing the concentration of IL-2 10- to 20-fold. TGFβ-2 also suppresses the cytotoxic response of TILs against autologous glioma by up to 100 percent. Whereas a positive blastogenic response to autologous glioma by peripheral blood lymphocytes can be demonstrated in 58 percent of patients with malignant glioma, a similar response can be demonstrated by TILs in only 25 percent of patients. The blastogenic response of lymphocytes to glioma can be increased by culturing lymphocytes with interferon-gamma (IfNγ), but other lymphokines, such as IL-2, do not affect it. In contrast, although patients with gliomas have about one-third the number of circulating mononuclear cells of healthy control subjects, the cytotoxic capacity of lymphokine-activated killer (LAK) cells derived from those patients is similar to that of LAK cells derived from control subjects.

A number of investigators have attempted to treat patients with malignant gliomas with immune adjuvants such as recombinant interferons (rIFN) or through adoptive transfer of immune components such as IL-2 and LAK cells systemically or into the tumor bed. The main limitation to the use of IL-2 as adjuvant treatment of brain tumors relates to its cerebral vasotoxic effects. Patients receiving IL-2 exhibit marked increases in systemic capillary permeability and develop weight gain, hypotension, pulmonary edema, and transient changes in mental status. Cats injected with IL-2 show an increased cerebrovascular permeability to horseradish peroxidase and IgG, although in some infusion with excipient alone also alters the cerebrovascular permeability. MR scans of patients with malignant gliomas and with systemic cancers without intracranial metastases reveal an increased cerebral water content after administration of IL-2. Patients with malignant glioma treated with IL-2 deteriorate neurologically and demonstrate increases in peritumoral edema and mass effect. Cancer patients without intracranial lesions treated with IL-2 experience minor (lethargy and confusion) changes in mental status. With appropriate supportive care, all neurologic changes related to IL-2 administration are transient. To date, IL-2 plus LAK cells applied to the immediate tumor bed offers no significant advantage over surgery alone in the treatment of patients with recurrent gliomas.

Patients with gliomas may be more susceptible to the vasotoxic effects of IL-2 because the tumors secrete a vascular permeability factor (VPF) that is, at least in part, responsible for the edema produced by gliomas. The paired insult of IL-2 plus VPF may ultimately limit use of this immunomodulator in brain tumor therapy. Although IL-2 modifies and penetrates the blood–brain barrier, its effectiveness against intracranial neoplasms remains to be determined. In that regard, it has been reported that several patients with melanoma who had been successfully treated with IL-2 all developed metastases to the brain. It appears that a sanctuary was provided to those metastases within the context of otherwise effective therapy.

OTHER TREATMENTS

Photodynamic therapy (PDT) benefits from the interaction between absorbed light and photosensitizing hematoporphyrin derivatives (HPD), which are selectively retained within cancer cells. The interaction between HPD and light generates short-lived intracellular cytotoxic molecules. After sensitization with rhodamine-123 (a HPD), cultured human glioma, but not normal cells, are killed by exposure to light from a blue-green laser. This suggests that rhodamine-123 (or some other HPD) might be useful for the treatment of malignant gliomas. Several groups report discouraging results from pilot studies using HPD. Future technical advances may succeed in bringing PDT into the mainstream of brain tumor treatment.

Advances in hyperthermia technology may lead to its addition to the armamentarium of useful treatments for patients with malignant brain tumors. In systemic hyperthermia, patients are heated to a temperature of up to 41.8° C in a radiant heating device. Both brain and tumor are homogeneously heated to this temperature. Local hyperthermia can be accomplished by the direct implantation of the tumor with microwave antennas. Small localized areas of the tumor may reach temperatures up to 43° C but the majority of the tumor is heterogeneously heated to between 40° C and 42° C. The development of drugs capable of synergizing with hyperthermia might augment the chances of clinical success with this technique.

TUMOR METABOLISM

Until such time as a new drug(s) or treatment modality with significantly greater activity against malignant gliomas is developed, one approach to the rational care of patients with brain tumors is to develop a means of identifying those with high probability of responding to a particular therapy. We used positron emission tomography with [18F]-fluorodeoxyglucose (PET-FDG) to study the effects of chemotherapy and stereotactic brain irradiation on brain tumor glucose metabolism. In comparison to a baseline PET-FDG scan, peak tumor glucose metabolism increased 20 to 100 percent within 24 hours of either treatment. Patient survival correlated inversely with the magnitude of the post-treatment increase in glucose metabolism, which suggests that post-treatment acceleration of intermediary metabolism correlates with the ability of the tumor to repair the damage produced by cytotoxic therapy. Thus, PET- FDG might be useful in identifying patients likely to benefit from a particular treatment. If PET-FDG proves to be as sensitive as indicated by those preliminary studies, scans acquired before and within 24 hours after treatment could help determine whether or not to continue a particular regimen prior to the development of toxic side-effects and while the patient remains a candidate for alternative therapeutic interventions.

PET is helpful in differentiating between tumor necrosis and tumor recurrence. As brain tumor treatment becomes more aggressive and multimodal, both tumor and adjacent brain are at increased risk of necrosis. The initial dilemma usually arises at the time a follow-up scan is obtained. That scan may show an increase in size or some other change in the character of the lesion; the clinical condition of the patient may or may not have changed. Although occasional debulking of a necrotic mass is required, in most cases, tumor necrosis is amenable to conservative treatment with dexamethasone; tumor progression or recurrence requires a change in the treatment strategy. Although the only way to be certain of the diagnosis is to obtain tissue (either from a biopsy or from a debulking procedure), a PET-FDG scan can be quite informative. A hypometabolic-appearing lesion most likely indicates necrosis, whereas a hypermetabolic lesion is most likely tumor. The large partial volume effects of PET still make this precise differentiation difficult, but the electronic superimposition of PET scans on MR or CT images will enhance the specificity of PET in that area tremendously.

Acknowledgements. The editorial comments of Drs. Henry Schutta, Timothy Kinsella, Minesh Mehta, and Allan Levin are appreciated. Also appreciated were discussions with Drs. Nicholas Vick and Jonathan Finlay.

SUGGESTED READING

Bloom HJG. Intracranial tumors: Response and resistance to therapeutic endeavors, 1970–1980. Int J Radiat Oncol Biol Phys 1982; 8:1083–1113.

Kornblith PL, Walker M. Chemotherapy for malignant gliomas. J Neurosurg 1988; 68:1–17.

Leibel SA, Sheline GE. Radiation therapy for neoplasms of the brain. J Neurosurg 1987; 66:1–22.

McComb RD, Bigner DD. The biology of malignant gliomas—a comprehensive survey. Clin Neuropathol 1984; 3:93–106.

Nazzaro JM, Neuwelt EA. The role of surgery in the management of supratentorial intermediate and high-grade astrocytomas in adults. J Neurosurg 1990; 73:331–344.

Rozental JM. Positron emission tomography (PET) and single photon emission tomography (SPECT) of brain tumors. Neurol Clin 1991; 9(2):287–305.

Rozental JM, Kinsella TJ. Brain tumors. In: Lokich J, Byfield J, eds. Combined modality cancer therapy. Chicago: Precept Press, 1991:215.

Walker AE, Robins M, Weinfeld FD. Epidemiology of brain tumors: The national survey of intracranial neoplasms. Neurology 1985; 35:219–226.

HYPERTHERMIA: AN ADJUNCT TO CANCER THERAPY

H. IAN ROBINS, M.D., Ph.D.

The intentional elevation of body temperature to treat various ailments, including cancer, has been used throughout history. During the past 25 years, laboratory research has provided unequivocal evidence to support the clinical use of hyperthermia in the treatment of neoplastic diseases. Various investigations have documented the ability of elevated temperatures to kill tumor cells, as well as the potential of hyperthermia to enhance the cytotoxic effects of both ionizing irradiation and certain drugs. Some cancer cells appear to be inherently more sensitive to the damaging effects of hyperthermia than their normal cell counterparts. In this regard, leukemia, lymphomas, and malignant gliomas may represent histologic groupings that deserve special consideration. The assumption of a universally increased sensitivity of all types of cancers to heat, however, is probably not warranted.

Temperatures in excess of 41°C kill cells *in vitro* exponentially as a function of time with increased sensitivity for cells in S-phase or in hypoxic or nutritionally restricted environments. The direct killing effects of heat alone, however, may have limited clinical utility. Proponents of hyperthermia are moving away from heat alone for the treatment of cancer patients; it has been observed that response durations have been short when hyperthermia was used as a single modality for spontaneous neoplasms. The full potential of hyperthermia resides in its use as an adjunct to other forms of therapy. Cell heterogeneity of various neoplasms appears to limit the effectiveness of any form of therapy (e.g., radiation, chemotherapy, hyperthermia, or immunotherapy). As hyperthermia is nonmyelosuppressive and can potentiate the tumoricidal effects of radiation, chemotherapy, and immunotherapy, its use in a multimodality treatment approach is attractive. A combined approach diminishes the chances of any subgroup of cells being resistant to all modes of therapy utilized.

In addition to the therapeutic role of hyperthermia with chemotherapeutic agents, it may be clinically advantageous to combine hyperthermia with another class of drugs called labilizers. These drugs are not active against neoplastic cells at normal body temperature, but they do promote neoplastic cell killing under hyperthermic conditions. Anesthetic agents represent one class of such drugs. Some labilizers (e.g., lidocaine and thiopental) seem to exhibit selective neoplastic cell killing at drug levels consistent with traditional use in a clinical setting.

This chapter reviews the three forms of hyperthermia that have been developed for clinical application (i.e., local, regional, and whole body) in terms of their current status and future potential.

LOCAL HYPERTHERMIA

Local hyperthermia is generally used to heat superficial tumors (41°C to 45°C) with minimal perturbation of normal tissue. Several different technologies have been developed that externally deposit heat to treatment areas. The methodologies most utilized to date include microwave and ultrasound, although capacitive and inductive approaches have also been studied. External hyperthermia has had clinical application in the treatment of recurrent breast cancer involving the chest wall, adenopathy related to head and neck cancer, and superficial metastatic or recurrent malignant melanoma. Other histologies that have been studied to a lesser degree include lymphomas, sarcomas, and gynecologic cancers metastatic to lymph nodes and skin. The use of local hyperthermia has generally been to enhance the effects of ionizing radiation. The goal of therapy is to improve the efficacy of palliative radiation (particularly in patients who have had previous radiation) while minimizing toxicity to normal tissues. Beyond this, studies continue to attempt to optimize the proper coupling of radiation and hyperthermia (i.e., sequencing of hyperthermia with radiation, and the duration and frequency of hyperthermia treatments) in order to improve the chances of permanent local tumor control. In broad terms, the response rates for the combination of radiation and local hyperthermia are similar in most histologies and are roughly double those observed for equivalent doses of radiation alone. Research combining local hyperthermia with chemotherapy with and without superficial irradiation has begun to only a limited extent in the past 2 years.

Technologic problems common to most forms of local hyperthermia include invasive thermometry and uneven heating. The nonhomogeneous heating produced with local hyperthermia systems makes controlled clinical investigations difficult, because the time-temperature profiles produced during a single treatment session may not be reproducible, even in the same patient. Further, results of clinical studies in both man and the dog support the concept that the lowest temperature achieved in a tumor mass is the most significant hyperthermia prognosticator for response. This concept is being refined further in ongoing research that incorporates more sophisticated thermal mapping as well as preclinical and clinical efforts to define a useful system for thermal dosing.

Despite these technologic problems, a series of controlled local hyperthermic studies using paired tumor lesions has resulted in the Food and Drug Administration recognizing (January 1, 1985) the proven efficacy of local hyperthermia in combination with ionizing irradiation.

Beyond the technologic difficulties inherent in local heating and thermometry, there is a biologic limitation. Cancer that is refractory to conventional therapy tends to be systemic in nature, often involving deeply seated disease. Thus, local hyperthermia, by its very objective (i.e., local heating), in most cases limits itself to a palliative role. A notable exception to this generalization is the potential use of local hyperthermia as an adjunct to other modalities (i.e., radiation or drugs) in the treatment of selected primary cancers, such as cervical, central nervous system, or head and neck cancer. In this regard, interstitial systems for local hyperthermia currently are being explored at several centers. With these systems, multiple invasive heating antennas are surgically implanted in a tumor mass along with a series of thermometers. Interstitial hyperthermia systems are ideally suited for use in combination with brachytherapy, i.e., interstitial irradiation. Potential advantages over other forms of local hyperthermia for the use of interstitial hyperthermia include improved homogeneity of heating, ease of temperature-probe placement via catheters, and the potential theoretical advantage of administering heat and ionizing irradiation simultaneously rather than sequencing them temporally.

An exciting new approach to locoregional hyperthermia for superficial and deep tumor masses involves the use of ferromagnetic thermoseeds. In this approach, thermoseeds consisting of wires typically 1 mm in diameter and 1 to 5 cm in length are placed in the neoplastic tissue to be treated. Following this, an externally applied electromagnetic induction field is applied in a "contactless manner"; the thermoseeds that are placed in an oscillating magnetic field become self-contained heaters for which no cable connections are required. These seeds can be made from specific alloys that lose their ferromagnetic properties at specific temperatures ("Curie point"), so that theoretically automatic temperature regulation can result. This new approach, which has been studied preclinically for several years, is now being introduced into phase 1 clinical trials.

REGIONAL HYPERTHERMIA

One approach to heating deep-seated tumors has been to apply various technologies for regional hyperthermia, including microwave, ultrasound, and electromagnetic induction by circumferential coil. Although various reports suggest the feasibility of the regional approach, controlled clinical trials are problematic. Regional hyperthermia requires invasive thermometry; heating sessions (i.e., time-temperature profiles) are not reproducible for a given patient, let alone among different patients. Thus, the next challenge for workers in this area is to deliver a defined thermal dose to a given anatomic area (e.g., the pelvis).

Limb perfusion (i.e., extracorporeal heating) has been used clinically for two decades. This form of regional hyperthermia does not suffer from the technical limitations of thermometry, uneven heating, or inability to reach target temperature. Impressive response rates combining perfusion, hyperthermia, and chemotherapy have been reported in numerous uncontrolled studies spanning 20 years. Randomized prospective multi-institutional trials are now in progress at several centers in Europe.

WHOLE-BODY HYPERTHERMIA

Because whole-body hyperthermia (WBH) addresses the issue of cancer as a systemic disease, its proponents argue that it has the greatest potential for curative intent when used as an adjunct to other therapeutic modalities. This section describes the past experience with WBH as well as its future potential as a treatment modality for cancer in the setting of experimental clinical trials.

A variety of methodologies for WBH are currently available. In published reports of WBH in humans, core temperatures have been maintained at 41°C to 42°C for several hours with variable morbidity and occasional mortality. Most systems for WBH require general anesthesia with endotracheal intubation as well as complex equipment to regulate patient temperature. The system most used to date worldwide has been extracorporeal or direct blood warming. This requires the surgical placement of vascular shunts. It has been feasible to use extracorporeal heating in combination with both radiation and chemotherapy. A hot-water suit system, developed at the National Cancer Institute, has also undergone extensive clinical trials. This system has been recently modified; it currently includes general anesthesia with mechanical ventilation.

Despite its potential utility, the use of systemic hyperthermia has not been widely applied as a treatment modality, either alone or in conjunction with other therapies. This is due to the following concerns: the need for endotracheal intubation and mechanical ventilation, the high morbidity experienced with some systems, the cost, the labor-intensive aspects, and the inability to deliver multiple treatment sessions per week to a given patient. To overcome these concerns, a team at the University of Wisconsin Clinical Cancer Center (UWCCC) has pioneered the use of a radiant heat system for WBH. This system does not require general anesthesia with endotracheal intubation; it allows for multiple treatments per week; it is cost-effective; and it lends itself to a multimodality approach. Following a phase I clinical trial with WBH alone, several second-generation studies at the UWCCC have been reported. These have included WBH and interferon, WBH and local radiotherapy for non–small-cell lung cancer, WBH and Lonidamine, WBH and carboplatin, WBH and low-dose total-body irradiation for favorable B-cell neoplasms, and WBH in the setting of allogeneic bone marrow transplantation. As of 1990, over 650 treatments have been performed by this group without significant clinical toxicity.

Responses to WBH alone have been described in a variety of tumor types. As mentioned earlier, lymphomas and leukemias may represent a category of disease with unusually high thermal sensitivities. Additionally, hepatic involvement with neoplastic disease seems to respond to hyperthermia in higher proportions than tumors (primary or metastatic) located in other anatomic areas. Initially, it was believed that this predisposition to hyperthermia induced responses related to superheating of the liver. However, recent canine experiments done at multiple institutions suggest that elevated hepatic temperatures (in comparison to core body temperature) do not account for this phenomenon. Thus, the response of hepatic metastases to WBH may relate, in part, to the interactions of hyperthermia and a unique metabolic milieu found in the liver. Clearly, this is one of many aspects of hyperthermia research that deserves further investigation.

Although the upper temperature limit for WBH appears to be 42°C, preclinical studies have shown that a synergistic interaction with radiation or chemotherapy clearly occurs at lower temperatures as well. In this regard, remarkable regressions of advanced malignancies have been described for extracorporeal heating when combined with radiation or chemotherapy. Similarly, in nonrandomized clinical trials at the University of Texas, a water-suit system has induced good tumor responses in combination with different chemotherapeutic regimens.

The first randomized study involving 40.5°C WBH has been conducted in Germany. Patients with small-cell lung cancer were randomized between chemotherapy versus chemotherapy plus WBH. Results from this study favored the WBH arm; however, a clear benefit for the future use of WBH in this setting can not be concluded. The chemotherapy doses, which were chosen for this protocol many years ago, are significantly lower than those that have now been shown to be optimal for small-cell lung cancer; hence, the response and survival data of the chemotherapy/WBH arm of this study do not compare well with modern small-cell lung cancer treatment regimens. It is of interest that WBH technology used in this study (i.e., a Siemen's box, which is a combination of hot air and diathermy heating) only allows for relatively modest elevations of core temperatures (approximately 40.0°C) in comparison to other WBH technologies (approximately 41.8°C). Despite the methodologic problems inherent in this study, the results obtained, taken collectively with studies at other centers, encourage continued research directed at the use of WBH as an adjunct to other forms of cancer therapy.

FUTURE PROSPECTS

It is inevitable that technologic advances will further improve the potential for hyperthermia in cancer treatment. Similarly, pharmacologic investigation of active antineoplastic drugs with the ability to synergize with both hyperthermia and radiation will increase the potential of new multimodality approaches with curative intent. Other classes of drugs, such as labilizers, may prove to be similarly useful. For traditional chemotherapeutic agents, key questions remain relating to their proper sequencing with hyperthermia, as well as optimal temperature and hyperthermia treatment duration. Research regarding alterations in pharmacokinetics and drug mode of action during hyperthermia could be translated into increased therapeutic gain clinically.

Although the use of WBH in a multimodality approach may prove therapeutic in a metastatic setting, it may be of greatest importance as an adjuvant therapy (i.e., sterilizing micrometastases in patients with a high risk of recurrence after primary surgical treatment for Duke's C colorectal cancer, stage II mammary carcinomas, and stage I and II malignant melanomas).

The clinical problem of curing stage II breast cancer (i.e., axillary node involvement) provides an interesting example of this possibility. Adjuvant chemotherapy in this disease therapeutically provides a delay in recurrence as well as an increase in patient survival. In spite of this, one-third of treated patients will relapse within 5 years with a significant manifestation of systemic disease. Although relapse after adjuvant chemotherapy suggests drug resistance, surprisingly this is not the case. Patients who have received adjuvant chemotherapy and subsequently develop metastatic disease will respond to the same drugs given in the adjuvant setting. One explanation for these results (i.e., kinetic resistance) may be inadequate microvasculature, thereby leading to a failure of drug penetration at the time when tumor burden is minimal and multidrug therapy should have its major impact. It is argued that hyperthermia, specifically

WBH, may be of value in this setting by increasing drug sensitivity (i.e., overcoming kinetic resistance as opposed to biochemical resistance), e.g., by increasing membrane permeability or by altering cellular metabolism. This theoretical proposal, that WBH and chemotherapy in the adjuvant setting may be most efficacious against microscopic disease, can be tested in both transplantable and spontaneous animal models. From the standpoint of clinical feasibility, the concept of delivering WBH with adjuvant chemotherapy could be translated into wide-scale, randomized, multi-institution clinical trials with the whole-body hyperthermia radiant heat system described previously. (Patients treated with this system who have no underlying problems require only 12 hours of hospitalization after hyperthermia.)

SUGGESTED READING

Angheleri LV, Robert J, eds. Hyperthermia in cancer treatment. Vol 3. Boca Raton, FL: CRC Press, 1986.

Engelhardt R. Hyperthermia and drugs. In: Streffer C, ed. Recent results in cancer research and drugs. Vol 104. Berlin: Springer-Verlag, 1987:136–203.

Hahn GM. Hyperthermia and cancer. New York: Plenum Press, 1982.

Lowenthal JP, ed. Conference on hyperthermia in cancer treatment. 1984; 44:47,035–49,085.

Steeves RA, ed. Hyperthermia. Radiol Clin North Am 1989; 27:3.

Sugahara T, Saito M, eds. Hyperthermic oncology. Vols 1 and 2. Taylor and Francis: London, 1988.

Valdagni R, ed. Proceedings of the International Consensus Meeting on Hyperthermia, Trento, Italy. Int J Hyperthermia 1990; 6:839–877.

INFECTIOUS COMPLICATIONS IN PATIENTS WITH CANCER

JAY J. REDINGTON, M.D.
DENNIS G. MAKI, M.D.

Infection shadows the patient with cancer. Whereas the outcome of the patient with cancer is ultimately determined by the primary malignancy, infection proves to be the final cause of death or a major factor in the fatal outcome in over two-thirds of patients dying with acute leukemia and in one-half of patients with lymphoma. Over the past two decades major advances have been made in our understanding of patterns of infection with various types of cancer and how to diagnose these infections quickly and accurately. Moreover, potent anti-infective drugs are now available to treat every type of bacterial infection, most fungal infections, and an increasing number of viral infections, especially those caused by the herpesviruses—herpes simplex virus (HSV), Varicella-Zoster virus (VZV), Epstein-Barr virus (EBV), and cytomegalovirus (CMV). And most importantly, the epidemiology of many infections in patients with cancer has been sufficiently delineated that preventative measures, designed to block infection by micro-organisms from the hospital environment as well as endogenous infections from the patient's flora, have been shown to be effective for preventing many life-threatening infections.

INITIAL EVALUATION

Because of the increasing effectiveness of treatment for many forms of cancer and the aggressiveness of therapeutic regimens currently used, a physician caring for patients with cancer can expect to encounter a wide range of infecting pathogens and manifestations of infection. In order to recognize and diagnose life-threatening infections as early as possible and provide the most effective therapy, the physician must keep several cardinal principles of management of infection in patients with cancer in mind:

Prevention. It must be re-emphasized that many infections in patients with cancer are now preventable and that successful prevention will invariably be more successful than the most effective treatment.

Low Index of Suspicion. It is extremely important to be very aware of the possibility of infection in the patient with cancer, who may present only with fever or nonspecific symptoms such as malaise or myalgias. Many patients with cancer, particularly those receiving high-dosage corticosteroids or who are profoundly granulocytopenic, do not exhibit the characteristic findings of local infection on careful examination.

Patterns of Infection. The spectrum of infectious complications encountered in the patient with cancer is heavily influenced by alterations in the patient's immunity, produced by the cancer or its treatment, and the state of the patient's disease, i.e., whether early, prior to intensive anticancer therapy and prolonged exposure to anti-infective drugs, or late, when antineoplastic therapy and heavy exposure to antibiotics can themselves cause syndromes that may mimic infection. The prevalent infecting pathogens encountered in most patients with cancer are characteristically associated with predictable immune defects (Table 1).

Multiple myeloma and chronic lymphocytic leukemia predictably result in hypogammaglobulinemia. Splenectomy, done for staging of lymphoma, greatly increases the risk of overwhelming infections with encapsulated bacteria, particularly *Streptococcus pneumoniae* and *Haemophilus influenzae* Type b. Lymphoreticular malignancies are associated with defects with cell-mediated immunity (CMI) and vulnerability to myco-

bacteria, fungi, viruses, and parasites. Patients with solid tumors are vulnerable to serious infections associated with tumorous obstruction of vital organs; e.g., cholangitis with pancreaticobiliary malignancy, urosepsis with obstructive pelvic cancer, or pneumonia or lung abscess associated with obstructing bronchopulmonary malignancies. Granulocytopenia, especially when profound (absolute granulocyte count <100 per mm^3) and prolonged, is associated with a greatly increased risk of bacterial infections caused by staphylococci and gram-negative bacilli and deep fungal infections caused by

Table 1 Infections in Cancer Associated with Altered Host Immunity

Host Defect	Pathogens Encountered at Sites of Infection			
	Bloodstream or Disseminated	Pulmonary	Central Nervous System	Gastrointestinal
Hypogammaglobulinemia	*Streptococcus pneumoniae* *Haemophilus influenzae* *Neisseria meningitidis*	*S. pneumoniae* *H. influenzae* *B. catarrhalis*	*S. pneumoniae* *H. influenzae* Type b Enteroviruses	*Giardia lamblia*
Splenectomy	as above, plus *Malaria, Babesia* spp. *Bartonella*	*S. pneumoniae* *H. influenzae* *B. catarrhalis*	*S. pneumoniae* *H. influenzae* Type b	
Cell-mediated immunity	*Listeria monocytogenes* *Salmonella* Varicella-zoster virus Herpes simplex virus *Coccidioides immitis* *Histoplasma capsulatum*	*Pneumocystis carinii* *Mycobacteria* *Legionella* *Nocardia*	*Cryptococcus neoformans* *Listeria* *Toxoplasma gondii*	*Salmonella* *Campylobacter* *Candida* Herpes simplex virus *Cryptosporidium* *Entamoeba histolytica* *Strongyloides stercoralis*
Tumorous obstruction	Cholangitis Gram-negative bacilli *Enterococcus* *Clostridia* Urosepsis Gram-negative bacilli *Enterococcus* Pneumonia *S. pneumoniae* *S. aureus* Oral anaerobes	*S. pneumoniae* *S. aureus* Oral anaerobes		Gram-negative bacilli *Enterococci* *Clostridium* spp. *Bacteroides fragilis*
Granulocytopenia	Gram-negative bacilli (especially *Pseudomonas aeruginosa*) Staphylococci *Candida* spp. *Aspergillus* spp.	Gram-negative bacilli Staphylococci *Aspergillus* spp.		*Candida* Herpes simplex virus *Clostridium difficile* Other clostridia
Latent infections	Malaria *Coccidiodes immitis* *Histoplasma capsulatum*	*Mycobacterium tuberculosis*	*Toxoplasma gondii* *M. tuberculosis* *C. immitis* *H. capsulatum*	*Strongyloides stercoralis*
Central venous catheter	*Staphylococcus epidermidis* *Staphylococcus aureus* Corynebacterium spp. (JK) *Bacillus* spp. *Candida* spp. *Trichophyton* spp. *Fusarium* spp. *Mycobacterium* spp.			

Candida and *Aspergillus* species. Latent infections, with *Mycobacterium tuberculosis, Coccidioides immitis,* or *Toxoplasma gondii,* may be reactivated with the occurrence of the acquired immunodeficiency syndrome (AIDS) or cancer, or during cancer chemotherapy. Percutaneous central venous catheters and subcutaneous central venous ports are used widely in cancer patients and are associated with bloodstream infection caused by a broad array of skin organisms.

These pathoimmunobiologic relationships are very useful and should be kept in mind when evaluating an immunocompromised cancer patient with fever or other signs that suggest infection.

Noninfectious Syndromes Mimicking Infection. It is important to be informed of the side-effects of the treatments used, particularly radiation therapy, which produces pneumonitis and enteritis, which can mimic infection; and cytotoxic drugs, which can produce drug-related pneumonitis, stomatitis, enteritis, or systemic erythroderma.

Diagnosis. *The importance of making every effort to diagnose suspected infection cannot be overstated.* Failure to obtain appropriate cultures before initiating empiric therapy of suspected infection may severely impair efforts to prove that infection was originally present in a patient responding poorly to empiric antimicrobial therapy and may prove deleterious over the long run: the true diagnosis may be masked and delayed because of empiric antimicrobial therapy; life-threatening nonbacterial processes such as fungal infection might not be recognized sufficiently early to institute needed therapy, or the patient may be subjected to unnecessarily broad-spectrum antimicrobial therapy, which increases the risk of superinfection or other complications of antimicrobial therapy, such as interactions between antimicrobial drugs and cancer chemotherapeutic agents or the development of *Clostridium difficile* antibiotic-associated colitis.

It is rarely justifiable to start anti-infective drugs for suspected or presumed infection in a patient with cancer without obtaining appropriate cultures, which in the critically ill patient must always include blood cultures, ideally drawn from separate sites by percutaneous venipuncture. Patients with cancer, particularly patients with profound granulocytopenia with bacterial pneumonia, peritonitis, or organ infections associated with obstruction (cholangitis or pyohydronephrosis) are highly vulnerable to bacteremia, as are all patients with surgically implanted central venous devices. Studies have shown that there is little additional benefit to obtaining more than two 10-mL blood cultures. The availability of the Isolator blood culture system (DuPont Chemical), which provides a quantitative culture on solid media, offers improved sensitivity for diagnosis of fungemia and also allows identification of central venous catheter–related infection without removing the catheter. With infected central venous catheters, the number of organisms per milliliter of blood cultured is usually 10-fold or more higher in blood drawn through the infected catheter than in blood cultures drawn percutaneously from a peripheral vein.

Confusion or headache associated with fever or other neurologic signs should raise suspicion of meningitis, which cannot be diagnosed without examination of the cerebrospinal fluid (CSF). It is beyond the scope of this review to discuss further the diagnosis of infection in the patient with cancer, but it must be strongly re-emphasized that every effort should be made to establish the diagnosis of infection by appropriate cultures and other laboratory tests at the outset.

Adjustment of Antimicrobial Therapy. The decision to initiate antimicrobial therapy is based on the clinical examination of the patient or laboratory studies available at the outset. In many instances, the physical examination and initial laboratory studies, such as roentgenograms or microscopic examinations of sputum and urine, will not identify a clearcut site of infection because the patient is ill or highly susceptible, and empiric antimicrobial therapy is begun, appropriately, on the presumption that the patient has primary bacteremia. When empiric antimicrobial therapy has been initiated, the need for continued therapy must be continuously reassessed, particularly if cultures and other diagnostic study results are negative and the patient has not shown significant change. On the other hand, if an infecting pathogen has been identified, the antimicrobial regimen should be adjusted specifically for the infecting pathogen or pathogens, permitting more focused and less broad-spectrum therapy, which not only improves the likelihood of therapeutic success but also reduces the risk of superinfection and antibiotic-associated colitis.

Continuous Reassessment of the Patient. The course of the patient with cancer is continuously evolving and changing. It is essential to reassess the patient's condition continuously, even when infection has been identified and is under therapy. Patients with cancer are commonly infected by multiple pathogens, and even if they are only infected by a single organism at the outset, are more vulnerable than patients without cancer to superinfection by resistant bacteria or fungi. *During treatment of infection in the patient with cancer, the daily assessment must include efforts to confirm response of the infection and to identify side-effects due to its treatment, particularly superinfection and drug toxicity.*

SELECTION OF ANTI-INFECTIVE THERAPY

General Considerations

Beta-lactams

It has become increasingly clear that when beta-lactam antibiotics with a short half-life (1 to 2 hours) are used to treat proven gram-negative infections, particularly in granulocytopenic patients, the drugs should be administered frequently to maintain therapeutic drug levels that exceed the infecting organism's minimum inhibitory concentration (MIC) for as much of the dosing interval as possible. Drugs such as penicillin; ampicillin; or the antipseudomonal penicillins, ticarcillin (Ticar) and ticarcillin-clavulinate (Timentin), mezlocillin (Mezlin), piperacillin (Piperacil), and azlocillin (Azlin), should be administered no less frequently than every 4 hours for proved gram-negative infections. For beta-lactam antibiotics with longer half-lives, such as cefaperazone (Cefobid) or ceftriaxone (Rocephin), or ceftazadime (Fortaz, Tazicef, Tazidime), the dosing interval can be extended without compromising therapeutic goals. Recommended dosing intervals for patients with normal renal and hepatic function are provided in Table 2.

A number of novel beta-lactam and related antibiotics have become available over the past 5 years, most notably, the combination of a beta-lactam with a beta-lactamase inhibitor, i.e., ampicillin-sulbactam (Unasyn) and ticarcillin-clavulinic acid; the very potent and broad-spectrum carbipenem, imipenem-cilastin (Primaxin); and the monobactam, aztreonam (Azactam). Aztreonam is a novel beta-lactam–like drug that has no gram-positive activity but excellent activity against most aerobic gram-negative bacilli, including *Pseudomonas aeruginosa,* and also has the unique feature that it can be used safely in patients who have had anaphylactic allergic reactions with penicillin. All of these drugs have an important role to play in the management of infections in patients with cancer, and recommended dosing schedules and indications for their use are provided in Tables 2 and 3.

Aminoglycosides

Aminoglycoside antibiotics are still important in the management of serious gram-negative infections in patients with cancer, particularly those with granulocytopenia. Studies suggest that with gram-negative bacteremia and other serious gram-negative infections in patients with profound granulocytopenia (< 100 per mm^3), the use of two drugs that show in vitro synergy, such as a beta-lactam and an aminoglycoside, substantially improves the therapeutic outcome. Thus, with profound granulocytopenia and *proved* gram-negative bacillary infections, it is strongly recommended that *two* antibiotics be used, combining a potent beta-lactam with an aminoglycoside. For patients who are not granulocytopenic, it is much less clear whether two drugs need to be used, or especially, whether synergism translates to an improved therapeutic outcome.

In terms of selecting an aminoglycoside for use for empiric therapy for treating a proved gram-negative infection in granulocytopenic patients, there are no data showing clearcut therapeutic superiority of one aminoglycoside over another (assuming all are effective in vitro) when the aminoglycoside is combined with a beta-lactam in the initial empiric regimen. However, with *Pseudomonas aeruginosa* infections, tobramycin is superior to gentamicin and should be the agent of choice. With gentamicin- or tobramycin-resistant organisms, amikacin is often effective in vitro and would be the agent of choice; however, there are no data to indicate that amikacin is superior therapeutically to gentamicin or tobramycin for infections with organisms susceptible to all of these drugs. Comparing gentamicin and tobramycin, other than for *P. aeruginosa,* gentamicin is generally more effective than tobramycin in vitro against the broad range of aerobic gram-negative bacilli.

Recent studies have shown that the outcome of treatment of serious gram-negative rod infections with aminoglycosides is most heavily influenced by the peak blood level at the outset of therapy: patients with a subtherapeutic level of gentamicin or tobramycin (< 5 μg per mL) are much more likely to show therapeutic failure than patients with a therapeutic peak level (> 5 μg per mL) immediately following the first dose. Recent studies in Europe have shown that the total daily dose of an aminoglycoside such as gentamicin (5 mg per kg) can be given once daily, with therapeutic results comparable to dosing every 8 hours as is the practice in patients with normal renal function in the United States. It is thus recommended that in patients with normal renal function, gentamicin or tobramycin be administered every 12 hours, giving doses of 2.5 mg per kg (for a 70 kg patient, approximately 180 mg). This approach to dosing is not associated with an increased risk of ototoxicity or nephrotoxicity, but assures therapeutic blood levels at the outset of therapy (10 to 15 μg per mL), when it is most critical. If twice-daily dosing is not used when treating serious infections, it is important that aminoglycoside blood levels be measured at the outset of therapy (e.g., after the first dose) to confirm that the peak blood level exceeds 5 μg per mL.

Vancomycin

Vancomycin has come into wide use with the enormous increase in infections caused by staphylococci that are resistant to methicillin. Vancomycin exhibits in vitro activity against nearly all gram-positive cocci,* including methicillin-resistant strains of *Staphylococcus aureus* and coagulase-negative staphylococci as well as enterococci. It is the drug of choice for treating serious staphylococcal and streptococcal infections in patients with penicillin hypersensitivity.

The major side-effect of vancomycin is the "red man" syndrome, diffuse erythroderma and hypotension, commonly associated with urticaria and bronchospasm, deriving from nonallergenic release of histamine from peripheral leukocytes. This syndrome occurs in as many as 15 percent of patients given intravenous vancomycin. The risk of the red man syndrome and vancomycin-related hypotension is affected by the rate of administration, and can be greatly reduced by administration of the drug in a solution containing not more than 5 μg per mL over an interval not less than 1 hour. With patients who have had the syndrome, pretreatment with an H$_1$-histamine receptor antagonist, such as diphenhydramine, appears to be highly effective at preventing vancomycin-related hypotension and the red man syndrome. If hypotension occurs during administration of vancomycin, stopping the infusion and giving supplemental intravenous fluids and, if necessary, dopamine, quickly reverses the hypotension; the patient also should

---

*Exceptions: Leuconostoc, occasional strains of *Enterococcus, Lactobacillus,* and *Pediacoccus.*

Table 2 Dosing of Common Parenteral Anti-Infective Drugs for Treatment of Infection in Patients With Cancer

Drug	Total Daily Dose	For 70 Kg Adult*	Side Effects (frequency)
Penicillin	200,000–300,000 U/Kg	2–3 Million Q 4 Hr	Rashes (1–5%), anaphylaxis, hypersensitivity nephritis (<1%)
Ampicillin	100–200 mg/Kg	1–2 Grams Q 4–6 Hr	Same plus diarrhea *Clostridium difficile* colitis, superinfection
Ampicillin-sulbactam†	170 mg/Kg	1.5–3 Grams Q 6 Hr	Similar to ampicillin
Nafcillin or oxacillin	100–200 mg/Kg	1–2 Grams Q 4 Hr	Rash, granulocytopenia (nafcillin), hepatitis (oxacillin)
Antipseudomonal penicillins			Rash, diarrhea/colitis, superinfection
Ticarcillin, mezlocillin, piperacillin, azlocillin	250 mg/Kg	3 Grams Q 4–6 Hr	
Ticarcillin-clavulinate‡	250 mg/Kg	3.1 Grams Q 4–6 Hr	
Cefuroxime	30–50 mg/Kg	750–1500 mg Q 8 Hr	Similar to ampicillin
Cefotaxime, ceftizoxime	100 mg/Kg	2 Grams Q 6–8 Hr	Rash, diarrhea/colitis, coagulopathy, superinfection (*Candida*, coagulase-negative staphylococcus, enteroccus)
Ceftriaxone	30–50 mg/Kg	1–2 Grams Q 12–24 Hr	Similar to other third-generation cephalosporins
Antipseudomonal cephalosporins			
Cefoperazone, ceftazadime	50–100 mg/Kg	2 Grams Q 8 Hr	Similar to other third-generation cephalosporins
Imipenem-cilastatin	30–50 mg/Kg	0.5–1.0 Grams Q 6 hr	Like third-generation cephalosporins plus seizures (increased risk in renal insufficiency)
Aztreonam	50–100 mg/Kg	1–2 Grams Q 8 Hr	Superinfection, rash (however, *no* cross-sensitivity in the patient with penicillin allergy)
Vancomycin	30–50 mg/Kg	1 Gram Q 12 Hr	"Red man syndrome," hypotension (common), nephrotoxicity or ototoxicity (rare)
Clindamycin	20–30 mg/Kg	600–900 mg Q 8 Hr	Rash, diarrhea/colitis
Metronidazole	30 mg/Kg	750 mg Q 8 Hr	Rash, nausea, antabuse-like reaction, neutropenia, neuropathy (rare); potentiates warfarin activity
Gentamicin, tobramycin	5–6 mg/Kg	180 mg Q 12 Hr	Ototoxicity, nephrotoxicity (3–5%), neuromuscular blockade (rare)
Amikacin	15 mg/Kg	500 mg Q 12 Hr	Similar to other aminoglycosides
Trimethoprim-sulfamethoxazole	10–20 mg/Kg (TMP component)	2–5 Ampules Q 6 Hr (ampule: 80 mg/400 mg)	Rash (common), Stevens-Johnson syndrome (rare), myelosuppression (primarily in AIDS)
Ciprofloxin		500–750 mg Q 12 Hr (oral dose)	Rash, superinfection by gram-positive cocci
		400 mg Q 12 Hr (IV dose)	Neuropsychiatric (<1%) SHOULD NOT BE USED IN CHILDREN
Antifungal drugs			
Amphotericin B	See Table 6	See Table 6	Fever, chills, phlebitis (frequent) Azotemia, renal tubular acidosis/hypokalemia (universal)
Flucytosine	See Table 6	See Table 6	Rash, diarrhea, myelosuppression (common)
Miconazole	See Table 6	See Table 6	Rash, hepatitis (rare); cardiotoxicity with bolus administration (rare)
Fluconazole	See Table 6	See Table 6	Rash
Antiviral drugs			
Acyclovir	See Table 7	See Table 7	Rash, mental status changes, myelosuppression, azotemia (rare)
Ganciclovir	See Table 7	See Table 7	Myelosuppression (common)
Anti-pneumoncystis drugs			
Pentamadine	4 mg/Kg	300 mg/d	Rash, azotemia, hypoglycemia; cardiotoxicity with bolus administration

*Assuming normal renal and hepatic function. Whereas the leading dose is unchanged, subsequent doses or during intervals must be modified appropriately in patients with renal insufficiency or hepatic failure.

†Combination of ampicillin and betalactamase inhibitor, sulbactam, in a ratio of 2:1.

‡3.1 g of ticarcillin-clavulinate contains 3 g of ticarcillin and 0.1 g of the beta-lactamase inhibitor, clavulinate.

Table 3 Initial Anti-Infective Therapy for Major Infectious Syndromes in Patients with Cancer

Syndrome	Pathogens	Suggested Initial Regimens
Fever without identified local infection Not granulocytopenic	Staphylococcus aureus Streptococcus pneumoniae Enteric gram-negative bacilli	Ampicillin-sulbactam and aminoglycoside Third-generation cephalosporin* Imipenem-cilastatin Aztreonam and vancomycin†
Granulocytopenic (<500 mg per mm³)	S. aureus Gram-negative bacilli, including Pseudomonas aeruginosa	Anti-pseudomonal beta-lactam and tobramycin Ceftazadime, cefoperazone, or imipenem-cilastatin alone‡ Aztreonam, vancomycin and tobramycin†
Suspected bacterial pneumonia, etiology unknown	S. aureus S. pneumoniae Oral anaerobes Enteric gram-negative bacilli P. aeruginosa Legionella spp.	Ticarcillin-clavulinic acid, tobramycin and erythromycin Imipenem-cilastatin, tobramycin and erythromycin Aztreonam and erythromcyin[2]
Sinusitis	S. pneumoniae Haemophilus influenzae S. aureus Gram-negative bacilli	Amoxicillin-clavulinate Ampicillin-sulbactam Ticarcillin-clavulinate Trimethoprim-sulfamethoxazole†
Suspected bacterial meningitis	S. pneumoniae H. influenzae type b Neisseria meningitidis Listeria monocytogenes	Third-generation cephalosporin* and ampicillin Third-generation cephalosporin* and trimethoprim sulfamethoxazole† Chloramphenicol and trimethoprim-sulfamethoxazole†
Granulocytopenia	Enteric gram-negative bacilli P. aeruginosa	Ceftazadime, tobramycin, and ampicillin Imipenem-cilastatin and ampicillin Chloramphenicol and tobramycin (IV and intrathecal)†
Intra-abdominal Cholangitis	Enteric gram-negative bacilli Enterococci Clostridium	Ampicillin-sulbactam and gentamicin Third-generation cephalosporin and ampicillin Imipenem-cilastatin and ampicillin Aztreonam and vancomycin†
Primary peritonitis	Gram-negative bacilli S. pneumoniae	As above
Secondary peritonitis, intra-abdominal abscess, pelvic sepsis	As above plus B. fragilis, other anaerobes	Clindamycin, gentamicin and ampicillin (vancomycin†) Metronidazole, gentamicin and ampicillin (vancomycin†) Ampicillin-sulbactam and gentamicin Imipenem-cilastatin and ampicillin
Urosepsis	Enteric gram-negative bacilli P. aeruginosa Enterococcus	Gentamicin or tobramycin and ampicillin (vancomycin†) Third-generation cephalosporin and ampicillin (vancomycin†) Aztreonam and vancomycin†
Skin and soft tissue Uncomplicated, without granulocytopenia	S. aureus Beta-hemolytic streptococci [H. influenzae Type b] (children)	Nafcillin Vancomycin† [Third-generation cephalosporin or trimethoprim-sulfamethoxazole†]
Granulocytopenic	S. aureus Gram-negative bacilli, including P. aeruginosa	Ticarcillin-clavulinate and tobramycin Ceftazadime and tobramycin Other antipseudomonal penicillins, nafcillin and tobramycin
Necrotizing fascitis	Gram-negative bacilli Clostidia and B. fragilis Staphylococci and Streptococci Vibrio vulnificans	Same as secondary peritonitis Doxycycline or trimethoprim-sulfamethoxazole
Enteric infection Bacterial pathogens	Salmonella Shigella Campylobacter Enteropathogenic E. coli	Norfloxacin or ciprofloxacin orally† Trimethoprim-sulfamethoxazole† Ceftriaxone or cefoperazone
Antibiotic-associated colitis	Clostridium difficile	Vancomycin orally (severe infection) Metronidazole orally (mild or moderately severe infection)

*Cefotaxime, ceftizoxime, ceftriaxone, cefoperazone, or ceftazadime.
†For the patient with major penicillin hypersensitivity.
‡See text for those settings in which monotherapy can be considered safe as an initial empiric regimen in the granulocytopenic patient with fever.

be given intravenous diphenhydramine. Vancomycin can be safely resumed following the occurrence of red man syndrome if the patient is treated with an antihistamine prior to subsequent doses and the concentration of infused drug and rate of administration are carefully controlled.

Quinolones

Ciprofloxacin is a recently released quinolone antibiotic that exhibits excellent activity against most gram-negative bacilli, including *Pseudomonas aeruginosa*. Although the drug is effective in vitro against many gram-positive cocci, there have been increasing reports of therapeutic failure when the drug was used as a sole agent for gram-positive infections and for gram-positive superinfections during ciprofloxacin therapy. In general, ciprofloxacin should not be considered a first-line agent for treating gram-positive infections. In compromised patients with cancer, oral ciprofloxacin should be reserved for treatment of gram-negative infections of the urinary tract or enteric infections.

Dosing

It is extremely important that the drugs used to treat bacterial infections in patients with cancer be dosed appropriately, especially the aminoglycosides and antipseudomonal penicillins, ticarcillin, mezlocillin, azlocillin, and piperacillin; in patients with normal renal function, antipseudomonal penicillins should be given in a total daily dose not less than 250 mg per kg to assure therapeutic efficacy when treating gram-negative infections.

Antifungal Drugs

Amphotericin B (Fungizone), which is given intravenously, is the most important drug for treatment of life-threatening fungal infections in the patient with cancer. Relatively few fungi exhibit primary resistance to amphotericin (e.g., *Pseudoallescheria boydii*), and with few exceptions, for most deep fungal infections in patients with cancer, amphotericin B is still the drug of choice. The doses of amphotericin necessary for treating various types of fungal infection vary widely (Table 4).

In general, many physicians are reluctant to use amphotericin B because of its formidable toxicity. The side-effects of amphotericin B—hyperpyrexic reactions, rigors, nephrotoxicity, and electrolyte imbalance syndromes—can be greatly reduced by a protocol approach to its use, the most essential features of which are measures to avert dehydration and to counter the renal tubular acidosis with hypokalemia that invariably occurs (see Table 2). Vigorous hydration and salt loading and early treatment of drug-induced renal tubular acidosis can significantly reduce nephrotoxicity. Moreover, administration of diphenhydramine, 50 mg intravenously, and acetaminophen, 10 grains orally or by rectal suppository, prior to each dose of amphotericin will reduce hyperpyrexic reactions; for patients who continue to experience rigors despite pretreatment, meperidine, 50 mg by intravenous bolus, immediately prior to beginning the infusion, is usually effective. If pretreatment with acetaminophen and diphenhydramine fails to prevent severe febrile reactions, administration of hydrocortisone, 35 to 50 mg given as a bolus immediately prior to beginning the infusion, is highly effective; hydrocortisone should not be added to the bottle or bag. There is no evidence whatsoever that addition of heparin or mannitol to the container of amphotericin is of any value for ameliorating side-effects.

Flucytosine (Ancoban) is a valuable antifungal agent for the treatment of cryptococcal and *Candida* infections, but is only available in an oral form. The drug should be used with great caution, if at all, in patients with renal insufficiency; life-threatening myelosuppression has resulted from the use of flucytosine in patients with renal impairment. In general, when flucytosine is used for treating deep fungal infections in critically ill cancer patients, blood levels should be monitored, especially if the patient has azotemia, striving for serum levels of 50 to 100 μg per mL.

Three imidazoles are available for treatment of systemic fungal infections, ketoconazole (Nizoral), which is only available orally; miconazole (Monistat), which is only available parenterally; and the new triazole, fluconazole (Diflucan), which is available in both an oral and a parenteral form. The superior activity of fluconazole against most fungi and its availability in both an oral and a parenteral form will probably result in its rapidly superseding the other imidiazoles for treatment of fungal infections in cancer patients. Fluconazole is highly active against most *Candida* species and many filamentous fungi, mainly the soil fungi, *Histoplasma capsulatum, Blastomyces dermatitidis,* and *Coccidioides immidis;* it is not reliably active against *Aspergillus* or *Zygomycetes.* The drug has been used successfully for treating all types of *Candida* infections, although published data on deep-seated infections is still limited. In general, until such information becomes available, intravenous amphotericin B should be regarded as the drug of choice for deep-seated *Candida* infections in patients with cancer.

Fluconazole, however, provides an important option for treating deep fungal infections in patients who are unable to tolerate amphotericin B, such as many patients with AIDS. The drug has been quite effective for treating cryptococcal meningitis in patients with AIDS. Studies have shown that fluconazole also is effective prophylactically in granulocytopenic patients with cancer for prevention of *Candida* infections. Fluconazole should not be used for treating infections caused by *Aspergillus* or *Zygomycetes.*

Antiviral Drugs

A number of effective antiviral drugs are available for treatment of the patient with cancer, most importantly acyclovir (Zovirax), which is active against HSV, VZV, and, in high doses, CMV; ganciclovir (Cytovene), for CMV and possibly EBV; ribavarin (Viramid, Vira-

Table 4 Recommended Therapy for Fungal Infections in Patients with Cancer

Agent	Syndrome	First Choice Regimen*	Alternate Choices/ Comment
Candida spp.	Oropharyngeal ("thrush")	Clotrimazole 10 mg troches, 5 times daily	Ketoconazole 200 mg/d PO
	Esophagitis	Ketoconazole 100-200 mg/d PO	Fluconazole 100-200 mg/d PO or IV
	Endophthalmitis	Amphotericin B intravitreal and IV amphotericin B IV 0.5 mg/kg/d, total dose 10-20 mg/kg *plus* flucytosine or fluconazole	Fluconazole 200-400 mg/d PO or IV
	Cystitis	Amphotericin B bladder irrigation (15 mg/L) through catheter for 3-5 days	Fluconazole 100-200 mg PO or IV Flucytosine 100 mg/ kg/d PO Amphotericin B IV 0.4 mg/kg/d, total dose 3-5 mg/kg
	Transient IV line-related candidemia	Amphotericin B IV 0.4-0.7 mg/kg/d, total dose: 3-5 mg/kg	Septic thrombosis of central great vein requires total dose > 20 mg/kg
	Deep infection	Amphotericin B IV 0.5-0.7 mg/kg/d, total dose: 5-20 mg/kg	Addition of flucytosine 100 mg/kg/d
Cryptococcus neoformans	Meningitis	Amphotericin B IV 0.5-0.7 mg/kg/d *and* flucytosine 100-150 mg/kg/d for 6-8 weeks	Fluconazole 400 mg/d PO or IV Intrathecal amphotericin B may be required for refractory infections
Geographic fungi†	Pulmonary or disseminated, without meningitis	Amphotericin B 0.5-0.7 mg/ kg/d total dose: 1.5-2 g	
Coccidioides immitis	Meningitis	Amphotericin B IV 0.7-1.0 mg/kg/d total dose ≥ 2 g	Intrathecal therapy also needed in most cases
Aspergillus, Zygomycetes,	Pulmonary or disseminated	Amphotericin B IV 0.7-1.5 mg/kg/d total dose ≥ 2 g	Surgical extirpation or débridement of isolated foci infection (e.g., sinusitis, pulmonary, brain) Many authorities add flucytosine and rifampin to IV amphotericin for *aspergillus* or zygomycetes infections
Trichophyton, Fusarium spp.	Pulmonary or disseminated	Amphotericin B IV 0.7-1.0 mg/kg/d total dose ≥ 2 g	
Pseudoallescheria boydii	Pulmonary or disseminated	Miconazole 200-4000 mg IV Q 8 Hr for 2-4 weeks	Triazoles may be effective but little published data to guide their use

*Doses for adults with normal renal and hepatic function. Whereas the leading dose is unchanged, subsequent doses or during intervals must be modified appropriately in patients with renal insufficiency or hepatic failure.

†*Coccidioides immitis, Histoplasma capsulatum, Blastomyces dermatitidis.*

zole), for respiratory syncytial virus; and amantadine (Symmetrel), for influenza A. Recommended dosing schedules for these drugs are provided in Table 5. It is important that these schedules be followed closely, especially when HSV-caused central nervous system infections and VZV infections are treated with acyclovir, to assure maximal benefit. Whereas acyclovir has been associated with minimal toxicity, ganciclovir, which is now available for treating CMV infections, produces myelosuppression and occasionally, hepatotoxicity;

monitoring for toxicity is extremely important, especially in patients receiving other potentially myelotoxic drugs.

Amantadine is effective prophylactically for prevention of influenza A in the setting of an epidemic. When given within the first 24 to 48 hours after the onset of presumed acute influenza A infection, amantadine may ameliorate the severity of illness in vulnerable elderly or compromised patients. However, amantadine is not effective against influenza B, parainfluenza viruses, or any respiratory viruses other than influenza A. It is

Table 5 Recommended Therapy for Viral Infections in Patients with Cancer

Virus	Setting	First Choice Regimen*	Alternate Choice/Comment
Herpes simplex virus	Prophylaxis	Acyclovir 200 mg PO QID	Acyclovir 5 mg/Kg Q 8 H IV
	Stomatitis	Acyclovir 200 mg PO QID for 7-14 days	Acyclovir 5 mg/Kg Q 8 H IV
	Encephalitis	Acyclovir 10 mg/Kg IV Q 8 Hr for 10-14 days	Foscarnet (experimental)
Varicella-zoster virus	Local zoster	Acyclovir 800 mg PO Q 4 Hr for 7-10 days	Acyclovir 10 mg/Kg IV Q 8 Hr
	Disseminated, visceral, or ophthalmic infection	Acyclovir 10 mg/Kg Q 8 Hr IV for 10-14 days	Foscarnet (experimental)
Cytomegalovirus	Prophylaxis	Acyclovir 400 mg PO Q 6 Hr or acyclovir 5 mg/Kg IV Q 8 H	Immune serum globulin or hyperimmune CMV globulin
	Pneumonitis, retinitis, colitis or disseminated infection	Ganciclovir 5 mg/Kg IV for 10-14 days	Indefinite suppressive therapy required in AIDS patients
	Pneumonia	Ganciclovir 5 mg/Kg Q 12 H and CMV hyperimmune globulin†	
Influenza A	Upper respiratory tract infection or pneumonia	Amantadine 100 mg PO Q 12 H for 14-21 days	Modify dose if renal insufficiency or patient > 60 years of age.

*In patients with normal renal and hepatic function. Duration of therapy may be prolonged, especially in patients with HIV infection.
†Not yet approved for the therapy of CMV infection although studies confirm benefit.

important that the dose of amantadine be modified in elderly patients and in patients with renal insufficiency to prevent seizures.

Selection of Antimicrobial Therapy for Common Infectious Syndromes

It is important to re-emphasize the importance of making every effort to determine the microbial cause of a cancer patient's presumed infection, to guide initial and long-term therapy and to minimize side-effects. In many cases, it is possible to select a specific regimen because data available at the time of the initial evaluation point clearly toward a source of infection, such as bacterial pneumonia (microscopic examination of sputum or a tracheal aspirate, or fiberoptic bronchoalveolar lavage fluid), urinary tract infection (gram-stain of the urine), or meningitis (gram-stain of the ultra-centrifuged CSF). More often, the initial clinical and laboratory information suggest strongly that the patient is infected at a specific site, and although the initial diagnostic studies have not revealed a clearcut pathogen or pathogens, it is likely that the cultures will ultimately disclose the infecting organism or organisms. In such circumstances, the clinician is forced to choose an empiric regimen that is based on the microbial pathogens that can be reasonably anticipated to be present at the presumed site of infection (see Table 3).

Sepsis Without Identified Local Infection

Despite intensive efforts to identify a local infection, patients with cancer often present with fever, rigors, or even septic shock without an identifiable site of infection. Many of these patients, especially those who are granulocytopenic, will have culture-proved bacteremia. Thus, it is appropriate, after obtaining diagnostic studies, to treat these patients empirically on the premise that they are bacteremic.

The selection of the initial antimicrobial regimen is generally influenced by whether or not the patient is granulocytopenic (<500 per mm^3). For the patient without granulocytopenia, the regimen should be effective against *Staphylococcus aureus, Streptococcus pneumoniae, H. influenzae* Type b resistant to ampicillin, and enteric gram-negative bacilli and can be easily achieved with one drug, a third-generation cephalosporin (e.g., ceftriaxone or ceftazadime) or imipenem. If, however, the patient has received recent antimicrobial therapy or has recently been infected with beta-lactam–resistant gram-negative bacilli or *P. aeruginosa,* it would be prudent to use two antibiotics in the initial regimen, adding an aminoglycoside such as gentamicin or tobramycin to ampicillin-sulbactam, a third-generation cephalosporin, or an antipseudomonal penicillin (see Table 3).

A granulocytopenic patient has often received prior antimicrobial therapy and is thus more likely to be colonized by resistant organisms; unless the episode represents the patient's first episode of fever and possible sepsis, a combination regimen should be given, such as an antipseudomonal penicillin or cephalosporin combined with an aminoglycoside (see Table 3). For the febrile granulocytopenic patient who is early in the stage of neoplastic disease (e.g., during the first course of induction therapy for acute leukemia) who does not have an identified pathogen and is not floridly septic, and who has *not* received prior antimicrobial therapy, monotherapy with a potent beta-lactam will provide reliable initial coverage, pending the results of culture studies; ceftazadime, cefaperazone, and imipenem have been studied in randomized, comparative trials, and each drug given alone has been shown to provide efficacy comparable to a combination regimen including an aminoglycoside. If monotherapy is chosen, it is essential that if cultures identify an infecting organism, the regimen be adjusted and tailored for that organism, e.g., administering two antibiotics effective against the organism if the infecting species is a gram-negative rod, to provide additive—ideally synergistic—activity will improve the outcome in patients with severe granulocytopenia.

Double beta-lactam regimens, combining an antipseudomonal penicillin with a cephalosporin (e.g., ceftazadime and piperacillin) also provide reliable coverage, comparable to the combination of an antipseudomonal penicillin and an aminoglycoside; however, the higher cost, development of resistant organisms, lack of documented synergy, and potential for antagonism have limited the use of these regimens. The combination of an antipseudomonal beta-lactam with an aminoglycoside remains the standard by which empiric antibacterial regimens for granulocytopenic patients are measured.

There has been considerable controversy regarding the inclusion of vancomycin in the initial empiric regimen for the febrile granulocytopenic patient to provide a drug active against beta-lactam–resistant coagulase-negative staphylococci, *Bacillus* species, and *Corynebacterium* species. Comparative trials have shown that inclusion of vancomycin does reduce the frequency of bloodstream infection with these organisms during therapy; however, a large study from the National Institutes of Health has shown that not including vancomycin in the initial regimen, but giving the drug when a gram-positive infection was identified, was not associated with increased morbidity or mortality rates, and gram-positive infections were effectively treated in 100 percent of instances. Thus, we do not recommend the use of vancomycin in the initial antimicrobial regimen for the febrile granulocytopenic patient unless there are reasons to suspect infection by methicillin-resistant staphylococci, such as the patient has had a history of resistant gram-positive infection or the patient has local signs of central venous catheter–related infection, or the patient is at risk for endocarditis (e.g., the patient has valvular heart disease or a prosthetic heart valve). In the majority of cases, vancomycin can be reserved for microbiologically confirmed infections with coagulase-negative staphylococci or other resistant gram-positive organisms.

The increasing effectiveness of antineoplastic therapy and antibacterial drugs has extended the life of most patients with cancer, and deep fungal infections are being encountered increasingly in most centers, particularly in patients with prolonged granulocytopenia who have received intensive antibiotic therapy. Studies indicate that in a granulocytopenic patient who has received empiric antibacterial therapy but continues to be febrile after 5 to 7 days, addition of intravenous amphotericin B, 0.4 mg per kg per day, to the empiric antibacterial regimen reduces mortality caused by deep fungal infections and may have prophylactic value as well. However, efforts should be made to identify deep fungal infection in such instances by use of Isolator fungal blood cultures, by biopsy of suspicious skin or pulmonary lesions, and by contrast-enhanced computed tomography scans of the chest or brain to identify necrotizing nodular lesions characteristic of invasive *Aspergillus* infection.

Pneumonia

Pneumonia poses the greatest threat to the cancer patient and the greatest challenge to his or her physician. Several points bear emphasis before discussing therapy. First, pneumonitis in the cancer patient often has a noninfectious cause; many antineoplastic drugs, such as methotrexate, cyclophosphamide, and bleomycin can produce pneumonitis. Second, the primary neoplastic disease, radiation therapy, pulmonary emboli, congestive heart failure, and hemorrhage can mimic infectious pneumonitis. Third, these processes may coexist in the setting of infectious pneumonitis. Fourth, it is especially important to strive to establish the microbial cause of presumed infectious pneumonia in vulnerable cancer patients, rejecting empiric therapy without diagnostic studies.

The initial therapy of pneumonia in the cancer patient should, in our judgment, be based on the results of microscopic examination of the sputum or other lower respiratory tract specimens that are considered to provide the best information as to the probable cause of infection. It is beyond the scope of this review to discuss diagnostic studies in detail; however, screened sputum specimens, assuring representativeness as to tracheal origin, will provide the microbial cause in up to 80 percent of patients with culture-proved bacterial pneumonia. Unfortunately, many patients with cancer are unable to produce sputum, and studies over the past decade have established the accuracy of culture and gram-stain of tracheal aspirates or specimens obtained by fiberoptic bronchoscopy. We believe that if a critically ill patient with cancer presents with a clinical picture suggestive of pneumonia, sputum or a tracheal aspirate should be obtained for gram-stain and culture. If the specimen shows many white blood cells but no bacteria, it is highly likely that the infecting agent is not a conventional bacterium and that the process represents *Legionella* infection, viral pneumonitis, fungal pneumonia, or noninfectious pneumonitis; proceeding directly to fiberoptic bronchoscopy is most likely to provide the diagnosis and allow the most specific and effective antimicrobial therapy.

Table 6 lists suggested regimens, and for patients with life-threatening penicillin hypersensitivity, alternative drugs, for the treatment of infections, including pneumonia, caused by the major pathogens encountered in the patient with cancer. In patients with acute pneumonia in whom the gram-stain shows large numbers of white blood cells but no bacteria, legionellosis, chlamydial, or mycoplasmal pneumonia must be suspected, and erythromycin should be included in the initial empiric regimen.

Table 6 Recommended Therapy for Life-Threatening Infection with Specific Bacterial Pathogens in Patients with Cancer

Pathogen	Syndromes	First Choice Regimen*	Penicillin Allergy/Alternate
Streptococcus pneumoniae	Pneumonia	Penicillin G	Erythromycin
	Meningitis		Chloramphenicol (meningitis)
Staphylococcus aureus	Bacteremia	Nafcillin (methicillin-sensitive)	Vancomycin
	Pneumonia	Vancomycin (methicillin-resistant)	Vancomycin
	Cellulitis		
Coagulase-negative Staphylococcus	Bacteremia	Vancomycin	Vancomycin
	Device-related infection	Nafcillin (methicillin-sensitive)	
Haemophilus influenzae	Bacteremia	Third-generation cephalosporin†	Trimethoprim-sulfamethoxazole
	Meningitis		
Clostridium difficile	Colitis	Vancomycin (oral)	Metronidazole (oral)
Listeria monocytogenes	Meningitis	Ampicillin and gentamicin	Trimethoprim-sulfamethoxazole
	Bacteremia		
Legionella species	Pneumonia	Erythromycin and rifampin	Doxycycline
Pseudomonas aeruginosa	Bacteremia	Anti-pseudomonas beta-lactam‡ and tobramycin	Aztreonam and tobramycin
	Pneumonia		
Enterobacteriaceae	Bacteremia	Third-generation cephalosporin† and gentamicin	Aztreonam and gentamicin
	Pneumonia		
Xanthomonas maltophilia	Bacteremia	Trimethoprim-sulfamethoxazole	Ticarcillin-clavulinate
	Pneumonia		Ceftazadime
Nocardia asteroides	Pneumonia	Sulfadiazine	Trimethoprim-sulfamethoxazole
	Brain abscess		
	Metastatic infection		Imipenem-cilastatin and amikacin
			Minocycline and ampicillin

*The above regimens are suggested initial therapy most likely to be effective, pending the results of susceptibility testing. The results of susceptibility testing must guide selection of the final regimen.
†Third-generation cephalosporins: cefotaxime, ceftizoxime, ceftriaxone, cefoperazone, ceftazadime.
‡Anti-pseudomonas beta-lactam antibiotics: ticarcillin, mezlocillin, azlocillin, piperacillin; cefoperazone, ceftazadime; imipenem.

Clinicians often encounter patients who decline invasive diagnostic procedures, or such studies may not be immediately available. In such circumstances, the combination of tobramycin with ticarcillin-clavulinate or imipenem, which provide excellent activity against *Pseudomonas aeruginosa* and other gram-negative bacilli, pneumococci, *Haemophilus influenzae*, *Staphylococcus aureus*, and anaerobes, and erythromycin, for *Legionella*, is recommended.

Sinusitis

Roentgenograms will provide an accurate diagnosis of sinusitis in most patients. Opacification, air-fluid levels, or marked mucosal thickening (> 12 m) denotes infectious sinusitis approximately 90 percent of the time. Whereas most cases of acute sinusitis, including in patients with cancer, have a bacterial cause (see Table 3), granulocytopenic patients are vulnerable to fungal sinusitis, especially mucormycosis; in the critically ill cancer patient, particularly one with periorbital inflammation associated with sinusitis, mucormycosis must be considered.

For empiric therapy of presumed bacterial sinusitis in the cancer patient without granulocytopenia, ampicillin-sulbactam or trimethoprim-sulfamethoxazole will prove effective in the majority of cases. In critically ill patients, especially granulocytopenic patients or patients who have received prolonged, intensive antimicrobial therapy, therapy should be guided by the results of diagnostic sinus aspiration or biopsy to determine the

use of a more intensive regimen with activity against *P. aeruginosa* and other gram-negative bacilli or fungi.

Meningitis

Treatment of meningitis should be guided by the results of the CSF fluid examination, particularly the gram-stained smear. If these results are negative, the results of antigen tests for *Streptococcus pneumoniae*, *Haemophilus influenzae* Type b, and *Neisseria meningitidis* should guide treatment. If these study results are negative but the CSF profile strongly suggests bacterial meningitis (i.e., neutrophils, hypoglycorrhachia), the initial regimen must provide activity against the three aforementioned pathogens and *Listeria monocytogenes*, an increasingly important cause of meningitis in patients with cancer. The combination of a third-generation cephalosporin (such as ceftriaxone) and ampicillin (for *Listeria*) is recommended (see Table 3); in patients with penicillin allergy, chloramphenicol and trimethoprim-sulfamethoxazole can be used. In patients with granulocytopenia, the regimen also must be effective against *P. aeruginosa* (e.g., ceftazadime should be used). These regimens also will provide adequate empiric therapy if lumbar puncture is delayed or cannot be done because of threatened herniation.

Intra-abdominal Infections

Intra-abdominal infections fall into three major categories with differing microbial profiles (see Table 3):

cholangitis, peritonitis and intra-abdominal abscesses, and primary peritonitis.

Cholangitis occurs primarily in the setting of biliary tract obstruction; in patients with cancer this is usually a pancreaticobiliary neoplasm. If the obstruction is not promptly relieved surgically, overwhelming endotoxic shock and death rapidly occur, even in young patients. Cholangitis with bacteremia occasionally occurs in the absence of obstruction with a functional choledochojejunostomy or following hepatic transplantation. Cholangitis is caused predominantly by aerobic gram-negative bacilli, enterococci and occasionally, *Clostridium* species; *Bacteroides fragilis* and other anaerobic bacteria are rarely encountered in ascending cholangitis without hepatic abscess.

Primary peritonitis is a well-defined syndrome in which *S. pneumoniae* or enteric gram-negative bacilli, particularly *Escherichia coli,* produce unimicrobial peritonitis, associated with bacteremia more than one-half of the time, without identifiable disruption of the integrity of the gastrointestinal tract or cholangitis. Primary peritonitis is seen almost exclusively in patients with pre-existent ascites.

Treatment of presumed cholangitis or primary peritonitis mandates a regimen effective against aerobic gram-negative bacilli and enterococci: ampicillinsulbactam and gentamicin; an antipseudomonal cephalosporin (e.g., ceftazadime or cefoperazone) and ampicillin; or imipenem and ampicillin (see Table 3).

Bacteroides fragilis and other anaerobic organisms, together with aerobic gram-negative bacilli and enterococci, are polymicrobial copathogens in most cases of peritonitis due to disruption of the gastrointestinal mucosa and in intra-abdominal abscesses stemming from focal intra-abdominal infections. Metronidazole or clindamycin combined with an aminoglycoside and ampicillin; ampicillin-sulbactam and gentamicin; or imipenem and ampicillin have all been shown to provide reliable coverage (see Table 3). Patients with cancer in most instances are immunocompromised, and *Enterococcus* must always be considered a potential copathogen; thus, the regimen should always include ampicillin or vancomycin.

Typhlitis

Patients with granulocytopenia are uniquely vulnerable to a syndrome characterized by abdominal pain and tenderness, particularly in the right lower quadrant, associated with ileus and accompanied by a clinical picture suggestive of systemic sepsis. Typhlitis appears to represent a localized ileus involving the distal small bowel and cecum, and it is commonly associated with enteric gram-negative bacteremia or fungemia. Treatment of typhlitis consists of bowel rest and empiric antimicrobial (and possibly, antifungal) therapy, similar to that which would be used for treatment of an intra-abdominal infection but with reliable activity against *Pseudomonas aeruginosa.*

Gynecologic Infections

Gynecologic infections in patients with cancer are caused by the same spectrum of microorganisms encountered in patients with peritonitis caused by disruption of the gastrointestinal mucosa, e.g., anaerobes, enteric gram-negative bacilli, and enterococci. Thus, the empiric regimen for pelvic infection in patients with cancer, most of whom have had extensive pelvic surgery, is the same as for treatment of peritonitis or intra-abdominal abscesses.

Urosepsis

Urinary tract infections in patients with cancer are often caused by resistant nosocomial organisms such as *Klebsiella-Enterobacter, Proteus* species, *Pseudomonas aeruginosa, Serratia,* or enterococci. The initial regimen, pending culture results, must take this into account (see Table 3); ampicillin and an aminoglycoside, ampicillin and a third-generation cephalosporin, and imipenem are all acceptable initial regimens for urosepsis in the patient with cancer.

Skin and Soft-Tissue Infections

Uncomplicated skin and soft-tissue infections in adult cancer patients are caused almost exclusively by *Staphylococcus aureus* and beta-hemolytic streptococci; in young children with cancer, Type b *Haemophilus influenza* also causes skin and soft-tissue infections.

Cellulitis in granulocytopenic patients is often caused by staphylococci or streptococci, but is more often caused by aerobic gram-negative bacilli, including *Pseudomonas aeruginosa.* Perianal cellulitis is a syndrome unique to granulocytopenic patients and, unlike the situation with perianal abscesses in nongranulocytopenic patients, is nearly always a unimicrobial gram-negative bacillary infection, most often caused by *P. aeruginosa;* surgical drainage is not beneficial or recommended.

Patients with granulocytopenia; who have undergone recent gastrointestinal or gynecologic surgery; or who have soft-tissue infections complicating decubital ulcers or occurring in the setting of antineoplastic chemotherapy, diabetes, or peripheral vascular disease are vulnerable to highly invasive, polymicrobial soft-tissue infections such as necrotizing fascitis or synergistic gangrene or deeper infections involving the muscles, such as beta-streptococcal infection or clostridium pyomyositis. These infections are usually polymicrobial, caused by aerobic gram-negative bacilli and anaerobic organisms, the same pathogens implicated in peritonitis. Bacteremia occurs in up to 40 percent of cases. Any soft-tissue inflammation occurring in a patient with cancer who is at risk for these complex infections must undergo a detailed diagnostic evaluation at the minimum with gram stain and culture of percutaneous aspirates or biopsy specimens. If necrosis is present or gas is apparent in the deep tissues roentgenographically, exploratory surgery and extensive debridement are imperative at the outset. The case fatality of these complex skin and soft-tissue infections encountered in compromised patients is exceedingly high unless surgical débridement is employed early in the course of the infection.

Recommended initial empiric regimens for skin and soft-tissue infections in patients with cancer are provided in Table 3.

Enteric Infections

Many patients with cancer are at increased risk for enteric infections with *Campylobacter, Salmonella, Shigella,* enteropathogenic *Escherichia coli* or enterocolitis caused by *Clostridium difficile.* With the exception of *C. difficile* enterocolitis, most enteric infections can be treated effectively with a quinolone, such as norfloxicin or ciprofloxacin, given orally. If bacteremia has occurred, a third-generation cephalosporin, such as ceftriaxone or cefoperazone, will be effective against the aforementioned pathogens.

Clostridium difficile enterocolitis is now an extremely common complication of broad-spectrum antimicrobial therapy. Any cancer patient who develops watery diarrhea, especially associated with cramps and fever, or who simply develops unexplained ileus should be suspected of having this syndrome. The diagnosis often can be established by flexible sigmoidoscopy, showing the characteristic pseudomembranes, but tests for the presence of cytotoxin in the stool are more sensitive diagnostic tools.

Antibiotic-associated colitis must prompt reassessment of the need for continued broad-spectrum antimicrobial therapy. Oral metronidazole appears to be as efficacious as oral vancomycin for mild or moderately severe cases; however, for severe antibiotic-related colitis or with severely compromised patients, vancomycin, 125 mg orally four times per day, should be considered the regimen of choice.

Intravascular Catheter–Related Sepsis

Stable vascular access is essential to the management of the patient with cancer, and a wide variety of surgically implanted devices are now widely used, including permanent, surgically implanted, cuffed central venous catheters (e.g., Hickman, Broviac, or Groshong catheters) and subcutaneous central venous ports (e.g., the Infusaport and Portacath).

The relative risk of bloodstream infection caused by the various intravascular devices available ranges widely with the type of device used. The highest risk is with short-term central venous catheters, in the range of 2 to 4 percent, and is much higher for temporary hemodialysis catheters, i.e., 5 to 10 percent. In contrast, the risk of septicemia with small, percutaneous, peripheral intravenous catheters is now very low (less than 0.2 percent). Permanent surgically implanted catheters are now associated with a relatively low risk of bloodstream infection with good care. The risk is in the range of 0.2 bacteremias per 100 catheter-days; however, the diagnosis of infection with permanently implanted devices is more difficult, as is the decision whether the device needs to be removed to cure presumed bloodstream infection.

Evaluation of the patient with suspected device-related sepsis should include a thorough examination to exclude all other sites of infection. The access site must be examined carefully, and any expressible purulence should be gram-stained and cultured. Peripheral percutaneous blood cultures should always be obtained; in patients with surgically implanted catheters, quantitative blood cultures should be obtained from each catheter lumen. Quantitative blood cultures using the DuPont Isolator system show improved sensitivity for diagnosis of fungemia and can be very helpful in the diagnosis of device-related sepsis. A marked quantitative increase in bacteremia or fungemia in a blood culture obtained from the central venous device, as compared with a percutaneously drawn peripheral blood culture specimen, is highly suggestive of infection of the device. With presumed infection of a temporary percutaneous catheter, the device should be removed. If continued access is necessary, a new catheter can be inserted at a new site.

The majority of bacteremias associated with permanent cuffed central venous catheters derive from intraluminal contaminants and can be successfully treated without removing the catheter, by administration of intravenous antibiotics through the presumably infected catheter. The catheter should be removed if clinical signs of sepsis do not resolve within 3 days or bacteremia persists despite antimicrobial therapy; the subcutaneous tunnel is infected at the outset; there is clinical or echocardiographic evidence of endocarditis, septic thrombosis, or septic emboli; or the patient is at high risk for endocarditis (e.g., has had prior endocarditis or has a prosthetic heart valve); or the infecting pathogen is a *Bacillus* species, a mycobacterium, or filamentous fungus (e.g., *Trichophyton*). Approximately two-thirds of uncomplicated catheter-related bacteremias associated with permanent cuffed catheters can be permanently eradicated with 7 to 14 days of antimicrobial therapy administered through the catheter.

Device-related candidemia usually can be treated successfully with a total dose of approximately 5 mg per kg of intravenous amphotericin B combined with device removal. Septic thrombosis of a central vein caused by *Candida,* characteristically associated with high-grade candidemia, on the other hand, usually requires a higher daily dose, in the range of 0.7 mg per kg and a total dose of approximately 20 mg per kg; the addition of flucytosine to the regimen should also be strongly considered.

Bloodstream infection originating from an infected subcutaneous port can be diagnosed by demonstrating large numbers of organisms in quantitative culture of material aspirated from the subcutaneous reservoir or the cutaneous soft tissues. Local cellulitis without bacteremia often can be treated successfully with antimicrobial therapy. If, however, the patient has bacteremia and the causative role of the subcutaneous port has been established by quantitative culture of fluid aspirated from the device, the port should be removed in toto, as it is extremely difficult to eradicate implanted device-related infections medically.

Specific Anti-infective Therapy

The results of cultures and other diagnostic studies identifying the infecting organisms and the results of susceptibility testing should form the basis for selection of a definitive antimicrobial regimen for treatment of the patient's infection. In nongranulocytopenic patients, this usually permits a regimen that includes less broad-spectrum agents, particularly if the infecting pathogen is a single gram-positive or aerobic gram-negative organism.

With granulocytopenic patients, on the other hand, particularly with profound granulocytopenia, even if a single pathogen is identified, it is usually desirable to continue a broad-spectrum regimen on the premise that the patient may be infected by other organisms and is highly vulnerable to superinfection caused by aerobic gram-negative bacilli. Thus, although it may be appropriate to add vancomycin to the regimen if coagulase-negative staphylococcal bacteremia is identified, the initial regimen of an antipseudomonal penicillin or cephalosporin, with or without an aminoglycoside, should generally be continued if the patient is profoundly granulocytopenic, especially if the patient continues to be febrile.

Specific regimens for the treatment of infections caused by the major bacterial pathogens encountered in patients with cancer are given in Table 6; recommended doses and dosing intervals are provided in Table 2.

Fungal Infections

Amphotericin B is rarely included in the initial empiric regimen of patients with cancer in the absence of histopathologic or culture evidence confirming infection by fungi. However, cutaneous lesions of deep fungal infection, the finding of characteristic retinal lesions of *Candida* retinitis in a patient with a central venous catheter, the occurrence of *Candida* esophagitis in a profoundly granulocytopenic patient, necrotizing nodular lesions on CT scans of the chest or brain, and the occurrence of a clinical picture of sepsis in a patient who has recently had a deep fungal infection are all acceptable clinical grounds for empiric amphotericin B therapy.

The addition of intravenous amphotericin B to the empiric antibacterial regimen of the granulocytopenic patient with cryptogenic fever that persists despite antibacterial therapy has been discussed.

Recommended drugs and dosing regimens for infection caused by the major fungal pathogens encountered in the patient with cancer are provided in Table 4.

Viral Infections

The herpesviruses, particularly HSV, VZV, CMV, and to a lesser extent, EBV, produce substantial morbidity and occasional mortality in patients with cancer. HSV and VZV produce localized infections (HSV, stomatitis; VZV, dermatomal herpes zoster), which represent reactivation of latent infections and are very frequent. Both HSV and VZV can produce disseminated cutaneous infection and even visceral infection; HSV produces devastating necrotizing encephalitis. Visceral infections with HSV or VZV have high mortality rates. CMV infection is often asymptomatic or associated with little more symptomatically than fever, but CMV also can produce hepatitis, interstitial pneumonitis, colitis, or retinitis, especially in bone marrow transplant patients or patients with AIDS and cancer. EBV is an important cause of a lymphoproliferative syndrome that can progress to a highly invasive B-cell lymphoma that responds poorly to chemotherapy; however, the EBV-related lymphoproliferative syndrome is rare in patients with cancer other than those who have undergone bone marrow transplantation and is more commonly seen after solid organ transplantation.

Acyclovir is highly effective for HSV and VZV infections, and doses appropriate for treatment of the various syndromes seen with these viruses are given in Table 5. It is important to emphasize that HSV encephalitis and all VZV infections should be treated with high-dose acyclovir, 10 mg per kg intravenously every 8 hours for at least 10 days.

Ganciclovir has recently become available for treating life-threatening CMV infections and is quite effective except for CMV pneumonitis in bone marrow transplant patients and patients with AIDS. It is recommended that CMV immune serum globulin, 400 mg per kg on days 1, 2, and 7; and 200 mg per kg on days 14 and 21, be given with ganciclovir for patients with life-threatening CMV pneumonitis.

Amantadine, which is only available in an oral form, can significantly ameliorate the severity of influenzae A infection in elderly or compromised patients if it is given within the first 24 to 48 hours of illness. In elderly patients or patients with renal insufficiency, the dose should be halved (i.e., 100 mg per day), to prevent drug-associated seizures.

Antiparasitic Therapy

The three parasites most commonly encountered in patients with cancer are *Pneumocystis carinii*, which produces a bilateral, interstitial pneumonitis; *Toxoplasma gondii*, which in most cases produces focal encephalitis; and *Strongyloides stercoralis*, which produces a peritonitis syndrome, with or without pneumonitis, in cancer patients given high doses of corticosteroids or other drugs impairing CMI.

Pneumocystis carinii pneumonia (PCP) can now be diagnosed in the majority of cases by fiberoptic bronchoscopic bronchoalveolar lavage; occasional patients require examination of lung biopsy specimens obtained bronchoscopically or by open thoracotomy. Two regimens are effective for treatment of PCP: high dose trimethoprim-sulfamethoxazole (TMP-SMZ) and intravenous pentamidine. In the patient without HIV infection, TMP-SMZ is associated with less toxicity, whereas in AIDS patients with cancer, TMP-SMZ produces cutaneous rashes or cytopenias in two-thirds of patients.

It is extremely important in treatment of PCP that TMP-SMZ be given in appropriate doses; in patients with normal renal function the dose is 20 mg per kg per day of the TMP component, in divided dosage, usually in an every-6-hour regimen. For patients with serious allergy to sulfonamides, intravenous pentamidine, 4 mg per kg per day in a single dose, is usually effective, but is associated with cardiotoxicity if the drug is given rapidly. Nephrotoxicity can be anticipated in 5 to 15 percent of treated patients and hypoglycemia commonly occurs hours or days after an infusion (see Table 2). PCP should be treated for at least 3 weeks to prevent recurrence, especially in patients with AIDS and cancer.

Toxoplasma gondii infection can be reliably diagnosed serologically in most patients with cancer who do not have HIV infection; nearly all patients will show a high titer of antibody, often IgM antibody, in association with a clinical picture of encephalitis and focal enhancing lesions seen on CT scan or MR imaging scan. In contrast, AIDS patients with *T. gondii* infection virtually never show IgM antibody, but usually show an elevated titer of IgG antibody against *T. gondii,* indicating past exposure to the organism. In the setting of focal encephalitis and AIDS, the diagnosis *T. gondii* infection is reasonably certain.

First-line therapy for *T. gondii* infection consists of the combination of a sulfonamide, 1.0 to 1.5 g every 6 hours for adults (75 to 100 mg per kg per day for children), combined with pyrimethamine, 50 mg per day (1 mg per kg per day for children), in patients with normal renal function; this combination is administered for at least 6 to 8 weeks. Patients with AIDS and *T. gondii* infection require suppressive therapy with lower doses of a sulfonamide and pyrimethamine for life to prevent recurrences. In patients with life-threatening allergy to sulfonamides, clindamycin, 900 mg given intravenously every 8 hours, combined with pyrimethamine appears to be effective.

Enteric infection with *Strongyloides stercoralis* is usually asymptomatic in the immunocompetent host. *Strongyloides* hyperinfection, invasion through the wall of the intestines, should be considered in any immunocompromised cancer patient, especially a patient who has received high doses of corticosteroids who develops abdominal pain with peritoneal signs, with or without respiratory symptoms and pulmonary infiltrates on chest radiographs; eosinophilia is frequently absent. Hyperinfection is encountered almost exclusively in cancer patients from Central or South America or third-world countries where intestinal helminthic infections are hyperendemic. The diagnosis is easily confirmed by demonstrating the characteristic vermiform larvae in microscopic examination of the stool. The treatment of

strongyloides hyperinfection is thiabendazole, 25 mg per kg per day P.O., given for 7 days, and antibacterial treatment for bacterial peritonitis (see Table 3).

ADJUNCTIVE THERAPY

In every patient with cancer who presents with signs of systemic infection, especially overwhelming infection, every effort must be made to identify the source of infection and if possible, to remove that source mechanically, by surgically draining an abscess, decompressing an obstructed common bile duct or obstructed ureter, or closing an intestinal perforation; removing an infected intravascular device, possibly even resecting a suppurative vein segment; or in the ICU patient, discontinuing an intravenous or intra-arterial infusion that may contain contaminants, or removing a heavily contaminated hemodialysis machine. Such measures are crucial to the patient's survival and in many instances, such as sepsis from a contaminated infusion, supersede antimicrobial therapy in therapeutic importance.

The importance of support of the circulation in the patient with hypotension also is critical. Studies have shown that administration of crystalloid solutions, such as Ringer's lactate, are just as effective as far more expensive colloids (albumin or plasma protein fraction). In patients with cardiorespiratory failure and hypotension who have not responded to 500 to 1,000 mL of crystalloid, the hemodynamic information provided by inserting a flow-directed, balloon-tipped pulmonary artery catheter can aid efforts to optimize gas exchange with associated respiratory failure and shock. For patients with frank septic shock and a suboptimal cardiac output, despite volume loading to a pulmonary capillary wedge pressure of 12 to 15 mm Hg, dopamine is the pressor of choice, starting with approximately 2 to 5 μg per kg per minute. Dobutamine is contraindicated in most patients with septic shock and can produce profound hypotension.

The role of high-dose corticosteroids for adjunctive therapy of septic shock now appears to have been satisfactorily resolved by two large prospective randomized double-blind trials: high dose methylprednisolone, 30 mg per kg per day, did not improve survival in either study. Several studies, however, have shown that in nongranulocytopenic patients with bacterial meningitis, administration of corticosteroids in this dosage range, *prior to beginning antimicrobial therapy,* substantially reduces morbidity and mortality rates, including in adults with pneumococcal meningitis.

Studies have shown that the use of narcotic antagonists such as naloxone or repletion of fibronectin with fresh-frozen plasma or cryoprecipitate does not improve survival in patients with septic shock.

The greatest promise in adjunctive therapy is based on prospective, randomized, double-blind trials that have shown that hyperimmune serum, with a high titer of antibody directed against the core antigens common to most enteric gram-negative bacilli and *P. aeruginosa,* given to patients with gram-negative bacteremia and septic shock improve survival two-fold. At the time of this writing, randomized trials have shown that monoclonal antibodies produced by recombinant technologies and administered to patients with gram-negative bacteremia also improve survival, and it can be anticipated that these products will become commercially available within the next 12 to 24 months.

Granulocyte transfusions are not recommended for most patients with serious infections and cancer, even patients with profound granulocytopenia. Whereas early studies showed a short-term advantage, the associated risks of transfusion-related CMV infection, alloimmunization, and pulmonary toxicity associated with concomitant use of amphotericin B have greatly dampened enthusiasm for the routine use of granulocyte transfusions as adjunctive therapy in infected granulocytopenic patients with cancer. The major occasion for granulocyte transfusion support at the present time is in the patient with profound granulocytopenia with reversible myelosuppression who has proved gram-negative bacillary infection or possibly, fungal infection unresponsive to intensive anti-infective therapy, especially pneumonia or soft-tissue infection.

Whereas the use of intravenous immune serum globulin (ISG) is clearly of value for prevention of infection in many patients with cancer, studies showing a therapeutic role for these preparations in the absence of documented hypogammaglobulinemia are less secure. However, in the patient with impaired CMI and severe CMV pneumonitis, particularly the patient who has undergone recent bone marrow transplantation, administration of hyperimmune CMV globulin, in conjunction with intravenous ganciclovir may improve the patient's chance for survival of this grave infection.

PREVENTION

It is beyond the scope of this review to consider in detail measures for prevention of infection in the patient with cancer; however, several important points warrant brief discussion.

Vaccines. Patients with cancer should be immunized at the outset against *Streptococcus pneumoniae* and should also receive the annual trivalent influenza vaccine; children should receive *Haemophilus influenzae* Type b vaccine as well. Patients' immunity against diphtheria and tetanus should be maintained by appropriate boosters after a primary series. Asplenic patients also should be given the *H. influenzae* Type b and meningococcal vaccines. Most adults with cancer have received the oral polio vaccine, but if they have not and it is considered desirable to provide immunity against poliomyelitis (e.g., an anticipated trip to a third-world country), the inactivated (Salk) vaccine should be used to avert rare vaccine-strain–related paralysis. In general, live virus vaccines should not be given to patients with cancer, especially those with impaired CMI.

Immune Serum Globulin. Patients with chronic lymphocytic leukemia, multiple myeloma, or lymphoma often have associated hypogammaglobulinemia. Patients with documented hypogammaglobulinemia (IgG < 200 mg per dL) or who have been vulnerable to recurrent bacterial infections and have subnormal levels of IgG, should receive supplemental ISG (400 mg per kg every 3 weeks). In general, immunoglobulin levels should be checked in any patient with cancer who develops recurrent bacterial infection, especially with encapsulated bacteria.

Patients with cancer who have never had chickenpox, especially children with acute leukemia, are vulnerable to overwhelming and often lethal infections with VZV. For immunocompromised patients who have been exposed to VZV and are susceptible, administration of zoster immune globulin can provide protection against lethal infection *if administered within 4 days after the exposure.* Administration of ISG to susceptible patients exposed to hepatitis A or measles may prevent or ameliorate otherwise severe infections.

Tuberculosis. Cancer patients with a positive tuberculin skin test result (> 10 mm of induration following a standard 5 TU PPD [>5 mm for patients with recent exposure to tuberculosis], HIV infection, or roentgenographic evidence of old tuberculosis) should receive prophylactic isoniazid, 300 mg per day (10 mg per kg per day for children), for a minimum of 6 continuous months, 12 months for the patient with HIV infection or an abnormal chest roentgenogram, to prevent reactivation of infection.

Antimicrobial Prophylaxis. Patients with acute leukemia who are undergoing induction therapy or patients undergoing bone marrow transplantation are highly vulnerable to bacterial infection during the 3 to 4 weeks of profound granulocytopenia. More than 20 randomized trials have shown that administration of TMP-SMZ, 160/800 mg twice daily, or norfloxacin, 400 mg, or ciprofloxacin, 500 mg twice daily, substantially reduces the incidence of bacterial infection during the limited period of severe granulocytopenia. The efficacy of these regimens for patients with chronic granulocytopenia is not established.

The use of drugs to prevent invasive fungal infection in patients with profound granulocytopenia has been disappointing until recently. Oral regimens such as nystatin, ketoconazole, or amphotericin B have been marginally effective at best. Recent studies with the potent triazole, fluconazole, however, suggest that in vulnerable cancer patients, particularly patients undergoing induction antileukemic therapy or bone marrow transplantation, fluconazole, 100 mg daily by mouth or intravenously, reduces the risk of *Candida* infections during the period of maximal vulnerability.

Antiviral Prophylaxis. Patients with profound granulocytopenia, especially patients undergoing bone marrow transplantation, are highly susceptible to reactivated infection caused by HSV. A number of trials have shown that acyclovir, 5 mg per kg intravenously every 8 hours, markedly reduces the incidence of severe necrotizing HSV stomatitis and disseminated HSV infection during the period of vulnerability.

During influenza A outbreaks, susceptible patients with cancer who have not been previously immunized should receive amantadine, 200 mg daily (100 mg in patients older than 60 years or with renal insufficiency), to prevent serious influenza A infection.

Protected Environments. Numerous studies have examined the efficacy of protected environments, e.g., laminar air flow room; and mandating use of sterile gowns, gloves, masks, and shoe covers for all individuals entering the room, for patients with cancer. Studies in patients with granulocytopenia have shown modest benefit for prevention of infection during the period of profound granulocytopenia; however, studies have shown that the use of nonabsorbable antibiotics or simply the use of orally administered TMP-SMZ appears to provide protection comparable to the use of these agents with a protected environment and clearly superior to the use of a protective environment alone. As such, few centers now routinely use extensive protective measures for the care of patients with cancer.

However, it is now very clear that patients with prolonged severe granulocytopenia are highly susceptible to pulmonary infection caused by airborne filamentous fungi, especially *Aspergillus fumigatus*. These infections have a high mortality rate. Studies have shown that the incidence of filamentous fungal infection during antileukemic therapy or bone marrow transplantation is greatly reduced by providing spore-free air—accomplished by use of high-efficiency particle (HEPA) filters. Inexpensive HEPA units for individual patient-care rooms are now available. Spore-free air must be considered a standard of care for treatment of acute leukemia or bone marrow transplantation.

Finally, it is very important that in all contacts with patients with cancer, maximal attention be paid to basic aseptic technique, particularly hand washing with an antiseptic-containing agent, such as 4 percent chlorhexidine, before all contacts with the patient and adherence to designated precautions in the management of urinary catheters, intravascular devices, and ventilatory support.

SUGGESTED READING

Emanuel D, Cunningham I, Jules-Elysee K, et al. Cytomegalovirus pneumonia after bone marrow transplantation successfully treated with the combination of ganciclovir and high-dose intravenous immune globulin. Ann Intern Med 1988; 109:777–782.

Hughes WT, Armstrong D, Bodey GP, et al. Guidelines for use of antimicrobial agents in neutropenic patients with unexplained fever. J Infect Dis 1990; 161:381–396.

Katz JA, Wagner ML, Gresik MV, et al. Typhlitis. An 18-year experience and postmortem review. Cancer 1990; 65:1041–1047.

Maki DG. Pathogenesis, prevention, and management of infections due to intravascular devices used for infusion therapy. In: Bisno AL, Waldvogel FA, eds. Infections associated with indwelling medical devices. Washington, DC: American Society for Microbiology, 1989: 161–177.

Mermel LA, Maki DG. Bacterial pneumonia in solid organ transplantation. Semin Resp Infect 1990; 5:10–29.

Rubin M, Hathorn JW, Marshall D, et al. Gram-positive infections and the use of vancomycin in 550 episodes of fever and neutropenia. Ann Intern Med 1988; 108:30–35.

Schimpff SC, Wiernik PH, Block JB. Rectal abscesses in cancer patients. Lancet 1972: 844–847.

Sickles EA, Greene WH, Wiernik PH. Clinical presentation of infection in granulocytopenic patients. Arch Intern Med 1975; 135:715–719.

Wade JC, Schimpff SC. Epidemiology and prevention of infection in the compromised host. In: Rubin RH, Young LS, eds. Clinical approach to infection in the compromised host. New York: Plenum Medical Book Company, 1988:5–40.

Young LS. Management of infections in leukemia and lymphoma. In: Rugin RH, Young LS, eds. Clinical approach to infection in the compromised host. New York: Plenum Medical Book Company, 1988:467–501.

ALLOGENEIC AND AUTOLOGOUS BONE MARROW TRANSPLANTATION

HILLARD M. LAZARUS, M.D.

In the late 1930s, the first attempts were made to transfer viable bone marrow cells from one individual to another as therapy for states of bone marrow failure (e.g., aplastic anemia and acute leukemia). In 1939, Osgood and co-workers reported a transient rise in peripheral blood counts after the use of massive marrow infusions for the therapy of a patient with aplastic anemia. These early attempts at marrow transplantation were unsuccessful for a variety of reasons, including a lack of knowledge regarding histocompatibility antigens and immunology and limited availability and understanding of the use of chemoradiation therapy. In the 1940s and 1950s, it was observed that radiation could be associated with significant damage to the bone marrow. The atomic age stimulated new preclinical investigations with marrow grafting in which many of the technical limitations were resolved. In 1960, Mathe and associates reported that two of three children with acute leukemia showed evidence of engraftment after conditioning with pretransplant total-body irradiation followed by allogeneic marrow infusion. In 1967, Thomas and colleagues successfully rescued a Gulf Oil worker accidently exposed to lethal doses of radiation (600 cGy) using marrow obtained from an identical twin (syngeneic graft), whereas a co-worker who also was acutely exposed to lethal irradiation (400 cGy) died of marrow failure in the absence of a marrow transplant. These dramatic cases ushered in the era of clinical bone marrow transplantation, spearheaded in the late 1960s by Dr. E.D. Thomas and colleagues at the Fred Hutchinson Cancer Research Center in Seattle, Washington. With the greater understanding of the major histocompatibility complex in humans, and advances in supportive care, clinical marrow transplantation was successfully undertaken. Bone marrow transplantation now occupies an important place in the treatment of cancer as well as in other marrow injury states, such as were incurred in the nuclear disaster at Chernobyl in 1986. As a result, the number of transplants performed has dramatically risen over the past decade. Through 1986, more than 15,000 allogeneic bone marrow transplants (>3,000 annually), and more than 4,000 autologous transplants (>1,500 annually) have been performed worldwide.

DOSE-RESPONSE EFFECT OF ANTINEOPLASTIC AGENT THERAPY

Chemotherapy and radiotherapy can be used successfully to treat patients who have advanced malignant disease, but the use of high doses usually is impractical owing to bone marrow toxicity. Dose-related injury to the hematopoietic stem cells (which reside predominantly in the bone marrow) is the most common and serious toxicity for the majority of chemotherapeutic agents and extensive radiotherapy. On the other hand,

significantly greater antitumor effects are noted when increasing quantities of drug are administered. Ionizing radiation and most drugs exhibit a log-linear relationship between tumor cell kill and dose over a certain range, and small changes in dose can produce significant changes in antitumor response. A great deal of laboratory and clinical data indicate that more intense cytotoxic drug treatment results in greater tumor reduction. Treatment with high doses of antineoplastic agents in leukemia and lymphoma results in improved antitumor effect and has led to cure in certain instances, whereas lower doses of the same agents did not. Hence, approaches that circumvent toxicity to the marrow during high-dose chemoradiation therapy are likely to be associated with improved antitumor effect. This idea is the aim of bone marrow transplantation. For example, in one of the earliest trials that was undertaken in a case of relapsed Burkitt's lymphoma, lower doses of an alkylating agent such as cyclophosphamide were ineffective in producing remission, but high doses were associated with significant antitumor effect. In fact, high doses of cyclophosphamide given in association with other agents (BACT therapy, BCNU, ara-C, cyclophosphamide, 6-thioguanine) and followed by infusion of bone marrow resulted in cure in 3 of 14 patients with end-stage Burkitt's lymphoma treated at the National Cancer Institute in the early 1970s. The infusion of hematopoietic stem cells, e.g., bone marrow transplantation, circumvents the problem of marrow suppression, permitting chemoradiation therapy doses to be escalated to the "myeloablative" range. Table 1 shows a comparison of the doses commonly used in conventional fashion versus those doses frequently used as part of a bone marrow transplant regimen. In both cases, the agents are usually used in combinations. Some agents, such as busulfan or thiotepa, are given at a more than tenfold dose increase above conventional regimens during transplant, whereas

Table 1 Comparison of Frequently Used Doses of Various Cytotoxic Agents: Conventional Doses Versus Bone Marrow Transplant (BMT) Doses

Agent	Conventional Dose	BMT Dose	Limiting Toxicity
BCNU (Carmustine)	100–200 mg/m^2	300–900 mg/m^2	Hepatic, pulmonary
Mitomycin-C	10–15 mg/m^2	40–60 mg/m^2	Hepatic, pulmonary, cardiac
Melphalan	20–30 mg/m^2	100–200 mg/m^2	Gastrointestinal
TBI	—	300–1,575 cGy	Pulmonary
Cyclophosphamide	15–38 mg/kg	120–260 mg/kg	Cardiac; genitourinary
Cisplatin	50–120 mg/m^2	150–200 mg/m^2	Renal
Cytarabine	700–1,000 mg/m^2	18,000–36,000 mg/m^2	Central nervous system, hepatic, gastrointestinal
Etoposide (VP-16)	300–500 mg/m^2	1,200–2,400 mg/m^2	Gastrointestinal
Carboplatin	200–400 mg/m^2	1,600–2,000 mg/m^2	Hepatic
Ifosfamide	4,000–8,000 mg/m^2	12,000–16,000 mg/m^2	Central nervous system, genitourinary
Thiotepa	30–60 mg/m^2	750–1,200 mg/m^2	Gastrointestinal, central nervous system
Busulfan	0.05–0.10 mg/kg (daily dose)	16 mg/kg	Hepatic, pulmonary
Mitoxantrone	14–30 mg/m^2	60 mg/m^2	Gastrointestinal, hepatic

TBI = Total body irradiation.

in other cases, only a two- to threefold dose increase is employed.

HEMATOPOIETIC STEM CELLS

Hematopoietic stem cells, which are usually obtained from the bone marrow, provide the ability to produce all of the circulating peripheral blood cell elements (red cells, white cells, and platelets). The data to support the concept of a hematopoietic stem cell was generated more than 30 years ago in experimental systems. Animals exposed to total-body irradiation, ablative to the immunologic and hematologic systems, could be rescued by infusion of bone marrow or spleen cells from littermates. Within 1 to 2 weeks, clonal colonies developed in the spleen, and later in the marrow cavity. When hematopoietic cell suspensions are separated into individual cells and grown in vitro using agar or methylcellulose, they give rise to small collections of progeny. These colony-forming units (CFUs) led to the concept of the hematopoietic stem cell, a multipotential cell that gives rise to all mature peripheral blood elements. This cell also has the capacity for self-renewal as well as the ability to restore hematopoietic and immunologic function after transfer to animals and persons deficient in these functions. Because it is not possible to identify the actual stem cell using morphologic or immunologic techniques, stem cells have traditionally been assayed using surrogate assays such as those for CFU-GM (colony-forming unit–granulocyte/macrophage) or CFU-GEMM (colony-forming unit–granulocyte, erythroid, macrophage, megakaryocyte). Recent data suggest that, with immunophenotyping studies, a more accurate estimate of stem cells can be made; marrow or blood cells that are simultaneously positive for the CD34 surface antigen and negative for the CD33 antigen using dual laser flow cytometry analysis may be the phenotypic stem cells.

These hematopoietic stem cells used for infusion or "rescue" after myeloablative therapy or bone marrow failure may be obtained from several sources: an identical twin (syngeneic transplant), an HLA-identical relative, usually a sibling (allogeneic transplant), or marrow previously obtained from the patient (autologous transplant). It also has been recognized for some time that hematopoietic stem cells are present in peripheral blood in small numbers. By using sophisticated leukapheresis technology, these cells can be collected and stored for later re-infusion to restore hematopoietic function after intensive chemoradiation therapy. Peripheral blood autologous stem cell transplants are being conducted with increasing frequency in patients who, because of marrow involvement with tumor, formerly would not have been considered candidates for intensive chemoradiation therapy programs. More recently, peripheral blood stem cell infusions are being used in conjunction with autologous marrow transplantation. Gianni and co-workers have reported that patients with breast cancer and lymphoma who were receiving combined marrow and peripheral blood stem cell infusions had almost complete elimination of the neutropenic period that accompanies transplantation (see section on hematopoietic growth factors). Two other unusual sources of stem cells include umbilical cord blood and fetal liver. Hematopoietic reconstitution using umbilical cord blood from an HLA-identical sibling as part of successful therapy for Fanconi's anemia was reported by Gluckman and colleagues. Rarely, fetal liver may be used as the stem cell source.

The bone marrow obtained from a normal donor contains lymphohematopoietic cells, which can be used to provide replacement cells in patients who have marrow failure (i.e., aplastic anemia) or congenital immunodeficiency states (i.e., severe combined immunodeficiency syndrome, or SCIDS). Similarly, infusions of these lymphohematopoietic cells can be used to correct the defect due to a congenital cellular enzyme deficiency (e.g., in storage diseases such as the mucopolysaccharidoses). The recent advances in genetic engineering technology eventually may make gene insertion via autologous bone marrow transplantation a future therapeutic option. Patients whose genetic defects (e.g., adenoside deaminase deficiency) could be corrected by providing a normal gene through the infused bone marrow theoretically could be cured with such procedures. Thus, bone marrow transplantation has a number of other potential applications, not only the treatment of malignant disorders (Table 2).

ALTERNATIVE BONE MARROW DONORS

In the past, allogeneic marrow transplants used only HLA-identical siblings as donors. More recently, the technique of employing unrelated HLA-identical or partially HLA-matched relatives as allogeneic bone marrow transplant donors has met with success in clinical trials and has resulted in a significant increase of activity in this area. Newer immunosuppressive agents such as cyclosporine, along with improved supportive care techniques (e.g., protective environment, more effective antimicrobial agents) and more effective in vitro purging techniques, have facilitated this strategy. The hope is to catalogue the HLA type of enormous numbers of normal persons so that more patients will have a potential donor. Donor registries have been developed that enroll pheresis donors and other persons. These registries have begun to interact with other registries in France, Great Britain, and Canada. Another, albeit more investigative approach is the ongoing research in developing cadaveric bone marrow banks. Cadaver marrow could be harvested, T-cell depleted, cryopreserved, and stored for potential later use. Such a strategy may be theoretically appealing, but many technical problems remain at present.

GOALS OF BONE MARROW TRANSPLANTATION

The first bone marrow transplants were attempted for aplastic anemia, but they were unsuccessful for a variety of reasons. Little was understood or appreciated regarding hematopoietic stem cell physiology, procurement, or administration, and supportive care techniques were extremely ineffective. In the mid-1960s, the stage was set for the clinical application of this modality. Sufficient preclinical data had been generated to guide investigators, and many advances in supportive care had been made (e.g., better antibiotics, improved blood banking practices, and so forth). It has been almost 20 years since the initial bone marrow transplants were performed successfully in patients who had advanced leukemia. The aim of these trials was to rid the patient of the diseased marrow and provide normal bone marrow from a sibling as replacement. It was recognized that the patient had to receive immunosuppressive therapy (as well as antineoplastic therapy) to prevent rejection of the foreign marrow (graft rejection). In addition to having refractory or unresponsive disease, many patients developed opportunistic infections that were very difficult to treat. Other patients succumbed to complications of the transplant, such as a regimen-related toxicity like interstitial pneumonitis. In addition,

despite matching at the major histocompatibility loci (HLA), many patients developed fatal graft-versus-host disease, a complex syndrome in which the immunocompetent lymphocytes of the donor (graft) marrow attack the patient (host) and result in a serious disorder (graft-versus-host disease). Despite these obstacles, about 10 percent of these patients with end-stage acute leukemia were cured of their disease. Seven of 56 patients with acute lymphoblastic leukemia and 6 of 54 patients with acute nonlymphocytic leukemias in relapse (13 of 110) transplanted at the Fred Hutchinson Cancer Research Center from 1970 to 1976 survived at least 10 years after transplant. This remarkable experience set the stage for more widespread use of this technique.

TOXICITIES AND TECHNIQUES OF BONE MARROW TRANSPLANTATION

All chemotherapeutic agents, radiation therapy, and biologic response modifier therapies can damage normal tissues to varying degrees. With increased doses administered in the course of transplantation, it is anticipated that there will be more organs affected and greater toxicity that approaches the tolerance of many normal tissues. The intense chemoradiation therapy used in preparing the patient to undergo allogeneic or autologous bone marrow transplantation (sometimes referred to as the conditioning regimen) causes many of the same complications observed with conventional-dose chemoradiation therapy. In addition, additional organ toxicities uncommonly associated with conventional therapy occur at a much increased frequency as a result of the significantly more intense treatment regimen. Table 3 shows some of the organ toxicities that develop as a result of exposure to high doses of chemoradiation therapy. Approximately 5 percent to 10 percent of patients may die as a result of early complications of the preparative regimen. Patients who have pre-existing organ dysfunction at the time of transplant (e.g., hepatocellular dysfunc-

Table 2 Potential Applications for the Use of Bone Marrow Transplantation in Both Malignant and Non-Malignant Conditions

Non-Malignant Disorders
Acquired
  Aplastic Anemia
  Paroxysmal noctural hemoglobinuria
  Myelofibrosis

Congenital
  Immunodeficiency syndromes (severe combined immunodeficiency syndrome, chronic mucocutaneous candidiasis)
  Hematologic defects
    Hemoglobinopathies (thalassemia, sickle cell anemia)
    Wiscott-Aldrich syndrome
    Fanconi's anemia
    Diamond-Blackfan anemia
    Gaucher's disease
    Congenital neutropenia
    Chediak-Hagashi syndrome
    Chronic granulomatous disease
  Osteoporosis
  Mucopolysaccharidoses (Hurler syndrome, Hunter syndrome)
  Mucolipidoses (metachromatic leukodystrophy)
  Lysosomal diseases (Lesch-Nyhan syndrome)

Malignant Disorders
  Acute leukemia (lymphocytic, non-lymphocytic)
  Chronic myelogenous leukemia
  Hairy cell leukemia
  Myelodysplastic syndromes (pre-leukemia)
  Lymphoma (Hodgkin's, non-Hodgkin's)
  Multiple myeloma
  Chronic lymphocytic leukemia
  Various solid tumors, including
    Breast cancer
    Small-cell lung cancer
    Germ cell tumors (testicular, extragonadal)
    Neuroblastoma
    Primary brain tumors
    Malignant melanoma
    Ovarian cancer

Table 3 Organ Toxicities That Can Occur During Bone Marrow Transplantation

Affected Organ	Potential Toxicity
Marrow	Pancytopenia, bacteremia, fungemia, hemorrhage
Gastrointestinal tract	Nausea, vomiting, oral mucositis, esophagitis, enterocolitis
Liver	Veno-occlusive disease, hepatitis
Lung	Interstitial pneumonitis, infectious pneumonia, bronchiolitis obliterans, intra-alveolar hemorrhage, pulmonary veno-occlusive disease
Heart	Hemorrhagic pericarditis, cardiomyopathy
Genitourinary tract	Tubular and glomerular injury, hemorrhagic cystitis
Central nervous system	Seizures, tremors, leukoencephalopathy
Eye	Cataracts

tion), advanced age (>60 years of age), poor performance status, active infection, or large, bulky tumor generally represent a significantly higher risk group for early mortality.

Technique of Bone Marrow Harvesting and Infusion Procedures

The technique of obtaining bone marrow for clinical use has been well developed. In many ways, the procurement of bone marrow differs little from the commonly used technique of performing a diagnostic bone marrow aspiration. Although in the past patients or normal donors generally were hospitalized for short periods to facilitate care, more recently some groups have reported that, in select cases, marrow harvest could safely be performed in an ambulatory surgical setting. The patient or normal bone marrow donor is taken to a sterile operating room, and general, spinal, or epidural anesthesia is administered. Then, the patient or normal bone marrow donor is placed in the prone position, and through a series of aspirations, bone marrow is harvested from the posterior (and sometimes anterior) iliac crests. These aspirations are accomplished by making three or four skin-puncture sites on each posterior hemipelvis using 10- or 11-gauge needles (which are considerably larger than those used for diagnostic testing). Also, multiple (rather than single) aspirations are performed. Usually 15 ml of bone marrow per kilogram of patient weight or more is removed in the course of a marrow harvest, which generally takes several hours to perform. In practice, over 1,000 to 1,500 ml of marrow is obtained. Intraoperatively, the marrow aliquots are continuously agitated gently in a vessel containing a balanced salt, amino acid, and glucose-containing solution (which provides a favorable environment for the cells) and heparin (to prevent marrow coagulation during the harvest procedure). At the completion of the harvest, the marrow is processed to produce a single-cell suspension.

In the case of an allogeneic marrow transplant, the marrow usually is processed and infused shortly thereafter, although rarely allogeneic marrow may be cryopreserved for later use. Allogeneic marrow may be manipulated in the laboratory for the purposes of removing incompatible red blood cells or plasma. The major histocompatibility loci (HLA-A, B, C, and D/Dr) are the important considerations in successfully completing an allogeneic marrow transplant. Red blood cell ABO incompatibilities between the patient and donor do not preclude performing a marrow transplant. The ABO incompatible bone marrow can be separated using centrifugation, hydroxyethyl starch sedimentation, or devices that employ the principles of affinity chromatography to remove the undesired or incompatible elements from donor marrow. The patient or recipient need not necessarily undergo specific therapy in preparation for a "minor" ABO incompatible graft (e.g., O-positive donor and A-positive patient). In this case, ABO incompatible donor plasma can easily be removed from the marrow prior to infusion. Conversely, in the case of a "major" incompatibility (e.g., A-positive donor

and O-positive patient), the patient must be protected from the consequences of receiving incompatible red blood cells. The patient may need to undergo a plasma exchange or plasmapheresis procedure in order to lower or remove plasma isoagglutinins. In some cases, the patient may receive infusions of donor-type ABO red cells (in small quantities) immediately before marrow infusion to adsorb isoagglutinins in order to prevent or reduce hemolytic transfusion reactions.

Autologous bone marrow, on the other hand, can be obtained, cryopreserved (frozen), and infused at a later date (days or even years after harvest). Marrow cryopreservation is a complex procedure designed to minimize cell damage during the freezing process. Freezing causes a change of state (e.g., liquid to solid phase) and will irreversibly damage cells unless a specific agent is used to protect cells. Dimethyl sulfoxide (DMSO), the most effective cryoprotective agent, is used at 5 to 10 percent final concentration along with patient plasma or human serum albumin. Glycerol, used to freeze red blood cells, is not an effective marrow cryopreservation agent. Recently, agents such as hydroxyethyl starch or pentastarch have been shown to be effective cryopreservative agents. The marrow mixture is frozen usually by using a controlled-rate liquid nitrogen freezing apparatus that minimizes the freezing injury by slowly lowering the temperature, and the marrow is stored in a liquid nitrogen refrigerator ($-196°C$). Recently, several investigators have demonstrated successful recovery of marrow progenitor cells without the aid of a controlled-rate freezer and a liquid nitrogen refrigerator for storage. Using special techniques, they showed that cells remained viable at $-140°C$ storage. It is unknown how long cryopreserved marrow will remain viable in long-term storage. Many centers have successfully transplanted marrow that has been in storage for many years. There is concern, however, that with prolonged storage (especially for marrow purged in vitro), stem cells may not be viable after thawing and re-infusion.

Because of the large number of cells and resultant highly viscous nature, allogeneic marrow (nonfrozen) or autologous bone marrow (which has been thawed in a 37°C water bath) must be infused intravenously via a large-bore central venous catheter. Marrow infusions usually take several hours to complete. In the case of an autologous marrow transplant, a total of at least 1.0×10^8 nucleated marrow cells (0.5×10^8 mononuclear cells) per kilogram of patient weight is required to ensure engraftment. Allogeneic transplant patients often require more cells in order to avoid engraftment failure. Therefore, at least 3.0×10^8 nucleated allogeneic cells per kilogram of patient weight usually are infused. Cryopreserved marrow takes somewhat longer to reconstitute in the recipient than infusions of fresh marrow. This finding is explained by suggesting that the cells first need to recover in vivo from the effects of the freeze-thaw injury.

Graft-Versus-Host Disease

This syndrome results from donor lymphocytes (graft) recognizing patient cell-surface antigens (host) as foreign. Although both the patient and the donor may be matched at the major histocompatibility loci, minor antigenic differences are not easily detected, which explains the development of this syndrome. Graft-versus-host disease (GVHD) may occur early after the transplant, in which case it is termed *acute GVHD*, or it can occur later, when it is termed *chronic GVHD*. These entities differ considerably in clinical characteristics (Table 4). Up to 40 percent of recipients of HLA-matched and 75 percent of HLA-mismatched recipients undergoing allogeneic bone marrow transplant will develop evidence of moderate to severe (grade ≥ II) GVHD (Table 5). Factors reported to increase the risk of GVHD include older age (of patient or donor) and sex-mismatched donor-recipient pairs, particularly female-to-male transplants. In the case of female-to-male transplants, the parity status of the female donor is an important factor; use of nulliparous women is not associated with any greater incidence of GVHD than the use of male donors, whereas an increase in parity results in a greater chance for the development of GVHD. These observations suggest in vivo sensitization by the fetus.

Although GVHD often is a life-threatening complication of bone marrow transplantation, patients who develop GVHD also may develop additional antitumor benefit in the form of graft-versus-tumor effect. Thus, bone marrow transplantation is effective because of direct antitumor activity of drugs and radiation and some contribution of graft-versus-tumor effect.

Acute Graft-Versus-Host Disease

Acute GVHD affects the skin (rash), gastrointestinal tract (diarrhea), and liver (hepatocellular injury). In up to 40 percent of those affected, the syndrome is relatively mild and involves only the skin. In 20 to 25 percent of patients, however, acute GVHD may be severe and lead to death. Graft-versus-host disease is graded on a scale of 1 to 4 using a complex system that takes into account the degree of impairment of the organs usually affected, e.g., skin, liver, and gastrointestinal tract (see Table 5). Some centers have also used lung injury in determining the grade of GVHD.

Graft-versus-host disease is mediated by donor immunocompetent T cells. To avoid the consequences of GVHD, various prophylaxis regimens are employed to prevent T-cell proliferation. Prophylaxis for GVHD is begun before and continued for long periods after the transplant. Usually a potent immunosuppressive agent

such as cyclosporine is given, frequently in combination with another agent such as prednisone or methotrexate. Cyclosporine plus prednisone, or cyclosporine plus methotrexate, appear to be the most effective regimens, and these preventative approaches have resulted in a reduction of acute GVHD morbidity and mortality. Graft-versus-host disease that is not prevented or attenuated by the prophylaxis regimen may become severe and unresponsive to therapy. A variety of agents have been utilized in an effort to attentuate acute GVHD, including high-dose corticosteroids and antithymocyte globulin, but in some patients (up to 20 percent of severely affected patients), the syndrome may remain refractory to therapy and result in death. More recently, immunoconjugates such as anti-CD5 monoclonal antibody conjugated to ricin have been shown to be effective therapy for acute GVHD in some patients.

Chronic Graft-Versus-Host Disease

In about 35 to 40 percent of patients who survive at least 100 days after transplant, chronic GVHD may develop. In these patients, chronic GVHD may occur de novo (without antecedent acute GVHD) or develop as a consequence of progression following unresolved acute GVHD. Chronic GVHD is a distinctive syndrome resembling a collagen-vascular disorder like scleroderma. Abnormalities may develop in the skin, liver, gastrointestinal tract, secretory glands (sicca syndrome), and immune system (excessive nonspecific suppressor cell activity, leading to severe immunodeficiency and recurrent infections). Some patients may develop joint contractures, muscle wasting, and progressive, destructive bronchiolitis. Chronic GVHD is classified clinicopathologically into limited or extensive stages. In the limited stage, there is localized skin involvement or hepatic dysfunction. Extensive chronic GVHD is defined as either generalized skin involvement, or localized skin involvement or hepatic dysfunction *plus* (1) marked hepatic derangement on liver biopsy; (2) involvement of lacrimal or salivary glands; or (3) involvement of any other target organ. Graft-versus-host disease usually is treated with immunosuppressive agents such as glucocorticoids, azathioprine, cyclosporine, or a combination thereof. More recently, thalidomide (the teratogenic agent) has been shown to be highly effective in the treatment of chronic GVHD.

Patients who develop acute or chronic GVHD are at increased risk to develop serious or life-threatening

Table 4 Comparison of Acute Versus Chronic Graft-Versus-Host Disease

	Acute GVHD	*Chronic GVHD*
Onset (days after transplant)	Days 20 to 100	After day 100
Organs involved	Skin, liver, gastrointestinal tract	Widespread, including skin, liver, musculoskeletal, gastrointestinal tract, lungs, eyes, salivary glands
Pathologic features	Primarily epithelial cell destruction	Mixed epithelial and mesenchymal destruction

Table 5 Staging of Acute Graft-Versus-Host Disease

Individual Organ Severity Due to Graft-Versus-Host Disease*
Skin

Stage	+1	Maculopapular eruption involving less than 25% of the body surface
	+2	Maculopapular eruption involving 25%–50% of the body surface
	+3	Generalized erythroderma
	+4	Generalized erythroderma with bullous formation and often with desquamation

Liver

Stage	+1	Moderate increase of the transaminase SGOT (150–750 IU) and serum bilirubin (2.0–3.0 mg/100 ml);
	+2	Bilirubin rise (3–5.9 mg/100 ml) with or without an increase in SGOT
	+3	Bilirubin rise (6–14.9 mg/100 ml) with or without an increase in SGOT
	+4	Bilirubin rise to >15 mg/100 ml with or without an increase in SGOT

Diarrhea

Stage	+1	>30 ml/kg or >500 ml of stool/day or positive biopsy for GVHD
	+2	>60 ml/kg or >1.000 ml of stool/day
	+3	>90 ml/kg or >1.500 ml of stool/day
	+4	>90 ml/kg with abdominal pain or >2,000 ml of stool/day

Cultures for cytomegalovirus and *Clostridium difficile*-toxin negative, or mucosal-positive biopsy for GVHD

Grading of Acute Graft-Versus-Host Disease

Based on the severity and number of organ systems involved, patients are placed into four categories:

Grade 1 is +1 to +2 rash without gut or liver involvement and no decrease in performance status or fever.

Grade 2 is +1 gastrointestinal involvement or +1 liver involvement, or both, or stage +3 skin alone.

Grade 3 is +2 to +4 gastrointestinal involvement or +2 to +4 liver involvement.

Grade 4 is skin bullae and desquamation with or without visceral disease, or performance score decreased to ≤40% because of GVHD.

*Blume KG, Petz LD, eds. Clinical bone marrow transplantation. New York, Churchill Livingston, 1983. Adapted from Glucksberg H, Storb R, Fefer A, et al. Clinical manifestations of graft-versus-host disease in human recipients of marrow from HLA-matched sibling donors. Transplantation 1974; 18:295–304.

infections. Graft-versus-host disease itself is a syndrome of disordered immunity in which the immunologic system has not yet fully reconstituted yet is directing its responses at host organs rather than defending the host from the danger of infiltration by microorganisms. In addition, the immunosuppressive agents used to suppress GVHD (e.g., cyclosporine, corticosteroids) are themselves potent agents that reduce host immunity. Thus, the majority of patients with severe GVHD develop infections or experience infections that trigger an increased response in the immune system and worsen GVHD.

In Vitro Tests to Predict Occurrence of GVHD

It had been thought that allogeneic bone marrow transplantation always required the use of GVHD prophylaxis therapy. Our group at the Ireland Cancer Center showed that, in some patients, GVHD prophylaxis was not necessary, because GVHD either was mild or did not occur in such patients. These observations were corroborated by the group at the University of Florida, leading to in-depth investigations into predicting which donor-recipient pairs are likely to develop GVHD.

Vogelsang and colleagues at Johns Hopkins Oncology Center have developed new techniques that may predict which individuals are likely to develop GVHD. These complex assays utilize a skin biopsy and lymphocytes from the patient and the prospective donor. Donor lymphocytes are reacted with host lymphocytes in vitro and then are incubated for several days with patient skin (termed a *skin explant assay*). The skin then is fixed, stained, and examined for infiltration by donor lymphocytes. The results of this test correlate well with the clinical development of GVHD if a transplant is performed later, i.e., those patients whose skin biopsy does not have donor lymphocyte infiltration usually do not develop GVHD. The individuals who have a positive skin explant test frequently will manifest GVHD. This work is in the process of being tested in a prospective trial using the results of this technique in treatment planning. Patients in whom the skin explant assay predicts that GVHD will not develop may undergo an allogeneic bone marrow transplantation without the use of GVHD prophylaxis therapy. Such an approach may be beneficial, because these patients will not be exposed to the risks of posttransplant immunosuppressive therapy.

CONTRASTING ALLOGENEIC VERSUS AUTOLOGOUS MARROW TRANSPLANTATION

Both allogeneic and autologous bone marrow transplantation have potential and practical limitations and benefits (Table 6). Autologous bone marrow transplantation offers much wider application, because each patient serves as the donor. This statement presupposes that the autologous marrow is not grossly contaminated by tumor and is adequate in terms of number of marrow stem cells. In contrast, because the major histocompatibility complex (located on chromosome 6) is inherited in co-dominant fashion, there is only a 25 percent chance that a patient's sibling will be HLA-identical and can be used as an allograft donor. In addition, owing to the posttransplant immunosuppression to prevent GVHD, patients usually tolerate the side effects of an autologous marrow transplant much better than those of an allogeneic transplant. In fact, many centers will not perform allogeneic transplantation for patients over the age of 45 to 50 years. This approach is based, in part, on data that show that the likelihood of developing GVHD increases dramatically with increasing age of the patient or donor. Autologous bone marrow transplant patients are not at risk for the development of GVHD (except in isolated situations). Thus, more patients are theoretically likely to be candidates for autologous bone marrow transplantation.

Table 6 Advantages and Disadvantages of Allogeneic Versus Autologous
Bone Marrow Transplantation

Donor Type	Advantage	Disadvantage
Autologous	More donors Rarely GVHD (see text) No graft rejection No pre- and posttransplant immunosuppression Better tolerated in older patients	Occult marrow tumor No graft-versus-leukemia Stem cell damage (from previous chemotherapy)
Allogeneic	Normal donor Graft-versus-leukemia	Fewer donors GVHD Graft rejection Pre- and posttransplant immunosuppression Increased risk for interstitial pneumonitis Less well tolerated in older patients
Syngeneic (identical twin)	Normal marrow No GVHD No graft rejection No pre- and posttransplant immunosuppression	Rare donor No graft-versus-leukemia

Autologous or Syngeneic Graft-Versus-Host Disease

Autologous or syngeneic GVHD can occur rarely owing to a complex regulatory phenomenon that arises between the host (who has undergone treatment) and the re-infused marrow cells. These autologous or syngeneic marrow cells may somehow recognize the treated host as different. This particular type of GVHD reaction generally is quite mild and self-limited, unlike allogeneic GVHD. Recent work from studies performed at Johns Hopkins Oncology Center has demonstrated that autologous GVHD can be induced by the use of low doses of cyclosporine for several weeks. It is hoped that inducement of mild, self-limited GVHD (usually confined to skin only) will provide additional antitumor response through the graft-versus-tumor effect. Of course, patients undergoing allogeneic or autologous bone marrow transplantation must receive only blood product transfusions that have been externally irradiated by 1,500 to 3,000 cGy to inactivate immunocompetent lymphocytes contained in the product that could mediate an inadvertent GVHD reaction, referred to as *transfusion-associated GVHD*. The problem of inadvertent GVHD is becoming increasingly appreciated in other severely immunocompromised patients who receive blood products, such as lymphoma patients, neonates, or solid-organ (heart, liver) transplant patients. Recently, cases have been reported in which surgical patients have developed a GVHD-like syndrome called *postoperative erythroderma*, which results from infusions of normal viable lymphocytes homozygous for one of the host HLA haplotypes.

Allogeneic Bone Marrow Purging

In an effort to reduce GVHD, allogeneic marrow may be manipulated to remove the immunocompetent lymphocytes that mediate the graft-versus-host reaction. This type of marrow treatment is referred to as in vitro purging or ex vivo treatment of allogeneic marrow. A variety of methods are in use and include physical (elutriation of lymphocytes), pharmacologic (agents that have antilymphoid effects, such as corticosteroids or deoxycoformycin), and immunologic (monoclonal antibodies linked to toxins, isotopes, or used with complement) procedures, to name a few. Although such lymphocyte-depletion techniques have been useful in reducing the number of infused immunocompetent T cells and reducing or eliminating graft-versus-host disease, three problems have emerged with this approach. First, some patients suffer graft rejection after T-cell depletion, in part because some specific T-cell subsets may be necessary to facilitate engraftment. Graft rejection is rare and occurs in less than 2 percent of patients receiving bone marrow transplants from HLA-identical donors, but it occurs in about 15 percent of recipients of HLA-nonidentical transplants. The risk of failure to engraft is substantially increased if in vitro T-cell depletion techniques are used to prevent GVHD (15 percent of HLA-matched and 30 to 50 percent of HLA-mismatched grafts). More intensive pre- or posttransplant immune suppression may be required to prevent this problem.

Second, patients who undergo a T-cell–depleted allogeneic bone marrow transplant have a higher relapse rate than those patients who receive an unmanipulated marrow graft. These data are similar to those obtained using syngeneic (twin) transplants in patients with acute myelogenous leukemia in first remission who have a threefold (60 percent) relapse rate compared to HLA-identical sibling transplants. The current belief is that the immunocompetent T cells of the donor contribute to the antitumor effect of the regimen, e.g., the so-called graft-versus-leukemia or graft-versus-tumor effect. In animals, GVHD can be separated from graft-versus-leukemia, and it is unclear whether this is the case in man. Graft-versus-host disease can be eliminated in gnotobiotic ("germ-free") mice without affecting graft-versus-leukemia effect. In man, the competing processes of reduced GVHD versus increased relapse and graft rejection appear to cancel out, so that lymphocyte-depletion techniques have not resulted in an overall improved patient survival.

Finally, recent data have emerged that indicate that patients may develop lymphoproliferative disorders after undergoing T-cell—depleted bone marrow transplants. This finding of B-cell neoplastic states is higher in patients who have received T-cell–depleted histoincompatible transplants.

Autologous Bone Marrow Purging

Autologous bone marrow may be purged in the laboratory after the marrow harvest in an attempt to remove any potential contaminating tumor cells. The question of whether purging is necessary is controversial; it is sometimes difficult to show an effect when attempting to remove undetectable tumor cells. More importantly, most patients relapse from tumor deposits that were not eradicated by the preparative regimen rather than from infusion of occult tumor in the marrow. Thus, it is hard to show that purging improves the therapy. A case in point are the data from several studies in Europe on acute myelogenous leukemia transplants using unpurged marrow. One study reviewed the data obtained from 263 patients undergoing autologous bone marrow transplant at many centers: in vitro purging using a variety of methods was performed in 80 patients, whereas 183 patients received unpurged marrow. Fifty-three percent of the group who received unpurged marrow (96 patients) remain alive and disease-free at least 2 years after transplant. In a large percentage of these patients, autologous bone marrow transplant was performed many months after a complete remission was attained. Consolidation or intensification therapy was continued for several cycles to these patients prior to enrollment on a transplant protocol. It is suggested that the use of additional chemotherapy prior to marrow harvest and transplant may just add a few logs of leukemic cell kill in a situation in which the leukemic cell population already is small and can be eradicated before it has regrown beyond a certain critical mass, e.g., that the marrow in these patients was purged in vivo.

As in the allogeneic situation, autologous marrow purging technology is quite advanced. Numerous methods are in use at many centers and include photoactive (merocyanin), pharmacologic (4-hydroperoxycyclophosphamide or mafosfamide, etoposide, methylprednisolone), and immunologic (monoclonal antibodies used in conjunction with complement or conjugated to toxins or radionuclides as immunotoxins, or use of lymphokine-activated killer cells [LAK cells]). One particularly interesting immunologic technique employs latex particles that contain minutely dispersed grains of iron oxide. These "magnetizable" microspheres or beads are coated with antimouse antibodies. To purge marrow, murine monoclonal antibodies directed against the tumor are added to the marrow suspension and mixed; later, the coated latex beads are added. The entire mixture is placed in a strong magnetic field that retains the tumor cells adherent to the magnetic beads, and the normal marrow progenitors can be collected.

Recent data have demonstrated that combinations of agents or methods are more likely to reduce tumor contamination by as many as 5 to 6 logs, compared to only 2 to 3 logs when only a single aspect of purging is utilized. For example, monoclonal antibody used in conjunction with 4-hydroperoxycyclophosphamide is considerably more effective than use of each purging agent individually. Such combination purging is extremely time-consuming and labor-intensive, and requires larger quantities of marrow to work with, because cell loss and cell damage are greater. Combinations of agents and techniques, however, likely will be required, because some tumor cells may be quite resistant to a single modality. For example, acute lymphocytic leukemia cells have been shown to be much more resistant in vitro to either 4-hydroperoxycyclophosphamide or radiation than acute myelogenous leukemia cells.

Long-Term In Vitro Marrow Growth

Another novel approach in the area of marrow purging is the use of marrow cultured in vitro for many days or weeks (long-term maintenance "Dexter cultures"). It has been noted that cancerous progenitor cells will lose their malignant phenotype in long-term culture (e.g., disappearance of the Philadelphia chromosome in chronic myelogenous leukemia). The normal stem cells may be expanded and the abnormal cells reduced in numbers, so that autologous marrow may be used for transplant in diseases such as acute or chronic myelogenous leukemia. This approach has been used most effectively, albeit in small numbers of patients, because of the ability to track the abnormal clone (Philadelphia chromosome), and because patients with chronic myelogenous leukemia receive less intense therapy in chronic phase. Small marrow samples are taken and cultured in vitro for 4 to 5 weeks. The goals are to determine if the Philadelphia chromosome-containing hematopoietic progenitors die out in culture, and if the patient's "normal" progenitors exceed at least 2 percent of progenitors present in cultures of marrow samples obtained from normal volunteers. Should these criteria be met, the patient likely may be a candidate for this type of autologous bone marrow transplantation procedure. Patients who have not been exposed to agents more toxic to stem cells (busulfan rather than hydroxyurea or alpha interferon) for long periods of time are more likely to have less stem cell damage and be eligible for such an approach.

TIMING AND RESULTS OF MARROW TRANSPLANTATION

The best results for transplantation are obtained in patients who are best able to withstand the intense nature of the treatment. In particular, this group includes younger patients, patients who have otherwise good visceral organ (heart, liver, lung, renal) function, and those patients who have a disease that has responded to cytotoxic therapy in the past or who have a low tumor burden or are in complete remission at the time of transplant. Older patients and patients with a history of remote or active cardiovascular, pulmonary, renal, or hepatic dysfunction may fare poorly or die during transplant owing to the recrudescence of organ dysfunction. Most importantly, patients who have never achieved a remission (primary refractory disease) or patients who had a responding disease that now is shown to be resistant to therapy immediately before transplant are much less likely to benefit from the intense antitumor treatment.

Allogeneic bone marrow transplantation has been shown to be associated with significantly better results than continued conventional chemotherapy in patients with acute nonlymphocytic leukemia in first complete remission. Appelbaum and colleagues at the Fred Hutchinson Cancer Research Center reported a series of 111 consecutive patients aged 17 to 50 years with acute myeloid leukemia. A total of 90 patients attained remission; 44 patients had an HLA-identical sibling and were assigned transplant, and 33 underwent transplant. The remaining 46 patients who did not have a donor were assigned to receive conventional chemotherapy. Five-year disease-free survival in the transplant group was 48 percent compared to only 21 percent in the chemotherapy group, which strongly suggests that transplant should be offered to patients who achieve remission, are of a suitable age and medical condition, and have a compatible donor. HLA status was not a factor. Other studies have suggested that such therapy be reserved for patients with acute myeloid leukemia in second complete response.

In a review by Singer and Goldstone, only 11 of 398 patients (2.8 percent) with non-Hodgkin's lymphoma were alive in complete remission 2 years after conventional salvage chemotherapy treatment. Similar data are available for patients with Hodgkin's disease who relapsed on therapy or within 1 year after completion of initial therapy. Recent data strongly suggest that autologous bone marrow transplantation is considerably more effective than conventional salvage therapy for relapsed lymphoma. Transplantation at first relapse or second remission results in a 2-year disease-free survival of 20 to 50 percent. Armitage and colleagues reported the experience of the Nebraska Lymphoma Study Group for patients with non-Hodgkin's lymphoma in first relapse who were under the age 60 years during the period from 1982 to 1987. Twelve of 17 patients achieved complete response after autologous marrow transplant, compared to only 3 of 17 conventionally treated relapsed patients in this nonrandomized study. Only one patient attained 2-year disease-free survival in the conventional salvage (cisplatin-containing) group, whereas nine autologous transplant patients achieved long-term disease-free survival. Gulati and colleagues at Memorial Sloan-Kettering Cancer Center designed a trial for patients with large-cell lymphoma who were believed to be at high risk for later relapse by comparing autologous transplant in remission versus conventional treatment as postremission therapy. Fourteen patients underwent autologous marrow transplant immediately after successful induction with the L-17M regimen, and 13 patients continued on conventional chemotherapy treatment. Eleven of 14 patients (79 percent) undergoing transplant after remission was attained remain alive and free of disease (31+ to 71+ months), compared to only 4 of 13 patients (31 percent) who continued to receive chemotherapy treatment (36+ to 64+ months). Of 17 patients (24 percent) undergoing transplant in relapse or after induction failure, only 4 patients remain disease-free (40+ to 64+ months). Thus, most investigators now favor transplant at first relapse, or, in selected patients, in first remission.

Allogeneic bone marrow transplantation may be performed in patients who have nonmalignant conditions or who have hematologic malignancies such as acute leukemia. In recent years, an increasing number of patients with diseases such as Hodgkin's and non-Hodgkin's lymphoma, multiple myeloma, myelodysplastic syndromes, and other disorders are undergoing allografting procedures. The best results are obtained in those patients transplanted in remission (Table 7).

Autologous marrow transplantation (with or without marrow purging) is performed most commonly for acute leukemia and lymphoma. There are striking

Table 7 Results of Allogeneic Marrow Transplantation for Various Disease Types and Stages

Disease	Stage	Probable Cure Rate (%)
Acute nonlymphocytic leukemia	First, second remission	40–60
Acute lymphocytic leukemia	First remission	50–60
	Second remission	20–40
Chronic myelogenous leukemia	Chronic phase	60–70
	Accelerated phase	30
	Blast crises	10

differences in the use of autotransplants between North America and Europe. Leukemia was the major indication for autotransplantation in Europe (59 percent), but leukemia accounted for only 6 percent of transplants in North America. On the other hand, lymphoma and solid tumors constituted 94 percent of the autologous transplants in North America.

Autologous transplantation is preferred for patients with acute leukemia who are older (aged 45 to 55 years for acute leukemia and aged 50 to 60 years for chronic leukemia) or for leukemia patients who do not have an HLA-A, B, C, or D/Dr compatible donor. It appears that the likelihood that GVHD will occur increases with increasing age of the patient (and donor). In addition, autologous marrow transplant does not require the use of posttransplant immunosuppressive agents (e.g., cyclosporine, prednisone), which can be associated with an increase in infectious complications that can have a high morbidity and mortality rate. Most autologous transplants have been performed in patients who have lymphoma or other diseases (Table 8).

AUTOLOGOUS MARROW TRANSPLANTS FOR SOLID TUMORS

Increasing numbers of patients with solid tumors are likely to benefit from this type of therapy. Such tumor types include breast cancer, neuroblastoma, and germ cell (testicular) cancers, and the early results are promising. The results of more than 750 autotransplants in breast cancer have been reported. Long-term survival has been observed in about 10 to 30 percent of patients with stage III or IV breast cancer when this therapy is administered early in the course of a patient with responding disease, but more striking results have been obtained in adjuvant fashion. Peters and co-workers at Duke have noted that 50 of 55 stage II or III patients with ten or more positive axillary nodes who underwent transplant as part of an adjuvant program remain alive and disease-free at least 1 year since transplant. These patients received four cycles of conventional adjuvant therapy (cyclophosphamide, adriamycin or doxorubicin, and 5-fluorouracil) that were followed by high-dose cyclophosphamide, BCNU, cisplatin, recombinant GM-

CSF, and stem cell re-infusion. Such an intriguing result needs to be corroborated in a multicenter trial.

Many centers are examining the role of intensive chemoradiation therapy and autologous bone marrow rescue for traditionally more resistant diseases such as brain tumors, colorectal cancer, lung cancer, and malignant melanoma. A unique approach that has recently been undertaken combines the high-dose therapy approach with the use of agents such as biochemical modulators. These agents increase the effect of alkylating agents by making the tumor cells more susceptible to attack or by interfering with the ability of the tumor cell to repair the chemotherapy-induced damage. For example, our trial using melphalan, misonidazole (a hypoxic cell sensitizer used as a biochemical modulator), and marrow re-infusion has shown dramatic antitumor effect in advanced colorectal cancer patients.

IMPROVED SUPPORTIVE CARE

The patient must be sustained through the time of chemoradiation therapy, the resultant injury to multiple organ systems, and the period of marrow recovery. This supportive phase is a critical component of successful transplantation. Advances in the blood banking sciences have enabled patients to receive relatively pure blood components (e.g., red blood cell transfusions virtually devoid of contaminating white blood cells), which reduces the chance for transfusion reactions. More compatible blood products also are available (e.g., HLA-identical platelet transfusions for the highly alloimmunized thrombocytopenic patient). The use of supportive care techniques, such as human intravenous immunoglobulin and newer antibacterial, antiviral, and antifungal agents, has reduced infectious deaths. For example, death due to cytomegalovirus (CMV) infections in the allograft (e.g., CMV interstitial pneumonitis) has been dramatically reduced using prophylaxis with serologically negative CMV blood products, intravenous immunoglobulin, and high-dose acyclovir. Similarly, overt CMV interstitial pneumonitis mortality has been reduced from 80 to 90 percent to 30 to 40 percent using hyperimmune CMV globulin or intravenous immunoglobulin and gancyclovir (DHPG) therapy.

Table 8 Results of Autologous Bone Marrow Transplantation for Various Disease Types and Stages

Disease	Stage	Probable Cure Rate (%)
Acute nonlymphocytic leukemia	First, second remission	35–50
Acute lymphocytic leukemia	First remission	30–50
	Second remission	20–25
Hodgkin's disease	Relapse	20–50
Non-Hodgkin's disease	Relapse	30–60
Breast cancer	Responding stage III or IV	10–30
	Adjuvant	Unknown
Germ cell tumor (testicular)	Refractory	20–30
Neuroblastoma	First remission	35–40

RECOMBINANT HEMATOPOIETIC GROWTH FACTORS IN MARROW TRANSPLANT

The use of newer cytotoxic agents, an improved understanding of pharmacokinetics and drug interactions, and improvements in marrow purging, processing and storage techniques, and supportive care (including newer antibiotics) have led to more widespread use of this therapy. Transplantation now is undertaken earlier in the course of a patient's illness. Another significant advance involves the use of recombinant hematopoietic growth factors to stimulate the growth of infused marrow after transplant. These products have been made available by the use of recombinant DNA technology. The normal human genes that control the production of marrow growth factors have been cloned and expressed in vitro in mammalian, bacterial, or yeast systems. This maneuver allows for the production of enormous quantities of these agents for clinical use. Normally, marrow reconstitution does not occur until several weeks after marrow infusion, at which time there is a rise in peripheral blood cell counts above critical levels; generally, this period is 2 to 3 weeks in allografts and 3 to 4 weeks in autologous transplants. Use of these growth factors in clinical transplant trials has resulted not only in earlier recovery of hematopoietic function but in a significant decrease in systemic infections (bacteremias, fungemias). These findings are due to recovery in marrow function in a quantitative sense as well as a qualitative sense, because the mature cells are activated by the growth factors and are more effective at antimicrobial killing. One of the most striking results of the use of recombinant growth factors is the observation that there was much less organ injury in patients who received these agents after transplant. Use of growth factors has led to significantly less renal, lung, and hepatic dysfunction, perhaps owing to effective eradication of an early undetected systemic infection.

Recombinant hematopoietic growth factors have been successfully used in conjunction with marrow transplantation. Brandt and colleagues reported a phase 1 trial in 48 patients with breast cancer and malignant melanoma who received daily infusions of mammalian-derived recombinant human GM-CSF beginning 3 hours after completion of marrow re-infusion. A dose of 2.0 to 32.0 μg per kilogram per day of glycosylated protein was given for up to 21 days, and a dose-dependent acceleration of myeloid recovery was noted. Compared to historic controls, bacteremia was decreased from 35 percent (8 of 23 historical patients) to 18 percent (9 of 48 patients receiving rhGM-CSF). Occurrence of bacteremia was limited to the first week of study. One of 47 and 1 of 46 patients experienced other documented bacterial infection during the second or third weeks, respectively. Although significant toxicity consisting of central catheter site thrombosis and a vascular leak-like syndrome ("capillary leak") was observed at the highest doses evaluated, the administration of rhGM-CSF was well tolerated at doses of 10 μg per kilogram per day or less of protein. In addition, considerably less renal, hepatic, and pulmonary dysfunction was noted in the study population compared to historic controls. In a phase 2 trial in patients with lymphoid malignancies, *Escherichia coli*–derived GM-CSF was infused at doses of 250 μg per square meter per day for 20 days after marrow transplant in a randomized placebo-controlled trial. Neutrophil count did not return significantly faster, but the group treated with GM-CSF had less renal dysfunction, fewer platelet transfusions, and faster platelet recovery. In addition, the group treated with GM-CSF was discharged significantly earlier (28 days versus 43 days), at a total cost of inpatient treatment of $79,000 versus $112,000. Similar findings have been noted in allogeneic marrow transplant trials; no increase in GVHD was noted.

One remaining problem is that the neutrophil count falls 30 to 60 percent within 24 to 72 hours of discontinuing growth factor infusions. Also, although the period of absolute neutropenia is shortened, severe neutropenia persists. A new approach is to combine marrow infusions with peripheral blood stem cell infusions obtained during growth factor stimulation of the patient. In a few small series of patients, infusions of these two cell preparations simultaneously and administration of recombinant growth factor have been shown to eliminate neutropenia almost completely. These intriguing results require corroboration in larger trials.

SUGGESTED READING

Santos GW. History of bone marrow transplantation. Clin Haematol 1983; 12:611–639.

Frei E III, Canellos GP. Dose: A critical factor in cancer chemotherapy. Am J Med 1980; 69:585–595.

Vogelsang GB, Hess AD, Santos GW. Acute graft-versus-host disease: Clinical characteristics in the cyclosporine era. Medicine 1988; 67:163–174.

O'Reilly RJ. Review. Allogeneic bone marrow transplantation: Current status and future directions. Blood 1983; 62:941–964.

Thomas ED. Marrow transplantation for malignant diseases (Karnofsky Memorial Lecture). J Clin Oncol 1983; 1:517–531.

Cheson BD, Lacerna L, Leyland-Jones B, et al. Autologous bone marrow transplantation: Current status and future directions. Ann Intern Med 1989; 110:51–65.

Kessinger A, Armitage JO, Landmark JD, et al. Autologous peripheral hematopoietic stem cell transplantation restores hematopoietic function following marrow ablative therapy. Blood 1988; 71:723–727.

Brandt SJ, Peters WP, Atwater SK, et al. Effect of recombinant human granulocyte-macrophage colony-stimulating factor on hematopoietic reconstitution after high-dose chemotherapy and autologous bone marrow transplantation. N Engl J Med 1988; 318:869–876.

Barnett MJ, Eaves CJ, Phillips GL, et al. Successful autografting in chronic myeloid leukemia after maintenance of marrow in culture. Bone Marrow Transplant 1989; 4:345–351.

Gorin NC. Collection, manipulation, and freezing of hematopoietic stem cells. Clin Haematol 1986; 15:19–48.

PAIN CONTROL IN CANCER

CHARLES S. CLEELAND, Ph.D.

For most patients most of the time, cancer pain can be adequately controlled with standard analgesics given by mouth. When this is not possible, a variety of supplemental pain-management techniques can provide control, and it is estimated that approximately 95 percent of patients could be free of significant pain. Unfortunately, smaller percentages of patients actually achieve adequate pain control. Estimates based on surveys in this country indicate that less than half of all cancer patients with pain obtain optimal pain control. Poorly controlled pain has such deleterious effects on the patient and the patient's family that its proper management must have the highest priority for those who routinely care for cancer patients. Not only do mood and quality of life deteriorate in the presence of pain, but pain can have adverse effects on such measures of disease status as appetite and activity. Severe pain may be a primary reason why both patients and their families decide to abandon treatment. An increasing awareness of when pain is liable to occur and how to evaluate and treat it will be of benefit for countless patients.

PREVALENCE

It is well known that the majority of cancer patients with end-stage disease will need careful pain management. It has been estimated that between 60 and 80 percent of such patients will have significant pain. Less attention has been paid to pain as a problem for patients before the terminal phase of the disease has been reached, in which case patients with months or years to live may have function compromised by poorly controlled pain.

Severe pain is rarely a problem before metastatic disease is present. Most immediate postoperative pain can be managed without difficulty. Only 5 to 10 percent of patients report persistent disease-related pain at this stage. When the disease has metastasized, however, the percentages increase dramatically. Fully 30 to 40 percent of hospitalized patients with metastatic disease report pain of a severity that significantly affects their mood and quality of life. Preliminary studies indicate that similar percentages are found among outpatients. Both the presence and severity of pain are dictated by several factors, including the primary site of the disease and metastatic location. Many cancers that were painless at onset have a high incidence of pain as the disease progresses. Breast disease is an excellent example: Although rarely painful in the early stages, half of those affected will report pain after metastatic disease is present. One survey study using analgesic requirement as a criterion found that 85 percent of patients with primary bone tumors, 52 percent of patients with breast carcinoma, and 45 percent of patients with lung cancer required analgesics. Patients who required analgesics less frequently included those with lymphomas (20 percent) and leukemias (5 percent).

It is important to consider the severity of cancer pain. Mild pain is often well tolerated with minimal impact on the patient's activities; however, there is a threshold of pain severity beyond which pain is disproportionately disruptive. This threshold has been reached when patients rate the severity of their pain at the midpoint or higher on any of the commonly used pain severity scales. By this index, one-fifth to more than one-third of patients with metastatic disease will have pain that significantly interferes with their quality of life. When pain is very severe, it becomes the primary focus of attention and prohibits most activity that is not directly related to pain.

PHYSICAL BASIS OF CANCER PAIN

In surveys of pain clinics, direct tumor involvement was the most common cause of pain in approximately two-thirds of patients with pain due to metastatic cancer, with tumor invasion of bone as the physical basis of pain in about one-half of patients who report pain. The remainder have pain due to nerve compression or infiltration, or involvement of hollow fiscus or soft tissue. Persistent posttherapy pain, due to long-term effects of surgery, radiotherapy, and chemotherapy, accounts for an additional 20 percent, with a small residual group having pain due to non–cancer-related causes. In patients with advanced disease, the majority have multiple pain mechanisms. A new complaint of pain in a patient with metastatic cancer should first be thought of as disease-related.

The sensation of pain is generated either by stimulation of peripheral pain receptor or by damage to afferent nerve fibers. Peripheral receptors can be stimulated by pressure, compression, and traction as well as by disease-related chemical changes (nociceptive pain). Damage to visceral, somatic, or autonomic nerve trunks produces neurogenic or deafferentation pain. Spontaneous activity in these damaged nerves is most probably responsible for the painful sensation. Damage to nerves can be caused by treatment or by the disease itself. Cancer patients often have both nociceptive and deafferentation pain simultaneously. The physical basis of the pain is especially important to determine, as deafferentation pain is less responsive to opioid analgesics.

EVALUATION OF THE PATIENT

A clear understanding of the characteristics of the pain and its physical basis is essential to proper management. The changing expression of cancer pain demands repeated assessment, because new causes for pain may emerge rapidly. In advanced cancer, pain due to multiple etiologies may be the rule and not the exception. A careful history includes questions concerning the location, severity, and quality of the pain as well as the impact the pain is having on the patient.

There are many barriers to optimal physician-patient communication about pain. Although a small minority of patients may complain of pain in a dramatic fashion, more patients with cancer underreport the severity of pain and lack of adequate pain relief. Several reasons for this have been suggested, and these include not wanting to acknowledge that the disease is progressing, not wanting to divert the physician's attention from treating this disease, and not wanting to tell the physician that pain treatments are not working. Patients may not want to be put on opioid analgesics because they do not want to become addicted, because they fear psychoactive components of opioids, because they are concerned that using opioids "too early" will endanger pain relief when they have more pain, or because they fear that being placed on opioids signals that death is near. Presenting information that addresses these concerns in a straightforward manner will allay most of these fears, and should be considered as an essential step in providing good pain control.

Communication about pain is greatly aided by having the patient use a scale to report his or her pain. A simple rating scale for pain severity has patients rate pain from 0 to 10, with 0 being no pain and 10 being pain "as bad as you can imagine." Other scales include categorical scales (where the patient picks a word characterizing pain severity) and visual analogue scales (where the patient picks the place on a straight line that best represents pain severity). Numeric scales are probably the easiest for patients to use. When patients are trained to use them, pain-severity scales can be invaluable in titrating analgesics and in monitoring for increases in pain due to progressive disease.

When pain is of moderate or greater severity, a negative impact on the patient's quality of life must be assumed and its expression evaluated. This includes the number of hours the patient is now sleeping compared with the last pain-free interval. Difficulties with sleep onset, frequent interruptions of sleep, or early morning awakening will suggest appropriate pharmacologic intervention, often adding an antidepressant HS. Similar to their hesitance to report severe pain, patients may hesitate to report depression. Having patients report how depressed or tense they are on a scale of 0 to 10 may help overcome some of this reluctance. Significant depression should lead to psychiatric or psychological consultation, especially if it persists in the face of adequate pain relief.

The physician who treats cancer patients should be familiar with the common pain syndromes associated with the disease. Having the patient shade in the area of pain on a drawing of a human figure may aid diagnosis. This may be particularly helpful in indicating areas of referred pain, which are common with nerve compression. Careful questioning concerning the characteristics of the pain is essential for physical diagnosis. In addition

to severity, these characteristics include the temporal pattern of the pain (is it constant or episodic?), its relationship to physical activity, and what seems to alleviate the pain. The physical examination of the patient includes examination of the painful area as well as neurologic and orthopaedic assessment. Because bone disease is a common etiology of pain, and because pain can occur with changes in bone density not detectable on radiographs, bone scans are often invaluable.

Computed tomography (CT) scan is especially useful in the evaluation of retroperitoneal, paravertebral, and pelvic areas as well as the base of the skull. Myelography may be necessary in determining the cause of pain. Finally, diagnostic nerve blocks can provide information concerning the pain pathway as well as determine the potential effectiveness of neuroablative procedures.

TREATMENT

The prompt relief of pain due to cancer frequently involves the use of simultaneously rather than serially administered combinations of drug and nondrug therapies. Identification of a treatable neoplasm as a factor in pain production will call for appropriate radiotherapy or chemotherapy or, in some instances, surgical debulking. Until such treatment can be effective (this may take days to weeks), the patient's pain must be managed with analgesics. In many instances, analgesics are the only pain treatment available because of the patient's condition, the physical basis of the pain, or limited treatment options. The principles of pharmacologic management of pain are evolving through studies of analgesic effectiveness and research on the use of combinations of palliative medications. There is a growing consensus concerning the types of drugs to use, their routes of administration, and how best to schedule them. The first step is the choice of analgesic drug to be used (opioid, nonopioid, or a combination of both). The second step is the choice of adjuvant drugs, which may increase analgesic effectiveness as well as produce other palliative effects to counter the disruptive consequences of pain.

The choice of an opioid analgesic as opposed to a nonopioid analgesic follows from an assessment of the severity of pain. The decision is relatively easy when pain is mild (choose nonopioid) or severe (choose opioid, usually in combination with a nonopioid). The choice is more difficult when the patient reports moderate pain, especially when there is reason to suspect that the patient may be underreporting pain severity. Several studies have documented that many cancer patients are inadequately managed because of the physician's reluctance to use opioids in dosages and with schedules known to be sufficient to relieve moderate pain.

Nonsteroidal anti-flammatory drugs (NSAIDs) constitute the majority of nonopioid analgesics. Their effect on the inflammatory process is a key to their analgesic property. By blocking prostaglandin synthesis, these drugs apparently block pain at the level of pain receptors. Their possible central effects are less well understood. Enteric-coated aspirin or acetaminophen is the first-choice drug for mild to moderate cancer pain. Other NSAIDs, such as ibuprofen, diflunisal, naproxen, and trilisate, have established their value in the management of clinical pain. In some patients, these drugs are better tolerated than aspirin. Individual differences in response to the various NSAIDs are not well understood at this time. Some reports indicate that NSAIDs are particularly effective for bone pain, most usually in combination with the opioids.

Opioid analgesics should be prescribed promptly as soon as there is evidence from continuing assessment that pain is not well controlled with nonopioid analgesics. Usually, nonopioid analgesics can be continued as a way of maximizing analgesia, as their site of action is different than that of the opioids. Oral morphine, either in immediate or sustained-release preparation, is the analgesic of choice for moderate to severe cancer pain. Except in a minority of patients whose pain is clearly episodic, analgesics should be given on an around-the-clock basis, with the time interval based on the duration of analgesic effectiveness of the particular drug (3 to 4 hours for immediate-release morphine) and the patient's report of the duration of effectiveness. Long-acting morphine preparations, either MS Contin or Roxanol SR, are currently available in the United States and are convenient for both patient and health care staff. MS Contin is approved for use every 12 hours, and Roxanol SR is approved for use every 8 hours.

A typical starting dose for immediate-release oral morphine is 10 to 30 mg every 4 hours. When switching from another opioid (usually codeine or oxycodone) to morphine, it is important to calculate the equioanalgesic morphine dose as a basis for determining what morphine-equivalent doses are currently ineffective in pain control. Once an effective dose of short-acting morphine has been established, the required dose for a long-acting preparation can be calculated. An additional supply of short-acting morphine, given as needed, will help the patient manage "breakthrough" pain. Consistent need for this additional morphine will dictate an upwards adjustment of the dose of sustained-release product. Orders for immediate-release morphine should allow for some upwards titration of dose by the patient or by the nurse.

There is evidence that total opioid requirement is lower when opioids are given on a scheduled basis, thereby preventing peaks of pain. Putting patients in the position of having to ask for medication or continually making a judgement about whether their pain is severe enough to take analgesics focuses their attention on pain, reminds them of their need for drugs, and allows pain to reach a severity not readily controlled by the same doses that would be effective with scheduled administration. It is important to remember that there may be large individual differences in the required dose of opioid, depending on such factors as the patient's prior opioid history, activity level, and metabolism. The patient's report of pain severity and pain relief is the best guideline for opioid titration.

The so-called "weak" opioids, including codeine and oxycodone, which are usually formulated in combination with acetaminophen or aspirin, can provide the active patient with good pain relief for long periods of time. As disease advances, oral administration of the more "potent" opioids provides the majority of patients with pain relief. There is considerable agreement that meperidine should not be used on a chronic basis because of its toxic metabolite normeperidine, which is a central nervous system (CNS) stimulant, has a long serum half-life, and has no analgesic properties. Although the oral route is preferred, the physician must remain flexible to changes in patient requirements that are dictated by the patient's ability to use orally administered drugs. This may include the use of opioid and nonopioid suppositories, and other alternate routes of administration.

Although the opioid agonist-antagonist analgesics have established their effectiveness in the control of acute (especially procedurally related) pain, their use in chronic cancer pain is limited by (1) the possibility of precipitated withdrawal in the patient who has been taking morphine-type drugs, (2) their analgesic ceiling effect, and (3) the lack of an oral form of administration (with the exception of pentazocine, which yields a relatively high proportion of patients reporting disturbing psychotomimetic effects).

An assessment of the impact of pain on the patient will help the choice of adjuvant drugs. These drugs include steroids and antidepressants, which have analgesic effects in addition to providing non–pain-specific palliative effects. Disturbed sleep and depressed mood call for the consideration of tricyclic antidepressants. An HS dose of 25 to 75 mg of amitriptyline may aid sleep and increase the analgesic effect of an opioid. Corticosteroids may also brighten mood in addition to potentiating opioid analgesia. Deafferentation pain is less responsive to opioid analgesia than is nociceptive pain. When pain is caused by an injury to nerve, the trycyclic antidepressants and the anticonvulsants may be helpful. Again, it is important to recall that multiple etiologies for pain are often present in advanced disease.

Opioid side effects should be anticipated and prophylactic treatment instituted. In this way, side effects will be less of a barrier to providing adequate pain protection. Constipation is the most common adverse side effect of opioid administration and calls for a regular bowel program, including dietary fiber and stool softening. Respiratory depression is less of a problem in the chronic, as opposed to the acute, use of opiates. If it does occur, it can be reversed by naloxone, a specific opioid antagonist. Excessive sedation may call for modification of drug dose or interval, an alternate route of administration, or reduction or elimination of hypnotics, anxiolytics, or antidepressants. Some have advocated the use of stimulants, such as methylphenidate, to counteract opioid sedation. Should a change in disease status or a neuroablative procedure allow an opiate to be discontinued, the physical dependence of the patient should be recognized and the dose tapered over several days to prevent withdrawal. Physical dependence is quite different from psychological addiction, the latter being extremely rare in the use of opiates for analgesia in cancer pain. The physician's reluctance to use opioid for analgesia in the treatment of cancer pain because of concern about addiction presents an unfortunate barrier to good patient care.

The evaluation of the physical basis of the pain may indicate that a neuroablative procedure would be of benefit for pain control. Destruction of the pain pathway can be accomplished surgically or through destructive nerve blocks using an agent such as phenol. The major barrier to the more widespread application of these techniques is the limited number of experts in their use. The most frequently used neurosurgical procedure is the anterolateral or spinothalamic cordotomy. This is often performed as closed percutaneous cordotomy by stereotaxically placing a radiofrequency needle in the anterolateral quadrant of the cervical cord. By achieving unilateral pain control, this procedure may unmask significant pain on the opposite side of the body. For pain of head and neck cancer, procedures such as percutaneous radiofrequency coagulation of the glossopharyngeal nerve may be used. Pituitary ablation via injection (hypophysectomy) has been reported to be of benefit for diffuse pain. It is important to remember that performance of such procedures does not eliminate the need to titrate analgesics. Because of afferent regeneration, neurosurgical procedures have had their greatest application in patients whose life span can be measured in months.

Destructive anaesthetic block of the celiac plexus had been used for several decades in the management of pain in the abdominal region. This block, which can be preceded by reversible diagnostic block, is especially useful in the pain syndrome accompanying cancer of the pancreas and may also be helpful for pain due to cancers of the liver, gallbladder, or stomach. If success is achieved with the diagnostic block, lasting disruption of the pain pathway can be achieved using alcohol or phenol. Pain due to rib metastases or tumors of the chest wall may be relieved with intercostal nerve blocks. Intrathecal and epidural nerve blocks have provided pain relief, but those procedures carry a risk of sensory and motor deficit.

Teaching patients specific skills to manage their pain may be of help to a majority of patients, especially those who face pain for months to years. Evaluation and prescription of the specific skills most beneficial to the individual can often be obtained through consultation with a behaviorally oriented psychologist, psychiatrist, or pain nurse specialist. The skills taught include relaxation, self-hypnosis, and other distraction and cognitive control techniques. These measures can affect the sensation of pain by reducing muscle tension on pain-generating lesions, as well as by maximizing the patient's ability to cope with the pain and remain as active as his or her disease permits.

SUGGESTED READING

Cancer pain relief. Geneva: World Health Organization, 1986.
Cleeland CS, Rotondi A, Brechner T, et al. A model for the treatment of cancer pain. J Pain Symp Manag 1986; 1(4):209.
Foley KM. The practical use of narcotic analgesics. Med Clin North Am 1982; 66(5):1091.
Foley KM. The treatment of cancer pain. N Engl J Med 1985; 33:384.
Payne R. Pathophysiology of cancer pain. In: Foley KM, Bonica JJ, Ventafridda V, eds. Advances in pain research and therapy. Vol 16. New York: Raven Press, 1990.
Portenoy RK. Cancer pain: Epidemiology and syndromes, Cancer 1989; 63:2,298.

TERMINAL CARE OF THE PATIENT WITH ADVANCED CANCER

LLOYD K. EVERSON, M.D.
NEIL IRICK, M.D.
KAREN ISEMINGER, C.R.N.P., M.S.N., O.C.N.

Many patients with cancer, despite our best efforts with surgery, radiation, chemotherapy, immunotherapy, and biologic response modifier therapy, progress to advanced metastatic disease that is incurable. Unfortunately, those procedures have limited usefulness in improving the quality of life in patients with terminal disease. As health care providers and specialists in cancer care, however, this does not relieve us of the responsibility to continue our efforts at support and palliation of the symptoms of advanced malignancy and to minimize cancer's impact on the various aspects of patients' and families' lives.

This chapter deals with a few of the many complex issues involved in the care of patients with terminal cancer. We have limited our discussion to four aspects of the care of the terminally ill patient: (1) the psychological dimension of terminal care, with specific emphasis on empowerment of the patient and family; (2) special needs of caring for the terminally ill patient, including symptom control; (3) an overview of the hospice philosophy of care; and (4) some aspects and challenges of the multidisciplinary team approach to terminal care.

WHAT IS TERMINAL CARE?

The most important principle in terminal care management of patients is the preservation of comfort and the quality of life, not the preservation of life. The definition of comfort and quality of life is that which is desired by the patient and the family.

Many of us have equated terminal care with the hospice movement and its philosophy. Hospice can be an excellent means of providing multidisciplinary care to both the patient and family in the terminal care situation. However, there are many patients who are never treated under the hospice "umbrella" but are treated with an extension of the already established supportive care programs that have been started during earlier parts of their chronic illness. Hospice, in our view, provides one alternative to the care of the patient with advanced cancer and should be considered in the total context of the multidisciplinary management of patients with cancer and their families.

The use of the phrase *terminally ill* came into common use in recent medical history. This was probably as a consequence of the increased use of the hospice movement as well as the increased visibility of death as an intriguing, if not popular, subject in the lay literature.

The phrase *terminally ill* has commonly been used to mean "a life expectancy of less than 6 months." An alternative definition, promulgated by Jennifer Pardoe, defines terminal illness "as an illness from which there can be no recovery as far as understood in the context of the current state of medical knowledge; and that its irrevocable progression will kill the unfortunate patient."

Part of the challenge of assessing the accuracy of the diagnosis of terminal illness is in weighing the individual prognosis of a particular patient within the context of other patients with a similar stage and extent of disease. Health care providers must be cognizant of the consequences of labeling someone as terminally ill and must make every attempt to determine that the presenting problem is in fact caused by the underlying diagnosis and is not a treatable and reversible condition. The diagnosis of a patient as terminally ill is, in many respects, a philosophical as well as a physical "reality" rather than an absolute statement of fact, knowing that there are some exceptions to the total predictability of any one patient's disease progression and physiologic condition. The philosophy of management of patients with terminal care, however, in no way releases the physicians and caregivers from the responsibility for care of the patient.

A multidisciplinary team approach can optimize care in the patient's best interests. It is essential that the team of physician, caregiver, patient, and family promote the sense of close communication and shared responsibility for the terminal patient care. Given the complex issues involved in the care of the dying patient, it is essential that there is an openness and sharing of the traumatic events that can occur in the lives of the entire team.

Some investigators and clinicians have suggested that psychotherapy, aimed at reducing levels of anxiety and depression in patients and families, may have a positive impact on survival. At the very least, reversing the trend to depression and anxiety can increase the strength of a patient's self-image and his or her ability to cope with the myriad of psychological and physical problems.

EMPOWERMENT OF THE PATIENT AND FAMILY

Administrators have used the concept of empowerment in the contexts of relationships with employees and staff for years. When incorporated into terminal and hospice care, the philosophy of empowering others is especially applicable to patients and their family members. Terminal illness destroys any self-image and control that a patient and family may have had, as the disease relentlessly progresses toward death.

It is our goal as caregivers to the patients and families of the terminally ill to do anything within our capabilities to lessen this experience of powerlessness through specific interventions. In this approach, the goal is to provide a heightened awareness in the patient and family of their own potential for control in the remaining days of their lives. There are at least eight specific ways that the health care team can utilize their roles in enabling the patient and family to regain some control of their lives.

Table 1 indicates some of the interventions that can be used to help this empowerment process. It is difficult to achieve all these goals with every patient; however, even partial success can be rewarding to patient, family, and the caregiver team.

As patients progress toward death with advanced cancer, they and their families' feelings of powerlessness, loss of control, and fear of the future become heightened with the unrelenting invasion of their lives of the cancer process. Adding to this are the numerous traumatic side effects of chemotherapy, surgery, financial burden,

Table 1 Empowerment Interventions

1. Accurately assess the physical, psychological, and spiritual needs of the patient and family.
2. Control the terminal disease symptoms (i.e., pain, nutrition).
3. Provide information on diagnosis, prognosis, and care plan to the patient and family.
4. Counsel and provide anticipatory guidance to the patient and family (i.e., sexuality, living will, grief, signs of impending death).
5. Facilitate communication between the patient and family with regard to the re-allocation of roles within the family.
6. Provide support for spiritual and philosophical guidance.
7. Promote a sense of belonging and encourage close relationships and honesty between caregivers, patient, and family.
8. Facilitate the patient's and family's ability to realize that a sense of pleasure is a vital component of living, even in the terminal stages of disease.

disability, and psychosocial insults that can accompany the support and treatment process throughout the early and late stages of the illness. The goal of the caregiver, in this milieu, is to assist the patient with progressive cancer to decrease his or her feelings of powerlessness in the life remaining. In the management of the patient with terminal cancer, one of our most difficult challenges as physicians, nurses, and caregivers is to help our patients find a balance between the reality of their terminal illness and the assurance that their worst fears will be addressed. In the diagnosis of a patient with cancer, a physical exam and assessment is performed before a specific intervention (i.e., chemotherapy, surgery, radiation therapy) is recommended. The same approach is needed for the case plan of a terminally ill patient. This involves assessment of the physical, familial, psychological, social, and spiritual needs and resources of the patient and the family.

The management of symptoms of patients with terminal care—whether these symptoms be pain, diarrhea, nausea, or vomiting—is of vital importance. Effective relief of these problems not only has the direct advantageous effect of helping with the physical problems of the terminal patient but also relieves the family's anxiety over their concern with the suffering of their loved one.

Inherent in the philosophy of empowering the patient and family to take part in their care is the premise that the patient, caregivers, and the family share the knowledge of the reality of the terminal nature of the disease. An honest and open interchange with the physician, caregiver staff, patient, and family with regard to type of cancer, stage of cancer, what vital organs are affected, the best estimate as to a reasonable prognosis, and what complications may ensue is essential in caring for patients with terminal disease. When this information is shared in this manner, guidance and counseling from the professional staff are often required. This is best handled with trained counselors or psychologists. Physicians and nursing staff can assume this role if they've had experience and training in counseling both staff and patients.

Often, a severe and chronic disease as life-threatening as cancer places tremendous stress on the family structure and necessitates the re-allocation of roles within the family. In longitudinal studies with families facing cancer, some investigators have concluded that open communication with flexible role reassignment within families provides less conflict and eventually a more cohesive family environment, especially as the terminal nature of the disease becomes increasingly evident. The psychological, financial, and spiritual impact on the family unit cannot be underestimated and should be part of the total approach to care of the terminal patient.

In addressing the total needs of the patient and family, one must offer acknowledgement of and assistance towards the patient's plight to understand existential concerns related to the meaning of suffering and death. As the health care team becomes more closely involved in the terminal care of patients and families, the meaning of suffering and death comes to the forefront of thinking, not only for the patient and family but for the caregiver as well. The caregiver has an enormous challenge in this environment, to assist the patient in realizing that his or her "value" is not related to his or her current level of functioning. Frankl stated this challenge in another way: "Life remains potentially meaningful under any circumstance, even sometimes in the most miserable environment."

Although the search for "meaning in life" is a cause for deep introspection, humor plays a significant role in giving the patient a sense of belonging and normalcy. Most patients long for a degree of normalcy with regard to events of everyday living. Through the provision of therapeutic humor, these types of interventions may in fact assist the patient to feel "normal," to bear life's burden, and to feel that life can still be pleasurable, even in the last full days of existence. Obviously, the timeliness of this type of intervention is an important concern.

Jacob Bronowski, in Kaufman's *The Dynamics of Power*, described mankind's desire for control in this manner: "We must feel ourselves as we are, shapers of the landscape, not merely figures of the landscape. Having choices in matters that affect us to maintain our role as architects in the landscapes of our life." This is the goal of successful implementation of palliative care of the patient with terminal disease.

CONTROL OF SYMPTOMS

Physicians and nurses have classically been trained in the fundamentals of pain control. In numerous studies, however, the contrast between what is known to be superior and even adequate pain control versus inadequate application and practice by many health care professionals presents us with some major challenges. Whether the symptom we are aiming to control is severe pain, or some other problem related to advanced cancer, such as ascites, the type of intervention that is used for control of these symptoms is not so much manipulation of the physiologic challenge as it is the appropriateness of the intervention that is being considered.

Table 2 lists some of the common symptoms that can be encountered in patients with terminal cancer. Although this list is by no means comprehensive, it does

Table 2 Some Symptoms Encountered in the Terminally Ill Patient

Pain
Nausea and vomiting
Anorexia and fatigue
Xerostomia and stomatitis
Diarrhea and constipation
Dyspnea and intractable cough
Bowel and urinary incontinence
Decubitus ulcers
Fluid retention with ascites and edema
Psychological depression

include some of the more common symptoms encountered in an oncology practice. Control of pain is considered in the preceding chapter. However, alleviation of nausea, vomiting, xerostomia, stomatitis, diarrhea, constipation, dyspnea, cough, incontinence, and psychological depression require just as much attention and care. Tables 3 through 8 summarize some of our approaches to the management of these symptoms.

In the palliative care of the terminally ill patient, aggressive interventions with radiation therapy, surgery, and chemotherapy have limited use. These modalities can play a role in symptom management when the procedure itself will not cause any additional pain or decrease in quality of life, and they will improve palliation of symptoms related to advanced cancer. The timing of these specific interventions is difficult and challenging under the best of circumstances, but in the terminal care situation, it is even more so. These decisions are best approached within the multidisciplinary team care approach, taking into consideration the needs and resources of the patients, families, and caregivers.

In the terminal care setting, the use of antibiotics,

transfusions, artificial respirator support, and cardiac resuscitation is inappropriate. Gastric tubes can be used in the care of patients but only, in our opinion, when they can contribute to the immediate comfort of the patient, such as for relief of gastrointestinal obstruction and uncontrolled vomiting.

"HOSPICE" PHILOSOPHY OF CARE

The philosophy of hospice has been intertwined with people's attitudes about death. These perceptions have

Table 3 Palliation of Symptoms Encountered in the Terminally Ill Patient

Pain (oral medications given regularly every 4 hr)
  Mild: aspirin or acetaminophen, 325 mg
  Moderate: acetaminophen and codeine, 30 mg
  Severe: acetaminophen and oxycodone, 5 mg, or morphine, 30 mg
Anorexia: In some cases, anorexia is benefited by corticosteroids. Cyproheptadine may prove effective in some patients
Xerostomia and stomatitis
  Treatment of choice: Moi-Stir for xerostomia; Peridex for stomatitis
  Antimicrobial: ketoconazole for oral moniliasis; acyclovir for oral herpes simplex

Table 5 Palliation of Constipation Encountered in the Terminally Ill Patient

Agents	Examples
Stimulants	
Senna	Senokot (2–8 tablets, bid)
Casanthrol (+ docusate)	PeriColace (1–4 capsules, bid)
Bisacodyl	Dulcolax (5–10 mg/daily)
Osmotic Agents	
Lactulose	Cephulac (10–30 cc qid)
Magnesium hydroxide	Milk of Magnesia (30–60 cc/hr)
Magnesium citrate	Citromag (4.5–9.0 oz)
Softeners	
Detergent — docusate sodium	Colace, Surfak (100–240 mg)
Lubricant — mineral oil	(30–60 cc bid)
Bulk Agents	
Diarrhea — Usually can be stopped by eliminating the offending agent, such as tube feedings or fecal impaction	
Kaolin — pectin (absorbent)	Kaopectate concentrate
	Imodium (2–4 mg prn)
	Lomotil (1–2 tablets prn)

Table 4 Palliation of Nausea and Vomiting in the Terminally Ill Patient

Stimulus	Area Affected	Treatment	Examples

Drugs, uremia, ketosis	Chemoreceptor trigger zone	Dopamine antagonists	Prochlorperazine
			  PO: 10–30 mg spansule bid
			  IM: 10 mg q3–4h prn
			  IV: 10 mg piggyback *slowly* in 100 cc of normal saline
			Haloperidol
			  PO: 5–10 mg tid
			  IM/IV: 2–5 mg tid
			Fluphenazine
			  IM: 1–2 mg tid

Gastric irritation, gastroparesis	Stomach/duodenum	Gastrokinetic agent	Metaclopromide PO: 10–20 mg q10

Psychological stimuli, increased ICP	Cerebral cortex		Lorazepam
			  PO: 1–2 mg q4–6h
			  IV: 0.5–1 mg q4–6h
			Cannabinol
			  PO: 2.5–5.0 mg tid
			Dexamethasone
			  PO: 0.5–4.0 mg qbh
			  IV: 0.5–1.0 mg qbh

varied throughout the years, but they seem to have come "full circle" with respect to care of the terminally ill (Table 9).

The concept of hospice originated during medieval times. Religious orders of that era developed the philosophy and created places where pilgrims from the Crusades and travelers could be "refreshed." Many of these travelers were helped by whatever healing and relief of pain that could be supplied by the meager resources available. Those who were dying received special care and honor, for in those days, they were also seen as pilgrims, and closer than many others to God.

As the science of medicine came to the forefront in the late 1800s and early 1900s, the philosophy of hospice became diluted. Later, in the 20th century, the initial groundwork for the public and professional recognition of the need for hospice was laid by Pfeiffer's *The Meaning of Death* and Kubler-Ross' *On Death and Dying*. Such a public groundswell of concern and support resulted that hospice was at times perceived as an antiphysician movement; this was not the case, however. In England in the 1940s, a remarkable woman and physician, Cicely Saunders, struggled over the ensuing 20 years to build a home for the care of others who were dying and to rekindle the spirit of hospice.

As hospice evolved in England and the United States, the philosophy of caring was considered to provide a service to the terminally ill, regardless of disease. Modern-day concepts embraced in the United States originated at St. Christopher's in England, the hospice established by Cicely Saunders. Much of the research in symptom control and pain relief that has shaped our current practice in terminal cancer care originated there.

In the United States, some hospices developed into large inpatient units, as had been established in England. However, most hospices in the United States typically function as a program of home care in liaison with other nonhospice agencies and inpatient facilities. Indeed, in many communities across the United States, hospice care has become synonymous with terminal care.

The TEFRA act was passed in 1982, and the hospice movement was institutionalized as a part of the Medicare benefit program in November, 1983. The five key components of the hospice Medicare-sponsored benefit programs are listed in Table 10.

Although the law and regulations have continued to evolve, this has had a multitide of far-reaching implications for cancer care in the United States. Some of the ramifications of this act include the following:

Table 6 Palliation of Dyspnea and Intractable Cough in the Terminally Ill Patient

DYSPNEA

Drugs	Examples
Anxiolytic	Valium (2–5 mg, tid)
Narcotics	Morphine (2–5 mg SC per EZ set)
Nebulized bupivacaine	Marcaine (0.5%, 1 cc)
Oxygen	

Nondrug measures
Relaxation therapy
Fan or draft
Reassurance

INTRACTABLE COUGH

Central
Narcotics
Dextromethorphan, 30–60 mg PO qid
Codeine, 15–30 mg PO q4h
Hydrocodone, 5–7.5 mg PO q4h
Morphine, 15–30 mg q4h
Methadone, 2.5–5.0 mg q4h

Peripheral

Benzonatate	Tessalon perles
Bupivacaine (nebulized) or as a hard sugar-based candy used as a lozenge	Marcaine

Table 7 Palliation of Urinary Symptoms Encountered in the Terminally Ill Patient

Symptom	Intervention
Irritated bladder or bladder spasm	Amitriptyline, 25–50 mg daily Propantheline, 15 mg, 1–2 times daily
Hesitancy	Bethanecol, 10–30 mg, 2–3 times daily
Incontinence	Foley catheter

Table 8 Palliation of Psychological Depression and Fatigue Encountered in the Terminally Ill Patient

Tricyclic antidepressants	Desipramine, 25–75 mg daily Nortriptyline, 25–75 mg daily
Fluoxitene	20–40 mg daily in morning
Bupropion	100 mg, 2–3 times per day

Table 9 History of Attitudes Toward Death*

Decade	Attitude Toward Death
1800s	Patient is "in God's hands" Physician is to comfort Death is part of life
1900–1920s	Physician response was "trust me, don't worry"
1930s	Death in hospitals Patient is "only sleeping"
1940s	Cancer = death Education on grief therapy
1950s	Fatal outcome of cancer revealed to family, but not to patient
1960s	More open discussion of death Concern for death and dignity Criticism of silence
1970s	First formal hospice unit "Right-to-die" issues
1980s	Right of "natural death" Study on ethical problems in medicine
1990	Palliation through increasing expertise in symptom management

*Information on 1800 to 1980s adapted from Holland JC, Rowland JH. Handbook of psycho-oncology: Psychological care of the cancer patient. Oxford, England: Oxford University Press, 1989.

Table 10 Components of Hospice Benefits Programs

1. Election and certification: Beneficiaries must elect hospice care and receive it in a Medicare-certified hospice.
2. Core services: Medicare-certified hospices must directly provide all home health care services, including physician, nursing, medical social work, counseling, and chaplaincy services.
3. Volunteerism: At least 5% of total working hours must be provided by volunteers.
4. Interdisciplinary team: Care must be planned and managed by a team composed of physicians, nurses, social workers, and counselors. Covered services include physical and other therapies, homemaker and home health aid services, drugs, supplies, equipment, and inpatient respite care.
5. Reimbursement: Every day of service the hospice provides is reimbursed according to the service delivered. The four per diem categories are routine home care, continuous home care, general inpatient care, and inpatient respite care.

Adapted from Health care financing administration extramural report: Medicare hospice benefits program evaluation. Washington, DC: US Department of Health and Human Services, 1987; with permission.

1. The recognition of the patient and family as the unit of service and their involvement in decision making
2. The delivery of care by the team approach, using, in addition to the doctor and nurse, a social worker, chaplain, and counselor
3. The provision of support for the staff giving the care for the use of volunteers to help provide care (at least 5 percent of total hours)
4. The continuation of care after the death of the patient by providing bereavement services to the family

Hospice care, especially as it has evolved in the United States, can best be described as a concern for management of "total pain and suffering of the patient and family." The hospice approach to care of the terminally ill patient necessarily involves a multidisciplinary philosophy, with the goals focusing on superior symptom control; improved caregiver, patient, and family communications; and family support.

Table 11 is an example of some of the admission criteria used in the Indiana Regional Cancer Center hospice program. It attempts to translate concept into reality in order to guide physicians, nursing personnel, caregivers, volunteers, patient, and family in delineating the appropriate types of patients for admission to a hospice program. It limits patient hospice admission to those who have no more than an anticipated 6-month survival. This emphasizes that the primary goal in the care of these patients is *not* to prolong life but to care for the physical, psychological, spiritual, social, and family needs of the patient during the terminal phase of their illness.

ROLES AND NEEDS OF MULTIDISCIPLINARY TEAM

Much has been written about the use of an integrated, multidisciplinary team in the care of patients

Table 11 Hospice Admission Criteria

1. The patient must be terminally ill with a life expectancy of less than 6 months.
2. The patient must understand that his/her medical care will be managed by his/her attending physician and/or the Hospice Medical Director.
3. There must be an individual in the patient's home who is available, able, and willing, and is primarily responsible for providing patient care.
4. Care must be provided in the patient's own home setting, unless his/her condition, as determined by the Interdisciplinary Care Group, warrants transfer to an alternate facility; i.e., nursing home or hospital.
5. The patient and primary caregiver must agree to hospice care as defined in a Hospice Admission Consent Form.

From 1990 IRCC Hospice Policies and Procedures Manual.

with cancer. Hospice philosophy mandates that a team of professionals and volunteers be included in the total care of the patient and family with terminal illness. Although not all patients and families are amenable to care within the hospice arena, the principles that we have discussed in terms of addressing the total needs of the patient, family, and caregiver, and empowerment of the patient and family are key elements in the delivery of quality care for terminal patients.

Professionals, whether they be primary care physicians, nurses, radiation oncologists, or medical oncologists, are trained to preserve and protect life "at all costs." In changing from the aggressive and acute care management of patients with cancer to palliation and support, major changes in the psychological and intellectual orientation of the health care team are required. Consequently, many of the same stresses that the patient and family experience are magnified in the physician, who is taught throughout medical school and residency to preserve life at all costs. In this setting, a key component of the multidisciplinary team is the counseling, psychological guidance, and support that are available to patient, family, and the caregiver team, which is composed of physicians, nurses, and volunteers.

Table 12 lists some of the key personnel in an integrated multidisciplinary team that focuses on the care of a terminally ill patient. The hospice is the ideal environment for the implementation of this philosophy of care. However, let us stress that this team approach can be applied to any situation in which a terminally ill patient needs continuing care.

CHALLENGES FOR MANAGEMENT OF TERMINAL CARE

The complexities of care for patients with terminal disease are huge, and the challenges impact all health care professions and the public. Within that context, some of the issues that require continuing attention and concern include the following:

1. The complex ethical issues that need to be addressed when considering withholding costly

Table 12 Multidisciplinary Team for Care
of Terminally Ill Patients

Physicians (hospice medical director, primary care physician, and
  oncologists)
Administrator or hospice director
Oncology nursing personnel
Counselors and/or psychologists
Social workers
Chaplains
Volunteers (respite and bereavement support)
Visiting home care nursing

and "ineffective" therapies versus those that are considered by some to be "life-sustaining"
2. The nature of the relationship between hospice (terminal care) in the United States and US Government Health Policy
3. The continued education of health care professionals in appropriate pain and other symptom management of patients with terminal disease

Ethical issues in the care of patients with terminal disease are now more openly discussed in public, medical, and legal forums. Public attitudes concerning the right of terminally ill patients have changed rapidly in the last few years. Even euthanasia is discussed openly and more favorably by some.

However, legal considerations are of increasing importance in our society, and even Living Wills statutes do not allow the withholding of nutrition and intravenous fluids in many states. Currently, 38 states now have legislation authorizing Living Wills. Fifteen states authorize the patient to appoint a "proxy" for them in the right to decide use or withdrawal of life support. Courts have also upheld the dying patient's right to refuse medical treatment.

However, the argument that physicians are not bound legally, morally, or ethically to preserve life "at all costs" does very little to increase the comfort level of those on the health care team when dealing with the numerous expectations of the patient, family, and the legal and medical professions in the United States. Nevertheless, the best interest of the patient and family necessitates that these issues be discussed in a frank and anticipatory manner with the patient and family.

There is increasing interest in research of the care of the terminally ill patient. Because of its impact on the psychosocial nature of terminal illness, research is best enhanced through the use of both quantitative and qualitative methodologies to provide a complete picture of the needs of the terminally ill patient.

There are many unique challenges to the psychological and social assessment of the cancer patient. Although a number of studies have focused on outcome measurement, only a few have concentrated on the processes involved. Further study is required in understanding and alleviating caregiver stress, comparison of symptom intervention approaches, and analysis of quality of life in the terminal cancer patient.

Of the multitude of questions that need to be addressed, at least four areas of concern lend themselves to further investigation:

1. What has been the impact on quality of care and reimbursement for hospice services with the advent of Medicare certification since the original National Hospice Study was done in 1981 or 1982?
2. What are the real effects of a formalized psychotherapy intervention process in the terminal illness context?
3. What are the long-term effects of the bereavement process and the total impact of the illness on the multidisciplinary caregiver team, both immediately and in the years after a patient's death?
4. What are the barriers to use of hospice care in the lower income and minority population?

Many studies have analyzed the cost and benefits of hospice care in the home versus traditional institutionalized care. In 1983, the National Hospice Organization published results that suggest that terminally ill patients and their families do equally well in hospices or more conventional arrangements, and hospice care can be less costly than an acute care setting for terminally ill patients.

SUGGESTED READING

Hospice in the United States: An overview by Sandol Stoddard. J Palliative Care 1989; 5(3):10–19.

Health care financing extramural report: Medicare hospice benefit program evaluation. Washington, DC: US Department of Health and Human Services, 1987.

Kaufman G. The dynamics of power. Rochester, VT: Schenkman Books, 1983.

The international bibliography on palliative care. The Palliative Care Foundation, Toronto, Canada, 1983.

Herth K. Contributions of humor as perceived by the terminally ill. Am J Hospice Care 1990; January/February.

Twycross R, Lack S. Therapeutics in terminal cancer. London: Pitman, 1984.

Kaye P. Notes on symptom control in hospice and palliative care. Hospice Education Institute, Essex, Connecticut, 1989.

Holland JC, Rowland JH. Handbook of psycho-oncology: Psychological care of the cancer patient. Oxford, England: Oxford University Press, 1989.

Wanzer SH, Federman DD, Adelstein SJ, et al. The physician's responsibility toward hopelessly ill patients: A second look. N Engl J Med 1989; 320(13):844–849.

SPECIAL APPLICATIONS OF RADIATION THERAPY

MINESH P. MEHTA, M.D.

Although external-beam radiation is the most commonly employed and best known form of radiation therapy, radiation has also been employed in several "specialized" situations, including brachytherapy, stereotactic radiosurgery, intraoperative radiation, thermoradiotherapy, and radioimmunotherapy. The well-established modality of brachytherapy and the emerging field of stereotactic radiosurgery are the subjects of this chapter.

BRACHYTHERAPY

The term *brachytherapy* refers to radiation delivered from a short distance, as opposed to teletherapy or external radiation, which is delivered at distances usually in excess of 80 cm. Five years after the discovery of natural radioactivity in 1896, Danlos began using radium to treat cancer. Although rapid initial strides were made in the early 1900s, including the elaborate physical principles of brachytherapy as espoused by Patterson-Parker and Quimby, the resurgence of brachytherapy in the 1970s and the 1980s had to await the discovery and modification of better radioisotopes such as iridium-192 and the creation of remote afterloading devices. Computerized treatment planning has permitted substantial refinements.

Unlike external radiation, brachytherapy permits the delivery of relatively high doses in a shorter time interval with substantial sparing of normal tissue as a consequence of rapid dose fall-off and the ability to tailor dose distribution to the geometry of the tumor. The radiobiologic effects of continuous low-dose radiation produce an improved therapeutic ratio. The major factor limiting the application of brachytherapy is the requirement to place carriers into or in close proximity to the tumor. This, therefore, limits the use of brachytherapy to surface application (plesiotherapy), intracavitary application, or interstitial brachytherapy, in which the radiation sources are directly imbedded into the tumor.

Radioisotopes

The ideal radioisotope employed in brachytherapy would combine the advantages of a modest half-life (several days to weeks), rapid fall-off, and physical characteristics that permit fabrication of a variety of different implantable physical forms. The initial efforts were limited by the availability of radium, which is considered too hazardous for most modern brachyther-

apy applications. A variety of different isotopes, including radon, cesium, cobalt, gold, iridium, palladium, and californium, have since become available, and their critical characteristics are illustrated in Table 1.

Techniques

Brachytherapy implants are labeled *permanent* when the radioactive sources are left in place, and *temporary* if the sources are removed after a fixed duration. When sources are placed within body cavities, the technique is referred to as *intracavitary brachytherapy*. Interstitial techniques employ insertion of sources within or around tumors without central cavities, either by placing radioactive "seeds" directly into the tumor or loading these sources into hollow needles or tubes placed within the target.

INTRACAVITARY BRACHYTHERAPY

Cancer of the Cervix

The primary application of intracavitary brachytherapy is in the management of cervical cancer. Numerous applicators, most bearing the names of their designers, exist, and a detailed discussion regarding these is beyond the scope of this chapter. A brief historical review, however, is useful. Cancer of the cervix was first treated with radium in 1908. The early experience centered around preloaded radium applicators. Working independently, Regaud, in Paris, and Forsell, in Stockholm, developed two independent techniques. In the 1930s, the Paris technique was modified by the group from Manchester, which laid down the current foundations of gynecologic brachytherapy. In principle, most systems combined the use of a central uterine stent or tandem and peripheral ovoids placed within both lateral fornices. The resultant "pear-shaped" isodose curves conformed well with the shape of the tumor. Preloaded applicators had numerous disadvantages, including excessive personnel exposure, bulky radium sources, a high-risk of radon leakage, and the requirement for heavy shielding. The lack of an interlock between uterine

Table 1 Characteristics of Common Isotopes Used in Brachytherapy

Isotope	Half-life	Type of Radiation	Energy (mev)
Radium-226	1,622 yr	Gamma	0.05–2.4
Radon-222	3.8 days	Gamma	0.5
Cesium-137	30 yr	Gamma	0.7
Cobalt-60	5.3 yr	Gamma	1.17–1.33
Gold-198	2.7 days	Gamma	0.41
Strontium-90	28.1 yr	Beta	2.3 (max)
Iridium-192	74 days	Gamma	0.3–0.47
Palladium-103	17 days	X-ray	0.02
Californium-252	2.7 yr	Neutron	2.35
Iodine-125	59.6 days	X-ray	0.03

and fornicial sources also resulted in substantial source displacement. By the late 1950s and early 1960s, cesium afterloading applicators had replaced radium preloaded applicators. In the United States, Suit and Henschke introduced two popular applicators almost simultaneously in 1959 and 1960. These applicators have since undergone numerous modifications and revisions.

As early as 1950, results on over 60,000 patients treated with these techniques were reported, with 5-year survival results for stages I, II, and III approaching 60 percent, 40 percent, and 22 percent, respectively. Modern 5-year survival rates are 90 percent for stage IB, 75 percent for stage IIA, 60 percent for IIB, and 30 percent for stage III.

Recent innovations have allowed for the development of high-dose-rate remote afterloading units that permit multifractionated brachytherapy on an outpatient basis without any exposure to personnel. Among their other clinical applications, these units are being used to manage cervical cancer. Preliminary results indicate equal tumor control, but long-term toxicity data must be awaited.

Uterine Carcinoma

Radical surgery remains the modality of choice for the management of cancer of the corpus. In stage I disease, no prospective, randomized trial has demonstrated a survival advantage using postoperative or preoperative radiation. In selected patients at high risk for local recurrence, brachytherapy techniques are employed to reduce cuff recurrences. Patients with inoperable stage I disease may be treated with intracavitary brachytherapy, with cure rates in the 75 percent range. The role of external radiation is outside the scope of this chapter. Patients with stage II disease are frequently treated with a combination of intracavitary radiation, external radiation, and surgery.

Endobronchial Radiation

With more than 150,000 cases every year, lung cancer represents today's major oncologic challenge. There are more than 120,000 deaths annually, and most therapeutic approaches result in a high incidence of local failure that frequently manifests as malignant airway occlusion. According to one estimate, 20 to 30 percent of newly diagnosed lung neoplasms present with atelectasis due to endobronchial disease. Because of a high rate of local failure following conventional therapy, up to 50 percent of patients with lung cancer will eventually develop symptomatic endobronchial disease. Death from airway occlusion is often a painful process of slow asphyxiation, frequently complicated by obstructive pneumonia and hemoptysis.

Endobronchial radiation is an extremely effective modality in achieving roentgenographic reaeration. A high complete response rate of around 73 percent is noted on endoscopic follow-up. We have recently published results of our series of 55 implants performed using fiberoptic bronchoscopy and manually afterloaded iridium-192 single-line seed sources. Our conventional practice has been to deliver 20 Gy at 2 cm from source center. We have also gathered preliminary experience with high-dose-rate remote afterloading brachytherapy for malignant airway occlusion. Both techniques produce symptomatic resolution in over two-thirds of patients. Therefore, endobronchial radiation is a highly effective palliative modality that provides excellent control of local symptoms for a significant duration of a patient's remaining life span. In the setting of recurrent disease, however, malignant airway occlusion results in a median survival of only 5 months, and endobronchial therapy does not significantly impact overall survival.

Other Sites

Endocavitary radiation has also been employed to deliver a boost to tumors of the urinary bladder, vagina, urethra, biliary tract, and esophagus.

INTERSTITIAL BRACHYTHERAPY

Practically any tumor that can be accessed or exposed surgically or localized clinically or radiographically may be amenable to interstitial brachytherapy. The list includes tumors of the head and neck region, brain, breast, lung, pancreas, prostate, bladder, recurrent pelvic neoplasms, soft-tissue sarcomas, vulvar cancer, pediatric tumors, cutaneous malignancies, and ocular melanoma. A comprehensive discussion of all these clinical applications is not feasible in this chapter.

Interstitial brachytherapy for brain neoplasms provides a good example of one of these applications. The conventional results of treatment of malignant gliomas have been universally disappointing. Survival appears to be correlated to radiation dose, but normal tissue tolerance limits external radiation to approximately 60 Gy. Selected malignant gliomas can be implanted stereotactically using Silastic catheters fixed to the outside of the skull. These catheters can be loaded with iodine-125 or iridium-192, and an additional boost of approximately 50 to 60 Gy can be delivered over 100 hours. In a series of 63 patients reported by Leibel and colleagues, the median survival for 42 patients with glioblastoma multiforme undergoing brachytherapy was 95 weeks compared with 52 weeks in matched controls. The median survival for 21 patients with anaplastic astrocytoma undergoing implantation was 223 weeks compared with 165 weeks in matched controls. This modality is currently being further evaluated in prospective, randomized studies.

STEREOTACTIC RADIOSURGERY

Stereotactic radiosurgery may be defined as the delivery of a highly focused beam of radiation to an intracranial target without delivering excessive radiation to surrounding normal brain. Stereotaxis, or the localization of a point in three-dimensional space, is essentially an engineering problem. The structures within the cranium, limited in terms of their mobility and generally unaffected by respiration and physical movement, can be localized in three-dimensional space with reference to an externally fixed device. Horsley Clark is credited with the development of the first stereotactic frame. Subsequently, several such frames were developed and found application in numerous neurosurgical procedures. In 1951, Lars Leksell coined the phrase *stereotactic radiosurgery*. The principles of his technique combined the immobilization and precise three-dimensional localization offered by stereotaxis and the use of multiple beams of ionizing radiation, all focused to the stereotactically selected site. Leksell originally employed 200 kVp photons, but these orthovoltage beams proved to have inadequate penetration. In the 1950s, proton beams became clinically available in Sweden and the United States. These beams, harnessed from high-energy physics research systems, exhibit the unique characteristics of depositing minimal dose along their entry path, culminating in the deposition of a large burst of energy, the so-called Bragg peak. These beams, as well as heavy-charged particles from synchrocyclotrons, which are available at a handful of centers in the world, have been employed for stereotactic brain radiation for several years.

GAMMA KNIFE

In the 1960s, Leksell and Larsson developed the first gamma knife, containing 179 cobalt-60 sources, all focused to a point. Originally employed for thalamotomies for intractable pain and capsulotomies for obsessive-compulsive disorders, the gamma knife was later redesigned for the treatment of inoperable arteriovenous malformations. The first United States gamma knife became operational at the University of Pittsburgh in 1987.

LINEAR ACCELERATOR–BASED RADIOSURGERY

Owing to the expense and source-replacement problems of the gamma-knife, work continued in Europe and in Argentina, leading to the development of linear accelerator–based radiosurgery. The first United States linear accelerator–based unit became operational in 1986. Currently, there are approximately a dozen centers in the United States engaged in this technique. Most of these institutions utilize either multiple noncoplanar converging arcs with a stationary couch or a combination of a simultaneously moving couch and gantry (or dynamic radiosurgery). All of the techniques employ an externally fixed stereotactic frame used for immobilization and localization. The various different radiosurgical procedures, although quite divergent in physical char-

acteristics, lead to the same end result—obliteration of a small intracranial target.

RADIOSURGERY VERSUS RADIOTHERAPY

Although both forms of radiation produce distinct biologic change as a consequence of the interaction of ionizing radiation and target tissues, several differences exist.

Whereas conventional radiation is fractionated over several weeks, with small daily increments that reduce the tumor cell population by a certain fraction, stereotactic radiosurgery involves delivery of extremely large doses, all in a single fraction. The toxicity of large fraction radiation is normally too prohibitive, but as long as the volume radiated remains small, it is possible to stay within the limits of normal tissue tolerance. In general, stereotactic radiosurgery is, therefore, not performed for lesions larger than 3.5 to 4 cm in diameter. Kjellberg has published data analyzing the dose-volume relationships, and these data are commonly used for prescribing radio-surgical doses. Because of the possibility of severe damage, it is critical that all radiosurgical systems employ very finely collimated radiation beams, absolute head immobilization, and precise localization and delivery systems.

CLINICAL APPLICATIONS OF RADIOSURGERY

Arteriovenous Malformations

Arteriovenous malformations are congenital vascular malformations of unknown incidence and prevalence, because the vast majority are only discovered when they become symptomatic. The lesion is characterized by a capillary tangle fed by hypertrophied arterioles and drained by distended venules. The low-pressure, high-flow system is prone to hemorrhage at a rate of approximately 2 percent per year after the first bleed. The lifetime mortality and morbidity approach 20 percent and 40 percent, respectively, in most series with long-term follow-up.

Single large doses of radiation produce endothelial thickening and proliferation, eventually obliterating the malformation over a 1- to 3-year period. Obliteration rates have ranged from 60 percent to 90 percent. Several thousand patients have been treated with this modality.

Benign Tumors

Acoustic Neuromas

Although microsurgical excision is the treatment of choice, radiosurgical ablation remains a viable alternative for patients who are deemed inoperable, those who have other significant medical problems, or those who refuse surgery. The largest reported study, from the Karolinska Institute, showed an overall control rate of 86 percent in 115 patients. In the series reported by Lunsford, an overall 97 percent control rate was achieved in a series of 92 patients. Facial neuropathy has been reported as a consequence of therapy in approximately one-fifth of patients. In most patients, this improves over the subsequent 5 to 12 months. Trigeminal neuropathy is also a potential complication.

Meningiomas

Surgery remains the mainstay of management for most patients with meningioma. Conventional radiation has been employed with good results whenever surgical resection is incomplete, the patient is inoperable, or if the tumor is recurrent. The use of stereotactic radiation is new and controversial. In a series of 50 patients reported by Kondziolka and colleagues, the 2-year actuarial tumor growth control rate was 92 percent. The 2-year actuarial complication rate was 9 percent. These initial data suggest a possible role for stereotactic radiosurgery in selected patients, although long-term follow-up data are necessary before one can draw firm conclusions.

Pituitary Adenomas and Craniopharyngiomas

The largest experience in the management of pituitary adenomas is the stereotactic Bragg peak proton-beam therapy trials. In a recent report of 791 patients with growth hormone– or adrenocorticotropic hormone (ACTH)-secreting intracellular pituitary adenomas treated over 27 years, follow-up information was available in 93 percent of the cases. In acromegalics, cure was defined as growth hormone levels of 5 μg per milliliter or less. Five- and 10-year cure rates of 60 percent and 100 percent were achieved in patients treated above the 95 percentile dose level. In patients with Cushing's disease, an overall cure rate of 100 percent was achieved by 4 years in patients treated above the 95 percentile dose level. Proton-beam therapy, therefore, is extremely effective in the management of intrasellar growth hormone– and ACTH-secreting pituitary adenomas.

The Karolinska Institute has reported on more than 100 patients with ACTH-secreting pituitary microadenomas who were treated with one to four radiosurgical treatments using up to 70 Gy. A 76 percent complete remission rate has been reported.

A 10 to 15 percent rate of hypopituitarism is expected in these patients. Approximately 2 percent of patients develop oculomotor disturbance. Complete or partial blindness may result if the optic chiasm receives more than 10 Gy; therefore, it is critical to select patients with adenomas that are small enough to prevent injury to the chiasm.

Coffey and colleagues have recently reported preliminary experience with craniopharyngiomas. These data are too preliminary to make firm conclusions or recommendations. The Karolinska group has treated the solid component of craniopharyngiomas in 36 patients and have achieved progressive tumor shrinkage and clinical improvement in the majority.

Malignant Tumors

Gliomas

Most high-grade gliomas are characterized by diffuse infiltration into surrounding brain, which prohibits the use of stereotactic radiosurgery. Data from several interstitial implant studies, however, suggest that when a course of external radiation is combined with an implant, which by its very nature is extremely localized, good results may be obtained. Stereotactic radiosurgery may, therefore, potentially be utilized as a boost technique, following external radiation, in selected patients.

Sturm and colleagues have treated 36 patients with two daily fractions of 30 Gy, each without any conventional external radiation. Their experience has not been very encouraging. Survival and local control were not improved, but complication rates appeared somewhat higher.

Loeffler and colleagues, as well as we, have used stereotactic radiosurgery both as a boost following external radiation in newly diagnosed patients and as sole therapy for recurrent lesions. The subjective impression of improved local control has been reported, but objective data are not yet forthcoming. In our series of 12 patients, a 25 percent objective response rate has been noted.

A small series of low-grade gliomas has recently been reported from Italy. Twelve of 14 patients had a partial or complete radiographic response.

The role of radiosurgery in gliomas is still being defined. It is unlikely to replace either surgery or conventional radiation, but it is likely to find application in the management of selected patients as a boost.

Metastases

Metastases to the brain from systemic malignancies are commonly seen in radiotherapeutic practice and represent an important cause of morbidity and mortality. Conventional management with steroids and whole-brain radiation yields a median survival of approximately 18 weeks. The most frequent cause of death (approximately 50 percent) in these patients is intracranial disease progression.

Given the poor outcome with conventional therapy, recent efforts have been directed at resecting solitary brain metastases in selected patients prior to whole-brain radiation. In one such recent prospective, randomized study (Patchell), the median survival improved from 15 to 40 weeks, and recurrence at the metastatic site decreased from 52 to 20 percent. Because most metastatic lesions in the brain are less infiltrative than gliomas, it is appealing to consider stereotactic radiosurgery for these patients. At least five groups (Sturm, Valentino, Loeffler, Lunsford, Mehta) have reported their preliminary experiences. In the largest series, reported by Valentino, 52 of 58 patients (90 percent) showed clinical and radiographic improvement. In most series, an approximate 15 percent complete response rate is documented. In our series of 19 patients with 23 lesions, 6 of 23 (26 percent) patients experienced a complete response and 9 of 23 (39 percent) had greater than 50 percent reduction in tumor volume, for an objective overall response rate of 15 of 23 (65 percent). In a selected subset of nine patients meeting Patchell's criteria, median survival has not yet been reached, with a median follow-up of 24 weeks. The recurrence rate at the metastatic site is only 11 percent. This compares favorably with conventional surgery and whole-brain radiation. Most patients have tolerated this treatment without undue toxicity and with good resultant quality of life as measured by Karnofsky performance score, neurologic functional status, and steroid dependence.

This exciting new technique deserves further investigation in the management of brain metastases. The Radiation Therapy Oncology Group has recently initiated a phase 1 dose-searching protocol, and a second study will be activated in the near future.

Pediatric Tumors

Brain tumors represent approximately 20 percent of all pediatric malignancies. They are the most common solid tumors of childhood. Although significant gains have been made in the treatment of these tumors with chemotherapy and hyperfractionation, failure at the primary site remains the major issue in the management of these patients. Only a handful of patients have been treated with stereotactic radiosurgery. Loeffler and colleagues have recently reported results of radiosurgery in 22 recurrent pediatric tumors, including ependymoma, astrocytoma, craniopharyngioma, medulloblastoma, dysgerminoma, and pineo-blastoma. Fifteen of 22 patients (68 percent) have been rendered free of disease, with dramatic responses seen as early as 6 weeks in some patients. Radiosurgery, therefore, appears to have the potential for retreatment of recurrent pediatric brain tumors and may also be considered in selected situations as a boost.

SUGGESTED READING

Hilaris BS, Nori D, Anderson LL. Atlas of brachytherapy. New York: MacMillan, 1988.

Kumar PP, Good RR. A new intracavitary cervix applicator: Review of existing intracavitary techniques. Endocurietherapy/Hyperthermia Oncol 1985; 1:247–256.

Leibel SA, Gutin PH, Wara WM, et al. Survival and quality of life after interstitial implantation of removable high-activity Iodine-125 sources for the treatment of patients with recurrent malignant gliomas. Int J Radiat Oncol Biol Phys 1989; 17:1129–1139.

Leksell L. The stereotaxic method and radiosurgery of the brain. Acta Chir Scand 1951; 102:316–319.

Loeffler JS, Alexander E. The role of stereotactic radiosurgery in the management of intracranial tumors. Oncology 1990; 4:21–31.

Lunsford LD, ed. Modern stereotactic neurosurgery. Norwell, MA: Martinus Nijhoff, 1987.

Lunsford LD, Flickinger J, Lindner G, et al. Stereotactic radiosurgery of the brain using the first United States 201 source cobalt-60 gamma knife. Neurosurgery 1989; 24:151–159.

Mehta M, Shahabi S, Jarjour N, et al. Effect of endobronchial radiation therapy on malignant bronchial obstruction. Chest 1990; 97:662–665.

CANCER MANAGEMENT IN THE ELDERLY

JEROME W. YATES, M.D., M.P.H.

Expected changes in population demographics, a continued reduction in mortality from heart disease, and limitations in available health care resources are all factors that have and will demand the development of a pertinent data base that will serve as the foundation for more reasoned approaches to cancer management in persons 65 years of age and older. Because age itself is the greatest risk factor for developing cancer and a previous history of cancer is a second major risk factor, cancer incidence (newly diagnosed cases) can be expected to increase continuously over the next 50 years. As the elderly proportion of the population increases and we achieve greater success in curing and controlling cancer, there will be an increase in the number of survivors requiring periodic follow-up and testing for second malignancies. Improved laboratory methods aimed at assessing the risk of developing cancer (e.g., oncogene expression) and improved family histories will require physicians ranging from pediatricians to geriatricians to expand their attention to cancer detection. Oncologists will be asked with greater frequency to act as informed consultants regarding management of the elderly. Continued governmental and private sector budgetary constraints will be working to limit health care, especially diagnostic testing and treatment for the elderly. Although government makes societal decisions through regulatory and reimbursement restraints, physicians will have to consider each patient and the impact of disease and treatment on quality of life. Physicians will be forced to consider other factors, such as institutional care requirements and probable need for other expensive health care resources, before embarking on costly diagnostic and treatment efforts in the elderly.

INCIDENCE

The incidence of cancers for both sexes in the elderly are listed with decreasing frequency as follows: lung, breast, prostate, colon, rectum, corpus uteri, stomach, and non-Hodgkin's lymphomas and leukemias. An expected reduction in the number of common cancers in the elderly can be predicted as some of the contributing causes are decreased or eliminated. Because smoking is the major cause of lung and head and neck cancers, the continued decrease in the number of smokers will have a beneficial effect. Improved nutrition should further reduce the incidence of stomach cancer. A reduction in the consumption of dietary animal fat, should the population heed present recommendations, could decrease the incidence of associated neoplasms (breast, prostate, colon, and rectal cancers). The epidemiologic evidence for this association between diet and cancer is highly likely, and a prudent approach would be to decrease by 50 percent the present fat intake, as suggested by the National Cancer Institute. The careful and limited use of exogenous estrogens in perimenopausal women should decrease the incidence of cancer of the corpus uteri. The trend toward women intentionally delaying pregnancies beyond the teenage years may propel future increase in breast cancer. Greater sexual activity at young ages with a large number of partners can be expected to increase the incidence of cancer of the uterine cervix. An artifactual increase in specific cancers can be expected to result from more aggressive diagnostic approaches in the elderly. Non-Hodgkin's lymphomas and leukemias are two such cancers that historically were ignored, particularly if the elderly patient was frail.

Comorbidity in the elderly can serve as a distraction that delays diagnosis and acts to complicate the treatment of cancer patients. The treatment of comorbid conditions may serve to focus the attention away from a potential cancer for both the patient and the health care provider. Delays in diagnosis and lack of early treatment will generally lead to disseminated cancer. Ignored or underappreciated comorbid conditions can increase the hazard of cancer treatment by the surgeon, radiotherapist, and medical oncologist. The most common chronic comorbid conditions encountered in the elderly population include arthritis, hypertension, hearing loss, heart disease, decreased physical mobility, sinusitis, visual impairment, and diabetes mellitus. Allowances for decreased senses (sight, hearing, touch, taste, and smell) as well as difficulty in accessing health care are important. Lack of mobility, poor nutrition, and decreased understanding may greatly limit their participation in self-care.

Decreased physiologic function with aging affects immunologic competence, physical reserve, and symptom tolerance, and delays resolution of physical and mental stress. Decreased awareness because of an age-related pain tolerance often blunts individual sensitivity to pain as an early sign of cancer. This may also occur with other repetitive symptoms and signs that patients experience. Decreased appreciation of the early signals of cancer can lead to life-threatening delays. Other obstructions to accessing medical care are often enhanced by the dependence of the elderly on others for transportation or their concerns about the costs of care. All of the elderly will experience varying reductions in cognitive function, mobility, and physical stability. Poor nutrition is a common change with aging as well as with certain kinds of cancer. The nutritional status of some patients may limit their ability to tolerate treatment. Polypharmacy from treatment for comorbid conditions requires the collection of a very careful medication history. Treatment for comorbid conditions should not be interrupted when patients are undergoing treatment for cancer and may require some modifications in drugs, dosage, or scheduling because of incompatibilities, metabolic interactions, or interruptions resulting from nausea and vomiting. The natural history of the patient with advancing cancer mimics an acceleration in the aging process. Decreased cognition, total loss of physical independence, social isolation, and often a diminishing quality of life can be minimized with careful management plans. The management of these people should be thought of as an active rehabilitation program.

PREVENTION

Preventing cancer in the elderly is possible for those well-known causal factors such as smoking or exogenous estrogen therapy in perimenopausal women. The diagnosis of premalignant disease (e.g., leukoplakia, erythroplakia, atypical hyperplasia) and their reversal using agents that block cell progression to malignancy may be possible, and encouraging investigations are underway that assess both retinoid and antiestrogen treatment. The prevention of breast cancer in the elderly may be possible by using an antiestrogen such as tamoxifen. In those at great risk of developing head and neck cancer, retinoids may have a role. A greater understanding of the risks of developing cancer and interventions to prevent or delay the development of cancer should be a reasonable expectation for the future. Scientists are developing biologic probes and improved pharmacologic interventions that will surely come to clinical application within the next decade.

EARLY DETECTION

The early detection of any disease generally relies on patient awareness and response to a set of specific symptoms. With age comes tolerance of a variety of symptoms that serve to warn younger persons who then seek immediate medical attention. Less individual concern about pain, blood in the stool, and soft-tissue lumps are examples of changes that are likely to be dismissed by the elderly as being relatively unimportant.

The value of early detection presupposes the availability of an effective treatment for local disease. For the common cancers occurring in the elderly, curative treatment usually means surgical excision. Early detection in lung cancer occurs generally by accident, because by the time lung cancer is clinically apparent, 90 percent of the patients have metastases and will succumb from this disease. Only about 20 percent of the cancers of the prostate are localized at the time of their diagnosis. Surgery or radiotherapy can offer survival prolongation and perhaps cure for some patients. Encouraging routine rectal exams by generalists and the added use of ultrasound examination in selected patients could contribute to detection of prostate cancer while it is still curable. Detection of small breast lesions has been greatly improved with mammography and becomes differentially more accurate as a diagnostic tool as women age. Breast self-examination is another general health education intervention that may also be helpful. Both techniques offer the greatest advantage for the early detection of lesions in the elderly, but the successful practice of breast self-examination assumes the woman has normal tactile and visual senses. This may not be the case in all elderly women. The early detection of colon and rectal cancer through regular endoscopic examinations and a sensitivity to the importance of blood in the stool or changes in bowel habits will only work if there is adequate access to medical care. Once diagnosed, the patient risk of undergoing surgery needs to be assessed and definitive treatment planned to include the amount of supportive care necessary to carry the patient through the acute phase.

TREATMENT

There is some controversy about whether cancers in the elderly have different growth characteristics than in their younger counterparts. The experimental animal evidence is in conflict, with both slower and faster growth suggested. Expected changes in host factors with aging should theoretically favor the early discovery of cancer because of their slower growth and longer period of potential discovery. Slowed growth from diminished circulation, nutrition, local oxygenation, and less angiogenesis are factors that suggest that the discovery of cancers during a more prolonged growth phase in the elderly should be possible. However, an examination of some data does not support this contention. When certain cancers are examined, the elderly are more likely to present at diagnosis with a more advanced stage of disease and have a higher age-associated mortality for the same stage. If age groups for the elderly who present with advanced disease at diagnosis are assessed for survival, age confers a survival disadvantage. This is not treatment-related, but it reflects the host's poorer age-related survival for cancers such as lung, colon, and prostate cancer. It is assumed that some combination of comorbidity and decreased physiologic reserve decreases their tolerance to both the cancer and its treatment. It is also possible that the cancers are more aggressive in the elderly, but an examination of differences in the rate of early deaths does not appear to support this assumption.

Of the three major modalities used in the treatment of cancer, only surgery and radiotherapy for selected localized cancer provide the opportunity for cure. It appears possible to expect that chemotherapy will cure selected elderly patients with non-Hodgkin's lymphoma. Regardless of the modality chosen, an assessment of the physiologic status of the elderly patient prior to the initiation of any aggressive anticancer therapy is necessary. If treatment complications are to be intercepted successfully, prevented, and treated, anticipation of problems by the physician is crucial.

Chemotherapy in the elderly most often causes acute problems related to diminished bone marrow function, which results in leukopenia and thrombocytopenia, and makes these patients susceptible to infection and hemorrhage. Organ-specific toxicities such as renal impairment with the platinum-related compounds, cardiotoxicity with the anthracyclines, and late leukemogenesis with the alkylating agents are all potential complications. In selecting chemotherapy, careful consideration of the treatment goals and their potential benefit and negative impact on quality of life must be considered.

SUGGESTED READING

Abrams WB, Berkow R, eds. The Merck manual of geriatrics. Rathway, NJ: Merck & Co., 1990.

Kane RL, Ouslander JG, Abrass IB, eds. Essentials of clinical geriatrics. New York: McGraw-Hill, 1989.

Yancik R, ed. Perspectives on prevention and treatment of cancer in the elderly. New York: Raven Press, 1983.

Zenser TV, Coe RM, eds. Cancer and aging. New York: Springer-Verlag, 1989.

CLINICAL TRIALS: GROUP C DRUGS

MICHAEL A. FRIEDMAN, M.D.
CLARENCE L. FORTNER, M.S.
MICHAEL J. HAWKINS, M.D.
DALE SHOEMAKER, PH.D.

In the mid-1970s the Division of Cancer Treatment (DCT), National Cancer Institute (NCI), and the Food and Drug Administration (FDA) recognized the need to establish a means for the distribution of an investigational anticancer agent that had demonstrated efficacy and safety for a particular type of patient prior to its approval by the FDA for commercial distribution. This new classification was termed Group C.

There is often an unavoidable delay between the time an investigational anticancer agent is confidently found to be effective in clinical trials and its approval for commercial marketing by the FDA of New Drug Applications (NDAs) for cytotoxic agents and Product License Applications (PLAs) for biologic agents. A number of factors may contribute to this delay:

1. If the agent was discovered and developed by the DCT, NCI, a pharmaceutical company must be identified to submit the application and subsequently market the agent. If the potential market is small (i.e., the indication is for a relatively rare malignancy or clinical situation) or there is no longer a patent position on the agent, it may be difficult to interest a pharmaceutical company in committing the considerable resources necessary to prepare and submit the application. These issues have been addressed somewhat by the Orphan Drug Act of 1983, which provides tax credits and periods of exclusivity for marketing.
2. Once the data that will be used to support the application have been collected, they must be reviewed by the sponsor and properly formatted for presentation to the FDA. Since the data on each patient in the pivotal clinical studies are of interest, this preparation is very often a time consuming process.
3. After the NDA or PLA is submitted, the application must undergo review by numerous staff members from the FDA, who examine not only the clinical data and statistical analyses but also the processing and manufacturing data. As this review progresses, the application also is reviewed by an FDA advisory committee in a public forum. This review process has become more rapid; however, some delay at this stage is unavoidable if public safety is to be maintained.

To place an agent in the Group C status, the DCT, NCI submits the data demonstrating the efficacy and safety to the FDA, and the data are reviewed by the FDA staff and the FDA's Oncologic Drugs Advisory Committee. Therefore, for an investigational anticancer agent to be classified as a Group C agent, there must be a consensus that patients with a specific malignancy have an appreciable chance of benefiting from treatment with the agent.

HISTORICAL BACKGROUND

Establishment of the Group C Classification

During 1975 and 1976, the Bureau of Drugs, FDA and the DCT, NCI held a number of meetings to discuss DCT's procedures for studying investigational anticancer agents and several proposed alterations in the investigational drug distribution system. The Group C mechanism emerged from these discussions. The procedures for this mechanism were formally addressed in a Drug Master File maintained by the DCT. A Memorandum of Understanding Relative to Anticancer Drug Development was signed by the FDA and the DCT, NCI in January 1979. Included in the Drug Master File is a detailed description of the overall plan of investigational anticancer drug development, the system of clinical monitoring, the system of drug distribution and data reporting, pertinent information on the DCT staff, and the background information normally included in individual Investigational New Drug (IND) applications. The Group C mechanism is currently described under the drug distribution and data reporting section of Drug Master File 2803 as follows:

Group C Drugs

During the evaluation of investigational drugs by the DCT, NCI certain drugs are found to have a role in the treatment of specific tumor types. There is often an appreciable time period before these drugs, sponsored by the pharmaceutical industry, receive NDA approval. In order to allow patients with these diseases to have the benefit of this drug therapy, a Group C drug classification has been developed. The purpose of this distribution is to allow access to beneficial therapy and to acquire information on safety in the context in which the drug is likely to be used in clinical practice after marketing.

Definitions

1. Group C Drugs: Drugs supported by evidence of reproducible relative efficacy in patients with a specific tumor type, which alter the pattern of care of the disease, and which are safely administered by properly trained physicians without requiring specialized supportive care facilities as judged by available abstracts, papers, and reports in the IND.

Modified Group C Drug: A drug which meets all the Group C criteria but requires an additional laboratory or safety-monitoring component.

2. Relative efficacy: A drug has relative efficacy in the treatment of a specific tumor if the frequency of objective responses (usually defined as a decrease of greater than 50 percent of the product of two perpendicular dimensions of a measurable tumor) is at least as good as the response rate produced by the most effective, commercially available agent for that tumor at a comparable point in the therapy of the disease. Response rates over 25 percent in refractory diseases qualify as showing evidence of relative efficacy, even if several other agents of similar efficacy are available.

Resources

Group C drugs are provided to properly trained physicians who have registered via an FDA-1572 Form for the treatment of individual patients who qualify under the conditions of "The Guidelines" for the drug.

Mechanism of Group C Classification

1. The Drug remains eligible for research studies, even when advanced to Group C.
2. "Guidelines for Clinical Use" and supporting data are submitted to FDA for review and approval.
3. Review of materials by FDA is conducted so that no more than 3 months elapse between the request and acceptance or rejection of the request.
4. Requests for approval of revisions of the Guidelines are handled in a similar manner.

Criteria For Group C Classification

1. Evidence of safety and relative efficacy in the treatment of patients with a specific cancer type in the form of published abstracts, papers, and reports to the NCI.
2. Impact on the pattern of care of patients with the specific cancer type.
3. Relative efficacy, demonstrable by schedule and doses that are safely administered by properly trained physicians without requiring specialized supportive care facilities. This review is to be based on available published or unpublished data and without the need for additional supportive survival data. It is not tantamount to formal FDA approval of effectiveness for this indication.

Establishment of the Treatment Protocol/IND

In the IND Rewrite published in the *Federal Register* on June 9, 1983, the FDA proposed a section to codify the procedures to authorize the treatment use of investigational drugs in an investigational context. The preamble to the proposal stated that the "FDA would only authorize use of a drug under a treatment protocol/IND if it found: (1) That the proposed use is intended for a serious disease condition in patients for whom no satisfactory approved drug or other therapy is available; (2) that the potential benefits of the drug's use outweigh the potential risks; and (3) that there is sufficient evidence of the drug's safety and effectiveness to justify its intended treatment use. These criteria would ordinarily mean that a drug would not be a candidate for a treatment use until it had gone through the kind of studies conducted during Phase 2. Thus, investigational drugs would ordinarily only become available for a treatment use at the end of Phase 2 or during Phase 3 of an investigation." The proposal went on to state that "The Group C system at the National Cancer Institute has followed these same principles and has achieved considerable success."

The final rule on treatment use published on May 22, 1987 included the following criteria for the treatment use of an investigational drug: "FDA shall permit an investigational drug to be used for a treatment use under a treatment protocol or treatment IND if: (i) the drug is intended to treat a serious or life-threatening disease; (ii) there is no comparable or satisfactory alternative drug or other therapy available to treat that stage of the disease in the intended patient population; (iii) the drug is under investigation in a controlled clinical trial under an IND in effect for the trial, or all clinical trials have been completed; and (iv) the sponsor of the controlled clinical trial is actively pursuing marketing approval of the investigational drug with due diligence."

Differences Between Group C and the Treatment IND

The Group C classification differs from the Treatment Protocol/IND in the following respects:

1. Because the DCT, NCI cannot actively pursue marketing approval for an agent, this is not a requirement for the placing of an agent into Group C.
2. Only agents that are to be used for the treatment of cancer patients are eligible for Group C status.
3. Agents cannot be placed into Group C status unless there is consensus agreement between the DCT, NCI, the FDA, and the FDA Oncology Advisory Committee.
4. Group C agents are always provided free of charge.
5. The Health Care Financing Administration (HCFA) provides full reimbursement for care associated with Group C therapy.

AGENTS CURRENTLY IN GROUP C

The first agents were approved under the Group C mechanism in April 1976. To date 19 agents have been

Table 1 Division of Cancer Treatment, NCI All Group C Agents Past and Current

Drug	Date of IND Submission	Date of Group C Approval	Date of NDA Approval
Carmustine	6/63	4/76	5/77
Lomustine	2/68	4/76	10/76
Azacytidine	1/71	8/76	–
Daunorubicin	12/65	8/76	5/80
Semustine	1/71	8/76	–
		(Withdrawn 7/83)	
Streptozotocin	3/67	8/76	1982
Asparaginase *E. coli*	1/68	10/76	4/78
Cisplatin	7/71	7/77	12/78
Hexamethylmelamine	6/63	7/77	12/90
Asparaginase *Erwinia*	3/71	2/78	–
Etoposide	9/72	5/78	10/83
Tetrahydrocannabinol	9/78	10/80	5/86
Amsacrine	8/77	12/81	–
Interleukin-2/LAK	2/84	5/87	–
Ifosfamide/Mesna	1/87	12/87	12/88
Deoxycoformycin	6/79	7/88	–
Teniposide	9/72	10/88	–
Levamisole	2/77	5/89	6/90
Fludarabine phosphate	11/82	10/89	–

sponsored by the Division of Cancer Treatment, NCI through Group C. A list of all the Group C agents and the pertinent dates of IND submission, Group C approval and NDA approval is included in Table 1. Lists of past (Table 2) and current (Table 3) Group C agents also are provided.

HOW TO OBTAIN GROUP C DRUGS

Clinicians may request a Group C drug by telephoning the Drug Management and Authorization Section, IDB, at 301-496-5725 Monday-Friday, 9:00 AM to 4:00 PM Eastern Standard Time. To receive the Group C drug the physician must be registered (one time only) with the National Cancer Institute as an investigator by having completed a Statement of Investigator, Form FDA 1572. Physicians not currently registered will be sent a Group C drug with the understanding that they will complete and return the registration form within 10 working days of its receipt.

During the initial telephone conversation, the Group C protocol requirements will be reviewed with the clinicians if they are not familiar with them. General information about the patient will be requested when a drug is ordered. This will include diagnosis, height, weight, body surface area, age, sex, and the patient's name. Medical information requirements will vary according to the drug requested. The use of a drug for a Group C indication will be fully described in the protocol. The indications, dosage, dosage modifications, precautions, warning, and known adverse effects of the drug will be described in the protocol.

The amount of data collected from the physician will vary with each drug. All life-threatening and lethal (grade 4 and 5 unknown reactions not listed in the protocol as known toxicities) adverse drug reactions must be reported by phone (301-496-7957) to the Investigational Drug Branch within 24 hours. A written report must follow within 10 working days. All grade 4 and 5 known reactions (except grade 4 myelosuppression) and grade 2 and 3 unknown reactions should be reported by mail within 10 days. An adverse drug reaction form for investigational drugs and the chart for common toxicity criteria are in the protocol appendices. All reports should be mailed to the Investigational Drug Branch, P.O. Box 30012, Bethesda, Maryland 20824.

Written informed consent must be obtained from the patient for the use of Group C drugs and kept on file. A copy of a model informed consent form is included in the protocol and must be used if there is no local institutional review board (IRB) review.

If the physician agrees to these FDA requirements and the patient meets the criteria of the protocol, the drug will be provided if the patient cannot be entered into an ongoing clinical trial. The drug will be supplied to the physicians for their patients until a New Drug Application has been approved by the FDA and the drug becomes commercially available. At that time, the NCI will discontinue distribution of the Group C drug.

The request for Group C drugs has greatly expanded over the past year. Requests for the older Group C drugs (amsacrine, azacytidine, and *Erwinia* asparaginase) have remained stable. However, requests particularly for deoxycoformycin, fludarabine phosphate, and levamisole (became commercially available in June 1990) have been extremely active. Deoxycoformycin and fludarabine phosphate are indicated for secondary use, and

Table 2 Past Group C Agents

Agent	Use
Carmustine	Brain tumors not amenable to surgical resection or radiotherapy; Hodgkin's disease refractory to standard therapy; Melanoma
Lomustine	Brain tumors not amenable to surgical resection or radiotherapy; Hodgkin's disease refractory to standard therapy
Daunorubicin	AML and ALL patients
Semustine	Carcinoma of the colon and stomach; Melanoma
Streptozotocin	Metastatic islet cell carcinoma of the pancreas; Metastatic carcinoid
Asparaginase *E. coli*	ALL patients
Cisplatin	Nonseminomatous carcinoma of testis; Ovarian carcinoma
Etoposide	Single agent therapy in patients refractory to standard therapy for small cell carcinoma of the lung
Tetrahydrocannabinol	Nausea and vomiting induced by antineoplastic chemotherapy
Ifosfamide/Mesna	Refractory germ cell carcinoma
Levamisole	Postoperative adjuvant for Duke's C c colon carcinoma
Hexamethylmelamine	Refractory ovarian carcinoma (single-use agent)

Table 3 Current Group C Agents

Agent	Use
Azacytidine	Refractory AML (single-use agent)
Asparaginase *Erwinia*	ALL patients sensitive to *E. coli* asparaginase
Amsacrine	Refractory adult AML (single-use agent)
Interleukin-2/LAK	Melanoma and renal carcinoma
Deoxycoformycin	Hairy cell leukemia refractory to alpha-interferon
Teniposide	Relapsed or refractory acute lymphoblastic leukemia
Fludarabine phosphate	Refractory chronic lymphocytic leukemia

levamisole is indicated for adjuvant therapy. The indications for Group C drugs are shown in Table 3. The number of requests for these drugs and for information about them is shown in Table 4.

Copies of Group C protocols may be obtained by calling 301-496-5725 or by sending a written request to the Drug Management and Authorization Section, IDB, National Cancer Institute, 9000 Rockville Pike, Executive Plaza North, Room 707, Bethesda, Maryland 20892.

All other nonresearch drug requests for clinical use from NCI will be considered under the "Special Exception Mechanism." Physicians with patients who are refractory to standard therapy, who are not eligible for ongoing research protocols, and who have a diagnosis for which an investigational drug has demonstrated activity may receive the drug under the "Special Exception Mechanism" by calling the same telephone number as for Group C Drugs.

SPECIAL CONSIDERATIONS

Paperwork

A survey of the NCI's Group C mechanism was conducted at the ASCO meeting in Washington, DC in 1990. This survey was conducted to obtain information that would assist the NCI in making Group C drugs easily available to physicians for their patients. The survey asked specific questions; however, the questions were open-ended to reveal unanticipated concerns. The survey was completed by 150 physicians. Most participants were satisfied with the program. Fifteen physicians were unaware of the program or were not familiar with the drugs available or the procedure to obtain these drugs.

According to the survey, the greatest concern of 35 of the participants was the quantity of paperwork or the amount of time required to complete this paperwork. These requirements of the Group C program primarily involve two areas: (1) FDA requirements and (2) scientific data collection.

The FDA requires each physician using investigational drugs to complete a Statement of Investigator form (Form FDA-1572), obtain IRB approval if indicated, have the patient review and sign an informed consent prior to administration of an investigational agent, and report adverse drug reactions.

The largest objection was to patient data collection. The NCI is asking the treating physician to assist in this data collection. It seems reasonable to obtain additional patient data from physicians for at least some of these Group C agents, because some agents were placed in this category before they were fully evaluated in Phase 3 clinical trials. If NCI did not collect this data, it would be a great loss of valuable medical information, because these agents are used in a large number of patients outside of clinical trials. Levamisole is an excellent example, 4,749 patients were treated with levamisole in approximately 9 months. The patient data response from the clinical trials was so compelling and the data submitted to FDA were from Phase 3 clinical trials; therefore, only a minimal amount of information was obtained. Another 1,196 patients have been treated with deoxycoformycin for hairy cell leukemia; teniposide has been used for acute lymphoblastic leukemia, and fludarabine phosphate has been used for chronic lymphocytic leukemia, and in these cases the data submitted to the FDA were not as mature. The amount of data collected for these agents has been greater than for levamisole. Thus, patient data collection appears to be prudent for these Group C drugs.

Table 4 Group C Distribution Analyses

Drug	Date Approved	Physician Information Requests	Group C Patients Registered	Number of Denials
Deoxycoformycin	7/88	N/A*	35	N/A
Teniposide	10/88	N/A	172	N/A
Levamisole†	5/89	13,762	4749	607
Fludarabine phosphate	10/89	2,659	979	–

*N/A = not applicable.
†Approximately 21,000 patients eligible to receive this agent.

Institutional Review Board Review

The Division of Cancer Treatment, NCI requests a waiver from the FDA for the IRB approval of the Group C protocols. The request for the waiver is based on the following review process for each Group C protocol:

1. The Group C protocol is reviewed by the Cancer Therapy Evaluation Program (CTEP) Protocol Review Committee from the investigational agent, disease, regulatory, and statistical aspects. The regulatory aspect includes a review of the informed consent form to ensure that it includes all the elements specified by the regulations of the FDA and the NIH Office for Protection from Research Risks (OPRR). The CTEP-approved Group C protocol is then reviewed by the NCI subpanel of the NIH Clinical Center IRB.
2. The approved Group C protocol is submitted to the FDA along with all supporting documentation. Although the FDA reviews the scientific and regulatory aspects of the protocol as do the other groups, their review also ensures that the protocol meets the criteria for a Group C agent, including reproducible antitumor activity by the agent in a particular tumor type as well as a satisfactory safety profile. The informed consent form is reviewed by a separate division to ensure that all elements required by federal regulations are included.

On the basis of the review by the CTEP Protocol Review Committee, the NCI IRB, and the FDA's own review, waivers have been granted for the current Group C agents (except the interleukin-2/LAK modified Group C). Each waiver must be renewed annually. It should be noted that the waiver does not preclude the right of a local IRB to review a Group C protocol. However, a local IRB need not review the Group C protocol for each patient.

Reimbursement

A consideration of growing importance is the successful reimbursement for the cost of clinical care associated with administering a Group C agent. For most of these agents and for most patients the therapy is delivered in the outpatient setting. Hence, private or federal insurers usually provide coverage. The picture is more heterogeneous for inpatient care. The Health Care Financing Administration (HCFA) is the largest Federal insurer, providing coverage for many elderly and indigent patients. Currently, HCFA recommends reimbursement for care associated with Group C therapy. However, both private and public carriers permit regional autonomy in decision making, so there is no national uniformity in enforcing reimbursement guidelines.

Even the threat of non-reimbursement is a powerful discouragement to the use of a Group C agent. Given the extensive documentation of safety and efficacy for these agents, such disincentives are inappropriate and indefensible. The Group C agent is provided free of charge and is certified as the best possible clinical option by both the NCI and the FDA. Consequently any additional financial obstacle should be vigorously challenged.

Delay to Full FDA Approval

The Group C mechanism was initially designed as a bridge between the identification of efficacy and commercial approval by the FDA. Clearly it is in everyone's interest to have a speedy transition. Unfortunately, some Group C agents have been parked in a holding orbit for long periods of time. There are now two drugs that have carried Group C designation for more than a decade while awaiting full NDA approval. These are azacytidine (8/76) and *Erwinia* asparaginase (2/78). When first studied, all of these drugs suffered from lack of an industrial sponsor, an imprecise development plan, and unsatisfactory clinical trials methodology. Happily these deficits have been largely recognized and corrected. Currently, the FDA is considering a formal application for *Erwinia* asparaginase. Since this agent has demonstrated meaningful antitumor effects and has copious clinical trials data, it should be approvable in the near future.

With the current sophistication of the NCI, investigators, and industry personnel, every effort will be made to limit the time that an agent spends in the Group C category.

SUGGESTED READING

21 CFR Part 312. Fed Reg 1983; 48(112):26720-26749.
21 CFR Part 312. Fed Reg 1987; 52(99):19466-19477.

Page numbers followed by f indicate figures; page numbers followed by t indicate tables.